Orthopedic and Sports Physical Therapy

Orthopedic and Sports Physical Therapy

THIRD EDITION

Edited by

Terry R. Malone, EdD, PT, ATC
Associate Professor and Director
Physical Therapy Division
University of Kentucky
Lexington, Kentucky

Thomas G. McPoil, PhD, PT, ATC
Professor and Co-Director
Gait Research Laboratory
Department of Physical Therapy
Northern Arizona University
Flagstaff, Arizona

Arthur J. Nitz, PhD, PT
Associate Professor
Physical Therapy Division
University of Kentucky
Lexington, Kentucky

with 462 illustrations

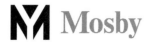 Mosby

St. Louis Baltimore Boston Carlsbad Chicago Naples New York Philadelphia Portland
London Madrid Mexico City Singapore Sydney Tokyo Toronto Wiesbaden

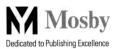

Mosby
Dedicated to Publishing Excellence

A Times Mirror
Company

Publisher: Don Ladig
Executive Editor: Martha Sasser
Developmental Editor: Kellie F. White
Project Manager: Dana Peick
Senior Production Editor: Stavra Demetrulias
Designer: Amy Buxton
Manufacturing Supervisor: Linda Ierardi

THIRD EDITION
Copyright © 1997 by Mosby–Year Book, Inc.

Printed in the United States of America
Composition by Graphic World, Inc.
Printing/binding by Maple-Vail

Mosby-Year Book, Inc.
11830 Westline Industrial Drive
St. Louis, Missouri 63146

Library of Congress Cataloging-in-Publication Data

Orthopedic and sports physical therapy. — 3rd ed. / [edited by] Terry
    R. Malone, Thomas G. McPoil, Arthur J. Nitz.
         p.   cm.
      Rev. ed. of: Orthopaedic and sports physical therapy / edited by
    James A. Gould III. 2nd ed. 1990.
      Includes bibliographical references and index.
      ISBN 0-8151-5886-6
        1. Orthopedics.   2. Physical therapy.   3. Sports physical therapy.
I. Malone, Terry, 1950–   . II. McPoil, Thomas G.   III. Nitz,
Arthur J.   IV. Orthopaedic and sports physical therapy.
      [DNLM: 1. Orthopedics—methods.   2. Physical Therapy—methods.
3. Sports Medicine—methods.   WB 460 077 1997]
RD736.P47078   1997
613.8′2—dc20
DNLM/DLC   96-20127
for Library of Congress   CIP
International Standard Book Number 0-8151-5886-6

    97 98 99 00 / 9 8 7 6 5 4 3 2

CONTRIBUTORS

Paul Beattie, PhD, PT, OCS
Assistant Professor
Ithaca College at the University of
  Rochester
Rochester, New York

James Bellew, MS, PT
Graduate Student
Physical Therapy Division
University of Kentucky
Lexington, Kentucky

Richard Bowling, MS, PT
CEO, CORE Network LLC;
Adjunct Assistant Professor
University of Pittsburgh
Pittsburgh, Pennsylvania

Mark W. Cornwall, PhD, PT
Associate Professor and Co-Director
Gait Research Laboratory
Department of Physical Therapy
Northern Arizona University
Flagstaff, Arizona

George Davies, MEd, PT, ATC, SCS
Professor
Department of Physical Therapy
University of Wisconsin-LaCrosse;
Director-Clinical and Research Services
Western Wisconsin Sports Medicine
LaCrosse, Wisconsin

Carl DeRosa, PT, PhD
Professor and Director
Department of Physical Therapy
Northern Arizona University
Flagstaff, Arizona

Todd S. Ellenbecker, MS, PT, SCS, CSCS
Clinic Director
Physiotherapy Associates
Scottsdale, Arizona

Tony English, MSEd, PT
Assistant Professor
Physical Therapy Division
University of Kentucky
Lexington, Kentucky

Ivan J. Gradisar, Jr., MD
Professor of Orthopaedics
Northeastern Ohio Universities
College of Medicine
Rootstown, Ohio

Captain Robert C. Hall, MS, PT
United States Air Force
Physical Therapy
Wilford Hall Medical Center
San Antonio, Texas

Anne Leath Harrison, MS, PT;
Assistant Professor
Division of Physical Therapy
Department of Clinical Sciences
University of Kentucky
Lexington, Kentucky

Charles Hazle
Graduate Student
Physical Therapy Division
University of Kentucky
Lexington, Kentucky

Dixie L. Hettinga, BS, PT
Director of Physical Therapy
Department of Physical Therapy
Wausau Hospital Center
Wausau, Wisconsin

Susan J. Isernhagen, PT
President
Isernhagen and Associates, Inc.
Duluth, Minnesota

James S. Keene, MD
Professor
Team Orthopedic Surgeon
University of Wisconsin Athletic Teams;
Section of Sports Medicine
Division of Orthopedic Surgery
University of Wisconsin Hospitals and
  Clinics
Madison, Wisconsin

Thomas G. McPoil, Jr., PhD, PT, ATC
Professor and Co-Director
Gait Research Laboratory
Department of Physical Therapy
Northern Arizona University
Flagstaff, Arizona

Terry R. Malone, EdD, PT, ATC
Associate Professor and Director
Physical Therapy Division
University of Kentucky
Lexington, Kentucky

Robert E. Mangine, MEd, PT, ATC
Director
Kentucky Rehabilitation Services
Fort Mitchell, Kentucky

Arthur J. Nitz, PhD, PT, OCS, ECS
Associate Professor
Physical Therapy Division
University of Kentucky
Lexington, Kentucky

James A. Porterfield, MA, PT, ATC
Rehabilitation and Health Center
Crystal Clinic
Akron, Ohio

Cheryl Riegger-Krugh, ScD, PT
Division of Physical Therapy
Department of Medical Allied Health
  Professions
School of Medicine
University of North Carolina
  at Chapel Hill
Chapel Hill, North Carolina

Paul A. Rockar, Jr., MS, PT, OCS
Vice President, CORE Network LLC;
Adjunct Assistant Professor
Duquesne University;
Adjunct Associate Professor
Slippery Rock University
Pittsburgh, Pennsylvania

Mark J. Rowinski, PhD, PT
Director and Associate Professor
Physical Therapy Program
University of Rhode Island
Kingston, Rhode Island

Barbara Sanders, PhD, PT, SCS
Director and Professor
Physical Therapy Program
Southwest Texas State University
San Marcos, Texas

Carolyn Thaxton Wadsworth, MS, PT, OCS, CHT
Owner, Practitioner
Heartland Physical Therapy
Cedar Rapids, Iowa

Lynn A. Wallace, PhD, PT, ATC
Director
Ohio Physical Therapy and Sports
  Medicine;
Consulting Athletic Trainer
Case Western Reserve University and
  Lake Erie College
Beachwood, Ohio

M. Elyse Wheeler, PhD
Assistant Professor
Director of Information Services
Dept. of Pathology & Laboratory
  Medicine
College of Allied Health Professions
University of Kentucky
Lexington, Kentucky

Kevin Wilk, BS, PT
Co-Director of Research
Health South Sports Medicine and
  Rehabilitation
Birmingham, Alabama

In Memoriam
James A. Gould, MS, PT
(1946 - 1995)

The entire physical therapy community mourned the passing of James A. Gould in August 1995. It is always important for students entering a discipline or career to be reminded of those individuals who have shaped the very profession they will inherit on graduation. Jim Gould was one of these individuals, and part of his legacy will live through his work as co-editor of the first edition of this text as well as the sole editor of the second edition.

Jim was recognized as a true leader in the area of orthopedic physical therapy and was considered a visionary who helped develop the current practice parameters used today by orthopedic/manual physical therapists. At the time of his death, Jim was

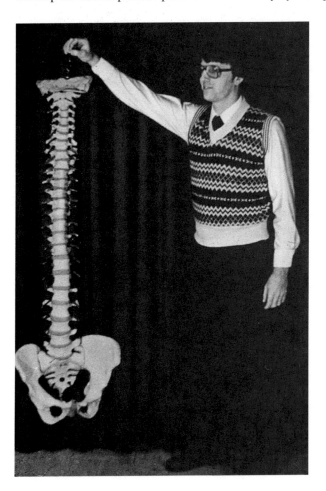

an Associate Professor of Physical Therapy at the University of Wisconsin at LaCrosse. While he had been a member of the Faculty at the University of Wisconsin at LaCrosse for 20 years, Jim remained actively involved in clinical practice during that entire time. It was Jim's belief that in order to teach the subject of orthopedic physical therapy, one had to also practice it! In recognition of his many achievements, Jim was the recipient of the Paris Distinguished Service Award from the Orthopedic Section of the APTA as well as the Robert Dicus Outstanding Service Award from the Private Practice Section of the APTA.

For all of Jim's many accomplishments, he surely had to be proud of his ability to teach. Having heard Jim lecture several times and having talked to many of his former students, it is obvious that Jim was a true teacher. It is because of his intense desire to "teach and prepare" his students to successfully enter the physical therapy profession that we believe Jim would be pleased with this third edition of *Orthopedic and Sports Physical Therapy*.

As Henry Adams said, "A teacher affects eternity; he can never tell where his influence stops." No doubt Jim's former students will continue to carry his thoughts and influence throughout their professional careers. Unfortunately, those students that follow will not have the opportunity to learn and be influenced directly by Jim! We, as well as all of those individuals who have had the privilege of being motivated and enlightened by Jim during his short time on earth, will miss him.

Terry R. Malone, EdD, PT, ATC
Thomas G. McPoil, PhD, PT, ATC
Arthur J. Nitz, PhD, PT, ECS, OCS

To my wife Becky and sons Matthew and Mark
whose love and understanding have provided more
than they will ever know.
TRM

To my wife Mary Anne and daughters Meredith and Molly
whose love, patience, and constant understanding have allowed
me to achieve so much!
TGM

To my wife Jane and children
whose encouragement has been a great source of strength.
AJN

Preface

The preface to the second edition of *Orthopedic and Sports Physical Therapy* indicated that the profession of physical therapy was in the midst of a tremendous revolution in both practice and theory. In 1990, when the second edition was published, physical therapists were just being certified as clinical specialists in the areas of both sports and orthopedics. Furthermore, the role of the physical therapist as a direct provider of patient care was evolving, placing an even greater emphasis on the need for sports and orthopedic physical therapy specialists. Thus, the second edition of this text was designed to assist the practicing physical therapist in developing the competencies necessary to assume the role of sports and orthopedic rehabilitation specialists.

Unfortunately, in 1990 no one could have predicted the dramatic changes that have occurred in the provision of health care in the United States: the advent of managed care, the proliferation of health maintenance organizations, and the reduction in "fee for service" based health insurance plans. These changes in the way that health care is delivered have yet to diminish the need for sports and orthopedic specialists. These changes have, however, markedly changed the level of expectation for the newly graduated physical therapist. Physical therapy graduates now find themselves in a position where they are expected to assimilate into the current health care workplace at a level of proficiency that was only an educational vision in 1990. It is because of these new demands placed on the "entry-level" physical therapist that the third edition of *Orthopedic and Sports Physical Therapy* has been developed. While the editors still believe that the text will be a tremendous asset to the practicing physical therapist, the third edition has been redesigned to assist the entry-level student in developing a sound foundation in the evaluation and management of clients with orthopedic- and sports-related problems.

To meet this goal, the third edition has been divided into four sections: Basic Sciences, Evaluation, Regional Considerations, and Special Areas. To assist the student and practicing clinician in applying the concepts presented in these various sections, case studies have been included in those chapters of the text devoted to regional considerations. The outstanding list of contributing authors have either revised or completely rewritten their respective chapters in order to provide the reader with the most current information available in the area of orthopedic and sports physical therapy.

We hope that this text will continue to be a valuable resource for both the entry-level student and the practicing physical therapist. The challenge presented to the physical therapy professional by an evolving managed health care system requires an extensive and current level of knowledge based on a strong scientific foundation. We believe that this new edition can assist in providing this foundation in the areas of orthopedic and sports physical therapy. In closing, we would like to thank Martha Sasser, Kellie White, Amy Dubin, and the staff of Mosby for all of their assistance in making this third edition possible.

Terry R. Malone, EdD, PT, ATC
Thomas G. McPoil, PhD, PT, ATC
Arthur J. Nitz, PhD, PT, ECS, OCS

Contents

PART ONE

Basic Sciences

1 Bone, 3
  • *Cheryl Riegger-Krugh*

2 Neurobiology for Orthopedic and Sports Physical Therapy, 47
  • *Mark J. Rowinski*

3 Biomechanics of Orthopedic and Sports Therapy, 65
  • *Mark W. Cornwall*

4 Inflammatory Response of Synovial Joint Structures, 81
  • *Tony English, M. Elyse Wheeler, and Dixie L. Hettinga*

5 Fracture Stabilization and Healing, 115
  • *Ivan A. Gradisar, Jr. and Arthur J. Nitz*

6 Ligament and Muscle-Tendon Unit Injuries, 135
  • *James S. Keene and Terry R. Malone*

PART TWO

Evaluation

7 Evaluation of the Musculoskeletal Disorders, 165
  • *Arthur J. Nitz, James W. Bellew, Jr., and Charles R. Hazle*

8 Basic Concepts of Orthopedic Manual Therapy, 191
  • *Robert C. Hall and Arthur J. Nitz*

9 Exercise and Rehabilitation Concepts, 211
  • *Barbara Sanders*

10 Assessment of Strength, 225
  • *George Davies, Kevin Wilk, and Todd S. Ellenbecker*

PART THREE

Regional Considerations

11 The Foot and Ankle, 259
  • *Thomas G. McPoil*

12 The Knee, 295
  • *Lynn A. Wallace, Robert E. Mangine, and Terry R. Malone*

13 The Wrist and Hand, 327
  • *Carolyn Wadsworth*

14 The Elbow Complex, 379
  • *Richard W. Bowling and Paul A. Rockar, Jr.*

15 The Shoulder, 401
  • *Kevin Wilk*

16 The Hip, 459
  • *Paul Beattie*

17 The Spine, 509
  • *Carl DeRosa and James A. Porterfield*

18 The Temporomandibular Joint, 555
  • *Anne Leath Harrison*

PART FOUR

Special Areas

19 Industrial Physical Therapy, 597
  • *Susan J. Isernhagen*

Orthopedic Sports and Physical Therapy

PART ONE

Basic Sciences

Bone

Cheryl Riegger-Krugh

OUTLINE

Strength (mechanical properties) of materials
Bone composition
Bone growth
    Sequential bone growth
    Membranous (intramembranous) bone growth
Strength (mechanical properties) of bone
    Stresses and strains related to bone shape
    Areas of bone strength and weakness
    Stresses at epiphyseal plates
    Bone yielding and failure
    Bone healing
    Differences in men's and women's bone strength
    Age-related differences in bone strength
    Adaptation of bone to exercise stress
Bone growth and loading patterns of the lower extremity
  bones
    Femur
    Tibia and fibula
    Foot
Common bone-related problems in older adults
    Osteoarthrosis and osteoporosis
Summary

LEARNING OBJECTIVES

After studying this chapter, the reader should be able to:
1. Describe the general structure of bone.
2. State the seven different categories of bone.
3. Describe the function and components of bone.
4. Discuss the relationship between bone strength and weakness in regard to functional adaptation of bone.
5. Describe the mechanical stresses imposed on bone during functional activities.
6. Explain why the term *strength* must be operationally defined.
7. Explain the purpose of bone modeling.
8. Describe how bone adapts to stresses caused by exercise.
9. Differentiate between beneficial versus harmful stresses caused by exercise.
10. Explain the role of bone remodeling in the pathology of osteoarthritis and osteoporosis.

KEY TERMS

bone	growth
stress	osteoporosis
strain	osteoarthritis
strength	

Bone is a living tissue that provides support and structure to the body. Through its attachments to bone, the muscular system initiates and sustains movement, which allows us to perform the activities of daily living. Often, bone is viewed as the dead, dehydrated, brittle material of skeletal models. In reality, bone is a dynamically adaptable material that undergoes constant remodeling. This fact is the key to understanding the mechanical properties and behavior of bone.[75] There are seven categories of bone[75,89]:

1. *Long bones* are tubular, usually longer than they are wide and having a shaft or body with convex or

concave articular ends. The shaft usually contains a hollow center, called the *medullary cavity.* Examples of long bones are the femur and humerus.

2. *Short bones* are generally small and cube-shaped. Of their six surfaces, no more than four are articular, and two or more serve as attachment sites for tendons and ligaments or as entry sites for blood vessels. Examples of short bones are the carpal and tarsal bones.

3. *Flat bones* consist of two plates of compact bone, with trabecular bone and marrow located between the plates. The skull, sternum, and scapula are examples of flat bones.

4. *Irregular bones,* such as facial bones and vertebrae, are usually composed of various nonuniform shapes and do not fit in the other categories.

5. *Pneumatic bones* contain air cells or sinuses with a cortical shell of bone surrounding the air spaces. The mastoid portion of the temporal bone is an example.

6. The round or oval *sesamoid bones* are located within tendons. They not only protect tendons from friction and compression, but also increase the muscle's mechanical advantage for producing strength. They do so by increasing the angle of application at the muscle attachment site. Examples of sesamoid bones are the patella and the bones connected to the flexor pollicis brevis and flexor hallucis brevis tendons.

7. *Accessory* or *supernumerary bones* develop when an extra ossification center appears in the main part of the bone or a normally occurring ossification center fails to fuse with the main part of the bone.

The main functions of bones are to support the body, facilitate joint movement, produce red blood cells (including some lymphocytes, granulocytic white blood cells, and platelets), protect various body structures and organs, and store calcium, phosphorus, and magnesium salts.

STRENGTH (MECHANICAL PROPERTIES) OF MATERIALS

The strength of inanimate objects and components of animate beings can be defined in terms of the mechanical properties of the materials within them. External forces can deform these materials. Strength is determined by comparing the effects of forces external to the material with the ability of the material to withstand those forces. The strength of total animate beings—people, animals—may also be defined in other ways, such as by functional performance.

The internal reaction of a material to the external forces imposed upon it is difficult to measure directly. The magnitude of the load experienced internally by the material is quantified as the load divided by the contact area of the load, called *stress,* symbolized by the Greek letter sigma σ, or by the magnitude of the external load itself. The deforming effect of the load experienced internally by the material is quantified as the deformation as a percentage of the original length, called *strain,* symbolized by the Greek letter epsilon ϵ, or by the magnitude of the deformation itself. Units of measure for load, deformation, stress, and strain are listed in Table 1-1. Types of stresses and strains are listed in Table 1-2.

A structure can be loaded, separately or in combination, with five different types of load: tensile, compressive, shear, bending, and torsion. Tensile loads tend to distract or pull apart. The structure tends to elongate, and tensile stress and strain result. Maximal tensile stress occurs on a plane perpendicular to the applied load (Fig. 1-1). If a force of equal tensile magnitude was applied at an angle to a surface instead of perpendicular to the surface, a reduced tensile stress would occur, as some of the force would cause sliding or shear. Compressive loads tend to shorten and widen a structure, resulting in compressive stress and strain (Fig. 1-2). Maximal compressive stress also occurs on a plane perpendicular to the applied load. Shear stresses occur when equal but not directly opposite loads are applied to opposing surfaces of structures. Normal shear strain is a linear deformation that occurs as molecules move past each other (Fig. 1-3). Shear stresses and strains result when either tensile or compressive loads are applied to a structure. At any point within the structure, tensile and compressive stresses are maximal in two perpendicular or orthogonal planes, one plane aligned with the external load and the plane perpendicular to it. The maximal tensile and compressive stresses are called the *principal stresses.* At the same point, the shear stress and strain are zero in the direction of the principal

Force	Deformation	Stress σ	Strain ε
Newton (N)*	Meters (m)	N/m² (pascal) MPa (megapascals) (mpa) Gpa (gigapascals) (gpa)	Percent (%) change in length Angular deformation in radians
Pound (lb)	Inch (in)	lb/in² (psi) (in pounds)	
	Feet (ft) Centimeters (cm)	lb/ft² (ft-pounds)	

Table 1-1. Units of measure for force, deformation, stress, and strain

*A newton is the force that, when applied to a mass of 1 kg, gives an acceleration of 1 m/sec².

stresses and maximal in a plane at a 45-degree angle to the principal stresses (Fig. 1-4). When a structure is loaded in tension or compression, angular deformation occurs as the shear stress is produced (Fig. 1-5). The other two types of load are bending and torsion, which are discussed later.

The strength of a material can be quantified by analyzing the relationship of loading a structure to the deformation caused by the load, and this relationship can be viewed as a load-deformation curve for that material. For comparison of the strength of different structures, loads must be normalized as loads per unit area and deformations as deformations per unit length or percentage of deformation. The result is a stress-strain curve.[94] Many important strength characteristics can be determined directly from this curve[14,94,99] (Fig. 1-6):

1. *Strength*—the maximal stress, maximal strain, or total area under the load-deformation or the stress-strain curve, which is also called the *energy storage* or *total energy absorbed.*

2. *Yield point*—the point (Y) at which the material no longer reacts elastically. With stress and strain combinations that occur to the left of the yield point on the stress-strain or load-deformation curve, the material reacts in an elastic manner; that is, no permanent deformation remains after the release of the load. At the yield point, the deformation or strain of the material can proceed without any additional increase in the external load. Deformation beyond the yield point identifies the *plastic deformation range* of the material. In this range, stress and strain are not linearly related, and permanent deformation remains when the external load is released.

3. *Ultimate failure point (U)*—the level of stress or load and strain or deformation at which failure occurs.

4. *Stiffness (modulus of elasticity, Young's modulus, or E)*—the slope of the elastic portion of the stress-strain curve for tensile or compressive loads. For an elastic material or, more likely, a material loaded within the *elastic deformation range*, stress and strain are fairly linearly related, such that stress equals E × strain (Hooke's law).

Table 1-2. Examples of stress and strain

Internal reaction	Symbol	Method of determination
Tensile stress	Tσ	Tensile force/ contact area
Tensile strain	Tϵ	Percentage increase in length
Compressive stress	Cσ	Compressive force/ contact area
Compressive strain	Cϵ	Percentage decrease in length
Shear stress	$\tau\sigma$	Shear force/contact area
Shear strain	$\tau\epsilon$	Angular deformation

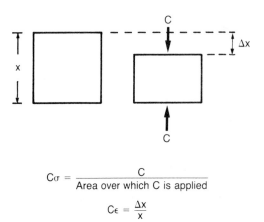

$$C\sigma = \frac{C}{\text{Area over which C is applied}}$$

$$C\epsilon = \frac{\Delta x}{x}$$

Fig. 1-2. Compressive stress and strain.

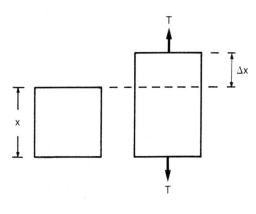

$$T\sigma = \frac{T}{\text{Area over which T is applied}}$$

$$T\epsilon = \frac{\Delta x}{x}$$

Fig. 1-1. Tensile stress and strain.

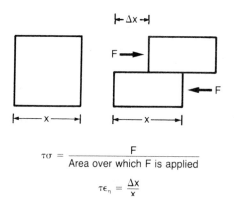

$$\tau\sigma = \frac{F}{\text{Area over which F is applied}}$$

$$\tau\epsilon_{\eta} = \frac{\Delta x}{x}$$

Fig. 1-3. Shear stress and strain.

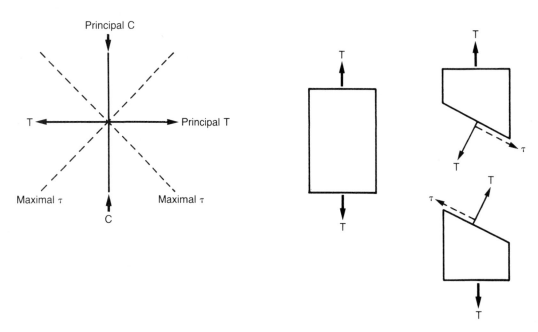

Fig. 1-4. Maximal shear occurs in a plane 45 degrees to the planes of principal tensile and compressive stress.

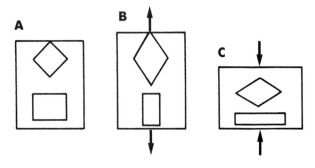

Fig. 1-5. Angular deformation occurs in a structure because shear strain is caused when loading in tension or compression occurs. The unloaded condition, **A,** can be compared to tensile loading, **B,** and compressive loading, **C,** with the resultant deformation in each case.

5. *Shear modulus of elasticity*—the slope of the elastic portion of the stress-strain curve for shear loads or, sometimes, the slope in the initial portion of the torque–angular deformation curve.
6. *Ultimate stress*—the stress at the point of failure.
7. *Ultimate strain*—the strain at the point of failure.

Materials are ductile, brittle, or on a continuum between the two, depending on the amount of deformation they can withstand before failure.[41] A ductile material deforms a great deal before failure and therefore has a long plastic deformation region. A brittle material has little or no plastic deformation region and deforms very little before failure. At the time of failure, the two ends of the brittle material, such as glass, can be approximated to conform to the original shape of the material, much like fitting together pieces of a jigsaw puzzle.

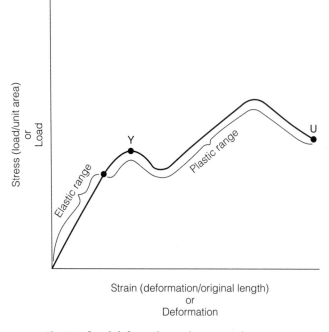

Fig. 1-6. Load-deformation and stress-strain curves.

Loading systems produce bending if two force pairs act at opposite ends of a structure (four-point bending), if three forces cause bending (three-point bending), or if an already bowed structure is loaded axially[31,94] (Fig. 1-7). Upon bending, the convex portion of the structure is subject to tensile stresses and is elongated, whereas the concave portion is subject to compressive stresses and is shortened. Because a structure may be asymmetrical, the tensile and compressive stresses may not be equal. Tensile and compressive stresses are maximal at the farthest point within the

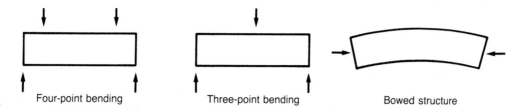

Fig. 1-7. Four-point bending, three-point bending, and axial loading of a bowed structure.

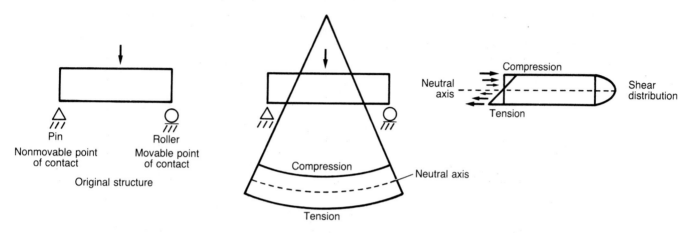

Fig. 1-8. Bending results in tensile, compressive, and shear stresses and strains.

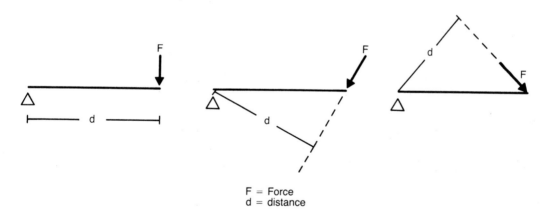

F = Force
d = distance

Fig. 1-9. Bending moment = (load) force × distance, which is the perpendicular distance from the action line of the force to the axis.

structure from the neutral axis and are proportional to the square of that distance. Shear stress is greatest at the neutral axis (Fig. 1-8).

The tendency of a force or load to cause a structure to move clockwise or counterclockwise around an axis is the *moment* produced by the force. The moment is determined by multiplying the force times the perpendicular distance from the action line of the force to the axis[111] (Fig. 1-9).

$$\text{Moment M} = \text{force} \times \text{distance}$$

In static equilibrium, the sum of the forces in any direction equals zero ($\Sigma F = 0$), and the sum of the moments around any axis also equals zero ($\Sigma M = 0$) for all three planes of motion. The force summation to zero mathematically represents the absence of translation of the structure, and the moment summation to zero mathematically represents the absence of rotation of the structure.

If accelerations are involved, the inertial resistance to such movements must be calculated. The inertial resistance to linear translation of an object is determined by the object's mass. The equation of force = mass × acceleration describes the relationship of a linear force (F) and a resultant linear acceleration (a) of a mass (m). The inertial resistance of an object to rotating around an axis is determined by the object's mass and the object's mass distribution relative to the axis. The mass moment of inertia (I) represents the inertial resistance to change of angular velocity of the object around the axis. The mass moment of inertia changes if the chosen axis of rotation changes. Mass moment of inertia, as the representation of inertial resistance to change in angular velocity, is analogous to mass as the inertial resistance to change in linear motion or translation.

The value I is determined about the axis of rotation by summing each particle of mass times the square of the distance of each particle of mass from the axis. This distance factor, the *radius of gyration,* is different from the center of mass and is specific to the axis of rotation. Summation of the moments related to a moving object would not sum to zero

but would sum to I times the angular acceleration (α) (ΣM = I × α). The meaningfulness of the mass moment of inertia is the comparative ease of the swing portion of gait for the person with a flexed hip and knee (less mass moment of inertia) compared to the relative difficulty of the swing phase for the person with maintained hip and knee extension (greater mass moment of inertia).

The strength of a structure in resisting loads that tend to bend the structure is called the *bending moment of inertia,* which is also abbreviated I. The value of I is determined about the axis of rotation by summing each mass times the square of the distance of each mass to the axis of rotation (Fig. 1-10). The equations show that I is minimal when rotation occurs about the center of mass and that mass that

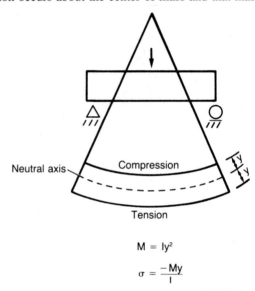

$$M = Iy^2$$

$$\sigma = \frac{-My}{I}$$

Fig. 1-11. Moments of inertia; equations that incorporate moment of inertia *(I)*, bending moment *(M)*, distance from the neutral axis *(y)*, and stress *(σ)*.

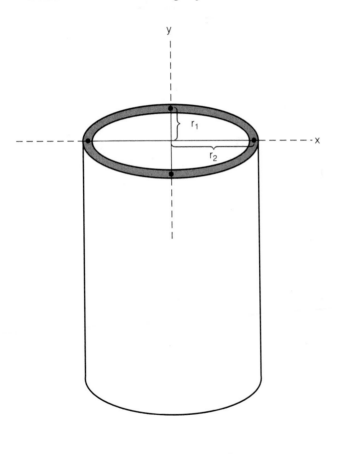

$$Iy = \int m r_2^2$$

I about the y axis = the sum of each particle of mass times the radius squared of each particle of mass to the axis

$$Ix = \int m r_1^2$$

m = each particle of mass
x = x axis
y = y axis
r = radius of particle of mass to
    the radius

Fig. 1-10. Moments of inertia *(I)* around the y and x axes.

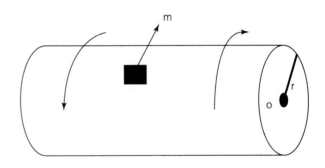

$$J_0 = \int m r^2$$

m = each particle of mass
r = radius of each particle of mass to the axis

Fig. 1-12. Polar moment of inertia *(J)*, or the resistance of a structure to torsion loads, is calculated by $J_o = \int r^2 dA$.

is close to the axis of rotation has little effect on I. The bending strength of a structure is maximized by adding mass to the structure and, more so, by distributing the mass farther from the center of cross-section of the structure.[134] Fig. 1-11 shows the equations that incorporate the bending moment (tendency for a structure to bend) and the bending moment of inertia (resistance to bending).

The strength of a structure in resisting loads that tend to twist the structure is measured by the polar moment of inertia (J). The polar moment of inertia represents resistance to torsional or twisting loads and is determined by the equation $J_o = mr^2$, where m is each small mass of the material and r is the distance of that mass to the center of rotation (o) (Fig. 1-12). For a cylinder, as shown in Fig. 1-12, o is the center of the cylinder, or the neutral axis. Polar moment of inertia represents the maximum strength in shear in terms of the material and dimensions of the structure. Shear stress results from torsional loads. The magnitude of the shear stress is directly proportional to the distance from the neutral axis (Fig. 1-13, A and B) and is maximal on planes parallel and perpendicular to the neutral axis (Fig. 1-13, C).

Tensile and compressive stresses resulting from tensile, compressive, and bending loads on structures are shown in Fig. 1-14. The net stresses for structures undergoing combined loads can be determined algebraically, as illustrated in Fig. 1-15.

BONE COMPOSITION

Bone is classified as a connective tissue, as are cartilage, ligaments, tendons, blood, fat, and fasciae. The connective tissues have three parts: a fiber component, a ground substance with a tissue fluid component, and a cellular component. The first two components form the extracellular matrix and make up the bulk of the connective tissue. Mechanical properties of a connective tissue are determined by the contents forming the tissue, the proportions of the three components, and the direction of the fibers.

The fiber component of connective tissues consists of collagen fibers, which are large and coarse and occur in bundles, and elastin fibers, which are smaller, thinner fibers. Collagen fibers resist tensile stresses, whereas elastin fibers, as the name implies, are elastic or resilient. Elastin fibers can be extended and recover their original shape when a stretching force of defined magnitude is removed. The stress-strain curves for collagen and elastin are shown in Fig. 1-16.

The second component is a ground substance composed of amorphous glycosaminoglycans (GAGs, formerly known as mucopolysaccharides), the constituents of which are protein-sugar combinations (proteoglycans, glycoproteins, chondroitin sulfate, and keratan sulfate) and hyaluronic acid (Fig. 1-17). The ground substance–tissue fluid component has many functions, including maintaining tissue water and electrolyte balance, controlling the diameter growth of

SHEAR STRESSES

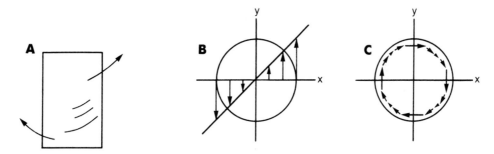

Fig. 1-13. A, The result of a torsion load is shear stress over the entire surface of the structure. **B,** The magnitude of the shear stress is directly proportional to the distance from the neutral axis. **C,** Shear stress is maximal on planes parallel and perpendicular to the neutral axis *(C).*

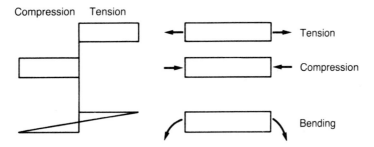

Fig. 1-14. Visualization of tensile and compressive stresses.

RESULTANT RELATIVE
COMPRESSION AND TENSION

LOADING PATTERN

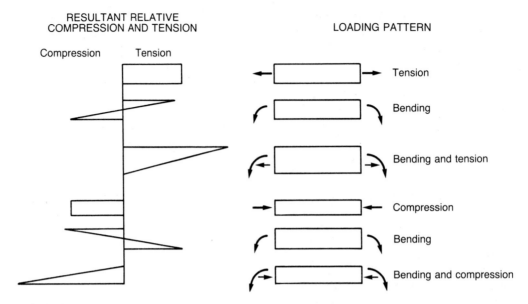

Fig. 1-15. Net stresses resulting from combined loading.

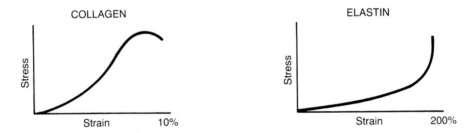

Fig. 1-16. Stress-strain curves of collagen and elastin.

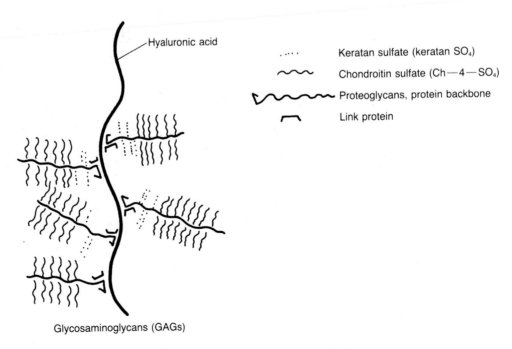

Fig. 1-17. Structure of glycosaminoglycans.

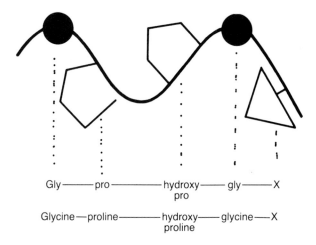

Fig. 1-18. Amino acid sequence of collagen.

collagen fibrils,[78] forming linkages with collagen fibers,[78] decreasing friction between fibers, resisting tissue compression, and helping transmit tensile loads between collagen fibers by filling in the spaces.

The third component of connective tissue, the cellular component, contains fibroblasts and fibrocytes, from which fibers are produced, as well as cells that are specific to a particular type of connective tissue.

Bone consists of a collagenous fiber component[1]; a ground substance of mostly calcium phosphate ($Ca^{++}P$), which is reordered to form hydroxyapatite, GAGs, and hyaluronic acid; general connective tissue cells; and the bone-specific cells: osteoblasts, osteocytes, osteoclasts, and osteoprogenitor cells. Bone is unique in that it has both an inorganic mineral component, mainly hydroxyapatite, and an organic component, mostly collagen but also GAGs and lipids.[75,99] Approximately 40% of bone is organic. Because the properties of bone differ significantly from the properties of either of the original components, bone is called a *composite material*.[75] Bone has been viewed as a two-phase material[129] in which the hydroxyapatite crystals are considered the high-modulus (or stiff) portion and collagen is the low-modulus (or deformable) portion. Others have represented bone with a three-phase model of mineral, organic, and fluid.[129]

Collagen has the general amino acid sequence glycine-proline-X and contains another amino acid, hydroxyproline (Fig. 1-18). In humans, only collagen contains hydroxyproline. Collagen exists in a greater relative amount in bone than in any other connective tissue or structure, and bone collagen has a shorter half-life than collagen of other areas of the body.[11] These facts suggest that detection of hydroxyproline in urine, for example, may yield valuable information about bone deposition and resorption during different states of growth, adaptation to exercise, and disease. Collagen originates from a precursor, tropocollagen, and has a triple alpha-helix formation[99] (Fig. 1-19). The stability of collagen is increased during maturation via crosslinkages formed

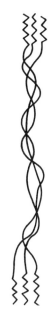

Fig. 1-19. Triple alpha helical chains forming tropocollagen.

between alpha-helices and various intramolecular and intermolecular bonds, including those of water, with the polar groups in the collagen backbone (Fig. 1-20).

Fibroblasts, if placed in tension and stretched as a result of muscle traction forces at a tubercle or because of bending that causes tension on one side of a bone, elongate and align to lines of tensile stress. Collagenous fibrils then appear along these lines to counteract the stress.[127,131] Water is attracted to and fills the intervening spaces between collagen fibrils, which allows the fibrils to develop even more of a parallel arrangement, thus increasing their structural stability. This parallel alignment allows collagen to resist tensile loads. However, collagen does not have equal mechanical properties when loaded in different directions and thus is termed *anisotropic* (Fig. 1-21). The ground substance portion of the organic phase of bone acts as a glue, lubricant, and shock absorber.[99]

The hydroxyapatite crystals of the inorganic or mineral phase of bone, composed of calcium and phosphorus, are slender rods 200 to 400 Å (angstrom = 10^{-10} m) long by 15 Å thick; they are located between and within the collagen fibrils.[99,107] Other mineral ions are citrate, carbonate fluoride, and hydroxyl ions.[99] The mineral phase gives stiffness (two-thirds that of steel), rigidity, and hardness to bone.[63]

New bone is formed by osteoblasts that mature to become osteocytes; bone is resorbed by osteoclasts. Osteoblasts synthesize enzymes that modify collagen fibrils and GAGs to produce osteoid or bone matrix.[107] Lysosomal, neutral pH phosphatase activity is unique to differentiated skeletal cells (i.e., osteoblasts, osteocytes, and osteoclasts) and to cartilage cells. A major difference between osteoblasts and osteoclasts is the tremendous quantity of lysosomal enzymes produced in the Golgi apparatus around the cell nucleus in osteoclasts.[107] Because osteoblastic activity causes bone deposi-

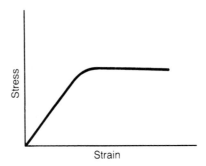

Fig. 1-20. The main collagen crosslink in bone is dehydrodihydroxylysinonorleucine.

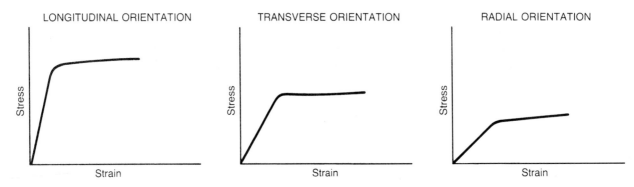

Fig. 1-21. *Top,* An isotropic material has a similar stress-strain curve independent of the direction of loading. *Bottom,* Different stress-strain curves result if nonisotropic material is loaded in different directions.

tion and osteoclastic activity causes bone resorption, more osteoclastic activity than osteoblastic activity results in bone loss. Osteoprogenitor cells are located in the endosteum (inside) and periosteum (outside) of bone. There is no periosteum at attachment sites for ligaments and tendons or on articular cartilage, and thus sesamoid bones, the subcapsular area of the femoral neck, and the talus lack osteoprogenitor cell activity.

BONE GROWTH

Bone can develop either by endochondral bone growth or ossification, which involves an intermediate cartilaginous model of the bone, or by membranous (intramembranous) bone growth, which involves direct bone formation from embryonic mesoderm, called *mesenchyme*.[10,30,32,72] Membranous bone growth occurs in bones that do not require a great magnitude of growth and in areas of the body that need protection early in life. The skull, sternum, and part of the clavicle are formed membranously. The rest of the bones grow in length by endochondral bone growth and often grow in width by membranous bone growth.[47] As one of the connective tissues, bone is derived from mesenchyme. Mesoderm is one of the three embryonic germ layers, the other two being ectoderm and endoderm (or entoderm). Bone from part of the face and jaw, formed from the pharyngeal arches, is mesectodermal (mesoderm and ectoderm) in origin. Mesenchyme differentiates into other connective tissues and into muscle, which is not connective tissue. Mesoderm forms lateral, intermediate, and medial portions called *somites* or *paraxial mesoderm*. Fig. 1-22 shows the three portions of mesoderm and their skeletal derivatives.

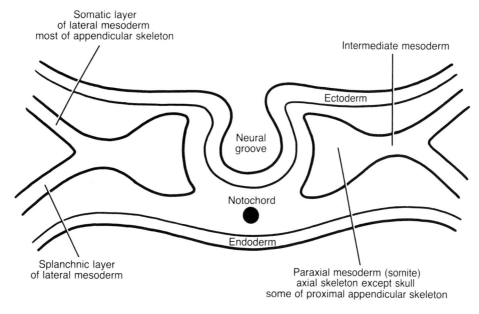

Fig. 1-22. Paraxial, intermediate, and lateral portions of intraembryonic mesoderm and their skeletal derivatives.

Sequential bone growth

The relative time schedule for bone growth follows.*
Prenatal period

Week 3 (after fertilization). Mesenchymal cells begin migration from the intraembryonic mesoderm to specific locations.

Week 4. The migrated mesenchymal cells aggregate and condense. Somites are formed from the paraxial mesenchymal cell aggregations. The somites consist of (1) a ventromedial portion, the sclerotome, which is the precursor for bone, cartilage, and ligament within the axial and the proximal appendicular skeleton, and (2) a dorsolateral portion, the dermomyotome, from which the dermis of the skin and skeletal muscle form, again for the axial skeleton plus the proximal portion of the appendicular skeleton.

The sclerotome migrates in three directions: ventromedially to surround the notochord and form the intervertebral disk, dorsolaterally to cover the neural tube forming the vertebral arch, and ventrolaterally toward the body wall to form the costal processes (future ribs) on the thoracic vertebrae and portions of the transverse processes on other vertebrae (Fig. 1-23).

Week 5. Mesenchymal models of future bones have now formed, with the upper extremity models at a slightly later stage of development than those of the lower extremities. The carpal bones have formed in the hand, but metacarpal bones and phalanges have not yet appeared.

Week 6. Mesenchymal cells differentiate into chondroblasts, resulting in cells that form hyaline cartilage models of future bones. Growth occurs by cell division in the middle of the cartilage (interstitial growth) and by proliferation and differentiation of new chondroblasts at the periphery of a

* References 30, 89, 90, 123, 128, 130.

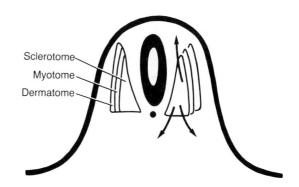

Fig. 1-23. Migration of cells from the sclerotome includes cells migrating ventromedially, dorsolaterally, and ventrolaterally.

cartilaginous mass (appositional growth). The deep part of the perichondrium contains cells capable of forming new chondroblasts, which can secrete ground substance and eventually become mature chondrocytes. Cartilaginous models are present in the hand for carpals, metacarpals, and proximal phalanges (Fig. 1-24).

Joints begin to develop at this time.[53] This development includes the start of differentiation of the interzone mesenchyme, between the mesenchyme of the future bones, into two dense laminae and one intermediate lamina. The dense laminae will form the articular cartilage at the ends of bone, and the intermediate lamina will form the area of cavitation, where synovial fluid will be found.

Embryological cartilage forms by the condensation of undifferentiated mesenchymal cells into centers of chondrification. In the vertebral column, five chondrification centers appear in each mesenchymal vertebra, two in the centrum, two in the vertebral arch, and one in the pedicle (Fig. 1-25).

Week 7. Three primary centers of ossification (bone) appear in the vertebrae, one in the anterior centrum and one

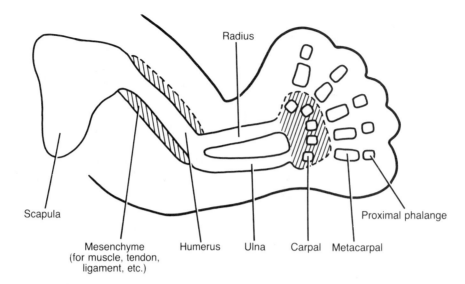

Fig. 1-24. The cartilaginous model of the hand bones includes metacarpals and proximal phalanges at 6 weeks of embryological development.

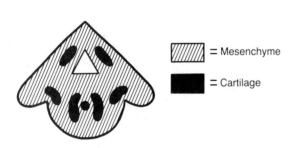

Fig. 1-25. Five chondrification centers in the vertebra at 6 weeks of embryological development.

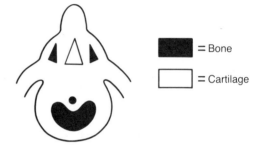

Fig. 1-26. Three primary centers of ossification in the vertebra at 7 weeks of embryological development.

in each pedicle area (Fig. 1-26). Primary ossification in cartilaginous models of the long bones of the limbs occurs as early as the seventh week. Cartilaginous models of the future hand bones include the proximal and middle phalanges of the hands. Joint development may end as early as week 7[96] but may extend to week 10.[53]

Week 8. Primary ossification begins in the diaphyses (shafts) of the future long limb bones (Fig. 1-27). The cartilaginous bone model, except at the articular surfaces, is enclosed in a dense, irregular connective tissue covering called the *perichondrium.* The deepest part of the perichondrium of the diaphysis contains osteoprogenitor cells that differentiate into osteoblasts, which form the bone collar on the shaft. As the bone collar forms, the connective tissue covering of the bone model is called the *periosteum* instead of the perichondrium, which covered the cartilaginous model of the bone. Blood vessels invade the bony collar first and then the central cavity, providing the pathway for osteoprogenitor and blood-forming stem cells to enter the bony interior (Fig. 1-28). As the blood vessels proliferate longitudinally in both directions, the invasion of vascular connective tissue and lysozymes stimulates cartilaginous

hypertrophy and degeneration, leaving calcified cartilage (bone mineral) at the ends of the bone.

Bone mineral is a complex calcium phosphate similar to hydroxyapatite [$Ca_{10}(PO_4)_6 OH_2$] and also contains calcium carbonate ($CaCO_3$), citrate, fluoride, Mg^{++}, and Na^+. The hydroxyapatite crystals become intimately related to the collagen fibers that have been carried in by the vascular connective tissue. Trabecular (primary spongiosa, spongy marrow, woven-fibered, cancellous, and interwoven) bone is formed as osteoblasts attach to the calcified cartilage spicules, break them down, and replace them with bony spicules, which then attach to other spicules (Fig. 1-29). Some osteoblasts become surrounded by the matrix and sit within lacunae, remaining connected to other cells by canaliculi. These cells are now called osteocytes.

Bony spicules with spaces among them are left as the vascular connective tissue from the deep periosteum carries osteoclasts as well as osteoblasts through the bone collar and into the central cavity. The bony spicules form medullary spaces. Calcified cartilage becomes covered with osteoblasts, which lay down osteoid matrix and develop into osteocytes if they become trapped in lacunae. Subperiosteal

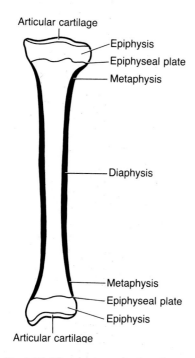

Fig. 1-27. The portions of a long bone.

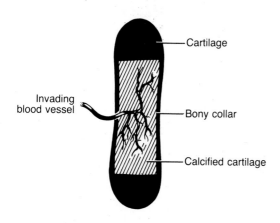

Fig. 1-28. Blood vessel invasion of bone.

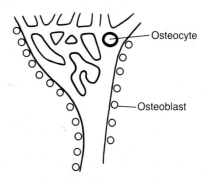

Fig. 1-29. Trabecular bone forms as osteoblasts break down calcified cartilage spicules and replace them with bony spicules.

trabeculae thicken and the space between them narrows. Collagen fibers from the matrix are secreted onto the walls of the spaces and become increasingly organized as parallel bundles, in either longitudinal or spiraled patterns. The osteocytes occupy roughly concentric rows around a central channel, the haversian canal, which contains nerves and blood vessels and usually capillaries or postcapillary venules, but only occasionally an arteriole.[9,10]

The haversian canal system forms the bone's nutritional source. The longitudinally coursing haversian canals are interconnected by the transversely and obliquely running Volkmann's canals (Fig. 1-30). These canals are unnecessary in cancellous bone, where nutrition can occur by diffusion. Haversian systems that are not fully developed but exist as sequential rows of osteocytes are called *primary osteons* or *atypical haversian systems.* These systems are eventually eroded and replaced by osteons characterized by layers of osteoid matrix around the osteocyte and a haversian canal. These are then called *secondary (lamellar) osteons* or *haversian systems.* Between the osteons are fragments of lamellar bone, organized into interstitial lamellae. There are also sharp demarcations, called *cement lines,* between the haversian system and the interstitial lamellae (Fig. 1-31).

The fibrovascular periosteum and endosteal tissue remain potentially osteogenic and contain cells that undergo mitosis and can secrete new matrix that is combined with collagen fibers. Bone modeling and remodeling occur through bone deposition and resorption by osteoblasts and osteoclasts, respectively, as growth progresses. Primary ossification centers extend throughout the bone shafts. The bony collar continues to thicken.

Postnatal period (years 1 to 2). Secondary centers of ossification begin to form with vascular invasion of the epiphyses, which proceeds as previously described.[123] Epiphyseal plates, or plates of cartilage, remain between the epiphyses (ends of the bone) and the metaphyses (areas of bone that connect the epiphyses and the diaphyses) (Fig. 1-27). Not all bones have two secondary centers of ossification.

Cartilaginous plates undergo interstitial growth, with the plate shape and cell orientation determined mostly by

bone is added and endosteal bone removed to form the primitive marrow cavity.

The main events of this eighth week include cartilaginous growth, formation of a central cavity via cartilaginous hypertrophy, degeneration, and calcification; formation of a bony collar, vascular invasion; cartilaginous changes toward the ends of the bone; and replacement of calcified cartilage spicules by bony spicules. Fetal movement is detectable by ultrasound imaging.[40,71]

Week 12 and after. Cartilage cells in the remainder of the bone model continue to grow by appositional and interstitial growth. Within the model, areas of reserve, proliferative, mature, and hypertrophic cartilage can be seen. As cancellous bone is formed, space develops around the bony spicules. As compact or cortical bone is formed, the

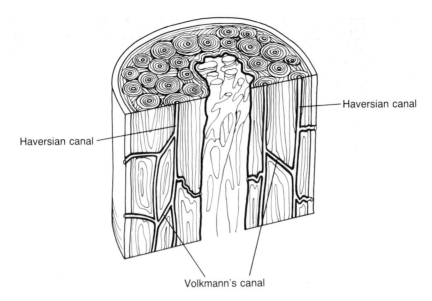

Fig. 1-30. Interconnection of haversian and Volkmann's canals.

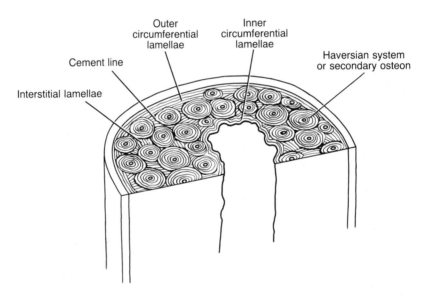

Fig. 1-31. Secondary bone with lamellar (secondary) osteons or haversian systems, interstitial lamellae, and circumferential lamellae with demarcating cement lines.

principal lines of tension and compression. Zones of cartilage within the epiphyseal plates include areas of cell reserve, proliferation, maturation, and hypertrophy. After the cells hypertrophy, they degenerate, and the walls of the empty lacunae fill with hydroxyapatite crystals. Bones lengthen by this process. The stimulus for bone growth in length is intermittent compression by weight bearing, muscle activation, and so forth.[47]

The stimulus for shape and growth of bony prominences is intermittent tension from ligaments or muscle-tendon units.[47] Cartilaginous growth plates also occur at concentrated areas of muscle attachment. Because muscle contraction causes the traction or tensile loading that stimulates bone growth at these areas, these epiphyseal plates are called

traction epiphyses or *apophyses*. A traction epiphysis is found at the greater trochanter of the femur, where many hip muscles are inserted.

Puberty and adulthood. When the epiphyseal plates have ossified, growth in length ceases. Most bones have ossified by the twentieth year. Table 1-3 lists bones that ossify by endochondral growth including the locations of the primary and secondary ossification centers.

Hyaline cartilage, which is avascular, aneural, and alymphatic, remains on the articular surfaces of bone. Therefore, periosteum is absent from the articular bone surfaces, from the attachment sites of tendons and ligaments, and from sesamoid bone surfaces (such as the patella). Wherever periosteum is absent, the connective tissue in

Table 1-3. Primary and secondary centers of ossification

Bone	Primary center	Secondary center
Humerus	Shaft	One proximal epiphyseal plate Apophysis at greater tubercle Apophysis at lesser tubercle One distal epiphyseal plate
Radius	Shaft	One proximal plate One distal plate
Ulna	Shaft	One proximal plate One distal plate
Metacarpals	Center	One proximal plate for thumb One distal plate for digits 2 to 5
Phalanges (hand)	Body	One proximal plate (begins to form in years 3 or 4)
Vertebrae	Centrum	One at spinous process One at each transverse process One at superior edge of body One at inferior edge of body, beginning at puberty
Femur	Shaft	One proximal plate Apophysis at greater trochanter Apophysis at lesser trochanter One distal plate
Tibia	Shaft	One proximal plate, one distal plate
Fibula	Shaft	One proximal plate, one distal plate
Metatarsals	Center	One proximal plate for hallux One distal plate for toes 2 to 5
Phalanges (feet)		One proximal plate (fused by years 11 or 12)
Clavicle	Growth is membranous in center and endochondral at ends	
Scapula	Body	Two at coracoid process Two at acromion One each at medial border, inferior angle, and lower rim of glenoid cavity
Sternum	Manubrium ossifies from one, two, or three centers—first and second sternebrae (one of four sections from which sternum develops) usually from one center and third and fourth usually from two centers; these centers appear in fifth intrauterine month; union between centers occurs at about puberty for the third and fourth sternebrae, 25 years of age for first and second, and 40 years of age for xiphoid process.	
Ribs	Rib 1 (shaft) Ribs 2 to 10 (angle of rib) Ribs 11 and 12 (shaft and head)	One at head, one at tubercle One at head One at articular part of tubercle One at nonarticular part of tubercle
Pelvis	Ilium (above greater sciatic notch) Ischial body (month 4) Superior ramus of pubis (months 4 or 5)	Two at iliac crest One at acetabulum One at acetabulum One at acetabulum

Modified from Tachdjian MO: *Pediatric orthopaedics*, Philadelphia, 1972, WB Saunders.

contact with the bone lacks the osteogenic potential to aid in the healing of fractures in the area. The tarsal and carpal bones are particularly lacking in periosteum.

Membranous (intramembranous) bone growth

Membranous bone growth[30] takes place earlier and more rapidly than endochondral bone growth. During the formation of the flat bones of the skull (frontal, parietal, temporal, and parts of the mandible and sphenoid bones), condensations of mesenchymal cells occur in proximity to blood vessels. Mesenchymal cells in some areas of the body begin to produce a mucoprotein (organic) matrix called *osteoid*, in which collagen fibers become embedded. Inorganic crystals of calcium phosphate accumulate around, inside, and on the collagen fibers. This accumulation results in a mineralization of the osteoid matrix (ossification). From the calcium and phosphate, a group of minerals called *apatites* are formed, the most abundant of which is hydroxyapatite.

In the membranous growth areas, mesenchymal cells differentiate into osteoblasts, which secrete osteoid. The osteoid quickly becomes mineralized, and osteoblasts embedded in it become osteocytes. Extensions from these osteocytes emerge and contact other cellular extensions via pathways called *canaliculi,* which carry ions and nutrients. The space around the nucleus of the osteocyte, the *lacuna,* is formed by the removal of osteoid. Spicules of bone form and unite with other spicules or trabeculae to form a meshwork of primary cancellous bone. A layer of osteoblasts forms deep to the superficial dense sheath of connective tissue and becomes the cambium layer of the periosteum.[33] These osteoblasts deposit subperiosteal layers of bone called *lamellae.*

Near the time of birth, the primary cancellous bone becomes compact in some locations. This process involves a thickening of trabeculae by the addition of concentric lamellae around osteocytes and trabecular rearrangement into haversian systems or secondary osteons. The bony trabeculae in the relatively large marrow spaces are called *primary osteons.* Eventually the original marrow space becomes only a small tubular pathway, a central osteonal or haversian canal, which contains a single capillary and nerve fiber. The haversian system is composed of 4 to 20 (usually 6 or less) concentric lamellae. The canal is about 50 μm in diameter, and the concentric lamellae are 3 to 7 μm thick. With formation of many secondary osteons, the cancellous bone becomes compact bone. Where trabecular bone remains, trabecular growth ceases and vascular tissue differentiates into hematopoietic tissue. Compact bone forms the outer portions of the membranous bone growth areas, surrounding marrow cavities called *diploës,* which are centrally located and surrounded by trabecular bone.

When the bone reaches its eventual size, the osteoblasts revert to resting osteoprogenitor cells. Bone modeling and remodeling occur by the same mechanism of osteoblastic-osteoclastic activity.

The secondary osteons in the compact bone usually course along the length of the bone. Cement lines, which are highly mineralized and devoid of collagen fibers, clearly mark the outer limit of each secondary osteon. Communication among the haversian canals and between the canals and the periosteum is by the transverse and obliquely coursing Volkmann's canals.

All bones have an outer shell of cortical or compact bone and an inner mass of trabecular bone, except where the latter is replaced by the medullary cavity or an air space.[89,90] Trabecular bone gradually becomes cortical toward the outer surface of the bone.[33,99] In long bones, the epiphyseal and metaphyseal areas are mostly trabecular, whereas the diaphyses are mostly compact bone. Cortical bone is distinguished from cancellous bone by the amount of mineralized tissue per total bone tissue volume. Measures of mineralized tissue include bone porosity (percentage of non-mineralized tissue), apparent density (mineral tissue/total bone tissue volume), and ash density (ash weight/total bone tissue volume).[21] Ash weight is a measure of the mineralized portion of bone. Advanced densitometric techniques have made possible accurate measurement of bone density and skeletal loss.[57]

Cortical bone is 5% to 30% porous—that is, 5% to 30% of the tissue is nonmineralized—whereas cancellous bone is 30% to 90% porous.[94] Interestingly, the term *cancellous* is derived from *cancelli,* the Italian word for the open lattice screens behind which Roman judges sat. Spongy bone is a three-dimensional lattice or meshwork of bony spicules (trabeculae or rods) and thin plates (lamellae).[64,118] The term *trabeculae* here indicates only the rod portion of cancellous bone, but it is often used loosely to indicate all elements of cancellous bone. Human cancellous bone may be of many types, varying in a composition as follows[117]:

1. Rods only in deeper parts of the ends and walls of the marrow cavities in the shafts of long bones
2. Rods and plates
   a. Large plates with rods, as in the pubis and lateral angle of the scapula
   b. Thick rods with irregularly shaped plates, as in the calcaneus
   c. Plates crossed by rods, as in the epiphyseal bone adjacent to some articular surfaces, such as in the patella or bodies of upper cervical vertebrae
3. Plates only, as in the ends of the tibia

The rod structure provides support along the medullary canals, whereas the plate structure provides support near articular surfaces. Because the plate structure exists at the tibial plateau area, which is subject to high shear stresses, this type of structure appears to offer strength to resist shear stresses as well.[117]

STRENGTH (MECHANICAL PROPERTIES) OF BONE
Stresses and strains related to bone shape

The loads placed on a bone can be seen as loads placed on a beam. Bone has an elastic deformation range and a yielding point that delineates the deformation range from a nonelastic or plastic range.[13,94] Bone is not entirely linearly elastic in the initial portion of its stress-strain curve.[94] Therefore, bone is subject to nonrecoverable deformation ("creep" or plastic flow) but can yield under stress and recover from deformation within a range (elastic range of the stress-strain curve). However, bone does not exhibit large recoverable deformations when significant energy loss or hysteresis occurs during loading and unloading.[5] Bone is neither ductile nor brittle but a combination of the two[94]; the mineral phase is more brittle and the organic (collagenous) phase more ductile. Because bone demonstrates time-dependent characteristics (changes in mechanical properties with altered rates and duration of load applications), it is considered a viscous material as well as a material with elastic qualities, which are not time dependent. Bone, like other connective tissues, is both viscous and elastic, or a viscoelastic material.[23,41,64]

Tensile loads on bone cause tensile stress and strain. A bone is strengthened in tension if the collagen fibrils (one fiber being composed of many fibrils) are aligned parallel to the tensile load.[105] The scanning electron microscope enables identification of the spatial orientation of the collagen fibrils in bone. The concentric rings in the osteons of cortical bone contain collagen fibrils that are arranged in parallel for each layer or lamella. However, the collagen fibrils in consecutive layers do not course in the same direction. Investigators have described fibril directions in consecutive layers as alternating in a longitudinal and then circumferential pattern in reference to the haversian canal[107] or in a longitudinal, then circumferential, and then oblique pattern, with most periosteal collagen fibrils oriented in the direction of the bone axis and additional fibrils interconnecting with the concentric lamellae.[63,75] Osteons with a predominantly longitudinal or predominantly oblique direction of collagen fibrils or a mixture were also observed.[44]

Bone organization with layers of collagen fibrils coursing in different directions allows bone to be strengthened by tension[72] in several planes because deformation from tensile loads is resisted when the load is applied parallel to the fiber direction. More and more layers of bone and increasing cross-sectional area lead to increased bone strength and stiffness as well. At bony attachment sites, collagen fibrils often become oriented parallel to large tensile stress from muscle-tendon units or ligaments. The primary orientation of the collagen fibrils in the tibial tuberosity is shown in Fig. 1-32. The fibrils have been aligned for the most part parallel to the pull of the patellar ligament.[117] The maximal tensile stress from any of these sources is located on a plane perpendicular to the tensile load (Fig. 1-33). Therefore, an increase in cross-sectional area increases bone strength and stiffness in tension, as long as the tensile loads are applied axially—that is, not as bending loads.

In periosteal, endosteal, and trabecular bone, most of the collagen fibers are oriented in the direction of the bone axis or along the axis of the trabeculae, indicating their function in resisting tensile or compressive stresses.[75] The hydroxyapatite crystals exist as rods and plates oriented with their long axes parallel to the local direction of the collagen fibrils.[63]

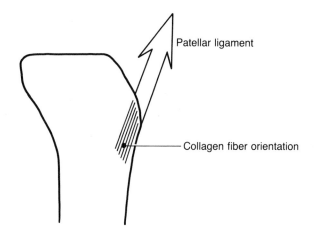

Fig. 1-32. Alignment of collagen fibrils parallel to the pull of the patellar ligament.

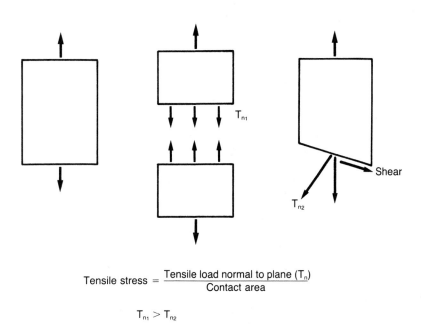

$$\text{Tensile stress} = \frac{\text{Tensile load normal to plane } (T_n)}{\text{Contact area}}$$

$$T_{n1} > T_{n2}$$

Fig. 1-33. Maximal tensile stress is located on a plane perpendicular to the tensile load.

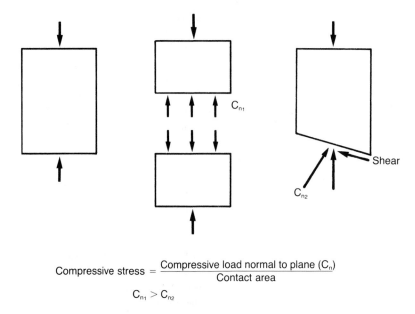

$$\text{Compressive stress} = \frac{\text{Compressive load normal to plane (C}_n)}{\text{Contact area}}$$

$$C_{n1} > C_{n2}$$

Fig. 1-34. Maximal compressive stress is located on a plane perpendicular to the compressive load.

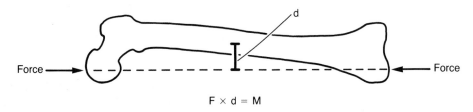

$$F \times d = M$$

Fig. 1-35. Calculation of the moment of force in an axially loaded bowed structure.

Like tensile loads, compressive loads on bone cause compressive stress and strain, with maximal compression occurring along a perpendicular plane to the applied load (Fig. 1-34). An increase in the cross-sectional area of bone increases the strength and stiffness of axially compressed bone. Vertebral bodies and inferior femoral neck regions receive the greatest compression loads.

Shear stress and strain occur with both tensile and compressive loads. Marked shear loads occur in cancellous bone. A specific anatomical area that receives great shear loads is the tibial plateau area.

Bending loads cause tension, compression, and shear stresses and strains. Increasing the moment of inertia of a bone in a particular direction by increasing the amount of bone or by displacing the bone farther from the axis of bending increases the resistance of bone to bending in that direction. An example of axial loading is the load placed on the bent femur during weight bearing. Fig. 1-35 shows that the bending moment caused by the loading force equals the loading force times the perpendicular distance from the action line of the force to the neutral axis (M = F × d).

Torsional loads caused by twisting result in large shear stresses over the entire surface of the bone, with maximal shear on planes that are perpendicular and parallel to the

applied loads and with maximal tension and compression on diagonal planes. Increasing the polar moment of inertia of a bone in any one direction increases the resistance of the bone to torsion or twisting, indicating an increased maximal shear stress strength of the bone.

Usually there are combined loads on bone. Combination loads serve useful functions in decreasing the net effect of a particular load. For example, the femoral neck sustains large compressive loads inferiorly and large tensile loads superiorly as a result of bending loads during weight bearing. However, the hip abductors, particularly the gluteus medius, are active during weight bearing, causing a compressive load superiorly on the femoral neck, which produces a marked decrease of the tensile load on the superior neck (Fig. 1-36). Because bone fails with lower tensile loads than compressive loads, preventing muscular fatigue can reduce the risk of fractures. Specifically in this case, prevention of hip abductor fatigue or loading when fatigue has occurred can reduce the risk of femoral neck fractures.

Bone is a living material. Although metabolically expensive to produce, it can be modeled (development of the initial shape) and remodeled (ongoing deposition-resorption modifications of the shape with time or after a fracture), which is in obvious and striking contrast to the analogy of bone as a

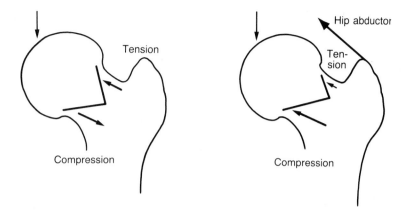

Fig. 1-36. Muscle contraction can decrease tensile loading on a bone.

simple beam. The approximate shape of bone is genetically determined, evidenced by protuberances (although underdeveloped) and bendings in newborns' bones.[71,92,120] However, much of the detailed form of bone is produced by stresses and strains caused by weight bearing and loading from muscle-tendon units and ligaments.[47,49,91] Frost proposed that the genetic factor was dominant until 8 weeks of intrauterine development, at which time mechanical forces on the bone became the overriding stimuli for bone remodeling.[47] The long weight-bearing bones resemble slightly curved beams, so that bending stresses can be minimized.[31] The geometry of the metaphyses allows the transfer of high loads applied at articular surfaces to the compact bone of the diaphyses.[64] Attachment sites of ligaments and tendons on bone provide a means to transfer joint loads to the cortical shaft.[115]

The purpose of bone modeling is to modify the shape and adjust the mass of a bone so that the stresses of everyday activities can be withstood. Bone strength can be altered by changes in the material and geometrical properties of bone. Material properties include the percentage of organic to nonorganic portions of bone, the number of crosslinks among the collagen fibrils, and the orientation of collagen fibrils in relation to the orientation of applied loads.[44] Geometrical properties, such as the amount of cortical and subperiosteal area, the plane of the maximal moment of inertia (the plane with the greatest resistance to bending), and the plane of the minimal moment of inertia (the plane with the least resistance to bending), represent the structural strength of bone. In some instances, changes in material properties that would weaken the bone may be compensated for by changes in geometrical properties. This topic is discussed in the section on age-related changes of bone.

Many theories have been proposed regarding the mechanism that stimulates bone modeling and remodeling. Bassett stated that bones subjected to mechanical strain develop electrical charges, with compressed regions (tending to be concave) having a negative charge and tensile regions (tending to be convex) having a positive charge.[6,7] Because

of this polarity, bone may be laid down in negatively charged regions by osteoblasts and resorbed by osteoclasts in positively charged areas. This linkage of mechanical strain and electrical polarization, called the *piezoelectric effect,* is a possible stimulus for bone modeling and remodeling. Bassett and Pawlick implanted a metal plate next to living femoral shaft bone in adult dogs and found that, when optimal amperage was used, new bone was laid down at the cathode (negatively charged plate), with a peak effect seen in 2 weeks.[7] No osteoclasis occurred at the anode. However, when Hert and Zalud measured negative potentials on compressed bone surfaces and positive potentials on surfaces subjected to tensile strain in rabbit tibiae undergoing intermittent bending loads, they found that appositional bone growth occurred on both surfaces.[68] They proposed an alternate hypothesis that negative and positive electrical potentials may constitute a nonspecific activator of osteogenic activity by inducing ion shifts in bone. Fukada identified the piezoelectric activity as caused by the collagen fibrils.[52] Becker and Murray reported that the electrical field resulting from stress within bone and observed at fracture sites is capable of activating protein-synthesizing organelles in osteogenic cells in frogs.[8] In addition, they claimed that the presence of the electrical field near polymerizing tropocollagen caused fibers to orient perpendicularly to lines of force.

Many researchers hypothesize that mechanical stresses modulate the growth, addition, or resorption of bone. Optimal stress within an appropriate range is essential for bone strength because understressed or overstressed bone can be weakened by resorption that overwhelms bone deposition.[54,64,99] Wolff's law (1884) relates bone growth to the stresses and strains placed on bone.[135] The ability of bone to adapt by changing size, shape, and structure depends on the mechanical stresses on the bone. Wolff's law can be paraphrased as follows: Where there is optimal stress within bone, bone deposition is greater than bone resorption; where there is nonoptimal stress due to either inadequate or excessive stress, bone resorption is greater

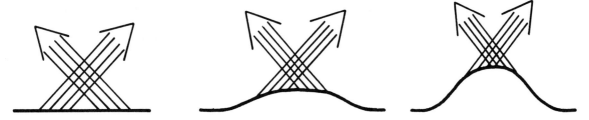

Fig. 1-37. Bony protuberances develop as a result of tensile stress.

than bone deposition.[106] Increased deposition results in increased bone density, strength, stiffness, and the like, and vice versa. Bone changes in external shape (external or surface remodeling) and in porosity, mineral content, radiographic opacity, and mass density (internal remodeling).[54] These changes can be rapid (several days because of increased output or uptake of mineral salts) or slow (months to years). Long bones increase in length from intermittent optimal compressive stress and develop protuberances from intermittent optimal tensile stress (Fig. 1-37).

Clinical manifestations of Wolff's law are abundant. Improper placement or tightening of plates, screws, nuts, or bolts in bone surgery may cause bone resorption because of either local stress concentration or decreased vascular perfusion.[15,29,54] Plates that are too rigid also may cause bone atrophy, as intermittent compressive stresses cannot be perceived by bone prevented from deforming.[112] Decreased stress on bones caused by weightlessness in space travel,[83] by immobilization from casting a portion of the body,[39] or by bed rest results in a net loss of calcium[39,83] and phosphorus[39] from the body. When volunteers were immobilized in bivalved casts from the waist down for 6 to 7 weeks, normal levels of calcium and phosphorus were not regained for more than 6 weeks after removal of the casts.[39] In an attempt to avoid massive bone resorption during space travel, astronauts utilize daily calcium supplements and simulated weight-bearing exercises.[83]

Currey stated that surface osteocytes received information via transient electrical fields or from the nerves entering the periosteum and initiated the adaptation or remodeling process.[31] However, direct innervation of bone may not be required for bone to react to stress, in that Hert, Liskova, and Landrgot found that compact bone reacted to intermittent stress by apposition of new bone regardless of whether the periosteum was innervated.[66] Roux, as quoted by Fung[54] and reviewed by Roesler[109] and Pauwels,[100] formulated in 1895 two principles of bone remodeling: (1) functional adaptation (adaptation to function by practicing the function) and (2) maximum-minimum design (maximum strength achieved with a minimum of material). Roux stated that compression and tension were the functional stimuli that controlled modeling and that bony deposition and resorption were connected with the absolute value of local stress.

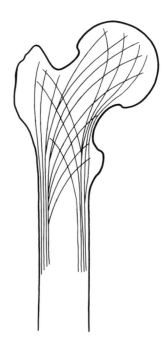

Fig. 1-38. Trajectorial design of trabeculae.

Wolff and Roux proposed a trajectorial design for the trabeculae of the femoral neck. This arrangement of trabeculae would result in the greatest strength of the femoral neck during weight bearing (Fig. 1-38). Hayes and Snyder supported this trajectorial theory of trabecular architecture with highly significant correlations between principal stress directions and trabecular orientation.[65] They suggested that trabecular bone was densest in regions of high shear stress (the principle of maximum difference in stresses causing shear), that trabeculae were aligned in the principal stress direction (45 degrees to the plane of maximum shear), and that trabecular orientation developed to minimize bending deformations in individual trabeculae. Lanyon has shown that the direction of trabeculae conforms closely to the direction of the greatest principal strains.[80]

Frost suggested that mechanical loads may control bone modeling in portions of bone between articulations and apophyses based on the amount of surface strain caused by the loads.[47,51] Osteoclastic activity would occur on the convex surface and osteoblastic activity would occur on the concave surface as bone drifted toward the load-induced concavity and therefore minimized bending and maximized compressive stress. Frost described this process as the flexural drift law. Because bone has greater strength with compressive loads than with other types of load, this process would strengthen the bone in general. Frost distinguished internal remodeling, which involves adding or removing bone on osteons already in existence, and surface remodeling, which involves the deposition of new bone on periosteal and endosteal surfaces.[51,109] Remodeling involves reduction of flexural unit strains of lamellar bone tissue to or below a threshold level of strain stimulus[110] called the *minimal effective strain* (MES).[47] Frost previously described this process as the minimum strain principle.[51]

Several studies have involved in vivo imposed loading of the bones of experimental animals.[29,80] The most optimal loading pattern is controversial, as compressive loading may have a greater remodeling effect than loading in bending,[29] and dynamic bending forces may have a greater remodeling effect than dynamic compressive or tensile forces alone.[47] Bone growth has been correlated with the magnitude of loading, the strain rate during each loading cycle (with the strain rate being more critical than the peak magnitude of strain),[80] the required number of consecutive loading cycles per day (which can be as few as 36[80]), and the strain range. The strain range varies from expected strains connected with walking (0.001), running (0.001 to 0.002), and vigorous exercise (0.002 to 0.004) to strains that are large enough to create considerable fatigue, microdamage, and a strong remodeling stimulus.[17] The optimal stresses, the optimal loading conditions to produce these optimal stresses, and the best way to determine when the optimal stresses have been attained have not yet been determined.

The biochemical activity of calcium may be involved in the modeling or remodeling process of bone. Justus and Luft in 1970 found that, when bone undergoes strain, there is an increased calcium concentration in the interstitial fluid.[74] This increased concentration is due to a change in the solubility of hydroxyapatite crystals in response to stress. The chain of events is shown in the following flowchart:

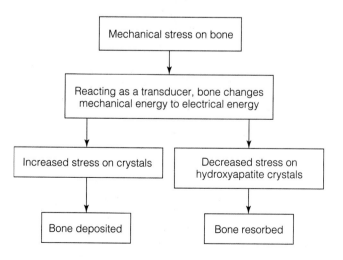

Altered strength of bone can be explained by one of the remodeling theories presented, by a combination of theories, or perhaps by some process not yet fully understood. Because collagen fibers provide tensile strength, stiffness, and ductility, GAGs provide compressive strength and bonding among collagen fibers; cells each have their own function, change in the percentage of these materials, and the direction of the fibers alter the strength properties of bone. The stress-strain curves of collagen and elastin (Fig. 1-16) demonstrate that collagen fibers can withstand 10% or less elongation, whereas elastin fibers can be elongated to 200% of their original length before they fail.[94]

Collagen fibers can vary a great deal in orientation within any connective tissue, including bone. Fibers can have a course parallel, perpendicular, oblique, or random to any applied load; they can course singly or in series; and they can be crimped (exist in a wavy state when relaxed and a straightened state when loaded). If all fibers are oriented equally in all directions, the structure is isotropic; that is, it possesses the same mechanical properties when loaded in all directions. However, the anisotropic nature of bone results in different mechanical properties of the bone with different load types and different directions of loading, depending on the orientation of the bone structure with respect to the applied load.[64]

Areas of bone strength and weakness

Mechanical stresses on bone (as well as on other biological materials, such as wood) more or less conform to engineering estimations. The stresses and strains on soft tissues, in contrast, seldom strictly obey Hooke's law. The strains measured in animal soft tissue can be 1000 times higher than the strains with which an engineer deals.

The strength of a composite material such as bone can be estimated by determining the stress-strain curves of the fiber and matrix materials.[63] If the fibers and matrix are well bonded and deform together, the load on the composite is shared between them in proportion to the cross-sectional area of each. Although the compressive strength of many composite materials is lower than their tensile strength, bone has a higher compressive strength.[54,63] The collagen fibers provide flexibility within bone, and the whole organic component allows bone to be a good energy absorber. The mineral component provides rigidity and stiffness, about two thirds of the stiffness of steel.[63,75] Most of the load in a normal loading situation is carried by the mineral phase because demineralized bone has only 5% to 10% of the strength of mineralized bone.[90] The microstructural organization of bone (i.e., the osteons and interstitial lamellae, bonded at cement lines with ground substance) is partly responsible for some of the viscoelastic properties of macroscopic bone. In torsional loading, cement lines contribute significantly to the viscoelastic properties of bone.[75]

Specific geometrical properties of bone indicate the strength of bone with specific loading patterns. Bone cross-sectional area is proportional to bone strength in axial loading, that is, loading in either tension or compression. With a bending or torsional load, the maximal and minimal moments of inertia indicate bone strength or resistance to bending in two planes or to twisting in a third plane of motion, respectively.

Cement lines around the osteons and the planes between the lamellae in the haversian systems are generally weak areas in bone.[88] Bone stiffness is inversely proportional to osteon size, the ratio of osteons to cement lines, and the size of haversian and Volkmann's canals.[33,75] Stiffness is the ratio of stress to strain, load to deformation, or force to length. Haversian bone has been reported to have 69% of the compliance of lamellar bone.[62,75] Compliance is the ratio of strain to stress, deformation to load, or length to force and is the inverse of stiffness.

Bone strength is increased by:

1. Increasing the bone density, with a correlation of $p = +.40$ to $+.42$[41,129]
2. Increasing the mineralization of bone to an optimal level[129]
3. Increasing the percentage of small particles within bone,[106] which increases the surface area that is available for bonding; small particles can account for as much as 30% of the total number of particles in bone, and their presence increases the tensile strength of bone
4. Increasing the stiffness of bone[129]
5. Increasing the length to diameter ratio (slenderness) of fibers within bone[129]; apatite crystals join end to end to increase fiber length
6. Increasing the cross-sectional area of bone,[94] which affects strength in tension, compression, bending, and torsion (proportionality does not always exist; for example, a decrease in diameter by 20% may decrease the bone strength in torsion by 60%[94])
7. Altering the distribution of bone tissue so as to increase the area moment of inertia,[94] which increases the bone strength in bending and torsion
8. Increasing the strain rate[34]

Bone stiffness can be increased by:

1. Increasing the density of bone[41,75,129]
2. Decreasing the water content of bone, which increases the viscosity[106] and degree of mineralization[75]
3. Increasing the speed at which bone is loaded[94] (during normal activity, a small percentage of the total energy storage of a bone is used; this energy storage capacity varies proportionally with the speed at which bone is loaded)
4. Increasing the strain rate[21,54]
5. Increasing the cross-sectional area of bone[94]
6. Increasing the area moment of inertia of the bone[94]

The shape of a bone as a whole and the orientation of trabeculae within it are determined genetically and according to the stresses to which the bone is subjected.[94,119] For any of the weight-bearing bones, compression is caused by weight bearing, and bending is produced if the compression is eccentric to the neutral axis of the bone. Reduction of bending in cortical bone and the tensile stress resulting from the bending can result from a number of factors:

1. Movement at joints eliminates the need for bone to bend as much within the shaft.[103] Decreased range of motion in a joint may lead to abnormal bending loads on the bone.
2. As mentioned previously, some muscles, such as the gluteus medius, contract to reduce bending and therefore tensile stress, in this case on the femoral neck. Bony protuberances, such as the greater trochanter in this example, increase the mechanical advantage and therefore the effectiveness of the muscles.[90]
3. The curve of a bone is in alignment with the predominant resultant force(s) acting on the bone, which increases the compressive stress on the bone but reduces the bending tendency and therefore the tensile stress. Bone fatigues at lower bending stresses than axial stresses, and bone is weaker in tension than in compression,[63] so reducing bending stresses[31] as well as tensile stresses is important (Fig. 1-39).
4. Bones are hollow, tubular structures.[99,103] The longer the bone, the greater the magnitude of the bending moment caused by application of a force. The stresses are proportional to the bending moment; that is, they are increased as the bending moment is increased. The tubular shape of bones and the increase in the moment of inertia therefore allow a lighter bone to have the

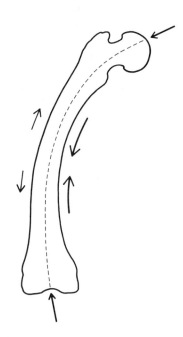

Fig. 1-39. Loading of a curved bone can result in decreased tensile stresses because of a decreased bending moment.

same bending strength as a solidly filled structure.[41,99] A bone can be protected against fracture by eccentric distribution of bone mass. Large bone mass also protects against fracture, but the bone then becomes unmanageably heavy.[31]

The polar moment of inertia is the mechanical property of bone that represents the strength of bone in resisting torsional or twisting loads, just as bending moment of inertia represents the strength of bone in resisting bending loads. Tubular bone allows even greater resistance to torsional loads than to bending loads. The resistance to the torsional load for circular sections such as long bones is proportional to the distance of the bone mass from the neutral axis raised to the fourth power. The magnitude of bone mass is important, but not as important as distribution of the bone mass.[103]

Activities such as standing, walking, carrying, throwing, and pounding produce mainly tensile stress on the convex side of long bones as a result of bending stresses within the bone. Regions where net tension in a skeleton occurs during such functions include[95]:

1. Bony crests where opposing muscles have linear attachments on opposite edges, as on the cranial crests or the crest of the scapular spine. The temporal muscles, for example, pull laterally on the sagittal crest of the cranium. Usually humans and other species chew alternately on each side of the mouth, so that the sagittal crest area is not in marked net tension for a long period of time. Another example is the pull of the middle trapezius muscle, opposing that of the middle and posterior deltoid muscles on the scapular spine and acromion process. These three muscles usually do not contract forcefully at the same time and thereby avoid a large net tension at this site.

2. Thin bony plates where opposing muscles have surface attachments on either side. The infraspinatus and subscapularis muscles are good examples as they attach to opposite surfaces of the scapula. Both have acute angles of application on the scapula, so that when they cocontract, as during shoulder stabilization, they do not have a great percentage of their pull applied perpendicularly (or normally) to the scapula. They have opposing rotation functions at the shoulder as well. As a result, there is seldom a great net tensile stress on the scapular surface.

3. When muscles pull on opposite sides of a structure, a fibrous sheet may exist between the muscles. An example is the obturator foramen, where the internal and external obturator muscles attach on opposite sides of the obturator membrane, as well as on the surrounding bone. Net tension occurs at the attachment site during external hip rotation, the main motion of both muscles, but the membrane instead of the bone resists some of the tension.

4. Bones, such as the patella, which is loaded in net tension when both the quadriceps tendon and patellar ligament are tight.

The mechanical properties of cancellous bone and diplöe depend on the orientation and distribution of trabeculae within the bone.[41] Trabeculae are arranged to provide maximal strength with a minimum of material. They are aligned according to the principal stress directions in a particular bone, taking into consideration the forces, quantities of forces over time, and direction of the forces, that is, according to physiological loading.[99] The trabeculae in the proximal femur have been closely studied regarding the thickness, spacing, and density of the trabeculae. The principal stress directions in the proximal femur may be compressive,[79] a combination of tensile and compressive stresses,[95] or predominantly shear stresses.[65]

The strength of trabecular bone is less than that of cortical bone. The relationship of trabecular direction and mechanical strength for cancellous bone appears in Table 1-4 and that for cortical bone appears in Table 1-5. The specimens that are compared include longitudinal bone sections (sections cut parallel to the longitudinal axis of the bone), transverse sections (cut perpendicular to the longitudinal axis), radial sections (cut in the direction of the center of the arc formed by the longitudinal axis), and tangential sections (cut at a tangent to the longitudinal axis). These sections are diagrammed in Fig. 1-40.

Longitudinal sections of cortical bone can absorb more energy before failure than transverse sections, which is consistent, for example, with the lines of weight bearing in the lower extremity bones. In general, the stress and strain characteristics of cortical bone in adult human long bones are influenced by the duration and magnitude of the load applied because the rate of plastic deflection of bone is proportional to the magnitude of the applied stress.[41] The measures of several mechanical strengths for different bones, as listed by Park,[99] are given in Table 1-6. Femoral strength has been reported as 160 MPa in bending and 54.1 MPa for ultimate shear as tested in torsion.[5,54]

The greatest strength overall of the weight-bearing bones of the lower extremities is in the longitudinal sections (Tables 1-4 to 1-6). External loading in these bones is closely aligned to the longitudinal axis more often than to any other axis. In the vertebral segments, external loading most often occurs along the longitudinal extent of the vertebral column but farther from the axis than in the lower extremities. In the upper extremities, the main load imposed on the major bones is in bending, characterized by such activities as throwing, pounding, lifting, and carrying. These loads cause primarily tensile stresses on the convex side of long upper extremity bones, which correspond to the posterior surfaces of the humerus, ulna, and radius. This loading pattern requires great strength in the upper extremity bones along the longitudinal axis to resist bending loads. Greater shear strength in the longitudinal sections of compact long bones

Table 1-4. The relationship of trabecular direction and mechanical strength in cancellous bone

	Compression	Tension	Shear
Strength	Trabeculae are aligned primarily according to compressive stresses[67]	Ultimate tensile strength is less than ultimate compressive strength[94]	Trabeculae may be aligned according to the direction of principal shear stresses[56] Longitudinal sections loaded normally are stronger than transverse ones loaded parallel
Strain	Sections cut and loaded in a lateromedial direction have the greatest amount of compressive strain	Ultimate tensile strain is less than ultimate compressive strain[94]	
Modulus of elasticity	Modulus is less with compressive loads than with tensile ones	Modulus is greater with tensile loads than with compressive ones; the E of trabecular bone is less than that of compact bone[94]	Sections cut and loaded in a lateromedial direction have the highest shear modulus
Energy absorbed to failure			Sections cut and loaded in a lateromedial direction have the greatest amount of energy absorbed to failure
Density			Sections cut and loaded in a lateromedial direction have the greatest amount of density

Based on data from Evans FG: *Mechanical properties of bone,* Springfield, Ill, 1973, Charles C Thomas.

is also required at the sites of muscle, tendon, and ligamentous attachment.

Compact bone can undergo less strain as the number of osteons increases because of the general weakness of cement lines, which increase as the number of osteons increases. This effect is particularly important to remember when a bone is loaded in shear because less strain will be tolerated before fatigue as the osteon number increases. Greater deformation is tolerated by compact bone loaded in torsion than by compact bone loaded in tension, which is beneficial because the initial failure of compact bone loaded in torsion is in shear.

The compressive strength and modulus of elasticity for different types of osteons have been tested.[130] Three types of osteons have been isolated. Type 1 osteons have lamellae with collagen fibers coursing predominantly in a transverse spiral direction. The collagen fibers in the lamellae of type 2 osteons course in a transverse direction in one lamella and a longitudinal direction in the next, whereas those in type 3 osteons had predominantly longitudinal fibers. Compressive strength was greatest for type 1 osteons and least for type 3 osteons. Tensile strength was greater in bone with osteons that had collagen fibers that coursed longitudinally (type 3) or were steeply spiraling (type 2) than in bone that had osteons with transverse (type 1) fibers.[75]

The modulus of elasticity of cancellous bone is less than that of cortical bone.[54] The modulus (E) for tensile loading is intermediate between the values of E for collagen or apatite alone.[54] Therefore, bone strength is greater than collagen or apatite strength individually, that collagen prevents apatite from brittle cracking and apatite prevents collagen from yielding. The modulus of elasticity and other mechanical properties, such as shear modulus, ultimate stress and strain, and viscoelastic properties, depends not only on the composition of bone—such as percentages of compact and cancellous bone, bonds between fibers, bonds between fibers and matrix, percentages of haversian and lamellar bone, and bone density—but also on bone structure and the geometric shape of different areas of bone.[2,3,54]

The mechanical properties of human bone can be affected by a number of other in vivo and in vitro factors, including the following[58,64]:

1. Storage method—formalin, freezing, storage time, freezing rate
2. Specimen preparation procedures—machining methods, temperature during preparation, irrigation medium
3. Testing procedures—grip method, type of testing machine, deformation rate, uniformity of stress applied, environment

Table 1-5. The relationship of trabecular direction and mechanical strength in cortical bone

	Compression	Tension	Shear	Bending	Torsion
Strength	Longitudinal sections are strongest, then transverse,[19, 84] tangential, and radial, in order Ultimate compressive strength is greater than ultimate tensile strength[94]	Longitudinal sections are 8 times stronger than radial or tangential sections Ultimate tensile is less than ultimate compressive strength[94]	Longitudinal sections loaded perpendicularly are twice as strong as transverse sections loaded in parallel		
Strain	Strain is greatest in transverse sections Ultimate compressive strain is greater than ultimate tensile strain[94]	Ultimate compressive strain is greater than ultimate tensile strain[94]			Torsional stress results in an initial short elastic region Torsional stress does not usually lead to strain
Breaking load	Ultimate compressive stress increases with increasing strain rates	Longitudinal sections have greater ultimate strain than transverse sections		Longitudinal sections can withstand more bending load than transverse sections and radial sections	
Deformation		Little plastic deformation occurs if the direction of a tensile load is perpendicular to the long axis of the bone[94]			
Modulus of elasticity	In the human femur, longitudinal sections have a greater modulus than transverse, tangential, and radial sections[63]; the modulus increases with increased strain rates of loading	In cattle bone, longitudinal sections have greater moduli than transverse sections The modulus is greater with tensile loads than with compressive loads[94]	A single osteon has the greatest shear modulus Adding osteons decreases the modulus	Longitudinal sections have a higher modulus than transverse sections	

Based on data from Evans FG: *Mechanical properties of bone,* Springfield, Ill, 1973, Charles C Thomas.

4. Individual characteristics—gender, age, height, weight, race, cause of death, activity before death, nutritional status before death, disease affecting the bone
5. Section of bone—right or left, variation in different portions of the bone

The mechanical properties of dried bone differ from those of embalmed bone, wet bone from a fresh cadaver, and bone in vivo. Drying affects all regions of the bone the same but affects each strength property differently.[3] Bone with the in vivo characteristic of being bathed in fluid can absorb more energy and elongate more before fracture than dry bone because, unlike brittle materials, bone undergoes creep and stress relaxation.[43,94,99,125] The ultimate tensile and compressive stresses and modulus of elasticity for tension and compression are increased by drying.[94,88] Compressive

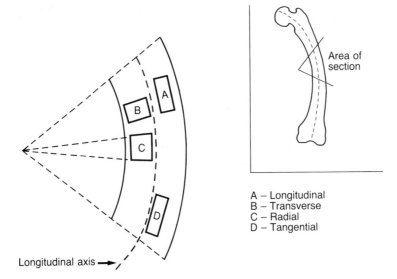

A – Longitudinal
B – Transverse
C – Radial
D – Tangential

Longitudinal axis →

Fig. 1-40. Different orientations of bone sections.

Table 1-6. Mechanical strengths for different bones

Bone	Test direction	Modulus of elasticity (Gpa)	Tensile strength (MPa)	Compressive strength (MPa)
Femur	Longitudinal	17.2	121	167
Tibia	Longitudinal	18.1	140	159
Fibula	Longitudinal	18.6	146	123
Humerus	Longitudinal	17.2	130	132
Radius	Longitudinal	18.6	149	114
Ulna	Longitudinal	18.0	148	117
Vertebrae	Longitudinal	0.23	3.1	10
Lumbar	Longitudinal	0.16	3.7	5
Cancellous		0.09	1.2	1.9
Skull	Tangential		25	

strength decreases and shear strength is altered with embalming.[3,94]

Stresses at epiphyseal plates

The stability of the epiphysis relative to the diaphysis depends on the relationship of the epiphyseal plate to the internal stress pattern created by the most stressful activity over a majority of the time. Generally, the most stable position for an epiphyseal plate is transverse to the long axis of the parent bone. However, other advantages may outweigh this basic rule, depending on the individual bone.

Most epiphyseal plates are oriented perpendicular to the lines of principal stress, tension, or compression, so that shear stresses on the plate can be minimized. Proliferative columns of cartilage cells, however, bear no relationship to the stress patterns. They are oriented instead in the direction of the bone growth they produce. Cartilage cell columns may be perpendicular or oblique to the plane of the epiphyseal plate. Only after primary diaphyseal bone trabeculae (those that form on the rods remaining after cartilage cell degeneration and erosion) have eroded and been replaced by secondary trabeculae can the structural alignment of the trabeculae according to stress patterns be seen. The epiphyseal plates have their characteristic forms at birth,[119] so much of their general form is genetically determined. However, until the secondary trabeculae develop, the plates are exposed to shear stresses that tend to displace the plate on the diaphysis. These stresses serve as stimuli for epiphyseal plate reorientation.

In areas of maximal compressive stress, plates are usually parallel to tensile stress lines and perpendicular to compressive stress lines. An exception is where the epiphyseal plate approaches the articular cartilage; there the plate often angles toward the diaphysis rather than remaining transverse to the long axis. When the epiphyseal plate deviates from its transverse course, muscles attaching near the joint attach to the epiphysis or apophysis instead of the diaphysis. If muscles attached to the diaphysis, the muscle attachment would have to move relative to the bone surface during growth, which is disruptive and destabilizing to the attachment site.[116]

Alteration of gravitational pull can markedly change the growth of the epiphyseal plates.[93] When 2-week-old chicks subjected to twice gravity's pull were compared with

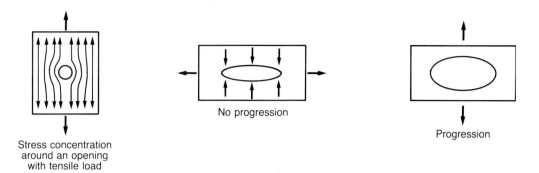

Fig. 1-41. Tensile stresses at the location of a crack progress the crack, whereas compressive stresses do not.

controls, they showed an increased width of cartilaginous layers in the proximal epiphysis and inhibition of both height and width of layers in the distal epiphysis.

Bone yielding and failure

Failure in bone can occur from trauma, degeneration, fatigue, or disease. Most fractures result from a combination of several loading modes occurring simultaneously.[94] The amount of energy absorbed before failure can be calculated by measuring the area under the stress-strain curve. Most fractures arise from high impact with inadequate energy absorption.[41,103] Because energy is released by the bone at the time of fracture, fractures can be differentiated as low energy, such as the simple torsional ski accident; high energy, as often occurs in auto accidents; or very high energy, such as a gunshot wound.[94]

Solid materials, including bone, have a great number of microscopic defects that usually do not progress into fractures unless available energy turns the defects into larger and larger cracks. These defects explain why the stress-strain curve for bone is not purely linear in the initial portion of the elastic deformation range of the curve.[5,94] To propagate a fracture, energy must rupture chemical bonds and create new surfaces. A propagating crack requires less energy to continue than a crack that has not begun to progress.[103] Fracture stress for crack growth in a brittle material is related to the initial crack depth by the following formula:

$$\text{Fracture stress}^2 \quad \frac{4 \times \text{Young's modulus} \times \text{surface energy}}{\text{Depth of the crack}}$$

where *surface energy* = energy to progress a crack (determined in units of ergs, calories, or British thermal units).

Because bone is a composite material, however, neither totally brittle nor totally ductile, the nonmineral components of bone can undergo a substantial plastic deformation before failure.[63] These components are compliant and have good energy-absorbing characteristics (toughness), although bone crystals themselves are rigid, stiff, and brittle and fracture easily.[74] The composite characteristics of bone, plus the fact that the microfractures lead to various changes in bone based on the particular load, result in a large fracture energy (toughness or ability to absorb energy without fracture) for

bone.[63,103] The somewhat plastic behavior of bone has a strengthening or toughening effect.

Maximal stress before bone failure can be approximated by the equation for maximal stress on a simple beam before failure:

$$\text{Stress} = \frac{-My}{I}$$

where

M = bending moment

y = distance from the neutral axis to the extreme fibers

I = moment of inertia

Tensile stresses in bone are particularly high at areas of stress concentration, called *stress risers,* such as where bone normally or pathologically suddenly narrows—at grooves, notches, or openings—or at any place where there is a change in the bone cross-section.[103] The more abrupt the change, the greater the concentration of tensile stress. In a sharp, deep crack, tensile stresses can be concentrated by a factor of 10,000. Only the component of the tensile stress that is perpendicular to the crack will progress the crack (Fig. 1-41).

When a crack appears in a bone, the weakest link within the bone fails. The weakest links for stress concentration are haversian canals, canaliculi, lacunae, and cement lines. As shown in Fig. 1-41, tensile stresses perpendicular to the crack pull these areas apart, whereas compressive stresses perpendicular to the crack discourage crack growth. The combined stress-strain curves for both tension and compression appear in Fig. 1-42.[14] More compressive stress than tensile stress is required to produce an equal amount of strain. A bone fails sooner under a tensile load because tensile stress causes greater disruption of weak link areas, thus causing more strain and earlier fracture than occur with a compressive stress of equal magnitude.

Microdamage may be the stimulus for bone remodeling.[18] If microfracture is produced by fatigue, bone remodeling cannot occur rapidly enough to manage the microscopic damage caused by repetitive loading stresses. Carter and Hayes have suggested that bone yielding may be due to

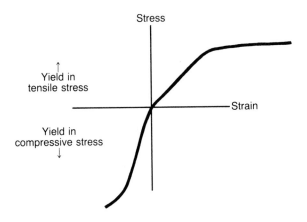

Fig. 1-42. Greater compressive stress than tensile stress is required to produce an equal amount of strain.

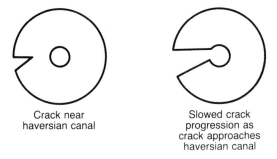

Fig. 1-43. Progression of a crack is slowed at the site of a haversian canal.

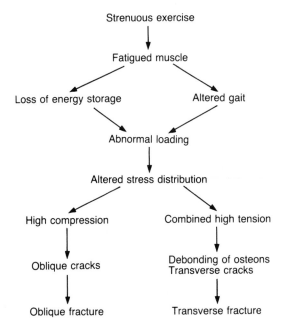

Fig. 1-44. Theory of muscle fatigue leading to fracture.

diffuse structural damage, such as debonding, microcracking, and fiber damage.[19-21] During repeated loading, bone progressively loses stiffness and strength.[18-20,45] Fatigue life shortens as stress amplitude or temperature increases.[17,22,24] The load (force), number of repetitions, and frequency of loading are important variables[94] in that an overuse syndrome can develop from a situation of high repetition and low load or from low repetition and high load.[108] An example of the former is a runner who suddenly increases his or her mileage per day. An example of the latter is the high jumper who jumps a few times per day but with great effort at each jump.[37]

Remodeled (secondary or haversian) cortical bone is more compliant than primary bone and has about 83% of the Young's modulus of elasticity for primary bone.[17,20,75] The decreased fatigue resistance of secondary bone may be the result of the decreased density of haversian bone[24] because a highly significant positive correlation exists between fatigue life and bone density.[17] Continuous strenuous activity not only fatigues muscle but also prevents neutralization of stress because the bone stores less energy when it is constantly stressed.[94] Fewer repetitions are required to cause a fracture as the stress per repetition approaches the point that corresponds to the yield point on the stress-strain curve.

Within haversian bone, there is increased resistance to fatigue at the edge of a haversian canal. Even though openings in bone increase stress concentration around the opening, cement lines and haversian canals can act at times to slow the propagation of a crack. The cement lines can guide a crack longitudinally, which may cause less damage. Because the haversian canal has an increased radius of curvature—that is, an edge that is not as sharp as the crack edge—higher stresses are required to progress the crack at the edge of the canal[103] (Fig. 1-43).

Speed of loading is important in determining fatigue. The higher the speed of loading, the more energy can be stored in the bone and the more load can be withstood before failure.[94] With increasing speeds, the load to failure can almost double, whereas the deformation changes little. The speed of loading not only influences the fracture pattern but also affects the amount of soft tissue damage at the fracture. When bone fractures after being loaded at a slow speed, energy can often dissipate by the formation of a single crack, and there may be little soft tissue damage or damage to the rest of the bone. If a fracture occurs when bone is loaded at a high speed, the release of the large amount of stored energy tends to shatter the bone and cause extensive soft tissue damage.[94] Cracks or fractures resulting from slow loading tend to propagate preferentially along osteon boundaries and not through osteons.[75]

Muscle fatigue tends to increase the possibility of fatigue fractures. As mentioned before, muscle contraction can decrease or even eliminate tensile stress resulting from a bending load by producing a compressive stress that partially or totally neutralizes the tensile stress. The resultant tensile stress can result in fracture because of the relative weakness of bone when loaded in tension. The theory of muscle fatigue leading to fracture as a sequential series of events is outlined in Fig. 1-44.[94]

Bone failure is controlled by strain magnitude and stress magnitude. Fatigue fractures can occur during military basic training; in ballet dancers, runners, or other athletes; or in people who abruptly begin a vigorous exercise program or too quickly progress through an exercise routine.[17,19,21] Military personnel may incur fatigue fractures at the metatarsal level when they are instructed to march long distances, hence the common term *march fracture.* Fatigue fractures of the upper third of the fibula may occur when basic training involves performing full deep knee bends and walking from that position.[122] During this maneuver, the soleus, posterior tibialis, peroneus longus, and flexor hallucis longus muscles pull forcefully on the fibula. A forceful contraction of the ankle plantarflexor and toe flexor muscles pulls the tibia and fibula together, which could be the mechanism for fibular fracture here and in runners as well.[101]

Fatigue fractures commonly occur in the elderly at the sites of the femoral neck region, the distal radius, vertebral bodies, and the surgical neck of the humerus. As bone density decreases with increasing age and osteoporosis occurs, the incidence of trabecular microfractures and fractures increases.[45] The earliest and most striking decreases in bone density occur in trabecular bone, with the trabeculae becoming thin and sparse.[114] Microdamage accumulation occurring at a faster rate than healing seems to be the main failure mechanism in that an increased number of trabecular failures have been located in the same site as the gross fractures in the subcapital femoral neck area.[45]

Cortical bone is stiffer than cancellous bone and therefore can withstand more stress before failure but less strain. Cortical bone fractures when the strain is greater than 2% of the original length of the segment, whereas cancellous bone fractures only after a strain of greater than 7%. As a result, cancellous bone is said to have a high-energy storage capacity.

Table 1-7 lists the ultimate strength properties and failure mechanisms of bone for different types of load. Whereas failure in tension results in debonding of osteons, failure in compression results in oblique cracking of osteons. Failure in bending occurs at maximal tensile stress. Failure in torsional loading occurs initially with maximal shear stress as a crack parallel to the neutral axis occurs at the bone surface and then proceeds along the plane of maximal tensile stress,[94,103] which is at a 30- to 45-degree angle to the axis of the torsional loading.[103]

Bone healing

The ability of bone to heal without scarring is unique to bone and possibly synovial membrane. The healing ability of bone is directly related to the vascularity of the bone, the abundance of periosteum, and the stability (maintained relative immobility) of the fracture site.[70] Cells that will proliferate and differentiate into fibrous connective tissue, fibrocartilage, hyaline cartilage, and bone are supplied by the torn ends of the periosteum, endosteum, and bone marrow.

Periosteum that is not severely torn is most able to assist in the healing process. The tearing of the periosteum strongly stimulates osteoprogenitor cell proliferation in the deeper periosteum. Without the formation of new cells, a femoral fracture could take a projected 200 to 1000 years to heal.[70] Because the life span of osteoblasts is only 2 to 3 months,[114] formation of new cells is critical.

New bone formation can begin within 48 hours in young people. Bone healing is rapid at birth (on the order of 3 weeks in the infant), slower with each year of childhood, and constant from early adulthood to older adulthood. Healing in elderly individuals may take longer if the bone is brittle and less able to deform with external loads. The time required for bone healing is directly proportional to the total volume of injured bone and the extent of the damage. If the fractured segments are in contact, bones such as the humerus, radius, and ulna may unite in 3 months; union of femoral and tibial fractures may require twice that time. Spiral fractures tend to heal more quickly than transverse fractures.

Healing has occurred when the strength of the bone equals the strength of the same bone before fracture.[12] The repair process progresses through several stages, which have been given different names by different authors.[12,46,70] The first stage (inflammatory response or phase, granulation stage, fracture stage, clot stage) involves the presence of a clot, except in stress fractures. Dead and injured cells from bone and soft tissue are the stimulus for the invasion of the clot by a loose meshwork of capillaries and fibroblasts.[16,70,132]

Prostaglandin release enhances healing by stimulating osteoclast action and modulating the inflammatory response. A number of mediators, such as interleukin 1, fibronectin, and the somatomedins, are involved in as yet vaguely understood ways to enhance tissue healing. This mechanism, named the *regional acceleratory phenomenon* by Frost,[46,48] is caused by the injury process and speeds up healing by about 2 to 10 times.

The second phase, or repair process, is known as the repair or reparative phase or process or the callus stage. The bridge between the fracture sites is made by internal callus from periosteal and endosteal cells, and the fracture site is closed by external callus from the mesenchymal cells from surrounding tissue.[70] The flexible, compliant callus is an unorganized meshwork of cartilage, which deforms easily with loading, allowing enhanced deformation or strain in response to mechanical stimuli and therefore enhanced stimulation for healing. Initially the callus is replaced by woven bone.[69] Adequate oxygen supply and relative immobility with adequate minimal effective bone strain enhance formation and growth of bone, whereas inadequate oxygen supply and a lack of relative immobility favor growth of cartilage. This stage can take 1 to 4 months.

The third phase, or reorganization process, is called the remodeling, modeling, or consolidation phase[46,114] and involves the replacement of woven bone by well-oriented

Table 1-7. Ultimate strength properties of bone

	Tension	Compression	Shear	Bending	Torsion
Ultimate strength	Failure of bone is closely associated with planes of maximal stress,[13] usually caused by bending or torsion[103] Tensile strength is greater in bending than axial loading[13] Load to failure in axial tension is proportional to cross-sectional area of bone[94] Cortical bone can withstand greater tensile than shear stress[94] Fatigue fracture from tensile stress results in transverse crack and may fracture rapidly and completely[94] Ultimate strength of wet bone is about 13,818 psi, whereas that of dry bone is about 19,939 psi (as compared to that of collagen—80,000 psi)[88]	Load to failure in axial compression is proportional to the cross-sectional area of bone[94] Cortical bone can withstand greater stress in compression than tension[94] Fatigue fracture due to compression stress proceeds more slowly than one due to tension[94]	Fracture from torsional stress begins with a crack parallel to the neutral axis due to shear[94]	Fracture begins on the tensile side and the crack proceeds across the bone[103]	Tensile deformation causes the crack[103] Fracture site is where the smallest moment of inertia is found[94]
Fracture healing				Callus increases area moment of inertia[94]	Callus increases polar moment of inertia[94]
Mechanism of failure	Widely distributed fractures accumulate; these lead to delamination of haversian systems and debonding at weak osteonal matrix interfaces (cement lines), with subsequent erosion of osteons[45,63,94] Bone fails in tension before it fails in compression[23]	Fracture occurs from oblique cracking of osteons[45,94]	Bone can deform by kinking[63]	Bone is stronger in bending than with uniaxial loads[23] More damage occurs on the side of compressive stress[17]	Strain results from deformation of collagen with shear between the collagen and the crystals Torsional stress results in failure in shear and then failure in tension[94,103]

lamellar bone. During this phase, lamellar bone becomes oriented to local peak longitudinal compressive and tensile stress and strain on the bone. An orderly sequence of bone deposition and resorption proceeds, as, for example, osteoclasts form tunnels for haversian canals, through which blood vessels flow. Mature cartilage callus is replaced by bone in a similar manner to initial endochondral ossification. Cancellous bone heals faster than cortical bone as the bone deforms more with loads and there is less bone to replace. Long oblique or spiral fractures of the shaft, with a relatively large fracture surface, usually heal faster than transverse fractures.

Conditions with a negative effect on bone healing include poor nutrition, alcohol abuse, smoking, and possibly general physical inactivity and old age. Massive soft tissue injuries may disturb the mediator-driven mechanism.

Nonunions or delayed unions may be pushed to fracture site union with use of an electrical stimulus at the area of the fracture site[87] or the transfer of a muscle graft to the site of the fracture.[70]

Differences in men's and women's bone strength

Bone strength is greatest in the direction of physiological loading, that is, where maximal loads occur for the most time. Bone strength increases to meet increasing demands. Bone strength in men is absolutely greater in most mechanical properties than bone strength in women because men are subject to higher physiological stresses from a more active life[99] and because of anatomical variations in body muscle mass and skeletal design. Relative bone strength in men and women is controversial. When Burstein and colleagues tested the mechanical properties of bone in men and women ages 21 to 86, they found no significant differences among tensile, compressive, and torsional test loads.[13,14] A comparison of the mechanical properties of bone for men and women is found in Table 1-8.

Age-associated differences in bone strength

The changes associated with bone strength are based primarily on the maturation of bone tissue, the physical activity status of the individual, and, to a lesser extent, the biological aging of the individual. For bone, as for most of the connective tissues, loss of strength in older people appears to be due more to physical inactivity than to biological age. This issue will be clarified as the bone strength of physically active older adults is compared to that of physically inactive older adults and the reversibility of bone weakness from physical inactivity in older adults is assessed.

Bone becomes relatively stronger during growth from childhood to adult life.[23] Subperiosteal bone grows rapidly postnatally by appositional growth, markedly decreases in growth rate at about 6 months, grows more rapidly during both juvenile and adolescent growth spurts, and continues to grow at a slow rate via appositional growth throughout life.[55]

Table 1-8. Comparison of mechanical properties of bone in men and women

Mechanical property	Comparison
Cortical human bone	
Tension	
Tensile strength	Greater in men or equal
Ultimate strength	Equal
Percentage of elongation	Equal or greater in women
Mean deformation at failure	Equal
Modulus of elasticity	Greater in men or equal
Compression	
Compressive strength	Greater in men
Modulus of elasticity	Equal
Bending properties	Equal
Torsion strength	Greater in men
Density	Increases in men longer than in women; the decline in density begins earlier in women
Cancellous human bone (vertebral bodies)	
Tension	
Tensile strength[14,41]	Equal
Tensile strain	Equal
Compression	
Mean ultimate compressive stress	Greater in men
Compressive strength	Controversial
Compressive strain	Equal or greater in women
Compressive modulus of elasticity	Greater in men
Torsion	
Torsional strength[14,41]	Equal
Breaking torsional moment	Greater in men
Energy absorbed to failure	Greater in men
Density	Greater in men

Based on data from Evans FG: *Mechanical properties of bone,* Springfield, Ill, 1973, Charles C Thomas.

An initial neonatal gain of cortical bone until the age of 6 months is followed by an infantile loss, a juvenile gain, an adolescent spurt, a slight adult gain to the fifth decade, and then a slow decline.[55] The reported decrease in cortical bone density (including subperiosteal bone) associated with advancing age is probably the reported increase in average bone porosity.[23]

Differences in osteon properties are seen with aging.[73] Children have increased bone formation and resorption and therefore an increased turnover rate of bone. (Density is comparatively low because the number of forming osteons and resorption cavities is high.) Most osteons are not fully mineralized by young adult age. Bone material strength decreases after age 30 because of increased porosity from an increase in the number of vascular channels. The osteonal picture parallels the general increase in endosteal resorption in the later years. From age 60 on, the number of osteons that are less than three-fourths closed or complete, especially in endosteal bone, sharply increases. From age 70 on, up to 25% of the bone surface may be occupied by resorption cavities.[73]

An infant cannot walk until Young's modulus is high enough—that is, until the bones have adequate stiffness (which is determined by stress and strain measurements) and until the bone is strong enough. The tensile strength, tensile strain, and failure in infant femoral bones are comparable to the same values determined for adult femoral bones, although the modulus of elasticity is considerably lower. The modulus may not develop until walking is attempted.[41] The stability of collagen fibers increases with age as more bonding occurs.[35]

A summary of the findings on various mechanical properties of bone with age as a variable is found in Table 1-9. In general, mechanical and material properties of bone tend to decrease with increasing age after 40 to 50 years,[38] but changes in the geometrical properties of bone may compensate for changes in intrinsic bone properties. Traditionally, static tensile strength has been used as the criterion in judging the overall quality of bone, whether to determine age effects on bone, effects of gender on bone quality, or effects of nutrition on bone.[58]

Ultimate tensile strength decline is altered with advanced age, and at times the decline is quite rapid. A rapid decline does not appear to be caused by properties of collagen fibers, which do not change quickly, or the degree of preferred orientation of the apatite crystals, which also changes little during life. The decline is more likely caused by differences in mineral particle size distribution within a bone. Any radius

Table 1-9. Mechanical properties of bone as a function of age

Mechanical property	Bone	Characteristics
Cortical bone		
Tensile strength	Femur Tibia Fibula	Tensile strength was less in those over 60 than in those under 60
	Femur, unembalmed	Mean strength decreased up to 10% with age except in women 15-19 years old; tensile strain maximal at 10-19 years old and minimal at 60-70
	Fibula	Microhardness of cortical bone increased to 30, then reached a plateau
	Tibia, embalmed	Mean tensile stress and strain maximal from 20-39, then decreased; Young's and shear moduli maximal at 40-59, then decreased gradually
	Femur	Shear modulus maximal at ages 20-39, decreased from 40 to 59
	Femur	Progressive loss of strength from 21 to 86[14]
	Tibia	Tensile strength did not decrease with age[14]
	Femur	Mean tensile stress and strain to failure for infants was in the adult range, while modulus of elasticity was lower[142]
Compressive strength	Femur (posterior shaft)	Mean ultimate strength maximal at 20-29, with a plateau to 39, then a decrease[142]
Bending strength	Femur	Bending strength maximal at 24-32 and minimal at 70-80; mean ultimate fiber strength, energy absorbed to failure, and modulus of elasticity decreased in elderly people
	Cortical bone	Bending strength was greatest from 20-29, with a plateau to 39, then a decrease[138]
	Femur	Bending strength decreased in elderly people[125]
Torsion	Embalmed bone	Maximal torsional strength at 20-39, then decreased to a minimum at 60-79
	Cortical bone	Torsional strength greatest at 20-29, followed by a plateau to 39, then a decrease[142]
Plastic deformation	Femur Tibia	From 20-80, the plastic part of the stress-strain curve increased with increasing age, in the femur more than the tibia
Elastic deformation		The femur had greater stiffness than the tibia
Cancellous bone		
Compressive strength	Femur	Maximal compressive strength, modulus of elasticity, and energy absorbed to failure decreased after 70; compressive strain to failure increased to 70

Based on data from Evans FC: *Mechanical properties of bone,* Springfield, Ill, 1973, Charles C Thomas.

change in particles affects bone strength because the effect of a particle on strength dimensions is a function of its distance cubed from the neutral axis of the bone.[106] The percentage of small particles in the mineral (apatite) phase of bone—the high modulus portion—increases on average to the fourth decade and then decreases.

The subperiosteal and endosteal changes in bone affect men and women differently. Both genders have endosteal resorption of bone with advanced age as the walls of cancellous bone become progressively thinner.[56] This endosteal resorption is greater in women, particularly after menopause. Men and women also have subperiosteal bone growth (men more than women), which could increase the moment of inertia[55,56] and bending stiffness.[111] However, the increase in subperiosteal diameter is later and longer in men.[55] Men also experience a larger subperiosteal change in their late teens.[55] This subperiosteal expansion may be a compensatory mechanism for bone loss caused by endosteal resorption and cortical thinning.[109] This expansion of the subperiosteum in men offsets endosteal resorption of cortical bone, whereas cortical bone in women undergoes a net decrease with advancing age (i.e., the subperiosteal expansion does not offset the endosteal resorption).[55,91] Therefore, there is a net decrease over time in the ability of women's bones to resist failure.[55,84,91]

In terms of femoral changes, the most profound differences between men and women are at the ends of the femur. Although femoral material strength decreases with increasing age for both men and women, the increased moment of inertia in men compensates for the decreased material strength.[84] In women the subperiosteal expansion is not significant enough, in view of the endosteal resorption, to increase the moment of inertia. There is an actual decrease in the moment of inertia, which, together with the decreased material strength of the bone with increasing age, weakens the femur.[84]

The strain characteristics of the older adult bone differ from those of younger bone. The decrease in ultimate strain relates to the inability of the bone as a whole to bend. Bones of elderly people can withstand about half the strain of the bones of younger adults. The bones of elderly people are less ductile and less able to store energy to failure.[94] From a structural viewpoint, the decrease in ultimate strain is the most important age change in bone.[13,14] The weakening of the femur in females because of decreases in the moment of inertia, material strength, and subperiosteal expansion in the femoral neck compared with the remaining femur,[121] coupled with the fact that women live longer than men and have marked hormonal change,[49,50] explains why elderly women have so many fractured femurs. Although many people with fractured femurs believe they caused the fracture by falling, many have spontaneous fractures while standing or walking and fall as a result.[45,121,125]

All of these changes associated with aging should be viewed in the context of the more sedentary lifestyle of most older people and the probability that many of the changes are, in fact, due to physical inactivity.

Adaptation of bone to exercise stress

Original bone modeling and remodeling involve the reaction of bone to stresses from gravity, joint position, dynamic motion, and genetic influences. Bone adaptation may be stimulated by microdamage, piezoelectricity, surface strain, some combination of stimuli, or an as yet unknown mechanism.[85,112] The extent to which exercise can maintain bone integrity in these areas may be inferred by comparing the percentage of hip fractures in women from nonindustrialized societies with the percentage in industrialized societies. Women in the former group have fewer hip fractures,[26] partially because of their more active lifestyles.

Women's physical inactivity in industrialized societies fails to stimulate the geometrical changes in bone that could help to compensate for the decreasing bone material strength with advanced age.[84] The subperiosteal apposition and therefore the increased moment of inertia that would be caused by the exercise stimulus do not occur in sedentary individuals.

Mechanical considerations, such as the moments produced around a joint, joint forces, the duration of exercise, and bony alignment (particularly of weight-bearing joints), are important in understanding the adaptation of bone to exercise. Mechanical characteristics are often discussed broadly in terms of multiples of body weight loads occurring at a joint. During normal walking, for example, forces 2 to 4 times body weight usually occur at the hip, with forces 6 to 9 times body weight occurring during a fast walk. Landing after a jump from a 1-meter height causes a compressive load of about 24 times body weight at the knee joint.

A number of variables must be considered when exercise is linked to the actual stress to bone. General exercise variables include the type of exercise (continuous or intermittent), the intensity (mild, moderate, or intensive), and the duration (times per day and number of weeks, months, and years), recognizing such factors as the person's age, health, and previous immobilization.[59,67,81,133] Exercise can have a specific effect—for example, increased cortical thickness in the forearm bones of the dominant side in tennis players[136,137]—or a generalized effect, such as an overall increase in bone mineral content in cross-country runners.[36] (The increase was measured in the forearm bones of the runners.) Because most of the experiments with different training intensities have involved animals, extrapolating exercise intensities to humans is difficult. However, Woo and colleagues have suggested that 40 km per week be considered moderate training for running, with additional distance constituting intense exercise.[137]

Bone responds differently to low or moderate exercise than it does to intense exercise. Goodship, Lanyon, and McFie[60] performed ulnar ostectomies on young male pigs and found that, within a 3-month period of free movement, the cross-sectional area of the radius of the operated side equaled that of the radius and ulna of the nonoperated side.[60] Chamay and Tschantz reported similar effects.[27] Woo and colleagues exercised 1-year-old pigs in a running routine that was gradually increased over a year to a moderate level.[137] Results on the exercised bone included an increase in cortical thickness (17%), increased energy absorbed to failure, increased bone mass, decreased endosteal bone, and increased calcium content in the bone, all of which added to bone strength. Bony adaptations in mice exercised by running at low or moderate levels have included increased bone mass in the limb bones,[77] longer bones,[76,77] and heavier bones.[76,77,116] Rats made bipedal at birth developed femurs with increased breaking strengths and densities.[115] Anderson, Milin, and Crackel reported that pigs exercised by running at a moderate level had a decreased hydroxyproline content in their urine, probably indicating an increased hydroxyproline retention in the bone and increased collagen synthesis.[4]

Intense exercise in experimental animals has been shown to inhibit the length and girth of bone growth. Although the operational definitions of mild, moderate, and intense exercise varied among investigators, the exercise intensities generally consisted of about 50 to 80 minutes of running a day as moderate exercise and more than 120 minutes per day as intense exercise, with speed varied according to the size of the animal. Kiiskinen and Heikkinen exercised mice with a running program to an intense level and reported shorter and lighter limb bones, decreased bone volume, and a decreased hydroxyproline content in bone as compared to controls.[76,77] The decreased hydroxyproline content probably indicated a reduced rate of collagen synthesis in the bone. These inhibitory effects on bone growth could reflect

a slower rate of the bone's repair of microdamage rather than the actual microdamage rate. The effects seen in varying exercise intensities may be altered by factors such as the age and size of the experimental animal.[11,124]

The differing effects of continuous and intermittent exercise were reported by Hert, Liskova, and Landrgot, who loaded rabbit tibial by inserting two wires through the metaphyses of the bone.[66] Long-term continuous bending of the adult bone resulted in an absence of reaction, even after 12 months of loading, although some effects were seen in growing animals.[66] Intermittent loading within physiological limits, along with freedom of movement by the rabbits, resulted in an increase of bone growth.[61,82] Maintenance of lower extremity bone structure has been attempted for people who are unable to stand or walk by using a tilt table. A person can be secured to the table, which is tilted vertically at a varying rate and to a varying extent. The stimulus to bone from simulated weight bearing is a continuous one. Although the tilt table may have other benefits, such as stimulation of mechanisms needed for blood pressure regulation, there does not appear to be value for maintaining bone integrity.

BONE GROWTH AND LOADING PATTERNS OF THE LOWER EXTREMITY BONES

The long bones of the lower extremities are the structural supports for the body.[75] The main function of the femur and tibia is weight bearing, whereas that of the fibula is to serve as an attachment for muscle.[41] Each of these bones is subjected to asymmetrical loading modes. A comparison of material strengths of the three bones is listed in Table 1-10. In general, the fibula is strongest in tensile loading, a result of the muscular traction forces imposed constantly. The

Table 1-10. Comparison of material strengths of the femur, tibia, and fibula (human, unembalmed bone)

Load	Mechanical property	Material strength
Cortical bone		
Tension	Average tensile strength	Adult men: fibula > tibia > femur > humerus
	Tensile strain	Adults 20 to 39 years old: fibula > tibia > femur[14,41]
	Young's modulus	Fibula > tibia > femur[41,119]
Compression	Average compressive strength	Tested along the long axis, tibia > femur,[14,41] or femur > tibia > fibula[14,41]
	Compressive strain	Tested along long axis in 20- to 39-year-old adults, fibula > tibia > femur[14,41]
Shear	Shear strength	Controversial
	Ultimate displacement	Fibula > tibia > femur
Bending	Strength	Femur > tibia in men; tibia > femur in women (no age ranges given)
	Young's modulus	Femur > tibia
Fatigue life (cycles to failure)	Strength	Femur = tibia = fibula
Cancellous bone		
Tension and compression	Young's modulus	Fibula = tibia > femur

Based on data from Evans FG: *Mechanical properties of bone,* Springfield, Ill, 1973, Charles C Thomas.

femur is able to withstand greater bending loads because it has a higher modulus of elasticity than the tibia. These findings are based on relatively few studies, some of which are controversial. Further data are needed to verify findings and clarify contradictions.

Femur

During weight bearing, the femur is subjected to compressive, bending, and tensile stresses. The bending stress from weight bearing tends to bow the shaft of the femur so that the tensile stress tends to occur on the lateral[103] and anterior diaphyseal regions of the femur[84] and compressive stress tends to occur on the medial and posterior shaft region (Fig. 1-45). Tensile stresses also occur at muscle attachment sites and are generally highest for the antigravity muscles, the hip extensors, knee extensors, and plantarflexor muscles. Compressive stresses are especially high at the medial aspect of the femoral neck (Fig. 1-46)[113] because of weight bearing on the bowed femoral neck. Compressive stresses also occur as a result of muscles pulling at an acute angle with the bone.

In Fig. 1-45, the bending loads from weight bearing produce the forces A and D and their respective components.

Forces E and B tend to bend the femur in one direction, whereas forces C and F tend to bend the femur in the opposite direction. Because the resultant forces D and A are aligned to the neutral axis of the femur, forces E and B can counter the bending moment caused by C and F. The material strengths of various portions of the femur are compared in Table 1-11.

Fracture of the femur can occur from lack of material strength and is often associated with planes of maximal tensile stress, which are usually the result of torsion or bending loads.[14,103] Femoral neck fractures may occur as a result of osteoporosis and muscle fatigue (especially that of the gluteus medius), which combined lead to high tensile stresses on the superior femoral neck.[94,121] Compressive fractures, by contrast, can occur near the hip joint when abnormally high compressive stresses are caused by strong cocontraction of the hip muscles. These stresses can be produced during electroconvulsive shock therapy to result in subcapital fracture of the femoral neck.[94] Shear fractures can occur at the femoral condyles.[94] As seen in Fig. 1-47, fractures from torsional stress exhibit initial bone failure in shear (*A*), parallel to the neutral axis. The fracture line then tends to follow about a 30- to 45-degree angle to the neutral axis (*B*), which corresponds to the plane of maximal tensile stress.[94,103]

Epiphyseal plates align perpendicularly to the major lines of compressive and tensile loading in a bone to decrease shear stress on the epiphyseal plates. The relevant lines and plates for the distal femur during weight bearing are viewed in Figs. 1-48 and 1-49. When the femur bears weight, the shaft tends to bend anteriorly and laterally and to subject the anterior and lateral portions of the femur to tensile stress and the posterior and medial portions to compressive stress. Muscle groups help reduce the tensile stress, as, for example, the quadriceps do in pulling anteriorly on the femur to reduce the tensile stress on the anterior surface from weight-bearing

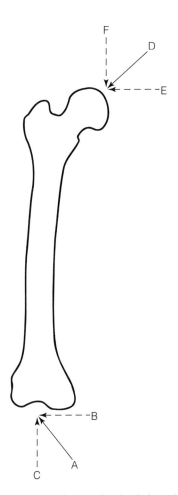

Fig. 1-45. Forces caused by bending loads in weight bearing.

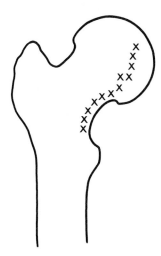

Fig. 1-46. In the femoral head and neck, the *x*s mark the areas of increased average compressive strength.

loads. This natural management of tensile stress by muscle activation occurs in a second example, as the gluteus medius tends to compress the femoral head and greater trochanter to reduce tensile stress on the proximal or superior femoral neck resulting from the bending loads caused by weight bearing.

The trabecular alignment in the femoral neck is perhaps the best example of how the trabeculae align with the major stresses. The trabeculae in the medial portion of the femoral neck, for example (Fig. 1-46), are aligned perpendicularly to the line of the compressive loading, which is the major load imposed on that region.

Tibia and fibula

The tibia is a weight-bearing bone, as is the femur. The tibia has mechanical properties similar to the femur but

Table 1-11. Material strengths of various portions of the femur

Load or characteristic	Mechanical property	State of human bone	Material strength
Cortical bone			
Tension	Average tensile strength	U	Middle third > distal third
	Tensile strain	E, wet	Middle third and lateral quadrant are strongest, proximal third and anterior quadrant are weakest
	Stiffness (Young's modulus)	E, wet	Middle third stiffest, proximal most flexible, with no quadrant differences
Shear	Average shear strength	E, wet, adult	Middle third > proximal third > distal third
			Medial and posterior quadrants > anterior and lateral quadrants
Bending	Bending strength	U, wet, adult	Lateral quadrant > medial > anterior > posterior
Torsion	Torsional shear stress	E, wet, adult	Middle third > distal; medial quadrant > lateral > posterior > anterior
	Shear modulus	E, wet, adult	Middle third stronger than distal third; medial quadrant > lateral > posterior > anterior[41,42]
	Energy absorbed to failure	E, wet, adult	Middle and proximal thirds absorb more than distal; medial and lateral quadrant absorb more than anterior[41,42]
Characteristic			
Complete osteons			Middle third has more than distal third and anterior quadrant[42]
Complete secondary osteons			Lateral quadrant has most[42]
Interstitial lamellae			Anterior quadrant and distal third has most; lateral quadrant and proximal third has least[42]
Cancellous bone			
Compression	Average strength	U, adult	Greatest in medial femoral neck (Fig. 1-46)
	Young's modulus (stiffness)	U, adult	From high to low modulus—femoral head, lateral condyle, medial condyle, greater trochanter
	Compressive strain	U, adult	From high to low strain withstood—lateral condyle, greater trochanter, medial condyle, femoral neck
	Energy absorbed to failure	U, adult	From most to least energy absorbed, femoral head, femoral neck, lateral condyle, medial condyle, greater trochanter

Based on data from Evans FG: *Mechanical properties of bone,* 1973, Springfield, Ill, Charles C Thomas.
E, Embalmed; *U,* unembalmed.

better mechanical stability than the femur.[13,14] Tibial bone has a faster turnover rate than the femur and, as a result, a better chance for faster bone repair when microfractures occur. The plastic portion of the tibial stress-strain curve is more consistent, which indicates more rapidly forming new collagen in the tibia than in the femur.[14]

Tibial fractures can occur as a result of many different mechanisms. The energy required to fracture the average tibia is about 1/10,000 of the kinetic energy of an 80-kg skier traveling at 10 ms (24 mph).[103] Fractures resulting from shear stress occur in the tibial plateaus. They can occur from three-point bending, such as when a skier falls forward so that the body weight at the proximal tibia and the ground cause a moment that tends to bend the tibia. The fracture is initiated posteriorly at the top of the boot, where maximal tensile stress occurs.[94] With torsional loads on the tibia, the distal part of the bone often fractures first because the distal bone is closer to the neutral axis. There is a decreased polar moment of inertia and less ability of the bone to resist the torsional stress at the distal tibia.

Material strengths of various portions of the tibia and fibula are given in Table 1-12. For the tibia, the middle third

of the bone is generally the strongest and stiffest, whereas the proximal third is the weakest and most flexible for the properties listed. For the fibula, the proximal or middle third of the bone is the strongest or stiffest. Significant differences have been reported between embalmed and unembalmed tested specimens. In either case, the fibula would logically have great tensile strength in the middle or proximal third and posterior quadrant because of the number of muscle attachments (as well as the interosseous membrane) that produce tensile stresses in those areas.

The proximal epiphyseal plate of the tibia corresponds to the lines of greatest tensile and compressive stress over time. In the standing position, the tibia is subjected to axial compression and forward bending, resulting in principal compressive stresses extending along the posterior shaft and mainly to either the lateral condyle or the region of the tibial tuberosity. These and the principal tensile stress lines in stance are seen in Fig. 1-50. The area marked 2 to 3 in Fig. 1-50, *B* is subject to shear stress because it courses obliquely to both axes. As a result, the epiphysis tends to displace proximally and posteriorly on the diaphysis. Areas between 1 and 2 are aligned with principal tensile stress lines and are subject only to compression. The distal dip of the anterior part of the epiphyseal plate allows adaptation of the plate to large tensile stresses.

The epiphyseal plates actually conform most closely to the lines of stress incurred during walking and running (Fig. 1-51).[119] As seen in Fig. 1-51, *A,* the plate is subject to shear stress at points 1 and 2. Because of tension in the posterior cruciate ligament, however, the central deflection of the plate adds to the stability of the epiphysis on the diaphysis. The existence of the central deflection suggests that the posterior cruciate ligament is significant in shaping the epiphyseal plate.

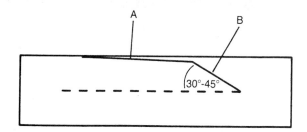

Fig. 1-47. Fractures from torsional stress exhibit initial bone failure in shear *(A)* and then follow the plane of maximal tensile stress *(B).*

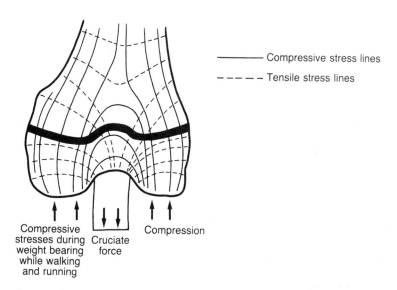

——— Compressive stress lines

– – – – – Tensile stress lines

Fig. 1-48. Compressive and tensile stresses on the distal femur in relation to the epiphyseal plates during weight bearing, anterior view. (Modified from Smith JW: *J Anat* 96:58, 1962.)

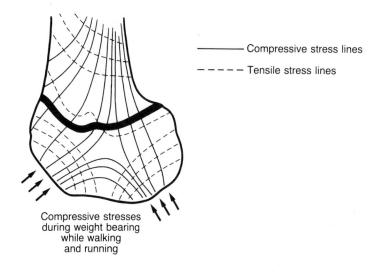

Compressive stress lines

Tensile stress lines

Compressive stresses
during weight bearing
while walking
and running

Fig. 1-49. Compressive and tensile stresses on the distal femur in relation to the epiphyseal plates during weight bearing, lateral view. (Modified from Smith JW: *J Anat* 96:58, 1962.)

Table 1-12. Material strengths of various portions of the tibia and fibula

Load	Mechanical property	State of human bone (if known)	Material strength
Tibia			
Tension	Tensile strength	E, wet, adult	Middle third and anterior quandrant > proximal third and medial quadrant
	Tensile strain	E, wet, adult	Middle third and anterior quadrant > proximal third and posterior quadrant
	Stiffness (Young's modulus)	E, wet, adult	Distal third and lateral quadrant stiffest; proximal third and anterior quadrant most flexible
Compression	Compressive strength	E, wet, adult male	Middle third and medial quadrant > proximal third and anterior quadrant
	Compressive strain	E, wet, adult male	Middle third and and posterior quadrant > distal third and lateral quadrant
	Stiffness (Young's modulus)	E, wet, adult male	Middle third and anterior quadrant are stiffest; proximal third and posterior quadrant most flexible
Fatigue life[14]	Strength		Middle third and posterior quadrant > proximal third and anterior quadrant
Fibula			
Tension	Tensile strength	E, wet, adult	Proximal third > distal third
	Tensile strain	E, wet, adult	Proximal third > distal third
	Stiffness (Young's modulus)	U, wet, adult	Anterior > posterior quadrant
		E, adult	Middle third stiffest; distal third most flexible
Shear	Shear strength	E, wet, adult	Middle third > distal third
Bending	Bending strength	U, wet, adult	Medial > lateral > anterior > posterior quadrant
Fatigue life	Strength	U, wet, adult	Middle third and posterior quadrant > lateral > medial > anterior quadrant and proximal third

Based on data from Evans FG: *Mechanical properties of bone,* Springfield, Ill, 1973, Charles C Thomas.
E, Embalmed; *U,* unembalmed.

STANCE

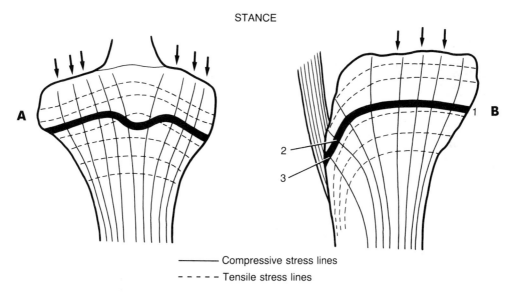

—— Compressive stress lines

- - - - - Tensile stress lines

Fig. 1-50. Compressive and tensile stresses on the proximal tibia in relation to the epiphyseal plates during stance. **A,** Anterior view; **B,** lateral view. (Modified from Smith JW: *J Anat* 96:58, 1962.)

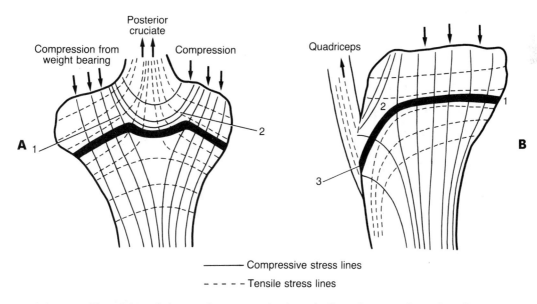

—— Compressive stress lines

- - - - - Tensile stress lines

Fig. 1-51. The epiphyseal plate conforms more closely to the lines of compressive and tensile stress during stance phase of walking and running. **A,** Anterior view; **B,** lateral view. (Modified from Smith JW: *J Anat* 96:58, 1962.)

Foot

The calcaneal epiphyseal plate orients to accommodate maximal stress on the calcaneus (Fig. 1-52, *2* to *3*). The plate of the calcaneus courses anteriorly on the inferior calcaneus and allows both the triceps surae tendon and the larger plantar muscles to attach to the epiphysis.[119] The relationship of the plate to principal tensile and compressive stress lines in stance can be seen in Fig. 1-52. The general forces on the foot in stance or in a simulated early support phase of gait also appear in Fig. 1-52. The epiphyseal plate lies parallel alternately to the principal lines of compression, then

tension, so that there is shear only at each bend point and not through most of the length (*3* through *5*) of the plate. The plate is allowed to adapt to the growth requirements of the epiphysis. When compared during stance and roll off in gait (heel off to toe off, Figs. 1-52 and 1-53), the plate corresponds to the principal stress lines in roll off. Roll off occurs when the forward motion of the body weight causes the longitudinal arch to flatten and plantar tissues to produce tension to stabilize the calcaneus.[119]

In stance, the more vertically directed body weight vector produces an equal and opposite ground reaction force

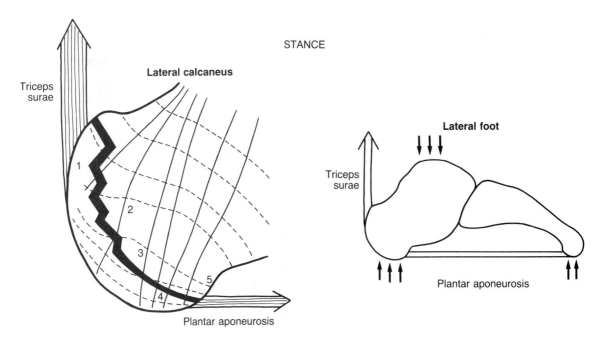

Fig. 1-52. Relationship of the epiphyseal plate of the calcaneus to the principal lines of tensile and compressive stress in stance. (Modified from Smith JW: *J Anat* 96:58, 1962.)

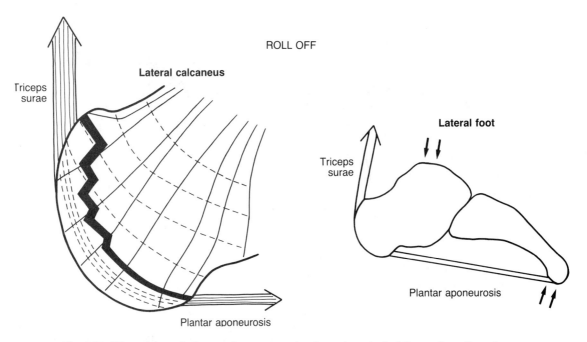

Fig. 1-53. The epiphyseal plate conforms more closely to the principal lines of tensile and compressive stress in the roll-off part of the gait cycle. (Modified from Smith JW: *J Anat* 96:58, 1962.)

through the calcaneal tuberosities, and the plantar aponeurosis tightens to resist depression of the longitudinal arch. These stresses are not as great as in roll off. In stance, the compression lines are more vertical because of the vertically directed ground reaction vectors, whereas those in roll off (in walking) or push off (in running) are obliquely directed to align parallel to the ground reaction vectors accompanying these actions.

COMMON BONE-RELATED PROBLEMS IN OLDER ADULTS
Osteoarthrosis and osteoporosis

Two bone-related pathologies that are problematic for older adults are osteoarthrosis (OA) and osteoporosis (OP). Osteoarthrosis is "wear and tear" joint degeneration that is primarily caused by abnormal joint mechanics and accompanied by very little joint inflammation.[102] The lack of significant joint inflammation makes the name *osteoarthro-sis* more representative of the pathological process than the name *osteoarthritis*. The abnormal mechanics may involve excessively fast heel loading with little absorption of the shock of heel contact[102,104] or excessive joint contact pressures due to joint malalignment or joint overloading.[25,97] Shock is normally absorbed with joint movements during loading (requiring well-timed eccentric muscle activation), deformation of trabecular bone near the joint surface, bending in the shafts of long bones, and deformation of periarticular soft tissue. Joint overloading can be traced to excessive body weight, especially during the twenties,[25] and large-magnitude loading of joints. Typically, the subchondral bone becomes denser or more sclerosed because of bone that has remodeled based on the excessive stress. The articular cartilage covering the subchondral bone wears away as the sclerosed subchondral bone loses its ability to help absorb the shock of joint loading. Pain with joint movement may inhibit joint motion as a mechanism to absorb shock; for example, people with knee OA may restrict knee flexion following heel contact. Although joint overloading has been linked to the cause of OA,[86] even extreme physical activity has not been shown to cause OA in biomechanically fit athletes[98] with no history of joint trauma or joint laxity.

Osteoporosis is loss of bone density to the extent that fracture risk is high. Fractures may occur with the impact of minimal trauma. Usually there is a direct link to Wolff's law. The fracture often results from insufficient bone mass due to overwhelming bone resorption from physical inactivity, hormonal changes, muscle fatigue, and other reasons. A fracture related to OP often occurs in the femoral neck and vertebrae, especially in elderly women.

Often, OA and OP are viewed as counterbalanced problems; that is, if a person is physically active throughout life, the person is likely to have OA but be spared OP, and vice versa. With insight into the parameters of mechanical stimuli that lead to the subchondral bone sclerosis in OA and the loss of bone density in OP, the harmful aspects of both ends of the spectrum can be avoided. Specifically, these parameters would include general life habits involving a physically active lifestyle with gradually increasing and consistent physical activity, avoiding joint loading on a malaligned joint, preventing overweight, and correcting harmful movement characteristics such as hard and fast joint loading with inadequate shock absorption. How we perform various movement activities may be more important than the activities chosen. Caspersen and colleagues integrate the results of several research studies in discussing the various clinical aspects of OA and OP.[25]

SUMMARY

Although the general shape of bone is genetically determined, bone itself is highly adaptable to the types of stresses imposed upon it. Genetic considerations affect bone strength throughout life, in men differently than in women. Researchers hope to reveal those stimuli that are required for optimal bone tissue growth, those that harm the musculoskeletal system and lead to bone-related pathology, and those that best help deformed or fractured bone heal and realign to the normal state.

ACKNOWLEDGMENTS

I would like to thank Dr. Christopher Ruff for guidance in the development of this chapter and my mentor, Dr. Whitney Powers, who guides, by example, all my professional efforts, either directly or indirectly. I also thank Teresa Friedel for her helpful critique from the viewpoint of readers, who we hope will benefit from the information in this chapter.

REVIEW QUESTIONS

1. What different strength characteristics of bone can be determined for the stress-strain curve?
2. How does bone develop during the prenatal period, the postnatal period, puberty, and adulthood?
3. How does bone strength differ between men and women? What is the rationale for these differences?
4. How are bone strength and stiffness increased?
5. What are the loading patterns of the lower extremity bones in response to weight-bearing forces?

REFERENCES

1. Albright JA, Skinner CW: Bone: structural organization and remodeling dynamics. In Albright JA, Brand RA, editors: *The scientific basis of orthopaedics,* ed 2, Norwalk, Conn, 1987, Appleton and Lange.
2. Amtmann E: The distribution of breaking strength in the human femur shaft, *J Biomech* 1:271, 1968.
3. Amtmann E, Schmitt HP: The distribution of density in compact human femoral shaft bone and its significance for the determination of the breaking strength of bone, *Z Anat Entwicklungsgesch* 127:25, 1968 (English abstract).
4. Anderson JJB, Milin L, Crackel WC: Effect of exercise on mineral and organic bone turnover in swine, *J Appl Physiol* 30:810, 1971.
5. Andrew EH: Fracture. In Vincent JFV, Currey JD, editors: *Mechanical properties of biological materials,* Symposia of the Society for Experimental Biology 34, Cambridge, 1980, Cambridge University Press.
6. Bassett CAL: Electrical effects in bone, *Sci Am* 213(4):18, 1965.
7. Bassett CAL, Pawlick RJ: Effects of electric currents on bone in vivo, *Nature* 204:652, 1964.
8. Becker RO, Murray DG: The electrical control system regulating fracture healing in amphibians, *Clin Orthop* 73:169, 1970.
9. Bjurholm A et al: Innervation of bone tissue by sensory nerve fibers, Proceedings from the Orthopaedic Research Society, *Trans Orthop Res Soc,* 12:179, 1987.
10. Bloom W, Fawcett DW: *A textbook of histology,* Philadelphia, 1975, WB Saunders.
11. Booth FW, Gould EW: Effects of training and disuse on connective tissue, *Exerc Sport Sci Rev* 83, 1975.
12. Brand RA, Rubin CT: Fracture healing. In Albright JA, Brand RA, editors: *The scientific basis of orthopaedics,* ed 2, Norwalk, Conn, 1987, Appleton and Lange.
13. Burstein AH, Reilly DT, Martens M: Aging of bone tissue, mechanical properties, *J Bone Joint Surg Am* 58:82, 1976.

14. Burstein AH et al: The ultimate properties of bone tissue: the effects of yielding, *J Biomech* 5:35, 1972.

15. Burstein AH, Wright TM: *Fundamentals of orthopaedic biomechanics,* Baltimore, 1994, Williams & Wilkins.

16. Carter DR, Blenman PR, Beaupre GS: Mechanical stress and vascular influences on fracture healing, Proceedings from the Orthopaedic Research Society, *Trans Orthop Res Soc,* 12:99, 1987.

17. Carter DR, Hayes WC: Fatigue life of compact bone: I, effects of stress amplitude, temperature and density, *J Biomech* 9:27, 1976.

18. Carter DR, Hayes WC: Compact bone fatigue damage: II, a microscopic examination, *Clin Orthop* 127:265, 1977.

19. Carter DR, Hayes WC: Compact bone fatigue damage: I, residual strength and stiffness, *J Biomech* 10:325, 1977.

20. Carter DR, Hayes WC: The compressive behavior of bone as a two-phase porous material, *J Bone Joint Surg Am* 59:954, 1977.

21. Carter DR, Hayes WC, Schurman DJ: Fatigue life of compact bone: II, effects of microstructure and density, *J Biomech* 9:211, 1976.

22. Carter DR, Schwab GH, Spengler DM: Tensile fracture of cancellous bone, *Acta Orthop Scand* 51:733, 1980.

23. Carter DR, Spengler DM: Mechanical properties and composition of cortical bone, *Clin Orthop* 135:192, 1978.

24. Carter DR et al: The mechanical and biological response of cortical bone to in vivo strain histories. In Cowin SC, editor: *Mechanical properties of bone,* Proceedings of the Joint ASME-ASCE Applied Mechanics, Fluids Engineering, and Bioengineering Conference, Boulder, Colo, June 1981, American Society of Mechanical Engineers.

25. Caspersen CJ, Kriska AM, Dearwater SR: Physical activity epidemiology as applied to elderly populations, *Bailliere's Clin Rheumatol* 8:7, 1994.

26. Chalmers J, Ho KC: Geographical variations in senile osteoporosis, *J Bone Joint Surg Br* 52:667, 1970.

27. Chamay A, Tschantz P: Mechanical influences in bone remodeling: experimental research on Wolff's law, *J Biomech* 5:173, 1972.

28. Cheal EJ et al: Stress analysis of compression plate fixation and its effects on long bone remodeling, *J Biomech* 18:141, 1985.

29. Churches AE, Howlett CR: The response of mature cortical bone to controlled time varying loading. In Cowin SC, editor: *Mechanical properties of bone,* Proceedings of the Joint ASME-ASCE Applied Mechanics, Fluids Engineering, and Bioengineering Conference, Boulder, Colo, June 1981, American Society of Mechanical Engineers.

30. Crelin ES: Development of the musculoskeletal system, *Clin Symp* 33(1):1, 1981.

31. Currey JD: The adaptation of bones to stress, *J Theor Biol* 20:91, 1968.

32. Currey JD: The mechanical properties of bones, *Clin Orthop* 73:210, 1970.

33. Currey JD: *The mechanical adaptation of bones,* Princeton, NJ, 1976, Princeton University Press.

34. Currey JD: Properties of bone, cartilage, and synovial fluid. In Dowson D, Wright V, editors: *Introduction to the biomechanics of joints and joint replacements,* London, 1981, Mechanical Engineering Publications.

35. Currey JD, Butla G: The mechanical properties of bone tissue in children, *J Bone Joint Surg Am* 57:810, 1975.

36. Dalen N, Olsson KE: Bone mineral content and physical activity, *Acta Orthop Scand* 45:170, 1974.

37. Davies GJ, Wallace LA, Malone T: Mechanisms of selected knee injuries, *Phys Ther* 60:1590, 1980.

38. Dhem A, Rober V: Morphology of bone tissue aging. In Uhthoff HK, Stahl E, editors: *Current concepts of bone fragility,* Berlin and Heidelberg, 1986, Springer-Verlag.

39. Dietrick JE, Whedon G, Shoor E: Effects of immobilization upon various metabolic and physiologic functions of normal men, *Am J Med* 4:3, 1948.

40. deVries JIP, Visser GHA, Prechtl HFR: The emergence of fetal behavior: III, individual differences and consistencies, *Early Hum Dev* 16:85, 1988.

41. Evans FG: *Mechanical properties of bone,* Springfield, Ill, 1973, Charles C Thomas.

42. Evans FG: Relations between torsion properties and histology of adult human compact bone, *J Biomech* 11(4):151, 1978.

43. Evans FG, LeBow M: Strength of human compact bone under repetitive loading, *J Appl Physiol* 10:127, 1957.

44. Evans FG, Vincentelli R: Relation of collagen fiber orientation to some mechanical properties of human cortical bone, *J Biomech* 2:63, 1969.

45. Freeman MAR, Todd RD, Pirie CJ: The role of fatigue in the pathogenesis of senile femoral neck fractures, *J Bone Joint Surg Br* 56:698, 1974.

46. Frost HM: The biology of fracture healing: an overview for clinicians, parts I and II, *Clin Orth* 248:283, 1989.

47. Frost HM: Mechanical determinants of skeletal architecture. In Albright JA, Brand RA, editors: *The scientific basis of orthopaedics,* ed 2, Norwalk, Conn, 1987, Appleton and Lange.

48. Frost HM: The regional acceleratory phenomenon, *Henry Ford Hosp Med* 31(1):3, 1983.

49. Frost HM: *Bone remodeling and its relationship to metabolic bone diseases,* Springfield, Ill, 1973, Charles C Thomas.

50. Frost HM: *The laws of bone structure,* Springfield, Ill, 1973, Charles C Thomas.

51. Frost HM: *Orthopaedic biomechanics,* vol 5, Springfield, Ill, 1973, Charles C Thomas.

52. Fukada E: Mechanical deformation and electrical polarization in biological substances, *Biorheology* 5:199, 1968.

53. Fulkerson JP, Edwards, CC, Chrisman OD: Articular cartilage. In Albright JA, Brand RA, editors: *The scientific basis of orthopaedics,* ed 2, Norwalk, Conn, 1987, Appleton and Lange.

54. Fung YC: *Mechanical properties of living tissues,* New York, 1981, Springer-Verlag.

55. Garn SM: The earlier gain and later loss of cortical bone. In *Nutritional perspective,* Springfield, Ill, 1970, Charles C Thomas.

56. Garn SM et al: Continuing bone growth throughout life: a general phenomenon, *Am J Phys Anthropol* 26:313, 1967.

57. Garnett ES et al: A photon scanning technique for the measurement of absolute bone density in man, *Radiology* 106:209, 1973.

58. Ghista DN: *Osteoarthromechanics,* Washington, DC, 1982, Hemisphere.

59. Goldstein SA et al: Experimentally controlled trabecular bone remodeling: effects of applied stress. Proceedings from the Orthopaedic Research Society, *Trans Orthop Res Soc,* 12:461, 1987.

60. Goodship AE, Lanyon LE, McFie H: Functional adaptation of bone to increased stress, *J Bone Joint Surg Am* 61:539, 1979.

61. Goodship AE et al: The effect of different regimens of axial micromovement on the healing of experimental tibial fractures. Proceedings from the Orthopaedic Research Society, *Trans Orthop Res Soc,* 12:98, 1987.

62. Gottesman T, Hashin Z: Analysis of viscoelastic behavior of bones on the basis of microstructure, *J Biomech* 13:89, 1980.

63. Harris B: The mechanical behaviour of composite materials. In Vincent JFV, Currey JD, editors: *Mechanical properties of biological materials,* Symposia of the Society for Experimental Biology 34, Cambridge, 1980, Cambridge University Press.

64. Hayes WC, Carter DR: Biomechanics of bone. In Simmons DJ, Klunin AS, editors: *Skeletal research: an experimental approach,* New York, 1979, Academic Press.

65. Hayes WC, Snyder B: Toward a quantitative formulation of Wolff's law in trabecular bone. In Cowin SC, editor: *Mechanical properties of bone,* Proceedings of the Joint ASME-ASCE Applied Mechanics, Fluids Engineering, and Bioengineering Conference, Boulder, Colo, June 1981, American Society of Mechanical Engineers.

66. Hert J, Liskova M, Landrgot B: Influence of the long-term, continuous bending on the bone, *Folia Morphol (Warsz)* 17:389, 1969.

67. Hert J, Sklenska A, Liskova M: Reaction of bone to mechanical stimuli: V, effect of intermittent stress on the rabbit tibia after resection of the peripheral nerves, *Folia Morphol (Warsz)* 19:378, 1971.

68. Hert J, Zalud J: Reaction of bone to mechanical stimuli: VI, bioelectrical theory of functional adaptation of bone [in Czech], *Acta Chir Orthop Traumatol Cech* 38:280, 1971.

69. Hettinga DL: Normal joint structures and their reaction to injury, *J Orthop Sports Phys Ther* 1(1):16, 1979.

70. Hulth A: Current concepts of fracture healing, *Clin Orthop* 249:265, 1989.

71. Ianniruberto A, Tajani E: Ultrasonographic study of fetal movements, *Semin Perinatol* 5:175, 1981.

72. Johnson KE: *Histology: microscopic anatomy and embryology,* New York, 1982, John Wiley.

73. Jowsey J: Age changes in human bone, *Clin Orthop* 17:210, 1960.

74. Justus R, Luft JH: A mechanochemical hypothesis for bone re-modeling induced by mechanical stress, *Calcif Tissue Res* 5:222, 1970.

75. Katz JL: The structure and biomechanics of bone. In Vinsant JFV, Currey JD, editors: *Mechanical properties of biological materials,* Symposia of the Society for Experimental Biology 34, Cambridge, 1980, Cambridge University Press.

76. Kiiskinen A: Physical training and connective tissue in young mice: physical properties of Achilles tendons and long bones, *Growth* 41:123, 1979.

77. Kiiskinen A, Heikkinen E: Effects of physical training on the development and strength of tendons and bones in growing mice, *Scand J Clin Lab Invest Suppl* 29:20, 1972.

78. Kobayashi TK, Pedrini V: Proteoglycans: collagen interactions in human costal cartilage, *Biochim Biophys Acta* 303:148, 1973.

79. Koch JC: The laws of bone architecture, *Am J Anat* 21:177, 1917.

80. Lanyon LE: The measurement and biological significance of bone strain in vivo. In Cowin SC, editor: *Mechanical properties of bone,* Proceedings of the Joint ASME-ASCE Applied Mechanics, Fluids Engineering, and Bioengineering Conference, Boulder, Colo, June 1981, American Society of Mechanical Engineers.

81. Lester GE et al: Relationship between physical activity and bone density in Caucasian women: a 1 to 2 year follow-up, Proceedings from the Orthopaedic Research Society, *Trans Orthop Res Soc,* 12:464, 1987.

82. Liskova M, Hert J: Reaction of bone to mechanical stimuli: II, periosteal and endosteal reaction of tibial diaphysis in rabbit to intermittent loading, *Folia Morphol (Warsz)* 19:301, 1971.

83. Mack PB et al: Bone demineralization of foot and hand of Gemini-Titan IV, V, and VII astronauts during orbital height, *Am J Roentgenol* 100:503, 1967.

84. Martin RB, Atkinson PJ: Age and sex-related changes in the structure and strength of the human femoral shaft, *J Biomech* 10:223, 1977.

85. Martin RB, Burr DB: A hypothetical mechanism for the stimulation of osteonal remodeling by fatigue damage, *J Biomech* 15(3):137, 1982.

86. McKeag DB: The relationship of osteoarthritis and exercise, *Clin Sports Med* 11(2):471, 1992.

87. McKibbon B: The biology of fracture healing in long bones, *J Bone Joint Surg Br* 60(2):150, 1978.

88. Melick RA, Miller DR: Variations of tensile strength of human cortical bone with age, *Clin Sci (Colch)* 30:243, 1966.

89. Moore K: *The developing human,* Philadelphia, 1977, WB Saunders.

90. Moore K: *Clinically oriented anatomy,* Baltimore, 1980, Williams & Wilkins.

91. Murray MP, Seireg A, Scholz RC: Center of gravity, center of pressure, and supportive forces during human activities, *J Appl Physiol* 23:831, 1967.

92. Murray PDF: *Bones,* Cambridge, 1936, Cambridge University Press.

93. Negulesco J, Kossler T: Responses of articular and epiphyseal cartilage zones of developing avian radii to estrone treatment and a 2-G environment, *Aviat Space Environ Med* 49:489, 1978.

94. Nordin M, Frankel VH: Biomechanics of bone. In Nordin M, Frankel VH, editors: *Basic biomechanics of the musculoskeletal system,* ed 2, Philadelphia, 1989, Lea & Febiger.

95. Oxnard CE: Tensile forces and skeletal structures, *J Morphol* 134:425, 1971.

96. O'Rilly R, Gardner E: The embryology of movable joints. In Sokoloff L, editor: *The joints and synovial fluid,* vol 1, New York, 1978, Academic Press.

97. Panush RS, Lane NE: Exercise and the musculoskeletal system, *Bailliere's Clin Rheumatol* 8:79, 1994.

98. Pascale M, Grana WA: Does running cause osteoarthritis? *Phys Sports Med* 17:157, 1989.

99. Park JB: *Biomaterials: an introduction,* New York, 1979, Plenum.

100. Pauwels F: *Biomechanics of the locomotor appatatus,* New York, 1980, Springer-Verlag.

101. Popov EP: *Mechanics of materials,* ed 2, Englewood Cliffs, NJ, 1976, Prentice Hall.

102. Radin E: Osteoarthrosis. In Wright V, Radin EL, editors: *Mechanics of human joints,* New York, 1993, Marcel Dekker.

103. Radin E et al: *Practical biomechanics for the orthopedic surgeon,* New York, 1979, John Wiley.

104. Radin EL et al: Relationship between lower limb dynamics and knee joint pain, *J Orthop Res* 9:398, 1991.

105. Reilly DT, Burstein AH: The mechanical properties of cortical bone, *J Bone Joint Surg Am* 56:1001, 1974.

106. Riegger-Krugh C: Relationship of mechanical and movement factors to prenatal musculoskeletal development. In Sparling JW, editor: *Concepts in fetal movement research,* New York, 1993, Haworth.

107. Robinson RA: Bone tissue: composition and function, *Johns Hopkins Med J* 145(1):10, 1979.

108. Rodahl K, Nicholson JT, Brown EM, editors: *Bone as a tissue,* New York, 1960, McGraw-Hill.

109. Roesler H: Some historical remarks on the theory of cancellous bone structure (Wolff's law). In Cowin SC, editor: *Mechanical properties of bone,* Proceedings of the Joint ASME-ASCE Applied Mechanics, Fluids Engineering, and Bioengineering Conference, Boulder, Colo, June 1981, American Society of Mechanical Engineers.

110. Rubin CT, McLeod KJ: Biologic modulation of mechanical influences in bone remodeling. In Mow VC, Ratcliffe A, Woo SL-Y, editors: *Biomechanics of diarthrodial joints,* vol 2, New York, 1990, Springer-Verlag.

111. Ruff CB, Hayes WC: Changes with age in cortical bone geometry and mineral mass in the human lower limb, *Trans Orthop Res Soc* 7:320, 1982.

112. Ruff CB, Hayes WC: Subperiosteal expansion and cortical remodeling of human femur and tibia with aging, *Science* 217:945, 1982.

113. Rybicki EF, Simonen FA, Weis EB Jr: On the mathematical analysis of stress in the human femur, *J Biomech* 5:203, 1972.

114. Salter RB: *Textbook of disorders and injuries of the musculoskeletal system: an introduction to orthopaedics, rheumatology, metabolic bone disease, rehabilitation, and fractures,* Baltimore, 1970, Williams & Wilkins.

115. Saville PD, Smith R: Bone density, breaking force, and leg muscle mass as functions of weight in bipedal rats, *Am J Phys Anthropol* 25:35, 1966.

116. Saville PD, Whyte MP: Muscle and bone hypertrophy, *Clin Orthop* 65:81, 1969.

117. Silver P: Personal communication (course in Biomechanics and Biomaterials), Spring 1981, Boston University.

118. Singh I: The architecture of cancellous bone, *J Anat* 127:305, 1978.

119. Smith JW: The relationship of epiphyseal plates to stress in some bones of the lower limb, *J Anat* 96:58, 1962.

120. Smith DW: *Recognizable patterns of human deformity: identification*

and management of mechanical effects of morphogenesis, Philadelphia, 1981, WB Saunders.

121. Smith RW, Walker RR: Femoral expansion in aging in women: implications for osteoporosis and fractures, *Science* 145:156, 1964.

122. Symeonides PP: High stress fractures of the fibula, *J Bone Joint Surg Br* 62:192, 1980.

123. Tachdjian MO: *Pediatric orthopaedics,* Philadelphia, 1972, WB Saunders.

124. Tipton CM, Matthes R, Maynard J: Influence of chronic exercise on rat bones, *Med Sci Sports Exerc* 4:55, 1972.

125. Torzilli PA et al: The material and structural properties of maturing bone. In Cowin SC, editor: *Mechanical properties of bone,* Proceedings of the Joint ASME-ASCE Applied Mechanics, Fluids Engineering, and Bioengineering Conference, Boulder, Colo, June 1981, American Society of Mechanical Engineers.

126. Vose GP, Stover BJ, Mack PB: Ouantitative bone strength measurements in senile osteoporosis, *J Gerontol* 16:120, 1961.

127. Wainwright SA et al: *Mechanical design in organisms,* Princeton, NJ, 1976, Princeton University Press.

128. Walker J: Musculoskeletal development: a review, *Phys Ther* 71:878, 1991.

129. Wall JC, Chatterji SK, Jeffrey JW: The influence that bone density and orientation and particle size of the mineral phase have on the mechanical properties of bone, *J Bioenerg Biomembr* 2:517, 1978.

130. Warwick R, Williams P, editors: *Gray's anatomy,* ed 35, Philadelphia, 1973, WB Saunders.

131. Weiss PA: Cellular dynamics, *Rev Mod Phys* 31:11, 1959.

132. Werntz JR et al: The osteogenic potential of bone marrow to heal segmental long bone defects, Proceedings from the Orthopaedic Research Society, *Trans Orthop Res Soc,* 12:441, 1987.

133. Whalen RT, Carter DR, Steele CR: The relationship between physical activity and bone density, Proceedings from the Orthopaedic Research Society, *Trans Orthop Res Soc,* 12:463, 1987.

134. Winter DA: *Biomechanics and motor control of human movement,* ed 2, New York, 1992, John Wiley.

135. Wolff J: *The law of bone remodeling* (translated by P Maquet and R Furlong), New York, 1986, Springer-Verlag.

136. Woo SL-Y: The relationships of changes in stress levels on long bone remodeling. In Cowin SC, editor: *Mechanical properties of bone,* Proceedings of the Joint ASME-ASCE Applied Mechanics, Fluids Engineering, and Bioengineering Conference, Boulder, Colo, June 1981, American Society of Mechanical Engineers.

137. Woo SL-Y et al: Effect of prolonged physical training on properties of long bone: a study of Wolff's law, *J Bone Joint Surg Am* 63:780, 1981.

138. Yamada H. In Evans FG, editor: *Strength of biological materials,* Baltimore, 1970, Williams & Wilkins.

CHAPTER 2

Neurobiology for Orthopedic and Sports Physical Therapy

Mark J. Rowinski

OUTLINE

Basic relevance of neural system concepts
General functional anatomy
Joint receptors
Primary afferent fibers: stimulus response relationships
    Fiber spectrum
    Receptive fields
    Force sensibility
    Neuron population response and across-fiber pattern
      coding
    Temporal response pattern
    Quantitative stimulus response functions
Efferent modulation of joint fiber afference: an influence
  of muscular activity
Functional implications
    Spinal reflex action: intrinsic stability and mobility
    Postural and equilibrium mechanisms
    Proprioceptive and kinesthetic awareness
Other clinical considerations
Summary

BASIC RELEVANCE OF NEURAL SYSTEM CONCEPTS

Orthopedic and sports clinicians treat a wide spectrum of conditions ranging from acute injury to the chronic impairment of function. From the mechanism of injury to the chronic inflammatory state, the clinician must focus on the factors controlling joint motion and stability, as well as those dependent on the musculotendinous length/tension relation. In the modification of the treatment plan, the regulatory function of the nervous system is a primary factor that the clinician must consider. Damage or other alterations of surrounding tissues may affect neural sensitivity and reactivity in a different way than direct injury to the neural tissue. It is therefore important in the assessment and rehabilitation of injury and impairment to distinguish the cause, nature, and impact of neural compromise of especially the periarticular tissues.

Reactions of the body to environmental forces are initiated through the cues provided by various proprioceptive and exteroceptive receptor systems that translate physical energies to impulse pattern codes. Proprioceptive receptors such as those in the joint tissues, muscles, and tendons receive their stimulation from some action, e.g., rotation of a joint, stretch of a muscle, or tension due to length change and voluntary contraction. The somatic exteroceptive receptors translate energies impinging on the cutaneous and protective tissues, e.g., heat, cold, or superficial mechanical forces, so that their information about the immediate environment may contribute to the program for subsequent action or posturing of the body. Reflexes arising from the proprioceptive channels become habitually attached and appended to certain reflexes excited by exteroceptive protective channels. Thus Sherrington, in the early part of this century, described an order to our motorsensory systems based upon governance of our internal movement control system by an external guidance and information seeking or "tracking" system.[72]

We now appreciate that much of the initiative for motion lies within us and is proactive rather than reactive and that skilled purposeful motion is highly dependent upon internal neuronal feedback and feedforward loops. These control elements act to execute motor commands, correct actions for accurate projection and placement, predict and eliminate redundant or expected information, and react to unexpected features of the force/mass field of the environment. The development of capacities and selected modes of operation through motor learning largely incorporates aspects of the environment in the patterning of motor commands and reactions. We continually seek to extend the "limits" of human locomotive performance. In actuality, the real limitations on motor skill performance are set by the anatomical and physiological constraints of the systems involved, such as the skeletal, muscular, and nervous systems. The biomechanical structures of the skeleton, joints, and muscles seem universally fashioned to optimally meet the organisms' needs for maintaining stability and producing motility.

The structural specialization of the joint provides for the interdependent requirements of rigid stability, shock absorption, and adaptable mobility, which are specific for survival of the species. The joints are adapted to the range of motion that is required of them in the characteristic activities of any particular animal form. In seeking to understand the relevant biomechanical-neuronal system transforms, scientific analyses have included invasive anatomical and physiological studies of tissue components and functional relations underlying freedom of action in some of our mammalian relatives, where functions and tissue relations are expected to be similar to those of humans. Highly controlled experimental efforts have yielded great insight into many features of normal and abnormal joint structure and function. In addition, psychophysical studies of human position sense under normal and pathological conditions have contributed much information regarding cognitive functions related to joint activity in the human. Gross morphological and detailed histological examinations of cadaver or amputated human articular structures have been accomplished, and detailed neuronal interrelations have been studied in order to achieve the basic understanding of how our articular systems function in normal and abnormal states.

Articular tissues are endowed by the nervous system with direct *afferent* innervation; that is, information about the degree of mechanical distortion of the articular structures is sent *toward* the central nervous system (CNS) through this innervation primarily to alert central neuron populations of current mechanical conditions for both perceptual experiences and nonperceptual reflexes and motor control. The status of articular tissues is conveyed in neural impulse code to many levels of the CNS so that information regarding static or dynamic conditions, equilibrium or disequilibrium, or biomechanical stress/strain relations may be ascertained. This information is used to influence muscle tone, motor execution programs, postural adaptation, and cognitive somatic perceptions.

Fine-grained analysis of receptor function through microelectrode recordings in the central and peripheral nervous systems have led to revisions in many of our long held, empirically derived beliefs regarding innervation of the joint and its role in biomechanical pathology. There has been a major revision in the commonly held view of the importance of joint versus muscular innervation with regard to kinesthesia and static position sense, and some critical reviews are available[7,10,58,74,75] (a selected reference list is also provided). Furthermore, more clinically relevant questions are being explored in view of the accepted notion that proprioceptive articular integrity is critical for rehabilitation and restoration of optimal musculoskeletal performance. It is apparent from behavioral studies that the human mind makes use of this information emanating from the articular tissues in a manner that can be used in the clinician's sculpting of the plastic changes that restore function after injury.

GENERAL FUNCTIONAL ANATOMY

The joint, or arthron, contains bone, cartilaginous inserts, and all the soft tissue structures between the rigid skeletal components and the adjacent pertinent muscular elements. Much of the early study of joint function has been reviewed in depth by Gardner, who included a review of the initial studies on joint innervation.[26]

The highly innervated soft tissues of the synovial joints include the fibrous and subsynovial capsule, the extrinsic and intrinsic ligaments, and the articular fat pads. Cartilaginous components of the joint such as the disks, menisci, and articular hyaline cartilage that covers the articular facets of the bone are commonly believed not to be innervated.[45] Earlier studies in the literature suggested that the outer edge of meniscal tissue receives direct innervation.[59,82] However, it now appears that only immediately adjacent perimeniscal capsular tissue is directly innervated.[45] There is also some disagreement in the literature regarding the afferent innervation of the synovial membrane. One group of investigators denies its existence,[18,25,83] whereas other studies[31,45] and practical clinical considerations attest to its importance in contributing to neural information emanating from the joint. It is known that subchondral bone is well innervated,[55,64] and there is increasing evidence that this innervation may be relevant in conditions such as patellofemoral pain syndrome. Shear stresses on the subchondral bone are thought to arise from abnormal tracking of the patella and the resultant focal compression during such activities as running.[24b]

The nerve supply to most appendicular joints occurs by way of specific articular nerves that proceed to the joint capsule region as independent branches of larger peripheral nerves and also by way of nonspecific articular branches of related muscle nerves that reach the joint by traversing the muscles and interfascicular connective tissue.[83] Some joints may also receive articular "twigs" from cutaneous and periosteal nerve branches.[63] The vertebral joints likewise appear to receive a dual innervation, with the primary innervation occurring via the posterior rami of the segmental nerves and an accessory innervation supplied by branches of nerves to the deep paravertebral muscles.[76,86] Significant reviews of specific joint anatomy with innervation described are available for major joints such as the knee.[58b] These articles demonstrate the relevance of regional localization and specialization for particular clinical conditions and for such mechanisms as motor learning and functional rehabilitation.

An example of the degree of spatial organization inherent in multi-innervated joints has been provided by Kennedy, Alexander, and Hayes[45] for the human knee joint. Their study consistently found that the knee was innervated by a posterior group of nerves (the posterior articular and obturator nerves) and by an anterior group (the articular branches of the femoral, common peroneal, and saphenous nerves). Each of the constituent nerves appears to have a particular spatial territory, and in some instances the territory includes diverse periarticular tissues such as the capsule and ligaments. Each nerve should therefore be considered multimodal and territorially specific. Nerve damage would necessarily result in spatially specific deficits across several modality or information channels emanating from a particular joint. This model serves as a guide to the multiple sources of innervation of a specific joint and is an excellent source of information for the orthopedic surgeon and therapist whenever procedures affecting specific periarticular innervations are considered. An example of specific relevance, again referring to patellofemoral pain, is the evidence presented recently that tight retinacular fibers demonstrate small nerve ending degeneration, suggesting the possibility of the retinaculum as a source of pain.[25b]

Generalized duality of innervation suggests that primary and accessory nerves to the joint may have different compositions and functional roles. It is therefore difficult to draw general conclusions about joint innervation based on a limited sampling of information transmitted via primary joint nerves or muscle nerves alone, without attending to the distinction between sensitivities and muscular- versus joint-originated signals. Such a caution, however, has not been heeded in many of the research endeavors in the past, and assumptions about functional implications have been subject to error.

Embedded in the connective tissue of the joints are mechanoreceptors or specialized neuroepithelial cell aggregates that transduce the mechanical distortion of the tissue into electrical activity belonging to the neural element of the receptor complex. Because these receptors are specifically sensitive to changes originating in the tissue rather than changes in external energies, they are appropriately categorized as proprioceptors. As mentioned previously, input from the receptors in itself does not imply the receptors participate in conscious appreciation of body sense. The typical mechanoreceptor ending is surrounded by specialized epithelial cells that are responsible for many of the response properties of the receptor complex.[4] However, some free nerve endings are not immediately "encapsulated" by epithelial cells, and these are believed to be either mechanically or chemically sensitive.

The intensity of mechanical distortion of the receptor ending or the concentration of the specific excitatory chemical agent coupled with such factors as the (1) previous history of such stimulations, (2) adaptability of surrounding tissue to distort,[12] and (3) specific sensitivity to the receptor ending itself, determine the amount of the electrical charge across the membrane of the receptor ending.

Thus distortion of the periarticular tissue triggers a change on the membrane of the specialized receptor ending whose amplitude is modulated by the previously listed factors. The potential change is referred to as the *receptor or generator potential* of the ending. As of this date, no recording of isolated joint receptor potentials has been reported, but it must be assumed that the mechanism of receptor potential generation does not differ significantly from the basic mechanism occurring in similarly configured somatosensory receptors in other body tissues.[71] The gradual receptor potential then excites the axonal portion of the peripheral primary afferent neuron, eliciting a barrage of the impulses in the parent axon. The rate of impulse production, termed the *discharge rate,* or response frequency, is mathematically related to the absolute amplitude of the generator potential, which in turn is directly proportional to the intensity of stimulation. The manner in which the afferent fiber's discharge rate is related to the overt activity of the joint is what determines the fiber's response type and serves as a convenient classification method of the receptor/primary afferent fiber complex.

Specific primary afferent fiber types have been distinguished through recent correlations of receptor structure and parent axon or primary afferent fiber response type. (Fig. 2-1 and Table 2-1). Anatomical classification according to general receptor morphology therefore should be used provisionally along with fiber response type to specify the innervation of discrete joint regions or specific tissue components. It is important to realize that classification of receptor/fiber morphology and physiology involves a simplification and reductionistic approach, which all too often ignores fine gradations in unit typology that have been elucidated by previous detailed studies.[63]

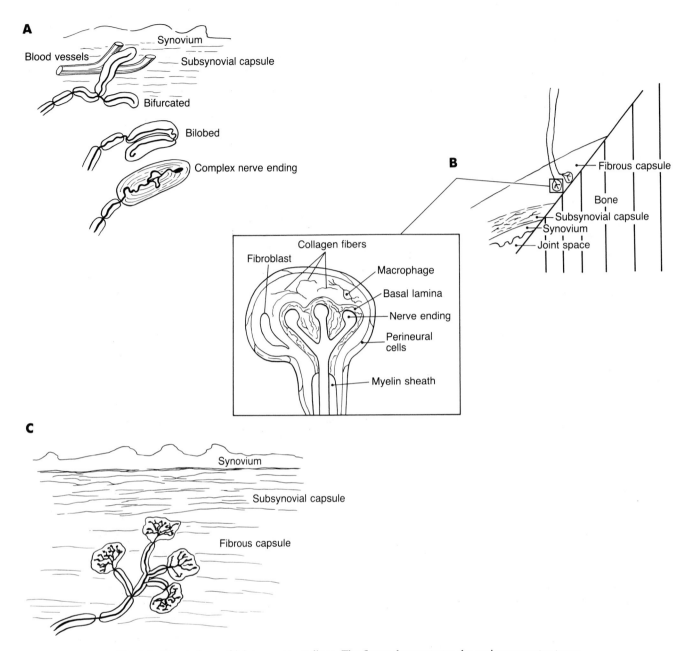

Fig. 2-1. Morphology of joint receptor endings. The figure demonstrates the various receptor types found in periarticular tissues, together with the initial segment of the parent axon and the typical ending cluster pattern: **A,** pacinian corpuscle; **B,** Golgi-Mazzoni corpuscle; **C,** Ruffini endings.

The articular soft tissue biomechanically stabilizes not only the bony structures of the joint but also the tissues. The extensive afferent nerve supply of articular soft tissue serves as a valuable and highly specific information source on which tissue property modification can be based.

JOINT RECEPTORS

Summaries of the type of neural receptors invested in periarticular tissues are available in the literature.[7,74,83] Most of the early studies that contributed to these reviews are based on indirect correlation between structure and function. More recent neurophysiological recording techniques involving single, peripheral afferent axon isolation have greatly clarified the concept of joint innervation and its purpose. Such microphysiological and histological scrutiny of the stimulated tissue has yielded important information on the specificity of the neural code, which arises from the periphery.

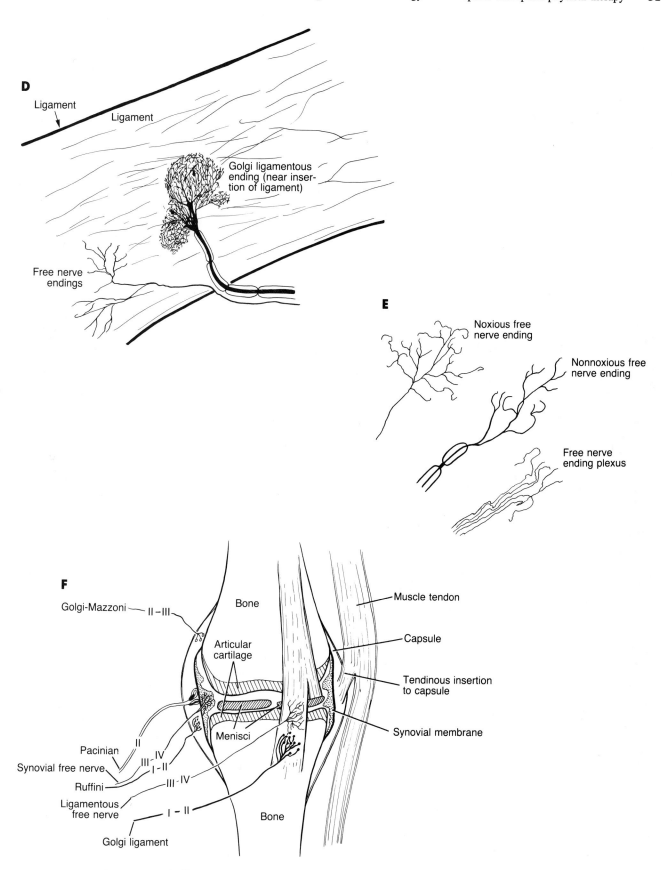

Fig. 2-1, cont'd. D, Golgi ligament ending; **E,** free nerve endings (noxious and nonnoxious); **F,** composite diagram of total joint innervation pattern, showing interrelations of afferent receptors.

Table 2-1. Joint receptors

Receptor	Location	Description	Sensitivity	Distribution (of receptor type)	Functional classification	Parent axon (fiber diameter, conduction velocity)
Pacinian corpuscles	Fibrous layer of capsule, on capsule-synovium border, close to small blood vessels	Single terminal within lamellated encapsulation; appears in clusters of five or less (20-40 × 150-250 μm cylindrical)	Sensitive to high-frequency vibration (>60 Hz), acceleration, and high-velocity changes in joint position; possible sensitivity to hemohydraulic, transient events and rapid contractile events of adjacent muscles	Found in all joints examined; sole corpuscular receptor in laryngeal and middle ear joints; greater density in distal than in proximal joints	Very rapidly adapting (RA); very low mechanical threshold	Group II (8-12 μM, 49 ms); terminal branch at 3-5 μm diameter
Golgi-Mazzoni corpuscles	Inner surface of joint capsule between fibrous layer and subcapsular fibroadipose tissue	Multiple terminating endings within thin encapsulation (30 × 200 μm cylindrical)	Sensitive to compression of joint capsule in plane perpendicular to its inner surface; insensitive to stretching capsule	Knee joint and many others likely; may have specific distribution within joint capsule	Slowly adapting (SA); response is linear function of compressive stress on capsule; low mechanical threshold	Group II-III (5-8 μm; estimate ≈ 30 ms)
Ruffini endings	Fibrous layer of capsule; few present in extrinsic ligaments	Spray-type terminal endings within thin encapsulation, having investment of collagen fibers (300 × 300-800 μm, two to six endings per axon)	Sensitive to capsule stretching along either of its long axes within capsular plane, direction and speed of capsular stretch, intracapsular fluid pressure change, amplitude and velocity of joint-position change	Few present in distal joints; greater density in proximal joints; concentrated in capsular regions of most stress	Slowly adapting (SA); low mechanical threshold; response is linear function of axial components of capsular plane stress	Group I-II (13-17 or 8-12 μm, 51 ms)
Golgi ligament endings (Golgi tendon organlike)	Extrinsic and intrinsic ligaments; adjacent to bony attachments of ligaments	Thick encapsulation, profuse branching (100 × 600 μm total terminal spread)	Sensitive to tension or stretch on ligaments	Present in most joints except cervical vertebral, laryngeal, and ossicular ligaments	Slowly adapting (SA); low-to-high mechanical threshold	Group I (13-17 μm; estimate ≈ 51 ms)
Free nerve endings (nociceptive and non-nociceptive)	Fibrous capsule, ligaments, subsynovial capsule, synovium, fat pads	Thin, bare nerve endings of small myelinated or unmyelinated axons; profuse branching	One type sensitive to nonnoxious mechanical stress; other type sensitive to noxious mechanical or biochemical stimuli	Present in all joints examined but density varies with joint component; most joints have relatively higher density in ligaments	Slowly adapting (SA); low-to-high mechanical threshold	Group III-IV (2-5 μm, <2 μm; 2.5-20 ms)

Based on data from references 2, 5, 6, 13, 25, 30, 37-40, 56, 63, 69, 70, and 88.

The periarticular receptors are subject to distortion by mechanical forces associated with soft tissue elongation, relaxation, compression, and fluid tension changes. Each type of nerve ending serves as a selective filter for a specific kind of stimulus energy and grades its activity within that energy spectrum according to the intensity of soft tissue distortion. The micromechanical status of the joint must be rapidly and accurately conveyed to the CNS so that such information (1) can influence the activity of those motor units that regulate the joint aperture, position, and angulation, (2) can influence upper motor neurons that govern the patterns and coordination of muscle activity at the joint, and (3) can influence the activity of those neural pathways that mediate perceptions associated with awareness of joint condition.

Functionally, this neural information protects the joint from damage by movement beyond its normal physiological range, (2) determines the appropriate balance of synergistic and antagonistic forces (i.e., muscular action necessary for voluntary smooth joint movement), and (3) participates with other proprioceptive afferent receptors from the tendons and muscles to generate a somatosensory image within the CNS. Most joint afferent receptors are active only near the end range of motion and thus probably contribute to only reflexive and motor control mechanisms of body movement and position, that is, a type of self "end feel."[10]

Table 2-1 incorporates the most recent findings available in the literature on receptor and primary afferent fiber functional relations and attempts to consolidate these data with previously presented classification schemes. Most of the properties of a receptor type are determined by assuming that the receptor is linked to a given primary afferent fiber and that response characteristics are learned from experimental invasive studies of the fiber's response to controlled mechanical stimulation of its assumed receptor ending. For this reason, most of the discussion of functional response properties is included in the following section on primary afferent fibers. Further clarification of the morphological appearance of joint receptors is provided in Fig. 2-1.

Several points regarding the localization of specific receptor types should be emphasized. First, Kennedy, Alexander, and Hayes[45] have traced free nerve endings into the synovial membrane of the human knee joint. These nerve endings are different from those innervating adjacent fat pads, capsular tissue, or intrinsic ligaments of the joint. The same study also emphasizes that meniscal tissue is not innervated as previously believed[82] but is surrounded by highly innervated perimeniscal tissue. A previous study of the cat has also confirmed the presence of fine nerve endings in the inner layer of the capsule, adjacent synovial tissue, adventitia of the large blood vessels, and arteriolar tissue.[68]

Other studies provide adequate evidence for the existence of highly sensitive vibratory receptors-pacinian corpuscles in close association with the blood vessels supplying the synovial membrane.[40] The receptors reside at the synovial-capsular border in the stratum synovium of the capsule. The exquisite mechanosensitivity of the pacinian receptors makes it very likely that they would discharge in response to rapid perturbations of the synovium and possibly to its perfusion pressure pulse under appropriate hydraulic conditions. This latter hypothesis, however, should not be taken as support of Grieve's suggestion[34] that the pacinian afferent receptors may subserve the function of throbbing joint pain, because a previous study[62] implicates pacinian afferent receptors in quite the opposite role of pain suppression. Detailed histological examination of the synovium reveals that it is highly vascularized, penetrated by lymphatic vessels, populated with adipocytes, and intimately bound to the subsynovial connective tissue and capsule.[4] It is therefore most probable that synovial mechanical distortion activates subsynovial mechanoreceptors as well. Thus the synovial membrane may be considered an important contributor to the arthroneural dependent behavior of the organism, and its dysfunction or removal may affect neural function of the joint.

A second point to be highlighted is that identification of the receptor type present in a joint region is not sufficient of itself to determine the neural information content contributed by that tissue. In other words, conclusions about structural and functional relations of joint innervation may be ambiguous if based only on information derived from histological examination of receptor density and typology. Physiological study must accompany histological identification. Two major findings support this contention. Grigg, Hoffman, and Fogarty[38] have determined that the Golgi-Mazzoni corpuscle, which resembles the rapidly adapting (RA) pacinian corpuscle in morphology, gives rise to a slowly adapting (SA) response (Fig. 2-2) when transcapsular compression forces are applied. This receptor type is virtually the only receptor type found on the anteromedial aspect of the cat knee capsule just anterior to the medial collateral ligament.[28] Many previous histological analyses of receptors in this region, which had not examined the exact physiological properties of the fibers innervating these receptors, may have actually attributed pacinian-like RA characteristics to these slowly adapting structures.[25,58] As a result, the responsiveness of this tissue to sustained compressive forces was largely ignored.

A further recent advance in our understanding of the relationship of structure and function in joint innervation comes from the work of Schaible and Schmidt,[69,70] who have studied small-diameter axons of articular nerves. These experiments have demonstrated that at least some of the previously assumed noxious stimulus detectors associated with small-diameter fibers[58,84,85] are actually fairly sensitive nonnoxious mechanoreceptors. In other words, not all free nerve endings in joint tissue are nociceptive, and some may actually be among the most sensitive mechanoreceptors of the joint. This situation is similar to the fact that the quality of light touch is mediated by some of the free nerve endings

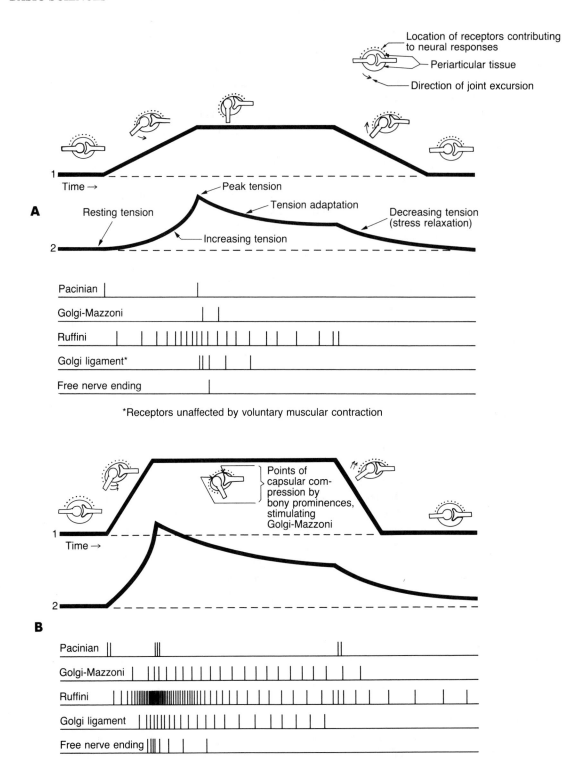

Fig. 2-2. Physiological response types of various joint afferent fibers. **A,** Typical responses of afferent fibers to moderate stimulation of the periarticular tissue. Excursion of joint is indicated by trace *1*, presumed tension generation in periarticular tissues by trace *2*, and neural responses by traces marked with appropriate afferent type. **B,** Same as **A** with the exception that more intense and rapid stimulus is applied to the joint.

of cutaneous tissue. Recent high-resolution experimental studies reveal that many of the classical assumptions about joint receptor function may have been overly generalized. Furthermore, the complexity and diversity of articular receptors match those reported for cutaneous mechanoreceptors.[2,13,39]

PRIMARY AFFERENT FIBERS: STIMULUS-RESPONSE RELATIONSHIPS

The mechanoelectrical transduction events taking place at the receptor level can be translated into the discharge rate of the primary afferent fibers, the parent axons that convey impulses to synapses in the spinal cord. Secondary afferents, whose cell bodies are in the dorsal horns or dorsal column nuclei, then transmit impulse coded information toward motorneurons, interneurons, brainstem, or thalamic nucleui. The activity of one peripheral primary fiber in isolation provides information about the mechanical events occurring in a very limited and discrete region of the joint, whereas the activity pattern of many afferent fibers describes the action of the joint as a whole. In other words, a single afferent fiber can signal to the CNS only what specific joint is moving and a very small bit of information about the distortion of a small portion of periarticular tissue of that joint. It is known that a single impulse may elicit a conscious perception, and that an entire barrage of impulses may be completely ignored or gated from consciousness. Some examples of the diverse response type characteristics of various articular afferent fibers as they relate to standard joint excursions are presented in Fig. 2-2. The figure demonstrates how different ranges of joint excursion can shift the neuron population response pattern by shifting into the sensitivity ranges of different types of receptors. It is generally held that we act on the basis of the *across fiber pattern* of impulses signaling tissue state to the brain.

Rossi and Grigg[65] have described a model for activation of capsular afferent receptors. In the hip joint, certain afferent receptors discharge only when the joint is rotated in a specific plane. The type of excursion that activates joint afferent receptors and their corresponding afferent fibers is determined by three factors: (1) location of the receptors in the capsule, (2) geometry of the joint, and (3) geometry of the capsule. For example, in the hip the most important movements appear to be internal/external rotation, which activates receptors of the posterior and anterior capsule, and abduction/adduction, which activates receptors of the inferior and superior portions of the capsule. Very few (2%) capsular receptors were found to be excited by flexion/extension of the hip. The study concluded that a joint's axis of rotation is signaled by the subpopulation of afferent fibers excited, whereas the extent of joint movement of excursion is signaled by the frequency of afferent fiber discharge. Capsular afferent fibers were generally not found to be active in neutral or intermediate limb positions.

Fiber spectrum

It has been reported that afferent fibers alone, among all of the traditionally defined afferent categories, innervate the periarticular tissues; that is, the fiber spectrum of joint innervation includes all fibers from the large group I myelinated range, the intermediate-diameter fibers, and the smallest unmyelinated group IV fibers. In Table 2-1 the fiber diameters and corresponding fiber classes are provided in relation to the receptors and tissues receiving the fibers. Note that the conduction velocity corresponds fairly well to Hursch ratio relating fiber size to impulse velocity, and the relation is closer to a factor of 6 m/sec per micron of axonal cross-sectional diameter for larger myelinated fibers, and closer to 1 m/sec per micron for the smaller nonmyelinated axons. It is important for the clinician to realize that more rapid conduction of impulses from the proprioceptors is necessary for nonnoxious reactivity of the motor and sensory systems of the CNS than for nociceptive reactions and perceptions.

Receptive fields

The area of the joint capsule, ligament, or other periarticular tissue whose mechanical distortion leads to excitation of a given joint afferent fiber is known as the receptive field (RF) of that afferent fiber. It has been determined that RFs of small-diameter fibers in groups III and IV are on the order of 25 mm^2, whereas larger diameter afferent fibers in group II may have smaller RFs or quite large RFs, ranging up to 100 mm^2.

The existence of joint afferent fibers with multiple RFs has been demonstrated by Schaible and Schmidt.[69] It is therefore possible that several receptor endings lying in spatially separate portions of a subregion of the joint capsule may be connected to one and the same parent afferent fiber. Alternatively, there may be regions of capsular heterogeneity that would contribute to differential sensitivity foci in a spatially compact receptor ending. The latter possibility may relate to posttraumatic periarticular receptor mechanisms, because scar tissue formation may be expected to cause significant distortion in the normal RF distribution of many joint primary afferent fibers.

Traditionally, it has been the custom to refer to the RF of a given joint afferent fiber in terms of the range of motion or joint excursion through which the afferent fiber is excited. For example, a given knee joint afferent fiber may begin to discharge only at 70° of flexion and may increase its discharge rate up to a maximum of 135° at the end of the range of joint flexion. The excursion RF of the neuron would therefore be considered to be 70° to 135°, and the unit would be referred to as a flexion-related unit and would be assumed to have its receptor ending located on the anterior aspect of the knee joint capsule. This type of categorization of joint innervation fields is perhaps more clinically useful than focal definition of the afferent RF (in terms of the area of joint capsule, ligament, or other periarticular tissue), but the spatial RF should not be totally ignored, especially in cases of spatially specific joint trauma. The clinician must be well aware that individual or small populations of joint afferent neurons are activated by mechanical events in only a specific locus of the joint tissue, that this locus determines the range of motion or static posture through which the afferent fiber will be active, and that a peak sensitivity of the unit or neuron population occurs somewhere within that range of motion.

Force sensitivity

The sensitivity of joint mechanoreceptors to tissue tension is within the same range as has been demonstrated for other force-transducing receptors of the somatosensory system. Controlled mechanical stretching of capsular tissue in various planes has been used recently to ascertain the sensitivity of joint afferent fibers.

Force-pressure or tissue-tension mechanical thresholds of activation have been determined for afferent fibers of medium conduction velocity originating from the Golgi-Mazzoni receptors of the medial knee capsule in the cat.[38] Thresholds range from 1.5 to 25 gm/mm² (6.4 gm/mm², mean) for these afferent fibers when oriented (compressive) stress is applied to mimic normal capsular activation conditions. Ruffini receptor endings have been investigated in other studies[37] and have been found to be much more sensitive. Thresholds can be detected with axially or longitudinally oriented loads applied to the capsule and range from 0.13 to 6.3 gm/mm² (0.2 to 0.3 gm/mm², mode).

Mechanical thresholds have also been determined for less sensitive afferent fibers by less controlled techniques of force application to capsular tissue. For example, focal application of force directly to the center of the RFs of afferent fibers has been used to investigate the mechanical sensitivity of small-diameter fibers.[44] This method, which involves the use of fine-tipped probes (aesthesiometers or von Frey hairs) to distort a punctate region of the total capsular RF of a unit under study, results in excitation of mechanoreceptors at lower than normal levels of force. Mechanical force thresholds determined in this manner for some group II and group IV joint afferent fibers have been found in the range of 0.3 to 22.5 gm, with the group IV fibers having the highest thresholds, that is, the lowest mechanical sensitivity.[69,70] It is expected that capsular loading under normal activity of the joint would have to be at least an order of magnitude higher than the above intensities to excite these fibers. The smaller diameter afferent fibers also tend to have a less steep slope (relating response to intensity or magnitude of force) than do the larger diameter fibers (Table 2-2). Because groups III and IV fibers represent the great majority of afferent fibers of a given articular nerve,[46] it is of great importance to understand their contribution to articular afferent mechanisms. Other major differences between groups III and IV joint afferent fibers relating to force sensitivity are given in Table 2-2.

Table 2-2. Comparison of groups III and IV joint afferent fibers

Parameter	III	IV
Conduction velocity	2.5 to 20 ms	0.3 to 1.1 ms
Rotation > flexion/ extension needed to excite	30.5%	13%
Nonnoxious stimulation weakly excites; noxious stimulation strongly excites	19.5%	7.5%
Only noxious stimulation excites	28%	26%
Insensitivity to joint movement	22%	43.5%
Discharge frequency/ stimulation intensity slope relation	Steep	Less steep
Mechanical threshold	Low (<3 gm)	Some low, most high (some >7.5 gm)

Based on data from Schaible HG and Schmidt RF: Activation of groups III and IV sensory units in medial articular nerve by local mechanical stimulation of knee joint, *J Neurophysiol* 49:35, 1983, and Responses of fine medial articular nerve afferents to passive movements of the knee joint, *J Neurophysiol* 49:118, 1983.

Desensitization of receptors is possible under certain conditions of repetitive activation.[69] An example of such desensitizing stimulation would be the application of a suprathreshold stimulus such as 20 gm for 30 seconds at 1-minute intervals for four repetitions. This type of stimulation has been shown to reduce responsiveness of some group III and IV fibers.

Neuron population response and across-fiber pattern coding

Functionally, the activity of an individual joint afferent fiber by itself may not be meaningful to CNS mechanisms, because its relation to the function of the joint as a whole may vary. It is the temporal and spatial response patterns of many joint afferent fibers discharging in concert that inform the CNS about what the joint is doing. The importance of this concept is emphasized by the fact that any single afferent fiber, discharging throughout a particular range of motion, may discharge differently when that motion is accomplished actively versus passively. Furthermore, the increased soft tissue tension that may be associated with a slight degree of torsion superimposed on a uniplanar joint excursion may significantly alter the stimulus response relation of a single unit. The former effect has been attributed to musculotendinous insertions into the capsule, which produce changes in capsule tension when muscle contraction occurs.[54] The latter effect is probably due to the increments or decrements in tissue tension arising from rotational tightening, deletion of slack, or the "windup" effect. Grigg and Hoffman[37] have demonstrated that many capsular afferent fibers respond to two or more directions of longitudinal capsular stress.

Therefore, evidence supports the argument that a somewhat tenuous relationship exists between single-unit discharge and the absolute excursion of the joint, whereas the neuron population response pattern must be considered the neural encoder of periarticular stresses and strains. The neuron population response therefore must clearly reflect the following aspects of joint function: (1) the static joint angle, (2) the velocity of joint excursion, (3) the planes in which the joint excursion occurs, (4) the activity of passivity of joint excursion (i.e., whether joint movement is elicited by muscular contraction), and (5) the nature of internal or external compressive forces on the articular soft tissue.

Sensorineural theory advocates the across-fiber pattern as the important factor in nonambiguous transfer of information to the CNS. However, more detailed study is required before a final verdict can be reached regarding the informational impact of a single afferent fiber input, because it has been determined in humans that activity in a single cutaneous peripheral afferent fiber is adequate to elicit a conscious perception.[78,79] When coupled with the knowledge of how many afferent fibers usually participate in a functional joint response, the sensitivity of individual afferent fibers becomes an important factor in determining the minimal afferentation necessary to evoke adequate function of the joint neuronal information system.

Temporal response pattern

Two general patterns of joint afferent receptor sensitivity exist in relation to the time domain. The RA response of the Pacinian afferent receptors consists of the occurrence of discharge of the receptor only during dynamic conditions involving rapid movement of the joint, that is, during high-velocity or accelerative phases of joint motion. It would be expected that very low amplitude vibrations (60 Hz or more) of the capsular or pericapsular tissue would be adequate to excite these afferent receptors.

Specific low-frequency vibration detectors such as the Meissner corpuscle of cutaneous origin[57] have not been found in periarticular tissues. However, SA articular afferent receptors such as the Ruffini, Golgi-Mazzoni, Golgi ligamentous, and free nerve ending type respond during both dynamic and static phases of stimulation. Therefore low-frequency vibration and low-stimulus velocities are likely to be signaled in the initial discharge rate of SA afferent fibers.[74] The traditional view has been that RA afferent receptors signal joint movement, and the SA afferent receptors specify static joint position. However, the neural code for static position and for low-velocity dynamic aspects of joint movement must rely heavily on the Ruffini, Golgi-Mazzoni, free nerve, and ligamentous afferent receptors and on different portions of their discharge pattern for unambiguity.

Grigg, Hoffman, and Fogarty[38] have determined that some SA afferent receptors of the knee joint capsule may present an RA-type response when stimulated off the focal point of their RF. This is analogous to what can be achieved by minimal stimulation of cutaneous afferent receptors at close to threshold strengths.[66] Large-amplitude movements to a given position therefore result in an entirely different sequence of neural information than does a sequence of small movements to the same position. Response variation as a function of the interplay of both intensity and stimulus sequence again requires that resolution of the mechanical events at the joint is encoded by the across-fiber pattern or spatial-temporal neural activity profile.[22] It is much too simplistic to relate joint movement detection to the RA afferent receptor channel and joint position to SA afference, especially because joint status is accompanied by status reports from the involved muscles and tendons. Whenever a joint assumes a particular position or is in the course of an excursion, it would be most fruitful to envision the myriad of impulses arising from muscular, fascial, tendon, and bony receptors, as well as from articular receptors.

Quantitative stimulus-response functions

Two major types of stimulus-response functions have been determined for joint afferent fibers. Skoglund[73] initially observed afferent fibers whose maximal discharge rates were elicited at some intermediate or "best angle" of joint positions. This type of stimulus-response relation, or "tuning" curve, is referred to as a nonmonotonic response function, because the response is maximal at some intermediate position of the range of motion curve and is submaximal on both sides of the best angle. This tuning curve is also referred to as "bell-shaped" and has been studied in great detail by McCall et al.[50] If this were the case for all joint afferent fibers, then each angle would be specified in a unique neuron subpopulation of the total spectrum of joint afferent fibers.[75]

On the other hand, Burgess and Clark[8,9] found that practically all the afferent fibers in their studies exhibited a maximal discharge rate at one or the other of the extremes of the range of motion. These same investigators found the tuning curves of many afferent fibers to be very flat throughout the intermediate angles of the range of motion, meaning that little or no information about changing joint conditions could be signaled at these angles by the joint receptors.[14] This type of stimulus-response relation is viewed as monotonic, because maximal response coincides with maximal stimulus intensity; that is, there is no diminution of response as either extreme of the range of motion is approached. Ferrell[23] concluded that the most common form of response function is in fact the monotonic form. Other authors have attempted to delineate the specificity of response function in terms of receptor types. The Golgi ligament ending, well studied by Andrew,[3] has been determined to have a monotonic type of relation, with an ever-increasing response toward the end range of motion, whereas Eklund and Skoglund[21] have attributed monotonic character to some Ruffini afferent receptors and nonmonotonic (minima or maxima and the end ranges of sensitivity) relations to other Ruffini receptors. Cohen[16] initially proposed that the monotonic type of relation for different joint afferent receptors helps to categorize each receptor as a flexion or an extension receptor.

EFFERENT MODULATION OF JOINT FIBER AFFERENCE: AN INFLUENCE OF MUSCULAR ACTIVITY

The relation between joint angle and excursion and joint afferent fiber discharge is in many instances subject to modification by the muscular tension exerted on the capsular tissue. Active muscular contraction resulting in joint angle change or isometric tension development is capable of inducing a response in the respective joint afferent neuron population. Millar[54] has suggested that one of the functions of muscle in proprioception may be to modulate joint afferent fiber discharge. Surely, certain muscles such as the articular muscles of the knee and elbow (articularis genu and articularis cubiti, respectively)[81] seem to be specifically designed to generate periarticular tissue changes. Other more diversified muscles such as the biceps, triceps, brachialis, pectoralis major, teres major, many of the forearm flexors, gluteus mimimus, vastus lateralis, and vastus medialis[54,81] also include tendinous insertions into joint capsules. These findings suggest that joint afferent fiber modulation by muscular tension development is a widespread and probably critically important physiological mechanism.

Grigg and Greenspan[36] demonstrated that few (<2%) of the primate knee joint afferent fibers tested in the posterior capsule (extension afferent fibers) were active at angles of more than 20° of flexion from full extension. Many of the tested afferent fibers were sensitive to muscular contraction and exhibited specific relation to the muscle group active around the joint. Force generation in the gastrocnemius muscle was primarily effective in activating 68% of the knee joint extension neurons, whereas force generation in the quadriceps muscle elicited activity in only 29% of these neurons. It was determined that torques on the order of 700 to 5000 gm-cm (2450 gm-cm, mean) were necessary to activate these capsular receptors. Muscular elicitation of knee joint activity was most likely at extreme joint extension, that is, in conditions of pronounced capsular leading, for afferent fibers that were generally sentient at intermediate joint angles. Evidence suggested a strong relation of joint afferent fiber discharge pattern to muscular force, because the decay rate of the SA discharge closely followed the rate of passive torque decay.

This modification of joint receptor activity may play a role in explaining the fact that accuracy of joint positioning is high for positioning a joint through active movement versus passive positioning of the joint as determined by subjective judgment testing.[60,61] Gandevia demonstrated significantly increased acuity with active motion. (See selected/recommended reference list.) Differences in joint afferent fiber activity with active and passive excursions may play a role in the postulated "sense of effort" or "feeling of innervation" that accompanies volitional muscular action.[52,53,67] Paillard and Brouchon[60,61] indicate that an accelerating afferent signal would be critical in the superior estimation of active displacement to that position. It has already been mentioned that articular Pacinian afferent receptors correspond to joint movement acceleration detectors. It would seem that this peripheral method for discrimination between active and passive body movements should complement any internal feedback mechanisms of motor command signal monitoring that provide the individual with knowledge regarding muscular contractions.[49,51,66]

One other mechanism to explain the increased receptor discharge that occurs between active and passive articular excursion lies in the additional receptor discharge from the component movements of rotation, roll, and glide, which occur with muscular control of the joint excursion, versus the lack of these component movement discharges when the joint is moved passively. The role and interplay of muscle input are fertile grounds for additional research.

FUNCTIONAL IMPLICATIONS

The most important contributions of primary joint afference to CNS mechanisms include three distinct actions. At the lowest level, joint afferent fibers converge on spinal interneurons and are responsible for the eventual reflex activation, facilitation, or inhibition of motor neurons. This regulation of motor activity constitutes a control over the coordination of antagonistic and synergistic patterns of muscular contraction, establishing functional joint stability or mobilization. At the next level, afference from the neck, trunk, and limb joints is required by brain stem neuronal circuits for interaction with vestibular afference to facilitate postural and equilibrium maintenance. Finally, at the highest level, joint afference can mediate some aspects of cognitive awareness of body position and movement or at least modulate the perceptual impact of other somatosensory afference.

Spinal reflex action: intrinsic stability and mobility

Although the exact spinal termination pattern of primary joint afferent fibers has not been elucidated, the functional roles of the fibers has been determined by study of reflex motor effects and actions on spinally mediated patterns of neural activity that subserve purposeful action. Periarticular tissue afference affects the following reflexes[74,77]: (1) a facilitatory effect on the ipsilateral flexion reflex,[27] (2) a facilitatory effect on the contralateral (crossed) extension reflex,[27] (3) effects opposite to the first two reflexes,[27] (4) facilitation of the ipsilateral group Ib or Golgi tendon organ reflex,[48] (5) modification of directional signs of cutaneous ambulatory reflexes, and (6) elicitation of reflex muscular splinting during conditions of abnormal stress about the joint.[11,45,80]

Kennedy, Alexander, and Hayes[45] have recently provided a scheme for understanding the manner in which posttraumatic abnormal joint afference can contribute to a loss of reflexive muscular splinting. They suggest that tonic or dynamic cocontraction of antagonistic muscles involved in dynamic stabilization of the joint may be inhibited by abnormal patterns of joint afference, resulting in an increased propensity for reinjury via destabilization.

Implied in the postulated loss of automatic motor control of a limb because of aberrant feedback from the articular receptors is the fact that therapeutic progression must incorporate a relearning paradigm, as well as a promotion of physical recovery factors. That is, joint injury represents a peripheral neurological dysfunction that triggers a new state of motor control factors in the nervous system. A portion of therapeutic recovery therefore must be devoted to reestablishment of an appropriate afference and development of motor skill on the basis of this new afference. This type of recovery program would seem to be most critical to avoid reinjury of the joint, primarily in the early stages of recovery. During the recovery/rehabilitation period, new sensory cues for motor guidance and retraining of appropriate muscle activation sequences may be required. It has been suggested that this relearning of normal function in an injured joint may involve several months.[29]

Less obvious but perhaps more important effects have been determined also regarding modification of motor neural activity patterns in the spinal cord and perhaps at higher CNS centers as well. Recent investigations have concluded that rhythmic limb movements, which occur in activities such as walking, depend upon a phase relationship between central neural activity patterns and feedback from the periphery.[1] According to this view, a centrally generated, locomotor neural activity pattern, primarily at local spinal levels, must be maintained by activity from periarticular receptors, which are stimulated by the locomotive actions. The relevant investigations have not, however, decisively determined whether joint afferent fibers from small muscles surrounding the joint (like the relationships of the pectineal muscle to the hip joint) are the major contributors to this input. It seems logical to conclude from these studies that joint afferent fiber response is necessary, if not sufficient, to "entrain" the central locomotive activity pattern and generate a dynamic equilibrium for the maintenance of a regular ambulatory activation pattern.

Aberrations in joint afferent fiber feedback may therefore serve to disrupt the phase relation between feedback and the central pattern and lead to secondary problems in gait. These problems may include increased sense of effort in the control of gait, deficiencies in developing high-velocity or accelerative components in the gait cycle, and an increased amount of total conscious involvement in ambulation. Because the CNS has been shown to be highly adaptable, it is reasonable to assume that abnormalities in the feedback and CNS pattern relations may require intelligently designed retraining exercises to foster more appropriate relations, especially in planning therapeutic programs.

Postural and equilibrium mechanisms

Joint afference is related to medullary and brain stem centers by way of the dorsal columns and the ascending somatosensory tracts of the dorsolateral fascicular, spinocerebellar,[47] and spinovestibular pathways.[24] Numerous studies have stressed the importance of this information for cerebral processing involved in motor control,[77] but its involvement in brain stem motor integration mechanisms is also critical. For example, the proprioceptors of the neck region include the cervical joint afferent receptors, which are involved in providing neck afference to the vestibular system of the head. The functional role of this afference includes (1) coordination of eye, head, and neck movements to stabilize retinal imagery for vision,[41,43] (2) maintenance of posture,[17,42] and (3) maintenance of coordinated movement patterns.[17,19]

Joint afferent fiber activity also assists the muscle spindle afferent fibers in inhibiting antagonist muscle activity under conditions of rapid lengthening and associated periarticular tissue distortion, both of which accompany unexpected postural perturbations. When simultaneous input arises from cutaneous, joint, muscle, and vestibular receptors, a unique pattern of afference is generated and elicits long-latency, nonvoluntary postural adjustments, acting to stabilize and bring the body center of gravity into a state of equilibrium.

It has not yet been determined to what extent joint afference responding to noxious stimulation impinges on brain stem neurons involved in the transmission and control of pain, but it is likely that the pathways and nuclei demonstrated for other afferent fibers are involved.[87] Patients frequently report that chronic pain localized to deep tissues of the spine or pelvis is alleviated or mitigated by movement, suggesting that the analgesic effect of joint mechanoreceptor stimulation may be quite powerful. The analgesia derived from selective activation of pacinian afferent receptors has been adequately demonstrated.

Proprioceptive and kinesthetic awareness

During the 1960s joint afferent receptors were viewed by man to be the unique determinants of position and movement sensation. The outright rejection of Sherrington's "muscular sensation" was fixed in vogue by numerous erroneous conclusions.[49] However, Burgess et al.'s[10] critical review of the literature together with their own experimental and clinical findings concluded that there is no valid evidence that the articular receptors of any joint are important for the conscious awareness of joint position. Two main types of studies contributed to this position: (1) local anesthetization of joint tissues did not reduce joint position awareness,[33,49] and (2) joint replacement surgery in humans in which most of the joint receptors were surgically removed resulted in little subsequent kinesthetic impairment.

The suggested role in perception for the articular receptors involves their contribution to the feeling of deep pressure experienced by an individual near the limits of the range of motion of a joint.[10] This concept is supported by the fact that most joints, with the exception of the hip, have very few receptors that are activated either statically or dynamically in the middle of the range of motion, yet conscious appreciation of this part of the range is no more inferior than that near the end of the range.

The receptors that seem to be the most suited for a crucial involvement in joint position sense are the muscle spindle receptors.[20,32,33,49] These receptors are supported in this junction by the activity of cutaneous and some joint receptors,[15] and all the afferent receptors together must be integrated with a corollary discharge from motor tracts in the brain at such centers as the cerebellum and the dorsal column nuclei.[49] Preliminary comparative investigations indicate that the joint afferent receptor channel may be subject to descending corticofugal modulatory influences to a greater extent than are other somatic afferent channels.[66] Readers are urged to peruse the selected/recommended references for further information.

OTHER CLINICAL CONSIDERATIONS

Taking into account the functional anatomy, tissue relations, sensitivities, peripheral and central nervous system response transformations, and the resultant perceptual and motor influences that involve periarticular and musculotendinous proprioceptors, it is critical for the clinician to apply concepts of function to the individual whose injury is in the controlled rehabilitative phase. Stabilization of the joint by varying degrees of cocontraction of muscle synergists and antagonists during static, dynamic, and reactive conditions depends heavily on the integrity of appropriate neural signal patterns. Reduction of deleterious effects of protective muscle spasm in painful and inflammatory conditions depends in part on the skillful application of mobilization techniques in concert with controlled driving of peripherally elicited impulses by mechanical or electrical forms of stimulation. In the formulation of treatment plans, intervention strategies must simultaneously attend to the reduction of pathological tone, reflex inhibition reduction, the facilitation of degrees of freedom in mobility, and the incorporation of optimal stabilization capacity for the injured region of the body. Enhancement of voluntary control and the focusing of healthful proprioceptive awareness and guided movements for capacity development should be the outcome and "take home message" from the clinician to the patient. Perhaps the conceptual basis for the efficacy of closed chain kinetic functional training and exercises in addressing such problems as ACL injury/reconstruction rests on the complex integration and linkage of periarticular information with that of active musculotendinous afferentation, while functional

motor activity commands are being demanded and formulated by the cerebral motor execution apparatus. (See selected/recommended references.)

SUMMARY

Knowledge of articular neurology is of prime importance in physical therapy in order to guide voluntary and preprogrammed motor activity associated with motor skills, the reflexive modulation of muscle tone, the sequential activation and coordination of synergistic and antagonistic muscle groups, and some limited features of somatic sensation and perception.

Knowledge of the relationship of structure and function in joint and musculoskeletal innervation is most critical for adequate prevention and treatment of maladaptation in the articular apparatus. Concentrating on the intricate balance of activity patterns arising from the joint and muscle-tendon afferent receptors, we can begin to appreciate the degree of focal specificity and varied complexity with which the nervous system operates. Physiological dissection of afferent channels of information emanating from each joint makes possible a new evaluative selectivity and provides the opportunity for new quantum leaps in therapeutic design. Decision making in the orthopedic and sports clinical setting must acknowledge the selective stimulation of specific afferent channels to facilitate appropriate biomechanical stabilization or mobilization processes. The interaction of muscular and soft tissue components of the articular system must be thoroughly understood as a basis for rational designs of therapeutic intervention and prevention of maladaptations and securing optimal rates of restitution of adequate function.

REFERENCES

1. Anderson O, Grillner S: On the feedback control of the cat's hindlimb during locomotion. In Taylor A, Prochazka A, editors: *Muscle receptors and movement,* New York, 1981, Oxford University Press.
2. Andres KH, von During M: Morphology of cutaneous receptors. In Iggo A, editor: *Handbook of sensory physiology,* vol 2, *Somatosensory system,* New York, 1973, Springer-Verlag.
3. Andrew BL: The sensory innervation of the medial ligament of the knee joint, *J Physiol (Lond)* 123:241, 1954.
4. Bloom W, Fawcett DW: *A textbook of histology,* ed 10, Philadelphia, 1975, WB Saunders.
5. Boyd IA: The histological structure of the receptors on the knee joint of the cat correlated with their physiological response, *J Physiol* 124:476, 1954.
6. Boyd IA, Roberts TDM: Proprioceptive discharges from stretch-receptors in the knee joint of the cat, *J Physiol (Lond)* 122:38, 1953.
7. Brodal A: *Neurological anatomy,* New York, 1981, Oxford University Press.
8. Burgess PR, Clark FJ: Characteristics of knee joint receptors in the cat, *J Physiol (Lond)* 203:317, 1969.
9. Burgess PR, Clark FJ: Dorsal column projection of fibres from the cat knee joint, *J Physiol (Lond)* 203:301, 1969.
10. Burgess PR et al: Signaling of kinesthetic information by peripheral sensory receptors, *Annu Rev Neurosci* 5:171, 1982.
11. Cailliet R: *Low back pain syndrome,* ed 3, Philadelphia, 1981, FA Davis.
12. Catton WT, Petoe N: A viscoelastic theory of mechanoreceptor adaptation, *J Physiol (Lond)* 187:35, 1966.

13. Chouchkov C: Cutaneous receptors, *Adv Anat Embryol Cell Biol* 54:1, 1978.

14. Clark FJ, Burgess PR: Slowly adapting receptors in cat knee joint: can they signal joint angle? *J Neurophysiol* 38:1448, 1975.

15. Clark FJ et al: Contributions of cutaneous and joint receptors to static knee-position sense in man, *J Neurophysiol* 42:877, 1979.

16. Cohen LA: Activity of knee joint proprioceptors recorded from the posterior articular nerve, *Yale J Biol Med* 28:225, 1955/1956.

17. Cohen LA: Role of the eye and neck proprioception mechanism in body orientation and motor coordination, *J Neurophysiol* 24:1, 1961.

18. Dee R: Structure and function of hip joint innervation, *Ann R Coll Surg Engl* 45:357, 1969.

19. deJong P et al: Ataxia and nystagmus induced by infection of local anaesthetics in the neck, *Ann Neurol* 1:240, 1977.

20. Eklund G: Position sense and state of contraction: the effects of vibration, *J Neurol Neurosurg Psychiatry* 35:606, 1972.

21. Eklund G, Skoglund S: On the specificity of the Ruffini-like receptors, *Acta Physiol Scand* 49:184, 1960.

22. Erickson RP: Parallel "population" neural coding in feature extraction. In Schmitt FO, Worden FG, editors: *The neurosciences: third study program,* Cambridge, Mass, 1974, The MIT Press.

23. Ferrell WR: The adequacy of strength receptors in the cat knee joint for signalling joint angle throughout a full range of movement, *J Physiol (Lond)* 299:85, 1980.

24. Fredrickson JM, Schwarz D, Kornhuber HH: Convergence and interaction of vestibular and deep somatic afferents upon neurons in the vestibular nuclei of the cat, *Acta Otolaryngol* 61:168, 1965.

24b. Fredrickson M: Patellofemoral pain in runners. *J Back Musculoskel Rehabil* 5:305-16, 1995.

25. Freeman MAR, Wyke B: The innervation of the ankle joint: an anatomical and histological study in the cat, *Acta Anat* 68:321, 1967.

25b. Fulkerson JP, Shea KP: Disorders of patellofemoral alignment, *J Bone Joint Surg Am* 72A:1424-29, 1990.

26. Gardner E: Physiology of moveable joints, *Physiol Rev* 30:127, 1950.

27. Gardner E: Reflex muscular responses to stimulation of articular nerves in the cat, *Am J Physiol* 161:133, 1950.

28. Gardner E, Noer R: Projection of afferent fibers from muscles and joints to the cerebral cortex of the cat, *Am J Physiol* 168:437, 1952.

29. Glencross D, Thornton E: Position sense following joint injury, *J Sports Med Phys Fitness* 21:23, 1981.

30. Godwin-Austen RB: The mechanoreceptors of the costovertebral joints, *J Physiol (Lond)* 202:737, 1969.

31. Goldie I, Wellisch M: The presence of nerves in patients synovecto-mised for rheumatoid arthritis, *Acta Orthop Scand* 40:143, 1969.

32. Goodwin GM, McCloskey DL, Matthews PBC: The contribution of muscle afferents to kinesthesia shown by vibration-induced illusions of movement and by the effects of paralysing joint afferents, *Brain* 95:705, 1972.

33. Goodwin GM, McCloskey DL, Matthews PBC: The persistence of appreciable kinesthesia after paralysing joint afferents but preserving muscle afferents, *Brain Res* 37:326, 1972.

34. Grieve GP: *Common vertebral joint problems,* New York, 1981, Churchill Livingstone.

35. Grigg P, Finerman GA, Riley LH: Joint position sense after total hip replacement, *J Bone Joint Surg Br* 55B:1016, 1973.

36. Grigg P, Greenspan BJ: Response of primate joint afferent neurons to mechanical stimulation of knee joint, *J Neurophysiol* 40:1, 1977.

37. Grigg P, Hoffman AH: Properties of Ruffini afferents as revealed by stress analysis of isolated sections of cat knee capsule, *J Neurolphysiol* 47:41, 1982.

38. Grigg P, Hoffman AH, Fogarty KE: Properties of Golgi-Mazzoni afferents in cat knee joint capsule, as revealed by mechanical studies of isolated joint capsule, *J Neurophysiol* 47:31, 1982.

39. Halata Z: The mechanoreceptors of the mammalian skin: ultrastructure and morphological classification, *Adv Anat Embryol Cell Biol* 50:1, 1975.

40. Halata Z: The ultrastructure of the sensory nerve endings in the articular capsule of the knee joint of the domestic cat (Ruffini corpuscles and pacinian corpuscles), *J Anat* 124:717, 1977.

41. Hikosaka O, Maeda M: Cervical effects on abducens motoneurones and their interaction with the vestibulo-ocular reflex, *Exp Brain Res* 18:512, 1973.

42. Igarashi M et al: Role of the neck proprioceptors for the maintenance of dynamic bodily equilibrium in the squirrel monkey, *Laryngoscope* 79:1713, 1969.

43. Igarashi M, et al: Nystagmus after experimental cervical lesions, *Laryngoscope* 82:1609, 1972.

44. Kanaka R, Schaible HG, Schmidt RF: Von Frey thresholds of mechanosensitive joint afferent units are related to conduction velocity, *Pfluegers Arch* 291:R44, 1981.

45. Kennedy JC, Alexander U, Hayes KC: Nerve supply of the human knee and its functional importance, *Am J Sports Med* 10:329, 1982.

46. Langford LA, Schmidt RF: The medial articular nerve: an electron microscopic examination, *Pfluegers Arch* 394:R57, 1982.

47. Lindstrom S, Takata M: Monosynaptic excitation of dorsal spinocerebellar tract neurons from low threshold joint afferents, *Acta Physiol Scand* 84:430, 1972.

48. Lundberg A, Malmgren K, Schomburg ED: Role of joint afferents in motor control exemplified by effects on reflex pathways from Ib afferents, *J Physiol (Lond)* 284:327, 1978.

49. Matthews PBC: Where does Sherringon's "muscular sense" originate? Muscles, joints, corollary discharges? *Annu Rev Neurosci* 5:189, 1982.

50. McCall WD Jr et al: Static and dynamic responses of slowly adapting joint receptors, *Brain Res* 70:221, 1974.

51. McCloskey DL: Knowledge about muscular contractions. *Trends Neurosci* 3:311, 1980.

52. Merton PA: Human position sense and sense of effort, *Symp Soc Exp Biol* 18:387, 1964.

53. Merton PA: The sense of effort. In Porter R, editor: *Breathing, Hering-Breuer Centenary Symposium,* London, 1970, Churchill Livingstone.

54. Millar J: Joint afferent fibres responding to muscle stretch, vibration, and contraction, *Brain Res* 63:380, 1973.

55. Miller MR, Kasahara M: Observations on the innervation of human long bones, *Anat Rec* 145:13, 1963.

56. Molina F, Ramcharan J, Wyke BD: Structure and function of articular receptor systems in the cervical spine, *J Bone Joint Surg Br* 58B:255, 1976.

57. Mountcastle VB et al: Neural base for the sense of fluttervibration, *Science* 155:597, 1967.

58. Newton RA: Joint receptor contributions to reflexive and kinesthetic responses, *Phys Ther* 62:22, 1982.

58b. Nyland J, Brosky T, Currier D, Nitz A, Caborn D: Review of the afferent neural system of the knee and its contribution to motor learning. *J Orthop Sports Phys Ther* 19:2, 1994.

59. O'Connor BL, McConnaughey JS: The structure and innervation of cat knee menisci and their relation to a "sensory hypothesis" of meniscal function, *Am J Anat* 153:431, 1978.

60. Paillard J, Brouchon M: Active and passive movements in the calibration of position sense. In Freedman SJ, editor: *The neuropsychology of spatially oriented behavior,* Homewood, Ill, 1968, The Dorsey Press.

61. Paillard J, Brouchon M: A proprioceptive contribution to the spatial encoding of position cues for ballistic movements, *Brain Res* 71:273, 1974.

62. Pertovaara A: Modification of human pain threshold by specific tactile receptors, *Acta Physiol Scand* 107:339, 1979.

63. Polacek P: Receptors of the joints: their structure, variability and classification, *Acta Fac Med Univ Brun* 23:1, 1966.

64. Reimann I, Christensen SB: A histological demonstration of nerves in subchondral bone, *Acta Orthop Scand* 48:345, 1977.

65. Rossi A, Grigg P: Characteristics of hip joint mechanoreceptors in the cat, *J Neurophysiol* 47:1029, 1982.
66. Rowinski MJ, Stoney SD Jr: Specificity of cortical efferent modulation of somatosensory neuronal activity in the raccoon cuneate nucleus, *Exp Neurol* (in press).
67. Rymer WX, D'Almeida A: Joint position sense: the effects of muscle contraction, *Brain* 103:1, 1980.
68. Samuel EP: The autonomic and somatic innervation of the articular capsule, *Anat Rec* 113:53, 1952.
69. Schaible HG, Schmidt RF: Activation of groups III and IV sensory units in medial articular nerve by local mechanical stimulation of knee joint, *J Neurophysiol* 49:35, 1983.
70. Schaible HG, Schmidt RF: Responses of fine medial articular nerve afferents to passive movements of the knee joint, *J Neurophysiol* 49:118, 1983.
71. Sheperd GM: *Neurobiology,* New York, 1983, Oxford University Press.
72. Sherrington CS: *The integrative action of the nervous system,* London, 1948, Cambridge University Press.
73. Skoglund S: Anatomical and physiological studies of the knee joint innervation in the cat, *Acta Physiol Scand Suppl* 36:124, 1956.
74. Skoglund S: Joint receptors and kinaesthesias. In Iggo A, editor: *Handbook of sensory physiology,* vol 2, Somatosensory system, New York, 1973, Springer-Verlag.
75. Somjen G: *Sensory coding in the mammalian nervous system,* New York, 1972, Plenum.
76. Stilwell DL: The nerve supply of the vertebral column and its associated structures in the monkey, *Anat Rec* 125:139, 1956.
77. Tracey DJ: Joint receptors and the control of movement, *Trends Neurosci* 3:253, 1980.
78. Vallbo AB, Hagbarth KE: Activity from skin mechanoreceptors recorded percutaneously in awake human subjects, *Exp Neurol* 21:270, 1968.
79. Vallbo AB et al: Somatosensory, proprioceptive, and sympathetic activity in human peripheral nerves, *Physiol Rev* 59:919, 1979.
80. Vrettos XC, Wyke BD: Articular reflexogenic systems in the costovertebral joints, *J Bone Joint Surg Br* 56B:382, 1974.
81. Williams PL, Warwick R, editors: *Gray's anatomy,* ed 36, Philadelphia, 1980, WB Saunders.
82. Wilson AD, Legg PG, McNeur JC: Studies on the innervation of the medial meniscus in the human knee joint, *Anat Rec* 165:485, 1969.
83. Wyke BD: The neurology of the joints, *Ann R Coll Surg Engl* 41:25, 1967.
84. Wyke BD: Articular neurology: A review, *Physiotherapy* 58:94, 1972.
85. Wyke BD: Morphological and functional features of the innervation of the costovertebral joints, *Folia Morphol* 23:296, 1975.
86. Wyke BD: Neurology of the cervical spinal joints, *Physiotherapy* 65:72, 1979.
87. Wyke B: Neurological implications of low back pain. In Jayson M, editor: *The lumbar spine and back pain,* New York, 1976, Grune & Stratton.
88. Wyke BD, Polacek P: Articular neurology: The present position, *J Bone Joint Surg Br* 57B:401, 1975.

SELECTED PROPRIOCEPTION/KINESTHESIA REFERENCES

General Overview

Schmidt R: *Motor learning and performance,* Champaign, Ill, 1991, Human Kinetics Publishers.
Lephart S, guest editor: Proprioceptive considerations for sport rehabilitation, *J Sport Rehabil* 3:1, 1994.

Skin Factors

Clark FJ, Burgess RC, Chapin JW: Proprioception with the proximal interphalangeal joint of the index finger: evidence for a movement sense without a static-position sense, *Brain* 109:1195, 1986.
Edin B: Quantitative analysis of static strain sensitivity in human mechanoreceptors from hairy skin, *J Neurophysiol* 67:1105, 1992.
Edin B, Abbs JH: Finger movement responses of cutaneous mechanoreceptors in dorsal skin of the human hand, *J Neurophysiol* 65:657, 1991.
Feurbach JW, Grabiner MD, Koh TJ, Weiker GG: Effect of an ankle orthosis and ankle ligament anesthesia on ankle joint proprioception, *Am J Sports Med* 22:223, 1994.
Moberg E: The role of cutaneous afferents in position sense, kinesthesia and motor function of the hand, *Brain* 106:1, 1983.
Nicholas J, Melvin M, Saraniti A: Neurophysiologic inhibition of strength following tactile stimulation of the skin, *Am J Sports Med* 8:181, 1980.
Vallbo AB, Olssen KA, Westberg K-G, Clark FJ: Microstimulation of single tactile afferents from the human hand, *Brain* 109:729, 1984.

Muscle Factors

Bastide G, Zadeh J, Lefebvre D: Are the "little muscles" what we think they are? *Surg Radio Anat* 11:255, 1989.
Buxton D, Peck D: Neuromuscular spindles relative to joint movement complexities, *Clin Anat* 2:211, 1989.
Gandevia SC, McClosky DI, Burke D: Kinesthetic signals and muscle contraction, *Trends Neurosci* 15:62, 1992.
Gandevia SC, Hall LA, McClosky DI, Potter EK: Proprioceptive sensation at the terminal joint of the middle finger, *J Physiol (Lond)* 335:507, 1983.
Gandevia SC, McClosky DI: Joint sense, muscle sense and their combination as position sense, measured at the distal interphalangeal joint of the middle finger, *J Physiol (Lond)* 260:387, 1976.
Hutton R, Atwater S: Acute and chronic adaptations of muscle proprioceptors in response to increased use, *Sports Med* 14(6):406, 1992.
Jozsa L, Balint J, Kannus P, Jarvinen M, Lehto M: Mechanoreceptors in human myotendinous junction, *Musc Nerve* 16:453, 1993.
Lalatta-Costerbosa G, Barazzoni A, Clavenzani P, Callegari E: Histochemical profile of articularis humeri muscle in the horse, *Boll Soc Ital Biol Sper* 66:767, 1990.
McClosky DI: Kinesthetic sensibility, *J Physiol* 58:763, 1978.
Nitz AJ, Peck D: Comparison of muscle spindle concentrations in large and small human epaxial muscles acting in parallel combinations, *Am Surg* 52(5):273, 1986.
Peck D, Buxton D, Nitz A: A comparison of spindle concentrations in large and small muscles acting in parallel combinations, *J Morphol* 180:243, 1984.
Rymer WZ, D'Almeida A: Jt. position sense: the effects of muscle contraction, *Brain* 103:1, 1980.
Snyder-Mackler L, Williams P, Eastlack ME: Reflex inhibition of the quadriceps femoris muscle after ACL reconstruction. Orthopaedic Research Society, Transactions of the 39th Annual Meeting, 18:309, San Francisco, 1993.
Solomonow M, Baratta R, Zhou BH, et al: The synergistic action of the anterior cruciate ligament and thigh muscles in maintaining joint stability, *Am J Sports Med* 15:207, 1987.

Capsule Factors (Classic Articles of Freeman/Wyke)

Freeman MAR, Dean MRE, Hanham IWF: The etiology and prevention of functional instability of the foot, *J Bone Joint Surg* 47B:678, 1985.
Freeman MAR, Wyke B: Articular contributions to limb muscle reflexes: an electromyographic study of the influence of ankle joint mechanoreceptors upon reflex activity in the gastrocnemius muscle of the cat, *J Physiol* 171:20P, 1964.
Freeman MAR, Wyke B: The innervation of the knee joint: an anatomical and histological study in the cat, *J Anat* 101:505, 1964.
Freeman MAR, Wyke B: Articular reflexes of the ankle joint: an electromyographic study of normal and abnormal influences of ankle-joint mechanoreceptors upon reflex activity in leg muscles, *Br J Surg* 54:990, 1967.

Ligament Information

Beard DJ, et al: Proprioception after rupture of the ACL, *J Bone Joint Surg Br* 75B:311, 1993.

Berchuck M, et al: Gait adaptations with ACL patients, *J Bone Joint Surg Am* 72A:871, 1990.

Fuss FK, Bacher A: New aspects of the morphology and function of the human hip joint ligaments, *Am J Anat* 192:1, 1991.

Halata Z, Haus J: The ultrastructure of sensory nerve endings in human anterior cruciate ligament, *Anat Embryol* 179:415, 1989.

Heppleman B, Heuss C, Schmidt RF: Fiber size distribution of myelinated and unmyelinated axons in the medial and posterior articular nerves of the cat's knee joint, *Somatosensory Res* 5:273, 1988.

Johansson H: Role of knee ligaments in proprioception and regulation, *J Electromyog Kinesiol* 1(3):158, 1991.

Receptors in knee joint ligaments, *Crit Rev Biomed Eng* 18(5):341, 1991.

Kraupse R, Schmidt M, Schaible H-G: Sensory innervation of the anterior cruciate ligament, *J Bone Joint Surg Am* 74A:390, 1992.

Michelson JD, Hutchins C: Mechanoreceptors in human ankle ligaments, *J Bone Joint Surg Br* 77B:219, 1995.

Pope MH, et al: Role of musculature with MCL, *J Bone Joint Surg Am* 61A:398, 1979.

Salo P, Tatton W: Age-related loss of knee joint afferents in mice, *J Neurosci Res* 35:664, 1993.

Schultz R, Miller D, Kerr C, Michelli L: *Mechanoreceptors in human cruciate ligaments, J Bone Joint Surg Am* 66A:1072, 1984.

Yahia LH, Newman NM, Rivard CH: Neurohistology of lumbar spine ligaments, *Acta Orthop Scand* 59:26, 1988.

Zimny M, Schutte M, Dabezies E: Mechanoreceptors in the human cruciate ligament, *Anat Rec* 214:204, 1986.

Role in Joint Protection

O'Connor BL, et al: Gait alterations in dogs CNS, reprogramming. *Trans Orthop Res Soc* 17:478, 1992.

O'Connor BL, et al: Neurogenic acceleration of osteoarthritis in dogs, *J Bone Joint Surg Am* 74A:367-376, 1992.

Shoulder Information

Guanche C, Knatt T, Solomonow M, Lu Y, Baratta R: The synergistic action of the capsule and the shoulder muscles, *Am J Sports Med* 23(3):301, 1995.

Lephart SM, Warner JP, Borsa PA, Fu FH: Proprioception of the shoulder joint in healthy, unstable and surgically repaired shoulders, *J Shoulder Elbow Surg* 3(6):371, 1994.

O'Brien SJ, Neves MC, Arnoczky SP, et al: The anatomy and histology of the inferior glenohumeral ligament complex of the shoulder, *Am J Sports Med* 18(5):449, 1990.

Sharkey NA, Marder RA: The rotator cuff opposes superior translation of the humeral head, *Am J Sports Med* 23(3):270, 1995.

Smith RL, Brunolli J: Shoulder kinesthesia after glenohumeral joint dislocation, *Phys Ther* 69:106, 1989.

Speer KP, Xianghua D, Torzilli PA, Altchek DA, Warren RF: Strategies for an anterior capsular shift of the shoulder: a biomechanical comparison, *Am J Sports Med* 23(3)264, 1995.

CHAPTER 3

Biomechanics of Orthopedic and Sports Therapy

Mark W. Cornwall

OUTLINE

Why biomechanics?
Basic terms and concepts
  Force
  Frictional force
  Strength
  Pressure
  Power
  Load, stress, and strain
  Strength of materials
  Resilience and toughness
  Creep
  Fatigue
Moments of force
  Torque
Kinematics
  Motion
  Measurement of motion
  Motion and injury
Kinetics
  Newton's first law
  Newton's second law
  Newton's third law
  Impulse and momentum
  Work
  Energy
Summary

LEARNING OBJECTIVES

After studying this chapter, the reader should be able to:
1. Define the term *biomechanics*.
2. Describe the four characteristics of force.
3. Explain the difference between a resultant force and a composition of forces.
4. Describe how the magnitude of frictional force is determined.
5. State the formula used to calculate pressure.
6. Describe the difference between force and power.
7. State how the terms *resilience, toughness,* and *creep* relate to the properties of a material.
8. Describe how mechanical advantage is used to determine the efficiency of a lever system.
9. State the difference between two-dimensional and three-dimensional motion analysis.
10. Describe Newton's three laws of motion.

KEY TERMS

biomechanics	motion analysis
kinetics	work
kinematics	energy
torque	

WHY BIOMECHANICS?

Mechanics analyzes forces acting on an object. Biomechanics, therefore, applies the principles of mechanics to human and animal tissues. It is the basis of musculoskeletal function. Whether recognized or not, biomechanical principles are an integral part of orthopedic and sport injury assessment and treatment. Radin[43] states that, of all the basic sciences, mechanics has the clearest direct application to injury therapy and functional recovery from musculoskeletal problems. Knowledge of mechanical principles, therefore, can be extremely helpful in understanding the prevention, diagnosis, and treatment of orthopedic and sport injuries. All body postures can be thought of as the result of forces, both internal and external. In addition, all body movements are caused by the net forces acting from inside and from outside the body. Within the body, muscles are the major structures controlling posture and movement. Ligaments, cartilage, and other soft tissues also aid in the control of joint movement and body position. Gravity is generally the single biggest external load the body experiences.

Muscles produce forces that act through the bony lever system. The skeletal system either moves or statically resists these forces. If a load is applied to the lever system, the muscles react to control the load. Muscles exert this control in a variety of different ways. The fiber arrangement of each muscle determines the amount of force the muscle can produce and the distance over which the muscle can contract. Muscles often act together to obtain a resulting force of the desired magnitude and direction. An individual muscle's attachment to the lever system also influences its lever arm length and angle of pull, which ultimately affect the magnitude of the force that is produced. The distance the muscle attaches from the joint axis determines the muscle moment of force, whereas the angle of muscular pull controls the rotatory and nonrotatory components of the force.

If the forces that cause an injury are known, steps can be taken to prevent or reduce the seriousness of the injury. The practitioner who knows the mechanism of injury is better able to evaluate the kind of injury involved and its extent. Several authors have emphasized the value of accurate evaluation of the injury-producing force in order to aid early detection and prompt diagnosis.* Every time an injury is evaluated, the practitioner uses procedures based on the principles of biomechanics. For example, several tests for knee joint laxity use the three-point principle to apply a graded distraction force. Tests for other joints also make use of mechanical principles.

In addition to evaluation, many procedures used to treat or rehabilitate musculoskeletal injuries are to a great extent based on biomechanical principles. Surgical procedures, casting, bracing, splinting, and exercise programs all depend on correct application of forces for satisfactory results. For example, successful surgical realignment of the patella either proximally or distally depends on the surgeon's knowledge of force application. Also, the effective use of foot orthoses in the conservative management of foot problems requires knowledge of foot mechanics as well as of the cushioning properties of various materials used in the construction of orthoses.

Finally, many types of exercise devices exist, each with their own unique advantages and disadvantages. Knowledge of the application of resisting force and its effect on the muscle and joint is essential for the professional to develop the best exercise program for each individual. Items such as headgear, padding, and footwear are designed to either protect or enhance performance. To accomplish these objec-

tives, biomechanical principles are frequently employed. Over the last several years, the dramatic drop in the cost of videotaping equipment has created great interest among clinicians in using videography to analyze abnormal movement. It has also sparked interest in demonstrating the efficacy of specific treatment techniques. Although these goals are worthwhile and realistic, the clinician needs to be aware of the limitations so that meaningful data can be gathered and interpreted correctly.

BASIC TERMS AND CONCEPTS

Many of the terms in biomechanics are often misused. Just like engineering, biomechanics uses words with precise meanings. Knowledge of the terms and concepts used in biomechanics is important to clinicians to ensure intelligent and accurate application of mechanical principles to patient care situations.

Force

The science of mechanics deals largely with forces. A force is merely a push or a pull. Just because a force exerts either a push or a pull on an object, the object is not obligated to move. When a force acts upon an object and it does not move, the object is said to be in equilibrium, which means that another force of equal magnitude is acting on the object in a way that cancels the potential effect of the first force. The study of such situations is a branch of engineering called *statics*. If the object is not in equilibrium, it begins to move; these situations are studied by the branch of engineering called *dynamics*. In orthopedics and sport therapy, dynamic situations are prevalent and therefore of greater interest to the clinician than static situations.

A force is typically described by four characteristics: (1) magnitude (the amount of push or pull), (2) the direction in which the force is applied, (3) the point at which the force is applied, and (4) the line along which the force acts. In many biomechanical texts, these properties of a force are depicted graphically (Fig. 3-1). The most common forces involved in orthopedic and sport therapy are muscular,

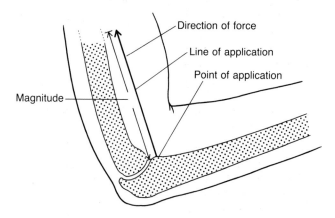

Fig. 3-1. The four characteristics of force.

---

* References 19, 24, 26, 41, 49, 50, 62.

gravitational, inertial, buoyant, and contact forces. The actual amount of force produced by a muscle depends upon several factors, such as the speed of muscle contraction and the length of the muscle fibers. Gravitational forces result from the weight of an object and are always directed vertically down. The concept of inertia maintains that a body remains at rest or in uniform motion until acted upon by an outside force. This concept happens to be Newton's first law of motion. By definition, inertia is not a true force. Inertia behaves like a force because it resists the change in motion (or lack of it) of an object. Buoyant force tends to resist the force of gravity while in water. In the water, the magnitude of this force equals the weight of the water that the object displaces. This principle of buoyancy force is effectively used during exercise programs in a pool. Because of the buoyancy force of water, individuals can exercise in the water while reducing the compressive forces of their body weight on affected joints.[32] Exercise in water up to an individual's waist typically reduces the weight-bearing forces of gravity by 50%. Exercise in chest-level water eliminates 75% of the weight-bearing forces. Finally, contact forces exist whenever two or more objects are in contact with each other. This type of force may be a reaction force or an impact force. In either case, the force can be thought of as composed of two separate forces. The first is a force perpendicular to the contacting surfaces, and the second is a shearing or frictional force that is parallel to the contacting surfaces.

Replacing a single force by two or more equivalent forces is referred to as the *resolution of force* (Fig. 3-2, *A*). As an illustration, forces acting on a bone, such as the pull of a muscle or the weight of a load, can be thought of as two separate forces. One force is perpendicular to the bone and tends to cause rotation or shearing of the body segment about the joint. The other force is parallel to the bone and causes either compression or distraction of the joint surfaces (Fig. 3-2, *B* and *C*). Although the force from a muscle contraction generally creates a compressive force at the joint it crosses, it can also create a distracting force. A compressive force usually enhances the stability of the joint. This compressive force component, however, can be detrimental, as in the case of degenerative joint disease, in which the compressive force may increase the pain felt by the patient.

Another example of the resolution of a force into two or more equivalent forces is illustrated in walking or running. As the foot strikes the ground, part of that resulting force is directed downward. Another portion of the force is directed parallel to the ground. Fig. 3-3 shows these two ground reaction forces during walking. The curve labeled F_z represents the perpendicular component discussed earlier; curve F_y is the parallel force component. Note that the magnitude of F_y is much smaller than that of F_z and that it changes direction during the course of the stance phase. The initial negative deflection of the F_y curve represents a retarding force of the ground on the individual's forward progression, whereas the positive

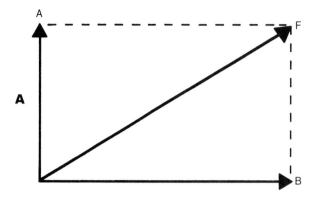

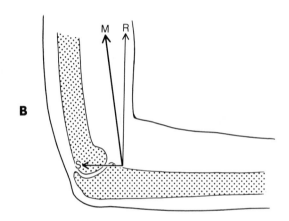

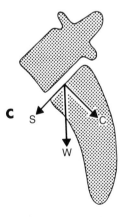

Fig. 3-2. A, *A* and *B* are rectangular components of force *(F)*. **B,** Rotary *(R)* and stabilizing *(S)* components of muscle force *(M)*. **C,** Compression *(C)* and shearing *(S)* force components of the superincumbent weight *(W)* at the lumbosacral junction.

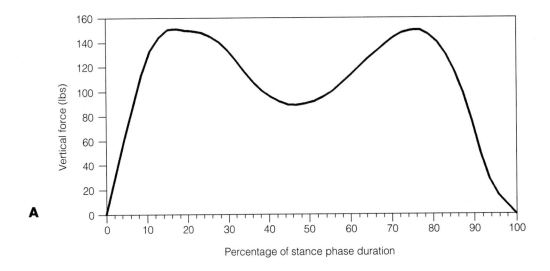

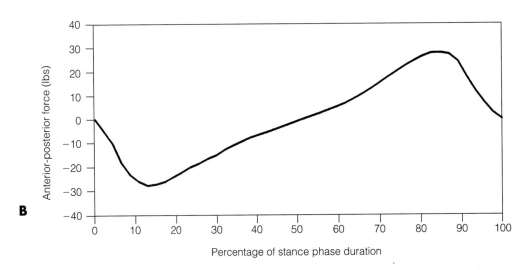

Fig. 3-3. Normal vertical (**A**) and anterior-posterior (**B**) ground reaction curves during walking.

portion of the curve indicates a propulsive force by the individual during the later portion of stance, during the advance forward for the next step (Fig. 3-4). The angle at which the foot strikes the ground determines the relative magnitude of each component. If the foot strikes nearly perpendicular to the ground, the parallel (F_y) force component is relatively small. If, however, the foot is extended farther in front of the person, the perpendicular (F_z) component is reduced and the parallel component (F_y) is increased. This action is exactly what happens in runners who are midfoot rather than rearfoot strikers.[7]

Often several forces combine like a single force to act on an object (Fig. 3-5, *A*). This singular force is called the *resultant force* because it is the "result" of the combination of all other forces. The process of finding a single resultant force from several individual forces is called the *composition*

of forces. There are many examples of the composition of forces in the human body, including the combined pull of the quadriceps muscles providing a single resultant force that acts upon the patella (Fig. 3-5, *B*).

The method of determining the magnitude of the force components is based upon simple trigonometry and algebra, which can be reviewed in most kinesiology and physics textbooks.[1,29,44] Calculating the magnitude of these components may provide valuable information, such as the exercise effect of a load, the hazardous effects of certain exercises, or the most advantageous placement of a body part to gain a maximal result. Injuries may also occur as a result of a combination of forces. For example, increased compression of the patellofemoral joint occurs as the forces from the quadriceps muscle group and the patellar tendon act on the patella at greater amounts of knee flexion.[29]

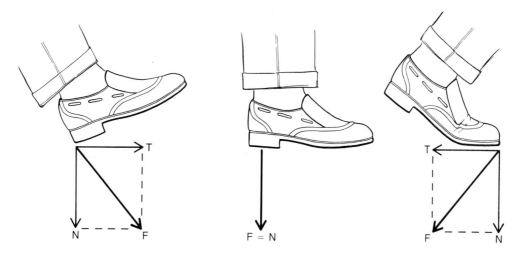

Fig. 3-4. Normal *(N)* and tangential *(T)* components of contact force *(F)* during gait.

Frictional force

Besides the force of gravity and that from muscle contraction, frictional force also plays an important role in the cause of injury as well as in its prevention. Frictional force is created when two objects are in contact with each other. The force of friction is that component parallel to the contacting surfaces that serves to keep an object at rest.[1,29,37] The magnitude of frictional force is determined by the product of the magnitude of the force pushing the two objects together and the properties of the two objects' surfaces. As either of these two factors increases, so does the force resisting the objects from moving relative to each other (frictional force). The factor dealing with the property of the objects' surfaces is represented by a value called the *coefficient of friction.* Coefficients of friction have been calculated for many conditions, including the human body. Brand reported that the coefficient of human joints is typically in the range of .005 to .01.[5] Most manufactured mechanical systems are in the range of 0.005 to 0.1, and total joint replacements have coefficients of friction between 0.142 to 0.163.[60] Therefore, joint movement in a healthy state is extremely efficient and difficult to reproduce. The presence of a disease process such as degenerative arthritis markedly compromises this efficiency.

Frictional force also plays an important role in many aspects of orthopedic and sport therapy. In specific situations, increasing or decreasing the coefficient of friction of the surfaces may reduce the chance of injury to the athlete. Frictional characteristics of athletic footwear are frequently measured to determine which type of outsole would be best for certain sports or playing conditions such as artificial turf, grass, and wood courts.*

* References 2, 37, 46, 47, 52, 57.

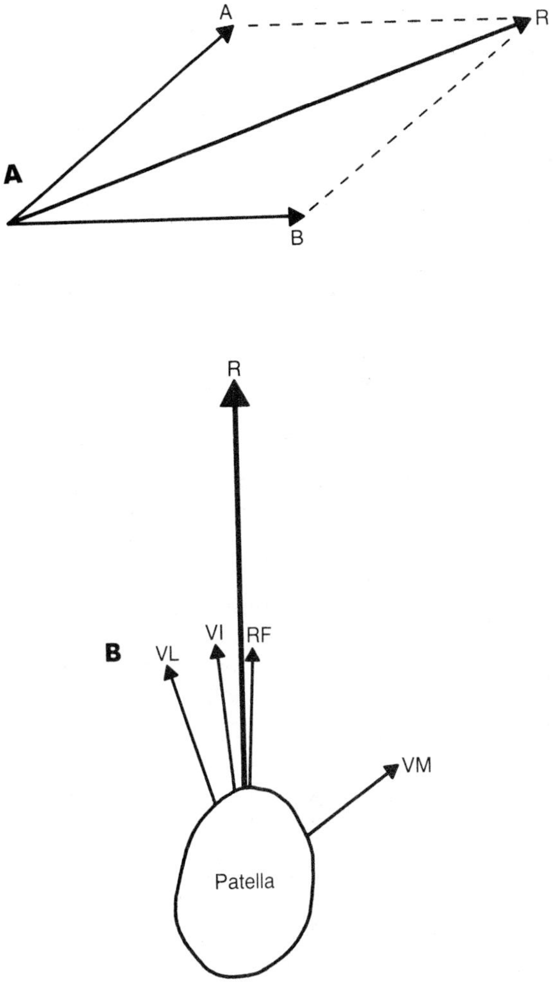

Fig. 3-5. A, Forces *A* and *B* acting together to provide a resultant force *(R).* **B,** Resultant force *(R)* of the quadriceps muscle on the patella terminating in the combined forces of the vastus lateralis *(VL),* vastus intermedius *(VI),* rectus femoris *(RF),* and vastus medialis *(VM).*

Strength

The term *strength* is frequently used to mean the ability of a muscle to produce or resist a force. The greater the force produced by a muscle, the greater the strength the muscle is said to have. Unfortunately, muscle strength, or the amount of force it can produce, cannot be measured directly. Instead, muscle strength is measured indirectly by the amount of resistance the muscle lever system can either overcome or maintain. These measurements include such factors as the muscle's angle of pull, the angle of application of the resisting force, the muscle's length, the speed of muscle contraction, and the speed of movement.

Pressure

Pressure is defined as the amount of force distributed over a specific area and is usually measured in terms of pounds per square inch (lb/in.^{2}) or newtons per square centimeter (N/cm^2). This definition of pressure illustrates that force and area are inversely related to each other; as one of the values increases, the other must decrease for pressure to remain the same. For example, a specific amount of pressure can be increased by either increasing the force applied or decreasing the area over which it is applied.

Pressure plays an important role in orthopedic and sport-related injury, treatment, and prevention. For example, protective pads reduce pressure by distributing impact forces over a larger area and thus reduce the chance of injury. Hip pads protect football players against hip pointer injuries, pads on the shoulders of lacrosse players and on the shins of soccer players protect against contusions, and helmets for children with cerebral palsy protect against concussions. Conversely, pads on braces and parts of casts and splints can cause the skin to break down if the area of contact is too small or the force over the contact area is too great. Also of concern is the effect of forces applied to an area, over an extended period of time. Such is the case with the development of decubitus ulcers (pressure sores) when a person lies or sits in one position for an extended period of time. Another example of the detrimental effect of pressure can be illustrated in Fig. 3-6, *A*. An individual with a plantar pressure pattern has extremely high pressure values under the heel and forefoot. Because of the repetitive nature of locomotion, the soft tissue in these areas is highly susceptible to breakdown, especially if the person's cutaneous sensation is compromised, which is very common in individuals with diabetes mellitus.[4,42,51] Modification of footwear is frequently indicated for these individuals to prevent soft tissue damage or to aid healing following injury.[31] Fig. 3-6, *B,* shows a pressure plot of the same individual, except with a layer of cushioning material under the foot. The scaling shows that the pressures have been reduced to less than 50% of the original values.

Power

The word *power* is often confused with force. Power, however, is the rate of doing work or dissipating energy.

Because work is force applied over a known distance, force is incorporated in the concept of power, but time is also a very important factor. The units of power are commonly foot pounds per second (ft-lb/sec) or newton-meters per second (N-m/sec). An individual may be able to produce a great amount of force, but, unless the force is produced rapidly, the amount of power is low. Some sporting skills require force to be produced without regard to time, but others emphasize the rate at which the force is produced and applied. Training for power activities can be quite different from training for events requiring strength.

The type of injury that may occur can also be related to the rate of energy dissipation. Any musculoskeletal activity that requires moving an object during a short period of time involves the concept of power. Common tests for determining power are the vertical jump, the standing long jump, and the softball throw. Each of these activities requires the movement of an object against resistance. Individuals who sprint, jump, or throw an object for speed or distance during a sport must have the strength to provide a large amount of force and the neuromuscular coordination to contract the muscles rapidly. Training for power is specific, and the individual must train the muscle to contract rapidly against a heavy load.[33,54]

Load, stress, and strain

An outside force or group of forces acting on an object is called a *load.* For example, a heavy box placed on a table provides an external force or load on the table. The contraction of muscles to resist an object placed in your hand creates a load on the bone. A blow to the thigh would also be considered a load, but to the soft tissues of the thigh. A load may act directly on a specific point or at some distance away from the point of application. As these forces are applied, there are internal forces that react to the external load. These internal forces are distributed across an area within the object and are defined in terms of force per unit area, which is similar to pressure. This internal reaction or resistance to the external load is called *mechanical stress.* Frequently, as an external load is applied to an object, deformation occurs. This deformation or change in the object's dimensions is called *mechanical strain.*[11]

The three principal mechanical stresses are tension, compression, and shear (Fig. 3-7). Tension occurs when the external forces (load) applied are collinear and act in opposite directions (away from each other). Compression is when the external forces applied are collinear and act toward each other. Shear stress results when two parallel forces, opposite in direction and not collinear, cause one point on a surface of an object to slide past a point on an adjacent surface.

Tension stress is very common in biological tissues. It is present in all tendons when their muscle contracts and in ligaments as they resist load and provide joint stability. Injury to ligaments and tendons is almost always a direct result of tension stress that exceeds the strength of the biological tissue. Health practitioners often apply a tensile load

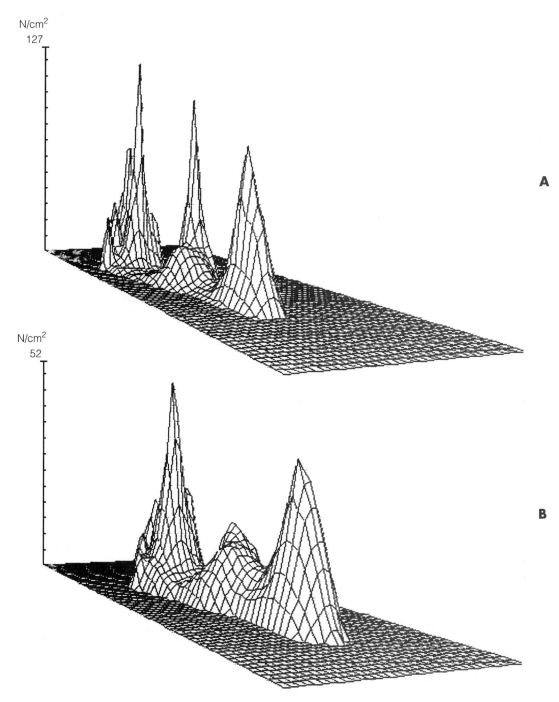

Fig. 3-6. A, Barefoot plantar pressure plot of an individual with extremely high pressure values; **B,** barefoot plantar pressure plot of the same individual with a cushioning material under the foot.

in order to obtain the elongation of muscle or connective tissue during stretching activities. Compression stress is also very common in the human body. Compression stress occurs at such places as the patellofemoral joint when the quadriceps muscles contract, between the articulating surfaces of all weight-bearing joints, and with many injuries, such as contusions. Examples of shear stress include spondylolisthesis and the formation of blisters and abrasions. Shear loads are often found following joint implants, and the implant can fail as a result of too much shearing.[61]

A common mechanical example of these stresses is a load placed on a horizontal beam that causes it to bend (Fig. 3-8). Compression stress develops parallel to the length of the beam in the concave portion, whereas tension stress develops parallel to the length of the beam in its convex portion. A neutral axis is located along the center of the beam, where neither compression nor tension occurs. Shear stress is also produced maximally in two directions within the bending beam. One maximal shearing stress is parallel to the load and perpendicular to the compression

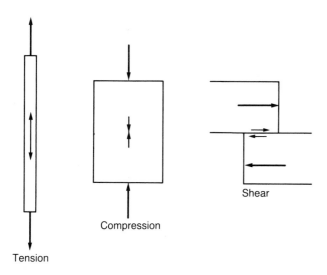

Fig. 3-7. The three principal stresses or strains.

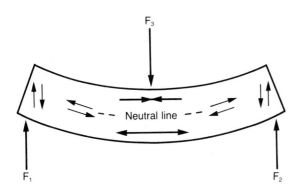

Fig. 3-8. Bending strain with tension (○), compression (→←), and shear (⇆). Examples are bracing, greenstick fractures, and knee injury. This is the basic three-point principle (three forces: F_1, F_2, and F_3).

and tension stress. The sum of this shearing stress results in the bending of the beam. A second shearing stress is parallel to the beam as the horizontal layers of the beam attempt to slide past each other.

Another illustration is cantilever bending. One end of a beam is fixed, and the free end is loaded (Fig. 3-9). In this situation, tension is created in the upper convex portion of the beam, whereas compression occurs in the lower concave portion. Shearing stresses are established parallel to both the load and the beam. In the supporting column, compression stress is added on the beam side to the compression caused by the load, and tension is created on the opposite side, which subtracts from the load's compression.

A final example is torsional loading of an object (Fig. 3-10). In torsional loading, compression and tension occur in a spiral pattern, which is at a 45-degree angle and perpendicular to the long axis of the object. The shear stresses lie in two planes: one parallel to the long axis of the object and the other parallel to the applied load. Common torsional injuries

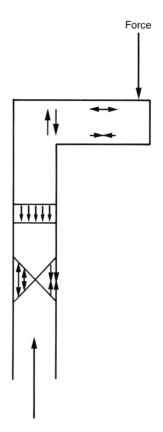

Fig. 3-9. Forces acting in cantilever bending, which result in strains of tension (○), compression (→←), and shear (⇆). An example is the femur and lower limb as a whole.

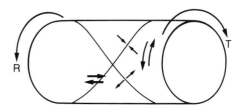

Fig. 3-10. Applied torque *(T)* and resisting torque *(R)* setting up resulting strains of tension (○), compression, (→←), and shear (⇆). Examples are spiral fractures and twisting fractures.

are spiral fractures, which can occur in the tibia during skiing and in the humerus during throwing.[56,63] Each of these examples illustrates that the principle stresses rarely occur in isolation. Combinations of tension, compression, and shear stresses are frequently found in biological tissue and contribute to the type and severity of the injury. Often, treatment is aimed at controlling these stresses by splinting or bracing the injured tissue.

Strength of materials

The strength of a particular material refers back to an important aspect of strength discussed previously. Because strength is related to stress, or the ability of an object to resist a load, the stronger a material, the longer it can withstand a load before it breaks. This general definition of material strength can be looked at from several different ways. Frankel and Nordin[20] present three different characteristics for determining the strength of an object: (1) the magnitude of the load an object resists before it breaks, (2) the degree of deformation that the object undergoes before it breaks, and (3) the amount of energy the object absorbs before it breaks.

Frequently, a graph called a *stress-strain curve* is used to illustrate the relationship between the internal resistance of a material to a load (stress) and the amount of elongation or deformation (strain) resulting from the load.[11,21,36] Although each type of material has its own unique curve, certain characteristics of the curve are similar from one material to the next. Fig. 3-11 depicts a typical stress-strain curve, in which the first portion of the curve is a straight line. Here, the strain is directly proportional to the ability of the material to resist the load. The elasticity of an object is measured by the slope of this straight portion of the curve, B, which is called the *elastic range*. If the load is released while the stress-strain curve is in the elastic range, the material returns to its original size and shape. Some ligaments contain more elastin than others and are therefore more extensible to allow increased range of movement. Other ligaments, however, have more collagen and elongate less, thus providing more stability. This difference in elasticity between materials is often referred to as *stiffness* and is characterized graphically by an increase in the slope of the elastic range. The higher the slope, the stiffer the material. The point at which the strain is no longer proportional to the load is called the *proportional limit,* A; the point beyond which the material does not return to its original size and shape is termed the *elastic limit.* These two points can be the same on a stress-strain curve. The region from the elastic limit to the point of rupture is called the *plastic range,* C. A material deformed within this region of the curve remains permanently deformed. Some materials, such as glass and metal, have either a small plastic range or none at all. Other materials, such as plastic and clay, have a relatively large plastic range. Such materials include a point at which an increase in strain occurs without an increase in stress, which is characterized by a plateauing or even a "dip" in the stress-strain curve and is termed the yield point (Y). Other points typically identified within the plastic range of a stress-strain curve is the ultimate strength (U), which is the greatest load that the object can resist, and the point of rupture or breaking strength (R).[9,38]

Knowledge of the strength characteristics of certain materials is very important in orthopedic and sports medicine. Biological materials such as muscle, bone, ligaments, tendons, and cartilage may need improved strength or plasticity to avoid breaking.[16] Knowledge of strength values and how much load brings about these stress levels within a material could be of great importance in understanding the mechanism of injury and in treatment.

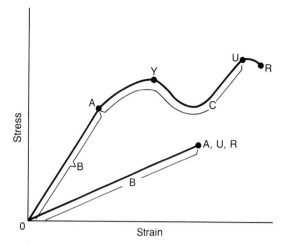

Fig. 3-11. Stress-strain curve showing elastic or proportional limit *(A),* yield point *(Y),* elastic range *(B),* ultimate strength *(U),* plastic range *(C),* and rupture or breaking strength *(R).*

Often treatment is performed to stretch joint tissues, break adhesions, or correct deformities. Important questions are, How much force should be applied? Where should the force be applied? For how long should the force be applied? Without some knowledge of material strength, these questions cannot be accurately answered. In addition, injury may be the result of tissue strain beyond the yield point. In these cases, treatment might include bracing or strapping to protect the stressed tissues and to prevent elongation outside of the elastic range. A knowledge of the stress-strain characteristics of various equipment and treatment materials is also needed to ensure that they are properly used for their intended purpose.

The strength of various biological tissues is dramatically influenced by such things as exercise, aging, and immobilization. The research in this area indicates that aging and immobilization result in a decrease in strength and in stiffness of bone tissue.[11,48] Similar findings have been reported for collagenous tissue such as ligaments and joint capsules.[11,45] With regard to articular cartilage, immobilization results in a reduction in the tissue's resilience and a softening of the cartilage.[11,12,27,39,40] These changes can lead to further damage from abnormal friction and pressure.[17] Physical exercise and activity, by contrast, lead to increases in strength of bone, cartilage, and ligaments.[3,6,11,55,58] The therapist should be aware of these changes in the mechanical properties of biological tissue and what can be done to minimize or reverse their effects.

Resilience and toughness

Most materials have a certain amount of resilience and toughness. These characteristics are related to the absorption and release of energy as a material is loaded rapidly. The resilience of a material is its ability to absorb energy within the elastic range.[21,25,36] The amount of work performed upon a unit volume of a material as it is loaded rapidly from zero to the proportional limit of the material defines the *modulus of resilience* for the material. As a resilient material is loaded, work is done on it and it absorbs energy. When the load is released, the energy is released and the material returns to its original shape. A good example of this concept is the resilience of a tennis ball. If it is highly resilient, it bounces back from a hard surface to approximately the same height from which it was dropped. Resilience also seems to be time-dependent. An object that is highly resilient tends to return to its original shape quickly and give off the absorbed energy quickly. A poorly resilient material tends to return to its original shape slowly and give off low-level energy as heat. Therefore, a common characteristic of resilience is the ability of an object to bounce back quickly.

The resilience of a playing surface can be of major concern and importance when determining the nature and severity of certain athletic injuries. Some materials are not resilient, but deform permanently when a load is applied. This type of material is called *analastic*—neither elastic nor resilient.[21] An example is a ball of bread dough dropped on a kitchen counter. The dough is deformed but does not bounce back. If a playing surface is analastic, it becomes permanently deformed and could easily be injurious to the athlete. A very muddy playing field covered with deep footprints is a good example of an analastic surface. Conversely, a playing surface such as pavement, concrete, or tile that returns energy very quickly may also cause injuries such as shin splints and stress fractures to the lower limb. Some surfaces, such as wrestling mats, landing mats for gymnastics, and jumping pits, should have limited resilience. They should absorb the energy and give it off slowly, but they should not become permanently deformed.

Toughness, by contrast, is the ability of a material to absorb energy within the plastic range.[21,25,36] The amount of work done on a unit volume of material as a load is applied rapidly from zero to the point of rupture defines the *modulus of toughness*. An important aspect of material toughness is its ability to absorb energy without breaking.[36] Quite often, practitioners in orthopedics and sports medicine are concerned with the toughness of a material. The ability of ligaments, cartilage, bone, muscles, and tendons to absorb energy without rupturing is important for the prevention of injury. If too much energy is absorbed, however, when the material finally does rupture, the absorbed energy is released violently, shattering the tissue. Such a situation can be seen in certain types of sprains, strains, and fractures.[40]

Creep

Material creep occurs when a low-magnitude load—below the yield point and usually within the elastic range—is applied over a long period of time. This process is most obvious in metals and viscoelastic materials such as biological tissue. Mechanical creep occurs in all types of materials and with any level of load; however, the greater the load, the more rapid the material creep. Increasing the temperature also tends to increase the rate of creep. A load placed on an object for an extended period of time causes the material to elongate. Eventually, permanent plastic deformation results or else the material breaks.[16] Therapists frequently apply this behavior of materials during stretching exercises in which a prolonged duration of sufficient load is applied to muscle or ligamentous tissue. Tissues that have been heated first are more easily stretched because the creep of the tissue is more rapid.

Fatigue

Material fatigue is also a characteristic process of all materials. A material may fail below the yield point from mechanical fatigue if the material is loaded cyclically. The greater the load applied, the fewer cycles needed for the material to break. A minimal load, however, is necessary. Below this specific minimal load, an infinite number of cycles are needed to cause the material to fail. This load is called the *endurance limit* of the material.[16] A common example of mechanical fatigue failure is the breaking of a plastic credit card by bending it back and forth rapidly several times. A great deal of heat is produced where the card is bent. Heat is also produced in biological tissue. This buildup of heat may result in further disruption of collagen cross-bridges[13] and therefore hasten the failure observed with cyclic loading. Fatigue fractures (stress fractures or stress reactions) in runners, dancers, and marching soldiers are all examples of mechanical fatigue in biological tissues. Fatigue fractures often develop in runners because of excessive mileage or poor running style. A jogger with a 2-m stride has 5000 cycles on one lower limb while traveling 10,000 m. A heavy athlete has an increased load and subsequent stress upon the lower limb. Daily jogging at this distance may cause a fatigue fracture in one of the bones of the lower limb. In such cases, footwear with midsole construction using materials that absorb the stress of impact loading of the lower extremity is extremely important. Additional absorption inside the shoe from accommodative orthoses or special insole material may also be necessary.[30,31] Fortunately, biological tissue can repair itself, providing the load is not too great, the number of cycles not too many, and the period between loading is sufficiently high.

MOMENTS OF FORCE
Torque

When a load acts upon an object, it frequently acts at a distance from a point where rotation can occur. This distance is often referred to as the *lever arm* of the load. Such a situation creates a tendency for movement to occur at the point of rotation. Whether movement happens depends upon the magnitude of the load applied and its distance from the rotational axis. The product of the distance from the axis and the magnitude of the force perpendicular to the lever arm (Moment [M] = Force [F] × distance [d]) is called the

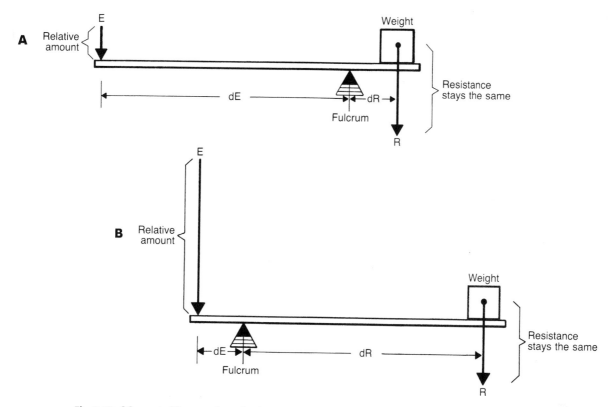

Fig. 3-12. Moment of force and mechanical advantage (MA) demonstrated with effort *(E)*, effort arm *(dE)*, resistance *(R)*, and resistance arm *(dR)*. **A**, MA > 1. **B**, MA < 1.

moment of force (Fig. 3-12). Moments are typically measured in foot-pounds (ft-lb) or newton-meters (N-m).

As can be seen from this equation, a greater amount of force or a longer lever arm increases the moment about the point of rotation. Such leverage may be set up so that a small force applied to a relatively long arm can produce the same moment (torque) as a large force at the end of a short lever arm (Fig. 3-12, *A*). The reverse situation is also true (Fig. 3-12, *B*). The efficiency of various lever systems is frequently measured in terms of their mechanical advantage (MA), that is, the ratio of the length of the effort arm (dE) to the length of the resistance arm (dR), or MA = dE/dR. The effort arm is the distance of the applied force to the fulcrum, and the resistance arm is the distance from the fulcrum to the resisting load. If the effort arm is greater than the resistance arm, the mechanical advantage is greater than 1. If the resistance arm is longer than the effort arm, the mechanical advantage is less than 1.

Although a gain in force is often a reason for using a lever system, other effects may also be important. If the effort arm is shorter than the resistance arm (MA < 1), the resisting load travels farther and faster than the point where the effort force is applied. This result may be more important than a gain in force. Most lever systems of the human body have the effort arm much shorter than the resistance arm, as in the example of the biceps brachii muscle acting at the elbow joint (Fig. 3-13). The biceps brachii attaches fairly close to the elbow

joint axis, and the resisting load (weight of the forearm and hand) is distal to the elbow. The brachioradialis muscle, by contrast, has its point of application at the wrist. Because of the anatomical arrangement of the two muscles, the biceps brachii has the advantage of speed and distance over the brachioradialis. Conversely, the brachioradialis muscle has the advantage of torque production over the biceps brachii.

Also implied in this example is the fact that more than one effort force and more than one resistance force may be involved in any situation—actually, the norm rather than the exception as far as the human body is concerned. The effort forces and resistance forces are not the only ones involved in the lever systems of the human body. A very important force is also found acting at the joint center (Fig. 3-13). It is a reaction force and typically resists the compressive forces produced by muscle contraction around the joint.

The length of an object and the force applied to that object are of great importance in musculoskeletal rehabilitation and injury prevention. Research on skiing injuries has shown that longer skis can result in more severe injuries.[15,34,63] The face mask in football may prevent facial injuries, but the length of the bars protruding from the helmet may also provide an increased lever arm from which severe cervical injuries may result.[24] Exercise programs also make use of the principle of moments for intensity grading. Bent-leg curls to strengthen the abdominal muscles may be made more difficult by having the individual move the arm position more distally

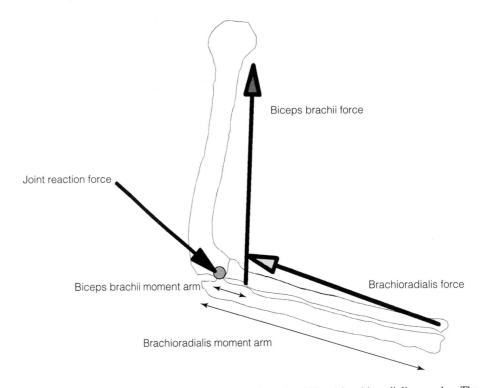

Fig. 3-13. Differences in the moment arms of the biceps brachii and brachiovadialis muscles. The joint reaction force is created in response to all other forces, including muscle and gravity.

from the hip, a maneuver that provides a longer resistance arm for the same force. Straight-leg exercises to strengthen the quadriceps muscle may be made more difficult by placing a weight at the ankle or easier by moving the weight proximal toward the knee. The principle of levers is also used extensively in the performance of manual muscle tests.[28]

KINEMATICS
Motion

Forces tend to cause objects to move. The description and study of the motion of an object is called *kinematics.* Kinematics is concerned with describing motion in terms of both translation (linear motion) and rotation (angular motion). Motion is generally described by four terms: time, displacement, velocity, and acceleration. The concept of time is often used in gait analysis, as well as in the analysis of movement in various sporting activities. Time is also a vital part of velocity and acceleration. Displacement is the change in an object's position. It refers both to the distance between the original position and the final position and to the direction of the movement. Velocity is the rate of displacement change; it is how rapidly the object is moved. Displacement may be calculated by dividing the amount of displacement by the amount of time that has elapsed. Velocity has both magnitude and direction. The term *speed,* however, has only magnitude. Often these terms are used interchangeably if direction is of no concern or is obvious. Acceleration is the rate of change in velocity. It also has magnitude and direction. *Deceleration* is the common term used for negative

acceleration. As the magnitude or direction of velocity changes, the object experiences acceleration and speeds up, slows down, or changes direction.

Measurement of motion

The measurement of dynamic motion is generally accomplished by the two-dimensional (2-D) or three-dimensional (3-D) recording of specific points on a subject's body while they move. There are both strengths and weaknesses inherent in both methods.

Two-dimensional analysis. By far, 2-D motion analysis has been the most common measurement technique. Two-dimensional analysis can be cinematography or the more popular videography. The principal reasons for the prevalence of 2-D analysis is the relatively low cost of the equipment and the short time required to perform the analysis. However, 2-D motion analysis is considered to be only moderately accurate. The greatest inaccuracies occur when the body segment being measured moves away from a position of being perpendicular to the camera's field of view. Because of these inaccuracies, many investigators have abandoned 2-D in favor of 3-D analysis. From a research point of view, this position is probably warranted. From a clinical perspective, however, the cost of 3-D analysis in terms of money, time, and space is prohibitive. For many movements, such as walking, the movement of interest is primarily perpendicular to the camera. In such cases, 2-D analysis yields essentially the same information as 3-D analysis of the same movement.

Three-dimensional analysis. As mentioned earlier, a problem with 2-D analysis is perspective error. Three-dimensional analysis corrects this problem and is therefore the method of choice in research settings. It uses two or more cameras positioned to observe the desired movement from different angles. Now that the exact position of the body segment being measured is known in all three planes, perspective error can be eliminated. In essence, rotation of a subject's extremity in any direction does not affect the size of the angle being calculated.

With the advent of microcomputers and their continual advance in power and capability, 3-D analysis has become less technically demanding and therefore more common. Despite its increased prevalence and ease of use, however, for the most part it is still impractical as a clinical tool. Although the cost of equipment and software has come down dramatically, it is still prohibitive for most clinical practice settings. In addition, it still requires a relatively large amount of space and time to film, digitize the images, and then manipulate the data into the desired format.

Motion and injury

The description of motion can be invaluable to practitioners for determining the cause or extent of the injury, as well as the effects of the treatment. Knowledge of the normal patterns of movement is therefore essential. If the practitioner knows normal movement, the presence of abnormal motion is easily determined. An abnormal running or walking pattern can cause injuries in several areas of the body, including the foot, knee, hip, and back.[14,53] Analysis of a person's gait pattern therefore provides information about the extent or possible cause of the injury. Because range of motion, velocity, and acceleration of the body are altered as a person moves, it is reasonable to think that treatment—certainly if bracing or foot orthoses are prescribed—will bring these movement characteristics to within normal values.[8,35] Another example is the study of the acceleration and deceleration of the head during football, which provides information about injuries to the head and neck.[15,24,25] Similar studies have been done for hockey injuries.[49]

KINETICS

The study of kinematics provides only limited information concerning movement. The study of kinetics, by contrast, provides information about the forces that affect the motion of the object, the same forces discussed in the previous section. The laws of motion developed by Isaac Newton form the basis for the study of kinetics.

Newton's first law

Force has often been defined as the entity that accelerates an object. This definition implies motion. This concept is presented in Newton's first law of motion, the *law of inertia,* which states that an object remains in its existing state of motion or nonmotion unless acted upon by an outside force. Therefore, a stationary object does not begin to move unless an unbalanced outside force acts upon it. Conversely, an object that is in motion remains in motion at the same speed and direction unless acted upon by an outside force.

Inertia can play an important role in understanding brain injury resulting from a blow to the skull. A blow causes the skull to accelerate rapidly, yet the brain inside stays relatively stationary because it is surrounded by cerebral spinal fluid. The moving skull therefore contacts the stationary brain and damages it without fracturing the skull. A similar situation occurs when the head is suddenly and rapidly decelerated. Although the skull stops moving, the brain, because of its inertia, continues moving until it contacts the skull. Mass movements of the brain in such instances can cause contusions on the blow side of the brain and tissue tearing on the opposite side.[25]

Another example of the effect of inertia occurs during sprint running. Once the muscles initiate hip flexion, inertia is a major cause of the continued motion of the forward swinging limb. An outside force is therefore needed to decelerate and stop the leg, which is accomplished by a strong contraction of the hamstring muscles just before the foot strikes the ground.[10] Hamstring strains result if the force needed for deceleration is greater than the strength of the hamstring muscles.

Newton's second law

Newton's second law of motion is the *law of acceleration:* If an outside force acts upon an object, the object changes its velocity or accelerates in direct proportion to the force that was applied. The object also accelerates in inverse proportion to its mass. Hence, mass tends to resist acceleration. The well-known formula of force equals mass times acceleration ($F = ma$) illustrates this relationship. According to Newton's law, this formula would be expressed as $a = F/m$. The application of this law is fairly common and well understood. Everyone understands that accelerating a heavy object requires more force than accelerating a lighter object.

Newton's third law

Gravity is an outside force that is always acting on an object on the earth. To balance this increasing force, a second outside force must be introduced. An object resting on a table is acted upon by at least two forces: the force of gravity and the force exerted by the table to resist gravity. Such an example illustrates Newton's third law of motion, the *law of reaction:* Any force acting on an object has another force of equal magnitude, but opposite in direction, acting on the same object. Thus, as the object on the table is acted upon by the pull of gravity, the table reacts to this force of gravity with an equal and opposite force. If the opposing forces are not equal and opposite, the object begins to move.

Impulse and momentum

The momentum of an object in either translatory or rotatory motion is the product of force or torque and the change in velocity per unit of time. When two objects collide, their combined momentum after the impact is equal to their combined momentum before the collision. This principle is called the *law of conservation of momentum.* Simply stated, the change of momentum of the first object is equal in magnitude and opposite in direction to the change in momentum of the second object. The product of force or torque and time is known as *impulse,* which is equal to the change in momentum. A greater force applied or a force applied over a longer period of time increases the momentum of an object. Less force is needed if more time is used to absorb or reduce the momentum of a moving object.

An egg toss at a summer picnic demonstrates the principle of impulse. The egg must be caught carefully by hands moving in concert with the moving egg. This action, if done properly, increases the amount of time it takes to catch the egg and therefore reduces the force imparted on the egg. If the catching time is not sufficiently long, the force on the egg is too great and it breaks. Another application of impulse is the use of padded dashboards to reduce the force on occupants during automobile accidents. The padded material allows more time for the impact force to be absorbed and thus reduces the likelihood of injury. The same principle is used with certain types of materials in foot orthotic design and fabrication for individuals with lower extremity stress fractures and stress reactions.[31] Such a person generally has difficulty dissipating the shock of body weight at the instant of foot contact, so cushioning materials are placed in the shoes to absorb these forces.[30,31] Another example is a person who lands on the ground abruptly with the joints in extension. Serious injuries may result because the body's momentum is stopped too quickly and a large force of impact occurs. A step from a stair or a curb or walking or running without a small amount of knee flexion can cause an increased load on the weight-bearing joints. The usual landing surfaces in jumping and gymnastic events require more time to absorb the momentum of the body, and thus less force is transmitted to the body.[59]

Work

If the force applied to an object results in its movement, the principles of work and energy come into play. In mechanics, work equals the product of the force exerted on an object and the object's displacement (Work [W] = Force [F] × distance [d]). Although this formula looks identical to that of moments, the concept is very different. Work is accomplished as the force overcomes a resistance and moves the object. A moment or torque, by contrast, is the force component perpendicular to the lever arm times the length of the lever arm. A force that produces torque may do work resulting in rotatory motion. If the moment generated is not sufficient to overcome the resistance of the object, however, no work is performed, despite the presence of the moment. During weight training, positive work is done as the weight is raised, and negative work is done as the weight is lowered.

Energy

Energy is the capacity to do work. Of the many forms of energy, only mechanical energy and heat are considered in this chapter. Heat is often a by-product of work. Increased heat occurs when molecules in the area increase their movement. Mechanical energy can be divided into two types: potential and kinetic energy. Potential energy (PE) is stored energy; it has the potential to perform work. When released, potential energy becomes kinetic energy (KE), which is the energy of motion. The most common example of potential energy in mechanics is related to the location of an object and the force of gravity exerted on that object. The formula to determine the potential energy of an object is PE = mgh, where m is the mass of the object, g is the value of gravitational acceleration, and h is the height of the object above a reference point, usually the ground. As the object begins to fall, it loses potential energy because the h is getting smaller.

Kinetic energy is determined by the formula KE = ½ mv^2, where m is the mass of the object and v is its velocity. A falling object gains kinetic energy as its velocity increases. When the object reaches the reference point, such as the floor, the height (h) equals zero, so that the object no longer has potential energy. However, the object's velocity is maximal, and therefore kinetic energy is at its maximum. If the object bounces, it regains some potential energy and loses some kinetic energy as it rises. When the object finally comes to rest, the total mechanical energy (PE and KE) will have been converted to heat.

Gainor and colleagues determined that the amount of energy that develops in the arm of a pitcher is about 27,000 in.-lb.[23] This magnitude of energy is sufficient to cause severe damage to part of the throwing mechanism. Similar calculations have been made for other activities: The energy developed at the hip and knee in kicking,[22] absorbed by the hip or upper limb in a fall,[18] created in the tibia as it is twisted by a ski, and produced on the hand by a karate blow all have sufficient energy to produce injury. Knowledge of how to prevent injury by absorbing the energy is therefore of major importance. For example, various helmets can be evaluated to determine their energy-absorbing abilities. Gurdjian, Roberts, and Thomas found a linear relationship between kinetic energy and the degree of brain injury resulting from head collisions during football practice and games.[25] They also found that helmet design and padding thickness affected the amount of energy absorbed by the head.

The energy involved in loading a tissue may also determine the type and degree of injury that result. A rapid rate of loading may produce a ligament rupture, whereas a slow rate of loading may result in an avulsion fracture. If a bone is loaded rapidly, more load is needed to fracture it and more energy is absorbed before it breaks. When the bone fractures, however, it is then probably a high-energy explosion. Slow loading generally produces a low-energy fracture.[40] During locomotion, the energy absorbed by the natural shock absorbers (bones, menisci, intervertebral disks, and joints) may be insufficient and therefore lead to overuse injuries. Methods that reduce the energy transmitted to these body parts would therefore be important to delay, reduce, or prevent damage.

SUMMARY

Many different biomechanical principles are involved in movement and sport activities. Most mechanisms of injury, evaluation, treatment, and prevention can be explained and understood with biomechanical principles. This chapter has discussed basic principles and has given examples of how they are involved in orthopedic and sports medicine. The practitioner should become familiar with them and able to apply them to be fully competent in sports medicine or orthopedic therapy.

REVIEW QUESTIONS

1. What are the most common forces involved in orthopedic and sports therapy? Describe each type of force.
2. How is the principle of buoyancy force used in designing pool exercise programs?
3. How does the use of soft, cushioned materials in shoes decrease pressures acting on the plantar surface of the foot?
4. What three different characteristics are used for determining the strength of an object?
5. How do Newton's three laws of motion apply to human walking? Explain the effect of each law on stance and the swing phase.

REFERENCES

1. Benedek GB, Villars FMH: *Physics: mechanics,* vol 1, Reading, Mass, 1973, Addison-Wesley.
2. Bonstingl RW, Morehouse CA, Niebel BW: Torques developed by different types of shoes on various playing surfaces, *Med Sci Sports* 7:127, 1975.
3. Booth FW, Gould EW: Effects of training and disuse on connective tissue. In Wilmore JH, Keogh JF, editors: *Exercise and sports science review,* New York, 1975, Academic Press.
4. Boulton AJM et al: Dynamic foot pressure and other studies as diagnostic and management aids in diabetic neuropathy, *Diabetes Care* 6:26, 1983.
5. Brand RA: Joint lubrication. In Albright JA, Brand RA, editors: *The scientific basis of orthopedics,* New York, 1979, Appleton-Century-Crofts.
6. Cabaud HE et al: Exercise effects on the strength of the rat anterior cruciate ligament, *Am J Sports Med* 8:79, 1980.
7. Cavanagh PR: Forces and pressures between the foot and floor during normal walking and running. In Cooper JM, Haven B, editors: *Proceedings of the 1980 Biomechanics Symposium,* Indianapolis, 1980, Indiana State Board of Health.
8. Clarke TE, Frederick EC, Hamill CL: The effects of shoe design parameters on rearfoot control in running, *Med Sci Sports Exerc* 15:376, 1983.
9. Cochran GVB: *A primer of orthopaedic biomechanics,* New York, 1982, Churchill Livingstone.
10. Cornwall MW: *Kinematic and kinetic analysis of sprint running,* masters thesis, Chapel Hill, 1981, University of North Carolina.
11. Cornwall MW: Biomechanics of noncontractile tissue: a review, *Phys Ther* 64:1869, 1984.
12. Cornwall MW, LeVeau BF: The effect of physical activity on ligamentous strength: an overview, *J Orthop Sports Phys Ther* 5:275, 1984.
13. Cummings GS, Tillman LJ: Remodeling of dense connective tissue in normal adult tissues. In Currier DP, Nelson RM, editors: *Dynamics of human biological tissues,* Philadelphia, 1992, FA Davis.
14. DeLacerda FG: The relationship of foot pronation, foot position, and electromyography of the anterior tibialis muscle in three subjects with different histories of shinsplints, *J Orthop Sports Phys Ther* 2:60, 1980.
15. Dubravcik P, Burke DL: Ski fractures above and below the boot top, *Can J Surg* 22:243, 1979.
16. Dumbleton JH, Black J: *An introduction to orthopedic materials,* Springfield, Ill, 1975, Charles C Thomas.
17. Evans EB et al: Experimental immobilization and remobilization of rat knee joints, *J Bone Jt Surg Am* 42:737, 1960.
18. Frankel VH, Burstein AH: *Orthopedic biomechanics,* Philadelphia, 1970, Lea & Febiger.
19. Frankel VH, Hang YS: Recent advances in the biomechanics of sports injuries, *Acta Orthop Scand* 46:484, 1975.
20. Frankel VH, Nordin M: *Basic biomechanics of the skeletal system,* Philadelphia, 1980, Lea & Febiger.
21. Frost HM: *Orthopedic biomechanics,* Springfield, Ill, 1973, Charles C Thomas.
22. Gainor BJ et al: The kick: biomechanics and collision injury, *Am J Sports Med* 6:185, 1978.
23. Gainor BJ et al: The throw: biomechanics and acute injury, *Am J Sports Med* 8:114, 1980.
24. Gurdjian ES, Lissner HR, Patrick LM: Protection of the head and neck in sports, *JAMA* 182:509, 1962.
25. Gurdjian ES, Roberts VL, Thomas LM: Tolerance curves of acceleration and intercranial pressure and protective index in experimental head injury, *J Trauma* 6:600, 1966.
26. Hirsch C: Biomechanics in motor skeletal trauma, *J Trauma* 10:997, 1970.
27. Inerot S et al: Articular-cartilage proteoglycans in aging and osteoarthritis, *Biochem J* 169:143, 1978.
28. Kendall FP, McCreary EK, Provance PG: *Muscles: testing and function,* ed 4, Baltimore, 1993, Williams & Wilkins.
29. LeVeau B: *Biomechanics of human motion,* ed 2, Philadelphia, 1977, WB Saunders.
30. McPoil TG, Cornwall MW: Rigid versus soft foot orthoses: a single subject design, *J Am Podiatr Med Assoc* 81:638, 1991.
31. McPoil TG, Cornwall MW: Effect of insole material on force and plantar pressures during walking, *J Am Podiatr Med Assoc* 82:412, 1992.
32. Michlovitz SL: *Thermal agents in rehabilitation,* ed 2, Philadelphia, 1990, FA Davis.
33. Moffroid MT, Whipple RH: Specificity of speed of exercise, *Phys Ther* 50:1692, 1970.
34. Mortiz JR: Ski injuries, *Am J Surg* 98:493, 1959.
35. Mueller K et al: Effect of a tone-inhibiting dynamic ankle-foot orthosis on the foot-loading pattern of a hemiplegic adult: a preliminary study, *J Prosth Orthot* 4:86, 1992.
36. Nash WA: *Strength of materials,* New York, 1972, McGraw-Hill.
37. Nigg B: The validity and relevance of tests used for the assessment of sports surfaces, *Med Sci Sports Exerc* 22:131, 1990.
38. Nordin M, Frankel VH: Biomechanics of whole bones and bone tissue. In Frankel VH, Nordin M, editors: *Basic biomechanics of the skeletal system,* Philadelphia, 1980, Lea & Febiger.

39. Noyes FR: Functional properties of knee ligaments and alterations induced by immobilization: a correlative biomechanical and histological study in primates, *Clin Orthop* 123:210, 1977.

40. Noyes FR et al: Biomechanics of ligament failure: II, an analysis of immobilization, exercise, and reconditioning effects in primates, *J Bone Jt Surg Am* 56:1406, 1974.

41. O'Donoghue DH: Injuries to the knee, *Am J Surg* 98:463, 1959.

42. Patil KM, Srinivasan H: Measurement of pressure under leprotic feet using a baragraph, *J Rehabil Res Devel* 24:9, 1993.

43. Radin E: Relevant biomechanics in the treatment of musculoskeletal injuries and disorders, *Clin Orthop* 146:2, 1980.

44. Rasch PJ, Burke RK: *Kinesiology and applied anatomy,* Philadelphia, 1974, Lea & Febiger.

45. Rasch PJ et al: Effect of exercise, immobilization and intermittent stretching on strength of knee ligaments of albino rats, *J Appl Physiol* 15:289, 1960.

46. Rheinstein DJ, Morehouse CA, Niebel BW: Effects on traction of outsole composition and hardness of basketball shoes and three types of playing surfaces, *Med Sci Sports* 10:282, 1978.

47. Schlaepfer F, Unold E, Nigg B: The frictional characteristics of tennis shoes. In Nigg B, Kerr BA, editors: *Biomechanical aspects of sport shoes and playing surfaces,* Calgary, 1983, University Printing.

48. Semb H: The breaking strength of normal and immobilized cortical bone from dogs, *Acta Orthop Scand* 37:131, 1966.

49. Sim FH, Chao EY: Injury potential in modern ice hockey, *Am J Sports Med* 6:378, 1978.

50. Slocum DB: The mechanism of some common injuries to the shoulder in sports, *Am J Surg* 98:394, 1959.

51. Stokes IAF, Faris IB, Hutton WC: The neuropathic ulcer and loads on the foot in diabetic patients, *Acta Orthop Scand* 46:839, 1975.

52. Stucke H, Baudzus W, Bauman W: On frictional characteristics of playing surfaces. In Frederick EC, editor: *Sport shoes and playing surfaces,* Champaign, Ill, 1984, Human Kinetics Publishers.

53. Subotnick SI: Podiatric aspects of children in sports, *J Am Podiatr Med Assoc* 69:443, 1979.

54. Thistle HG et al: Isokinetic contraction: a new concept of exercise, *Arch Phys Med Rehabil* 48:279, 1967.

55. Tipton CM et al: Influence of exercise on strength of medial collateral knee ligaments of dogs, *Am J Physiol* 218:894, 1970.

56. Tullos HS, King JW: Lesion of the pitching arm in adolescents, *JAMA* 220:264, 1972.

57. Van Gheluwe B, DePorte E, Hebbelinck M: Frictional forces and torques of soccer shoes on artificial turf. In Nigg B, Kerr BA, editors: *Biomechanical aspects of sport shoes and playing surfaces,* Calgary, 1983, University Printing.

58. Viidik A: Biomechanics and functional adaptation of tendons and joint ligaments. In Evans FG, editor: *Studies of the anatomy and function of bone and joints,* New York, 1966, Springer-Verlag.

59. Voloskin A, Wosk J: Influence of artificial shock absorbers on human gait, *Clin Orthop* 160:52, 1981.

60. Walker PS: *Human joints and their artificial replacements,* Springfield, Ill, 1977, Charles C Thomas.

61. Wilkins KE: The uniqueness of the young athlete: musculoskeletal injuries, *Am J Sports Med* 8:377, 1977.

62. Williams JGP: Wear and tear injuries in athletes: an overview, *Br J Sports Med* 12:211, 1979.

63. Zernicke RF: Biomechanical evaluation of bilateral tibial spiral fractures during skiing: a case study, *Med Sci Sports Exerc* 13:243, 1981.

CHAPTER 4

Inflammatory Response of Synovial Joint Structures

Tony English, M. Elyse Wheeler, and Dixie L. Hettinga

OUTLINE

Synovial joint structure and functions
The inflammatory responses
  Cause of inflammation
  Definition of trauma
  Types of trauma to the joints
  Effects of trauma
  Phagocytosis
  Repair
The synovial membrane
  Morphology
  Synovial lining or intima
  Type A and B cells
  Subsynovial tissue
  Functions
  Joint lubrication
The synovial membrane and its reaction to injury
  Posttraumatic synovitis
  Pigmented villonodular synovitis
  Solitary nodular synovitis
  Regeneration of synovium
Synovial fluid
  Composition and characteristics of synovial fluid
  Synovianalysis
  Viscosity of synovial fluid
  Functions of synovial fluid
Synovial fluid and its reaction to injury
  Synovial fluid in posttraumatic synovitis
  Synovial fluid in hemorrhagic effusions
  Synovial fluid containing fat globules
  Cloudy synovial fluid
  Reabsorption of traumatic effusions

The joint capsule
  Composition
  Nerve and blood supply
  Functions
The joint capsule and its reaction to injury
  Sprains
  Enthesitis
Intraarticular fibrocartilage and fat pads
  Menisci
  Fat pads
  Functions
Intraarticular structures and their reaction to injury
  Meniscus injury
  Injury to fat pads
  Intraarticular damage and osteophytes in osteoarthritis
  Joint bodies
Articular cartilage
  Composition
  Nutritional supply
  Zones of articular cartilage
  Metabolic activity of articular cartilage
  Functions of articular cartilage
Articular cartilage and its reaction to injury
  Capacity for repair
  Partial-thickness and full-thickness defects
  Complete fracture of articular cartilage
  Osteoarthritis
  Pathology and pathogenesis
  Symptoms and treatment
  Traumatic arthritis
Summary

After studying this chapter, the reader should be able to:
1. Describe the structural elements of a synovial joint.
2. List six causes of injury to a synovial joint that can lead to inflammation.
3. Describe the morphology of the synovial membrane.
4. State three ways in which synovium provides physiological support to a normal joint.
5. Describe the composition and characteristics of synovial fluid.
6. List the five classifications used to categorize synovial fluid when a synovianalysis is performed.
7. List the eight functions of menisci.
8. Describe the composition and nutritional supply of articular cartilage.
9. State the four zones of adult articular cartilage that are observed in a histological examination.
10. Describe the difference between primary and secondary osteoarthritis.

KEY TERMS

inflammation	synovial membrane
joint capsule	articular cartilage
synovial fluid	intraarticular fibrocartilage

The framework of the human body is essentially composed of a series of bones that articulate at joints and are moved by muscles. The joints form an integral part of this complex system because they allow motion to take place, hold parts of the bony skeleton together, or perform both functions.

Joints are frequently classified according to the type of motion they allow. Three groups are recognized: (1) synarthroses or immovable joints, (2) amphiarthroses or slightly movable joints, and (3) diarthroses or movable joints. Diarthroses—also known as synovial joints—comprise the majority of the body's articulations.[32]

SYNOVIAL JOINT STRUCTURE AND FUNCTIONS

The *synovial joint* is constructed to allow movement in one or more directions between two or more major segments of the human skeleton under either weight-bearing or non–weight-bearing conditions or both. The joint provides a low-friction articulation to enable movement of the body with minimal effort.[46,47,70] The articulating bony surfaces—termed *articular endplates*—are thin plates of dense cortical bone that overlay cancellous bone. Tightly adherent to the bony endplates is the *hyaline cartilage,* specialized connective tissue that acts as a bearing and gliding surface. The *joint cavity* is a tissue space lined with the synovial membrane that contains only a few milliliters of synovial fluid.[32]

Joint mobility is provided by movement of the cartilaginous surfaces on one another. Joint stability, necessary to prevent movement in abnormal planes or excessive slippage under load, is provided by the bony configuration of the joint, the ligamentous and capsular support systems, the muscles controlling the joint, atmospheric pressure, and, for many joints, gravity. Each joint has unique load and positional requirements, which are reflected in its individual design. Uniaxial, biaxial, or polyaxial joint motion is possible, depending on the fit of the component at the various ranges.[24,32] To a certain extent, maximal strength and mobility are incompatible, and joints typically represent a compromise in which strength is somewhat sacrificed for mobility (e.g., at the shoulder) or mobility is somewhat sacrificed for strength (e.g., at the hip).[24]

The range of motion possible at joints is restrained by apposition of soft tissue, by limitations in the articular surface (impingement of bone against bone), and by muscles that are not long enough to allow an extreme movement in a direction opposite to which they normally act.[24] Accessory structures that maintain the integrity of the joint are the fibrous capsule and the ligaments. The *fibrous capsule* consists of dense connective tissue, which is invested in the entire joint and inserted into the bone, usually close to the articulating surfaces. Within the capsule are parallel bands of collagen fibers called *ligaments.* These, too, insert in the bony parts and vary in their tension from anatomical site to site, depending on the position of the joint.[32]

Within the joint capsule and defining the intraarticular space is the *synovial membrane* or *sac,* composed of *synoviocytes,* a specialized layer of connective tissue cells. Beneath this layer are varying amounts of highly vascular adipose, fibrous, or areolar tissue supporting the synoviocytes and allowing the sac to be appropriately loose in certain ranges of motion, without permitting the synovial folds to become entrapped between the joint surfaces. The synovial membrane replicates the inner surface of the capsule but is reflected at the capsular insertion into the bone, and then extends along the bone to the margin of the articular cartilage but does not cover the cartilaginous surfaces.[24]

The subsynovial tissue is endowed with nerve endings, which, along with those in the capsule and with spindles in the muscles and tendons, are responsible for proprioception and deep pain perception that protect the joint.[24] The nerve supply to a synovial joint is usually derived from several nerves, the general rule being that each nerve that innervates muscles acting across a joint gives at least one branch to that joint. Some of the nerves follow blood vessels and are apparently vasomotor.[24]

Some joints have a complete or incomplete fibrocartilaginous discoid partition known as a *meniscus.* The

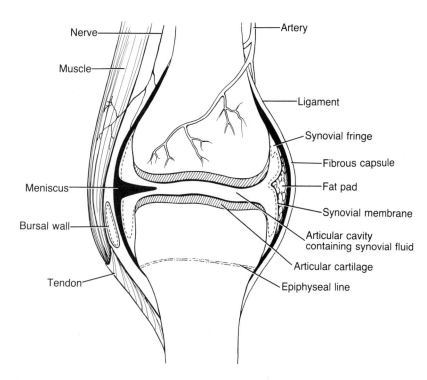

Fig. 4-1. A typical synovial joint. (From Wright V, Dowson D, Kerr J: *Int Rev Connect Tissue Res* 6:105, 1973.)

synovial membrane does not cover the avascular, aneural meniscus, which is firmly fixed to the joint margin by attachment to bone and to the ligaments or capsule, preventing abnormal movement or intraarticular displacement during joint function.[32]

Thus the essential components of a synovial joint are the synovial membrane, synovial fluid, articular cartilage, the joint capsule with associated ligaments, and, in some cases, intraarticular structures (Fig. 4-1). In the following discussion, the normal composition and function of each of these tissues will be delineated so that the structure's specific response to injury can be better appreciated.

THE INFLAMMATORY RESPONSE
Causes of inflammation

The body's response to injurious agents—inflammation—is almost always the same regardless of the location of the injury or the nature of the agent. Injurious agents can include physical injury; injury from heat, light, and laser beams; bacterial and viral effects; endotoxin shock; effects of antigen-antibody reactions; and chemical injury.[25] Joints are most often affected by physical trauma (direct or indirect), infections, metabolic disease (gout), neuropathies (tabes dorsalis, syringomyelia), systemic diseases (hemophilia, serum sickness), and local joint disturbances (aseptic necrosis).[66] For the purpose of this chapter, discussion will be limited to joint inflammatory responses initiated by physical injury.

Definition of trauma

The types of trauma that can cause insults to joints are as varied as the resulting injuries. Trauma can result from a direct blow to the joint area by an object or by a fall. This type of trauma may produce a sprain, subluxation, dislocation, fracture, or any combination of these injuries, depending on the force of the blow. Indirect trauma—from forcing a joint beyond its normal range of motion or causing an abnormal motion of the joint—may result in some degree of sprain, or it may result in a more severe injury, depending on the type, duration, and direction of the force.[11]

Types of trauma to the joints

The mildest form of joint injury is either a simple sprain of the ligaments, the joint capsule, or both with no displacement of articular surfaces. A *sprain* is defined as the partial or complete rupture of the fibers of a ligament. In a first-degree sprain, the mildest form of ligamentous injury, a few fibers are torn but integrity of the ligament is maintained and the joint remains stable. In a second-degree sprain the fibers are torn in sufficient quantity to diminish the ligamentous function, but joint stability is still maintained. Some excessive joint motion is evident when compared with the contralateral joint, and some discomfort is elicited. Complete tearing of fibers with loss of integrity and evidence of joint instability constitutes a third-degree sprain.[11,46]

In more severe injuries there is not only excessive joint motion, but the articular surfaces are also displaced from their normal positions. If there is no contact between the surfaces, the joint is said to be *luxated* or completely dislocated. If there is some contact between articular surfaces, the joint is said to be *subluxated* or partially dislocated. Severe injury can also result in intraarticular fractures or a combination of a fracture and a dislocation.[46]

Acute inflammation in the joint demonstrates the same characteristic cellular responses of inflammation (the accumulation of fluid and leukocytes in extravascular tissue) seen in other body cavities or tissues. Upon injury to the joint, chemical, metabolic, and vascular changes occur, resulting in increased vascular permeability, leukocyte infiltration, and cellular repair.[28,54] The goal of the inflammatory process is to rid the area of the results of the injury such as cellular debris and necrotic tissues, which may be accompanied by bacteria or toxins in the presence of a penetrating wound, and to promote repair.

Effects of trauma

Trauma causes both direct and secondary injury. Trauma, whether produced by a blow or by stretching and tearing of joint tissues, results in direct damage to the cells of both structural tissues (muscles, tendons, and ligaments) and associated tissues (nerves, capillaries, and blood vessels). The torn vessels allow bleeding into the interstitial spaces of the injured area. The release of cellular debris and exposure of the subcellular matrix promote adhesion and activation of blood platelets. The activated platelets not only form a platelet plug in an effort to contain the bleeding but also provide a surface for the activation of the classic clotting cascade, resulting in the stabilization of the clot by the deposition of insoluble fibrin matrix. The result is the formation of a hematoma.

Also as a result of trauma, tissue cells undergo structural changes that may lead to cell death. When cells degenerate, they release substances capable of producing vascular changes. These substances, known as vasoactive amines, include *serotonin* and *histamine* (which are also released from the activated blood platelet), which cause rapid increases in vascular permeability. This effect occurs rapidly after exposure and is usually reversible and short-lived (15 to 30 minutes). The endothelial cells in the vessel wall contract, leaving gaps through which fluid and blood cells can escape. While blood vessels that are torn by the initial injury allow hemorrhage into the immediate area, increased permeability occurs in nondisrupted blood vessels in the areas adjacent to the injury. The increase in permeability results in the passage of plasma proteins, colloids, and water, primarily from the venules, into the interstitial spaces, producing swelling and edema.[52] Within the blood vessel, the result is an increase in the concentration of red and white cells and an increase in viscosity of the blood, producing a slowing of blood flow. The histamine-mediated response is an immediate reaction to injury that appears within minutes and wanes within hours. Additionally, products of the

coagulation cascade activated during clot formation, specifically fibrinopeptides, can induce immediate increases in vascular permeability.

In contrast, cytokines such as interleukin-1 and tumor necrosis factor (α and β) and the interleukin-8 family produce prolonged permeability by inducing structural changes in the endothelial cells, causing retraction of the cells or cell death and detachment. These changes are mostly regulated at the level of gene transcription and are referred to as endothelial activation. These effects have a delayed onset (4 hours or more post injury) and may last 24 hours or more.[22,52]

The goal of the postinjury vascular events is to mobilize and transport the defense components of the blood—the white blood cells or leukocytes—to the injury site. For the white cells or leukocytes that circulate in the vascular system to move to the site of injury, the cells must exit the bloodstream and enter and transit through the extracellular spaces of the tissue. The first step by which this movement is accomplished is *margination,* or the process by which the cells in the middle of the flowing blood move to the side of the stream, contact the endothelial lining of the vessel, and adhere to the endothelial cell.[21] Margination is facilitated by the slowing of blood flow in the area of the injury as a result of the fluid movement into the tissue. The adhesion of the leukocytes to the endothelial cell is mediated by the binding of complementary adhesion molecules on the leukocyte and the endothelial cell surface (a lock and key interaction similar to the recognition of antibody and antigen). The expression of the binding sites has been shown to be mediated by the cytokines, tumor necrosis factor, and interleukin-1. The physiologic importance of the leukocyte and endothelial adhesion molecules in this process has been illustrated by the characterization of clinical genetic deficiencies in the leukocyte adhesion proteins. In these patients, the leukocytes do not migrate to sites of injury and infections are a serious clinical problem.[3,18]

The second step is transmigration or *diapedesis* in which the leukocyte inserts the leading foot or pseudopod into the junction between two endothelial cells and moves through the vascular wall into the extravascular space. The third step is the migration through the extravascular space toward the site of injury. Directed movement toward the site of injury is a process known as *chemotaxis,* which is simply defined as locomotion oriented along a chemical gradient.[52] A number of different chemical substances in the tissues cause the leukocytes to move either toward or away from the source of the chemical. Degenerative products of injured tissues, especially tissue polysaccharides, platelet factor 4 (released from the activated blood platelet) cytokines, and components of the complement system, can cause white blood cells to move toward the area of inflammation. Chemotaxis depends on the existence of a concentration gradient of the chemotaxic substance. The concentration is greatest near the source, and as the substance spreads by diffusion from the source, its concentration decreases approximately in proportion to the square of the distance. Therefore, the concentration of the chemotactic substance is greater on one side of the white blood cell than on the other. Binding of the chemotactic agent to specific receptors on the cell surface activate the cell to assemble contractile elements that are responsible for cell movement. This results in the extension of a pseudopodia toward the source of the substance.[63]

Phagocytosis

When the white blood cells arrive at the site of injury, they begin the process of removing the cellular debris caused by the injury. This cleanup is accomplished by *phagocytosis.* In early acute inflammation, the predominant leukocyte type involved in this process is the polymorphonuclear leukocyte PMN, while the monocyte is the predominant cell type present in chronic inflammation (longer than 48 hours).

PMNs, which compose 60% to 70% of the circulating white cells, are formed in the bone marrow and released to peripheral circulation in the bloodstream. The lungs are known to be a large reservoir due to the extensive vascularization of the tissue. The PMNs *marginate* or park in the lungs and are mobilized (or demarginated) under a variety of conditions including stress, acute infection, or strenuous exercise. In chronic inflammation, especially that associated with infection, other factors increase the rate of maturation and release of the neutrophil cells from the bone marrow. This can be seen by the increase in white blood cell count as a component of a total blood count (e.g., CBC or hemogram).

Neutrophils entering the tissues are already mature cells that can immediately begin phagocytosis. On approaching a particle to be phagocytized, the neutrophil projects pseudopodia to surround the particle. When the pseudopodial leading edges meet, they fuse, encapsulating the particle with membrane. The capsule then invaginates into the inside of the cellullar cytoplasmic cavity, and the portion of the cellullar outer membrane that surrounds the phagocytized particle breaks away from the outer membrane to form a free-floating phagocytic vesicle in the cytoplasm of the neutrophil. Once a particle has been phagocytized, lysosomes in the cell move into contact with the phagocytic vesicle and their membranes fuse. Acid hydrolase enzymes contained within the lysosomes are released into the phagocytic vesicle. The digestion of the phagocytized particle begins. Neutrophils and macrophages both have an abundance of lysosomes filled with proteolytic enzymes especially designed for digesting bacteria, cellular proteins released upon necrosis, and other protein matter recognized as foreign matter.

Monocytes compose about 5% of white blood cells in the peripheral circulation. They are released from the bone marrow as immature cells. In addition to circulating in the bloodstream, they often migrate into the interstitial spaces and take up residence as tissue histiocytes. Alternately, under the influence of a chemotactic stimuli, monocytes will migrate into the tissues and mature into *macrophages.* The macrophage is five times larger than the immature monocyte form and contains large numbers of lysosomes. The macrophages are more efficient than neutrophils in cleaning up the injury site, often engulfing as many as 100 bacteria each before undergoing necrosis. They also have the ability to engulf much larger particles including whole red blood cells and necrotic tissue. The monocyte is the predominant cell type under conditions of chronic inflammation.[52]

Obviously, the neutrophils and macrophages must be selective in the target for phagocytosis; otherwise, some of the normal tissues would be ingested. The process of phagocytosis is enhanced by two factors. Most natural substances of the body have electronegative surface charges; so they repel the phagocytes, which also carry electronegative surface charges. Dead tissue and foreign particles, on the other hand, are usually electropositive, making them more susceptible to phagocytosis. Microorganisms are not recognized efficiently unless they are coated with *opsonins,* which are factors found in normal plasma. The two major opsonins are a fragment of immunoglobulin G (IgG) and opsonic fragment of C3 generated by the activation of the complement system.

When an injury occurs and results in damage to the cells, the first cells to respond are the tissue histiocytes, which are monocytes that have migrated into the tissue under normal conditions (noninflammatory) and have become attached in the subcellular matrix. The release of chemotactic stimuli from the injured tissues stimulates the histiocytes to release from the point of attachment and migrate to the site of injury. They are few in number but provide the primary response within the first hour. The first motile white blood cells to arrive are the neutrophils. Contribution of the neutrophils reaches maximum between 6 and 12 hours. At that point, large numbers of monocytes have begun to enter the tissue. The monocytes evolve into macrophages and begin the process of phagocytizing cellular debris (injured tissue as well as the remains of the exhausted neutrophils), fibrin, red blood cells, and any other particles, clearing the joint space for repair.

While the inflammatory response to trauma in a joint cavity is the physiologic process for the removal of damaged tissue and of toxic or foreign materials, prolonged continuation of this response may also cause damage to surrounding joint structures. The process of chemotaxis and phagocytosis results in the release of products within the phagocytic vesicle and into the extracellular space. The most important of these materials are lysosomal enzymes, oxygen-derived metabolites, and products of arachidonic acid metabolism. All of these products can produce injury to normal tissues and thereby increase the inflammatory stimulus. Therefore, if the inflammatory process is not curtailed, the leukocyte infiltration becomes the injurious agent. Leukocyte-dependent tissue injury is a significant hallmark of several inflammatory diseases such as rheumatoid arthritis.

Repair

The healing process begins very early during inflammation. As early as 24 hours, while the macrophages are continuing the cleanup of the injured areas, fibroblasts and vascular endothelial cells begin proliferating. New vessels sprout from existing vessels to bring new blood supply to healing tissue. The immature vessels are leaky, which prolongs the edematous condition of the injury site. Fibroblasts secrete collagens, elastin, and proteoglycans into the healing wound to provide extracellular support to the regenerating tissues. Repair of the injured tissue occurs by two distinct processes, which are *regeneration,* the formation of new tissue of the same type as the old with no evidence of injury or *replacement,* in which connective tissue replaces the normal cell type producing a scar formation. The type of repair is determined by the type of tissue involved in the injury and the extent of the injury. The cells of the body can be classified into one of three types: (1) labile cells, which are continually growing and exfoliating such as squamous cells, lining mucousa, and columnar cells of the gastrointestinal tract; (2) stable cells, which demonstrate a low level of normal replication but can be stimulated to a rapid reconstitution such as fibroblasts, smooth-muscle cells, and vascular endothelial cells; and (3) permanent cells, which have limited capacity for regeneration such as neurons and skeletal and cardiac muscle cells.[52]

It is possible for there to be four outcomes of the inflammatory process: (1) resolution when the injury is limited and short-lived, (2) replacement occurs with the normal cell type being replaced by connective tissue (fibrosis), (3) the formation of an abcess, which occurs primarily when infection is present, and (4) the progression to chronic inflammation, which may be influenced by persistent injury or predisposing factors in the individual's general condition.

Other factors known to influence the inflammatory/healing process include nutritional status, diabetes, use of corticosteroids, hematologic diseases such as a deficiency of neutrophils *(neutropenia),* or defects in leukocyte function such as chemotaxis and phagocytosis. All of these conditions can prolong healing and increase the likelihood of infection or chronic inflammation. Another significant influence on the healing process is the location of injury. Under circumstances where extensive exudates fill the spaces but there is no associated necrosis of the tissue, healing can be initiated by the digestion of the exudate (initiated by the proteolytic enzymes released by the neutrophils and macrophages) and subsequent reabsorption of the exudate. This process of resolution of injury may be observed in peritoneal and pleural cavities and in joint spaces. However, it is more common for healing to involve some level of tissue necrosis resulting in a degree of connective tissue proliferation and scarring. The amount of exudate present is directly related to the total healing time. If the size and amount of exudate can be minimized, the total healing time is decreased.[28]

THE SYNOVIAL MEMBRANE

The synovial membrane, also referred to as the synovium, represents a condensation of connective tissue that covers the inner surface of the fibrous capsule and forms a sac enclosing the synovial cavity. The synovial membrane invests tendons that pass through the joint as well as the free margins of intraarticular structures, such as ligaments and menisci. The synovium is thrown into folds that surround

---

Clinical application

When one suffers an inversion injury to the ankle, the anterior talofibular ligament is frequently sprained. There may be involvement of other ligamentous tissues. Direct damage to the ligament occurs and initiates the inflammation process. Structural damage to the ligament is accompanied by damage to blood vessels and capillaries. Hemorrhaging occurs, which allows fluid composed of cellular debris, enzymes, and red blood cells to fill the interstitial spaces. In the case of the ankle, this includes the joint space as well as the sinus tarsi. If the process is allowed to continue unchecked, increased permeability to larger fluid particles forces a reversal of the normal reabsorption process and may lead to further edema. Repair follows the tissue damage and phagocytosis periods of inflammation but can only occur after inflammatory debris has been destroyed or removed.[16,19,51]

This is where the clinical physical therapist's choice of modality becomes critical. The use of cryotherapy is well accepted as a tool to reduce and prevent edema. Cryotherapy in the form of ice packs, cold packs, ice massage, and cold whirlpool are readily available. Cryotherapy in the form of intermittent compression devices is also available.[10,51]

In addition to cryotherapy, compression has been found to help control edema by increasing hydrostatic pressure within the interstitial fluid. Fluid is forced toward areas of lower hydrostatic pressure in the capillaries and lymph vessels. Compression can be applied via elastic bandages, mechanical intermittent compression units, elastic or neoprene sleeves, taping techniques, stockinette, or soft cast.[10,34,51,68] Elevation of the injured limb has been shown to be an effective method of reducing the edema, which can limit healing. Elevation of the edematous area above the heart facilitates fluid return.[10,51]

Rest is also considered an important tool used to reduce edema. Rest is defined as limiting motion and function in a way that helps the client avoid movements that are painful and that can cause reinjury to fragile healing tissue. Rest can be augmented by bracing, taping, and orthotics that limit injury producing motions.[10,51]

the margin of the articular cartilage, but it does not cover the bearing surface of the cartilage.[7,51] In joints where the fibrous membrane of the capsule attaches some distance from the edges of the articular cartilage, the synovial membrane leaves the fibrous layer to be reflected back along the periosteum to the edge of the cartilage (Fig. 4-2).[24]

Morphology

Recent research on the synovial membrane has concentrated on its cellular structure, with emphasis on the cells found lining the inner synovial surface. The lining cells, called *synoviocytes,* are not in close proximity to each other, and there is no basement membrane separating the cells from subjacent cells and capillaries.[53,58] Cell processes that may interdigitate project from the cells toward the surface. Thin branching filaments, probably of reticular origin, rather than collagen fibers (which are usually absent), appear to serve as a supportive membrane for the cells.[31] This makes the synovium different in character from the mesothelium found lining the major serous cavities (pleural, pericardial, and peritoneal). The cellular lining of the joint cavity is therefore discontinuous; the interior of a synovial joint should be looked upon as a large tissue space rather than as a membrane-lined cavity.[7]

The absence of a basement membrane in the synovium ensures a continuation of morphology as well as function. The change from the highly cellular outer synovial lining to the subsynovial layer, which is relatively acellular and formed to thick intertwining bands of collagen fibers, is not abrupt. The cells below the synovial layer resemble lining cells, but there is more connective tissue. Underlying these, the cells appear more fibroblastic. Next, fat cells increase in number, and larger blood vessels are seen. Then dense bands of collagen appear. The ligaments that span joints and confer stability on them are continuous with the outer layers of the capsule in many joints.[26]

Synovial lining or intima

The synovium can be divided into two layers: (1) the *intima* or synovial lining and (2) the *subsynovial tissue.*[26,32] The intimal portion of the synovial membrane consists of a layer of specialized fibroblasts known as synoviocytes, averaging one to three cells in depth (Fig. 4-3). These cells must be able to synthesize hyaluronic acid, which becomes a major component of synovial fluid. They must also be able to phagocytize particulate debris and pinocytize soluble products of cellular and macromolecular catabolism. The debris diffuses through the synovial fluid to the borders of the joint space. (*Pinocytosis,* a process similar to phagocytosis, refers to the uptake of extracellular fluid and solutes into membrane-bound vesicles.)

The normal synovial lining is a thin, fine, cellular aggregate overlying more dense subsynovial and capsular connective tissue. Grossly, the synovial membrane presents

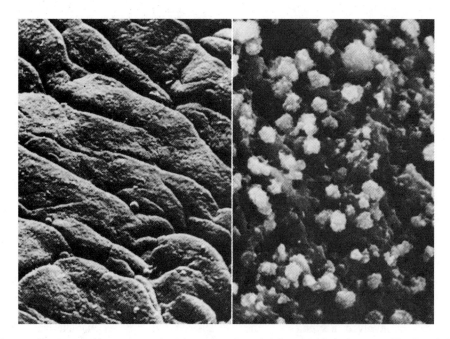

Fig. 4-2. Near normal human synovium (scanning electron microscopy). At low magnification *(left),* the surface topography is arranged in a series of shallow folds that are capable of expanding during joint movement. At higher magnification *(right),* individual synoviocytes are seen randomly distributed over the synovial surface. They are separated by wide areas, appear to be partially embedded within the intercellular matrix, and their surface exhibits folds and projections—the morphological expression of pinocytotic activity. (Courtesy Dr. C.R. Wynne-Roberts. Reprinted from *The primer of the rheumatic diseases,* ed 8, copyright 1983, The Arthritis Foundation.)

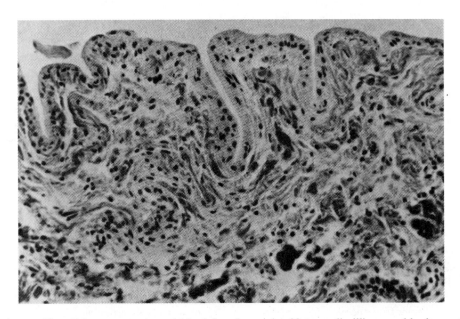

Fig. 4-3. Normal human synovium obtained from knee joint. Note small villi covered by layer of specialized synovial lining cells (synoviocytes), one to three cells in depth. The more superficial portion of the lining (stratum synoviale) consists of loosely textured, fibrous, connective tissue containing numerous capillaries, while the deeper portion approaching the capsule (stratum fibrosum or subsynovialis) is made up of more compact fibrous tissue. (Courtesy Dr. C.R. Wynne-Roberts. Reprinted from *The primer of the rheumatic diseases,* ed 8, copyright 1983, The Arthritis Foundation.)

a relatively smooth surface with a variable number of villi and folds that project into the joint cavity and that are especially numerous in the region near the attachment of the capsule.[7,26,56] The normal membrane rarely contains blood vessels visible to the naked eye; these appear only when inflammation is present.[26]

Type A and B cells

Electron microscopy of the synovial lining cells reveals two functional types of cells based on ultrastructural and cytochemical characteristics.[7,46,57] *Type A cells,* which are more numerous, contain many mitochondria and are characterized by the presence of a richly variegated collection of cytoplasmic organelles, including lysosomes, smooth-walled vacuoles, and micropinocytic vesicles. They have a prominent Golgi complex situated near the apical aspect of the nucleus. Frequently, the cell processes stretching into the adjacent matrix are seen. Type A cells have little endoplasmic reticulum and are active in phagocytosis and secretion (Figs. 4-4 and 4-5). *Type B cells* possess an abundant endoplasmic reticulum and Golgi apparatus but relatively few mitochondria, vacuoles, vesicles, and cell processes. These cells are believed to be involved in synthesis of the hyaluronoprotein of synovial fluid (Figs. 4-5 and 4-6).[7,26,58]

However, attributing distinct functions to the A and B cells may be an oversimplification. It ignores the fact that one cell may have more than one function and that, in response to different stimuli, cells can modulate their internal structure as their function changes. A number of observations support this view:

1. *Type C cells,* representing an intermediate type of cell, have been described. They have both an endoplasmic reticulum and Golgi complexes and vacuoles (Fig. 4-7).
2. The use of stains for RNA on ribosomes (an acceptable index of synthetic function in cells) indicates that only a few cells stain positively in the normal synovium. Staining increases in intensity and appears in an increased number of cells only if a joint has been traumatized, and in severe inflammatory states no cells without a developed endoplasmic reticulum are observed.
3. Synovial cells, which appear morphologically to be fibroblasts, will nevertheless demonstrate macrophage-like function in response to certain stimuli.
4. Evidence suggesting that type A cells may synthesize and secrete hyaluronic acid is mounting. The most convincing data are demonstrations by ultrastructural studies that hyaluronic acid is found both in the Golgi complex and in large secretory vacuoles of these cells.[26]

It may be reasonable to consider the synovial lining cell as one with multiple phenotypical possibilities and to resist categorizing it by its morphological resemblance at certain stages to other, better characterized cells. The A and B cells probably represent different functional phases of the same basic cell structure.[7,26,53]

Subsynovial tissue

Beneath the synovial lining is a loose meshwork of richly vascularized fibrous connective tissue, known as *subsynovial tissue.* The cells of this tissue are more spindle-shaped

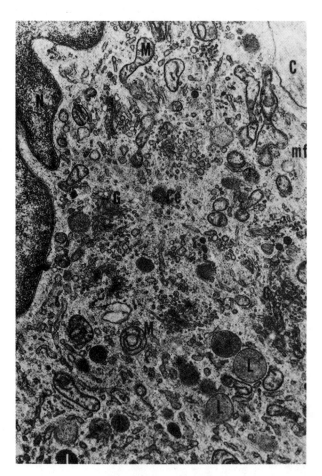

Fig. 4-4. Human syovium, type A cell. Cytoplasm of a type A synoviocyte demonstrating nucleus *(N)*, mitochondria *(M)*, a small centriole cut in cross section *(Ce)*, and several lysosomes *(L)*. The Golgi apparatus *(G)* is extensive and consists of lamellae and vesicles occurring in groups. Interspersed between the cytoplasmic organelles are fine microfilaments *(mf)*, and outside this cell lie a few collagen fibrils *(C)*. (Courtesy Dr. C.R. Wynne-Roberts. Reprinted from *The primer of the rheumatic diseases,* ed 8, copyright 1983, The Arthritis Foundation.)

than the lining cells and are spaced farther apart amid collagen fibrils, some fatty tissue, and a fine capillary network. These cells produce matrix collagen in moderate quantities. This subintimal portion of the synovial membrane differs in thickness and appearance from place to place within joints, being variously more or less fibrous, fatty, or areolar with elements of the reticuloendothelial system interspersed. This layer merges with the periosteum covering the bony components of the joint that lie within the confines of the capsule. At the margin of the articular cartilage, the conjoined tissue becomes continuous with the cartilage by means of a transitional zone of fibrocartilage.[7,26,32]

The synovium is richly endowed with a network of capillary vessels in the subsynovial layer. The vessels include some with thin walls and fenestrations that are adapted for rapid exchange of fluid and solutes (Fig. 4-8). Other vessels have thick walls with endothelial cells that can separate, producing gaps for the escape of cells and large

particles.[4] Because there is no basement membrane separating the lining cells from the capillaries, the exchange of waste products and nutrients is facilitated (Fig. 4-9).[70]

The subsynovial layer is also supplied with lymphatics and nerve fibers. The nerve endings are few and are mostly in the capsule surrounding the outside of the synovial membrane.[55]

Functions

The synovium supports the normal joint in at least three physiological ways:

1. It provides a low-friction lining in itself and produces hyaluronic acid, which is the mucin component of synovial fluid.
2. It transports needed nutrients into the joint space while it removes metabolic wastes through its capillary and lymphatic systems.
3. It plays an important role in maintaining joint stability.

In addition, the membrane, as a whole, regulates the entry of nutrients into the synovial fluid and inhibits the entry of serum proteins. The plasma in the capillaries is the source from which the dialysate fraction of the synovial fluid (synovial fluid except for hyaluronate) is derived, and the type A cells help keep the joint clear of debris by their phagocytic action.[57,64,70]

Joint lubrication

Motion is the main function of synovial joints. This means the synovium must be able to adapt to the full range of positions permitted by the surrounding tendons, ligaments, and joint capsule. When a joint flexes and extends, for example, the synovium must correspondingly expand and contract. This process appears to be more consistent with a folding and unfolding than with an elastic stretching of the tissue.[57]

This expansion and contraction of the synovium takes place over unopposed surfaces of articular cartilage. For any joint to function as more than a simple pivot, there must be a disparity in the configuration of the surface areas of opposing cartilages. When the joint moves, the smaller area glides across or around the larger one. Cartilage not in contact with opposing cartilage will be temporarily covered by the synovium. As the cartilaginous surfaces return to their original positions, an effective lubrication system must prevent pinching of the highly vascular synovial tissue. Were this system to fail, repeated hemarthroses would rapidly incapacitate the affected individual. The hyaluronate molecules that render synovial fluid viscous may find their major role in lubricating the synovium, thus permitting the tremendous changes of internal geometry that occur within synovial joints during normal activity. This process is easiest when the volume of synovial tissue and fluid is at a minimum, because the synovium must expand and contract within the confines of the joint capsule.[57]

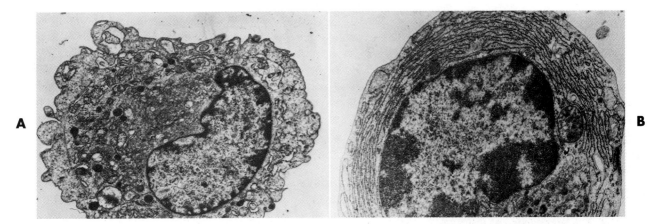

Fig. 4-5. A, Type A human synovial cell with many undulations in the cell membrane, vacuoles, and inclusions. This cell presumably has phagocytic capabilities and is thought of as a macrophage (× 11,200.) **B,** Type B human synovial cell with a very well-developed endoplasmic reticulum. This cell presumably has capabilities for synthesis of protein (× 17,500.) It must be emphasized that there are many synovial cells with organelles developed for both synthetic and phagocytic function. In addition, it is possible that individual cells may be modulated from cells with synthetic function to ones with phagocytic function. (From Kelley W, Harris ED, Ruddy S et al: *Textbook of rheumatology,* Philadelphia, 1981, WB Saunders.

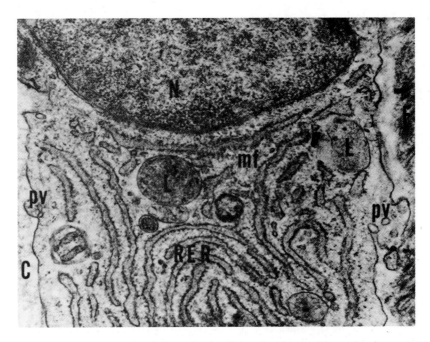

Fig. 4-6. Human syovium, type B cell. Part of a type B (synthetic) synoviocyte showing nucleus *(N),* well-developed lamellae of rough endoplasmic reticulum *(RER),* lysosomes *(L),* a few pinocytotic vesicles at the edge of the cell *(pv),* and a small group of microfilaments *(mf).* Some fibrin *(F)* and a small amount of collagen *(C)* lie outside the cell. (Courtesy Dr. C.R. Wynne-Roberts. Reprinted from *The primer of the rheumatic diseases,* ed 8, copyright 1983, The Arthritis Foundation.)

Synovial transport. Synovial permeability or transfer of molecules across the synovium involves two processes— passage through an endothelial wall as well as diffusion through the intercellular spaces of the synovial membrane. After leaving the vessels, all molecules must traverse the synovial interstitium before they enter the synovial fluid. The tissue space appears to offer the most significant resistance, limiting the overall transsynovial exchange of most small molecules. For most compounds, synovial permeability is inversely related to the size of the permeant molecule. This proportionality suggests that most small molecules cross the synovium by a process of free diffusion. A specific transport system accelerates the entrance of glucose into normal joints, probably by facilitated diffusion. In the case of proteins, the microvascular endothelium is probably the major barrier blocking equilibration of plasma and synovial fluid protein

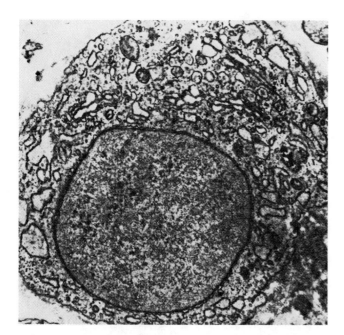

Fig. 4-7. Normal synovial cell, showing both prominent Golgi systems and abundant rough endoplasmic reticulum (intermediate type). (From Roy S, Ghadially FN, Crane WAJ: *Ann Rheum Dis* 25:259, 1966.)

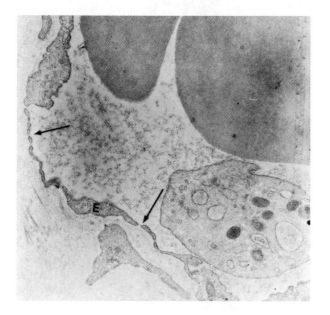

Fig. 4-8. Normal superficial synovial blood vessel. The endothelium *(E)* is thin and in some regions contains fenestrations *(arrows)* bridged only by a very thin diaphragm. (Electron micrograph.) (From Schumacker HR: *J Sports Med* 3:108, 1975.)

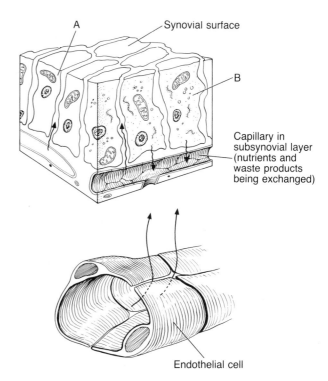

Fig. 4-9. Schematic representation of synovium. *A,* macrophage type of cell. *B,* hyaluronate-synthesizing type of cell. (From Sledge CB: *Orthop Clin North Am* 6[3]:619, 1975.)

Role in joint stability. Only a film of synovial fluid separates the moving surfaces in normal joints. The intraarticular cavity is primarily a potential space with a subatmospheric intracavity pressure. Several investigators have actually measured intraarticular pressures in normal knee joints, with the average pressure being -4 mm Hg.[57]

This pressure differential may play a significant role in stabilizing joints. In concert with the action of tendons and ligaments, the suction will draw articulating surfaces into the best possible fit and will help to guide the surface contacts as the joint moves through its range of motion. Simple atmospheric pressure, aided by the surface tension of synovial fluid, is able to contribute tremendously to the stabilization and congruent articulation of large joints, especially in the shoulder and hip, where ligaments play only a minor role in maintaining joint stability.[57]

THE SYNOVIAL MEMBRANE AND ITS REACTION TO INJURY

The basic inflammatory response in the synovial membrane is a proliferation of the surface cells, an increase in vascularity, and a gradual fibrosis of the subsynovial tissue. This can be seen as a gross thickening and development of a granular surface, while the effect of the changes is seen as an alteration of the synovial fluid.[31,46]

Posttraumatic synovitis

A clinical entity known as *posttraumatic synovitis* can be differentiated from other inflammatory and degenerative

(plasma contains large molecules, which are excluded from synovial fluid). In normal joints there is continual turnover of synovial fluid proteins. In contrast to the selectivity shown for entering proteins, all large molecules appear to leave the joints at equal rates. This clearance is thought to occur by lymphatic drainage.[57]

changes of the synovial membrane.[61] This represents the simplest response of the synovial membrane to minor trauma, such as might occur from a mild blow or a forced inappropriate movement. If such a simple mechanical disturbance occurs without too much bleeding, the synovial membrane is not microscopically disturbed, but it may have a severe vasomotor reaction. The capillaries of the synovial membrane dilate and filtration increases.[9] Protein leaks into the interstitium. As the extravascular concentration of protein rises toward the plasma level, there is a progressive diminution in the colloid osmotic pressure gradient between the two spaces. Because it is this pressure gradient that normally drives venular reabsorption of water, increased vascular permeability leads to edema in tissues and a traumatic exudate in the joint.[57]

Microscopically, there is only slight hyperemia of the synovial membrane and a slight cellular infiltration around the dilated capillaries. Later, the intima may multiply from three to five layers to eight or ten. This reaction of the synovial membrane disappears very quickly if the trauma occurs only once. The exudate disappears as the protein molecules are cleared by lymphatic drainage and the normal colloid osmotic pressure gradient is restored. The hyperemia lasts the longest but eventually decreases. The synovial lining then decreases to its original size.[9]

If the mechanical irritation is repeated, it can produce a characteristic posttraumatic synovitis. Studies by Bozdech[9] have revealed that, microscopically, the synovial lining becomes thicker and may contain up to 10 to 15 rows of cells. The synovial membrane is more infiltrated with lymphocytes, especially around the vessels, and the deeper cells of the synovial membrane show stronger activity. There is evidence of increased protein synthesis by the synovial cells, perhaps accounting for a portion of the excessive protein content in posttraumatic effusions.

Electron microscopy also reveals changes that occur in A and B cells. There are fewer A cells than are usually present in the normal synovial membrane because the A cells move into the synovial fluid as free macrophages. The synovial lining is also filled with fibroblasts that are usually deeper in the synovial membrane. These fibroblasts change into type B cells. A study by Roy, Ghadially, and Crane[53] confirmed this reversal of the normal A:B cell ratio. Electron microscopy of the remaining cells in the synovial lining revealed that the distinction between type A and B cells was almost completely lost. The majority of cells instead contained rough endoplasmic reticulum in large amounts with dilated cisternae and complex Golgi systems. Of the remaining cells, the majority contained large amounts of rough endoplasmic reticulum (type B cells), while only an occasional cell had abundant Golgi systems and smooth endoplasmic reticulum (type A cells). The general impression was one of marked hyperplasia of the rough endoplasmic reticulum system (Fig. 4-10).

Changes in the synovial fluid, occurring as a result of these alterations in the synovial membrane, will be discussed

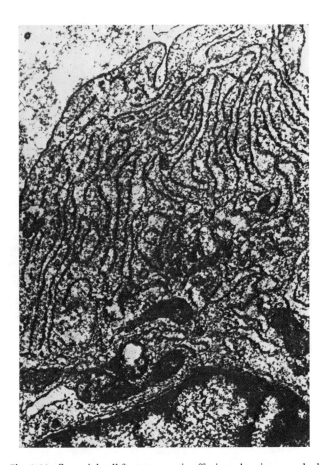

Fig. 4-10. Synovial cell from traumatic effusion, showing a marked hyperplasia of the rough endoplasmic reticulum. (From Roy S, Ghadially FN, Crane WAJ: *Ann Rheum Dis* 25:259, 1966.)

in a following section. After the inflammatory reaction, synovitis can remain reactive for a long time. When the type A macrophages are destroyed by the neutrophils and monocytic macrophages, the latter cells ingest the lysosomes and proteolytic enzymes. The white blood cells, especially the neutrophils, die quickly in the transudate and release proteolytic enzymes. These enzymes attack normal joint structures that are in close approximation. This results in a vicious inflammatory cycle. The process can keep a reactive synovitis alive for some time, even without further trauma.[9]

In studies by Soren et al.[60,61] comparative light-scanning and transmission electron microscopic examinations were carried out in 35 cases in which trauma had occurred at least 4 months previously. In the first 6 months after trauma, a slight hyperplasia of the synovial lining was noted. During this early phase of posttraumatic synovitis, there was only a moderate polymorphy of the synovial cells and enlargement of the synovial surface by closely apposed tentacular cell processes (Fig. 4-11). A progressive sclerosis of the synovial membrane, starting about 4 to 6 months after trauma, was exhaustively demonstrated. A rather particular feature of posttraumatic synovitis became evident in a few instances when *hemosiderin* (the product of phagocytic digestion of iron derived from the blood) was observed and *siderosomes*

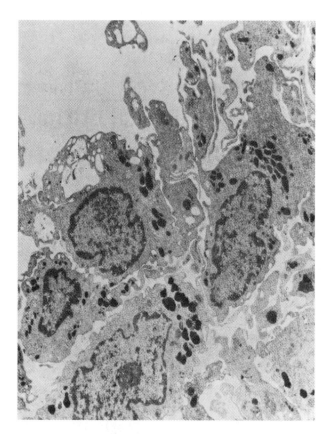

Fig. 4-11. Slightly polymorphic synoviocytes with siderosomes in posttraumatic synovitis. (From Soren A, Klein W, Huth F: *Clin Orthop* 121:191, 1976.)

(cells containing hemosiderin) were detected. The siderosomes were presumably partly dissolved and partly eliminated by the physiological desquamation of synovial cells. Without additional hemorrhages, the siderosomes vanished from the synovial membrane after about 6 months, and proof of previous hemorrhage due to trauma disappeared. However, when posttraumatic joint symptoms continued beyond the first 6 months, a smooth rounding of synovial cells with loss of the tentacular processes was observed. A deviation of the previously outlined course of posttraumatic changes was noted in those cases in which the injury caused either a secondary laxity of ligaments with instability of the knee, hypermobility of the meniscus, or avulsions from the articular surfaces with formation of free joint bodies; these caused a chronic traumatization of the synovial membrane with resulting proliferative synovitis.[61]

Changes in blood vessels may be regarded as relatively characteristic for the posttraumatic reaction of the synovial membrane. In tissues removed in the first 6 to 12 months after trauma, changes usually consisted of swelling of the endothelium, proliferation of adventitial cells and extravasation of erythrocytes (observed by light microscopy), increased phagocytic activity, and formation of siderosomes in the endothelium and perithelium (observed by electron microscopy). With longer duration, sclerosing alterations of the vascular wall occurred, which were not observed as frequently in any other type of synovitis.[50,51] Also, fibrosis of the synovial membrane was noted with formation of mature, densely packed collagen fibrils up to the synovial surface. This sclerosis was associated with atrophy of the remaining synovial cells.[61]

For purposes of diagnosis it should be pointed out that inflammatory cell infiltrates rarely appear in the chronic posttraumatic synovial reaction. Therefore the concept of posttraumatic "synovitis" is justified only with some limitation. Also, aspirates of joint fluid rarely contain a significant increase in the number of inflammatory cells. The chronic posttraumatic joint effusions should be considered not as primarily inflammatory exudates but more probably as a sequel of the progressing sclerotic alterations of the synovial membrane.[61]

Clinically, onset of symptoms in uncomplicated posttraumatic synovitis occurs 12 to 24 hours after the trauma. The effusion is usually not associated with much warmth, erythema, or tenderness. Often the main complaint is a tight sensation. Effusions may linger 1 to 2 weeks.[55] The effusion should be aspirated to determine whether hemarthrosis is present and to aid in further examination of the joint. Hemarthrosis is usually present if fluid appears within 2 hours after injury; in about half the cases, swelling occurs within 15 minutes. With hemarthrosis there is usually more pain and at times a low-grade fever. Fractures, internal derangements, or major ligamentous tears must be ruled out by examination and radiographs, which should include stress, skyline, and intercondylar views. (In one series of clients with traumatic knee joint hemarthrosis, 66 had fractures or ligamentous rupture and 20 did not.)[55] There may be detachment or laceration of cartilage or capsular tears; however, they are not discovered in this manner. It has been suggested, on the basis of calcification that sometimes develops later in the median parapatellar area, that lateral subluxation of the patella and tearing of the medial retinaculum may be the source of joint hemorrhage in some cases.[44]

Minor joint trauma, causing initially slight symptoms that do not require medical care, may nevertheless be responsible for significant symptoms months afterward, even without additional traumatization.[60,61] This can be attributed to the phenomenon of reactive synovitis, which can keep the inflammatory process going for some time.

The subjective tight sensation felt after a joint has been subjected to mild trauma usually results from the presence of a joint effusion that causes the normally negative intraarticular pressure to become positive. Effusions deprive the joint of the stabilizing effects of subatmospheric pressure and substitute instead a distending force that increases stress on ligaments and the joint capsule. In contrast to normal joints, the pressures of effusions are greatest in joints in full flexion and extension, with minimal intraarticular pressures occurring at 30° flexion.[57]

Conservative treatment with application of ice packs (or some other form of cryotherapy), rest, and elevation of the affected joint when possible during the acute inflammatory

Table 4-1. Treatment of posttraumatic synovitis

Time elapsed after injury	Clinical therapeutic techniques	Home management techniques	Medical interventions
21-48 hours	Ice, mechanical intermittent compression, high-voltage galvanic stimulation, isometric exercise, patient education.	Ice, elastic bandage, neoprene sleeve, elevation, isometric exercise.	Analgesics or antiinflammatory medications, diagnostic aspiration of large effusion.
3-5 days	Ice, mechanical intermittent compression, high-voltage galvanic stimulation, contrast bath, isometrics, gentle range of motion exercise in painfree range. See 1-2 times per week.	Ice after activity, elastic bandage/ neoprene sleeve, elevation after activity, isometrics and gentle ROM exercises in painfree range.	Continued use of analgesics or antiinflammatory medications as needed.
5-14 days	Whirlpool, moist heat, functional electrical stimulation, ice after activity, ROM, concentric and eccentric strengthening, PRE, progress to functional activities. See 1-2 times per week.	Moist heat, ROM, concentric/ eccentric strengthening, PRE, functional progression in both open and closed chain activities, ice after activity, compression PRN.	
If symptoms persist >3-4 weeks	Moist heat, functional electrical stimulation, mechanical intermittent compression and exercise may continue. Educate patient to manage at home, recheck biweekly.	Ice, compression, elevation, modification of activities to avoid painful ROM, isometrics, painfree ROM.	Repeated aspirations, corticosteroid injections.
>6-8 Weeks			Possible synovectomy

stage, followed by contrast baths or heat treatment in the form of whirlpools or hot packs, seems to be effective in most cases. Studies have shown that high-voltage galvanic stimulation is also effective in reducing edema, increasing circulation, and increasing tissue healing in acute injuries.[66] Compression dressings or posterior splints are also sometimes helpful. Graded quadriceps muscle exercises, in the case of the knee joint, can help reduce edema by muscle-pumping action, which also minimize muscle atrophy.

It is also important to follow clinical therapeutic sessions with a home program. Clients should augment the clinical sessions with a program to manage edema and speed the healing process while at home. The physical therapist must assume the role of educator to explain the procedures to the patient and teach the techniques to be used at home. This helps the client become more responsible for the rehabilitation and should speed recovery to independent functional ability.

Repeated aspiration after the initial diagnostic aspiration may be necessary if significant volumes of fluid reaccumulate.[44] Analgesics and antiinflammatory medication (e.g., aspirin) can be used. This synovitis is usually self-limiting, but if it continues, intraarticular corticosteroid injections (one to three in number) can be given.[9,55] If the inflammatory process continues and the transudate becomes

more inflammatory, a synovectomy will reduce the symptoms (Table 4-1).[9]

Pigmented villonodular synovitis

The synovium responds in a slightly different manner to recurrent hemarthroses. The most striking feature of synovial response to the injection of blood in experiments by Volz[67] was the production of a proliferative synovitis, known as *pigmented villonodular synovitis*. This synovial reaction was characterized by a villous and nodular hyperplasia of the synovial cells. Long villous projections of synovial tissue were seen extending into the joint. Associated with these changes was a prominent degree of subsynovial fibrosis. Also noted within the subsynovial layer were focal aggregations of round cells arranged in a pattern suggesting germinal follicles. Here and there giant cell formation was noted. Tissue stained with Prussian blue revealed moderate amounts of siderin pigment in the synovial layer (Figs. 4-12 and 4-13). The extent of these histological changes was observed to be roughly proportional to the number of injections of blood within the joint space. In no instance was there any suggestion of an inflammatory response.

Young and Hudacek (as cited by Volz[67] and Boyes),[8] in an experiment with dogs, demonstrated the correlation between blood injected into joints and the production of

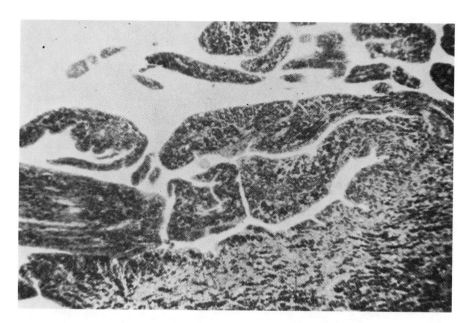

Fig. 4-12. Synovium displaying villonodular proliferative changes. Synovium was processed from a rabbit receiving 30 injections of iron. Note diffusely scattered multinucleated giant cells and siderin pigment. (From Volz R: *Clin Orthop* 45:127, 1966.)

solitary nodular and pigmented villonodular synovitis characterized by an increased vascularity and hyperplasia of the synovium, diffuse depositions of siderin pigment, scattered giant cells, and subsynovial fibrosis. They observed blood clots floating free in the fluid, some of which were attached to the lining surface in varying degrees of organization. They theorized that the nodules were formed by the attachment of blood clots or by fusion of adjacent villi and concluded that once villi are formed, the crushing of the nodule in joint motion may cause additional hemorrhage. Volz,[67] in a study on the effects of repeated experimentally produced hemarthroses on the rate of absorption of blood from the rabbit's knee joint, discovered that the rate of absorption is related to the degree of reactive change in the synovium. The absorption rate after several closely spaced hemarthroses is delayed initially as the synovium finds itself unable to clear the joint of blood. As the synovium proliferates in response to repeated hemarthroses, the rate of absorption of blood markedly increases. With advanced reactive changes after repeated hemarthroses, the rate of absorption becomes greater than normal. The stimulus for the production of the proliferative synovitis would appear to be the iron released from the red blood cells. Iron has been shown to possess definite irritative properties, which attack the synovium and stimulate the production of a villous and a nodular synovitis. The histological features of this condition closely resemble those of pigmented villonodular synovitis.[64]

Solitary nodular synovitis

Cytological findings in *solitary nodular synovitis* are similar to those described for pigmented villonodular synovitis except in the degree of synovial cell proliferation and villous formation. Gross findings in an experiment by

Boyes[8] revealed a solitary pedunculated nodule bathed in a serous effusion with associated lesions of the articular surfaces indicative of direct trauma. Within this vascular lesion were seen four basic cells: the giant cell, a polyhedral stroma cell, the lipophage, and the hemosiderin cell. Beneath the lining membrane of synovial cells in varying degrees of proliferation were masses of chronic inflammatory cells. Fibrin was seen in sheets, interspaced between the stroma cells, and undergoing necrosis.[8]

Regeneration of synovium

Synovial tissue has a remarkable capacity for regeneration, possibly stemming from its excellent blood supply and its origin from a single undifferentiated mesenchymal cell type. Within several months synovium completely regenerates into tissue that is indistinguishable from normal tissue. Synovial regeneration is actually the result of metaplasia of mesenchymal elements within the joint cavity rather than a hyperplasia of the residual synovial cells in the area. Further biochemical studies are needed to determine whether new synovium is metabolically identical to the original tissue.[63]

SYNOVIAL FLUID

Synovial fluid, also called *synovia,* is essentially a dialysate of blood plasma with the addition of proteins and a mucopolysaccharide—hyaluronic acid *(hyaluronate).*[71] The entry of proteins is regulated by the synovial membrane, and the synoviocytes secrete hyaluronate.

Composition and characteristics of synovial fluid

Normal synovial fluid is clear and pale yellow in color. It does not clot because it lacks fibrinogen as well as prothrombin. Synovial fluid is quite sparse in normal joints;

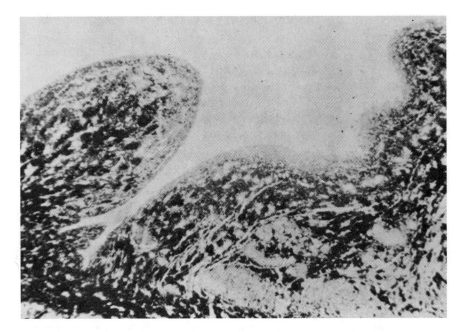

Fig. 4-13. Synovial tissue stained with Prussian blue. Darkly stained areas represent iron pigment deposits. (From Volz R: *Clin Orthop* 45:127, 1966.)

only about 0.5 to 4 ml can be aspirated from large joints, such as the knee. Menisci, intraarticular disks, fat pads, and synovial folds assist in joint lubrication by evenly spreading fluid throughout the joint and taking up dead space, thus economizing on the amount of joint fluid necessary.[64]

Synovial fluid is a viscous substance. Its viscosity is related to the presence of hyaluronoprotein, which is a complex macromolecule containing a large amount of hyaluronic acid. The other constituents of synovial fluid appear to be derived from plasma. Certain larger proteins, including fibrinogen, are normally absent; if present, they are in markedly reduced concentration compared with plasma. Synovial fluid contains slightly less total protein than plasma but has an albumin:globulin ratio of about 4:1.[46] Molecular charge and shape, as well as molecular weight, appear to be important in determining the permeability of the synovium to different plasma proteins.[7]

Synovial fluid normally contains only a few white blood cells, numbering less than 200 per ml.[3] These consist chiefly of mononuclear cells believed to be derived from the lining tissue. Inflammation, trauma, and other pathological processes affecting the system can alter the composition, cellular content, and physical characteristics of synovia. Examination of this fluid plays an important role in the diagnosis of joint problems.[7]

Synovianalysis

Synovianalysis or laboratory examination of synovial fluid serves to divide the fluid into one of five categories: (1) normal, (2) noninflammatory (group I), (3) inflammatory (group II), (4) purulent (group III), or (5) hemorrhagic (group IV). Table 4-2 gives the range of values found for various tests performed on the first four categories.

Table 4-3 lists some of the possible etiologies of the various types of synovial fluid. Trauma produces a noninflammatory (group I) type of synovial fluid, which will be discussed in the next section.[36]

Viscosity of synovial fluid

Synovial fluid exhibits a property common to all mucinous solutions in that its viscosity varies in a non-Newtonian fashion: when the rate of shear is low, it is highly viscous, and as the shear rate increases, the viscosity decreases.[4,16,31] Synovial fluid acts as a viscous fluid in the low-frequency region (corresponding to the slowly moving joint) but assumes the properties of an elastic material in the high-frequency region (corresponding to a rapidly moving joint). Synovial fluid is essentially a liquid whose relaxation time falls in the range between normal motion and motion that is rapid enough to induce trauma.[38]

The viscosity of synovial fluid results from the presence of hyaluronic acid, also called hyaluronate or mucin. Hyaluronate polymerizes into long-chain polysaccharides of high molecular weight and high viscosity.[64] A solution of hyaluronic acid is particularly suitable for lubricating joints required to carry load at varying rates of movement. The viscosity is high at the lowest rates to shear so that the joint is able to support a high load even at a low rate of movement. At higher rates of movement, the viscosity falls so that the drag of the joint is lessened, but the load that it will bear is not reduced because the greater rate of movement more than offsets the fall of viscosity. Hyaluronic acid produces high

Table 4-2. Gross analysis of joint fluid

Criteria	Normal	Noninflammatory (group I)	Inflammatory (group II)	Purulent (group III)
1. Volume (ml) (knee)	<4	Often >4	Often >4	Often >4
2. Color	Clear to pale yellow	Xanthochromic	Xanthochromic to white	White
3. Clarity	Transparent	Transparent	Translucent to opaque	Opaque
4. Viscosity	Very high	High	Low	Very low, may be high with coagulase-positive staphylococci
5. Mucin clot*	Good	Fair to good	Fair to poor	Poor
6. Spontaneous clot	None	Often	Often	Often

From McCarty DJ: Synovial fluid. In McCarty DJ, editor: *Arthritis and allied conditions,* Philadelphia, 1979, Lea & Febiger.
*Recent effusions do not give firm clot because of serum admixture.

Table 4-3. Examples of diseases producing fluids of different groups

Noninflammatory (group I)	Inflammatory* (group II)	Purulent* (group III)	Hemorrhagic (group IV)
Osteoarthritis	Rheumatoid arthritis	Bacterial infections	Trauma, especially fracture
Early rheumatoid arthritis	Reiter's syndrome	Tuberculosis	Neuroarthropathy (Charcot joint)
Trauma	Crystal synovitis, acute (gout and pseudogout)		Blood dyscrasia (e.g., hemophilia)
Osteochondritis dissecans	Psoriatic arthritis		Tumor, especially pigmented villonodular synovitis or hemangioma
Aseptic necrosis	Arthritis of inflammatory bowel disease		
Osteochondromatosis	Viral arthritis		Chondrocalcinosis
Crystal synovitis, chronic or subsiding acute (gout and pseudogout)	Rheumatic fever		Anticoagulant therapy
Systemic lupus erythematosus†			Joint prostheses
Polyarteritis nodosa†			Thrombocytosis
Scleroderma			Sickle cell trait or disease
Amyloidosis (articular)			

From McCarty DJ: Synovial fluid. In McCarty DJ, editor: *Arthritis and allied conditions,* Philadelphia, 1979, Lea & Febiger.
*As disease in these groups remits, the exudate (fluid) passes through a group I phase before returning to normal.
†May occasionally be inflammatory, usually when clinical picture is that of rheumatoid arthritis.

viscosity at a low concentration without a large osmotic effect. These properties result from its high molecular weight and its random chain structure.[40]

Functions of synovial fluid

One of the functions of synovial fluid is to assist in lubrication of the joints. Weight-bearing tends to squeeze lubricant out from between the contacting surfaces of opposing articular cartilages. This is resisted by the tenacious quality of the viscous synovial fluid and by the incongruent surfaces of diarthrodial joints. The latter effect allows contact of adjoining cartilage structures at a limited but changing number of regions as the joint moves through its range of motion. In the intervening area where the fit is not exact, synovial fluid forms films of greater thicknesses. The next result is the creation of a series of wedge-shaped fluid layers that act to force fluid over the entire cartilage surface. Thus a fluid film constantly separates the joint surfaces, thereby holding attrition of joint cartilage to a low level.[47,54] The film is probably composed mainly of hyaluronic acid. The voluminous, randomly coiled particles

may be thought of as being trapped and squeezed, like sponges, between the two articular surfaces (Figs. 4-14 and 4-15).[4,40]

Hyaluronate, besides lubricating the surfaces of the articular cartilage, has been shown to lubricate the periarticular soft tissues. The rubbing surfaces of synovial joints are made up of cartilage, synovial membrane, and soft tissues. The soft tissues around a joint are actually responsible for over 99% of the joint's resistance to movement.[47]

Another function of the synovial fluid is to provide nourishment for about two thirds of the avascular articular cartilage bordering the joint space.[55] (The role of synovial fluid in stabilization of joints has already been indicated.)

SYNOVIAL FLUID AND ITS REACTION TO INJURY

In general, nonhemorrhagic synovial fluids show relatively little change from normal after trauma. Typical fluids, aspirated less than 3 months after injury, are clear and do not clot. The total nucleated cell count is usually below 1000 per mm^3, sugar concentration is essentially the same as that of

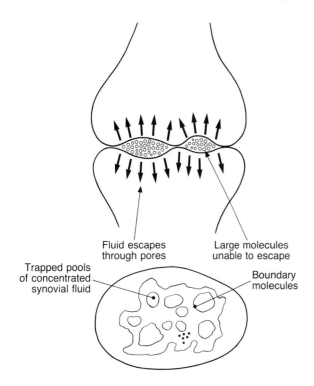

Fig. 4-14. Pictorial representation of the lubrication of cartilage with synovial fluid. (From Dowson D, Wright V, Longfield MD: *Biomed Eng* 4:160, 1969.)

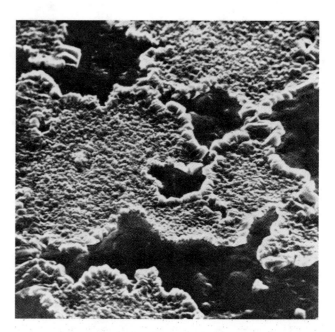

Fig. 4-15. Scanning electron microscope visualization of trapped pools of synovial fluid on the surface of articular cartilage. (From Dowson D, Wright V, Longfield MD: *Biomed Eng* 4:160, 1969.)

serum, and there is good mucin precipitate.[5] In reactive synovitis, the percentage of protein is slightly elevated (from 2.7% to 3.4%), and the number of white blood cells is only slightly increased (from 100 or 150 to 300/mm^3).[5]

Synovial fluid in posttraumatic synovitis

In synovitis of slightly longer duration or in posttraumatic synovitis, there is an increase in the white blood cell count to 600 to 2000/mm^3 (some sources say 5000[10]).[5] The white blood cells, mostly mononuclear macrophages, compose 80% to 90% of all cells. The amount of protein is about the same as mentioned for reactive synovitis. This transudate is typical for posttraumatic synovitis and can be used for diagnosis.[55,62] If the posttraumatic synovitis lasts for a long time, more and more neutrophils are seen in the exudate, where they can reach up to 20% of all cells.

The synovial fluid reflects the inflammatory reactions going on in the synovial membrane. Thus the increased protein is probably derived from the synovial-lining cells, because one of the responses of the synovial membrane to trauma is an increase in type B cells that synthesize protein.[53] Also, as mentioned earlier, entry of small molecules into synovial fluid can be explained by diffusion between synovial-lining cells, whereas factor-limiting protein entry is probably caused by the number and size of the fenestrations in the subsynovial capillaries. With inflammation and increased synovial blood flow, protein entry may often increase out of proportion to the entry of small molecules. Therefore virtually all protein molecules found in plasma

enter the joint; with increasing inflammation their concentration in synovia approaches the concentration of the plasma.[36] There is an increase in synovial fluid volume (often 10 to 20 times normal), resulting from increased production of exudate. The increase in white blood cells is a result of the inflammatory process, and the increase in total cell count also reflects the hypertrophy of the synovial membrane and the migration of type A cells into the synovial fluid.[46] There is also a decrease in viscosity due to a fall in the concentration of hyaluronate.[13]

After minor trauma, the joint shows only increased fluid volume with normal hyaluronic acid concentration and molecular weight. As the severity increases, the rate of fluid transfer to the joint surpasses the synthetic capacity of the synovial lining cells, and hyaluronic acid concentration falls below normal. When the inflammatory process becomes sufficiently disruptive, joint-lining cells not only fail to maintain hyaluronic acid concentration but also fail to maintain normal polymer weight.[13]

Synovial fluid in hemorrhagic effusions

Traumatic effusions that are hemorrhagic present a somewhat different picture. Sugar concentration is generally lower, the total nucleated cell count is higher, and the mucin precipitate is generally poorer. It is not uncommon to find small blood clots in a hemorrhagic effusion, but the majority of the blood remains fluid. Fibrinogen is not found in normal synovial fluid but occurs when there is bleeding into a joint. Because thromboplastic activity is absent or only slight in synovial and fibrous capsular tissue, it appears that local hemostasis after injury to a joint is effected chiefly by activation of the plasma thromboplastic system that enters the joint along with blood after injury.[15] With a grossly bloody fluid, there is the possibility of bleeding diathesis, pigmented villonodular synovitis, or tumor, as well as the suspected trauma. Bone marrow spicules or immature red blood cells in the fluid are often the first clue to a fracture. Blood is absorbed quickly by phagocytic cells in the synovial membrane so that blood may not be evident in the fluid if several days have passed after a hemarthrosis. However, an iron stain may show hemosiderin in synovial cells released into the synovial fluid.[44]

Synovial fluid containing fat globules

A recent traumatic effusion may also contain globules of free fat. When fractures are intracapsular, fat is liberated from the bone marrow; when there is cartilage and ligament injury, fat reaches the joint from the intracapsular, extrasynovial adipose tissue through a tear in the synovium.[6,15] In fractures of the knee, the joint may serve as a reservoir for fat so that the fat is absorbed slowly rather than discharged into the circulation in harmful amounts.[6]

Cloudy synovial fluid

If the aspirated fluid is cloudy, a variety of diseases should be considered. Cloudy fluids are usually caused by leukocytes (although cartilage fragments, crystals, red blood cells, fibrils, and "rice bodies" can occasionally be the cause). Leukocyte counts of greater than 2000 per mm^3 require careful evaluation for evidence of inflammatory joint diseases, such as gouty arthritis and rheumatoid arthritis. In the young, one should especially consider Reiter's syndrome, ankylosing spondylitis or colitis, viral or bacterial arthritis, as well as the collagen vascular diseases. Commonly, persons in the early stage of rheumatic disease associate the first swollen joint with trauma. Trauma can be shown to accentuate the severity of experimentally induced arthritis in rats and dogs.[55]

Reabsorption of traumatic effusions

The rate of absorption of solutions from the joint space is inversely proportional to the size of the particles—the larger the molecules, the slower the clearance. Diffusion and absorption are increased if the synovial fluid pressure is increased by intraarticular injection or movement. Small molecules are rapidly removed by osmosis and diffusion via the blood capillaries. Lymphatics remove larger molecules, such as proteins and colloidal solutions, from the joint space with minimal aid from the blood vessels. Solutions have been shown to be removed within a few hours from the knee joint of rabbits, but colloid particles larger than the globulin molecule, such as carbon, require up to 10 days to be removed by the regional lymphatics.[64] These larger particles are often ultimately deposited in the regional lymph nodes on the flexor surface of the joint. Large particles, such as iron and bismuth, are removed from the joint space and deposited in the subsynovial tissues where they remain. Clinically, absorption from a joint is increased by active or pas-

sive range of motion exercises, massage, and injections of intraarticular hydrocortisone for acute inflammation, whereas the effect of external compression is variable.[64]

THE JOINT CAPSULE
Composition

The joint capsule consists of two parts—*the stratum fibrosum* and the *stratum synoviale.* The outer layer (stratum fibrosum) is made up of dense fibrous connective tissue.[7,24] Specific thickenings, *ligaments,* may be contained within this part of the capsule. The ligaments assist the external musculature in maintaining the joint's mechanical integrity. The ligaments along with the rest of the joint capsule securely join the bones forming the articulation and serve to maintain the bones in apposition and influence the range of joint movement.[46] The stratum fibrosum also serves to protect and enclose the finely structured synovial membrane that lies within it.

Although there is some variation, the periarticular ligaments and capsule are fairly uniform in histological appearance, chemical composition, and tissue organization. The structures consist principally of parallel bundles or fascicles of collagen, sparsely populated with fibrocytes. Blood vessels traverse a tortuous course between the fascicles, and an occasional nerve fiber is noted, most frequently perivascular but occasionally free in the ligament or capsule. Together the fibrous proteins (collagen and elastin) account for 90% of the dry weight of the tissue.[28,59] The tough outer layer blends into the perichondrium and periosteum but does not extend over the surface of the articular cartilage within the joint. The ligaments and fibrous tissue are firmly united to the bone by collagen fibers, demonstrating a zonal organization. Parallel bundles of collagen first become invested with a fibrocartilaginous stroma and, as they near the bone, become calcified. The collagen fibers, continuous with the ligament, then enter the cortical osseous tissue in a manner analogous to Sharpey's fibers. The gradual transition of ligaments to mineralized fibrocartilage and then to bone enhances the ability of the insertions to distribute forces evenly.[32,46] The inner layer (stratum synoviale) consists of loose, highly vascularized tissue—the synovium (discussed in the first section of this chapter).[7,24]

Some joints are partially or completely subdivided by fibrocartilaginous disks or menisci that are attached at their periphery to the fibrous capsule. Fascia and other periarticular connective tissues blend with the joint capsule, adjacent ligaments, and the musculotendinous structures that pass over the joint, as well as investing the nerves and blood vessels entering the joint.[7]

Nerve and blood supply

The blood supply of the joint arises from vessels that enter the subchondral bone at or near the line of capsular attachment and form an arterial circle around the joint. These vessels subdivide into a rich capillary network that is especially prominent in the portions of the synovium immediately adjacent to the joint cavity.[7] Both capsules and ligaments have a poor blood supply but a very rich nerve supply with proprioceptive and pain endings.[37] Articular nerves carry both fibers derived from several spinal segments and autonomic and sensory fibers. The larger sensory fibers form proprioceptive endings that are sensitive to position and movement. Most of the smaller sensory fibers terminate in pain endings in the capsule, ligaments, and adventitia of blood vessels. The free nerve endings are particularly sensitive to twisting and stretching of these structures.[7] The capsule is thus the most generally receptive component of the joint tissues and is particularly sensitive to being stretched.[7] However, pain arising from the capsule or the synovium tends to be diffuse and poorly localized.[7]

Functions

Several functions of the joint capsule have already been mentioned. The stratum fibrosum, especially the ligaments, aids in holding together the bones that compose the joint. Besides maintaining the bones in alignment, the ligaments serve to check movement occurring at a joint. Ligaments and capsular structures vary considerably in thickness and position, depending on the joint studied and the site within that joint. Structures range from the thin, redundant capsule of the shoulder joint to the thick, collagenous collateral ligament of the knee. In some joints, ligaments are condensations within the capsule, while in others, they are discretely separated from the capsule by an areolar layer. Capsular redundancy is an important aspect of joint function, particu-

larly in relation to range of motion. The inferior medial portion of the shoulder joint capsule is a loose, redundant sac that becomes tense only when the shoulder is fully abducted or flexed. The posterior capsule of the knee is loose in flexion but so tight in extension that it becomes an important stabilizer. Ligaments that check movements often do so as the joint reaches the most stable position, and, as a consequence of being taut at that point, they frequently play a very important role in stabilizing the joint. Ligaments also sometimes guide movement at the joints. The stratum fibrosum protects and encloses the synovial membrane. The function of the stratum synoviale or the synovium has already been discussed.

THE JOINT CAPSULE AND ITS REACTION TO INJURY

The fibrous joint capsule reacts to trauma in a manner similar to the synovial membrane, showing an increase in vascularity and eventually the development of more fibrous tissue, resulting in a very thick capsule. The thickening of the joint capsule can often be palpated.[37]

Effusion into the joint cavity may lead to stretching of the capsule and associated ligaments. The elastic properties of the joint capsule can be expressed in terms of compliance. This compliance is given by relating the magnitude of a change in intraarticular volume to the associated change in intraarticular pressure (dV/dP). In general, a low-pressure effusion has been found to be associated with a hyperplastic synovial lining and a high-pressure effusion with an attenuated synovial surface. The physical properties of a particular effusion seem to be reflected in the changes in the synovium of the individual joint. The higher the hydrostatic pressure and volume of an effusion, the faster fluid reaccumulates after aspiration. This indicates that higher rates of transudation occur from synovial capillaries of such joints.[34,42]

A significant rise in intraarticular hydrostatic pressure contributes to joint damage by stretching the capsule and associated ligaments. In some cases the pressure level can be sufficient to exceed the elastic limit of the joint capsule.[34,42]

Sprains

Excessive or abnormal joint motion may cause injury to the ligaments or a sprain. Sprains are classified as first-, second-, or third-degree and may vary from minor tearing of a few fibers without loss of integrity of the ligament to a complete tear of the ligament. Tears may be longitudinal, transverse, or oblique, each causing elongation of the remaining ligamentous fibers. Strain may be considered to be the physical force imposed on the ligamentous tissues, which exceeds normal stress but does not cause deformation or damage to the tissues. Physiological recovery can be expected. Experimentally, it has been shown that ligaments in which some fibers remain and in which there is good circulation regenerate well. With poor circulation, there is scar tissue formation rather than ligamentous growth.[11]

Clinical application

Joint capsule redundancy is illustrated well in the shoulder. The inferior joint capsule is loose and the fibers are oriented in a twisting position. The redundancy not only allows full abduction and flexion, but the twisted fiber orientation assists in the necessary external rotation motion needed during abduction or flexion to allow the greater tubercle to clear the acromion process and avoid impingement.

In the case of one who has had the shoulder immobilized for several weeks, the redundant joint capsule will undergo the typical soft-tissue adaptations that occur with prolonged immobilization. The connective tissue becomes disorganized and shows a decrease in water and proteoglycan content. The tissue shortens, further limiting the range of motion and prolonging recovery.[23,39]

Stretch to these tissues is essential in recovering the proper fiber alignment and redundancy. The inferior joint capsule can be stretched via grade IV mobilizations with a hold applied at the end of the available range. Inferior glide mobilizations can be utilized at varying angles of abduction or flexion to provide the maximum tension on the joint capsule in the position of function.[23]

Clinical application: sprains

Adequate circulation in the presence of ligamentous injury leads to proper regeneration of the tissue. Compression, ice, elevation, and active exercise within a painfree range of motion promote improved circulation by reducing and limiting edema in the area of the injury. This will help speed healing/regeneration of tissue through proper nutrition and removal of inflammatory waste. By promoting regeneration of connective tissue, scar tissue, which is weaker and less organized, is minimized after injury.[39,68]

Clinical application: enthesitis

The proximal supraspinatus tenoperiostial junction is a common area of enthesitis. If both superficial and deep aspects are involved, a painful arc is likely to be present on full passive elevation. Usually in a case like this, calcification of the tenoperiosteal junction is present. This junction is one of continuous stress when the arm is unsupported. The supraspinatus tendon is under constant stress and tension as a primary superior supporting structure at the shoulder leading toward fibrosis and calcification as a result of the inflammatory reaction that develops.[39,41]

Enthesitis

Muscular insertions may also serve as reinforcing fibrous bundles in the joint capsule (as well as from tendon to ligament or between tendons). A continually recurring concentration of muscle stress at these points may provoke an inflammatory reaction known as enthesitis. There is a strong tendency toward fibrosis and calcification with this condition. Enthesitis can be differentiated from traumatic arthritis and periarthritis because only movements that bring into play the affected muscle are painful. Also, there is usually radiographic evidence of calcification at the insertion.[29]

INTRAARTICULAR FIBROCARTILAGE AND FAT PADS
Menisci

Fibrocartilage disks or menisci consist of a very dense, interwoven fibrous tissue with a scattering of mature fibrocytic cells. They are composed of complete or incomplete flattened, triangular, or somewhat irregularly shaped disks firmly attached to the fibrous capsules and often to one of the adjacent bones. Menisci normally occur only in the knee, temporomandibular, sternoclavicular, distal radioulnar, and acromioclavicular joints. Examination of menisci of the knee under polarized or light microscopy has shown that the collagen fibers are arranged circumferentially, presumably to withstand the tension of load bearing.[32,46,70]

The blood and nerve supply is from the joint capsule peripherally, and near the center of the joint, the menisci are virtually avascular. They presumably derive their nutrition from synovial fluid but also by diffusion from vascular plexuses, which are present in the soft tissues adjacent to their attachment to bone or fibrous capsule.[33,46,70]

Fat pads

Fat pads have a copious blood supply and consist of closely packed fat cells surrounded by fibrous tissue septa. These fibrous septa contain a considerable amount of elastic tissue. Besides the capillary network of the circulatory system, fat pads are liberally supplied with nerve endings. The fat pad as a whole is covered by a flattened layer of synovial cells.[69]

Functions

The menisci perform numerous functions.[32,70]

1. They help to fill in "dead" space between badly conforming bones. Serving in this way as physiological "packing," they tend to reduce the amount of play in the joint. They also provide better geometry for the appropriate wedge-shaped film of synovial fluid, characteristic of hydrodynamic lubrication, to be formed.
2. They act as shock absorbers, possibly because of the elastic nature of the disk, and serve to protect the articular surface (increasing area of surface contact).
3. They increase the congruity between articular surfaces, thereby improving joint stability.
4. They permit motion of bones relative to a joint-dividing disk as well as relative to each other.
5. They act as a chock to prevent undue forward gliding.
6. They provide a ball-bearing action (i.e., rolling of the lateral femoral condyle at the end of knee extension).
7. They improve weight distribution by enlarging effective contact area between the bones.
8. They also protect the joint margin.

Fat pads may act as packing—filling dead spaces in joint cavities—or as cushions, receiving the bony processes during extremes of movement. They may also assist in the generation of the lubrication wedge required for fluid-film or hydrodynamic lubrication.[70]

INTRAARTICULAR STRUCTURES AND THEIR REACTION TO INJURY
Meniscus injury

Mechanisms causing meniscus injury in the knee are numerous, but meniscus injuries are predominantly caused by compression, traction, or both. The usual injury mechanism is rotatory stress on the weight-bearing leg. The stress is imposed by violation of internal rotation during flexion or external rotation during extension. Another mechanism that frequently causes injury to menisci is a forced valgus of the knee during flexion and an external rotation that opens the joint space and consequently entraps the meniscus.[11,12]

Symptoms are not caused by the cartilage tear per se but by stretching or tearing of peripheral attachments, which results in an acute synovial reaction within the joint space. Synovial effusion invariably accompanies meniscus tears and results from injury to the synovium, the capsule, or the ligaments. Tears in the substance of the avascular portion of the cartilage do not heal. Tears in the peripheral zones heal by invasion of fibrous tissue. If part of the meniscus is removed, it is replaced by dense collagen fiber from the remaining portion of the meniscus.[11,12]

Injury to fat pads

Fat pads may be impinged on by internal hemorrhage or increased effusion after trauma to a joint. Pain results and, in the knee, tenderness is felt just medial (or lateral) to the patellar tendon. Examination may reveal a hypertrophied fat pad. Bilateral injury to the fat pads in the same knee occurs more often when there is a concomitant degenerative arthritis. Injection of the pad with corticosteroids may be both diagnostic and momentarily therapeutic, but usually surgical removal is necessary.[12]

Intraarticular damage and osteophytes in osteoarthritis

Tissues not injured in the original trauma can be damaged as the inflammatory process in the synovial membrane progresses. In osteoarthritis there may be splitting and shredding of the menisci, especially the medial meniscus.

Osteophytic proliferation occurs as the result of increased vascularity of the bone adjacent to the joint, including bone beneath the articular cartilage and at the articular margins. It is at the latter site that the osteophytes are most significant because they can be palpated there at an early stage and give the earliest indications of osteoarthritis that can be seen on radiographs. They contribute significantly to the overall increase in girth of osteoarthritic joints in addition to the thickened joint capsule, the inflamed synovial membrane, and other periarticular fibrosis.[46]

The periarticular *osteophytes* arise at the fibrocartilaginous transition zone between the synovial membrane and the joint capsule on one side and the articular cartilage on the other. The development is nodular at first, but as the disease progresses, the nodules coalesce to form large strips of cancellous bone usually covered with fibrocartilage, although grossly this often has the appearance of hyaline cartilage.[44]

The precise reason for the gross periarticular proliferation of osteophytes is not known. It would appear to be a logical response to locally increased blood flow and oxygen tension, but many theories advanced for the location of this reaction are either unsatisfactory or very difficult to prove.[46]

If their origin is obscure, then the clinical significance of osteophytes in the pathogenesis of the diseased joint is even more uncertain, apart from being an aid in diagnosis. They may be simply an indication of degenerate articular cartilage or generally increased blood flow. Occasionally, fragments of an osteophyte can become free in the joint and exacerbate the clinical signs, but this is rare. It is customary to remove the osteophytes when debriding a badly diseased joint to reduce stretching of the joint capsule and therefore irritation and pain.[46]

Joint bodies

Injury to joint regions may also cause formation of "free joint bodies," whose long-term effect is to enhance articular damage (like foreign bodies in a closed gearbox). Such joint "mice" may represent detached bits of articular cartilage, small osteoarticular fracture fragments, or marginal osteophytes. There are other sources of joint bodies—osteochondromatosis of the synovium or a focus of osteochondritis dissecans of the knee that has loosened and become free. Whatever the origin of joint bodies, they are nourished by the synovial fluid and grow slowly by the accumulation of layers of cartilage on their surfaces. Eventually, they become several times their original size. The cartilage component can become calcified, but ossification does not occur because this would require a blood supply.[31]

ARTICULAR CARTILAGE

The actual load-carrying surface of the synovial joint is covered by a thin overlay of specialized connective tissue referred to as hyaline cartilage. This layer is only about 1 to 7 mm thick in healthy joints.[70] The chief components of articular cartilage are collagen, protein-polysaccharides, and water. The physical properties of cartilage are determined by the chemical nature of its constituents as well as by their interactions and physical arrangement.[58]

Composition

The articular cartilage contains small numbers of chondrocytes, housed in lacunae, surrounded by a resilient, three-dimensional lattice of collagen fibrils that provides a large degree of the mechanical strength of the tissue. Between the collagen fibers lies the ground substance, composing all of the noncellular and nonfibrous material present. This ground substance is a gel-like interstitial medium composed of sulfated polysaccharides associated with protein and an aqueous solution of electrolytes.[46,65,70]

The matrix of articular cartilage is hyperhydrated, with a water content varying from 65% to 80% of the total weight. This water plays an important role in joint lubrication inasmuch as about two thirds is extracellular and provides the vehicle for diffusion of metabolic substrates and products of the chondrocytes.[57] The solid matter of the matrix consists chiefly of two macromolecules that are synthesized by the chondrocytes—collagen and proteoglycans (protein-polysaccharides). Collagen fibers form over half the dry weight of the matrix. These fibers play a major role in the elasticity of articular cartilage. The remainder of the solids are made up largely of protein-polysaccharides, a family of molecules consisting of a protein core to which are attached long chains of negatively charged, repeating units of sulfated disaccharide. The protein-polysaccharides are highly viscous and strongly hydrophilic, properties that are of key importance in the resiliency of articular cartilage and the lubrication of its bearing surfaces under compressive loads.[7]

Nutritional supply

Articular cartilage is distinguished by a relatively low concentration of cells and a corresponding preponderance of intercellular material. Normal articular cartilage is devoid of blood vessels, lymphatic channels, and nerves. The tissue derives its nourishment largely from the synovial fluid that bathes its surface and to a lesser extent from the diffusion of blood substrates coursing through vessels in the underlying bony endplate.[2,7,46,65] Isolation from the body's vascular system dictates that nutrients must pass through a double diffusion process to reach the chondrocytes. Normally, materials in the bloodstream destined to reach the chondrocytic cells must first diffuse across the synovial membrane into the synovial fluid and then across the matrix of the articular cartilage to traverse the cell membrane. Diffusion of nutrients across the synovial membrane is a relatively simple process, and the constituents of synovial fluid are an ultrafiltrate of plasma to which the B cells have added hyaluronate. Diffusion across the articular cartilage surface is considerably limited not only by the electrical charge of the nutrient but also by the theoretical "pore size."[1] Because of the high degree of entanglement of protein-polysaccharide molecules, the tight packing of collagen, and the large amount of bound or structured water, cartilage behaves as a molecular sieve, with an effective pore size of about 60 Å in diameter. This excludes large molecules, such as hyaluronate, plasma proteins, and immunoglobulins in the joint fluid, and retains the chondroitin sulfate and other matrix components.[58]

The movement of fluid into and out of articular cartilage appears to be produced by diffusion and osmosis. Joint mobility and agitation of the fluid increase the rate of diffusion. In a mature joint there is no transfer across the bone-cartilage interface, whereas in an immature joint there is some diffusion. Investigation into the effect of alternate compression and relaxation on diffusion shows that such alternation adds very little to the normal diffusion rate.[33,71] At low pressures intermittent loading (compression) contributes little to the material transfer into cartilage, while at high pressures intermittent loading does lead to the transport of solutes into cartilage, but it cannot significantly increase the rate of transfer above that attributable to normal diffusion. Loading cartilage surfaces for prolonged periods without allowing intermittent relaxation can be expected to lead to a decreased diffusion, without any absorption of fresh fluid attributable to the action of a pump, and this would

Clinical application

If complete immobilization is the treatment of choice after an injury, cartilage may lose fluid and become less able to attenuate energy as a primary shock absorber within the joint. Cartilage nutrition is dependent upon the movement of fluid in and out of the cartilage.[27,51]

Abnormal, constant weight-bearing through cartilage will also limit the flow of fluid in and out of the cartilage. In the case of a severe genu valgus, the deterioration that is manifested in the lateral joint space is a direct result of excessive compressive forces that result in deterioration of the articular cartilage and ultimately the degeneration of the joint surfaces.[27,51]

Active ROM within the painfree ROM will promote fluid exchange in the cartilage, leading to better nutrition and maintenance of the function of the cartilaginous structures within an injured joint.[27,51]

result in an overall decrease in the rate or penetration of substances into cartilage. A consistently maintained compression of cartilage results in the loss of fluid, which is taken up again on removal of the load.[33] The sloshing back and forth of fluid in and out of cartilage is essential for cartilage nutrition. Chondrocytes die in the face of absolute immobilization, excessive pressure, or lack of pressure on the joint, all of which prevent fluid flow.[57]

Zones of articular cartilage

Histological and ultrastructural examination of cartilage has revealed four zones: a *tangential* or *gliding zone* (zone 1), a *transitional zone* (zone 2), a *radial zone* (zone 3), and a *calcified zone* (zone 4) (Fig. 4-16).[66]

Zone 1, immediately adjacent to the joint space, consists of a very thin layer of small collagen fibers, lying parallel to the surface and covered by a fine, acellular, afibrillar membrane. The collagen fiber bundles are densely packed with little intervening ground substance, and the cells are small and of an elongated, elliptical shape with their long axes parallel to the articular surfaces.[46,58,70,71] At the periphery, the fibrous components merge with the fibrous periosteum of the adjacent bone.[66]

Zone 2, the intermediate or transitional zone, has collagen fibers that form a coiled, interlacing, open network. Ground substance is more abundant. Cells are more numerous than in the tangential zone and are spheroidal and dispersed but equally spaced.[66]

In the deep or radial zone, zone 3, the collagen fibers are thicker, form a tighter meshwork, and tend to run radially to the subchondral bone. The fibers are coiled and S-shaped with large spaces between, while the spheroidal cells are arranged in columnar fashion, often in groups of two to eight cells. The radial zone is separated from the calcified zone by a wavy, basophilic, irregular line called the "tidemark."[66]

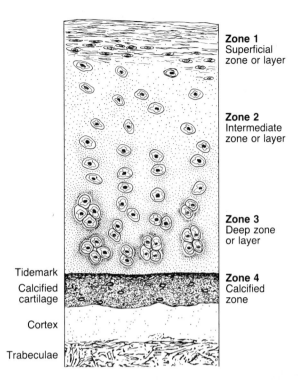

Zone 1
Superficial
zone or layer

Zone 2
Intermediate
zone or layer

Zone 3
Deep zone
or layer

Tidemark
Calcified
cartilage

Zone 4
Calcified
zone

Cortex

Trabeculae

Fig. 4-16. The zones of adult articular cartilage. (From Turek SL: *Orthopaedics: principles and their application,* Philadelphia, 1977, JB Lippincott.)

The deepest collagen fibers are embedded in the zone of calcified cartilage, zone 4, above the subchondral bone and help to secure the cartilage to the bone. The cells are sparser and smaller, and the matrix is heavily impregnated with calcium salts.* The fibers are of larger size and oriented perpendicularly with the meshwork more closely packed.[69]

The surface layer of circumferentially arranged fibers and featureless membrane remains very thin in all the joints studied, whereas the deeper zones vary in thickness from joint to joint and even at different points on one articular surface. This is reflected in a variation of thickness of the articular cartilage.[46]

Under static compressive loading, it appears that zone 1 provides a load diffusion effect in addition to a relatively smooth bearing surface.[69] Zone 2 and, to a lesser degree, zone 3, act as an area of deformability and energy storage—open meshwork becomes disrupted and the collagen fibers tend to orient perpendicularly to the direction of loading and to uncoil.[69,70] Zone 4 binds the tissue to the underlying bone and provides a degree of constraint.[69] The arrangement of collagen fibers and ground substance can account for the elasticity and compressibility of articular cartilage, which is essential for the pumping of nutrients through the tissue to the chondrocytes and aids in proper joint lubrication.[46]

Taken as a whole, the collagen fibers are arranged at right

* See references 33, 43, 50, 53, and 54.

angles to the surface of the subchondral bone to which they are attached, and they curve near the articular surface so as to run parallel to the surface (Fig. 4-17). This curve results in the formation of arches arranged to resist both shearing and direct compression forces. The collagen fibers add strength, whereas the ground substance provides firmness and smoothness to the surface. The gently curved shape of the bearing surface of the joints further provides for rapid, uniform dissipation of stress.[2]

Metabolic activity of articular cartilage

The articular cartilage in the adult is not simply a lining surface responsible for joint motion and tissue resiliency, but it is also an actively metabolizing tissue. Specifically, the chondrocytes synthesize the proteoglycans and collagen matrix. Turnover of at least a portion of the proteoglycans (estimated half-life, 8 to 17 days) is so rapid that it suggests the existence of an internal remodeling system. There is also ample evidence that the chondrocytes synthesize lysosomal enzymes presumably necessary for this internal remodeling system.[1,7,58] Normally, the cells cease their DNA synthesis at maturity but under a variety of circumstances may reinitiate this process, presumably to repair defects or respond to the chronic stress of osteoarthritis.[1]

Chondrocytes are metabolically very active cells, continuously utilizing both aerobic and anaerobic pathways. The chondrocytes from zones 2 and 3 of articular cartilage have extensive networks of rough-surfaced endoplasmic reticulum, dilated cisternae, vacuoles, and Golgi apparatus—suggesting that they actively synthesize protein, polysaccharides, collagen, and other components of the matrix. Metabolic studies using radioisotopes demonstrate that the chondrocyte cell synthesizes the components of macromolecules of proteoglycans and collagen, assembles them intracellularly, and then rapidly extrudes them into the surrounding matrix. The synthesis of proteoglycans is rapid, but the turnover rate of collagen is much slower.[59]

Functions of articular cartilage

Load carriage. *Load carriage* is the capacity of cartilage to sustain loads to which it is subjected without failing mechanically to compensate for the gross incongruities and small asperities at the subchondral bone surface and to reduce stress on the subchondral bone from dynamic loads. Cartilage compensates for bony incongruities by increasing the area of contact in the joint, thereby reducing the contact pressures on the bone.[66]

Articular cartilage seems to act primarily as a bearing surface and to distribute load rather than acting as a shock absorber.[1] The major contribution to peak force attenuation comes from the soft-tissue structures and bone rather than from cartilage and synovial fluid.[47,48] Articular cartilage is about 10 times as effective in reducing peak loads as is an equivalent amount of subchondral bone. However, because the amount of articular cartilage present in joints relative to

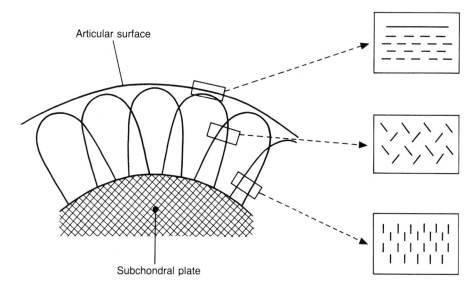

Fig. 4-17. Schematic representation of collagen-fiber orientation in articular cartilage. (From Sledge CB: *Orthop Clin North Am* 6[3]:619, 1975.)

bone is so small, even with its greater efficiency, cartilage contributes a minor share to peak force attenuation.[49] The important role played by periarticular soft tissues, such as the joint capsule, in force attenuation is probably due to their elastic nature.[48] Active contraction of muscle against tension can also absorb tremendous amounts of energy and is normally the major functioning shock absorber.[1,47]

Articular cartilage is structured to resist the repetitive rubbing and considerable deformation that its surface is subjected to in a lifetime. The cartilage matrix is composed of a systematically oriented fibrous network of collagen and a set of highly charged proteoglycan molecules. The collagen fibers at the surface run parallel and act as a membrane holding the matrix together. The collagen fibers in the calcified zone run vertically and actually connect the articular cartilage with its underlying calcified bone, preventing shear failure during joint motion. The fibers in the midzone of the cartilage appear to be randomly oriented, but when the cartilage is subjected to axial compression, the fibers tend to line up perpendicular to the compressive force, the most advantageous arrangement in resisting a compressive load. The lack of vessels in articular cartilage appears to be of significant functional advantage. Under physiological conditions, articular cartilage can be compressed to as much as 40% of its original height. If blood vessels traversed it, they would be rendered useless.[33]

Stress applied to articular cartilage is dependent not only on the magnitude of the applied force but also on the rate of application of the force. When load is applied to articular cartilage, an instantaneous deformation occurs and is followed by a time-dependent creep phase, in which the indentation increases continuously with time, although a constant load is maintained. The first stage of instantaneous deformation causes a change in contour but not in volume and results

from a simultaneous bulk movement of the matrix and collagen fibers rather than from a flow of water through the matrix. During the second stage, cartilage deforms increasingly with the passage of time, even though the applied pressure is held constant. This is known as *creep* and is related to the flow of water through the matrix. This property determines the description of cartilage as a viscoelastic material. The ability of cartilage to deform elastically and then flow under load is followed by a reabsorption of fluid when the load is removed. These viscoelastic properties enable cartilage to perform one of its vital functions in the diarthrodial joints—that of limiting the stresses transmitted to the bone ends.[66,70,71]

When the load is removed, cartilage recovers its original thickness as a result of an initial instantaneous (elastic) recovery followed by a time-dependent recovery phase (reimbibition of water). Cartilage is considered to be capable of displaying an elastic or "springlike" deformation within 2 seconds after application of a load. Approximately 90% or more of the instantaneous deformation is instantaneously recoverable when the load is quickly removed. During the normal walking cycle the duration of the applied load is between 0.5 second and 1 second, and peak loads are applied for less than 0.5 second.[66]

Most weight-bearing joints are subjected to loads applied rapidly and high loads of short duration. Cartilage assists in protecting the bones from these stresses by acting as a shock absorber (i.e., damping and attenuating dynamic loads by deforming to a substantial extent in a viscoelastic fashion). Two components of cartilage contribute to its load-carriage properties: proteoglycans, which retain water in the matrix and regulate its flow, and collagen, which resists tensile forces within the matrix and retains the proteoglycans in place.[66]

Lubrication. The extremely low coefficient of friction between joints is partly the result of the nature of articular cartilage—which is elastic and extremely smooth—although the surface roughness is about 10 times greater than conventional engineering bearing surfaces.[16,17] Its surface irregularities are elastic, becoming deformed and flattened with joint motions.[58] There is no one model available to describe lubrication at each point of the articulating cycle. There are basically two mechanisms involved in cartilage-on-cartilage lubrication.[32,66] *Boundary lubrication* means that each bearing surface is coated with a thin layer of molecules that slide on the opposing surface more readily than they are sheared off the underlying one. This is necessary for lowering frictional effects of cartilage on cartilage, but it ceases to function when loads are excessive.[66] Boundary lubrication functions primarily when joints move under a relatively light load. It involves the binding of a special glycoprotein found in synovial fluid, which is then affixed to the cartilage surfaces and keeps them from touching.[32] The second mechanism, *fluid lubrication,* produces synovial fluid film completely separating the opposing bearing surfaces, with resistance to motion arising from the viscosity of the fluid. A fluid film forms on the articular surfaces when cartilage is rubbed against cartilage under load in the presence of a lubricant. In the early phases of loading, fluid is trapped in the existing depressions in the surface of cartilage. The cartilage surface under load, because of its elasticity, undergoes deformation, creating a depression narrower at its periphery than at its center, trapping the fluid so that a phenomenon called *squeeze-film lubrication* results. *Squeeze-film lubrication* occurs when the approaching surfaces generate pressure in the lubricant as they squeeze it out of the area of impending contact between them. The resulting pressure keeps the surfaces apart. A fluid exudes from the cartilage and forms a film, termed the "squeeze film," in the transient area of impending contact.

Compressed articular cartilage also "weeps" fluid, mainly water and small ions. This fluid film produces *weeping lubrication,* a form of hydrostatic lubrication in which the interstitial fluid of hydrated articular cartilage flows onto its own surface when a load is applied to it.[66] Although the major part of water in cartilage is in the form of a proteoglycan-collagen gel, it is freely exchangeable with synovial fluid, and a significant portion can be liberated by pressure on the cartilage. Because in the adult there is little or no traversal of water through the subchondral plate nor a flow through the substance of the cartilage, the water displaced by cartilage compression will be expressed onto the surface of the cartilage, preferentially peripheral to the zone of impending contact. When the compression is released, the matrix within the cartilage contains enough of a fixed charge to osmotically attract the water and small solutes back into the matrix, and the cartilage regains its original height. The fluid film that exists between moving cartilage layers, therefore, consists of cartilaginous intersti-

tial fluid, which is squeezed onto the surface as the cartilage compresses the already present synovial fluid trapped in the contact zone.[32] The cartilage acts as a self-pressurizing sponge; when the pressure is released, the fluid flows back into the cartilage. "Weeping" probably occurs beyond the area of contact, where counteracting pressure is lower. This mechanism has also been termed *self-pressurized hydrostatic lubrication.*[66]

The hydrostatic mechanism functions best under substantial loads, because under small loads there is little cartilage compression and little weeping of fluid onto the surface. Cartilage weeping may well be the most important mechanism for protecting the articular cartilage from damage in certain high-load situations.[50]

Cartilage lubrication is supplemented when hydrostatic pressure buildup in the interstitial fluid in cartilage during loading counteracts the pressure in the lubricant that has been trapped in the area of deformation at the surface. This prevents the lubricant from entering the pores in the cartilage, and the hyaluronate molecules left behind become concentrated and supposedly enhance lubrication *(boosted lubrication).*[17,66,70]

There is also a theory that in cartilage-on-cartilage bearings the surfaces are elastic enough so that the lubricant pressure that is generated by motion under a given load depresses the surfaces a distance greater than the height of their asperities. Consequently, fewer asperities come into contact, and the fluid film is more easily maintained. This is termed *elastohydrodynamic lubrication,* a form of fluid lubrication. This concept of cartilage lubrication, however, is not universally accepted.[66]

Thus synovial joints are lubricated by two complementary systems—a hydrostatic (fluid lubrication) system that functions primarily at high loads and a boundary system that is most effective at low loads.[32] Hyaluronate appears to have little place in cartilage-on-cartilage lubrication but does play an important role as the boundary lubricant for synovial tissue. Because the friction of cartilage rubbing on cartilage is very low (measured as little as .002 coefficient of friction), the preponderance of frictional resistance in joint movement is in the periarticular soft tissues, which also usually make up the bulk of the articulating area within the joint capsule. Resistance to motion is the result of stretching of soft tissues (ligaments, muscles, tendons) and of soft-tissue fractional resistance (synovium-on-synovium, synovium-on-cartilage, cartilage-on-cartilage). Hyaluronate serves as a boundary lubricant in this system.[32]

ARTICULAR CARTILAGE AND ITS REACTION TO INJURY
Capacity for repair

Cartilage cells are quite active metabolically. The chondrocytes produce considerable amounts of collagen and mucopolysaccharides after injury. The numbers of chondrocytes and their metabolic rate may also increase. When an injury to cartilage is in an area close to some viable source of cells that are capable of metaplasia—such as synovium, subchondral bone, or perichondrium—cartilage heals by forming fibrocartilage, which is capable of maturing under appropriate circumstances.[47]

Substantial evidence exists to suggest that chondrocytes mitotically divide and that adult cartilage is capable, under certain circumstances, of repairing itself.[47] Experiments have shown that chondrocytes, isolated from mature individuals, grow readily and synthesize phenotypical glycosaminoglycans and collagen under proper conditions of culture in vitro. There is evidence for this in the release of the chondrocytes from their imprisoning matrix by enzymatic or other means. The matrix thus serves ordinarily to switch off the cell replicative mechanism. Although the rate of repair of articular cartilage is low, it may not be negligible over a period of time.[59] Whether the surface of articular cartilage continues to be slowly worn off in life and continuously replaced is still controversial.[47]

It has been suggested that the major shock absorber protecting cartilage is a reflexive neuromuscular response. Even in the presence of an intact neuromuscular system, the skeleton can be subjected to enough shock loading to microfracture the subchondral bone. Unexpected loads that present themselves in less then 65 msec (the natural response time) are not well dampened by the neuromuscular system. Substantial loads of a severe nature—such as might occur from auto accidents or skiing—can fracture bone. However, fracture is an excellent shock-absorbing mechanism, and, if the bone heals without malalignment and the break is distant from the joint, the cartilage is spared.[1]

Partial-thickness and full-thickness defects

Even when stress on a joint is insufficient to cause clinical fracture to the subchondral bone, damage may be found on microscopy. Articular cartilage—consisting of an elastic surface layer over a thin, calcified, brittle one—is likely to slip at a plane between these layers, and the existence of such a plane of weakness at this level has been proven. Moreover, if there is a gap in the deeper tissue, the elastic cartilage may be expected to herniate into the opening. Such changes can be seen in sections without any other structural abnormality, sometimes near complete fractures but also independent of them; therefore it is reasonable to suggest that the changes are mechanical. Three stages, short of complete fracture, can be described: (1) splitting at the *tidemark* (a wavy line that marks the junction between calcified and uncalcified cartilage), (2) depression of cartilage into bone, and (3) fissuring of both calcified cartilage and bone along a vertical plane that permits blood vessels from the marrow to reach the cartilage.[30]

A trauma-induced defect in articular cartilage possesses a variable potential for repair. *Partial-thickness defects,* limited to the articular cartilage, adjacent to the synovial attachment or perichondrium, can undergo some degree of

healing by proliferation and invasion from soft tissue. However, cartilage wounds at some distance from soft tissue do not heal well, although there is evidence of an intense biochemical response. Instead there is heightened synthesis of matrix components in such injuries and increased mitotic activity that is short-lived and ineffectual for healing. Nevertheless, there is complete repair in approximately 20% of the defects induced in experimental animals, involving a period of extraordinary cellular proliferation and cartilage growth. At first the surface is bridged by the layer of elongated compacted cells in a collagenous stroma. Then the defect is filled rapidly by cellular fibroblastic tissue that changes, as it extends deeply, into chondroid tissues with cells irregularly arrayed in a homogeneous matrix. The reparative tissue consistently forms hyaline cartilage, which blends with preexisting cartilage.[66] However, in general, experimentally induced gaps in articular cartilage that do not penetrate into the subchondral vascular marrow show little tendency to be filled by new cartilage.[59]

Repair of *full-thickness defects* (extending through the subchondral bone) takes place by proliferation of cellular tissue originating from the superficial layer that has bridged the defect at the surface and by rapidly invading osteogenic cells and granulation tissue from the narrow spaces at the base, resulting in a mixture of bony trabeculae, cartilage, and mostly fibrous tissue.[66]

The process begins when capillaries grow directly into the uncalcified cartilage without the mediation of any other cell to destroy the matrix ahead of them. There is physical splitting of the calcified cartilage behind them but no invasion or dissolution of it. The shape of the intruding mass into the cartilage is smoothly rounded. There is well-marked zonation around this mass—first, a chondrin-free ring next to the untouched cartilage; next, a ring where there is a gathering together of fine fibers to form a coarser set of strands; and finally, among the capillaries, the development of large and irregular fibers and the disappearance of cartilage cells (Fig. 4-18). When the process has gone on further, the degeneration of the hyaline cartilage is more complete. The hyaline cartilage loses its chondrin and reverts to fibrous tissue. The chondrocytes revert to fibrocytes, and there is much more than normal collagen in the margin of the intrusion; this process represents not only the removal of one component of cartilage but includes excess production of another.[30] The final healed defect is represented by a slightly discolored and roughened pit or a superficial linear defect on an otherwise smooth surface of hyaline cartilage. This implies that full-thickness defects will heal but only with fibrocartilage, a mechanically inferior tissue.[66]

However, the usual sequel of intrusion by capillaries in full-thickness defects includes early sealing off by ossification. This results in the formation of a nodule of bone in the deeper cartilage that, by fusion of adjacent foci, advances the bony articular lamella and thins the overlying cartilage in the middle of the joint; this impairs the cartilage's

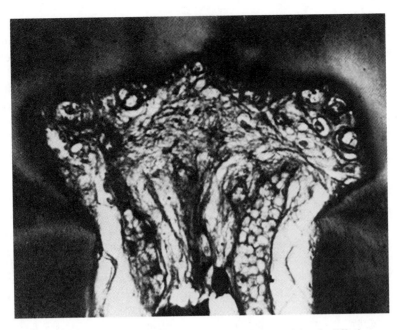

Fig. 4-18. Invasion of cartilage by capillaries from the bone below, with pale diffusion zone limited by a dark basophil ring. Cartilage cells and the aggregation of collagen fibers are well marked in the next zone; no adventitious cells. Process mechanically checked in the calcified zone but expands in the soft uncalcified zone; chemical changes stop abruptly at the tidemark. (From Landells JW: *J Bone Joint Surg Br* 38[2]:548, 1957.)

elasticity and favors further injury. At the edge of the cartilage, the process results in osteophyte formation.[30]

Cartilage formation is directly related to the nature of the stress that the tissue undergoes.[47] When a partial-thickness defect confined to the articular cartilage is subjected to constant joint motion, the differentiation toward hyaline cartilage is more pronounced. The main cartilaginous constituent forms nearer the surface. However, if the joint is immobilized, the defect fills with primitive connective tissue that includes little cartilage. When a full-thickness defect extends into the subchondral bone, granulation tissue rapidly invades from the vascular marrow spaces and healing is predominantly fibrous or fibrocartilaginous. Under conditions of continuous motion, the reparative tissue becomes more cartilaginous and restores a smooth articular surface, and the intercellular matrix fuses with the original cartilage.[66]

Complete fracture of articular cartilage

The changes in articular cartilage after complete fracture can be divided into three stages. Immediate changes may include a transverse fracture at the tidemark; vertical fractures elsewhere through the cartilage, calcified cartilage, and bone; and a narrow zone of dead cells around the injury site. Intermediate changes (3 to 14 days after injury) reveal no tendency of the cartilage to flake around the margin of the injury and little multiplication of cartilage cells exposed by the breach. The late stage of change and repair includes two events: (1) replacement of gaps left in the articular cartilage

Clinical application

With the effects of immobilization on cartilage well described, early motion should be used when speeding the healing process and strengthening the newly repaired tissue are desired. Continuous passive motion has been shown to have positive effects on cartilage healing. Active ROM within the painfree range and in a gravity eliminated situation can provide the needed motion without stressing the cartilage through weight-bearing and shearing forces.[35,39]

and (2) determination of the fate of the displaced fragments of such cartilage. Replacement is invariably by fibrous tissue, derived from granulation tissue emerging from the depths of the bone if the gap is central or from the synovial membrane if the gap is peripheral, or both. This fibrous tissue, if exposed to synovial fluid, is eventually impregnated with polysaccharides and may in several years come to resemble fibrocartilage and present a remarkably smooth surface, but the internal structure remains different from the original hyaline cartilage. Displaced fragments of cartilage change in several ways. When fibrous tissue grows over the surface of displaced cartilage and is itself nourished by synovial fluid, a new stratum of fibrocartilage may bury the old, which survives almost unchanged beneath it. More usually, however, cartilage perishes wherever it comes into contact with granulation tissue. The cells die and the chondrin is dissolved away before the actual invasion has gone far. Later, migrant fibrocytes penetrate the matrix and replace it with fibrous tissue, which may ossify.[30]

No specialized phagocyte appears to remove uncalcified cartilage. It is possible that the collagen is not removed but that the solution of the surrounding chondrin so changes the physical state of collagen that the fine fibrils dispersed in the gel come to form tight bundles. These take up little room, compared with their immediately adjacent pale diffusion ring, possibly because of the loss of much bound water as well as the acquisition of fresh interfibrillary bonds. In this vascular digestion, the adjacent calcified cartilage undergoes no internal change; its removal is always associated with the presence of multinucleate giant cells.[30]

The reaction that occurs in articular cartilage after trauma shows the importance of the normal balance between articular cartilage and its blood supply. The normal nutrition of cartilage is mainly synovial, although there is evidence of some vascular diffusion from bone. The presence of occasional blood vessels in the subarticular plane has been interpreted as important in the normal nutrition of cartilage, but such vessels are few in number and are insulated by a thin sheet of bone. If there are blood vessels present that do not have this sheet, abnormalities are visible in the cartilage. Examples of such contact may arise in several ways: (1) trauma may displace fragments into callus, (2) vascular tissue may grow over the cartilage surface, or (3) there may be intrusion of blood vessels through the articular lamella from trauma or erosion. In each case cartilage is being destroyed. A good blood supply is rapidly followed by complete disorganization of hyaline cartilage and its replacement by fibrous tissue, fibrocartilage, or bone.[30]

Osteoarthritis

Results of trauma to synovial joints can lead to subsequent development of some degree of a condition known variously as *osteoarthritis,* osteoarthrosis, hypertrophic arthritis, or degenerative joint disease. It is essentially a degenerative condition of articular cartilage with subsequent formation of marginal osteophytes, subchondral bone changes, bone marrow changes, inflammatory reaction of the synovium, capsular thickening, alteration of the synovial fluid, and damage to intraarticular structures.[11,46] Most authors distinguish between *primary* (idiopathic) *osteoarthritis* and *secondary osteoarthritis* (secondary to an infectious, traumatic, inflammatory, metabolic, or aging process). Often, however, the etiology of one type cannot be delineated from that of the other.[11,66]

Pathology and pathogenesis

The proteoglycan component of articular cartilage is readily susceptible to enzymatic degradation. This may occur after acute inflammation, synovectomy, immobilization, or even seemingly minor insults.[58] When subjected to increasing stress, the limiting effect of the pore size of articular cartilage is probably destroyed, and the ground

substance (proteoglycan) leaks out. Lysosomal activity becomes marked.[47] The protease implicated is probably a cathepsin derived from the damaged cartilage cells. Enzymatic degradation of the ground substance and abrasive forces then release cartilage debris and mucopolysaccharide materials, which can lead to the secondary changes of osteoarthritis—spurs, cysts, and synovitis.[14] When the proteoglycan content is depleted, the physical properties of the cartilage change, rendering the collagen fibers susceptible to mechanical damage. Along with degeneration of the mucopolysaccharide ground substance, there is loss of the fine superficial membrane and superficial cellular layer. When the disruption is confined to the tangential layer of the surface, the process is referred to as flaking; when the process extends to the deeper radial zone, it is described as fibrillation. The collagen fibers are thus exposed ("unmasked"), elasticity is impaired, and minor trauma is able to produce fissures and more fibrillation. This cracking of the surface is the earliest change visible to the naked eye and is followed by erosion of the tissue, often through to the subchondral bone, which may become smooth and shiny. There is no evidence of healing around areas of erosion and fibrillation.[46,59] Predilection for destruction of the joint surface is exhibited by those sites subject to the greatest load-bearing or shearing stress. Earliest fibrillation, however, is often present in regions that presumably carry low compressive stress.[59]

Where the cartilage is denuded and blood vessels reach the surface, there is a localized advance in the line of ossification.[31] New bone formation takes place in two separate locations in relation to the joint surface: in exostoses (osteophytes) at the margins of the articular cartilage and in the marrow immediately subjacent to the cartilage.[59]

The marginal osteophytes generally have one of two patterns of growth. One of these is a protuberance into the joint space; the other is a development within capsular and ligamentous attachments to the joint margins. In each circumstance the direction of osteophytic growth is governed by the lines of mechanical force exerted on the area of growth and generally corresponds to the contour of the joint surface from which the osteophytes protrude. Osteophytes consist in large part of bone that merges imperceptibly with cortical and cancellous tissue of subchondral bone. Osteophytic growth is frequently capped by a layer of hyaline cartilage and fibrocartilage that becomes continuous with the adjacent synovial lining.[59]

The proliferation of bone in the subchondral tissue is most marked in areas that have been denuded of their cartilaginous covering by osteoarthritic erosion. In these regions the articulating surface consists of bone that has been rubbed smooth. The glistening appearance of this polished sclerotic surface is the result of this process, termed *eburnation.* Most of the osteocytes in the eburnated surface undergo gradual degeneration, indicated by empty lacunae. This may result from frictional heat. In addition to this alteration, two other variants of new bone formation are seen in relation to the articular cartilage.[59]

"Cystic" areas of rarefaction of bone can be seen in radiographs immediately beneath the eburnated surfaces, most frequently in the hip joint. However, these lesions only infrequently contain pockets of mucoid fluid and thus are not truly cystic. The trabeculae in the affected areas disappear, and the marrow undergoes fibromyxoid degeneration. Fragments of dead bone, cartilage, and amorphous debris often are interspersed within them. In time, the entire area is encircled by a rim of reactive new bone and compact fibrous tissue. Minute gaps in the overlying articular cortex, resulting from microfractures, are commonly seen at the apices of the pseudocysts.[59]

The other type of new bone formation is a local ossific metaplasia of the base of the articular cartilage. This should be regarded as part of a general remodeling of the joint contour in which bone is added to a portion of the articular cortex, while other areas in the joint surface display focal resorption of the bone. What exactly happens to the subchondral bone depends on whether there is motion in the affected joint or not—if there has been motion, the subchondral bone tends to become sclerotic; if there is no appreciable motion, the bone undergoes atrophy.[31]

Although degenerative joint disease by definition is not inherently inflammatory, focal areas of secondary chronic synovitis are usually present in advanced cases. This is generally characterized by small infiltrates of lymphocytes and mononuclear cells in the synovium. Occasionally the infiltration is sufficiently severe to raise a question of rheumatoid arthritis or the possibility of inflammation arising through autosensitization to joint detritus. A foreign-body reaction to detached fragments of cartilage also occurs and is probably responsible for pain and effusion in acute cases. Secondary synovial osteochondromatosis usually is minimal. However, villous hypertrophy and fibrosis of the synovium occur frequently in clinically obtrusive osteoar-

thritis. In the knee joint, cruciate ligaments and menisci become frayed and a degree of instability results. Fibrillation and fibrosis of the synovial surface and even mild cartilaginous metaplasia of the patellar tendon may occur in such cases. Minute tears in the capsular tissues appear as slender fibrous or vascular seams disrupting the principal axis of the collagen bundles.[59]

Under clinical conditions, there is little chance of protecting the defects from further wear and tear, and healing of the articular cartilage appears to be unlikely. Also, because degeneration of the ground substance leads to a loss of compressibility and elasticity, the normal pumping mechanism for the passage of nutrients through the articular cartilage is impaired and chondrocyte metabolism is decreased.[14,46] The ability of the tissue to manufacture enough permanent matrix to keep up with the increasing loss is reduced. Cartilage debris and excess ester sulfates released into the joint continue to produce synovitis.[14] Differentiation of the synovial changes in posttraumatic synovitis from those in osteoarthritis is possible to a very limited extent because similar changes with a similar rate of incidence can be observed in both conditions. This suggests that similar etiological agents, possibly macrotrauma and microtrauma, are the common pathogenetic factors.[60]

Trauma can be implicated in several ways in the pathogenesis of osteoarthritis. Trauma may cause injury directly to the cartilage cells, initiating a cycle of cartilage degeneration. Trauma alone may also cause degenerative changes in healthy cartilage, and frequently repeated minor injuries in ordinary life can so affect the vascularity of cartilage that the degenerative changes of osteoarthritis will follow.[30] The events of cartilage degradation and repair can also be set off when there is loss of capacity to absorb impact energy. In this case overload is dissipated by fracturing of the trabeculae of the subchondral bone with consequent marginal joint remodeling and exposure of the articular cartilage to insult (Fig. 4-19).[1,43,61] Finally, in primary osteoarthritis minor traumatic effects will have a more serious impact if the cartilage has already degenerated.[30]

Clinical application

Someone with an acute exacerbation of pain due to osteoarthritis has pain with weight-bearing activities as well as movement of the joint involved. Pain deters movement and activity. As activity decreases, so does the process of new bone formation. This leaves the bone underlying the articular cartilage atrophied and weaker, unable to attenuate the energy applied to it during function. To help prevent the effects of inactivity on joints with osteoarthritis, active ROM exercises should be performed daily. The patient should use pain as a guide, avoiding the range that reproduces pain. Active ROM provides movement at the joint and, along with isometric exercises and resisted ROM with minimal resistance, provides the joint activity that may help to avoid atrophy of the bone.[51]

Clinical application

Muscular strength and ligamentous and cartilaginous integrity all play a role in attenuating energy applied through joints. As energy or force is applied, these structures play a role in absorbing and dissipating the force. It is the rehabilitation specialist's role to assist the patient's ability to attenuate the energy applied to the body during activity. Muscular strength and extensibility are key components of energy attenuation. Strengthening and stretching exercises help improve the motor function, strength, and power of the muscles, which help in absorbing the forces applied through the joints during functional, work, and recreational activities.[27,51]

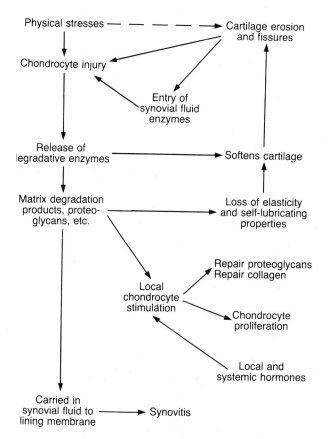

Fig. 4-19. A postulated final pathway of cartilage degeneration. (From American Academy of Orthopaedic Surgeons: *Symposium on osteoarthritis,* St Louis, 1976, Mosby.)

Symptoms and treatment

Clinically, early degenerative changes may be asymptomatic until synovitis develops with effusion, stiffness, capsular thickening, and formation of marginal osteophytes. The osteophytes may cause excessive deformity of the articular bone ends, pain because of stretching of the periosteum, and limitation of movement. Other sources of pain include bony changes at sites of ligamentous attachment and protective muscle spasms that occur to immobilize the joint.[11]

Treatment includes heat application in the form of hot packs, diathermy, or ultrasound. During the initial acute exacerbation of synovitis, some form of cryotherapy may also prove effective. If the patient is overweight, weight reduction is mandatory. Evaluation of daily activities must be undertaken—low chairs should be avoided and sustained postures should not be maintained. Active flexion and extension exercises of the joint (e.g., the knee) should be done every morning before weight-bearing is attempted. Walking is encouraged for daily activities but not forced for the sake of prolonged exercise as therapy. Deep knee bends should be avoided, and faulty posture that places a strain as

a result of stance should be corrected if the involved joint is the knee or any other joint in the lower extremity or the back. In the case of knee involvement, exercises should include those to strengthen the quadriceps muscle group, hamstrings, and gastrocnemius-soleus muscles.[11] However, if 6 to 8 weeks of such therapy is not beneficial, analgesic and antiinflammatory drugs can be used, but the regimen of restricted exercise must be maintained. If conservative treatment is unsuccessful, surgical debridement of the joint is indicated. Osteophytes are removed along with any damaged intraarticular structures and/or villous projections of the synovial membrane.[46]

Traumatic arthritis

In some cases trauma may lead to a form of arthritis known as *traumatic arthritis.* Because trauma causes cracking or fibrillation of the intraarticular cartilage with subsequent atrophy, it may scar or weaken the intraarticular and extraarticular supporting structures, thereby decreasing the ability of the joint to withstand the physiological trauma that results from motion or weight-bearing or both. Although it is relatively rare, arthritis may be precipitated by trauma.[20] More commonly, preexisting rheumatoid arthritis is aggravated by injury.[7,37]

SUMMARY

The synovial membrane, articular cartilage, joint capsule, and intraarticular structures each react to trauma in a characteristic way. Trauma to the synovial membrane, usually produced by a mild blow or overstretching of the joint capsule, may result in posttraumatic synovitis or pigmented villonodular synovitis, depending on whether the effusion is hemorrhagic or not. Repeated trauma to the articular cartilage may lead to osteoarthritis. All of these reactions can be observed by changes in the synovial fluid. The joint capsule can be injured directly (by overstretching) or indirectly (from effusion). Intraarticular structures can be damaged from a direct force or secondarily as a result of inflammatory processes occurring in nearby associated structures.

Beside gross, obvious damage in any injury to a joint (meniscus tear, sprain, subluxation, or dislocation), which may lead to decreased range of motion, increased temperature, edema, and decreased strength, one should be aware of changes that occur on a microscopic level and the clinical effects that can result. For example, the phenomenon of reactive synovitis can be responsible for damage to surrounding joint structures that were not involved in the initial injury.

Seemingly minor trauma can have its effect on the joint structures also and, if repeated or aggravated, can have serious consequences. There is an obvious implication to avoid mobilization techniques (which involve passive movements of the joint at the limit of its range) and vigorous exercising of an acutely injured or inflammatory joint.

REVIEW QUESTIONS

1. What is the effect of joint trauma on the pathogenesis of osteoarthritis?
2. What are the differences in the potential for repair between partial-thickness versus full-thickness defects in articular cartilage?
3. How is the process of phagocytosis initiated following trauma to the joint?
4. What are the inflammatory and degenerative changes associated with posttraumatic synovitis?
5. How does posttraumatic synovitis differ from pigmented villonodular synovitis in regard to histologic and morphologic changes?

REFERENCES

1. *Symposium on osteoarthritis,* American Academy of Orthopaedic Surgeons: St Louis, 1976, Mosby. pp 1-7, 34-47.
2. Anderson CE: The structure and function of cartilage, *J Bone Joint Surg Am* 44A:777, 1962.
3. Arnout AM: Leukocyte adhesion molecule deficiency, *Immunol Rev* 114:145, 1990.
4. Barnett CH: Wear and tear in joints: an experimental study, *J Bone Joint Surg Br* 38B(2):567, 1956.
5. Bennett JS, Shattil SJ: *Platelet function in hematology.* In William WJ, Beutler E, Erslev AJ, Lichtman MA, editors: p. 1233, New York, 1990, McGraw-Hill.
6. Berk RN: Liquid fat in the knee joint after trauma, *N Engl J Med* 277(26):1411, 1967.
7. Biology of connective tissue and the joints, *JAMA* 224(suppl 5):669, 1973.
8. Boyes JG: Solitary nodular synovitis: a traumatic lesion? *South Med J* 59:1212, 1966.
9. Bozdech Z: Posttraumatic synovitis, *Acta Chir Orthop Traumatol Cech* 43(3):244, 1976.
10. Brosky T, Nyland J, Nitz A, Caborn DNM: The ankle ligaments: consideration of syndesnotic injury and implications for rehabilitation, *JOSPT* 21(4):197, 1995.
11. Cailliet R: *Knee pain and disability,* pp 40-44, 62-68, 97-99, Philadelphia, 1972, FA Davis.
12. Cailliet R: *Soft tissue pain and disability,* p 234, Philadelphia, 1977, FA Davis.
13. Castor CW, Prince RK, Hazelton MJ: Hyaluronic acid in human synovial effusions: a sensitive indicator of altered connective tissue cell function during inflammation, *Arthritis Rheum* 9(6):783, 1966.
14. Chrisman OD: Biochemical aspects of degenerative joint disease, *Clin Orthop* 64:77, 1969.
15. Curtiss PH: Changes produced in synovial membrane and synovial fluid, *J Bone Joint Surg Am* 46A:873, 1964.
16. Dowson D: Lubrication and wear of joints, *Physiotherapy* 59(4):104, 1973.
17. Dowson D, Wright V, Longfield MD: Human joint lubrication, *Biomed Eng* 4:160, 1969.
18. Etzioni, A et al: Brief report: recurrent severe infections caused by a novel leukocyte adhesion molecule deficiency, *N Engl J Med* 327:1789, 1992.
19. Evans P: The healing process at the cellular level, *Physiotherapy* 66:256, 1980.
20. Gelfand I, Merliss R: Trauma and rheumatism, *Ann Intern Med* 50:999, 1959.
21. Guyton A: *Textbook of medical physiology,* p 72, Philadelphia, 1976, WB Saunders.
22. Habicht GS, Beck G: *The role of interleukin-1 in increased vascular permeability in inflammation in leukocyte emigration and its sequelae.* In Movat HZ, editor: p 51, Basel, 1987, S Karger AG.
23. Hertling D, Kessler RM: *Management of common musculoskeletal disorders: physical therapy principles and management,* p 177, Philadelphia, 1990, Lippincott.
24. Hollinshead WH: *Textbook of anatomy,* p 32, New York, 1974, Harper & Row.
25. Irwin JW, Way BA: Inflammation, *Bibl Anat* 17:72, 1979.
26. Kelly WN, Harris ED, Ruddy S et al: *Textbook of Rheumatology* p 271, Philadelphia, 1981, WB Saunders.
27. Kisner C, Colby LA: *Therapeutic exercise: foundations and techniques,* p 369, Philadelphia, 1990, FA Davis.
28. Knight K: The effects of hypothermia on inflammation and swelling, *Athletic Training* 11(1):7, 1976.
29. LaCava G: Enthesitis-traumatic disease of insertions, *JAMA* 169:254, 1959.
30. Landells JW: The reactions of injured human articular cartilage, *J Bone Joint Surg Br* 38(2):548, 1957.
31. Lichtenstein L: *Disease of bone and joints,* p 266, St Louis, 1975, Mosby.
32. Mankin HJ, Radin E: Structure and function of joints. In McCarty DJ, editor: *Arthritis and allied conditions,* p 151, Philadelphia, 1979, Lea & Febiger.
33. Maroudas A, Bullough P, Swanson SAV et al: The permeability of articular cartilage, *J Bone Joint Surg Br* 50(1):166, 1968.
34. Matsen FA, Krugmire RB: The effect of externally applied pressure on postfracture swelling, *J Bone Joint Surg* 56(12):1586, 1974.
35. McCarthy MR, Yates CK, Anderson MA, Yates-McCarthy JL: The effects of immediate continuous passive motion on pain during the inflammatory phase of soft tissue healing following anterior cruciate ligament reconstruction, *JOSPT* 17(2):96, 1993.
36. McCarty DJ: Synovial fluid. In McCarty DJ, editor: *Arthritis and allied conditions,* p 51, Philadelphia, 1979, Lea & Febiger.
37. McCracken WJ: The role of trauma in arthritis, *Industrial Med Surg* 24:327, 1955.
38. Myers RR, Negami S, White RK: Dynamic mechanical properties of synovial fluid, *Biorheology* 3:197, 1966.
39. Norkin CC, Levangie PK: *Joint structure and function: a comprehensive analysis,* pp 87, 88, 220, 221, Philadelphia, 1992, FA Davis.
40. Ogston AG, Stanier JE: The physiological function of hyaluronic acid in synovial fluid: viscous, elastic and lubricant properties, *J Physiol* 119:244, 1953.
41. Ombreght L, Bisschop P, ter Veer HJ, Van de Velde T: *A system of orthopedic medicine,* p 256, London, 1995, WB Saunders.
42. Palmer DG: Dynamics of joint disruption, *NZ Med J* 78:166, 1973.
43. Pathophysiology of arthrosis: a review, *Tidsskr Nor Laegef* 96(32):1687, 1976.
44. Pinals RS: Traumatic arthritis and allied conditions. In McCarty DY, editor: *Arthritis and allied conditions,* p 986, Philadelphia, 1979, Lea & Febiger.
45. Pober JS, Cotran RS: Overview: the role of endothelial cells in inflammation. *Transplantation* 50:537, 1990.
46. Pond MJ: Normal joint tissues and their reaction to injury, *Vet Clin North Am* 1(3):523, 1971.
47. Radin EL: The physiology and degeneration of joints, *Semin Arthritis Rheum* 2(3):245, 1972-1973.
48. Radin EL, Paul IL: Does cartilage compliance reduce skeletal impact loads? The relative force-attenuating properties of articular cartilage, synovial fluid, periarticular soft tissues and bone, *Semin Arthritis Rheum* 13(2):139, 1970.
49. Radin EL, Paul IL: Importance of bone in sparing articular cartilage from impact, *Clin Orthop* 78:342, 1971.

50. Radin EL, Paul IL, Pollack D: Animal joint behavior under excessive loading, *Nature* 226:554, 1970.

51. Richardson JK, Iglarsh ZA: *Clinical orthopedic physical therapy*, pp 408-411, 430, 431, Philadelphia, 1994, WB Saunders.

52. Robbins: Pathologic basis of disease. In Cotran RS, Kumar V, Robbins SL, editors: p 51, Philadelphia, 1994, WB Saunders.

53. Roy S, Ghadially FN, Crane WAJ: Synovial membrane in traumatic effusion: ultrastructure and autoradiography with tritiated leucine, *Ann Rheum Dis* 25:259, 1966.

54. Schmid FR, Ogata RI: The composition and examination of synovial fluid, *J Prosthet Dent* 18(5):449, 1967.

55. Schumacher HR: Traumatic joint effusion and the synovium, *J Sports Med Phys Fitness* 3(3):108, 1975.

56. Sherman MS: The non-specificity of synovial reactions, *Bull Hosp J Dis* 12:110, 1951.

57. Simkin PA: Synovial physiology. In McCarty DJ, editor: *Arthritis and allied conditions,* p 167, Philadelphia, 1979, Lea & Febiger.

58. Sledge CB: Structure, development, and function of joints, *Orthop Clin North Am* 6(3):619, 1975.

59. Sokoloff L: Pathology and pathogenesis of osteoarthritis. In McCarty DY, editor: *Arthritis and allied conditions,* p 1135, Philadelphia, 1979, Lea & Febiger.

60. Soren A, Klein W, Huth F: Microscopic comparison of the synovial changes on posttraumatic synovitis and osteoarthritis, *Clin Orthop* 121:191, 1976.

61. Soren A, Rosenbauer KA, Klein W et al: Morphological examination of so-called posttraumatic synovitis, *Beitraege Pathol* 150:11, 1973.

62. Sternbach GL, Baker FJ: The emergency joint: arthrocentesis and synovial fluid analysis, *JACEP* 5(10):787, 1976.

63. Stossel TP: On the crawling of animal cells, *Science* 260:1045, 1993.

64. Stravino VD: The synovial system, *Am J Phys Med* 51(6):312, 1972.

65. Tallquist G: The reaction to mechanical trauma in growing articular cartilage, *Acta Orthop Scand* 53(suppl):1, 1962.

66. Turek SL: *Orthopaedics: principles and their application,* pp 17-29, 147-169, 327-348, Philadelphia, 1977, JB Lippincott.

67. Volz R: The response of synovial tissues to recurrent hemarthroses, *Clin Orthop* 45:127, 1966.

68. Wilkerson GB: External compression for controlling traumatic edema, *Phys Sportsmed,* 13(6):97-104, 1985.

69. Wright V, editor: *Lubrication and wear in joints,* pp. 19, 41-48, Proceedings of a symposium organized by the Biological Engineering Society and held at the General Infirmary, Leeds, on April 17, 1969, Philadelphia, 1972, JB Lippincott.

70. Wright V, Dowson D, Kerr J: The structure of the joints, *Int Rev Connect Tissue Res* 6:105, 1973.

71. Wright V, Dowson D, Seller PC: Bio-engineering aspects of synovial fluid and cartilage, *Mod Trends Rheumatol* 2:21, 1971.

CHAPTER 5

Fracture Stabilization and Healing

Ivan A. Gradisar, Jr. and Arthur J. Nitz

OUTLINE

Significance of soft tissue damage
Pathomechanics of fracture
Brief review of fracture healing
Emergency fracture care
    Emergency splinting
Types of fractures
    Fractures in children
    Fractures in the elderly
    Stress fractures
Definitive fracture management
    Closed reduction
    Traction
    Open reduction
    Rigid external fixation
    Bioelectrical stimulation
    Fracture rehabilitation
Complications of fracture healing
    Nonunion fractures
    Edema
    Joint stiffness
    Neurologic complications
Summary

LEARNING OBJECTIVES

After studying this chapter, the reader should be able to:
1. Define a fracture.
2. Describe the significance of soft tissue injury that accompanies fractures.
3. Describe those factors that contribute to the pathomechanics of fractures.
4. List twelve types of fractures.
5. List those factors that may affect fracture healing.
6. List the basic principles of emergency fracture care.
7. Describe the special concerns associated with fractures that occur in children.
8. Describe the various approaches to definitive fracture management.
9. Describe the treatment for a nonunion fracture.
10. List the four major complications that can affect fracture healing.

KEY TERMS

fracture	fracture types
healing	rehabilitation treatment
pathomechanics	complications

A *fracture* has been defined as a severe soft tissue injury with an underlying bony defect.[11] This definition is unusual in its emphasis on the soft tissue rather than on the bone, but it is particularly useful to those whose job it is to get the patient back to full function within a reasonable period of time.

In the past 10 years, sophisticated advances have been made in some areas of fracture management. Despite these advances, the clinician can do little to increase the rate of fracture healing. Instead, efforts must be made to remove significant deterrents to the healing process, and in this endeavor the clinician needs to understand the ramifications of not only the bony lesion but also the associated soft tissue injury.

SIGNIFICANCE OF SOFT TISSUE DAMAGE

Whereas damage to bone is often immediately obvious in the shortening or deformity of the fractured limb, severe, permanent damage to the soft parts, such as skin, muscle, tendon, ligament, vessels, and cartilage, is much subtler and can easily escape attention in the early phases of fracture management. Damaged soft tissue can impede fracture healing in two important ways: First, it produces an increased metabolic burden, a poor source for vascular ingrowth, and thus a serious impediment to the process of repair because the tissues immediately surrounding the fracture act as a conduit for the new blood supply necessary to support the entire fracture-healing process. Second, it can prevent full recovery of function regardless of how well the fracture itself heals because the soft tissue elements, particularly muscle and tendon, are important musculoskeletal elements in their own right. In the long run, the soft tissue injury is a main determinant of the speed of recovery and the ultimate functional level of the recovered patient.

Some soft tissue injuries are immediately apparent, as in cases of compound fracture in which bleeding or skin defects clearly signal damage to tissue. In other cases, however, soft tissue damage may not become apparent until the rehabilitation process has begun. In the early stages of rehabilitation following a long period of immobilization in traction or a cast, a therapist sometimes discovers that a patient's fractured femur has been accompanied by a previously unnoticed disruption of the medial collateral ligament or tear of the meniscus. In 1980 Kennedy and Walker reported on 26 cases of knee ligament damage associated with femoral shaft fractures and recorded a latency of 12.8 months before the ligament damage was noted. They found that 30% of 54 patients with femoral shaft fractures had "severe" ligament disruption in the ipsilateral knee.[14]

Belated discovery of soft tissue damage, which is sometimes unavoidable, often forces downward revisions of the rehabilitation timetable and ultimate recovery potential. Thorough appreciation of soft tissue damage surrounding a fracture at the time of the first evaluation can prevent such downward revisions and forestall the disappointment they cause.

Soft tissue injury has serious implications for health and function long after a fracture has healed. A look at the pathomechanics of a fracture can be helpful in developing greater appreciation of the distribution of damage between bone and soft tissue when fracture occurs.

PATHOMECHANICS OF FRACTURE

The energy imposed on the human body by the forces of impact must be dissipated—preferably by non–injury-producing methods of absorption. Fig. 5-1 shows an idealized load-deflection curve generated in the laboratory

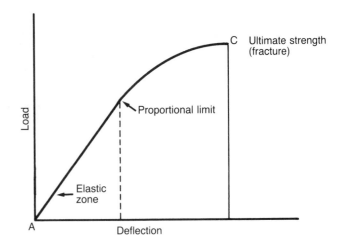

Fig. 5-1. Load-deflection curve representing idealized mechanical behavior of bone under slow loading. Point *C* represents fracture.

by applying a load to bone and recording the deformation or bending that occurs as the load is increased.

The test begins at point A, where load and deflection are assigned a value of zero. As the load increases, the bone deforms along a portion of the curve designated as the "elastic zone." In this region, the bone can absorb energy elastically and then spring back to shape promptly when the load is removed. Bones normally operate in this loading range. However, when load is increased beyond point B, which marks the "proportional limit," tiny failures in bone substance begin to occur, creating permanent deformity as a consequence. Throughout the portion of the curve designated as the "plastic zone," progressive destruction occurs. If the load were removed at any point in the plastic zone, the bone would not return to its normal, healthy state but would continue to contain small infarctions requiring repair. These defects, even when too small to be seen radiographically, may produce pain. During the repair process, the elaboration of callus can be seen radiographically even when frank fracture had not been observed at the time of first analysis and treatment of injury. This phenomenon often occurs in cases of stress fractures or march fractures—common among athletes.[23] In laboratory tests or actual occurrences, if the load applied to bone is increased to point C on the curve, the ultimate strength of bone is reached, and the bone fails. This failure results in a classic bone fracture accompanied by all the clinical manifestations, including pain, deformity, false motion, and swelling.

Bone has a tremendous capacity for load bearing, often reaching 10 to 20 times body weight or up to 2000 to 4000 lb.[27] In most instances of sudden impact, a portion of the load to be borne by the bone is external—applied by something outside the body, such as the ground or an athletic opponent—while another portion is internal—generated by the contractile forces of an individual's own muscles acting across the bone to control body position, as in jumping or falling. The total energy load imposed is usually applied only briefly, sometimes for no more than a fraction of a second. Nevertheless, the accumulated load of both external and internal forces must be absorbed to keep the load in the elastic zone, if possible, but below the ultimate strength load that causes fracture.

Forms of protective gear designed for athletic use, such as helmets, pads, and bindings that release, are meant to help absorb impact and reduce the load on bone, and sports like hockey, fencing, and tackle football cannot be played safely without them. Protective gear alone, however, is not adequate to absorb all the forces of impact imposed on the body. Load is transmitted through protective materials and absorbed in part by the body's own padding in the form of muscle bulk or fat but also by harder body components, such as cartilage and bone.

The principal energy-absorbing mechanism in the human body, however, is a eccentric (lengthening) contraction of muscle. This phenomenon can be conceptualized by comparing the difference between jumping from a table and landing with hip, knee, and ankle locked in a fully extended position to landing in a flexed position so that an eccentric contraction of the gluteus muscle, quadriceps muscle, and gastrocnemius muscle can absorb the energy. In the former instance, the impulse is delivered almost directly to the large bones and axial skeleton. When the energy is too great for the bone, articular cartilage, or intervertebral disks to absorb, overload occurs, resulting in cellular damage. In its milder forms, such damage may affect the articular cartilage, resulting in chondromalacia and other minor destructive changes clinically manifested by joint achiness or swelling and minimal pain. However, if overload is extreme, damage can be severe, producing such injuries as vertebral compression fractures. When one lands from a jump with hips, knees, and ankles flexed, energy is absorbed by muscle, creating a much broader margin of safety and a far smaller incidence of injury. Here, the leap from table to floor amounts to jumping to the squat position and "catching the force" with a lengthening contraction of the quadriceps and gastrocnemius muscles. This mechanism of protection is often recognized and encouraged by such phrases as "roll with the punch," "let your body 'give' with the fall," and "bend your knees when you ski."

Understanding the role of muscle in energy absorption forms the basis for today's strong emphasis on preparticipation conditioning in athletics. Clearly, many of the serious injuries that occur "out of bounds," during a "late hit," or to a "fatigued athlete" can be directly attributed to the player's inability to use muscle contractions appropriately to absorb energy. This principle holds true for the general population as well. Strong muscles provide good protection from fracture.

Internally applied forces produced by voluntary or involuntary muscle contractions can be massive. Because bone is best able to withstand compressive forces, the safest loading configuration is one in which the bone is symmetrically loaded by its accompanying musculature. If agonist and antagonist muscles are equally stressed, bending or torsional loads can be avoided. Unfortunately, a person cannot always accomplish symmetric muscle loading, particularly in movements requiring rapid acceleration, deceleration, or turning. If bending or twisting exceeds the strength of the bone, a fracture can result, even in the absence of a collision or fall. The most common injuries of this kind are a "pulloff" fracture of the base of the fifth metatarsal, an "avulsion" fracture of the medial epicondyle of the elbow, and a spiral humeral fracture. In fact, some element of asymmetric loading is usually a factor in the pathomechanics of all fractures, especially those of long bones. Muscles, by contrast, can play opposing roles when people are injured. They can be protective agents in eccentric muscle contractions, but causative agents in avulsion and other fractures. In either case, the role of soft tissues in the prevention and rehabilitation of fractures cannot be overemphasized.

If the energy at the moment of impact is more than can be absorbed by protective gear or eccentric contraction, injury occurs—first to the soft tissue in the form of ecchymosis or muscle strain and then to bone and ligaments in the form of fracture or rupture. If the impact is severe enough and deformity occurs, vital soft tissues, such as arteries or nerves, can be damaged or destroyed. As an example, the extent of neurologic involvement (motor denervation) following proximal humeral fracture was recently reported by DeLaat and colleagues to represent 54% of such cases in their series of 101 patients.[12] This and other fracture complications are described in more detail later in this chapter. The energy of impact is ultimately totally dissipated, whether that outcome is achieved by protective gear and eccentric muscle contraction or by bony and soft tissue disruption.

The reason why soft tissue injury so often accompanies fracture can be better appreciated by considering the resemblance between the edges of a fractured tibia or humerus and the sharp, jagged edges of a broken piece of hardwood. Because the fractured bone may angulate 90 degrees or more at a high rate of speed during the injury process and then return to a more normal position either spontaneously (due to soft tissue elastic recoil properties) or as a result of deliberate repositioning, it is easy to imagine how soft tissue can be damaged. The rapid movement of fracture ends through adjacent muscle traumatizes the soft tissue and often leads to extensive bleeding and swelling in the area surrounding the fracture. The extreme destructiveness of these events makes it easy to understand why volumes have been written on the emergency care of the fracture patient.

BRIEF REVIEW OF FRACTURE HEALING

Salter has referred to fractures as "wounds of bones" in relation to their healing.[24] The initial effects of the fracture are, in many ways, an elaboration of the standard inflammatory response to soft tissue injury. These effects include blood vessel disruption, fracture hematoma, and tissue necrosis, which occur during the first 5 days following fracture. The early response to the fracture prepares the surrounding tissues and cells to support the proliferation or granulation stage. This stage involves recruitment of undifferentiated fibroblasts and osteoblasts, primarily from the periosteum, which proceed to form the soft callus and then the hard callus of woven bone. The proliferation stage actually begins during the latter period of the inflammation stage and continues for up to 3 months following the date of fracture.

Finally, bone remodeling begins during the end stage of hard callus formation and may continue for several years as osteoclasts continue their activity of altering the endosteal bone. As this maturation phase continues, woven bone of the hard callus stage is gradually converted into lamellar bone, which is functionally more efficient in load-bearing.[24]

EMERGENCY FRACTURE CARE

As with any musculoskeletal injury, identification of a fracture is dependent on as thorough a history and physical examination as the patient's condition allows. Information derived from the clinical examination establishes the presence and extent of any obvious deformity, tissue swelling and/or ecchymosis, and bony crepitus during palpation or limb movement.

Radiographs are indicated when bony disruption is suspected and should include no fewer than two standard views: anterior-posterior (A-P) and lateral. At times, an "oblique" view is required to provide the necessary clarity to identify bony discontinuity. Although physical therapists are not generally tasked with specifically identifying a patient's radiographic abnormalities, it behooves all members of the health care team to be familiar with basic features of the radiographic examination as well as typical findings. The reality in health care delivery today is that patients often bring their radiographs to the initial physical therapy evaluation for review by the physical therapist. In cases of direct access to physical therapy or of patients who have not yet had the opportunity to have their radiographs definitively evaluated by an orthopedic surgeon or radiologist, the physical therapist may need to identify basic radiographic elements. In such circumstances, the physical therapist must be able to identify obvious radiographic abnormalities and note any previously overlooked subtle changes, such as radial head bony irregularity. (See Chapter 7, which includes a brief review of standard elements of the radiographic examination.) Physical therapists are obligated to communicate immediately with the patient's physician upon identifying a previously overlooked bony abnormality or fracture.

Fracture management begins at the moment of first contact with the patient. The emphasis should be on *gentle*, nonforceful manipulation of the limb with immediate splinting to restore circulation and minimize the motion of the sharp fracture ends. This practice avoids additional soft tissue damage due to movement.

Emergency splinting

First-aid efforts involving splinting should be carried out or at least supervised by a physician or experienced technician.[13] A brief but thorough survey of all body parts through hands-on palpation and inquiry should be carried out first. Throughout this initial on-site evaluation, the guiding principle is that "fractures hurt." If squeezing or gently moving a body part does not produce pain, it can be safely assumed that the part is not fractured.

To be thorough in the use of the squeeze technique, the examiner should begin at the injured person's head and gently squeeze or palpate the skull, neck, shoulders, upper extremities, and so on, including the chest, pelvis, legs, and feet. Examination concludes with running fingers down the victim's spine. The squeeze technique is reliable and fast: A complete examination can be completed in less than 10 seconds. A positive response is recorded when the victim complains of pain in response to a squeeze, deformity in the bone is palpated, or when crepitation or false motion caused by a fracture is observed.

If a fracture is found, emergency splinting is necessary before the patient can be transported elsewhere for medical attention. If possible, the deformed part should be gently returned to its proper anatomic position. If significant resistance to this return is met, however, the part should be splinted in the position in which it was found.

Sometimes emergency splinting in athletics calls for considerable ingenuity, as, for example, when an injured athlete is still wearing protective equipment, such as pads, boots, or helmet. In many such instances, it is best to transport the patient with the protective gear still in place so as not to risk inflicting further injury.

Many kinds of devices are available to facilitate emergency splinting (Figs. 5-2 and 5-3), including inflatable splints, cardboard splints, backboards, litters, slings, and portable traction devices, such as the Thomas splint and traction splints. If none of these happened to be available, improvisation is in order, and items such as skis, ski poles, pillows, or even rolled-up magazines can be used to fashion crude but effective emergency splints. In extreme cases, the fractured leg can be splinted by binding it to the patient's uninjured leg; a fractured upper arm can be temporarily strapped to the chest.

Injuries to the neck require exceptional care. The patient with significant neck pain must, for safety's sake, be presumed to have suffered a neck fracture. In such cases, splinting the injured area is necessary, and the patient should be transported as quickly as possible to a medical facility where a definitive evaluation can be made. The safest transport device for the neck- or back-injured victim is a backboard and sandbags or straps. A complaint of even mild or localized numbness, flaccidity, or any other neurologic deficit—even if only of short duration—must always be interpreted as a contraindication to resuming activity until a complete evaluation of the injury has been made. This should

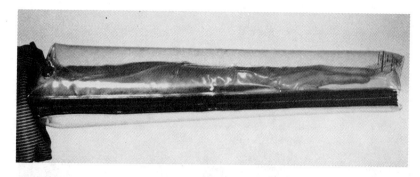

Fig. 5-2. Inflatable (air) splint for emergency immobilization of a fractured forearm.

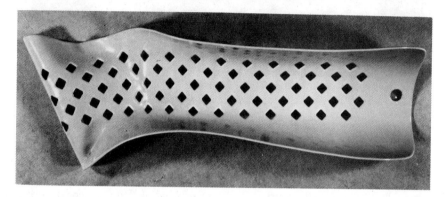

Fig. 5-3. Fixed forearm splint for emergency immobilization of fractured left forearm.

include radiographs followed by careful neurologic examination.

When the injured person is transported, the primary care group or the family must send relevant information with the patient, either in writing or by word of mouth. It should include:

1. A report of associated or secondary injuries
2. A description of the mechanism of injury
3. A list of relevant prior injuries or medical conditions

Some of these observations can be made only by the acute care group, but all are crucial to achieving complete and safe management of the patient. Too often a significant contributing factor to the seriousness of an injury has been ignored or poorly evaluated.

TYPES OF FRACTURES

Fractures may take any one of several forms (see the Box for a list of types of fractures), depending on the position of the limb when fractured, the velocity of the injury, the position of protective pads or equipment, and the duration of impact. For example, a high-energy, twisting injury that occurs to an alpine skier can produce a severely *comminuted* fracture. *Compound* fractures occur when sharp ends of broken bone protrude through the victim's skin or when some projectile penetrates the skin into the fracture site.

The presence of a compound fracture significantly alters fracture management and may negatively influence the

Types of fractures
Perforating (e.g., gunshot-bullet penetration)
Depressed or fissured
Greenstick
Spiral
Oblique
Transverse
Avulsion
Segmental
Comminuted
Stellate
Stress
Pathologic:
• Carcinoma
• Infection
• Osteoporosis

likelihood of complete healing because it often signifies the presence of extensive soft tissue damage or contamination. A compound fracture that has become infected does not heal until the infection has been eliminated. Therefore, to prevent infection, a limb with protruding bone ends should be covered with a sterile dressing and transported as is, without returning the bone end to its normal position inside the skin. This type of emergency treatment prevents the introduction of additional dirt and debris into the wound before the bone

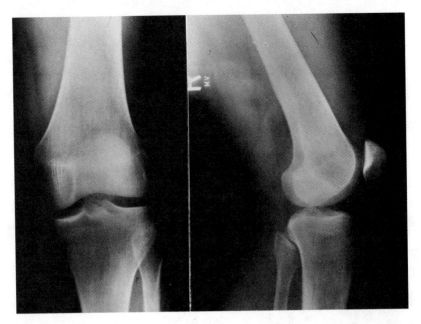

Fig. 5-4. Anteroposterior and lateral radiograph of an adult knee. Note articular cartilage interval between bones.

end can be cleansed and also alerts the surgeon to the need for cleansing the injured area thoroughly. Fractures that involve joints and disrupt the "load-bearing surface" demand special attention. In the management of these fractures, it is essential to reduce the joint surface to its original smooth condition. Severely damaged articular cartilage or a residual step-off of bone at the joint may lead to premature degenerative arthritis.

Fractures in children

Growth plates are disks composed of cartilage located close to the ends of long bones near all the major joints. Normally, this zone proliferates bone and causes the limbs to elongate, a process that accounts for normal bone growth throughout childhood and adolescence. After an individual reaches about 16 years of age, the growth plate closes solidly with bone and becomes less vulnerable. Until that time, however, damage to the cartilage cells in the growth plate—in the form of a fracture, infection, or some other incident or process—may disturb growth and causes, for example, a crooked limb or even complete cessation of growth.

Although fractures in children's bones are common and growth disturbances rare, the outcome of fracture through the growth plate is important. Unfortunately, a growth disturbance due to a fractured growth plate is difficult to diagnose. It reveals itself only gradually in the months following the injury as growth becomes increasingly and noticeably abnormal. The Salter-Harris system for classification of epiphyseal plate injuries has proven to be very useful for identifying potential growth plate disturbances following fractures in children and establishing a prognosis for such injuries.[24]

The growth plate appears on a radiograph as a lucent line near the joint, and a fracture through that line can easily be missed unless there is some disturbance in the alignment of the bone (Figs. 5-4 and 5-5). A special case occurs at the knee, where a fracture through the distal femoral or proximal tibial growth plates may be misdiagnosed as a ligament rupture. This kind of error can be avoided by a gentle stress radiograph when a growth plate fracture is suspected even though initial radiographs have been negative. If the knee opens at the growth plate rather than through the joint, a knee ligament injury should be ruled out, and a growth plate fracture can be diagnosed.

When a fracture occurs in a growth plate, the patient's family should be alerted to the possibility of growth disturbance, and the health professional should take special care to follow the healing process until the risk of growth disturbance has passed—at least 1 year, especially if a fracture has been somewhat refractory to healing and before definitive bone remodeling has occurred. The younger the patient, the greater the growth potential remaining and, concomitantly, the greater the danger of significant growth disturbance. Compliance with the necessary period of immobilization is difficult for most children, and special precautions are mandatory in the supervision of the very young fracture patient.

Fractures in the elderly

Significant fractures, such as femoral neck or trochanteric, in the elderly population carry with them an unusually high incidence of morbidity and mortality. Many predisposing factors may account for the incidence of fractures in the elderly, but the most important seems to be the presence of osteoporosis, whether senile or postmenopausal. Osteoporo-

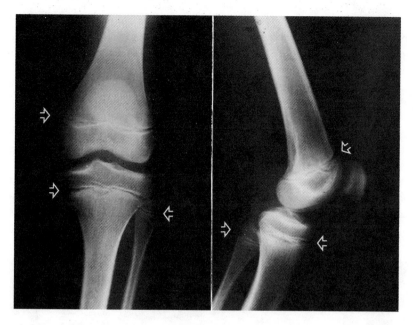

Fig. 5-5. Anteroposterior and lateral radiograph of a child's knee showing "open" epiphyseal growth plates *(arrows).* These are disks of epiphyseal cartilage that produce longitudinal growth.

sis is a process of demineralization resulting from osteoclastic activity out of proportion to bone deposition. It may occur during a period of prolonged immobilization, because of reduction in bone stress due to sedentary lifestyle, or following menopause in women. Osteoporosis affects an estimated 15 to 20 million postmenopausal women in the United States and may account for the devastating effects following bone trauma in women.[1] The need to minimize the postfracture period of immobilization (in an effort to diminish the incidence of morbidity) is one major reason why open reduction with internal fixation is often the treatment of choice for elderly individuals who have sustained a fracture of a weight-bearing bone.

Stress fractures

A stress fracture is the reaction of bone (usually in the lower extremity) to accelerated, unaccustomed, repetitive, submaximal stresses. Physical therapists should be especially alert to the possibility that their patients may develop fatigue or stress fractures because, in many cases, they represent a "training error." When strenuous exercise is imposed on easily fatigued muscle, that muscle has a diminished ability to dampen the skeletal system loading forces (Fig. 5-6). If such abnormal bone loading persists unrelieved, microscopic changes in the bone begin that result in the signs and symptoms of a stress reaction or fracture. The signs include exquisite point tenderness to palpation, localized edema and tissue temperature, antalgic gait, and significant relief of symptoms with rest. Initial radiographs taken shortly after the onset of symptoms are usually normal, although a bone scan can identify the focal area of bone reaction (elevated metabolic activity).

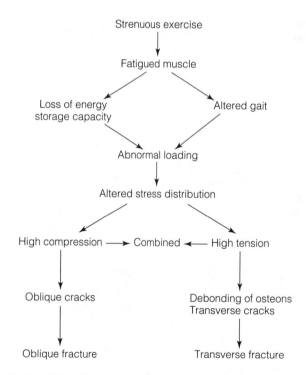

Fig. 5-6. Flow diagram showing sequence of factors leading to stress fractures. Loss of energy storage capability of muscle (fatigue) leads to microscopic bone failure (stress fracture).

Failure to identify a developing stress reaction may have devastating effects for highly motivated athletes as they attempt to "play through" their pain. Treatment usually consists of rest from running or walking and may necessitate the use of crutches for approximately 3 weeks as the bone heals. Maintaining cardiovascular fitness through alternative exercise protocols (for instance, running in the water) and a *gradual* resumption of prestress fracture activity to avoid further training errors are effective in returning most patients to full activity.

DEFINITIVE FRACTURE MANAGEMENT

The definitive management phase of fracture care usually begins in the hospital or clinic with a decision as to the most appropriate type of immobilization for the fracture in question. The selection process can be influenced by a number of variables, including the nature of the fracture (closed or open), its anatomic location, the physician's preference and skill in treatment, and the needs and preferences of the patient.

Today, such variables can usually be accommodated in several different ways, but occasionally an injury mandates a single treatment method. For example, a fracture that disrupts the joint surface requires that the bone fragments be held together to produce a smooth joint surface, which allows the fracture to heal and prevents the later development of degenerative arthritis. Therefore, the fracture must be treated either *closed,* by means of casting or traction, or *open,* by surgical intervention using plates, screws, or other internal fixation devices. The advantages of the closed method of reduction are obvious: avoidance of surgery,

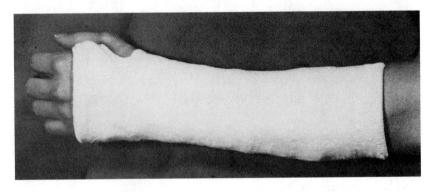

Fig. 5-7. Conventional plaster-of-Paris cast for wrist fracture.

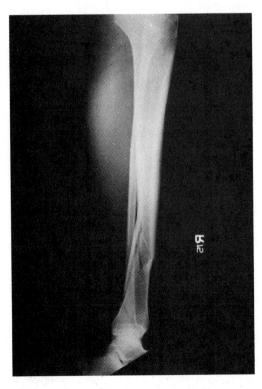

Fig. 5-8. Lateral radiograph of comminuted spiral distal tibial fracture.

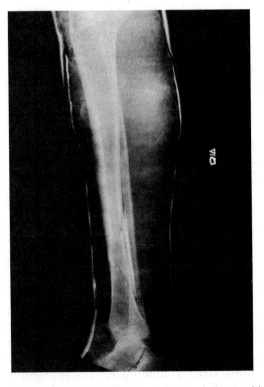

Fig. 5-9. Fracture, illustrated in Fig. 5-8, in excellent position in long-leg plaster cast.

reduction of the fracture, and usually (except in the case of traction) a shorter hospital stay. Open reduction, by contrast, may require subsequent removal of the metal devices, increases the possibility of infection, and usually requires hospitalization time. Regardless of the technique selected, however, premature return to the patient's prior activity level is never a good idea. The risk of permanent pain or deformity is simply too great.

Closed reduction

Closed reduction is the process of manually aligning the fracture, usually while the patient is under local or general anesthesia, and encasing the limb in a cast (Figs. 5-7 to 5-9). The plaster cast is the most common fracture immobilization device and offers several advantages over other techniques: It is easily applied and removed, inexpensive, "breathable" (that is, not airtight), nonallergenic, and noncombustible. The plaster cast consists of plaster-impregnated cloth rolls or sheets, which, when soaked in water, begin a heat-producing curing processing lasting from 2 to 10 minutes. Usually the cast is applied over several layers of cotton sheeting laid directly on the skin. When dry, the plaster can be cut and wedged or angled to align the fracture or split to expand and accommodate a swelling limb. It can be safely removed with an oscillating cast saw, and it can be fitted with hinges to allow the joint to move.

Today, however, despite its numerous advantages, the plaster cast is only one of several forms of immobilizing devices available for the treatment of fracture. Casts made of resin and Fiberglas tend to be more durable than plaster, are sometimes used to facilitate bathing, and permit the patient to continue exercising all body parts except the injured limb (Fig. 5-10).

Usually the patient can safely begin gentle range-of-motion exercises several weeks before the fractured limb is strong enough to return to normal weight-bearing function (in the case of lower extremity fractures) or to withstand resistance at the fracture site (in the case of upper extremity fractures). For this purpose, some casts are fitted with a metal or plastic hinged joint to permit early joint motion. Hinged casts are called *cast braces* and are extremely useful in shortening patient "downtime" as well as in facilitating early mobilization (Fig. 5-11).

In the later stages of fracture healing, prefabricated splints of plastic or fabric may be used. They can be worn to protect the fractured limb and taken off at intervals to permit joint mobilization or bathing (Figs. 5-12 and 5-13). The range of immobilizing devices available to today's health profes-

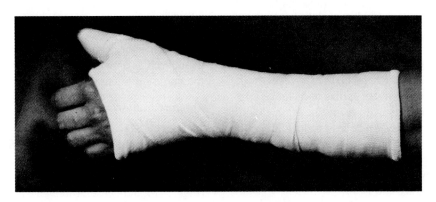

Fig. 5-10. Waterproof Fiberglas cast.

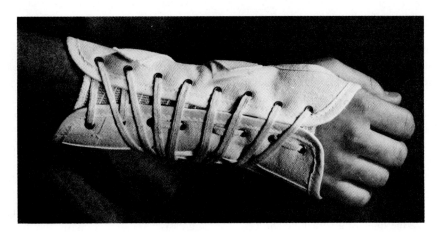

Fig. 5-11. Removable canvas wrist-splint used to treat wrist sprain or as protection during rehabilitation of wrist fracture.

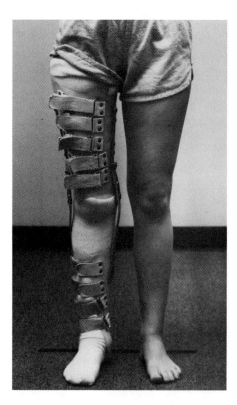

Fig. 5-12. Cast brace for fractured femur. Note adjustable thigh and calf bands and knee hinges. Note freedom of motion at knee and ankle.

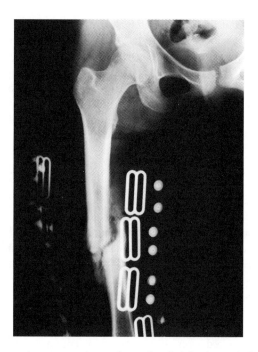

Fig. 5-13. Anteroposterior radiograph of right femoral fracture incurred by patient in Fig. 5-12. Note metal brace buckles and "cloud" of fracture callus.

sional permits the fracture-healing process to be staged. Rigid plaster immobilization for the first few weeks can be followed by a period of removable splints to facilitate joint mobilization. When the patient is ready to return to full activity, the chance of reinjury can be lessened by fitting the limb with a light protective splint or a brace. Even with a young person, 2 years or more may elapse before a seriously fractured bone is completely restored to its original, energy-absorbing functional level.

Traction

Traction is a very old but effective method of fracture management. It involves keeping the patient in bed with the fractured limb immobilized and influenced by a system of weights and pulleys. Skeletal traction is usually established by percutaneously drilling a pin through the distal fracture fragments and employing a U-shaped clevis device that permits ropes and weights to pull the pin and bone in a direction that aligns the fracture. The patient's own weight supplies the counterforce. The alignment process is assisted with a padded metal frame that gently supports the fractured limb.

The traction method takes advantage of the mass of soft tissues surrounding the injured limb. By pulling longitudinally on the limb, these surrounding muscles, ligaments, and tendons become taut (like the lines of a parachute shroud), thus correctly aligning the fractured bone they encircle.

Traction is maintained throughout the healing process,

which usually takes several months. When the patient's injury is particularly complex (such as head trauma or abdominal injury), so that other forms of fracture management, such as surgery, are contraindicated, traction may be the only safe fracture management option available.

Open reduction

Open reduction is the process of surgically opening the fracture site in order to align and secure the broken bone. This procedure has been known since medieval times, but only in the past 50 years has it been commonly employed (Figs. 5-14 and 5-15). Although there are disadvantages of open reduction and internal fixation (ORIF), as mentioned previously, they are often outweighed by the advantages, which include precise bony reduction, early mobilization of joints, and immediate stability, allowing earlier return to full function.

Bone-compression plating. One type of open reduction, bone-compression plating, was developed by the Swiss team of surgeons and engineers who founded the Association for the Scientific Investigation of Fractures (ASIF). In the 1960s and 1970s, the ASIF team designed plates, screws, and instruments to permit plating the fracture with metal and splinting the fracture so as to compress the bone ends together. Their approach was broadly inclusive, drawing attention to important issues such as the proper care of soft tissue, reestablishment of the contour of joint surfaces, and aggressive rehabilitation of the patient (Fig. 5-16). The techniques they described are especially valuable in cases of joint fractures or very complicated shaft fractures, and their

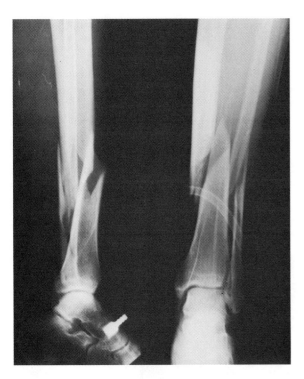

Fig. 5-14. Lateral and anteroposterior radiograph of distal tibial and fibular fracture. Note valve from air splint in lateral view.

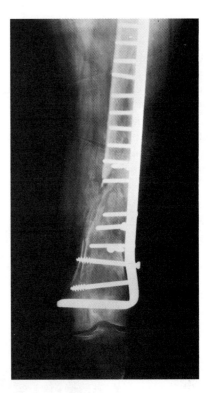

Fig. 5-16. Anterior radiograph of comminuted distal femoral fracture, secured with a condylar blade compression plate and multiple screws.

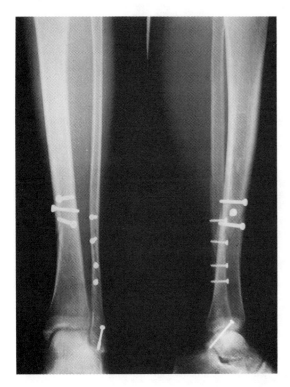

Fig. 5-15. Fractured lower leg illustrated in Fig. 5-14, repaired with interfragmentary screw fixation. Note: Short-term plaster cast was also used.

contributions have played a major role in the advances made in fracture care around the world over the past 20 years. A principal goal of the ASIF group was to encourage early return of function, a concept important to all patients but especially to athletes and the elderly.

Compression plating involves the direct securing of the injured bone with metallic internal fixation devices, such as plates or screws. They are constructed of modern surgical-grade metals, such as stainless steel, cobalt chrome, and titanium alloys, which are well tolerated by the body and produce a very low incidence of tissue reaction. The fracture-reduction procedure is undertaken by an orthopedic surgeon, usually on an elective basis after the fracture has been given a thorough preoperative assessment aided by radiographs. An appropriately shaped and sized device is selected, sterilized, inserted through a surgical incision, and secured to the bone with drilling and tapping techniques familiar to every experienced machinist. The main objectives are to restabilize the bone to its proper length and rotation, restore proper alignment, and, if a fracture has disrupted the joint, restore the joint surface to its normal smooth contour.

The normal joint is covered with a thin layer of articular cartilage, a highly specialized tissue that acts as a "biologic bearing." Cartilage can withstand immense loads for many years, but, once disrupted by a step-off irregularity, it roughens and can degenerate in a few months or years. This kind of joint destruction *(degenerative arthritis)* and its prevention is one reason why smooth reestablishment of a fractured joint surface is so essential to the health of the joint.

Sometimes, particularly in the case of metal plates, the inserted metal must be removed after the fracture has healed (1 to 3 years) because the end of the plate becomes a stress concentration or a focus for the forces of subsequent load on the bone at the end of the plate and increases the chances of a new fracture. When plates and screws are removed, the bone experiences a temporary weakening until the screw holes fill in and the bone remodels. This process may last from 6 to 12 weeks or longer, and during this period the patient may need to use crutches or a splint and begin a reconditioning process (Figs. 5-17 to 5-19).

Intermedullary rodding. Intermedullary rodding is another form of open reduction that is particularly useful in fractures of long hollow bones, such as the humerus, radius, tibia, and femur. In this technique, the surgeon places a solid or tubular metal rod down the endosteal canal of the bone. In the case of the femur—the bone for which this technique is most often used—fixation can be secure enough to preclude the use of a cast, although crutches are often necessary until the fracture unites. After the fracture heals,

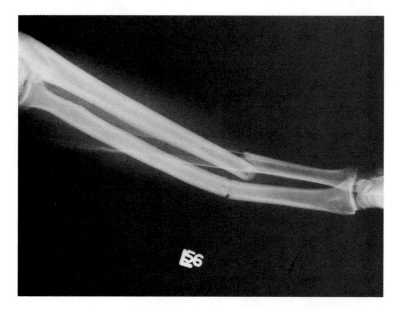

Fig. 5-17. Double bone fracture of distal forearm.

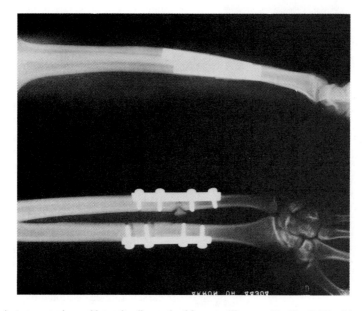

Fig. 5-18. Anteroposterior and lateral radiograph of fracture illustrated in Fig. 5-17, with compression plates in place.

the rod can be safely removed through a small incision at the hip (Fig. 5-20).

Rigid external fixation

Rigid external fixation involves the securing of each fracture segment with two or more metal pins percutaneously drilled through the limb and fracture fragment. Once in place, the pins first manipulate the fragments into correct alignment and then connect them to each other in a rigid external frame or a plaster casing. The injured limb looks as if it has been pierced with several arrows, but no incision need be made except for insertion of the pins. Thus, the patient can be treated out of the hospital with the pins left in place until the fracture has healed. Rigid external fixation is especially useful in cases involving extensive damage to the skin because the orthopedic surgeon and the plastic surgeon can work simultaneously on the patient (Figs. 5-21 and 5-22).

A specific form of rigid external fixation, the Ilizarov external fixator, has recently gained considerable attention. The Ilizarov device makes of the law of tension stress on bone through bifocal compression-distraction and has been particularly successful for treatment of high-velocity bone trauma, such as gunshots and car and motorcycle accidents.[4] High-velocity fractures are usually associated with significant bone loss and often become severely infected, which leads to delayed healing or nonunion. The Ilizarov method of external fixation has been especially helpful for this specific category of bone lesion.[21]

Bioelectrical stimulation

Bioelectrical stimulation is a relatively new fracture management technique that makes use of electrical stimu-

lation to help heal the fracture. To appreciate the particular value of this technique, it must be realized that sometimes a nonunion is really a fibrous connective tissue rather than bone. This fibrous tissue can be converted to bone by electrical stimulation.[5]

One method of bioelectrical stimulation surrounds the entire limb at the fracture site with an electrical coil and induces a pulsed electromagnetic field (PEMF) for 12 or more hours each day. This equipment is custom-designed and calibrated for each patient. A second method consists of surgically implanting tiny electrodes in the fibrous tissue at the nonunion site and connecting these to a power source, usually a lithium battery buried under the skin. A third method requires percutaneous insertion (under x-ray control) of Teflon-coated electrical wires into the nonunion site.[10] The tips of the electrodes are bare, and the wires are connected to a battery pack outside the skin. The fracture is then continuously electrically stimulated in the 2-nm range for 12 weeks (Figs. 5-23 to 5-25).

Most bioelectrical methods require the concomitant use of a cast and crutches throughout the process. The success rate of these methods applied to difficult cases of nonunion has been very good, approaching 80%,[15] although the validity of these results has been questioned by other investigators.[9] To date, bioelectrical methods have been used to treat nonunions alone (primarily tibial) and are not currently indicated in the treatment of acute fractures.

Fracture rehabilitation

The rehabilitation phase is the last stage of fracture management. The primary rationale for physical rehabilitation of the patient following fracture is the intuitive premise that loss of joint and overall movement is a major contributor

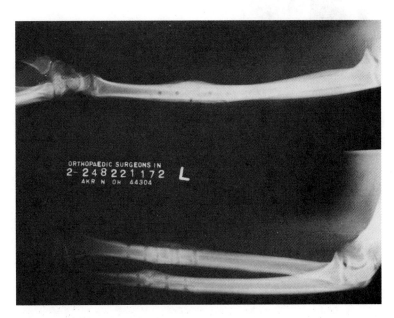

Fig. 5-19. Early remodeling phase of fracture seen in Figs. 5-17 and 5-18. Note: Compression plates have been removed, but drill holes are still evident 1 year after fracture.

to postfracture morbidity and, in some cases, mortality. Therefore, the goal of rehabilitation efforts is to restore functional movement in order to allow the patient to resume occupational, athletic, and/or social activities as quickly as possible. Research indicates that return to early motion and weight bearing (accelerated rehabilitation) results in better motion,[2] shorter hospital stays and less mortality,[6] less overall postfracture morbidity,[8] and less overall cost to the health care system than a no rehabilitation approach.[7]

Adequate rehabilitation is usually determined by analysis of a combination of factors, including swelling, pain, joint mobility, and muscle strength. Much of the uncertainty in determining completion of this phase is eliminated by direct objective measurements and, in the case of fractured limbs, by comparison of the injured limb with its uninjured

counterpart. Comparable limb diameter and joint swelling can be determined by circumferential measurements. Torque-generating capabilities of skeletal muscle may be measured by manual muscle testing or with an isokinetic dynamometer (when available) (Figs. 5-26 and 5-27) in

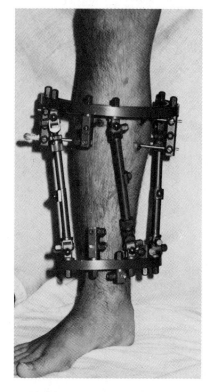

Fig. 5-21. External-fixation fracture device. Note percutaneous pins passing through bone.

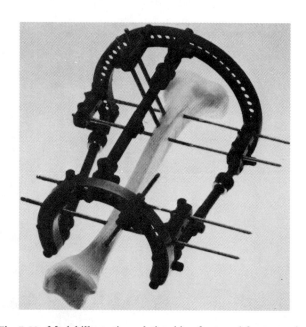

Fig. 5-22. Model illustrating relationship of external fixator to pins that pass through bone to maintain bone alignment.

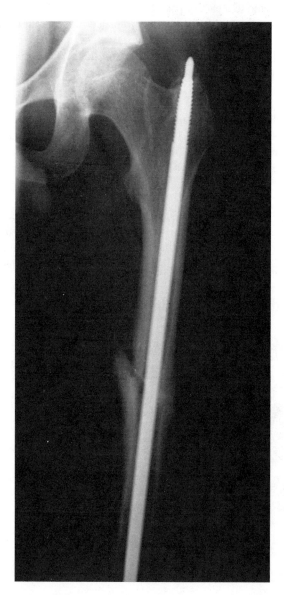

Fig. 5-20. Anteroposterior radiograph of a femur showing an intramedullary rod in the endosteal canal to secure a fracture.

radians per second or ft-pounds (Newton-meters) at varying testing rates. The patient's fractured limb is compared to its healthy counterpart (or, if necessary, to measurements of limb characteristics in a population of uninjured persons of similar age and body mass).

The decision to return a patient to his or her normal activity level is usually arrived at gradually with the return of strength and motion. The general rule of thumb is that vigorous activity can be resumed when the strength deficit is 15% or less, but today the decision is usually arrived at by discussion among surgeon, therapist, and patient. It is modified immediately in the event of any regression during the early stages of the patient's return to full activity.

The patient's own assessment of readiness is usually evident in level of confidence. Confidence is based on a constellation of factors that are internally, unconsciously weighed on a daily basis and can be evaluated by comparison with the patient's preinjury confidence level. A therapist can and should help the injured person establish a realistic level of confidence by helping the patient minimize or eliminate obscuring elements such as peer or family pressure, inordinately intense desire to overachieve, or fear that is out of proportion to reality. Even after careful measurement and management, determining the patient's confidence level is difficult and may be likened to determining whether someone's new shoe fits—only the person wearing it can be sure it is right. Failure to help the patient honestly develop confidence on the basis of good scientific rehabilitation principles

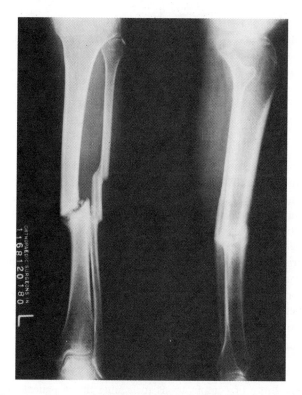

Fig. 5-23. Anteroposterior and lateral radiographs of a midshaft fractured tibia that has failed to heal because of tibial nonunion.

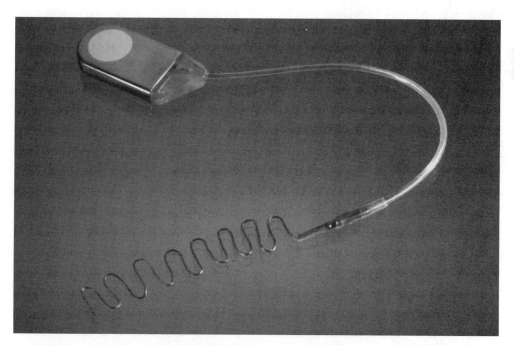

Fig. 5-24. OsteoGen™ implantable stimulation device for treating delayed union or nonunion of long bones. (Courtesy of EBI Medical Systems, Inc., Parsippany, N.J.)

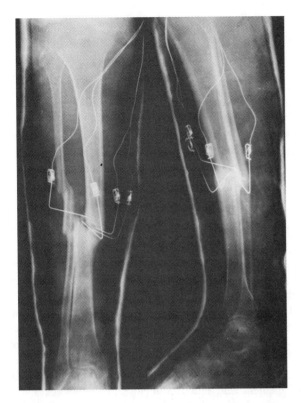

Fig. 5-25. Tibial fracture seen in Fig. 5-23 with percutaneous electrodes in place and electrode tips in fracture site.

can leave him or her in the perilous position of either never attaining full potential or plunging back into activity too quickly, thus performing inadequately or inviting reinjury.

Measurements of limb size or strength during the rehabilitation phase of fracture management tell much more about muscle strength and soft tissue repair than about bone strength. Even radiographic analysis provides only indirect information about the strength of the bone. The observation of a defect or failure in the bone is clear evidence of its weakness, of course, but the strength of bone under repair remains difficult to judge, and extensive experience is necessary before one develops confidence in accurate analysis of this important aspect of healing. Because of such considerations, motion, muscle strength, and atrophy are the principal determinants of the progress of healing, coupled with the patient's own level of confidence.

Although the fracture site begins to demonstrate microscopic histologic evidence of healing as early as 15 hours following injury, radiographic evidence of fracture healing in the form of callus is rarely seen before 4 weeks. In some bones, such as the carpals and the cervical vertebrae, the appearance of callus is often skimpy, even in a fracture healing normally. The first radiographic evidence of callus appears about the fourth week following injury and continues for 10 weeks or more, to be followed by months of remodeling.

Remodeling is best defined by Wolff's law, which states: "Bone remodels along the lines of stress according to certain mathematical principles."[26] During the months of remodeling, the abundant callus is replaced by a progressively stronger remodeled bone. It may be several years following the injury before the radiographic evidence of a fracture is no longer visible.

The time factors related to fractures present an interesting, if sometimes frustrating and disheartening, pattern. A fracture occurs in a matter of milliseconds, needs weeks of immobilization in a cast, requires months of rehabilitation time, and takes years to complete the remodeling process. Throughout the rehabilitation process, a patient's return to activities and subsequent degree of participation are dependent on range-of-motion measurements, assessment of strength, pain, swelling, and, finally, the health professional team's best estimation as to the strength of the healing bone. Fortunately, accumulated clinical experience and modern methods of treatment and evaluation make this studied estimation a reasonably safe procedure.

COMPLICATIONS OF FRACTURE HEALING

All members of the health care team must be alert to the possibility of complications to healing that a patient may experience following fracture. Potential complications are numerous and have been grouped, for classification purposes, in a variety of ways.[24] Complications range in severity from those that are life-threatening (fat embolism, pulmonary embolism from deep vein thrombosis), to those that are deformity producing (Volkmann's ischemic contracture), to those that are mostly nuisance (minor joint stiffness). Some of the more common and important complications follow.

Nonunion fractures

Age, general health, degree of violence, and location of the fracture are all important factors influencing the rate of fracture healing. In an infant, a fractured femur may heal in 4 weeks. The same fracture in a teenager may require 12 to 16 weeks to heal and, in a 60-year-old person, 18 to 20 weeks. The presence of diabetes or some other medical problem, such as osteoporosis, prolongs the healing period, increases the incidence of fracture—or both. Certain medications, such as steroids for allergy or other conditions, may have a similar slowing effect on the fracture-healing process.

When fractured bone has failed to reunite after 5 months, a *nonunion* is said to exist. In addition to the factors just described that are known to slow the healing process, two other factors often influence the development of a nonunion: (1) contamination of the fracture site through a break in the skin and (2) motion at the fracture site. Contamination is caused by foreign material, devitalized tissue, or bacteria (endogenous and/or exogenous), all of which inhibit the repair process and may prevent healing. Careful handling of tissue, thorough cleansing of the wound, surgical removal

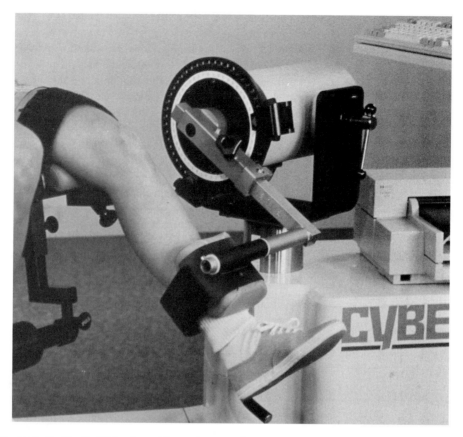

Fig. 5-26. Isokinetic (Cybex) machine testing muscle strength and endurance of the leg. (Courtesy Cybex, Ronkonkoma, NY.)

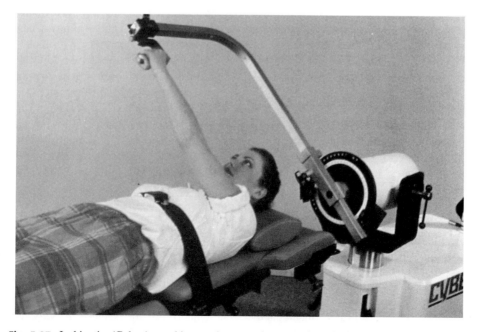

Fig. 5-27. Isokinetic (Cybex) machine testing muscle strength and endurance of the shoulder. (Courtesy Cybex, Ronkonkoma, NY.)

of devitalized tissue (debridement), and appropriate use of antibiotics reduce the incidence of nonunion in compound fractures.

Motion at the fracture site is another leading cause of nonunions. Motion can occur within a poorly applied cast, with certain internally applied devices such as rods or plates, or with a fracture close to a joint, such as the proximal humerus. Therefore, a basic tenet of fracture management is to immobilize the fractured bone one joint below the fracture site long enough for the fracture to heal. Prolonged immobilization, however, usually results in loss of muscle strength (atrophy) and bone strength (disuse osteopenia), and therefore the period of immobilization must last no longer than the time needed to produce a structurally safe union. This period is determined by radiographic evaluation and from experience. Immobilization promotes healing by allowing the swelling to subside and permitting formation of a healing "vascular swamp" around the broken bone that can bring in a rich blood supply to nourish callus first and then new bone.

A fracture management protocol must be individualized for each patient based on the type of fracture, the fracture location, and the method of stabilization. The healing process is monitored radiographically and by clinical examination based on experience. Such planning and diligence minimize the incidence of nonunion, but this unfortunate complication continues to occur, even in the face of expert care and optimum circumstances.

Nonunions are prone to occur in bones where the blood supply is precarious. Two notorious examples are the femoral neck and the carpal navicular bone. When a nonunion is identified, treatment consists of clearing an infection (if it exists), immobilizing the fracture (either by casting, plates and screws, rods, or other mechanical fixation techniques such as the Ilizarov device), electrically stimulating the bone, and often bone grafting. Bone grafting consists of harvesting small quantities of bone from an area, such as the pelvis, in a manner that does not seriously weaken the site. This bone is then transferred to a location immediately around the nonunited fracture site. Bone taken from the patient is called an *autograft,* and that taken from others or a cadaver is called an *allograft.* The use of allographic bone requires very careful technique to avoid transferring infection or disease to either the donor or the recipient. Nonunion sites thus stimulated by bone graft usually go on to heal.

Edema

Limb edema from extravasated interstitial fluid or lymph fluid often follows a fracture of the extremities. It is usually a self-limited complication and may be properly treated by instruction in appropriate limb positioning, gentle joint movement, and static muscle contractions to encourage muscle pump activity. Pressure gradient garments and intermittent pneumatic compression therapy have also been effective in reducing postfracture edema.[3]

Joint stiffness

Loss of joint movement may result from intraarticular fibrous adhesions, capsular fibrosis (such as adhesive capsulitis of the glenohumeral joint following proximal humeral fracture), or tendinous adhesions, which are common following hand fractures. Other postfracture complications that may result in loss of movement include reflex sympathetic dystrophy and myositis ossificans. Although these conditions are different in many ways, one common aspect of treatment is restoration of joint mobility through early joint mobilization, active range of motion, isometric muscle contraction, and continuous passive motion (CPM).[17,25] Electromodality application has been used with varying results based on the specific condition treated and the choice of device used (transcutaneous electrical nerve stimulation or TENS, high-amplitude muscle stimulation, high-voltage pulsed stimulation, iontophoresis, ultrasound).

Neurologic complications

The actual incidence of all nerve injuries associated with fractures is not known, although it has been reported that 80% to 90% of nerve injuries following fractures occur in the upper extremity.[20] Pollock and colleagues reported in 1981 that humeral fractures injure the radial nerve most often, with an incidence of 16%.[22] By contrast, a recent report documenting careful electrodiagnostic testing of 101 patients following proximal humeral fracture identified an incidence of nerve injury in 54% of these individuals.[12] Interestingly, the pattern of denervation involved the axillary nerve most often, followed by suprascapular nerve injury. We have found a similar pattern of denervation (confirmed by electromyography) following proximal humeral fracture.[19] Although the authors attributed the injury to infraclavicular brachial plexus lesion, it may also be due to neurogenic inflammation following trauma, an observation documented in other clinical studies,[18] and laboratory investigations.[16]

Although members of the health care team must be alert to immediate neurologic injuries like those described, they should also be aware that some nerve lesions are delayed in their development and manifestation. Ulnar nerve palsy may develop years or decades following a fracture about the elbow, whereas carpal tunnel syndrome may gradually develop over a period of weeks or months following a Colles' fracture of the wrist. In both cases, treatment involves surgical release of the compressed or constricted neurologic structure.

SUMMARY

Great strides have been made in the diagnosis and management of fractures since Wilhelm Conrad Röntgen first showed the world a roentgen ray of the hand in 1896. However, such advances have brought with them myriad new questions, for instance, Exactly how are bioelectrical and mechanical factors mediated? What is the precise mechanism by which nutrition affects bone healing and remodeling? How can the detrimental effects of postmenopausal hormonal changes on bone be minimized or reversed safely and conveniently? These questions are currently topics of ongoing research. Further improvements in the quality of care for fracture patients should result from the findings of such research.

REVIEW QUESTIONS

1. What is the purpose of bioelectrical stimulation in the management of fractures?
2. What are the basic stages of fracture healing and the general time frame for each stage?
3. How does bone compression plating differ from rigid external fixation?
4. What special steps should be followed when a child has a growth plate fracture?
5. What are the differences between an open versus a closed reduction of a fracture in regard to planning the rehabilitation program?

REFERENCES

1. Agnostini R: *Medical and orthopedic issues of active and athletic women,* Philadelphia, 1994, Hanley & Belfus.
2. Ahl T, Dalen N, Selvik G: Mobilization after operation of ankle fractures. Good results of early motion and weight bearing, *Acta Orthop Scand* 59:302, 1988.
3. Airaksinen-O: Changes in post-traumatic ankle joint mobility, pain and edema following intermittent pneumatic compression therapy, *Arch Phys Med Rehabil* 70:341, 1989.
4. Alonso JE, Regazzoni P: Use of the Ilizarov concept with AO/ASIF tubular fixator in the treatment of segmental defects, *Orthop Clin North Am* 21:655, 1990.
5. Bassett CAL, Valdes MG, Hernandez E: Modification of fracture repair with selected pulsing electromagnetic fields, *J Bone Joint Surg Am* 64:888, 1982.
6. Cameron ID, Lyle DM, Quine S: Accelerated rehabilitation after proximal femoral fracture: a randomized controlled trial, *Disabil Rehabil* 15:29, 1993.
7. Cameron ID, Lyle DM, Quine S: Cost effectiveness of accelerated rehabilitation after proximal femoral fracture, *J Clin Epidemiol* 47:1307, 1994.
8. Cimino W, Ichtertz D, Slabaugh P: Early mobilization of ankle fractures after open reduction and internal fixation, *Clin Orthop* 267:152, 1991.
9. Colson DJ et al: Treatment of delayed- and non-union of fractures using pulsed electromagnetic fields, *J Biomed Eng* 10:301, 1988.
10. Cundy PJ, Paterson DC: A ten-year review of treatment of delayed union and non-union with an implanted bone growth stimulator, *Clin Orthop* 259:216, 1990.
11. Curtiss PH Jr: Personal communication, May 15, 1967.
12. DeLaat EA et al: Nerve lesions in primary shoulder dislocations and humeral neck fractures: a prospective and clinical EMG study, *J Bone Joint Surg Br* 76:381, 1994.
13. Hoyt WA Jr et al: *Emergency care and transportation of the sick and injured,* ed 3, Chicago, 1981, American Academy of Orthopaedic Surgeons.
14. Kennedy JD, Walker DM: Occult knee ligament injuries associated with femoral shaft fractures, *J Sports Med Phys Fitness* 8:172, 1980.
15. Khasigian HA: The results of treatment of nonunions with electrical stimulation, *Orthopedics* 31:32, 1980.
16. Levine JD et al: Reflex neurogenic inflammation: I, contribution of the peripheral nervous system to spatially remote inflammatory responses that follow injury, *J Neurosci* 5:1380, 1985.
17. McAuliffe TB et al: Early mobilization of Colles' fractures. A prospective trial, *J Bone Joint Surg Br* 69:727, 1987.
18. Nitz AJ: Limb denervation following anterior cruciate (ACL) reconstruction without tourniquet application, *Phys Ther* 68:822, 1988.
19. Nitz AJ: Incidence of EMG abnormalities following proximal humeral fracture, Manuscript in preparation, 1995.
20. Omer GE: Injuries to nerve of the upper extremity, *J Bone Joint Surg Am* 56:1615, 1974.
21. Paley D et al: Ilizarov treatment of tibial non-unions with bone loss, *Clin Orthop* 241:146, 1989.
22. Pollock FH et al: Treatment of radial neuropathy associated with fractures of the humerus, *J Bone Joint Surg Am* 63:239, 1981.
23. Radin E et al: *Practical biomechanics for the orthopaedic surgeon,* New York, 1979, John Wiley.
24. Salter RB: *Textbook of disorders and injuries of the musculoskeletal system,* ed 2, Baltimore, 1983, Williams & Wilkins.
25. Soffer SR, Yahiro MA: Continuous passive motion after internal fixation of distal humerus fractures, *Orthop Rev* 19:88, 1990.
26. Wold J: *Das Gesets der Transformation den Knochen,* Berlin, 1892, A. Hirschwald.
27. Yamada H: *Strength of biological materials,* Baltimore, 1970, Williams & Wilkins.

CHAPTER 6

Ligament and Muscle-Tendon Unit Injuries

James S. Keene and Terry R. Malone

OUTLINE

Definition of terms
    Strains
    Sprains
Classifying instability
Diagnosis
    History
    Mechanism of injury
    Symptoms, sounds, and swelling
    Loss of function
    Physical examination
    Radiographic evaluation
    Magnetic resonance imaging
    Arthroscopy
    Summary
Treatment
    General principles
    Muscle-tendon unit injuries
    Ligament sprains
    Contusions
    Tendinitis
    Collateral ligament injuries
    Intraarticular ligament injuries
Summary

LEARNING OBJECTIVES

After studying this chapter, the reader should be able to:
1. List the components of the muscle-tendon-unit.
2. Explain the difference between a sprain versus a strain.
3. State the three classifications of instability and the types of instability associated with classification.
4. List the four principles or steps that are required for diagnosing ligamentous and muscle-tendon-unit injuries.
5. Describe the use of arthroscopy in evaluating ligamentous injuries.
6. State the four goals in the treatment of muscle strains and ligament sprains.
7. Describe the running-functional progression program that can be used in the rehabilitation of a muscle strain.
8. State and describe the three steps used in the rehabilitation of ligament sprains.
9. State the three classifications of tendon injury.
10. Describe the difference in the evaluation and treatment of extraarticular ligament injuries versus intraarticular ligament injuries.

KEY TERMS

ligament	sprain
muscle	instability
tendon	diagnosis
strain	treatment

The functional stability of the many joints in the body is due, in part, to the intricate ligament systems and muscle-tendon units associated with each joint. This chapter details the basic principles of defining, classifying, and treating injuries to the ligament and muscle-tendon units of the musculoskeletal system. The objectives of this discussion are to (1) define the terms that describe soft tissue injuries, (2) detail the process of detecting and diagnosing these injuries, and (3) discuss operative and nonoperative methods of treatment.

DEFINITION OF TERMS

Tendons are connective tissue structures that attach muscle to the bones. *Ligaments* are similar connective tissue structures, but they arise from and insert into bone. Despite their similarity, these two structures are quite distinct. Ligaments stabilize joints and serve to connect two bones but lack a motor component to move the joint; tendons are integral parts of the body's muscle-tendon units. A *muscle-tendon unit* refers to a complex unit formed by the muscle arising from bone, the muscle-tendon junction, and the tendon or tendons that insert into bone. Muscle-tendon units not only stabilize joints but also provide the motor power to move them and to absorb forces to protect them. Therefore, injuries to muscle or tendons should not be considered isolated entities because they affect the muscle-tendon unit as a whole. Injuries to muscle-tendon units are referred to as *strains,* whereas injuries to ligaments are called *sprains.*

Strains

An injury described as a *strain* indicates some degree of disruption in the muscle fibers, the muscle-tendon junction, the tendon, or the body insertion of a muscle-tendon unit. This disruption may be caused by (1) a direct blow (contusion), (2) excessive stretching (acute strain), (3) repetitive loading (chronic strain), or (4) a laceration.

The term *contusion* refers to an injury caused by a direct blow to the muscle belly of a muscle-tendon unit. This injury results in capillary rupture and bleeding into the muscle, followed by an inflammatory reaction. This inflammatory event is strongly related to extravascular blood elements. The severity of a contusion may be determined by the degree to which it limits the motion of the joint(s) that the muscle-tendon unit crosses. Acute and chronic strains occur when the muscular or tendinous portion of a muscle-tendon unit lacks the flexibility, strength, or endurance to accommodate the demands placed on it. Appreciating and evaluating these three qualities of the muscle-tendon unit are important to understanding the rationale for treatment and rehabilitation of these injuries. Acute strains are the result of a single violent force applied to the muscle-tendon unit. When the force is greater than the strength or exceeds the flexibility of the muscle-tendon unit, the muscle, muscle-tendon junction, or tendon tears. In some instances, the disruption occurs at the bony attachment of the muscle-

tendon unit, resulting in an avulsion fracture (Fig. 6-1), but the vast majority are at the muscle-tendon junction.[21,48] Chronic strains occur when reptitive forces exceed the endurance of the muscle-tendon unit. If the muscle or tendon has not been conditioned for repetitive loading, a tear occurs. The tear propagates to adjacent portions of the muscle or the tendon if the precipitating activity is not curtailed. The term *tendinitis* is used to describe injuries to the tendinous portion of the muscle-tendon unit. Tendinitis is, in fact, a tear of the tendon that varies from microscopic to macroscopic. With acute tendinitis, microscopic tears appear in the tendon, causing only localized swelling and tenderness. Frequently, chronic cases reflect a degenerative process and are thus better described as *tendinosis,* which typically is at the tendon-bone interface. In chronic cases, the tears may coalesce, causing a complete disruption of the tendinous tissue. The continuity of the tendon is then maintained only by inflexible scar tissue.

Strains are graded as mild (first degree), moderate (second degree), or severe (third degree). With first-degree strains, there is no gross disruption of the muscle-tendon unit. There is localized swelling and tenderness but no loss of strength in the injured unit or loss of motion in the adjacent joints. However, stretching and contractions of the injured muscle-tendon unit against resistance elicit pain at the site of injury. With second-degree strains, there is some degree of gross disruption of the muscle-tendon unit, resulting in loss of strength in the muscle and limitation of active motion in the adjacent joints, but clinical testing reveals that the muscle-tendon unit has not been completely disrupted. In third-degree strains, one or more of the components of the muscle-tendon unit are completely disrupted, and motion in the adjacent joints is severely

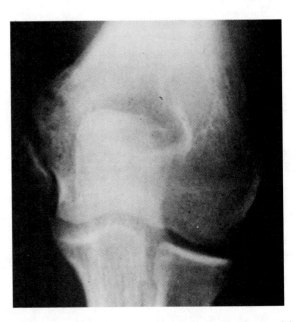

Fig. 6-1. Anteroposterior radiograph of elbow showing avulsion fracture at origin of extensor tendons.

restricted. Often, the site of the disruption is visibly evident. At other times, the defect may be palpated or documented by means of specific clinical tests. In ruptures of either the proximal or distal insertion of the brachial biceps muscle in the arm, the site of the disruption is usually evident (Fig. 6-2). Although a palpable defect is often present with third-degree strains of the Achilles tendon, these strains are best documented by the Thompson test, which is performed with the client in prone position with both feet extending past the end of the examination table. The examiner squeezes the calf muscles of the affected side (Fig. 6-3). If the tendon is intact, the foot demonstrates plantar flexion. If the tendon is ruptured, the foot does not flex. Clients with this injury can still actively flex their ankles because the function of their posterior tibial, flexor digitorium, and flexor hallucis longus tendons is not impaired.

Sprains

The term *sprain* describes injuries to the ligaments. Sprains are caused by forces that stretch some or all of the ligament's fibers beyond their elastic limit, producing some degree of rupture of the fibers and/or their bony attachments. As mentioned previously, ligaments are connective tissue structures that have no motor component to move joints but function to stabilize and prevent abnormal motion of a joint, particularly at the extreme of available joint range of motion (ROM). The classification and grading of ligamentous injuries are based on two factors: (1) the numbers of fibers

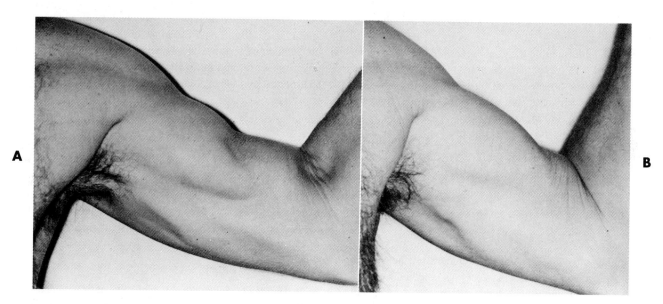

Fig. 6-2. Rupture of distal attachment of biceps muscle in right arm, **A**, is clearly evident when right and left arms, **B**, are compared.

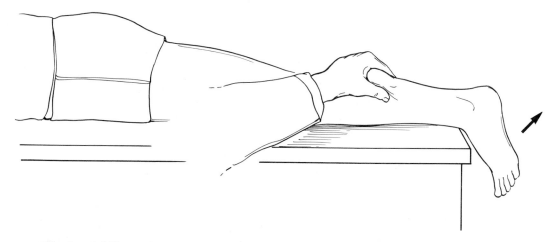

Fig. 6-3. Achilles tendon rupture diagnosed by Thompson test. If tendon is ruptured, foot does not plantar flex when calf muscles are compressed. If tendon is intact, foot flexes *(arrow)* with calf compression.

disrupted and (2) the subsequent instability of the joint involved. The severity of the injury depends on the magnitude, direction, and duration of the forces applied.

Like musculotendinous injuries, ligament injuries are graded as mild (first degree), moderate (second degree), and severe (third degree). First-degree sprains produce localized tenderness and swelling over the injury site. Some ligament fibers are torn, but there is no demonstrable clinical or functional loss of the integrity of the ligament. With second-degree sprains, many, but not all, of the ligament fibers are torn, and there is clinical evidence of joint instability. However, stress-testing does not demonstrate complete functional loss of the integrity of the ligament. Third-degree sprains disrupt the ligament completely. This disruption occurs at the bony attachments or within the substance of the ligament.

Joint instability resulting from ligamentous injury is designated as 1+, 2+, 3+. The degree of instability is determined by comparing the joint excursion permitted by an injured ligament and that permitted by its uninjured counterpart in the other extremity. Zero instability indicates no difference between the amount of joint excursion permitted by the injured and uninjured ligaments. In a 1+, 2+, or 3+ instability, the difference between the laxity of the injured and uninjured ligaments is less than 0.5 cm, 0.5 to 1 cm, or greater than 1 cm, respectively. These "schemes" are not as precise in the clinical realm as we would desire, even with the development of joint arthrometers to better quantify these motions.[12]

CLASSIFYING INSTABILITY

In addition to grading scales, a standardized nomenclature and several classification systems have been developed to describe ligament injuries and instabilities.[26,27,50,59] In hinge-type (ginglymus) joints, the instability is described as anterior, posterior, medial, or lateral. In joints that also have rotatory motion, the nomenclature and classification systems of ligament instability are more complex. The most elaborate classification systems of ligament instability have been developed for the knee by Hughston and colleagues[26,27] and by Noyes and Grood.[50] The Hughston system is based on clinical tests and operative findings, with knee instabilities classified as either straight (nonrotatory) or rotatory (simple or combined). The classification of straight instability is similar to that used for hinge-type joints and includes medial, lateral, anterior, and posterior instabilities. The classification of rotatory instability involves either anterior and posterior rotation of the lateral tibial condyle. There are three types of simple rotatory instability: anteromedial, anterolateral, and posterolateral. Of the various combinations of the three types of rotatory instability, the two most common combinations were (1) anterolateral and posterolateral rotatory instability and (2) anteromedial and anterolateral rotatory instability. The clinical tests and stability are summarized in Table 6-1. Several of these tests are discussed in detail in subsequent sections of this chapter. The Noyes and Grood concepts are based on six degrees of freedom (three dimensions) in knee function:

The diagnosis of a ligament injury must be expressed as a specific anatomic defect.

The clinical examination recognizes the three-dimensional motions of the knee.

Rotatory actions are characterized by specific tibial subluxations.

Selected assessments of specific primary and secondary restraints are utilized.

This system has been further integrated through the International Knee Documentation Form (Fig. 12-9).

DIAGNOSIS

There are several important principles and aids for diagnosing ligament and muscle-tendon unit injuries: (1) obtaining a detailed history, including the description of the mechanism of the injury; (2) performing a comprehensive physical examination; (3) using various radiographic techniques; and (4) evaluating the contents of the joint with an arthroscope.

History

A thorough history is often the key to understanding and appreciating which ligaments or muscle have been injured. Certain types of information should always be sought. Details of (1) the mechanism of the injury, (2) the timing and location of pain and swelling, and (3) the loss of function associated with the injury often provide important data necessary for developing a differential diagnosis.

Mechanism of injury

In the case of ligamentous injuries, it is important to determine the direction and/or angle of the forces that caused the injury. Often, if the examiner is present when the injury occurs, the mechanism of injury can be observed directly. In a sport such as football, the mechanism of injury can be determined from game films. If first-hand observation is not possible, the patient can be questioned regarding causes of the injury (e.g., contact with another person or an object) and angle of the impact. If the force was applied to the lateral aspect of the knee, for example, the examiner should carefully evaluate the medial ligaments and meniscus. If the injury was caused by a blow to the anterior tibia, there should be careful examination of the posterior cruciate ligament and posterior capsule. If the injury occurred as the person fell or changed direction while running, an anterior or posterior cruciate ligament tear is suspected.

Symptoms, sounds, and swelling

The client's localization of pain is another key to determining the site of injury. Is the pain experienced acutely, or had there been some pain in the same area prior to the acute episode? The chronic intermittent pain of

Table 6-1. Classification, positive stress tests, and injured ligamentous structures associated with various instabilities of the knee; an example of a ginglymus joint pattern

Classification of instability	Type of instability	Positive stress tests	Injured ligamentous structures
Straight	Medial	Abduction at full extension	Medial compartment Posterior cruciate
	Lateral	Abduction at 30° flexion Adduction at full extension	Medial compartment Lateral collateral Posterior cruciate
	Anterior	Adduction at 30° flexion Lachman's test Anterior drawer	Lateral collateral Anterior cruciate Anterior cruciate
	Posterior	Posterior drawer	Medial compartment Posterior cruciate Posterior oblique Arcuate complex
Rotatory	Anteromedial	Abduction at 30° flexion Anterior drawer at 15° external rotation	Medial compartment Anterior cruciate Posterior oblique
	Anterolateral	Pivot-shift or jerk Anterior drawer at neutral rotation Adduction at 30° flexion	Lateral capsular Anterior cruciate
	Posterolateral	Adduction at 30° flexion External-rotation recurvatum	Arcuate complex
Combined	Anterolateral and Posterolateral	Reverse pivot-shift Pivot-shift or jerk Adduction at 30° flexion Anterior and posterior drawer at neutral rotation	Lateral capsular Arcuate complex Anterior cruciate
	Anterolateral and Anteromedial	Reverse pivot-shift Pivot-shift or jerk Anterior drawer at neutral and 15° external rotation Adduction at 30° flexion Abduction at 30° flexion	Medial capsular Lateral capsular Anterior cruciate

tendinitis or tendinosus that culminates in an acute episode may signify that a complete rupture of the tendon has occurred. Is the pain diffuse, or can the client point to the site of the pain with one finger? Diffuse pain suggests a muscle contusion or intraarticular ligament tear. Point tenderness is more commonly reported with disruption of the superficial ligaments and tendons. Did the client hear or feel a snap or pop when the injury occurred? These sounds and feelings often occur with cruciate ligament injuries of the knee and subluxating peroneal tendons at the ankle. Did the injured joint immediately swell up, or was the onset of swelling slow? Immediate swelling of a joint, within the first hour of injury, is a hemarthrosis. An immediate, tense, bloody effusion in the knee (Fig. 6-4), for example, usually signifies a rupture of the anterior cruciate ligament.[13,14] Lesser effusions over a period of many hours indicate a synovial effusion and are experienced with meniscal and collateral ligament injuries.

Loss of function

Often the severity of the injury can be determined by its effect on a client's performance. After the injury occurred,

could the athlete continue playing and bear full weight on the injured extremity, or did the extremity give way? First- and second-degree ligament injuries may allow the athlete to continue playing or to walk off the field unaided, whereas third-degree injuries cause sufficient instability that the injured extremity buckles when weight is applied to it. Did the person experience locking and become unable to move the injured joint through a full range of motion? Medial collateral, anterior cruciate ligament, and meniscal injuries of the knee often cause locking and the loss of 10 to 45 degrees of extension. Quadriceps muscle strains and contusions often limit flexion.

The importance of asking the appropriate questions and obtaining a thorough history cannot be overemphasized. The history of the injury-producing event is the foundation on which physical examination of the various ligament and muscle injuries is based.

Physical examination

Ideally, ligament and muscle-tendon unit injuries should be evaluated immediately after they occur; otherwise, instability associated with the injury may quickly be masked

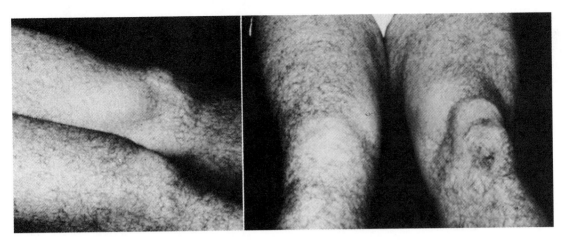

Fig. 6-4. Immediate, tense effusion is often associated with a third-degree anterior cruciate ligament disruption.

KNEE: LIGAMENTOUS INJURIES

Client's name History number	Preoperative		Anesthesia	
	R	L	R	L
Anterior drawer test				
External tibial rotation				
Neutral tibial rotation				
Internal tibial rotation				
Posterior drawer test				
External tibial rotation				
Neutral tibial rotation				
Internal tibial rotation				
Lachman's test				
Pivot-shift test				
Reverse pivot-shift test				
Abduction stress test				
Hyperextended				
0 degrees				
30 degrees				
Abduction stress test				
Hyperextended				
0 degrees				
30 degrees				

Diagnosis

Fig. 6-5. Evaluation form for recording clinical findings of examination of knees with ligamentous injuries.

by muscle spasm and joint tightness due to swelling. The examiner should first ascertain if the tenderness is localized or diffuse. Diffuse tenderness suggests more extensive soft tissue disruption. Next, the examiner should perform clinical tests for the suspected specific joint instability involved (Table 6-1). If these test are performed immediately after the injury, the degree of joint laxity can usually be accurately determined. If the examination is delayed, then stress testing becomes increasingly unreliable because of rapid onset of protective muscular resistance. If there is a suggestion of laxity but the examination is unsatisfactory because of muscular resistance, the injured joint should be examined with the client under a local or general anesthetic. The stability of the injured joint should always be compared to its uninjured counterpart. In this matter, the client's normal physiologic laxity is not mistaken for laxity caused by the current injury. The results of the initial examination should be carefully recorded (Fig. 6-5) so that the findings of subsequent examinations and other examiners can be compared (also see International Knee Documentation Form, Fig. 12-9, p. 311).

Radiographic evaluation

Although clinical tests for instability usually subjectively document (from the examiner's point of view) that laxity is present, standard radiographs should always be taken. They indicate if the laxity is caused by an avulsion of the ligament with its bony attachment or by an epiphyseal separation. They also demonstrate whether any fractures are associated with the ligamentous injury. The standard radiographic evaluation should always include two exposures that are right angles (90 degrees) to each other. If radiographs are taken in only one plane (e.g., only anteroposterior or lateral), the actual amount of displacement or malalignment of a fracture or joint cannot be ascertained. Ideally, all of the individual bony structures of the joint being examined should be radiographed in two planes, 90 degrees apart. The ancillary radiographic methods for evaluating ligament and cartilage injuries include stress radiographs, arthrograms, and magnetic resonance imaging (MRI). Although MRI is an effective method for documenting injuries to tendons, ligaments, and cartilage, because of its current cost, the two ancillary methods often used to evaluate ligament injuries are stress radiographs and arthrograms.

Stress radiographs. Stress radiographs are obtained by applying the appropriate varus-valgus or anteroposterior stress to a joint as a standard radiograph is taken. Although stress radiographs are not routinely required for evaluating joint laxity, they are useful in documenting instabilities of the ankle and in evaluating epiphyseal injuries of the knee (Fig. 6-6). Accurate information from stress studies requires close attention to the positioning of the joint to be examined. Also, comparative views of the opposite uninjured joint should always be obtained. Specific devices to allow standardization of this process are available as described by Staubli.[60]

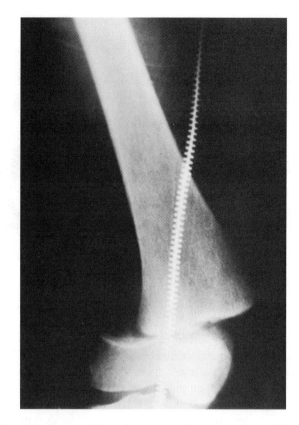

Fig. 6-6. Stress radiograph demonstrating separation of distal femoral epiphysis. Clinical stress testing may suggest a medial collateral ligament injury rather than epiphyseal injury.

Arthrography. Arthrography is often helpful in evaluating soft tissue injuries. Arthograms are used when the clinical history, physical examination, and standard radiographs do not clearly define the location and severity of the injury. Arthrography is performed by injecting a joint with either a radiopaque liquid (Renografin) and/or room air. The procedure is called a *double-contrast arthrogram* when both air and liquid are injected and a *single-contrast arthrogram* when only liquid is injected. After liquid, air, or both have been injected into the joint, serial radiographs can be obtained at many different angles.

Although this technique has been applied to many joints in the body, it is most often used to evaluate meniscal and ligamentous injuries in the knee. A single-contrast arthrogram of the knee is performed by injecting the joint with 10 ml of Renografin. An elastic bandage is wrapped around the knee to force the dye out of the suprapatellar pouch and popliteal space, thus thoroughly coating the menisci and cruciate ligaments. Anteroposterior radiographs are then taken to evaluate the integrity of the medial and lateral capsular and ligamentous structures. Lateral radiographs with the knee flexed to 90 degrees are done with and without anterior stress on the tibia to evaluate the cruciate ligaments. Subsequently, serial tangential views of the medial and lateral meniscus are taken (Fig. 6-7).

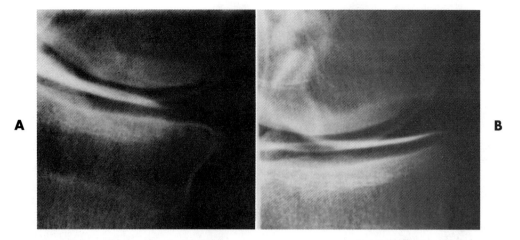

Fig. 6-7. Right knee arthrogram. **A,** Tangential views of medial meniscus demonstrate vertical tear. **B,** Normal meniscus.

Arthrography of the knee is employed for evaluation of knee injuries because of its accuracy in documenting meniscal lesions. Clinical accuracy in diagnosing meniscal injuries is usually reported to be approximately 70%.[34,54,57] Single- and double-contrast arthograms, in conjunction with a physical examination and a client's history, have improved the accuracy rate to 95%.[44,47,63,65] Single-contrast arthrography is usually the most effective technique for documenting cruciate and collateral ligament injuries (Fig. 6-8).

There are at least three significant limitations to the accuracy of knee arthrograms: The first occurs in diagnosing collateral ligament injuries. If the arthrogram is not performed immediately after a third- or second-degree collateral ligament tear, the site of the disruption may be sealed by synovium or a clot, and the dye does not leak out of the joint and does not localize the injury. The second limitation concerns the evaluation of the lateral meniscal lesions. Evaluation of the posterior third of the lateral meniscus is extremely difficult because the popliteal tendon sheath, which crosses this area, fills with dye and obscures the outline of the meniscus. In addition, the posterior fifth of the lateral meniscus cannot be visualized on an arthrogram because it is obscured by the interior cruciate ligament. The third limitation concerns evaluation of the anterior cruciate ligament. When this ligament is completely disrupted but its synovial sheath remains intact, the arthrogram usually appears normal, even under stress. In general, whenever there are overlapping structures within a joint, the arthrogram is of limited value in assessing the integrity of either one or both of the structures.

Magnetic resonance imaging

Magnetic resonance imaging allows a significant review of multiple joint structures and thus provides a great deal of information. When performed in an appropriate fashion and interpreted by a judicious and qualified clinician, MRI is

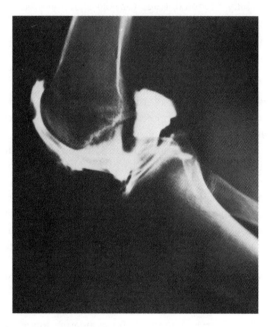

Fig. 6-8. Lateral view of single-contrast arthrogram of knee, demonstrating normal anterior and posterior cruciate ligaments.

invaluable to the surgeon in both evaluation and appropriate surgical or nonsurgical management decisions. It also allows fairly specific evaluation of bony responses.[55] As mentioned previously, cost is a significant impediment to the greater utilization of the modality.

Arthroscopy

Arthroscopy is another adjunctive diagnostic procedure that often is employed for the assessment of intraarticular soft tissue injuries. With this technique, an arthoscope, a cylindrical stainless-steel tube with a diameter ranging from 2 to 5 mm and optical lenses at both ends (Fig. 6-9), is inserted into a joint. With the aid of a continuous flow of

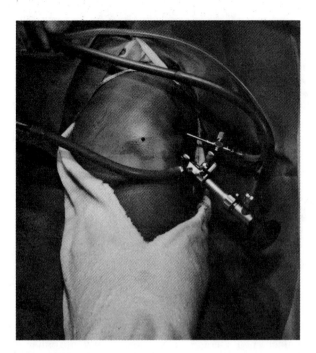

Fig. 6-9. A 170-degree, 5-mm arthroscope. The arthroscope is shown within the knee with fiberoptic light source and irrigation tubing in place.

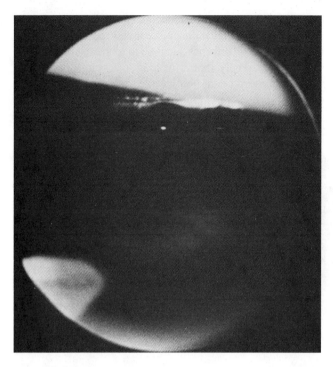

Fig. 6-10. Undersurface of normal patella as viewed through the arthroscope. Drainage cannula is evident beneath articular surface of patella.

sterile saline solution through the tube, a fiberoptic light source attached to the scope, and a small television camera, the structures within the joint can be examined directly. State-of-the-art arthroscopy has progressed to the point where most joints in the musculoskeletal system can be examined in this manner. The scope often has to be inserted at multiple sites (the polypuncture technique) for complete examination of the larger joints.

In a study of 100 clients with internal derangements of the knee, DeHaven and Collins found that (1) the correct diagnosis could be made arthroscopically in 94 of the cases; (2) clinically and arthrographically, diagnoses were incorrect or conflicting in 39 of the cases; and (3) arthroscopy demonstrated unexpected disorders instead of the expected lesions in 25 of the cases. However, they concluded that clinical examination, arthrography, *and* arthroscopy in combination provided a more accurate diagnosis than any modality did individually.[14]

My (JSK) experience has been that arthroscopy has particular advantages over arthrography in the evaluation of patellar, anterior cruciate, and lateral meniscal injuries. The articular surface of the patella can be clearly visualized and manipulated arthroscopically, but it is difficult to evaluate arthrographically (Fig. 6-10). In addition, the patellar articular surface can be debrided and abraded as necessary by inserting the appropriate instrument through another portal in the knee and then observing the surgery directly through the scope. Third-degree anterior cruciate ligament

injuries are also better evaluated with arthroscopy. The ligament may appear to be continuous on an arthrogram because of an intact synovial sheath. With arthroscopy, however, the ligament can be readily visualized and evaluated.

The integrity of the ligament is determined by placing a probe (Fig. 6-11) into the joint through another portal and then manipulating the ligament under direct visual inspection. Similarly, lateral meniscal tears that are obscured on the arthrogram because of dye in the popliteal tendon sheath are easily evaluated with the arthroscope (Fig. 6-12). The lateral meniscus can be seen in its entirety, including the posterior attachment, which, as mentioned previously, cannot be visualized on the arthrogram. In addition, most meniscal surgery is now performed with the arthroscope. As with the other procedures discussed, various cutting and grasping instruments can be inserted into the joint through separate portals or through the scope itself. All (total meniscectomy) or part of the torn meniscus (partial meniscectomy) can then be freed from any remaining soft tissue attachment or, when indicated, repaired under direct visualization. Excised fragments are removed from the joint through one of the puncture wounds (Fig. 6-13).

These arthroscopic procedures can be performed with local anesthesia. As can be imagined, the cost savings to both the client and the health care delivery system are remarkable. Also, the client does not need to be hospitalized, is not exposed to the risks of general or spinal anesthesia, and requires lower levels of narcotic analgesia in the postoperative period. The rehabilitation-recovery period—possibly including time on crutches and time to return to work and/or sports—is markedly shorter with arthroscopic surgery than with arthrotomy of the joint. Following partial meniscectomy, most clients use crutches minimally, and many have completed a rehabilitation program within 3 weeks. This

rapid recovery appears to be, in part, a result of less postoperative joint pain and swelling.

Summary

The key to establishing a diagnosis of ligament or muscle-tendon unit injury includes (1) obtaining a detailed history, (2) performing a thorough physical examination, and (3) utilizing, when appropriate, the adjunctive radiographic and/or arthroscopic techniques that are currently available. The importance of a detailed history must be stressed because certain points in the history—most often the mechanism of injury—help the examination form a provisional diagnosis and direct attention to specific aspects of the physical examination. The physical examination, if performed immediately after the injury or with anesthesia, usually localizes the site of the injury and documents the resulting loss of function and/or the joint instability. If the location and the severity of the injury cannot easily be determined from the history and physical examination, arthrography and/or arthroscopy should be performed. The examiner should not, however, rely solely on either the history, the physical examination, or the radiographic and arthroscopic findings when evaluating ligament and soft tissue injuries. These methods complement each other, and only by using them in combination can the most accurate diagnoses be achieved.

TREATMENT
General principles

The basic goals in the treatment of muscle strains and ligament sprains are to (1) regain full motion and stability of the joint involved; (2) facilitate normal neuromuscular patterns of movement; (3) restore the strength, flexibility, and endurance of the muscle involved; and (4) return the

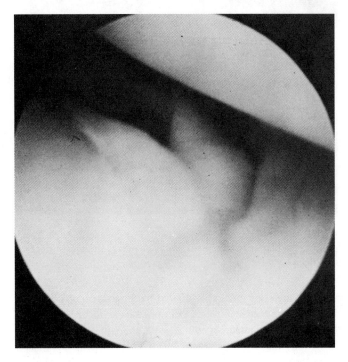

Fig. 6-11. Normal anterior cruciate ligament as viewed through the arthroscope. Ligament is the structure running obliquely along left side of photograph. Femoral articular surface is evident in upper right-hand corner.

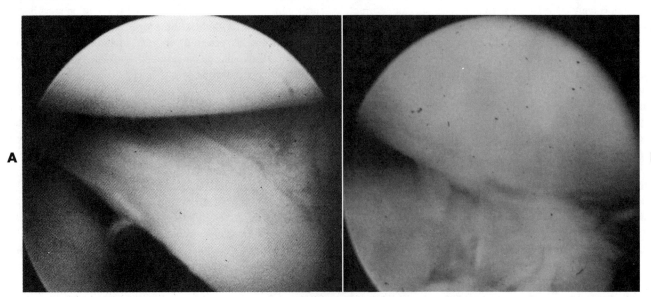

Fig. 6-12. Arthroscopic evaluation of lateral meniscus. **A,** Normal meniscus. **B,** Flap tear.

client to full function with minimal risk of reinjury. The method of achieving these goals is determined, in part, by the severity of the injury.

Muscle-tendon unit injuries

In general, first- and second-degree strains are treated nonoperatively. Third-degree strains in the tendinous portion of the muscle-tendon unit are treated operatively. (The term *nonoperative* is more descriptive than the term *conservative* because nonoperative treatment of some injuries, particularly third-degree strains, would be considered very radical and certainly not conservative.)

As mentioned previously regarding muscle strain, not only muscle and tendinous tissue but also the adjacent blood vessels are torn. Therefore, the initial goals of treatment are to stop the interstitial bleeding and prevent further tearing of the muscle fibers. They are frequently accomplished by applying a compression dressing, elevating and immobilizing the injured extremity, and placing ice on the injured area (five times per day for 20 minutes). This treatment is continued for 48 hours. During this period, only minimal weight bearing should be permitted. Some clinicians use pain-free ROM activities during this time but with the caveat that it is pain-free.

Generally, after 48 hours, gentle passive stretching of the injured muscle group is initiated. Subsequently, the individual is started on a more aggressive stretching program.[7,61]

Stretching program. Three basic forms of stretching activities are seen clinically: static stretching, ballistic stretching, and proprioceptive neuromuscular facilitation (PNF) techniques. Following injury, we recommend gentle, controlled static and PNF actions. Low load with prolonged deformation appears to be effective in both isolated tissues[38,66] and in intact muscle-tendon units.[1,39] We also use heat prior to and during stretch activities.[39,62,66] The stretching program is performed individually or with a partner.

The following exercises to stretch the knee are used as an example. If the affected muscle group is the quadriceps, adductors, or hamstrings, the stretching is performed in the following manner.

Step I—quadriceps stretch. The individual lies prone on a firm surface and flexes the knee on the injured side as far as possible. The partner kneels beside the individual's injured side and places one hand around the ankle and the other hand on the buttocks (Fig. 6-14, *A*). The individual then extends the knee against the resistance of the partner and holds the muscle contraction for a count of 6. The partner then stretches the quadriceps muscle by gently pushing the individual's heel toward the buttocks (Fig. 6-14, *B*)—holding a 10- to 15-second stretch. This sequence is repeated three times.

Step II—adductor (groin) stretch. The individual sits on a firm surface, spreads his or her legs, and grasps the partner's wrists (Fig. 6-15, *A*). The partner sits facing the individual with knees bent, places his or her feet just above the individual's ankles, and grasps the wrists. The injured person then contracts the adductors by pressing his or her legs against the partner's resistance for a count of 6 (Fig. 6-15, *B*). The individual then relaxes as the partner pulls him or her forward while slowly and evenly spreading his or her legs and holding a 10- to 15-second stretch. The sequence is repeated three times.

Step III—hamstring stretch. The individual lies supine on a firm surface with the knee of the injured extremity fully extended and the hip flexed to its limits. The opposite knee is also fully extended and the hip is extended so that it rests on the firm surface (Fig. 6-16, *A*). The partner then places the ankle on the individual's injured leg on his or her shoulder and grasps the anterior thigh, just above the knee, with both

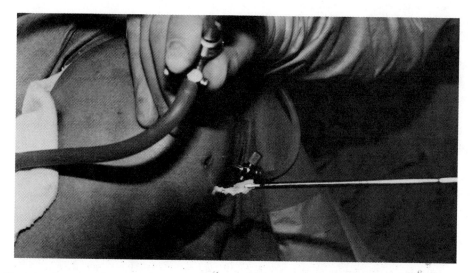

Fig. 6-13. Segment of torn lateral meniscus is removed through one of the puncture wounds. Excision of the meniscal tear was accomplished arthroscopically.

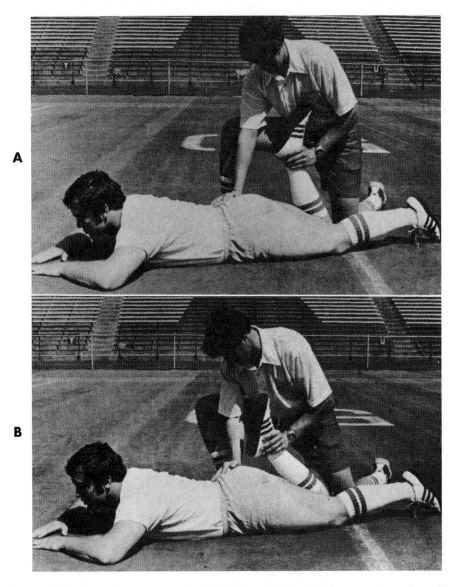

Fig. 6-14. Proprioceptive neuromuscular facilitation (PNF) stretching exercises of quadriceps muscles. **A,** Resistance-contraction phase. **B,** Stretching phase. (Steps of exercise are explained in text.)

hands. The partner's opposite knee is placed on the individual's extended leg. The individual then extends the injured leg downward at the hip against the partner's resistance for a count of 6 (Fig. 6-16, *B*). The individual then relaxes as the partner stretches the hamstrings by pushing the leg upward toward the individual's head and holding a 10- to 15-second stretch. This sequence is repeated three times.

Each stretch should be controlled and held "on stretch" 10 to 15 seconds for three repetitions (thus for a total stretch of 30 to 45 seconds), and the entire set of exercises should be performed three times per day until the individual can return to full activity.[1] These exercises should evoke minimal pain. Bouncing at the limits of the stretch (ballistic stretching) should be avoided because this type of stretching may cause further tearing and will not in-

crease flexibility of the muscle. The bouncing may cause muscle contraction because it stimulates the muscle-tendon stretch reflex.

When the injured muscle group is able to move the adjacent joint(s) through a full range of motion without producing pain, running-functional progression and weight programs can be started. We normally sequence activity with stretching performed immediately *before* and weight training immediately *after* the individual works on the running-functional progression program.

Running-functional progression program. The five-step running program described hereafter and summarized in Table 6-2 is an example used in an intercollegiate environment.

The individual performs the running program daily, beginning at step I, until he or she can complete all five steps

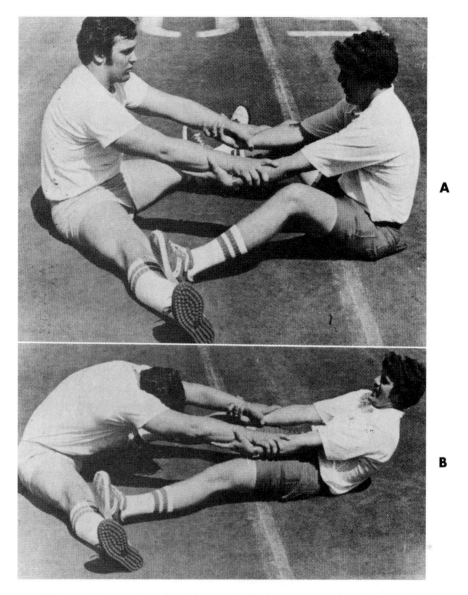

Fig. 6-15. PNF stretching exercises for adductors. **A,** Resistance-contraction phase. **B,** Stretching phase. (Steps of exercise are explained in text.)

Table 6-2. The running program

Step	Activity	Conditions
I	Jog ¼ to ½ mile/day; add ¼ mile every 2 to 3 days, until jogging at least 1 mile	No pain or limp
II	Run six to eight 80-yard sprints at ½ speed	Able to jog 1 mile with no pain or limp
III	Run six to eight 80-yard sprints at ¾ speed	Completion of step II with no pain or limp
IV	Run six to eight 80-yard sprints at full speed and do six fast starts	Completion of step III with no pain or limp
V	Run six to eight 80-yard sprints, cutting right or left every 10 yards to ¾ speed and then back up to full speed	Completion of step IV with no pain or limp

without developing pain or a limp. An individual who develops pain or a limp during any phase of the program must start the next day at step I. After completing the program, the individual, if an athlete, is put through various agility tests that are specific for the sport and position. This functional progression sequence is required to prepare the patient for return to the functional environment. These tests may include running figure eights, the carioca, back padding, hopping, lateral crossover running, and cutting around cones. The last progression includes the drills of sport or job, yet in a controlled fashion prior to full participation (see the Box).

Weight program. The weight-training program summarized in Table 6-3 is an intercollegiate example. It is started when an individual begins the running-functional sequence and should be done every other day immediately after running. The weight- and strength-training program is best accomplished in an integrated format including all forms of exercise: isometric, isotonic (concentric and eccentric), and isokinetic (multiple speeds and concentric/eccentric). Patients with muscle-tendon injury frequently respond well to an eccentric emphasis during strength training. To provide maximal-level eccentric forces, the patient must raise the weighted limb (concentrically) in a bilateral or assistive pattern of some nature followed by a single limb-lowering (eccentric) action. Isokinetic eccentrics may be integrated when available, using both the active eccentric mode or asking the patient to resist the moving lever arm in the "passive" motion mode.

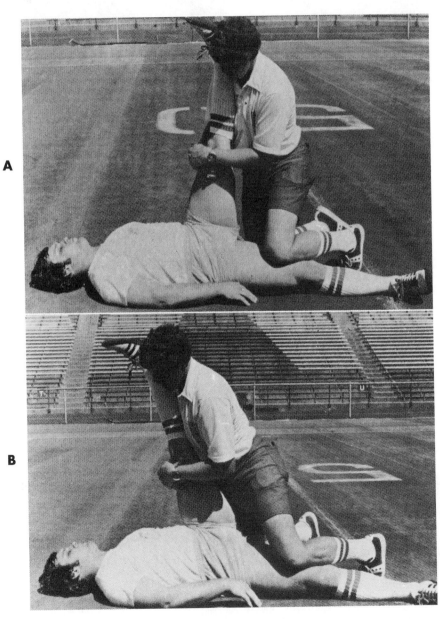

Fig. 6-16. PNF stretching exercises for hamstrings. **A,** Resistance-contraction phase. **B,** Stretching phase. (Steps of exercise are explained in text.)

We frequently recommend the application of ice packs to the injured area for 20 minutes or ice massage until the injured area is numb (usually 5 to 8 minutes) after completion of the weight program. When the single maximum lift (SML) of the injured and uninjured muscle comes within 10% of being equal, the individual has completed the weight-training program. We use a similar goal of 10% to 15% with isokinetic valves right to left when these data are available.

Summary. Muscle strains occur because the muscle-tendon unit lacks the strength, flexibility, and/or endurance to withstand the forces applied to it. Clinicians must appreciate the absorptive eccentric pattern of muscle function and use it as a part of the rehabilitation sequence. The stretching, running, and weight- and strength-training programs outlined minimize these deficiencies. The individual who has completed all three programs may return to normal function or, if an athlete, to competition with a minimal risk of reinjury.

Ligament sprains

In contrast to muscle strains, ligament injuries or sprains may cause some degree of joint instability. For this reason, the treatment of ligament disruptions requires a specific

---

Functional progression—lower extremity

Immobilization (primary healing)
ROM (protected)
Strengthening exercise—all forms
Progressive weight bearing
Proprioceptive activities
Functional strengthening
Walk-jog sequence
Jog-run sequence
Hop-jump sequence
Sprinting program
Cutting sequence
Agility drills
Specific activities
Return to sport

---

period of immobilization. The length of immobilization is determined by the severity of the injury and the type of ligament. In first- and second-degree sprains of the collateral ligaments, the length of immobilization may be only a matter of days. With third-degree sprains (ligament rupture), the ligament is usually either surgically reconstructed (cruciate ligaments) or immobilized for several weeks if a medial collateral injury. Although a period of immobilization is necessary for the injured or repaired ligament to heal, it is detrimental to the injured ligaments of the joint involved.

Noyes and colleagues' classic work has demonstrated that in monkeys an 8-week period of immobilization decreases the maximum failure load and the ratio of energy absorption to failure of uninjured anterior cruciate ligaments by 39% and 32%, respectively. They also found that, after 20 weeks of reconditioning after immobilization, the maximum failure load and ratio of energy absorption to failure had recovered, respectively, to only 86% and 84% of the normal range.[51] Their results suggest that the functional capacity of healing ligaments remains impaired for much longer than previously realized and evoke the question of whether the length of time allowed for ligament healing, particularly in athletes, is long enough. In many cases, athletes return to full competition before their injured ligaments have reached even 90% of normal strength.

Rehabilitation program. The basic rehabilitation program for first- and second-degree sprains is described in the following steps and summarized in Table 6-4. Individuals with healed or repaired third-degree sprains should start the program at the warm whirlpool phase of step II.

Step I. Immediately after the injury and for the ensuing 48 hours, the injured joint should be elevated and immobilized. Cryotherapy is applied to the injured area multiple times a day for 20 minutes (many protocols recommend five sessions daily). As previously mentioned, radiographs should be obtained to rule out avulsion fractures and epiphyseal injuries.

Step II. After 48 hours and for the next 2 to 3 days, the injured joint should be placed in a cold whirlpool for 20 minutes and range-of-motion exercise should be performed as tolerated. After 4 to 5 days, warm whirlpool treatment is initiated and continued until full range of motion is achieved.

Table 6-3. Muscle-strengthening program (accomplished with free weights)—concentric patterns

Step	Activity	Goal
I	Determine single maximum lift (SML) of muscle(s) in *uninjured* extremity	Establishes strength to be obtained by *injured* muscles
II	Determine SML of muscle(s) in injured extremity	Establishes weight to be used in steps III and IV
III	Do three sets of 10 repetitions with the weight equal to SML, minus 10 pounds	Builds muscle strength
IV	Do one set of 20 repetitions with the weight equal to SML, minus 20 pounds	Builds muscle endurance

Step III. When the client (1) achieves full range of motion, (2) has minimal swelling, and (3) can bear full weight and jump up and down on the injured extremity without pain, a running-functional program and a weight- and strength-training program, as described previously, are instituted. An individual, particularly an athlete, who completes these programs, is able to return to full competition.

The following sections of this chapter deal with the diagnosis and treatment of specific ligament and/or muscle-tendon unit injuries.

Contusions

Contusions most commonly occur in the biceps muscle of the arm and the quadriceps muscle of the thigh. They are produced by a direct blow to the muscle, causing localized bleeding and edema but not complete disruption or total loss of function of the involved muscle. Quadriceps muscle contusions are most commonly caused by direct blows from either an athletic opponent's headgear or knee or from an individual striking the thigh against a fixed object. The individual may not appreciate the severity of the injury until the next day, when knee motion is restricted and the quadriceps muscle is sore and swollen.

Quadriceps muscle contusions are graded as mild, moderate, and severe. Because these injuries take at least 24 hours to stabilize, the severity of the injury is determined from clinical findings after 48 hours. Mild contusions are characterized by local tenderness, at least 90 degrees of knee motion, and no alteration in gait. The person can perform a deep knee bend. Moderate contusions cause diffuse swelling and tenderness of the muscle mass, permit only 45 to 90 degrees of the knee motion (Fig. 6-17), and alter one's gait. The person cannot perform a deep knee bend and experiences severe pain while climbing stairs or rising from a sitting position. Severe contusions produce such marked tenderness and swelling that the contour of the muscle is difficult to define. Also, knee motion is restricted to less than 45 degrees, and a severe limp develops.

Treatment. Moderate and severe contusions are treated in three phases: During the first phase, the goal is to minimize the interstitial bleeding. It is accomplished by applying ice and compressive wrap to the affected area and by immobilizing and elevating the injured extremity.

This phase of treatment usually lasts 24 hours for mild contusions and 48 hours or more for moderate to severe contusions. During this phase of treatment, isometric quadriceps muscle exercise is permitted, but massage, heat, and range-of-motion exercise are not recommended.

After the swelling has stabilized and the person has regained quadriceps muscle control, the range-of-motion exercises of phase II are initiated. The goals of this phase of treatment are, first, to gain full extension of the muscle and then to restore flexion slowly. Active flexion and extension exercises are started in the prone position (Fig. 6-17), and the rate of progress is determined by the pain experienced by the individual. During this phase of treatment, crutch ambulation with touch weight bearing is permitted. If swelling recurs, the person is immediately returned to phase I of the treatment program. Phase II is completed when knee motion is at least 90 degrees and the individual has a normal gait.

In the final phase of treatment, progressive resistance exercises are performed until there is full motion and strength. During this phase, the person is required to complete the running-functional program and weight-and strength-training program outlined previously. When full motion, strength, and agility have been restored, the individual, if an athlete, can return to full competition.

The variable outcomes for clients with contusion injuries have been determined by Jackson and Feagin.[31] During a 9-month period, they diagnosed and treated 65 quadriceps muscle contusions in 65 male military academy cadets. They found that the average time of disability for the 47 cadets

Table 6-4. Rehabilitation program for first- and second-degree sprains

Step	Activity	Duration
I	Ice, elevation, and mobilization	48 hours
II	Cold whirlpool for range-of-motion exercise	Days 2-3
	Warm whirlpool until full range of motion attained	Days 4-5
III	Running, strength and weight training, and functional progression programs (Tables 6-2, 6-3, Box 6-1)	Days 7-21

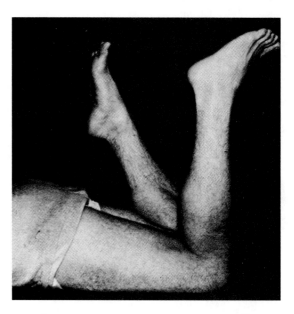

Fig. 6-17. Quadriceps contusions. Active knee motion is measured in the manner shown 48 hours after contusion occurred to determine severity of injury.

with mild contusions was 6½ days and the average time for the 7 cadets with moderate contusions and the 11 with severe contusions was 56 and 72 days, respectively. They also found that 13 of the 18 cadets with moderate or severe injuries developed heterotopic bone formation (myositis ossificans) in the injured quadriceps muscle within 2 to 4 weeks of the injury. However, all 13 returned to athletic competition in an average of 73 days, none required surgery, and their return was not dependent on resorption of the heterotopic bone. Lipscomb, Thomas, and Johnson reported similar results in treating this injury. However, they found it necessary to operatively excise the heterotopic bone in four individuals who had limited motion and persistent pain 5 to 7 months after the contusion. All four returned to athletics after surgery 5 to 7 months after the contusion.[40]

Summary. Improperly treated quadriceps contusions can severely disable a person. To treat these injuries properly, prevent reinjury, and shorten the period of disability, the examiner must (1) recognize and accurately classify these injuries, (2) admit individuals with severe contusions to a hospital for phase I of treatment, and (3) educate injured persons regarding the severity of the injury and temper their enthusiasm to return to normal function too rapidly.

Tendinitis

Although many persons participating in sports are prone to developing tendinitis, runners and other track athletes have a particularly high incidence of this injury. The most commonly affected tendon is the Achilles tendon. Brubaker and James[2] and Clancy[6,7] have reported that of 109 and 310 track injuries treated, respectively, 12% were tendinitis, and in 69% of these cases the Achilles tendon was involved.

Achilles tendinitis usually has an insidious onset. The person first notices a dull, aching pain in the Achilles tendon after running. The individual who continues running without treatment experiences pain in the Achilles tendon that is present on the initiation of running and increased with sprinting. Eventually, the individual has pain when walking and is unable to run. These three phases of symptoms represent the acute, subacute, and chronic stages of Achilles tendinitis and tendinosis. Table 6-5 outlines this process in detail for tendinitis and tendinosis. In the acute stage—symptoms of less than 2 weeks' duration—the pain resolves rapidly with rest. On examination, the tenderness is limited to a 1-in. area, 1 to 2 in. above the calcaneal attachment of the Achilles tendon (Fig. 6-18).

The soft tissue around this area may be slightly edematous, suggesting an increased width of the injured tendon with respect to its uninjured counterpart. This stage of Achilles tendinitis is usually resolved with 2 weeks of rest, oral antiinflammatory agents, and a heel lift. When the acute inflammation subsides, the individual is placed on an Achilles stretching program (Fig. 6-19) and allowed to return to running when there is no localized tenderness and full flexibility has returned.

In the subacute stage—symptoms of 3 to 6 weeks' duration—the pain is more diffuse and occurs during running. The clinical symptoms are similar to those of the acute stage, with the addition of crepitus noted during active dorsiflexion and plantar flexion of the ankle. Treatment is similar to that for acute tendinitis, but this stage of Achilles tendinitis requires at least 6 weeks of rest before the person can resume running.

In the chronic stage—symptoms over 6 weeks in duration—the pain is present over an even larger area, and the person is unable to run effectively. On clinical exami-

Table 6-5. Classification of tendon injury				
Injury	**Description**	**Histology**	**Signs and symptoms**	**Treatment**
Paratenonitis	Inflammation of *only* the paratenon	Inflammatory cells in paratenon "tissues"	Cardinal inflammation	Antiinflammatories controlled activity
Tendinosis	Intratendinous degeneration without macrotrauma; minimal symptoms	Noninflammatory degenerative lesion; "failed" healing response	Tender areas of tendon when palpated; often asymptomatic at low function	Stretching/strengthening (eccentric emphasis); progressive exercise demands; slow recovery (10-12 weks)
Tendinitis	Symptomatic degenerative lesion; macrotrauma in origin; inflammatory response/repair	Dependent on "degree"; pure acute inflammation; inflammation with pre-existing degeneration; inflammation with existing tendinosis	Class of inflammation and duration of symptoms important	Dependent on symptom duration, antiinflammatories, maintenance of function, progressive exercise, stretching/strengthening with eccentric emphasis; slow recovery in chronic, 10-12 weeks

Information in this table was combined from multiple sources. The primary source is Clancy WG: Tendon trauma and overuse injuries. In Leadbetter WB, Buchwalter JA, Gordon SL, editors: *Sports induced inflammation,* Park Ridge, Ill, 1990, American Academy of Orthopedic Surgeons.

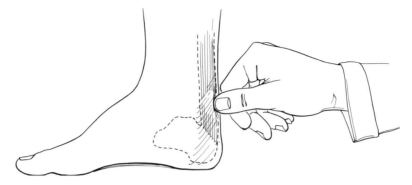

Fig. 6-18. With acute Achilles tendinitis, there is tenderness to palpation over a 1-inch area, 1 to 2 inches above proximal tip of calcaneal bone.

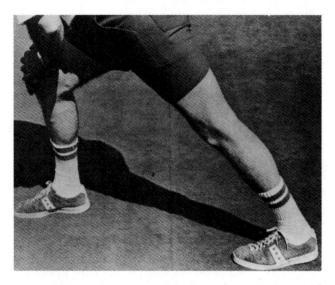

Fig. 6-19. Achilles tendon is stretched by keeping heel of side to be stretched on ground while the opposite knee is progressively flexed. The stretch should be performed in stocking feet and also with lower extremity rotations if a particular portion of the posterior muscle complex is implicated.

nation, the tendon is markedly thickened and often nodular. The treatment program outlined for the acute and subacute stages may not be effective. Clancy,[6-8] Fox and colleagues,[19] and Snook[58] have documented surgical findings in chronic Achilles tendinitis. The pathologic changes range from thickening and microscopic disruption to partial- and full-thickness tears. Clancy concluded that surgical intervention should be considered when symptoms persist after 6 to 8 weeks of nonoperative treatment. He recommended releasing the tendon sheath, excising the scar tissue, and repairing the tear. He has performed this surgery in 22 cases of chronic Achilles tendinitis; in all cases but one, clients have returned to running without symptoms.[6]

Collateral ligament injuries

The collateral ligaments of the knee and ankle are those most commonly injured by athletes. This section deals with current concepts regarding the diagnosis and treatment of medial and lateral collateral ligament injuries of the knee. However, the rationale for the clinical stress testing used in diagnosing these injuries can be understood only with a basic understanding of the normal anatomic and biomechanical properties of these structures. The knee here illustrates these points.

Medial ligamentous stabilizers of the knee. The ligaments that provide medial stability for the knee include (1) the superficial (medial) ligament, (2) the deep capsular ligaments (meniscofemoral and meniscotibial), and (3) the posterior oblique fibers. However, as Warren, Marshall, and Girgis have demonstrated, these ligaments should be considered only as consolidations within tissue planes and not as discrete structures (such as the cruciate ligaments).[68]

The superficial tibial collateral ligament is a broad, triangular ligament that is attached proximally to the medial epicondyle of the femur and distally to the tibia as far anterior as the tibia tuberosity. The posterior fibers of the superficial ligament blend with the deep ligament and are firmly attached to the posterior horn of the medial meniscus. The deep medial ligament lies beneath the superficial tibial collateral ligament and is divided into a meniscofemoral component that originates on the femur, just distal to the origin of the superficial ligament, and inserts in the midportion of the peripheral margin of the meniscus. The meniscotibial component, the coronary ligament, originates from the midportion of the peripheral margin of the meniscus and inserts on the tibia. The anterior and midmedial parts of the deep medial ligament are separated from the superficial ligament by one to three bursae. The posterior portion of the deep medial ligament, designated as the *posterior oblique ligament* by Hughston and Eilers,[25] blends with the superficial ligament as described previously.

The superficial medial side of the knee. Warren and Marshall have demonstrated that the anterior portion (parallel fibers) of the superficial against valgus and rotary stress from 0 to 90 degrees of flexion.[67,68] Grood and colleagues found that the superficial ligament provided 57% of the total medial restraint at 5 degrees of knee flexion and 78% at 25 degrees of knee flexion. In contrast, they reported that the deep medial ligament (including the posteromedial portion) provided 25% of the total medial restraint at 5 degrees of flexion and only 8% at 25 degrees of knee flexion. In addition, they found that the combined restraint of the anterior and posterior cruciate ligaments was only 15% and 13% of the total at 5 degrees and 25 degrees of flexion, respectively.[23]

Lateral ligamentous stabilizers of the knee. The ligaments that stabilize the lateral aspect of the knee include the (1) lateral (fibular) collateral ligament, (2) short collateral (fabellofibular) ligament, (3) lateral capsule, and (4) iliotibial tract.

The lateral (fibular) collateral ligament extends from the lateral femoral epicondyle to the fibular head. Unlike the posterior portion of the superficial medial ligament, the lateral collateral ligament has no attachments to the lateral meniscus. The short collateral ligament lies deep to the lateral collateral ligament and also extends from the femur to the fibular head. This ligament is of significant size only in individuals with a lateral fabella (8% to 16% of the population). It is often called the *fabellofibular ligament.*[33] The lateral capsule can be divided into three components. The anterior third originated from the lateral border of the patellar tendon and is reinforced by the lateral patellar retinaculum of the quadriceps tendon. The anterior portion of the capsule inserts into the articular margin of the proximal tibia and has no femoral attachment. The middle third of the capsule attaches proximally to the lateral epicondyle of the femur and distally at the anterior margin of the proximal tibia. The middle third of the capsule, like the deep medial ligament, has meniscofemoral and meniscotibial components. The posterior third of the capsule has femoral, meniscal, and tibial attachments that are similar to the middle third, but it also has an area of condensed and thickened fibers, which is called the *arcuate ligament.* This ligament reinforces the posterolateral corner of the knee. The femoral-tibial portion of the iliotibial tract supplies static support and reinforces the middle third of the capsule. The tract inserts proximally into the lateral femoral epicondyle and distally into Gerdy's (lateral tibial) tubercle.

The lateral (fibular) collateral ligament is the primary lateral restraint to varus forces. Grood and colleagues have demonstrated that the lateral collateral ligament provided 55% of the total lateral restraint at 5 degrees of knee flexion and 69% at 25 degrees of flexion.[23] The anterior and midlateral capsule provided only 4.1% and 3.7% of the restraint at 5 degrees and 25 degrees of flexion, respectively. The values for the posterior third of the capsule at the same degrees of flexion were 13% and 5%, respectively. The combined restraint of the anterior and posterior cruciate ligaments was 22% at 5 degrees of flexion and 12% at 25 degrees of flexion.

Medial and lateral ligament injuries. Medial collateral ligament injuries occur when there is an excessive *external* rotatory and/or abduction force applied to the flexed, weight-bearing knee. Lateral collateral ligament injuries are caused by excessive *internal* rotatory and/or adduction forces. In the case of a medial collateral ligament injury, the individual has pain to palpation over the medial epicondyle of the femur, the middle third of the medial joint line, and/or the tibial insertion of the ligament beneath the pes tendons. With lateral collateral injuries, the pain is localized to the fibular head or lateral femoral epicondyle. With first- or second-degree sprains, an athlete is usually able to walk off the field unaided. The amount of swelling and pain that ensues usually varies with the severity of the injury. In third-degree sprains, the complete disruption of the capsule and ligaments allows the fluid and blood to run out of the joint and thus lessens the swelling and the pain. With medial collateral injuries, the athlete may be unable to fully extend the knee. This represents pseudolocking of the knee because the block is not caused by a displaced meniscus but occurs because the medial collateral ligament is put on greatest stretch (tension) in the last 10 to 15 degrees of extension. Thus, fully extending the knee greatly increases the individual's pain. If the blocking is not a result of a meniscal lesion, full extension can often be obtained by injecting the femoral attachment of the medial collateral ligament with 1% solution lidocaine (Xylocaine).

The severity of medial and lateral collateral ligament injuries is best determined by performing adduction and abduction stress tests, respectively. These tests should first be performed on the uninjured knee to establish the individual's normal physiologic laxity. The abduction stress test is performed with the individual supine (Fig. 6-20). The extremity to be examined is abducted at the hip so that the thigh rests on the examining table and the quadriceps and hamstrings muscles are relaxed. The knee is then flexed to 30 degrees over the side of the table as the leg is grasped with one hand about the lateral aspect of the knee and one hand on the foot or ankle. Abduction stress is then slowly and gently applied to the knee up to the point of pain. If the test is performed in this manner, the examiner can accurately document the amount of instability. The adduction stress test is performed with the individual in the same position, but one hand is placed around the medial aspect of the knee, and adduction stress is applied. These tests do not accurately evaluate the integrity of the medial or lateral collateral ligament if they are performed with the knee in full extension because the cruciate ligaments and the medial and lateral capsular structures provide 43% and 45% medial and lateral restraint, respectively, to straight varus and valgus testing.[23]

One interesting situation occurs with lateral collateral ligament injuries. On occasion, the meniscotibial portion of the midlateral capsule is avulsed from the tibia, with part of the tibial bony attachment included. The fragment varies in size from a faint fleck to several millimeters in size and is evident on a routine anteroposterior radiograph (Fig. 6-21). This radiographic finding, which has been called the *lateral capsule sign,*[69] has great clinical significance because it not only indicates a severe lateral capsular injury but also is

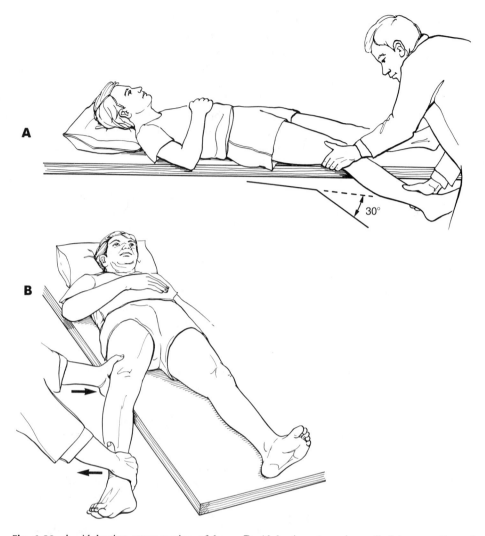

Fig. 6-20. A, Abduction stress-testing of knee. **B,** Abduction stress is applied in a gentle and controlled fashion.

usually associated with a third-degree anterior cruciate ligament injury and varying degrees of medial collateral ligament injury.

Treatment. When the abduction or adduction stress testing reveals that the athlete has sustained a first- or second-degree collateral ligament disruption, the injury is treated nonoperatively. Third-degree medial collateral sprains can also be successfully treated nonoperatively if there is no anterior cruciate injury.[28]

Many therapists have found that operative treatment of second- and third-degree collateral ligament injuries does not improve stability. The medial laxity associated with second- and third-degree injuries is not altered by surgical attempts at tightening the ligament. Therefore, recommended treatment of first-, second-, and third-degree medial collateral ligament injuries involves a therapy program following the tenets presented in Tables 6-2 through 6-4, but the emphasis is a functional progression (see the Box on p. 149).

The athlete may return to competition when (1) no local tenderness is apparent, (2) full range of motion has been restored, (3) quadriceps and hamstring muscle strengths are approximately 80% to 90% of the normal leg, and (4) the running program has been completed. This process requires a few days up to several weeks.

Intraarticular ligament injuries

The most commonly injured intraarticular ligaments of the musculoskeletal system are the anterior and posterior cruciate ligaments of the knee.

Anatomy. The anterior and posterior cruciate ligaments are strong, rounded connective tissue cords located within the knee joint capsule between the femoral condyles, but they lie outside the synovial cavity of the joint. They are positioned between the medial and lateral synovial compartments and behind the posterior wall of the anterior synovial cavity.

The detailed anatomy of the cruciate ligaments has been

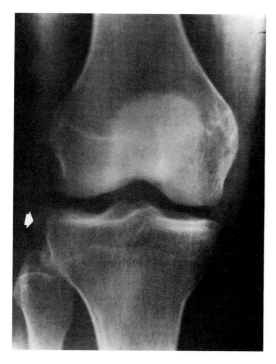

Fig. 6-21. "Lateral capsular sign." This anteroposterior radiograph demonstrates avulsion of bony attachment *(arrow)* of meniscotibial portion of lateral capsule. (Significance of this sign is explained in text.)

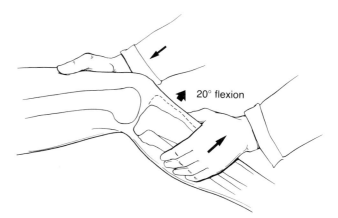

Fig. 6-22. Lachman's test shows position of examiner and examiner's hands with knee in 15 to 20 degrees of flexion. Anterior stress is applied to tibia. If test is positive, tibia slides forward on femur and examiner experiences no, or a "mushy," end feel.

documented by Girgis, Marshall, and Monajem.[22] The anterior cruciate ligament arises from depression on a 30-mm-long nonarticular area of the tibia, anterior to the intercondylar eminence. Its origin blends into the anterior attachment of the lateral meniscus. The ligament passes posteriorly and laterally to insert on the posterior nonarticular aspect of the medial surface of the lateral femoral condyle. The posterior cruciate ligament arises from a 13-mm-wide depression behind the posterior articular surface of the tibia and is attached to the posterior horn of the lateral meniscus. The ligament passes anteriorly and medially to insert on the posterior aspect of the lateral surface of the medial femoral condyle. These ligaments cross each other between their femoral and tibial attachments and thus are called *cruciates*. They are also named for their tibial attachments.

Girgis and colleagues[22] and Kennedy, Weinberg, and Wilson[37] have demonstrated that, except for the anterior medial portion, the majority of the fibers of the posterior cruciate are taut in flexion. In extension, the posterior fibers are taut, but most other fibers are lax. This variation in tension of the various parts of these ligaments may occur because they are multifascicular structures. The individual fasciculi are either directed in spiral fashion around the long axis of the ligament or pass directly from their femoral to tibial attachments. The major blood supply to the anterior and posterior cruciate ligaments comes from branches of the middle genicular artery.

The biomechanical functions of the cruciate ligaments have been best documented by Butler, Noyes, and Grood.[3] They found that the anterior cruciate ligament was the primary restraint to straight anterior stress placed upon the knee joint. The ligament provided 85% and 87% of the total restraint at 90 degrees and 30 degrees of flexion, respectively. The posterior cruciate ligament was the primary restraint to straight posterior forces placed on the knee joint. The posterior cruciate ligament provided 94% of the total restraint at 90 degrees and 30 degrees of flexion.

Anterior cruciate ligaments injuries. Anterior cruciate ligament injuries are caused by a variety of mechanisms: (1) external rotation, abduction, and straight anterior forces applied to the tibia; (2) internal rotation of the femur on the tibia; and (3) hyperextension of the knee. Injuries most commonly occur in noncontact situations.[50,52]

Diagnosis. Regardless of the mechanism of the injury, the patient is usually (85% of the time) unable to continue activity and experiences immediate swelling of the knee, posterolateral knee pain, and varying degrees of knee instability. The effusion becomes tense within 24 hours and pseudolocking (as described previously) occurs. Presence of a tense bloody effusion (hemarthrosis) (see Fig. 6-4) and a positive response to Lachman's test (Fig. 6-22) are the keys to diagnosing acute injuries. DeHaven[13] and Noyes and colleagues[52] have arthroscopically evaluated athletes with hemarthroses from acute knee injuries. They found partial or complete anterior cruciate tears in 72% of such cases, two thirds of which also had associated meniscal lesions. DeHaven also documented solitary meniscus tears in 15%, osteochondral fractures in 6%, posterior cruciate tears in 3%, and no demonstrable lesion in 4%. In arthroscopically evaluating several hundred athletes with hemarthrosis, I (JSK) have observed similar findings and percentages.

On clinical examination, the knee with an anterior cruciate disruption has a tense effusion. Stress testing of the knee, with adequate muscle relaxation, reveals a positive response to Lachman's test but only occasionally produces a positive anterior drawer test.

Lachman's test, as described by Torg, Conrad, and Kalen,[64] is performed as shown in Fig. 6-22. After the knee is gently flexed 20 degrees, the examiner pulls the tibia forward on the femur. The test is positive when the tibia can be subluxated forward with no end feel or a mushy end feel. The injured knee must be compared with the uninjured knee, and the hamstrings must be relaxed. When the uninjured knee is tested, the examiner should experience a solid ropelike end feel as the tibia is pulled forward. If the hamstrings of the injured knee are adequately relaxed, the test accurately (greater than 90+%) documents third-degree tears of the anterior cruciate ligament.[13,64]

However, the anterior drawer test is often negative with acute injuries because of a ball-valve action of the menisci, hamstring spasm, or a hemarthrosis.[64] The anterior drawer test is positive only when other ligamentous structures are acutely disrupted or when these secondary restraints become lengthened, as seen weeks to months after an anterior cruciate ligament injury.

Standard radiographs of the acutely injured knee usually demonstrate only hemarthrosis because the great majority of the anterior cruciate ligament tears occur within the substance of the ligament, not at their bony attachments. Kennedy and Fowler reported that 72% of 50 clients with anterior cruciate disruptions documented by arthrotomies had midsubstance tears.[36] Noyes, Delucas, and Torvik concluded from primate studies that the high strain rates experienced with athletic trauma should cause midsubstance tears. They found that lower strain rates produced tibial and, to a much lesser extent, femoral bony avulsions.[49]

These findings reflect my (JSK) experience with this injury. Often clients are evaluated in an emergency room, and, when radiographs are negative, they are told that they have a "sprained knee." The diagnosis is partially accurate in that they often have a sprain of the anterior cruciate ligament. However, the initial instability caused by this injury deserves further investigation and, more importantly, proper treatment.

The individual with an acute third-degree anterior cruciate injury should be examined to determined if there is also anterolateral rotatory instability. This is important because McDevitt and Muur[45] and Marshall and Olsen[42] have demonstrated in dogs and Slocum and colleagues[56] and Jacobsen[32] have shown in humans that anterior cruciate insufficiency and anterolateral rotatory instability of the knee are associated with the development of degenerative arthritis.

The many diagnostic tests for detecting anterolateral rotatory instability include (1) the pivot-shift, (2) the jerk, (3) flexion-rotation drawer, and (4) Losee. The original test was described by Galway, Beaupre, and MacIntosh[20] (Fig. 6-23). During this maneuver, the examiner feels and the client experiences a sudden shift (jerk) of the tibia on the

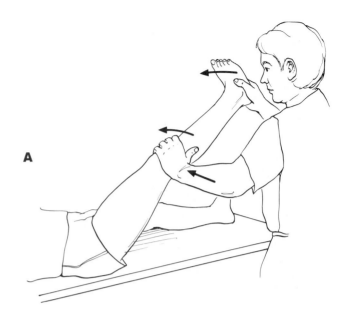

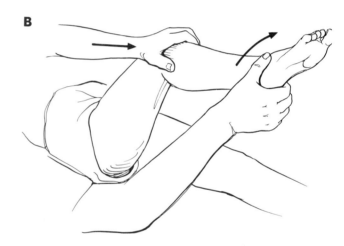

Fig. 6-23. Pivot-shift test performed on right knee. **A,** With knee in full extension, examiner's left hand grasps tibia at level of tibial tubercle and applies a valgus stress. Then examiner's right hand grasps and maximally internally rotates ankle and foot. This subluxates tibia anteriorly. **B,** Right hand then slowly flexes knee. If test is positive, examiner and client note a sudden posterior "shift" of the tibia on femur.

femur if the test is positive. The validity of this test for anterior cruciate and anterolateral rotatory instability has been confirmed by Fetto and Marshall.[18] They found that sectioning of the anterior cruciate produced a positive pivot-shift sign in 33 of 37 cadaver knees. However, they also observed that excessive physiologic soft tissue laxity may cause a false-positive result.

Treatment. When the diagnosis of a third-degree anterior cruciate ligament injury has been confirmed, there are several avenues of treatment. First, the examiner should ascertain if there is an associated meniscal injury. An MRI or a single-contrast arthrogram is usually obtained for this purpose. Second, the examiner should determine the degree of anterolateral rotatory instability by performing one or more of the tests previously listed. If muscle spasm or a loss of knee motion occurs, the examination should be performed with the patient under general or spinal anesthesia. If the client is anesthetized for the examination, the joint should be arthroscopically evaluated to assess, particularly, the lateral meniscus because it is not well evaluated by an arthrogram. Also, the arthroscopic examination should determine whether the torn cruciate is blocking knee motion when a patient's ROM does not return over 2 or 3 weeks after the injury. It has been my experience (JSK) and that of others that the torn cruciate can become lodged under the medial or lateral femoral condyles and block knee extension.[46] As a general rule, surgical intervention is used only after the patient has regained essentially a normal ROM, thus minimizing the likelihood of postoperative loss of motion.[24] Surgical intervention has become the norm, with reconstructive procedures using the patellar tendon graft the most common (see in recommended Readings the books edited by Daniel and colleagues, Feagin, and Scott). Anterior cruciate ligament reconstruction is recommended because the results of primary repair have been quite discouraging. Feagin and Curl found that fewer than 10% of 32 clients had an asymptomatic stable knee 5 years after a primary repair.[17] Many surgical procedures for correcting anterior cruciate ligament insufficiency have been proposed. However, these procedures can be classified as either extraarticular,[15,20,41] intraarticular,[5,16,30,53] or both.[10,43] A procedure that includes an intraarticular reconstruction of the ligament is preferred. My experience and that of others,[4] show several advantages to using part of the patellar tendon as the substitute: (1) It is the strongest of the biologic substitutes proposed to date, (2) it has been shown to revascularize and attain sufficient tensile strength,[9] and (3) its use does not require sacrificing other significant structures that are important to knee-joint function. Anterior cruciate reconstruction is demonstrated by Figs. 6-24 and 6-25. The procedure is primarily accomplished through arthroscopic actions and the stabilization of the bone blocks in the tunnels by either suture over screws (as shown) or via interference (wedging) screws.

Postoperative care is described in detail in several of the recommended readings. The "phased" approach to rehabilitation is highly recommended. Phases have been described by many authors (see *Journal of Orthopedic and Sports Physical Therapy* recommended reading volume) and typically include immediate postoperative phase (activities goals: pain modulation, quadriceps control, partial weight-bearing gait, patellar mobility, full extension, flexion to 90 degrees), maximal protection phase (activities and goals:) progressive ROM, bicycle, pool walking, normalization of gait, (weight bearing to tolerance to full weight bearing), moderate protection phase (activities and goals: light functional progression, middle ROM, open- and closed-chain exercise at controlled level of effort, proprioception

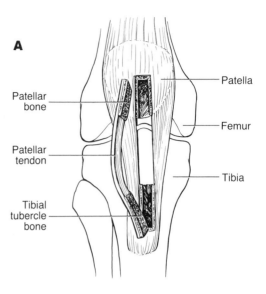

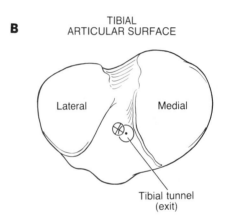

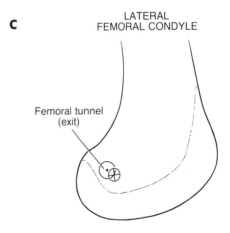

Fig. 6-24. Anterior cruciate ligament reconstruction. **A,** Harvesting of patellar bone, patellar tendon, tibial bone graft. Intraarticular location of the tibial, **B,** and femoral, **C,** tunnels.

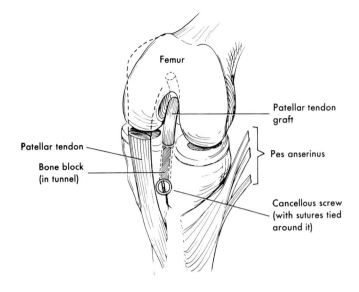

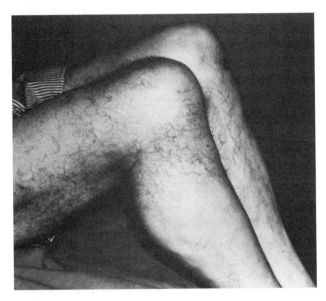

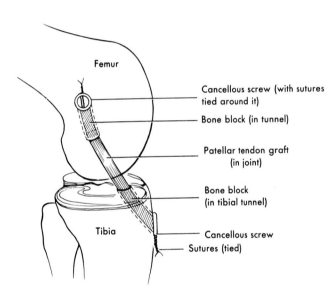

Fig. 6-25. Anterior cruciate ligament graft passed through bony tunnels and positioned within knee joint. Graft is put under tension and secured by tying sutures from bone blocks around cancellous screws. Many surgeons use an interference screw to wedge the bone plug in the tunnel.

activities, pool running), light activity phase (activities and goals: initiation of functional progression, running, middle ROM open- and closed-chain exercises at maximal effort level), and return to function phase (activities and goals: return to activity of choice through progression of controlled to uncontrolled patterns, continued strengthening, criteria referenced return to "sport" or "activity," which often include normal joint exam [ligamentous], ROM, effusion and/or swelling, muscle performance [approximately 70+% for running or 80+% return to contact actions], running, hop test).

Fig. 6-26. Posterior cruciate ligament insufficiency. With third-degree posterior cruciate ligament injuries, there is posterior sag of involved tibia on femur. It is best assessed by viewing client's knees from side with both knees in 90-degree flexion.

Individuals commonly move through these phases in approximately 4 to 6 months. We recommend using a range of weeks and specific criteria to monitor patient progression. Individual variation must be taken into account, and "time" must not become the primary determinate. In fact, progression should reflect multiple pieces of clinical data, not a single piece of information. The final activities must be functionally based.

Posterior cruciate ligament injuries. The majority of posterior cruciate injuries are caused by one of two mechanisms: (1) the individual either falls on one knee with the ankle in forced plantar flexion, or (2) the individual is struck on the anterior aspect of the tibia, which is forced posteriorly. Regardless of the mechanism of injury, a patient with an acute injury is usually able to continue activity and may experience only minimal swelling, some posterior knee pain, and varying degrees of knee instability. The effusion does not become tense within the first 24 hours, and the individual does not experience the pseudolocking that is associated with anterior cruciate ligament tears, but often there is marked posterior pain. Individuals with chronic posterior cruciate insufficiency frequently complain of pain and disability with activities of daily living.

Diagnosis. In the acute and chronic posterior cruciate injuries, the clinical examination is diagnostic. Individuals with acute injuries have (1) a very mild bloody effusion but definite posterior pain; (2) a posterior subluxation of the involved tibia, seen best from the side with the knee flexed to 90 degrees (Fig. 6-26); (3) loss of normal anteromedial and anterolateral prominence of the tibial plateau, beneath the femoral condyles, determined by palpation with the knee at 90 degrees of flexion; (4) a posterior drawer sign with the

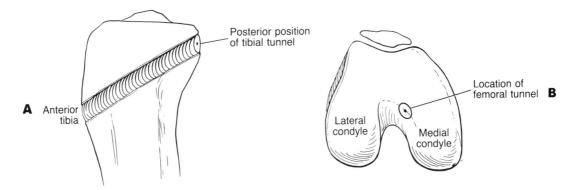

Fig. 6-27. A, Tibial tunnel created for posterior cruciate ligament reconstruction. **B,** Intraarticular location of femoral tunnel.

tibia in neutral and external rotation; and (5) a negative Lachman's test. Individuals with chronic injuries usually do not have an effusion but have greater posterior subluxation and laxity with stress testing. The examiner must pay close attention to detail when performing the posterior drawer test. With the knee flexed to 60 to 90 degrees, the tibia of the knee with a posterior cruciate ligament injury usually sags posteriorly. However, if the examiner does not recognize the subluxation, the anterior drawer test may be falsely interpreted as positive as the tibia is pulled forward and reduced. This mistake can be avoided by observing the relationship of the tibia and femur from the side and documenting the absence of the normal anterior tibial prominence before the stress testing is performed.

Standard lateral radiographs of the acutely injured knee may demonstrate the posterior subluxation of the tibia on the femur if they are taken with the knee in 90 degrees of flexion. An arthrogram also displays the posterior sag, particularly if a posterior stress is applied to the tibia when the lateral views are obtained. The posterior cruciate, like the anterior cruciate, usually sustains an interstitial tear. Therefore, standard radiographs rarely display an avulsion of one or the other of its bony attachments.

Treatment. When operative treatment of a third-degree posterior cruciate ligament injury is performed, a reconstruction, not a repair, is recommended. This recommendation is based on my (JSK) experience and that of others.[9,11,35] In 1980, Kennedy reported on 57 clients who had been treated nonoperatively for third-degree tears of their posterior cruciate ligament. Twenty-five of these 57 clients (44%) had developed degenerative changes in the knee joint within an average of 61 months from the injury.[35] Although Hughston and colleagues reported good results in 13 of 20 knees (65%) that had primary repairs of acute interstitial posterior cruciate, 9 of these cases required excision of the frayed ligament and reconstruction with a medial meniscal substitution.[27]

The procedure I (JSK) prefer for reconstructing the posterior cruciate ligament uses the middle third of the patellar tendon as the substitute. I believe that the middle

third of the patellar tendon is the best substitute for reconstruction purposes, based on the reasons discussed in the section on anterior cruciate ligament (ACL) reconstructions. Posterior cruciate reconstruction is demonstrated in Figs. 6-27 and 6-28.

Postoperative care is similar to that described for the ACL reconstruction patient except that greater care is taken in the early postoperative phases, as these patients tend not to maintain the reduction in ligamentous laxity as well as the ACL reconstructed patients. Clancy and colleagues reported on the results of 20 clients, 11 with acute and 9 with chronic instability, who were followed for at least 2 years. The 11 clients with acute instability had clinical findings similar to the posterior cruciate ligament injury described previously, and all had at least a 2+ on the posterior drawer test. Postoperatively, none exhibited posterior sag or loss of the tibial plateau step-off that they had preoperatively. Four clients had 0, four clients had a trace, and three clients had a 1+ result on the posterior drawer test. All returned to their previous level of athletic activity, including three who returned to intercollegiate football and one who returned to professional baseball. The results were similar for the nine clients with chronic instability.[11]

Summary. The anterior and posterior cruciate ligaments of the knee are the most commonly injured intraarticular ligaments. The anterior cruciate ligament is the primary restraint against abnormal anterior displacement of the tibia on the femur. The clinical history (immediate, tense, bloody effusion) and positive results on clinical stress (Lachman's, pivot-shift) are usually diagnostic. If the results of a clinical examination are not conclusive, the client's knee should be examined under general anesthesia, arthroscopically evaluated, or an MRI obtained. Anterior cruciate ligament reconstructions with a patellar-tendon, bone-block graft have been very successful.

The posterior cruciate ligament is the primary restraint against abnormal posterior displacement of the tibia on the femur. Clinically, individuals with this injury have a mild effusion, 2+ to 3+ result on a posterior drawer test, and posterior subluxation (loss of the normal tibial plateau

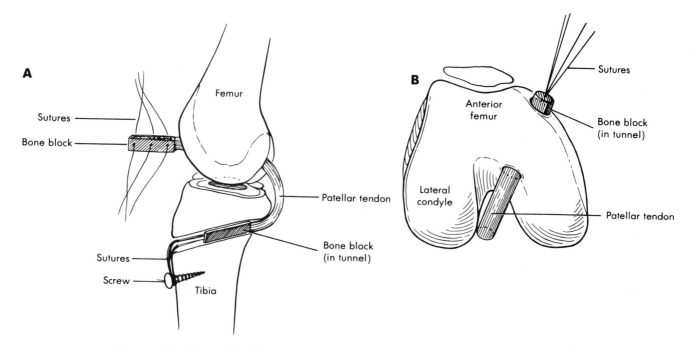

Fig. 6-28. Posterior cruciate ligament substitute has been passed through tibia, **A**, and femur, **B**. Tension is placed on graft by tying sutures over buttons.

prominence) of the tibia. The clinical examination is diagnostic. Posterior cruciate reconstructions with a patellar-tendon, bone-block graft have either eliminated the instability or improved stability to the extent that individuals with this injury have been able to return to recreational and even intercollegiate athletics.

SUMMARY

The diagnosis of ligament and muscle-tendon unit injuries is predicated on the accuracy with which one (1) obtains a detailed history, (2) performs a thorough physical examination, and (3) documents and classifies the instability and disability caused by the injury. A basic understanding of the normal anatomic and biomechanical properties of an injured ligament or muscle-tendon unit is of paramount importance for understanding the various operative and nonoperative treatment regimens that have been discussed. Rehabilitation of these injuries can be successfully accomplished with programs that are based on the scientific data currently available. These programs must be structured so that they (1) restore full joint motion, (2) facilitate normal neuromuscular patterns of movement, and (3) correct deficiencies in the strength, endurance, and flexibility of the muscles involved. Athletes with ligament and muscle-tendon unit injuries can be returned to full competition with a minimal risk of reinjury if those treating them are dedicated to applying and expanding the diagnostic and therapeutic principles that have been presented.

REVIEW QUESTIONS

1. How would a muscle stretching program be implemented following a muscle-tendon-unit injury using proprioceptive neuromuscular facilitation techniques?
2. What activities or drills should be considered when planning a functional progression following a muscle-tendon-unit injury?
3. How would the treatment program for a muscle contusion differ from the treatment program for tendinitis?
4. What ligaments provide stability to the medial and lateral aspects of the knee complex? What specific tests would be used to assess the integrity of these ligaments following injury?
5. What is the difference between Lachman's test in comparison to the anterior drawer test when assessing a possible injury to the anterior cruciate ligament?

REFERENCES

1. Bandy WD, Irion JM: The effect of time of static stretch on the flexibility of the hamstring muscles, *Phys Ther* 74:845, 1994.
2. Brubaker CE, James SL: Injuries to runners, *J Sports Med Phys Fitness* 2:189, 1974.
3. Butler DL, Noyes FR, Grood ES: Ligamentous restraints to anterior-posterior drawer in the human knee, *J Bone Joint Surg Am* 62:259, 1980.
4. Butler DL et al: Mechanical properties of transplants for the anterior cruciate ligament, *Orthop Trans* 3:180, 1979.
5. Cho KO: Reconstruction of the anterior cruciate ligament by semitendinosis tenodesis, *J Bone Joint Surg Am* 57:608, 1975.

6. Clancy WG: Lower extremity injuries in the jogger and distance runner, *Phys Sports Med* 2:46, 1974.

7. Clancy WG: Tendon trauma and over use injuries. In Leadbetter WB, Buchwalter JA, Gordon SL, editors: *Sports induced inflammation*, Park Ridge, Ill, 1990, American Academy of Orthopaedic Surgeons.

8. Clancy WG Jr, Neidhart D, Brand RL: Achilles tendonitis in runners: a report of five cases, *Am J Sports Med* 4:46, 1976.

9. Clancy WG Jr et al: Anterior and posterior cruciate ligament reconstruction in Rhesus monkeys, *J Bone Joint Surg Am* 63:1270, 1981.

10. Clancy WG Jr et al: Anterior cruciate ligament reconstruction using one-third of the patellar ligament augmented with extraarticular tendon transfers, *J Bone Joint Surg Am* 64:352, 1982.

11. Clancy WG Jr et al: Posterior cruciate ligament reconstruction: preliminary report of a new technique, *J Bone Joint Surg Am* 65:310, 1983.

12. Daniel DM, Stone ML: Instrumented measurement of knee motion. In Daniel DM et al, editors: *Knee ligaments: structure, function, injury, and repair,* New York, 1990, Raven.

13. DeHaven KE: Diagnosis of acute knee injuries with hemarthrosis, *Am J Sports Med* 8:9, 1980.

14. DeHaven KE, Collins R: Diagnosis of internal derangements of the knee: the role of arthroscopy, *J Bone Joint Surg Am* 57:802, 1975.

15. Ellison AE: Distal iliotibial band transfer for anterolateral instability of the knee, *J Bone Joint Surg Am* 45:905, 1963.

16. Erickson E: Sports injuries of knee ligaments: their diagnosis, treatment, rehabilitation, and prevention, *Med Sci Sports Exerc* 8:133, 1976.

17. Feagin JA Jr, Curl WW: Isolated tear of the anterior cruciate ligament: 5-year follow-up study, *Am J Sports Med* 4:95, 1976.

18. Fetto JF, Marshall JL: Injury to the anterior cruciate ligament producing the pivot-shift sign, *J Bone Joint Surg Am* 61:710, 1079.

19. Fox JM et al: Degenerating and rupture of the Achilles tendon, *Clin Orthop* 107:221, 1978.

20. Galway RD, Beaupre A, MacIntosh DC: Pivot shift: a clinical sign of symptomatic anterior cruciate insufficiency, *J Bone Joint Surg Br* 54:763, 1972.

21. Garrett WE, Almekinders LC, Seaber AV: Biomechanics of muscle tears in stretching injuries, *Trans Orthop Res Soc,* 9:384, 1984.

22. Girgis FG, Marshall JL, Monajem A: A cruciate ligaments of the knee joint: anatomical, functional, and experimental analysis, *Clin Orthop* 106:216, 1975.

23. Grood ES et al: Ligamentous and capsular restraints preventing straight medial and lateral laxity in intact human cadaver knees, *J Bone Joint Surg Am* 63:1257, 1981.

24. Harner CD et al: Loss of motion after anterior cruciate reconstruction, *Am J Sports Med* 5:499, 1992.

25. Hughston JC, Eilers AF: The role of the posterior oblique ligament in repairs of acute medial (collateral) ligament tears of the knee, *J Bone Joint Surg Am* 55:923, 1973.

26. Hughston JC et al: Classification of knee ligament instabilities: I, the medial compartment and cruciate ligaments, *J Bone Joint Surg Am* 58:159, 1976.

27. Hughston JC et al: Classification of knee ligament instabilities: II, the lateral compartment, *J Bone Joint Surg Am* 58:173, 1976.

28. Hughston JC et al: Acute tears of the posterior cruciate ligaments: results of operative treatment, *J Bone Joint Surg Am* 62:438, 1980.

29. Indelicato PA: Non-operative treatment of complete tears of the medial collateral ligament of the knee, *J Bone Joint Surg Am* 65:323, 1983.

30. Insall J et al: Bone-block iliotibial band transfer for anterior cruciate insufficiency, *J Bone Joint Surg Am* 63:560, 1981.

31. Jackson DW, Feagin JA: Quadriceps contusions in young athletes, *J Bone Joint Surg Am* 55:95, 1973.

32. Jacobsen K: Osteoarthritis following insufficiency of the cruciate ligaments in man: a clinical study, *Acta Orthop Scand* 48:520, 1977.

33. Kaplan EB: The fabellofibular and short lateral ligaments of the knee, *J Bone Joint Surg Am* 43:169, 1961.

34. Keats TE, Scaatz DS, Bailey RW: Pneumoarthrography of the knee, *Surg Gynecol Obstet* 94:361, 1952.

35. Kennedy JC: Posterior cruciate injuries. Paper presented at the interim meeting of the American Orthopedic Society for Sports Medicine, Atlanta, February 1980.

36. Kennedy JC, Fowler PJ: Medial and anterior instability of the knee: an anatomical and clinical study using stress machines, *J Bone Joint Surg Am* 53:1257, 1971.

37. Kennedy JC, Weinberg JW, Wilson AS: The anatomy and function of the anterior cruciate ligament, *J Bone Joint Surg Am* 56:223, 1974.

38. Kottke FJ, Pauley DL, Ptak RA: The rationale for prolonged stretching for correction of the shortening of connective tissue, *Arch Phys Med Rehabil* 47:345, 1966.

39. Lentell G et al: The use of thermal agents to influence the effectiveness of a low-load prolonged stretch, *J Orthop Sports Phys Ther* 5:200, 1992.

40. Lipscomb AB, Thomas ED, Johnson RK: Treatment of myositis ossificans traumatic in athletes, *Am J Sports Med* 4:111, 1970.

41. Losee RE, Johnson TR, Southwick WO: Anterior subluxation of the lateral tibial plateau: a diagnostic test and operative repair, *J Bone Joint Surg Am* 60:1015, 1978.

42. Marshall JL, Olsen S: Instability of the knee: a long-term experimental study in dogs, *J Bone Joint Surg Am* 53:1561, 1971.

43. Marshall JL et al: The anterior cruciate ligament: a technique of repair and reconstruction, *Clin Orthop* 143:97, 1979.

44. McBeath AA, Wirka HW: Positive-contrast arthrography of the knee, *Clin Orthop* 88:70, 1972.

45. McDevitt CA, Muur H: Biochemical changes in the cartilage of the knee in experimental and natural osteoarthritis in the dog, *J Bone Joint Surg Br* 58:94, 1976.

46. Monaco BR, Noble HB, Bachman DC: Incomplete tears of toe, anterior cruciate ligament and knee locking, *JAMA* 247:1582, 1982.

47. Nicholas JA, Freiberger RH, Killoran PJ: Double-contrast arthrography of the knee, *J Bone Joint Surg Am* 52:203, 1970.

48. Nikolaou PK et al: Biomechanical and histological evaluation of muscle after controlled strain injury, *Am J Sports Med* 15:9, 1987.

49. Noyes FR, Delucas JL, Torvik PJ: Biomechanics of anterior cruciate ligament failure: an analysis of strain-rate sensitivity and mechanisms of failure in primates, *J Bone Joint Surg Am* 56:236, 1974.

50. Noyes FR, Grood ES: Diagnosis of knee ligament injuries. In Daniel DM et al, editors: *Knee ligaments: structure, function, injury, and repair,* New York, 1990, Raven.

51. Noyes FR et al: Biomechanics of ligament failure, *J Bone Joint Surg Am* 56:1406, 1974.

52. Noyes FR et al: Arthroscopy in acute traumatic hemarthrosis of the knee, *J Bone Joint Surg Am* 62:687, 1980.

53. O'Donoghue DH: A method of replacement of the anterior cruciate ligament of the knee: report of twenty cases, *J Bone Joint Surg Am* 45:905, 1963.

54. Sach MD, McGaw WH, Rizzo RP: Studies in the scope of pneumography of the knee as a diagnosis aid, *Radiology* 54:10, 1950.

55. Schils JP, Resnick D, Sartoris DJ: Diagnostic imaging of ligamentous injuries. In Daniel DM et al, editors: *Knee ligaments: structure, function, injury, and repair,* New York, 1990, Raven.

56. Slocum DB et al: Clinical test for anterolateral rotatory instability of the knee, *Clin Orthop* 118:63, 1976.

57. Smillie IS: *Injuries of the knee joint,* ed 4, Edinburgh, 1970, Churchill Livingstone.

58. Snook GA: Achilles tendon tenosynovitis in long distance runners, *Med Sci Sports Exerc* 4:155, 1972.

59. *Standard nomenclature of athletic injuries.* Madison, Wis, 1968, Committee on the Medical Aspects of Sports of the American Medical Association.

60. Staubli HU: Stressradiography. In Daniel DM et al, editors: *Knee ligaments: structure, function, injury, and repair,* New York, 1990, Raven.
61. Strickler T, Malone T, Garrett WE: The effects of passive warming on muscle injury, *Am J Sports Med* 18:141, 1990.
62. Stoddard GA: The Stoddard warm-up: a preventive exercise program for increasing strength and flexibility, Madison, Wis, 1978, Guild Printing.
63. Tongue JR, Larson RL: Limited arthrography in acute knee injuries, *Am J Sports Med* 8:1923, 1980.
64. Torg JS, Conrad W, Kalen V: Clinical diagnosis of anterior cruciate ligament instability in the athlete, *Am J Sports Med* 4:84, 1976.
65. Wang JB, Marshall JL: Acute ligamentous injuries of the knee single contrast arthrography—a diagnostic aid, *J Trauma* 15:431, 1975.
66. Warren CG et al: Elongation of rat tail tendon: effect of load and temperature, *Arch Phys Med Rehabil* 52:465, 1971.
67. Warren LR, Marshall JL: The supporting structures and layers on the medial side of the knee: an anatomical analysis, *J Bone Joint Surg Am* 61:56, 1979.
68. Warren LR, Marshall JL, Girgis F: The prime static stabilizer of the medial side of the knee, *J Bone Joint Surg Am* 56:665, 1974.
69. Woods GW, Stanley RF, Tullos JS: The lateral capsule sign: x-ray clue to a significant knee instability, *Am J Sports Med* 7:27, 1979.

RECOMMENDED READINGS–PCL

Journals

Clancy WG Jr et al: Treatment of knee joint instability secondary to rupture of the posterior cruciate ligament: report of a new procedure, *J Bone Joint Surg Am* 65:310, 1983.

Cross MJ, Powell JF: Long-term follow-up of posterior cruciate ligament rupture: a study of 116 cases, *Am J Sports Med* 12:292, 1984.

Degenhardt TC, Hughston JC: Chronic posterior cruciate instability: non-operative management, *Orthop Trans* 5:486, 1981.

Fowler PJ, Messieh SS: Isolated posterior cruciate ligament injuries in athletes, *Am J Sports Med* 15:553, 1987.

Hughston JC: The absent posterior drawer test in some acute PCL tears of the knee, *Am J Sports Med* 16:39, 1988.

Hughston JC et al: Acute tears of the posterior cruciate ligament: results of operative treatment, *J Bone Joint Surg Am* 62:438, 1980.

Hughston JC, Degenhardt TC: Reconstruction of the posterior cruciate ligament, *Clin Orthop* 164:59, 1982.

Loos WC et al: Acute posterior cruciate ligament injuries, *Am J Sports Med* 9:86, 1981.

Parolie JM, Bergfeld JA: Long-term results of nonoperative treatment of isolated posterior cruciate ligament injuries in the athlete, *Am J Sports Med* 1435, 1986.

Roth JH et al: Posterior cruciate reconstruction by transfer of the medial gastrocnemius tendon, *Am J Sports Med* 16:21, 1988.

Books

Daniel DM, Akeson WH, O'Connor JJ, editors: *Knee ligaments: structure, function, injury, and repair,* New York, 1990, Raven.

Feagin JA, editor: *The crucial ligaments,* New York, 1988, Churchill Livingstone.

Hughston JC: *Knee ligaments: injury and repair,* St Louis, 1993, Mosby.

Scott WN, editor: *The knee,* St Louis, 1994, Mosby.

RECOMMENDED READINGS–ACL

Journals

DeHaven KE: Diagnosis of acute knee injuries with hemarthrosis, *Am J Sports Med* 8:9, 1980.

Feagin JA, Curl WW: Isolated tear of the anterior cruciate ligament: 5-year follow-up study, *Am J Sports Med* 4:95, 1976.

Fetto JF, Marshall JL: The natural history and diagnosis of anterior cruciate ligament insufficiency, *Clin Orthop* 147:29, 1980.

Giove TP et al: Non-operative treatment of the torn anterior cruciate ligament, *J Bone Joint Surg Am* 65:184, 1983.

Hawkins RJ, Misamore GW, Merritt TR: Follow-up of the acute nonoperated isolated anterior cruciate ligament tear, *Am J Sports Med* 14:205, 1986.

Lynch MA, Henning CE, Glick KR Jr: Knee joint surface changes: long-term follow-up meniscus tear treatment in stable anterior cruciate ligament reconstructions, *Clin Orthop* 172:148, 1983.

Noyes FR et al: The symptomatic anterior cruciate deficient knee, part I: the long-term functional disability in the athletically active individuals, *J Bone Joint Surg Am* 65:154, 1983.

Noyes FR et al: The symptomatic anterior cruciate deficient knee, part II: the results of rehabilitation, activity modification, and counseling on functional disability, *J Bone Joint Surg Am* 65:163, 1983.

Books

Clinical Orthopedics and Related Research Vol 172, Jan/Feb, 1983.

Daniel D, Akeson W, O'Connor J, editors: *Knee ligaments,* New York, 1990, Raven.

Drez D, Jackson DW: *The anterior cruciate deficient knee,* St Louis, 1987, Mosby.

Feagin JA, editor: *The crucial ligaments,* New York, 1994, Churchill Livingstone.

Journal of Orthopedic and Sports Physical Therapy: ACL Surgery and Rehabilitation Vol 15, No 6, June 1992.

Mangine R, editor: *Physical therapy of the knee,* New York, 1995, Churchill Livingstone.

PART TWO

Evaluation

CHAPTER 7

Evaluation of Musculoskeletal Disorders

Arthur J. Nitz, James W. Bellew, Jr., and Charles R. Hazle

OUTLINE

Evaluation schemes
Documentation
Standard examination procedure
   Case history
   Measurement of pain
   Planning the examination
   Clearing examination
"Objective" examination
   Observation
   Function
   Palpation
   Neurologic tests
   Additional medical examinations
Musculoskeletal diagnosis
Trial treatment
Interpretation of test procedures
Conclusion

KEY TERMS

evaluation	musculoskeletal disorder
examination	documentation
assessment	neurologic tests
diagnosis	

LEARNING OBJECTIVES

After studying this chapter, the reader should be able to:

1. List the five major components of the Frisch "5-5" evaluation scheme.
2. Develop pertinent questions necessary for obtaining a complete patient history.
3. Describe several effective methods for measuring a patient's perceived level of pain.
4. Describe how to plan the examination based on information obtained in the patient history.
5. List those tissues that are classified as *inert* structures.
6. List those tissues that are classified as *contractile* structures.
7. Define a clearing examination and state three anatomical reasons for the clearing examination.
8. State and define the five classifications of "end-feel."
9. List the five types of structures that should be considered in the palpation component of the examination.
10. List the five types of neurologic tests that should be performed in the examination.

Effective treatment of patients with musculoskeletal disorders requires carefully evaluating the patient. The need for accurately identifying a patient's condition is heightened by the current health care environment that includes, for many clients, direct access to physical therapy services or generic physician prescriptions such as "evaluate and treat." The physical therapist's knowledge of anatomy and patho-mechanics should enable him or her to analyze loss of functional movement, which is the primary loss for most patients with musculoskeletal disorders.

The principal goals of musculoskeletal evaluation are to identify the tissue(s) involved in the patient's complaint of pain or dysfunction and to establish the severity (acute, subacute, chronic) of the lesion. Once these factors have

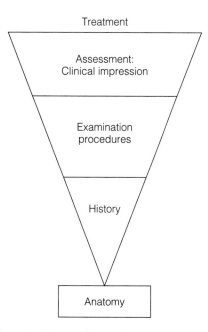

Treatment

Assessment:
Clinical impression

Examination
procedures

History

Anatomy

Fig. 7-1. The goal of appropriate patient treatment is dependent on executing various steps in the evaluation process and, ultimately, ability to make use of anatomic knowledge.

been identified, a coherent plan of treatment can be developed and implemented to address the problems posed by the lesion. Assessment of the patient's response to treatment then serves as the basis for further modification of the rehabilitation plan. The foundational role of anatomic knowledge is depicted in Fig. 7-1; according to Cyriax, "Diagnosis is only a matter of applying one's anatomy."[6]

The physical therapist usually has multiple opportunities to evaluate and observe the patient's response to treatment, which is of great value for refining the diagnosis and guiding further treatment. The successful clinician develops technical evaluation skills and becomes adept at critically analyzing information derived from the examination.

EVALUATION SCHEMES

Various approaches to patient examination for musculoskeletal dysfunction have much to commend them,[8] particularly the contributions of Cyriax, Maitland, Kaltenborn, and McKenzie. Physical therapists owe a debt of gratitude to these individuals for their willingness to systematize their approaches for evaluating patients with musculoskeletal disorders. Most evaluation frameworks have the same basic elements and are rooted in theory and a great deal of clinical observations.[8] However, little research is available to validate the various approaches objectively, a shortcoming that currently challenges the physical therapy professional community.[7,10]

Although no clear scientific evidence warrants any particular evaluation format, physical therapy students ought to adopt one evaluation scheme or another and adhere to it consistently to ensure that the examination process yields the most accurate and complete information possible. Although intuition may provide valuable information for the experienced practitioner,[7,12] radical departure from one's evaluation format may lead to examiner confusion because important elements of the history or physical examination results may be forgotten or overlooked and therefore unavailable for the clinical decision-making process. In the absence of scientific evidence that one evaluation scheme is clearly better than another, practitioners and academics often recommend an eclectic approach with important examination concepts from many different contributors.[8,14,16,27] Although most experienced clinicians develop an eclectic approach, Kaltenborn's "five-five scheme" evaluation framework (developed by H. Frisch) is recommended to the therapist in the early stages of training because it is systematic, lends itself to ready recall, and includes much of what other approaches advocate.[13] The five-five scheme, the basic elements of which are noted in the Box, is described in this chapter.

Sometimes the patient's condition requires modification of the evaluation scheme. For example, a patient who is experiencing severe pain cannot tolerate the various positions and examination procedures undertaken during the course of a typical evaluation. A patient with an acute episode of excruciating low back pain is not likely to tolerate a complete motion analysis. In such circumstances, the therapist should attempt to complete as much of the examination as is feasible and then develop a tentative diagnosis and treatment plan with the available information. As the clinical situation permits, the examination can be completed later, resulting in refinement of diagnosis and appropriate modification of the treatment program. Evaluation of moderately or severely debilitated in-hospital patients may require similar modifications of the evaluation scheme. The recommended evaluation scheme, when appropriately modified, is useful in examining musculoskeletal disorders in patients with primary neurologic (central nervous system or peripheral nervous system) conditions.

DOCUMENTATION

The most common documentation system used by clinicians today is the problem-oriented medical record method and the SOAP—Subjective, Objective, Assessment, and Plan—note format. This organized and useful means of recording information derived from the examination process tends to be substituted for the evaluation scheme itself, however, which may pose a problem. Previous investigators have noted shortcomings with the SOAP system when this format becomes the evaluation scheme.[7] Specifically, information supplied by the patient, falling under the "subjective" category, is by its nature not usually measurable and tends to be judged (wrongly) by many clinicians as less valuable than "objective" (measurable) information.[25] On many occasions, however, a carefully taken history provides overwhelming evidence of a patient's true condition while

Basic outline of the Frisch 5-5 evaluation system
A. Case history
B. Physical examination
1. Observation (inspection)
2. Function
3. Palpation
4. Neurologic tests
5. Special tests

the objective physical examination may provide little or no additional information upon which to make clinical judgments. Physical therapy students ought not curtail the examination process or minimize its importance but rather should be aware of the value of the subjective patient history.

In addition to these shortcomings, as an evaluation scheme the SOAP format tends not to comport with the realities of the clinical decision-making process. The SOAP type of system may lead the observer to conclude (incorrectly) that the diagnostic process is mechanistic and should only follow completion of the history and physical examination. Experience, however, indicates that the diagnostic process is much more fluid, as clinical data from the patient are analyzed in the light of the practitioner's previous experience and general knowledge base. Consequently, an expert clinician may entertain numerous possible diagnostic entities while going through the history, physical examination, and trial treatment components of evaluation.[7,12] Physical therapy students are especially challenged to be aware of how dynamic the diagnostic process is and to continually expand their didactic information and clinical experiential base.

From a practical standpoint, physical therapy students and practicing clinicians alike are encouraged to record clinical data from the history and physical examination while it is being obtained rather than waiting until some later time to write or dictate such information. This practice tends to ensure that important elements of the examination process are not forgotten. A prepared worksheet may be especially useful for the novice clinician to guide the history-taking and physical examination process.

STANDARD EXAMINATION PROCEDURE

"Ex nihilo nihil fit" ("out of nothing, nothing comes") is a good reminder to the examiner that there is no record of any uncaused event in the real world. The patient's condition has a cause to be carefully sought out by a proper case history and physical examination. The cause may not be immediately obvious, but the reminder that the cause exists encourages both the student and the experienced practitioner to persevere in the examination process until an appropriate explanation of the patient's symptoms and signs is identified.

Case history

If the clinician listens carefully and long enough, the patient generally tells the clinician what is wrong; that is, the clinician is, in essence, told (in layperson's terms) what the patient's diagnosis is. There are two basic approaches to obtaining a patient's history: examiner-directed (closed-ended) and patient-directed (open-ended). Both have advantages and advocates, and the therapist must determine how best to balance the more efficient examiner-directed style and the more relationship-oriented patient-directed format of history taking. Regardless, a therapist with a genuine interest in exploring a patient's complaint of pain rarely fails to establish the kind of rapport with the patient that is fruitful in developing and executing an appropriate treatment protocol.

Before obtaining a detailed history of the patient's present complaint, certain background information is helpful. Gender should be noted to remind the examiner to be alert to conditions more prevalent among men or women. As an example, gouty arthritis is more likely to be suspected among men when the patient's complaint is multiple joint arthalgias with a predilection for the great toe metatarsophalangeal joint. By contrast, sacroiliac joint dysfunction is more likely in women complaining of back pain than among men. In addition, the influence of monthly hormonal changes among women of menstrual age and the impact of postmenopausal osteoporosis among older women are important considerations for the clinician.

The patient's age should also be noted, as conditions tend to occur within generalized age ranges. Osteochondritis dissecans of the knee is more likely in well-developed young men than in older individuals. An exaggerated thoracic kyphosis is likely to be associated with an entirely different disease process in an adolescent (Scheuermann's disease) and in a 70-year-old woman (dowager's hump of osteoporosis). The examiner is encouraged not to stereotype by the patient's age, however, as some conditions that are unlikely in certain age groups do occasionally occur; for example, teenagers do occasionally herniate a spinal disk.

A patient's occupation, whether in or out of the home, should be given full consideration as an associated factor that may contribute substantially to the cause of the complaint. A description and, preferably, a demonstration of the patient's typical work activity and habitual postures may provide valuable insight into the likely explanation for musculoskeletal complaints.

For developing a protocol of questions to ask patients, a basic outline adopted largely from Kaltenborn is presented.[13]

   I. Immediate case history
      A. Chief complaint. The therapist must determine what brought the patient to seek attention. Patients who have more than one complaint, such as those with pain of spinal origin, should rank them in

priority. Although patients occasionally seek attention for stiffness or some other joint-related complaint, the vast majority of patients with musculoskeletal conditions do so for their pain. Consequently, the better part of history taking concerns identifying and characterizing the source and nature of the patient's complaint of pain.

1. Localization. Where is the pain or dysfunction? Although this item seems straightforward, it is not always the case. Pain often is referred to a site distant from the actual lesion. A good example is the common observation of pain referred from a cervical spine lesion to a site such as the inferior angle of the scapula. Referred pain is further confounded, in some cases, by the fact that the patient may have no awareness of cervical spine involvement. Another typical example occurs among patients with adhesive capsulitis of the shoulder. Often patients with this musculoskeletal condition complain of a primary site of pain at the distal attachment of the deltoid muscle to the humerus. Examination, however, reveals no true palpable tenderness at this site, and no real muscle or muscle attachment lesion exists.

These examples are just two among many such cases of referred pain. The therapist needs to be aware of both radicular and nonradicular patterns of pain location. A radicular pattern of pain referral generally follows an anatomic dermatomal distribution. By contrast, nonradicular pain is more likely to be distributed in a sclerotomal pattern. A patient with a C7 nerve root compression is likely to have a distribution of pain that corresponds to the dermatome (neck to shoulder, back of the arm and forearm and extending to the dorsal and volar aspect of the long finger). By comparison, a patient with a C7 facet lesion often complains of pain that is referred to the inferior angle of the scapula and can be reproduced by attempts to compress or otherwise distort the facet joint or its capsule.[2] Because no known pattern of dermatomal arrangement extends from the cervical spine to this distant scapular site, it is usually taken as evidence of a joint lesion (sclerotomal pattern) rather than a nerve root injury. An examiner needs awareness of not only the standard dermatomes but also the sclerotomes.

In addition to sclerotomal distribution of referred symptoms, the clinician must be alert to the possibility of retrograde referral of neuromusculoskeletal symptoms. Conventional wisdom indicates that the usual pattern of referral of pain or other neural mediated symptoms is from a proximal structure to a more distally located one. However, nerve compression at a distal site, such as the median nerve at the carpal tunnel, has been known to cause pain directed proximally to the elbow and even to the shoulder. In the absence of any local musculoskeletal pathology or any orthograde referral of neurologic symptoms from a proximal structure, consideration should be given to the possibility of retrograde referral of symptoms to explain a patient's complaints.

In an effort to localize the pain as accurately as possible, the patient should be encouraged to point with one finger to the area where the pain is the worst. The patient's usual inclination is to locate a diffuse area rather than a discrete region of pain, but with further questioning and thought most clients are able to refine their sense of the location of the pain.

2. Time. When did the condition begin? How did the pain begin? The schematic in Fig. 7-2, is useful for compiling information related to when and how the patient's pain or condition began.[18] It makes distinctions between conditions that began suddenly versus those that began insidiously or gradually. A condition that began suddenly because of trauma is rather straightforward, but important insight can be gained by determining the precise mechanism of injury. If the patient can actually demonstrate how the injury occurred, attention may be directed more easily to the tissues most likely involved.

Patients are at times confused and frustrated because a musculoskeletal condition arises rapidly and without any apparent external cause. Patient conditions that arise spontaneously may reflect the tissue inflammatory effect of accumulated, repetitive microtrauma. Careful questioning of patients about possible predisposing occupational factors or habitual postures often is helpful for delineating the actual cause of the lesion.[26] Alternatively, a spontaneously acquired joint manifestation may represent an underlying disease process. As an example, a patient with an obvious knee effusion who has no history of major trauma or repetitive microtrauma may be demonstrating the initial sign of one of the inflammatory arthritides such as systemic lupus erythematosus (SLE). Clearly, this patient requires further medical workup directed by his or her physician.

Many patients presenting with musculoskeletal complaints relate a history of gradual onset, with or without previous injury or trauma. Most of these patients have connective tissue conditions that often respond nicely to physical therapeutic intervention. However, a patient who complains of insidious onset of pain unrelated to any injury or precipitating cause should cause the therapist to proceed with great caution, as this history is often typical of a neoplasm. Again, given any suspicion of such a process in a patient who presents with other musculoskeletal complaints, the therapist should refer this patient for further medical evaluation.

3. Characteristics. What type of pain is present? One of

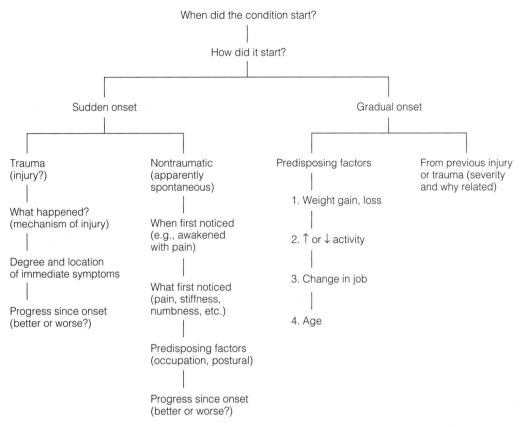

Fig. 7-2. Schematic for organizing information derived from the patient history. (Modified from Maitland GD: *Vertebral manipulation,* ed 5, Butterworth, 1986, London.)

the primary tasks of the evaluator is to determine whether the pain or other primary symptom is truly arising from a neuromusculoskeletal structure or is of systemic origin. A deep, boring, unrelenting pain, unrelieved by rest or position, that wakes the patient at night is likely to be serious and may have a systemic origin. However, not all pain that wakes a patient at night is so serious. Patients with a connective tissue disorder affecting the glenohumeral joint (adhesive capsulitis) often are consistently awakened at night by pain. Similarly, nocturnal wakening due to hand or arm pain or numbness is considered by many clinicians to be the sine qua non for a soft tissue, neurologically mediated condition located at the wrist (carpal tunnel syndrome).

Among the variety of terms patients use to describe pain, several major descriptors are particularly helpful for characterizing the pain and discovering its underlying cause.

- Dull, aching pain is considered by many clinicians to arise from deep joint or other somatic structures.
- Sharp, well-localized pain may represent a superficial joint condition. Cyriax's "painful twinges" are described as sharp, although they often arise from articular structure (i.e., not superficial cartilage).

- Sharp pain that is referred along a dermatomal pattern usually indicates nerve root compression. Patients with nerve pain often have difficulty getting to sleep.
- Other symptoms such as tingling and numbness usually indicate neurologic or vascular involvement. Their distribution should be carefully identified.

4. Influence. What causes or affects the pain? This category is related to the behavior of the patient's symptoms apart from treatment. We have found the schematic in Fig. 7-3 very useful for eliciting information that often identifies the tissue (e.g., disk versus joint structure) and the level of involvement (acutely versus chronically inflamed).[18]

Pain arising from most musculoskeletal disorders is aggravated by activity and relieved by rest, despite exceptions such as diskogenic low back pain, which is usually exacerbated by sitting and relieved by upright movement. Another exception to this rule may occur among patients with moderately severe osteoarthritis who experience pain and stiffness following long periods of rest (e.g., in the morning) and relief of these symptoms once joint movement begins.

A patient who contends that the pain does not vary

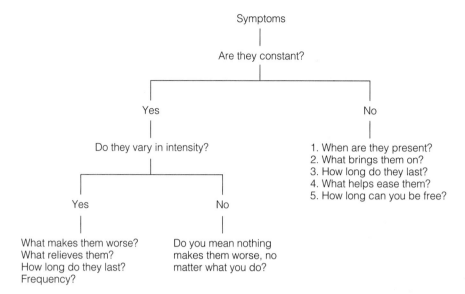

Fig. 7-3. Schematic depicting behavior of patient's symptoms related to posture and activity. (Modified from Maitland GD: *Vertebral manipulation,* ed 5, Butterworth, 1986, London.)

in intensity regardless of rest or activity should be referred to the family physician for further evaluation as this patient may have a serious underlying cause, such as neoplasm, for the pain. The patient may also be malingering or magnifying symptoms but should be given the benefit of the doubt and referred back to a physician for further testing.

5. Association. What other symptoms are associated with the pain? Other important symptoms may be present in association with or in lieu of pain. For example, a patient's primary complaint may be "numbness or tingling" in a particular distribution, usually implicating the neurologic system. A complaint of "weakness" may also indicate involvement of the peripheral nervous system or may be the result of tissue inflammation, whereby pain does not allow maximal contraction of the muscle-tendon complex (e.g., impingement syndrome of the shoulder). Joint injuries often result in loss of stability so that the patient experiences episodes of giving way, which may be the predominant complaint.

B. Previous history

1. This episode of symptoms. Of primary importance is discovering what attempts have been made to treat the present condition. These attempts may have been made by the patient alone, by the patient's physician (medical management), by other practitioners, or by previously ineffective physical therapy. This information may refine the examiner's perception of possible diagnoses and aid in planning the subsequent treatment for the condition.

2. Previous episodes of a similar nature. Inquiring about previous similar episodes of pain is valuable for multiple reasons. First, the sheer number of occurrences of the condition over a given length of time

provides the examiner with awareness of the nature of the malady in terms of its severity (minor versus major recurrent episodes) and chronicity. If a patient is currently seeking medical attention for a recurrent condition of a similar nature that previously resolved uneventfully (without medical intervention), then the condition may be becoming more severe with each episode.

Second, determining what precipitating causes may have led to previous episodes of a similar nature may prove helpful for the clinician. Again, this information allows insight into the rate of progression (if any) of the condition and some hint of the severity of the current episode.

3. Current medical status. A variety of general medical conditions have profound impact on the neuromusculoskeletal system. As an example, diabetes is often associated with fragility of connective tissue and less responsiveness of connective tissue to joint-stretching procedures. In addition, the likelihood of neurologic symptoms superimposed on a musculoskeletal condition is far greater if a patient has a metabolic condition, such as diabetes, which affects the health of peripheral nerves. Patients with generalized joint inflammatory conditions, such as rheumatoid arthritis, are more likely to be vulnerable to localized nerve compression (e.g., carpal tunnel syndrome).[21,30] Awareness of the impact of general health status on a patient's vulnerability to neuromusculoskeletal conditions alerts the examiner to be cautious during the evaluation and treatment planning process.

4. Family history. Particularly important for musculoskeletal conditions are any family history of chronic diseases and whether the patient's parents or siblings have had any specific history of neuromuscular

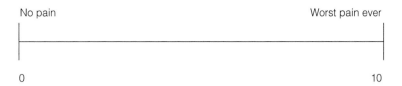

On the line below, place a mark indicating your pain level today.

No pain   Worst pain ever

0   10

Fig. 7-4. Visual analog scale for objective pain measurement.

conditions. Familial diseases of concern include rheumatoid arthritis, diabetes, and inherited neuromuscular diseases such as Charcot-Marie-Tooth. These conditions often have a musculoskeletal component to the overall presentation of signs and symptoms.

Measurement of pain

Although the topic here is the so-called subjective examination, which relates to the patient's complaints of pain, every effort should be made to *objectify* the patient's report. Measurement tools such as the Visual Analog Scale (Fig. 7-4), which has been shown to be both reliable and valid for examining a patient's pain, and the McGill Short Form Questionnaire (Fig. 7-5) have been helpful for pain measurement in a clinical setting.[20,23] Another helpful aid is the Forgione-Barber pain production device (Fig. 7-6), an instrument that stimulates pain endings through pressure of the fingernail bed using a discrete amount of weight for an indeterminant length of time. The patient's responsivity to the amount of pressure and ability to withstand this discomfort for a measured amount of time give an index of the patient's pain responsiveness. Another measurement tool developed over the last decade is the Oswestry Disability Index for Low Back Pain (Fig. 7-7). Similar instruments have been developed for cervical spine pain and are useful for identifying the relationship between the patient's pain and functional concerns (Fig. 7-8).

Planning the examination

Once the patient's history has been obtained, additional thought must be given to how the examination process will proceed. Geoffrey Maitland has referred to this process as "planning the examination," which is especially important for the "novice," according to his description.[18] Maitland's assertion is that, especially for developing therapists, appropriate consideration should be given to those structures that are likely to cause the pain. In his scheme, three major anatomic areas are given consideration:

1. Joints that lie under the painful area
2. Joints that refer pain into the area
3. Muscles that lie under the painful area

From this description, the clinician can perceive that Maitland gives considerable attention to structures whose sclerotomal distribution refers pain into the area. However, no category in his scheme is related directly to the radicular types of spinal nerve symptoms that are so often found among patients with musculoskeletal disorders. We believe the therapist must carefully consider and examine neurologic structures that are able to refer pain into the painful area, in addition to the joints and muscles advocated by Maitland.

The considerations outlined by Maitland are all directed toward identifying the cause of the pain. Often patients are referred for physical therapy intervention with the cause of their pain quite clearly delineated by the referring physician. For example, a patient is sent to the physical therapist for an impingement syndrome of the shoulder, and clearly rotator cuff inflammation (e.g., supraspinatus tendinitis) is the cause of the pain. Less clear, however, is the "cause of the cause of the pain." We assert that, more often than not, an astute physical therapist can fill this niche. Using the example of supraspinatus tendinitis, the therapist must identify not only the cause of the pain but also what might be leading to that particular tendon lesion. Is some muscle imbalance present between the various rotator cuff components? Often, capsular stiffness, especially loss of glenohumeral joint internal rotation, accompanied by weakness of the external rotators, has been associated with such inflammatory conditions as impingement syndrome. Even if the patient and therapist are successful in eliminating the acute inflammatory condition that brought the patient to the physical therapist in the first place, if no consideration is given to the underlying muscle imbalance or connective tissue tightness, then the likelihood of recurrence is greatly increased. Such underlying causes for the patient's condition are also relevant when patients with pain of spinal origin are examined. Often, postural dysfunction and other evidences of trunk muscle weakness and connective tissue tightness are the underlying, precipitating cause for the patient's condition.

Inert and contractile tissue (Cyriax). Prior to beginning the "objective" examination process, the therapist needs to give further thought to the neuromusculoskeletal anatomic entities to be examined. The various anatomic structures can be divided into those that are *inert* (no contractile capabilities) and those that exhibit *contractile* capabilities (originally formulated by Cyriax).[6]

These two major tissue divisions, listed in the Box, are discussed in additional detail concerning the actual examination procedures. For now, these anatomic entities focus the therapist's attention during the planning process and provide

1	2	3	4
1 Flickering	1 Jumping	1 Pricking	1 Sharp
2 Quivering	2 Flashing	2 Boring	2 Cutting
3 Pulsing	3 Shooting	3 Drilling	3 Lacerating
4 Throbbing		4 Stabbing	
5 Beating		5 Lancinating	
6 Pounding			

5	6	7	8
1 Pinching	1 Tugging	1 Hot	1 Tingling
2 Pressing	2 Pulling	2 Burning	2 Itchy
3 Gnawing	3 Wrenching	3 Scalding	3 Smarting
4 Cramping		4 Searing	4 Stinging
5 Crushing			

9	10	11	12
1 Dull	1 Tender	1 Tiring	1 Sickening
2 Sore	2 Taut	2 Exhausting	2 Suffocating
3 Hurting	3 Rasping		
4 Aching	4 Splitting		
5 Heavy			

13	14	15	16
1 Fearful	1 Punishing	1 Wretched	1 Annoying
2 Frightful	2 Grueling	2 Blinding	2 Troublesome
3 Terrifying	3 Cruel		3 Miserable
	4 Vicious		4 Intense
	5 Killing		5 Unbearable

17	18	19	20
1 Spreading	1 Tight	1 Cool	1 Nagging
2 Radiating	2 Numb	2 Cold	2 Nauseating
3 Penetrating	3 Drawing	3 Freezing	3 Agonizing
4 Piercing	4 Squeezing		4 Dreadful
	5 Tearing		5 Torturing

Fig. 7-5. McGill Short Form Pain Questionnaire for objective pain measurement. Words commonly used to describe pain. (Reprinted by permission from Melzack R: The McGill Pain Questionnaire: major properties and scoring methods, *Pain* 1:277, 1975.)

a framework for an organized approach to the various tissues that may be involved in the patient's musculoskeletal condition. All of these structures have some measure of elasticity. Even bone, which is primarily inorganic and a somewhat rigid structure, has a certain amount of elasticity, which should not be forgotten as the examination process proceeds. This particular delineation by Cyriax has served as a major contribution for those attempting to develop their diagnostic acumen in a systematic and ordered manner.

Clearing examination

Before a detailed examination of the involved area, standard procedure includes a *clearing examination* (also known as a *screening* or *scan* examination), undertaken to

identify more carefully the exact location of the patient's source of complaint. The purpose for the upper- and lower-quarter screening examination is to identify the major area of involvement and eliminate confusing information from the *clarifying examination* that could cloud the eventual diagnosis. From the standpoint of history taking, the clearing examination is necessary because a patient does not always reliably delineate the problem source to a single region. The screening examination proceeds prior to the clarifying exam for a number of anatomic reasons:

1. The extremities are developmentally derived from the sclerotome. Consequently, pain of deep somatic origin may be referred to any or all of the sclerotome (i.e.,

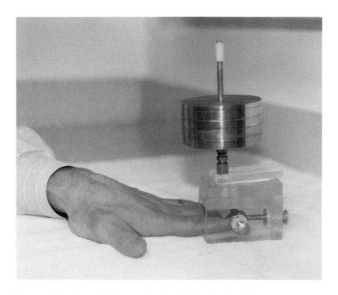

Fig. 7-6. Forgione-Barber pain stimulation device for measuring an individual's responsivity.

joints, bones, muscle, skin) when a deep musculoskeletal structure is the origin of the patient's pain.
2. Pain patterns often overlap, with both distal and proximal referral noted. Both spinal and extremity biomechanical disorders may coexist and therefore confuse the eventual diagnosis if the examiner fails consider this possibility (best delineated by use of a clearing or screening examination).
3. Finally, degenerative joint disease (DJD) of the spine, particularly of the facet and intervertebral disk joints, leads to hyperexcitability of the entire sclerotomal segment. Consequently, pain may be felt in the wrist joint, for example, when, in fact, the cause is located in the cervical spine (spondylosis). During the clearing examination, the examiner should look for the following:

• A related biomechanical derangement giving rise to pain
• Coexistent conditions causing summation of segmentally related afferent input
• Potential sources of error in evaluation

Standard examples of upper- and lower-quarter screening examination format (from Cyriax) are listed in the Boxes. These screening examination schemes include some consideration of postural assessment and of ROM of both the spinal element and the peripheral joints. In addition, neurologic structures are covered by inclusion of resisted muscle testing (myotomal screening) and sensory testing (dermatomal screening). Brief examination for Tinel's sign at various sites

in the upper quarter and deep tendon reflex (DTR) exam of both the upper and lower quarters are included in this standard screening examination process. In addition, one or two simple neurotension tests (e.g., straight leg raise) and one upper motor neuron test such as Babinski's reflex have been included.

This scheme is generally adequate for identifying a confounding factor or a spinal explanation for a patient's complaint of pain in the extremity, whether upper or lower quarter. Because the clearing examinations for both the upper and lower quarters include some objective examination of each anatomic element of that quarter, the entire screening examination process is unlikely to fail to yield any evidence of a musculoskeletal disorder. If a therapist's screening examination is entirely normal, then thought should be given to reexamination or possibly to a nonorganic or nonmusculoskeletal cause for the patient's complaint.

"OBJECTIVE" EXAMINATION

Following careful documentation of the patient's history and of the other information derived from the clearing examination, the therapist should be prepared to continue the clarifying examination process with "objective" evaluation procedures. The scheme used here (advocated by Kaltenborn and modified from Frisch) is generally referred to as the *5-5 examination scheme*.[13] This examination format is divided into five groups of tests, each of which is subdivided into five parts.

The five basic elements of the *observation* component of the examination process are delineated next.

Observation (inspection)

1. **Functional movements—gait patterns, general activities of daily living (ADL)**
2. **Posture—habitual postures, compensatory positions for avoiding pain (muscle guarding)**
3. **Shape—any deformity present, swelling, atrophy, muscle asymmetry**
4. **Skin—color (circulation), evidence of scar tissue, calluses, cyanosis**
5. **Assistive devices—canes, crutches, walker, use of corset, splint, sling, wheelchair, or other aid**

Although the objective examination formally follows the history taking, in reality, some of these objective examination procedures actually come first. Specifically, the manner in which the patient walks to the examination table, how the patient undresses prior to examination, and how the patient gets on and off the examination table all contribute to the database and generally precede taking the history. In addition, some observation activities are ongoing during history taking. For example, while listening to various responses, the physical therapist notes such obvious abnor-

Name: _____ Today's Date: _____

How long have you had back pain? _____ Years _____ Months _____ Weeks _____
How long have you had leg pain? _____ Years _____ Months _____ Weeks _____

PLEASE READ:
This questionnaire has been designed to give the physical therapist information as to how your back pain has affected your ability to manage in everyday life. Please answer every section, and mark in each section *ONLY THE ONE BOX* that applies to you. We realize you may consider that two of the statements in any one section relate to you, but please just mark the box that most closely describes your problem. **All information provided is confidential.**

SECTION 1—PAIN INTENSITY
- [ ] My pain is mild to moderate, I do not need pain killers.
- [ ] The pain is bad, but I manage without taking pain killers.
- [ ] Pain killers give complete relief from pain.
- [ ] Pain killers give moderate relief from pain.
- [ ] Pain killers give very little relief from pain.
- [ ] Pain killers have no effect on the pain.

SECTION 2—PERSONAL CARE (Washing, Dressing, etc.)
- [ ] I can look after myself normally without causing extra pain.
- [ ] I can look after myself normally but it causes extra pain.
- [ ] It is painful to look after myself and I am slow and careful.
- [ ] I need some help but manage most of my personal care.
- [ ] I need help everyday in most aspects of my care.
- [ ] I do not dress, wash with difficulty, and stay in bed.

SECTION 3—LIFTING
- [ ] I can lift heavy weights without extra pain.
- [ ] I can lift heavy weights but it gives extra pain.
- [ ] Pain prevents me from lifting heavy weights off the floor, but I can manage if they are conveniently positioned.
- [ ] Pain prevents me from lifting heavy weights, but I can manage light weights if they are conveniently positioned.
- [ ] I can lift only very light weights.
- [ ] I cannot lift or carry anything at all.

SECTION 4—WALKING
- [ ] I can walk as far as I wish.
- [ ] Pain prevents me walking more than one mile.
- [ ] Pain prevents me walking more than ½ mile.
- [ ] Pain prevents me walking more than ¼ mile.
- [ ] I can walk only if I use a stick or crutches.
- [ ] I am in bed or in a chair for most of everyday.

SECTION 5—SITTING
- [ ] I can sit in any chair as long as I like.
- [ ] I can sit in my favorite chair only, but for as long as I like.
- [ ] Pain prevents me from sitting more than 1 hour.
- [ ] Pain prevents me from sitting more than ½ hour.
- [ ] Pain prevents me from sitting more than 10 minutes.
- [ ] Pain prevents me from sitting at all.

Fig. 7-7. Oswestry Disability Index for Low Back Pain

SECTION 6—STANDING

☐ I can stand as long as I want without extra pain.
☐ I can stand as long as I want, but it gives me extra pain.
☐ Pain prevents me from standing more than 1 hour.
☐ Pain prevents me from standing more than 30 minutes.
☐ Pain prevents me from standing more than 10 minutes.
☐ Pain prevents me from standing at all.

SECTION 7—SLEEPING

☐ Pain does not prevent me from sleeping well.
☐ I sleep well, but only by using tablets.
☐ Even when I take tablets I have less than 6 hours sleep.
☐ Even when I take tablets I have less than 4 hours sleep.
☐ Even when I take tablets I have less than 2 hours sleep.
☐ Pain prevents me from sleeping at all.

SECTION 8—SEX LIFE

☐ My sex life is normal and causes no extra pain.
☐ My sex life is normal but causes some extra pain.
☐ My sex life is nearly normal but is very painful.
☐ My sex life is severely restricted by pain.
☐ My sex life is nearly absent because of pain.
☐ Pain prevents any sex life at all.

SECTION 9—SOCIAL LIFE

☐ My social life is normal and causes me no extra pain.
☐ My social life is normal but increases the degree of pain.
☐ Pain affects my social life by limiting only more energetic interests (dancing, etc.).
☐ Pain has restricted my social life and I do not go out as often.
☐ Pain has restricted my social life to my home. I have no social life because of pain.

SECTION 10—TRAVELING

☐ I can travel anywhere without extra pain.
☐ I can travel anywhere but it gives me extra pain.
☐ Pain is bad, but I manage journeys over 2 hours.
☐ Pain restricts me to journeys of less than 1 hour.
☐ Pain restricts me to short necessary journeys under 30 minutes.
☐ Pain prevents me from traveling except to the doctor or hospital.

Fig. 7-7, cont'd. For legend see opposite page.

malities as gross deformity, major joint swelling, or severe muscle atrophy, so often seen following trauma or surgery. Some of the activities described as observational may also be measured. For example, joint swelling or muscle atrophy can be evaluated objectively through circumferential girth measurements, which do not always provide the full story but are helpful for identifying objective differences between joint structures when a patient has a musculoskeletal complaint. Following completion of the five elements of the *observation* aspect of the inspection, the therapist should be prepared to proceed with what may be the heart of the examination, the assessment of movement and *function*.

Function

1. **Active movements**
2. **Passive movements**
   a. **Delineations of end feel**
   b. **Identification of capsular pattern**
3. **Resisted movements—standard interpretation (Cyriax)**
4. **Traction/compression—to test anatomic joint and intraarticular structures**
5. **Gliding—translatoric movement tests anatomic joint and intraarticular structures**

Name: _____ Today's Date: _____

How long have you had neck pain? _____ Years _____ Months _____ Weeks _____

How long have you had arm pain?_____ Years _____ Months _____ Weeks _____

PLEASE READ:

This questionnaire has been designed to give the physical therapist information as to how your neck pain has affected your ability to manage in everyday life. Please answer every section, and mark in each section *ONLY THE ONE BOX* that applies to you. We realize you may consider that two of the statements in any one section relate to you, but please just mark the box that most closely describes your problem. All information provided is confidential.

SECTION 1—PAIN INTENSITY
- ☐ I have no pain at the moment.
- ☐ The pain is very mild at the moment.
- ☐ The pain is moderate at the moment.
- ☐ The pain is fairly severe at the moment.
- ☐ The pain is very severe at the moment.
- ☐ The pain is the worst imaginable at the moment.

SECTION 2—PERSONAL CARE (Washing, Dressing, etc.)
- ☐ I can look after myself normally without causing extra pain.
- ☐ I can look after myself normally, but it causes extra pain.
- ☐ It is painful to look after myself and I am slow and careful.
- ☐ I need some help but manage most of my personal care.
- ☐ I need help everyday in most aspects of self care.
- ☐ I do not get dressed, I wash with difficulty, and I stay in bed.

SECTION 3—LIFTING
- ☐ I can lift heavy weights without extra pain.
- ☐ I can lift heavy weights, but it gives extra pain.
- ☐ Pain prevents me from lifting heavy weights off the floor, but I can manage if they are conveniently positioned (for example, on a table).
- ☐ Pain prevents me from lifting heavy weights, but I can manage light to medium weights if they are conveniently positioned.
- ☐ I can lift very light weights.
- ☐ I cannot lift or carry anything at all.

SECTION 4—READING
- ☐ I can read as much as I want to with no pain in my neck.
- ☐ I can read as much as I want to with slight pain in my neck.
- ☐ I can read as much as I want to with moderate pain in my neck.
- ☐ I cannot read as much as I want because of moderate pain in my neck.
- ☐ I can hardly read at all because of severe pain in my neck.
- ☐ I cannot read at all.

SECTION 5—HEADACHES
- ☐ I have no headaches at all.
- ☐ I have slight headaches that come infrequently.
- ☐ I have moderate headaches that come infrequently.
- ☐ I have moderate headaches that come frequently.
- ☐ I have severe headaches that come frequently.
- ☐ I have headaches almost all the time.

Fig. 7-8. Neck Disability Index. (Modified from Oswestry instrument, Fig. 7-7.)

SECTION 6—CONCENTRATION
- ☐ I can concentrate fully when I want to with no difficulty.
- ☐ I can concentrate fully when I want to with slight difficulty.
- ☐ I have a fair degree of difficulty in concentrating when I want to.
- ☐ I have a lot of difficulty in concentrating when I want to.
- ☐ I have a great deal of difficulty in concentrating when I want to.
- ☐ I cannot concentrate at all.

SECTION 7—WORK
- ☐ I can do as much work as I want.
- ☐ I can only do my usual work, but no more.
- ☐ I can do most of my usual work, but no more.
- ☐ I cannot do my usual work.
- ☐ I can hardly do any work at all.
- ☐ I cannot do any work at all.

SECTION 8—DRIVING
- ☐ I can drive my car without any neck pain.
- ☐ I can drive my car as long as I want with slight pain in my neck.
- ☐ I can drive my car as long as I want with moderate pain in my neck.
- ☐ I cannot drive my car as long as I want because of moderate pain in my neck.
- ☐ I can hardly drive at all because of severe pain in my neck.
- ☐ I cannot drive my car at all.

SECTION 9—SLEEPING
- ☐ I have no trouble sleeping.
- ☐ My sleep is slightly disturbed (less than 1 hour sleepless).
- ☐ My sleep is mildly disturbed (1-2 hours sleepless).
- ☐ My sleep is moderately disturbed (2-3 hours sleepless).
- ☐ My sleep is greatly disturbed (3-5 hours sleepless).
- ☐ My sleep is completely disturbed (5-7 hours sleepless).

SECTION 10—RECREATION
- ☐ I am able to engage in all my recreation activities with no neck pain at all.
- ☐ I am able to engage in all my recreation activities, with some pain in my neck.
- ☐ I am able to engage in most but not all of my usual recreation activities because of pain in my neck.
- ☐ I am able to engage in a few of my usual recreation activities because of pain in my neck.
- ☐ I can hardly do any recreation activities because of pain in my neck.
- ☐ I cannot do any recreation activities at all.

Fig. 7-8, cont'd. For legend see opposite page.

The functional component of the examination begins with *active movements* for a number of reasons. First, a patient's willingness to tolerate required movement analysis is noted by his or her performance of active movements. In addition, beginning the examination with active movements is sometimes useful for allaying apprehension about the nature of the physical examination if the patient senses some ownership of the process. A technique we have found useful for enhancing the validity of the movement examination is to examine the uninvolved extremity (in cases of nonspinal abnormality) for documenting a patient's normal available range and ability to undertake active movements. When the involved limb is being moved, it is sometimes helpful to begin the examination at a joint distal or proximal to the involved joint, which indicates to patients that they can undertake meaningful movement that is, in some cases, far more extensive than they had thought possible, given the nature of the particular injury. This procedure may also allow the therapist the opportunity, early in the examination, to compare involved with uninvolved extremity movement to determine departures from the normal situation. Active movement can take the form of standard, cardinal plane

Inert and contractile structures

Inert

Bone
Joint capsules
Ligaments
Bursae
Fascia
Duramater
Nerve roots

Contractile

Muscles
Tendons
Musculotendinous attachments

Mofidified from Cyriax J: *Textbook of orthopaedic medicine, vol 1, diagnosis of soft tissue lesions*, ed 8, London, 1982, Bailliere Tindall.

Sample lower quarter clearing examination

Posture assessment
Active forward, backward, and lateral bending of lumbar spine
Toe walking (S-1)
Heel walking (L-4, L-5)
Active rotation of lumbar spine
Twisting-hyperextension (Spurling maneuver)
Overpressure if spine is symptom free
Straight leg raise (L-4 to S-1)
Sacroiliac spring/gap tests
Resisted hip flexion (L-1 to L-2)
Hip quadrant position
Passive range of motion of hip
Resisted knee extension (L-3 to L-4)
Knee flexion, extension
Femoral nerve stretch
Babinski reflex test for upper motor neuron involvement
Deep tendon reflex (knee/ankle)

Sample upper quarter clearing examination

Postural assessment
Active range of motion of the cervical spine
Passive overpressure if spine is symptom free
Resisted shoulder shrug (C-2 to C-4)
Resisted shoulder abduction (C-5)
Active shoulder flexion and rotation
Shoulder impingement test
Resisted elbow flexion (C-6)
Resisted elbow extension (C-7)
Active range of motion of elbow
Resisted wrist flexion (C-7)
Resisted wrist extension (C-6)
Resisted thumb extension (C-8)
Resisted finger abduction (T-1)
Phalen, Tinel tests at wrist
Babinski reflex test for upper motor neuron involvement
Deep tendon reflex (biceps, brachioradialis, triceps)

movements (sagittal, horizontal, frontal) or movements that would be described as more functional in nature (e.g., impure swing—MacConaill description).[13]

Active range of motion (AROM) analysis may be very helpful in identifying areas in the range where pain is present and where crepitus and muscle guarding occur. Often during this component of the examination, the patient describes symptoms that are reminiscent of the pain that caused them to seek medical attention (Maitland's "comparable sign"[18]), and the remainder of the evaluation process serves simply to refine the precise movement abnormality encountered during this early stage of the examination. When no restriction in ROM is noted and standard ROM activities are painless, other techniques, such as overpressure of the joint and application of compression and distraction to the joint during motion, must be applied to provoke the movement abnormality.

A *painful arc* may be identified during the active movement portion of the functional examination. This clinical entity was first described by Cyriax as a pain felt by the patient at the midrange of motion that then disappeared after that portion of the range of motion was exceeded in either direction.[6] The interpretation, according to Cyriax (by implication), was that a tender, inflamed structure was impinged (pinched) between two bony or "unforgiving" structures.[6] A standard example of this particular condition is the shoulder impingement syndrome in which the supraspinatus tendon evokes a painful arc during active range of motion in flexion and abduction as the inflamed tendinous structure is impinged between the acromion and the greater tuberosity of the humerus.

Passive movements are designed to test all inert structures related to the particular joint examined. The movements undertaken are generally identical to those examined during active range of motion and may include pure, cardinal plane motions, as well as functional movements. The passive range of motion (PROM), like the AROM, is measured goniometrically and recorded for future reference. The difference in ROM between active and passive movements is the basis for one major interpretive concept in the field of musculoskeletal examination.

Cyriax referred to the three following primary situations and their respective interpretations:

1. Active and passive movements that are restricted or painful in the *same* direction indicate an *arthrogenic* lesion (structures belonging to the anatomic joint). An example would be a case of capsular restriction of the glenohumeral joint in which both active and passive

movements are equally restricted, in essentially an identical direction. Some contend that this observation actually indicates a capsular restriction rather than an arthrogenic lesion. A less ambiguous example would be a case of an osteochondral fragment (e.g., osteochondritis dissecans) of the knee in which the articular cartilage defect causes loss of both active and passive motions in the same direction and essentially at the same point in the range.

2. Active and passive movements that are restricted or painful in the *opposite* direction indicate a soft tissue lesion, and a contractile structure is usually considered to be the *cause*. An example would be a patient who has sustained a lesion of the primary hip flexor (iliopsoas muscle), resulting in a loss of active hip flexion due to the contractile structure's incompetence. In addition, there is restriction in passive hip extension as a result of the scar or muscle defect being stretched and pain or shortened connective tissues restricting the patient's range in this direction.

3. *Relative* restriction of passive movements in various directions indicates a *capsular* pattern, which may present as a sequence of lost motions that are quite consistent from patient to patient. Most of the following chapters related to specific joints include a standard capsular pattern description. Interestingly, a recent study challenging the Cyriax (interpretive) scheme of motion loss in a musculoskeletal condition has been published, and it does not appear to be entirely valid in all cases.[10]

At the extreme limit of each passive movement, the quality of sensation the examiner perceives has been referred to as *end feel*.[6] The standard end-feel categories and their generally accepted interpretations follow:

1. **Bone-to-bone:** an abrupt halt to movement when two hard surfaces meet (e.g., full passive extension of the normal elbow). Once this sensation is identified, further forcing of the joint is not indicated.

2. **Capsular end feel:** a "leathery" or "hardish" resistance to movement with a slight amount of give at the very end of the range. An example characteristic of capsular end feel is the glenohumeral joint in full external rotation.

3. **Springy block:** This usually pathologic end feel is generally thought to represent an intraarticular displacement such as is noted with a meniscus lesion in the knee. A rebound is both seen and felt at the end of range and is the result of the displaced cartilage being impinged between two articular structures of the knee and producing a recoil of movement. The therapist is cautioned that this movement is often painful for the patient and should not be undertaken on a repeated basis.

4. **Tissue approximation:** No further joint movement is available because of interposed soft tissue (engagement of one muscle component against another). An example would be an inability to flex the knee further because of contact of the gastrocsoleus complex with the hamstring muscles of the posterior thigh. The range of motion in such cases is full and painless.

5. **Empty feel:** Almost always pathologic. This movement may or may not be associated with joint effusion and disrupted intraarticular structures such as a completely torn anterior cruciate ligament. More pathologic yet is articular cartilage destroyed by joint-destructive lesions such as rheumatoid arthritis or by certain forms of carcinoma, resulting in an extremely hypermobile joint that renders an empty end feel.

In addition to end-feel analysis, examination of the peripheral joints for ligamentous laxity, or in some cases intraarticular cartilaginous lesions, is often undertaken at this point. The chapters that follow spell out the importance of ligamentous stability tests and the various joint provocative examination procedures.

The third major component under *function* is *resisted movements*—designed to test all contractile structures including the muscle, tendon, and musculotendinous interface. Standard resistive testing is initially limited to isometric contractions and generally proceeds from the three anatomic planes to more functionally related muscle groups or synergistic activities about a joint. Testing proceeds from gross muscle group testing to specific manual muscle testing of individual muscles when indicated to further delineate the origination of a particular condition of a contractile nature. Further delineation can be made between phasic muscle (fast twitch) fibers, by testing strength without reference to endurance, and tonic muscle (slow twitch) fibers by emphasizing endurance characteristics of the muscle contraction.

Cyriax is credited with providing the interpretive scheme that is most commonly accepted for muscle contraction. It is enumerated as follows:

1. Painful and strong = minor lesion of muscle or tendon (irritated bursae may also be uncomfortable and indicated by a painful and strong muscle contraction)
2. Painful and weak = major lesion of the muscle or tendon; this may also indicate a fracture close to the attachment site
3. Painless and weak = neurologic injury or complete rupture of the musculotendinous attachment
4. Painless and strong = normal

Instrumented muscle-testing procedures such as those offered by isokinetic devices may be included during this portion of the examination. They have proven to be reliable, although each of the various units has their drawbacks, especially when joint compression and translatoric gliding movements are unwanted during muscle testing procedures.

Special consideration should also be given to the *resistance* component of the examination, when a patient with musculoskeletal complaints has a coincidental upper motor neuron lesion, such as some children with cerebral palsy or adults who have sustained a cerebral vascular accident resulting in hemiplegia.

Maitland was the first to identify the importance of traction and compression designed to test joint and intraarticular structures during the functional part of the examination in an effort to elicit the *comparable sign*.[18] This procedure may be particularly useful when an intraarticular structure is the cause of the patient's pain, and standard range of motion and resistance movements have not elucidated the underlying cause. We have especially found this helpful in cases of triangular fibrocartilage lesions of the wrist, when compression of the ulnar half of the joint often reproduces the "comparable" painful sign of this particular condition. A joint pain relieved by traction typically points to an intraarticular lesion as the cause of the patient's symptoms.

Finally, *gliding* is an externally applied translatoric movement of one joint partner on the other, usually undertaken in the plane of treatment (parallel to the allowed joint play or component motion permitted by the joint). This particular motion assessment is useful as the therapist prepares for intervention by means of manual joint movement techniques such as anterior-posterior gliding procedures and other similar joint mobilization or manipulative treatment procedures. Assessment of passive intervertebral movements of spinal accessory motions might also be undertaken at this point in an effort to identify any restrictions of motion in one or more of the standard planes of motion allowed by the particular region of the spine under examination. After completing the assessment of movement and muscle-joint function, the examiner turns to the *palpation* portion of the examination.

Palpation

1. **Skin and subcutaneous tissue—Kibler's test (rolling of the skin), temperature, hypesthesia, hyperhydrosis, muscle splinting (guarding, spasm, and so on)**
2. **Muscles and tendons with attachments to muscle and bone—tenderness noted in both anatomic rest position and also various extremes of range of motion**
3. **Tendon sheaths and bursal—thickness, crepitus (especially silken/snowball crepitus), and tenderness**
4. **Joints—all anatomic components of the synovial joint to include bones, capsule, ligaments, any specialized structures, swelling, a change of shape or deformity, positional deficits, and tenderness**

5. **Nerves and blood vessels—identifying integrity of peripheral nerves where they lend themselves to palpation and also establishing normal circulation integrity**

Placing the *palpation* component of the examination at this point in the scheme allows the examiner to establish an acceptable level of credibility and confidence of the patient. By means of experiences during the *observation* and *functional* portion of the examination, the patient has developed some sense of the examiner's thoroughness and competence. At the same time, the examiner can gather some information about the patient's reactivity to pain and the likelihood of positive or negative response during the palpation exam. Because palpation seems somewhat simplistic and unsophisticated in that little or no instrumentation augments this part of the exam, palpation might be thought to be less valuable than some of the more sophisticated components of the examination. However, in a classic 1976 article regarding the value of palpation in identifying various entities following knee injury, Hughston and colleagues found that careful palpation examination identified the precise site of tissue at fault (verified thereafter by surgical exploration) with 76% accuracy.[11] That is, a noninstrumented, manual palpation examination indicated 76% accuracy in sensitivity to identifying the structure involved.

Having the patient identify the site of greatest palpation tenderness is extremely important, as this information goes a long way toward establishing the diagnosis. An example relates to medial knee pain. The discrete anatomic site of tenderness for a medial collateral ligament proximal attachment tear versus a medial meniscus tear versus a mid-substance ligamentous tear versus a distal medial collateral ligament tear is an extremely important distinction that can usually be made by careful palpation. Additionally, medial knee pain may be perceived in the area of the proximal tibia at the pes anserinus (bursitis) or the medial tibia plateau in the case of a runner who is in the process of developing a stress reaction in the tibia. These anatomic distinctions are crucial for the clinician who is attempting to identify by palpation the anatomic structure(s) of likely involvement. This kind of information underscores the value of a careful and competent palpation examination and reemphasizes Cyriax's statement, "Diagnosis is only a matter of applying one's anatomy."[6]

The examiner is encouraged to be as gentle as possible during the palpation examination. Whenever appropriate, the examiner should attempt the various palpation procedures on their own structures of the same region to determine what level of palpation pressure is necessary to elucidate the information and yet avoid overly aggressive palpation applied to the patient's body.

Although palpation activities are generally not considered to be very quantitative, joints that are effused can be assessed by circumferential girth measurement, and other qualitative descriptors can be used. For example, a patient who is demonstrating muscle guarding or in some other way splinting a particular motion can have the nature of that muscle contraction described in a fair amount of detail. The patient who has lost a good deal of quadriceps femoris musculature following a knee injury is noted to have a certain measurable amount of circumferential girth loss. However, *quantitative* measurements often do not accurately describe the *qualitative* loss, which is best perceived by palpation; as the patient contracts the normal quadriceps femoris muscle, it is compared to the injured-side muscle contraction. Here the differences are profound, whereas in many cases the circumferential girth differences, although significant, are not nearly as pronounced. In this case, the palpation examination, from a *qualitative* standpoint, may offer more useful information than the more "objective" girth measurement. Student therapists, in particular, are encouraged to develop their palpation skills by repetitive practice, dexterity exercises, and palpation-enhancing challenges such as attempting to palpate a piece of hair underneath various layers of paper. Manual therapists have been encouraged to continue refining their palpation skills by accurately identifying various structures on a coin without looking at it (e.g., palpating a specific site on a coin in the examiner's pocket).

Therapists need this kind of palpation skill to identify very important clinical information, such as capsular thickening noted with chronic or protracted periods of joint effusion and scar thickness in certain posttraumatic or postsurgical cases. The palpation examination has the potential of becoming the least systematic component of the evaluation because of the examiner's interest in immediately palpating the structure of greatest focus (the presumed injured structure). By so doing, the therapist often misses some of the more valuable data that can be derived from the remainder of a palpation examination that is undertaken in a more deliberate and systematic fashion. Consequently, both practicing therapists and students who are developing their examination skills are strongly encouraged to remain deliberate and thorough in their approach to palpation in the knowledge that the information derived from such diligence provides data that add to the examiner's ability to identify the involved structure. Following the first three major components of the physical examination, the next part is the *neurologic examination.*

Neurologic tests

1. **Nerve trunk—pain on stretching or on pressure; adverse neural tension**
2. **Reflexes—deep tendon reflexes (muscle stretch reflex), superficial reflexes, pathologic reflexes**
3. **Sensation—superficial modalities and deep pressure kinesthesia**
4. **Motor examination—central and/or peripheral muscle weakness, paresis**
5. **Cranial nerve examination**

Some consider this portion of the examination to be the exclusive domain of physicians, but physical therapists are required to conduct a competent neurologic screening examination, from a physical therapy viewpoint, in order to treat the patient knowledgeably and effectively. The outline for the neurologic testing procedures is relatively straightforward, but there is a fair amount of subtlety and overlap due both to an anatomic and physiologic organizational complexity and to an interplay between various body systems. Consequently, the body's response to one form of injury may be to include other biologic tissues in the condition (e.g., connective tissue injury leads to neurologic involvement). The section dealing with this portion of the examination includes examples of this process.

One aspect of a patient's response to neurologic compression that makes this portion of the examination somewhat more difficult to interpret is the possibility of a "double crush" phenomenon. This term was coined in 1973 to describe patients who had identified compression neuropathy in the periphery (e.g., carpal tunnel syndrome—compression neuropathy of the median nerve at the wrist) and who were also found, in a high percentage of cases, to have a concomitant compression of those cervical nerve roots that eventually give rise to the median nerve.[29] This phenomenon led the authors of the study to conclude that compression of the nerve root and trunk is often associated with—and, in fact, may serve as a precursor to—ease of compression of the nerve arborization at its various distal sites in the periphery.[29]

Another subtle aspect of the neurologic examination that bears mentioning is the fact that nerve injuries are known to lead to other musculoskeletal compromise and, potentially, further injury. Patients with known neurologic injuries develop musculoskeletal system injuries with greater ease because they do not have the necessary motor control of a particular joint segment to prevent compression forces, which ultimately lead to soft tissue breakdown either at the articular cartilage level or in the associated joint structures such as musculotendinous units and/or ligament structures.[3]

In addition, a number of studies have shown that musculoskeletal injuries may result in neurologic involvement through a process known as *neurogenic inflammation.* This particular neurologic response does not follow any strictly anatomic distribution. The typical sequence is that the joint region involved in the musculoskeletal injury is subtended by a number of key muscles and other neurally innervated structures in the area developing denervation, most likely through a process of inflammation in the neurologic structures themselves. This process is believed to be mediated by neurotransmitters such as substance P or histamine. As a result of these circumstances (denervation), the patient experiences prolonged muscle weakness much like that seen with known neurologic conditions as a result of denervation-like changes in the muscle. These changes have been identified electromyographically (EMG) and also in anatomic studies of laboratory animal models.[15,22]

A final complicating factor that makes interpretation of the neurologic examination more difficult is the presence of "redundancy" in the neuromuscular skeletal system. It has been shown that a 50% loss of motor units is necessary before a clear manual muscle testing weakness is noted during standard manual examination.[1] This particular observation brings to light the need for two clarifying components of the neurologic examination that have been fruitful in identifying this particular aspect. First, in undertaking the motor examination, the therapist must remember that more than one or two maximal contractions of the various basic muscle groups should be undertaken. A patient who actually has a C7 nerve root injury (e.g., disk compression) may be able to maximally contract the elbow extensors one or, at most, two times and thereby obscure any evidence of muscle weakness. However, further muscle testing with multiple repetitions usually reveals an increasing muscle weakness that appears to result from the inability of the neuromuscular system to repeatedly produce a maximal contraction of these key muscle elements. It is indicative of what is referred to as a "fatiguing muscle weakness" phenomenon. A further clarification of the motor exam can be accomplished with simple EMG testing in which an electrode is inserted into the key muscle(s) in question and the presence of denervation potentials or loss of motor unit recruitment can be identified to clarify the clinical presentation. This procedure properly falls under the heading of *special tests,* to be covered in more detail later.

Examination of the nerve trunk (nerve root). Nerve trunks are generally examined by an attempt to produce neurotension. The standard nerve root stretch technique in the lower extremity is referred to as the *straight leg raise test,* and a similar stretching technique is referred as the *femoral nerve stretch.* These tests are useful for identifying major nerve root irritation and compression (presumably from disk pressure against the nerve root) resulting in pain that is transmitted from the site of pressure down through the entire pattern of nerve distribution relevant to the nerve root in question. In the upper extremity, a series of neurotension techniques, such as the compression-distraction test, brachial plexus tension tests, neck hyperextension test, and a more recently described test entitled *brachial plexus compression test,*[27] have been quite helpful in elucidating similar nerve root pressure arising in the cervical spine.[28]

Other tests, including the slump test, Kernig's test, and Brudzinski's test, identify a combination of connective tissue and neurologic tension in the covering of the spinal cord (dura mater) and are referred to as *dural stretch* signs. Each involves stretching the spine in the cervical, thoracic, or lumbar regions to highlight connective tissue or neural restriction that gives rise to neurologic symptoms and signs into the arms, back, or lower extremities. The whole concept of adverse neural tension has recently caught the attention of the physical therapy community, and some very interesting theoretical work has been published on this topic in the last several years.[4]

Further testing in this category includes applying pressure in the form of tapping the nerve to elicit a Tinel's sign and compressing the nerve to identify an entrapment neuropathy, such as Phalen's test for median nerve compression at the wrist. Tinel's sign was originally described as an indication of nerve regeneration and was believed to be clinical evidence of nerve regrowth. Reinnervation is often characterized by a report of burning or numbness and tingling in the autonomous distribution for the nerve in question when it is tapped. Each of the major nerves in the upper extremity lends itself to this kind of modification of palpation testing. Specifically, the median nerve at the wrist (carpal tunnel syndrome) and the elbow (pronator teres syndrome), the ulnar nerve at the elbow (cubital tunnel syndrome), and the radial nerve also at the elbow (radial tunnel syndrome) are sites for nerve compression where a positive Tinel's sign might be elicited. Again, knowledge of the anatomic course of these various biologic structures is absolutely critical for meaningful neurologic examination.

Phalen's test was also designed to identify median nerve compression at the wrist (e.g., carpal tunnel syndrome). In this particular peripheral nerve compression test, the wrist is maximally flexed; in the presence of median nerve compromise in the carpal tunnel, the patient usually complains of neurologic symptoms of numbness and tingling or pain into the median nerve distribution. Other tests for compression of neurologic structures (e.g., brachial plexus) include the thoracic outlet syndrome tests such as the Adson, Allen, Halstead, and costoclavicular space compression tests.

Reflexes. The terms *muscle stretch reflex* (MSR) and *deep tendon reflex* (DTR) are usually interchangeable and reflect the fact that a monosynaptic reflex can be elicited by tapping virtually any tendon or muscle in the body. The standard upper extremity deep tendon reflexes are the biceps, triceps, and brachioradialis; in the lower extremity, the typical reflexes tested are at the knee (quadriceps) and the ankle (gastrocsoleus). Each of these reflexes is reflective of a nerve root or a number of nerve root or a number of nerve root levels, and interpretation of various findings requires the examiner to know the particular nerve root level(s) from which the reflex arises.

Standard interpretation of DTRs include *hyperreactivity,* which suggests central nervous system involvement (at or above the anterior horn cell). *Hyporeactivity* of the standard deep tendon reflexes generally indicates nerve entrapment or impingement anywhere along its course from the spinal nerve root on down to the individual peripheral nerve itself. Because of the variability among individuals in DTR responsivity, the examiner should develop an appreciation for this variance by consistently examining each patient and by including DTR reactivity as a part of the standard neurologic examination. This practice is likely to minimize any tendency on the part of the examiner to overinterpret or underinterpret patient DTR responses. On occasion, eliciting a particular reflex is difficult, and the therapist should be reminded of distraction techniques that are helpful in such situations. For example, if less than normal reactivity is encountered in the lower extremities and the patient is asked to perform an isometric contraction in the upper extremities (Jendrassik's maneuver), a normal reaction often results shortly thereafter upon attempts to elicit either knee or ankle reflexes. It is helpful to grade reflex responses, and a commonly accepted grading scheme is as follows:

0 = absent
1 = diminished or hyporeactive
2 = average
2+ = slightly exaggerated (hyperreactive)
3 = exaggerated (hyperreactive)
4 = associated with myoclonus

Although superficial reflexes are included as a matter of course in this particular outline of the neurologic examination, quite frankly they are rarely undertaken for most patients complaining about standard neuromuscular skeletal conditions. However, stroking the abdominal skin to evoke an umbilical reaction through contraction of the abdominal wall musculature is a useful procedure for identifying a patient with lower thoracic or thoracolumbar nerve root irritation. A comprehensive neurologic examination, which includes the entire gamut of superficial reflexes, is best undertaken by the patient's neurologist.

Pathologic reflexes are indicative of upper motor neuron involvement and may include gross hyperreactivity to tendon tapping (greatly exaggerated deep tendon reflex responses) or the standard pathologic reflexes such as Babinski's or Chaddock's sign in the lower extremity and Hoffmann's sign in the upper extremity. Beyond these standard procedures, undertaken with most neuromusculoskeletal screening examinations, more precise neurologic testing is generally best undertaken by the patient's neurologist. Interpretation of these clinically elicited reflexes is dependent on comparing the responses of both sides of the body, and therefore asymmetry is the finding most often indicative of significant neurologic involvement.

The examiner should be reminded that sometimes a combination of neurologic findings is actually related to an underlying musculoskeletal condition but has its primary abnormality in the neurologic system. An example is a case of cervical myelopathy in which bony hypertrophy or significant osteophyte involvement causes cervical spinal cord compression. This results in upper motor neuron signs below the level of the lesion as well as lower motor neuron signs such as sensation changes and motor weakness at the level of the lesion. This condition presents a somewhat contradictory clinical picture initially. However, when the underlying cause is identified, the composite clinical findings do make a great deal of sense.

Sensation. The examiner is reminded to review the concept of dermatome as most of the *sensation* examination is undertaken by comparing a patient's response in individual dermatomal segments to those from the autonomous distribution of the individual peripheral nerves. Most therapists recommend examining one, two, or possibly three sensory modalities. Most physical therapists typically examine the patient for pain, light touch or crude touch, and sharp-dull discrimination. In cases of distal peripheral nerve compression (e.g., carpal tunnel syndrome), two-point discrimination testing is also helpful. Many physical therapists have derived a great deal of benefit from their occupational therapy colleagues who often conduct an extensive battery of tests of sensory modalities in their standard screening examination of patients. Patients with "posterior column" involvement often manifest abnormalities related to position or vibration sense, which should be included in routine neurologic screening. When information derived from the sensory exam is ambiguous and raises concerns, the patient may be referred back to a neurologist for further evaluation procedures.

Motor examination. The motor examination to identify a peripheral neurologic involvement (anterior horn cell and below) generally follows a myotomal screening pattern. Specifically, all the muscles innervated by key segmental spinal levels are tested to identify whether a muscle weakness conforms, more or less, to a nerve root level, an extrasegmental distribution (such as multiple root levels), or a specific peripheral nerve distribution. The therapist should be reminded that the screening examination undertaken prior to beginning the clarifying exam includes a number of muscle-testing procedures. Information derived from the screening examination may allow the therapist to proceed with simple verification by briefly examining a few key muscle groups and let the previous screening examination stand as the primary source of information regarding muscle involvement. Identifying any upper motor neuron component by examining the patient for coordination difficulties or any evidence of intention or resting tremor is included in this portion of the exam. Evaluation of ambulation is, at times, a key element of the motor coordination exam, and it is often possible to identify an individual with a mildly spastic gait resulting from cervical myelopathy as an example of a musculoskeletal condition resulting in neurologic involvement.

Cranial nerve examination. When major cranial nerve involvement is suspected or identified with initial screening procedures, a physical therapist should refer the patient back to the original referring physician or recommend further examination by a medical specialist (usually a neurologist). However, simple screening procedures of the basic enumerated cranial nerves is certainly within the purview of the physical therapist. Eye movement, undertaken appropriately upon command, is generally reflective of normal status for the third, fourth, and sixth cranial nerves. The fifth (trigeminal) cranial nerve, among many other functions, supplies the muscles of mastication. Ability to clench the jaw (masseter muscle) powerfully usually indicates normal trigeminal nerve innervation. The muscles of expression, supplied by the seventh cranial nerve (facial), are easily tested for symmetry of response for the right and left halves of the face and is an important element of this portion of the examination. A patient's auditory acuity is a simple test of the eighth cranial nerve, and a standard gag reflex is reflective of normalcy of the ninth cranial nerve. Normal status of the upper trapezius and sternocleidomastoid muscles indicates normal health of the eleventh (spinal accessory) cranial nerve, and ability to project the tongue and move it about in a normal fashion is indicative of absence of abnormality for the twelfth (hypoglossal) cranial nerve. Once again, any major abnormalities identified during cranial nerve examination call for consulting with the physician, possibly referring the patient back to the original source of referral, or recommending further medical evaluation as indicated.

Cranial nerve involvement is noted infrequently during examination for most patients with musculoskeletal conditions. On occasion, however, patients with temporomandibular joint or orofacial pain have some involvement of the cranial nerve distribution, and it is therefore prudent to examine the patient for the extent of neurologic involvement. Patients with flexion-extension cervical spine injuries often have involvement of neck muscles, including the sternocleidomastoid and, in some cases, the upper trapezius muscle, suggesting stretch injury to eleventh cranial nerve. Some patients with forms of amyotrophic lateral sclerosis (ALS, Lou Gehrig's disease) may show a presentation of cranial nerve (bulbar) involvement. The cranial nerve examination completes the neurologic assessment and brings the examiner to the fifth and final component of the evaluation process: *additional medical examinations*.

Additional medical examinations

1. **Radiography—standard radiographs, other imaging techniques**
2. **Laboratory tests—blood, laboratory studies**
3. **Electrodiagnosis—electroencephalography, EMG, nerve conduction velocity studies, cronaxie, reaction of degeneration**
4. **Punctures—biopsies, aspiration**
5. **Special examinations—by other medical specialties (gynecology, urology, internal medicine, otolaringology, neurology) for referred pain evaluation**

In most instances, the patient's physician makes the determination to obtain the appropriate battery of tests when indicated. Because referring physicians sometimes seek input from the therapist regarding any additional test that might be helpful, however, acquaintance with the standard tests available in these five basic areas and some of the abnormalities that can be identified with such testing is useful.

Although the physical therapist is not expected to become an expert in radiographic examination and all the subtle nuances of interpretation, the therapist should take the time necessary to become familiar with the standard features of imaging techniques. In this way, at a minimum, the therapist can become conversant regarding any results that such testing has provided. Although patients, especially those with spinal pain, rarely avoid having back radiographs taken, standard radiographic films are usually taken to confirm a clinical opinion rather than establish one. Except for cases of trauma, in which radiographs are quite helpful in identifying subtle bony changes and documenting the extent of obvious deformity identified during the clinical examination, the main purpose of radiographic examination, especially of the spine, is to rule out serious underlying causes of back pain, which represent less than 1% of all patients with spinal pain. These causes fall into one of three categories of disease: infection, tumor, and ankylosing spondylitis.[9]

Information from the radiologic examination is certainly more useful if the therapist has been introduced to the whole field of radiography regarding the place that roentgen rays occupy on the electromagnetic spectrum, their energy per unit area, and the concept of relative radiolucency to radiopacity. Film positioning considerations are useful when viewing x-rays, and a methodical and deliberate approach to examining radiographs is important. The following is not meant to be an exhaustive list of considerations, but we do believe these points are useful guidelines for identifying important elements derived from radiologic examination:

1. Attempt to set the film in the anatomic position on the view box. This tends to decrease confusion regarding right and left side of the body and helps to keep the therapist oriented regarding likelihood of identification of abnormalities.
2. Identify the body part and the particular view taken: anterior-posterior, posterior-anterior, oblique, lateral, or a special view. This is particularly important in identifying abnormalities on spinal films.
3. Assess bone density at both the local and general levels in an effort to determine whether it is normal, increased, or decreased. Changes from the normal are seen following trauma, disease, or the normal aging process.
4. Examine the cortex for continuity, irregularity, or thickening.
5. Examine the medulla of the bone for destruction or sclerosis.
6. Examine the joints for narrowing or irregularity of joint space (seen with joint destructive processes such as osteoarthritis or, in some cases, the rheumatoid arthritides).
7. Finally, examine the joint area for any evidence of osteophyte development or osteochondral defect (loose bodies).

"Plain" radiographs are one of a number of diagnostic imaging procedures. Beyond familiarization with standard radiographs, therapists should avail themselves of the opportunity to become familiar with the value of fluoroscopy, tomography, nuclear medicine techniques (bone scan), and other nonionizing radiation forms of energy such as magnetic residence imaging (MRI).[19]

Laboratory tests are often ordered and prove very useful for identifying the underlying metabolic or medical cause for a patient's condition. Specifically, blood studies may be obtained to identify the rheumatoid arthritides (e.g., RA factor). Testing for a genetic marker, *HLA-B27,* may identify the presence of ankylosing spondylitis. An increased sedimentation rate identified during standard laboratory testing is generally reflective of some kind of inflammatory process; although fairly sensitive, it has limited specificity. The presence of infectious agents in cases of osteomyelitis may also be identified with standard blood cultures, especially those looking for the evidence of white blood cell count elevation.

Electrophysiologic testing. Standard testing, from a physical therapy standpoint, includes establishing chronaxies and the reaction of degeneration, although these two areas of testing have largely fallen from the list of testing procedures performed by physical therapists. They have been largely replaced by EMG and nerve conduction velocity (NCV) studies, which provide a great deal of information regarding the neuromuscular system and, in particular, the motor unit. The EMG and NCV procedures are especially helpful for identifying sites of peripheral or nerve root compression and can actually establish whether a neurologic condition is characterized primarily by axonal degeneration or by a myelin lesion. Results from electrophysiologic testing provides information about the extent of muscle-nerve abnormality present (severity) and any attempt at recovery (reinnervation potentials), which serve as useful prognostic information for the clinician. Rehabilitation procedures can be more knowledgeably developed with such information available, as the extent of neurologic involvement with a musculoskeletal condition is included in the information used to establish the treatment regimen.

The remainder of the special tests and referral to other medical specialists would generally occur in concert with the patient's referring physician (in most cases, the family practice physician). The physical therapist often has the benefit of seeing the patient on numerous occasions and observing the response to physical and medical treatment. Consequently, physical therapists are, in many cases, likely to pick up the need for any additional testing and can relay this information to the patient's physician and thus provide a real service to the patient.

MUSCULOSKELETAL DIAGNOSIS

Each of the five major categories and their five major subdivisions in the Frisch 5-5 evaluation scheme have been identified. Because this approach is systematic and sufficiently thorough, we recommend it as the primary evaluation format. However, a patient undergoing this examination would clearly, by necessity, be required to change position multiple times as the examiner takes the patient through the various test procedures and positions throughout the course of the examination. Unfortunately, these changes often lead to additional patient discomfort. Practicing clinicians and students are encouraged to warn the patients following the evaluation procedure that their symptoms may increase over 12 to 24 hours because of the increased irritative movements undertaken during the examination. In an effort to obtain the most information from the examination procedures while minimizing additional patient discomfort, clinicians are encouraged to develop a sequence that limits the number of times that a patient must change positions during the evaluation procedures. In this way, all those test procedures that require the patient to be standing, sitting, or lying down can be undertaken during a single component of the exam.

After all aspects of the examination procedure and the history have been completed, the clinician reviews the signs and symptoms found and thoughtfully determines the likely clinical impression or diagnosis. Some therapists prefer to simply draw up a list of problems (signs and symptoms) and allow these to direct their treatment procedures in an effort to address that list. Then again, some therapists believe it is best to identify the involved tissue and establish a clinical impression or provisional diagnosis. Because professional communication plays such a vital role in successful health care delivery, we recommend that physical therapists at least become familiar with the range of named diagnostic entities for each of the major musculoskeletal joint regions.

The diagnostic process is admittedly a complicated exercise involving integration of information derived from the history, the clinician's own academic and didactic background, and the data derived from the clinical test procedures themselves. As a clinician goes through the examination process, a variety of hypotheses are being generated and tested to look for "goodness of fit" to determine the tissue most likely to be involved and the severity and irritibility of the tissue involvement. The signs and symptoms identified during the examination should begin to fit a pattern that the student and the practicing clinician recognize. At times, patients may have a combination of signs and symptoms that do not clearly indicate the patient's diagnosis. When which of two conditions a patient may have is not clear, further testing of either a clinical nature or a more instrumented and diagnostic nature may be needed (special test components such as imaging studies or electrophysiologic testing). This approach usually results in additional information, which confirms one or another provisional diagnoses as the therapist attempts, as accurately as possible, to determine the clinical impression and the precise tissue involved.

The usual situation for most patients with musculoskel-

Guidelines for assessment of pain

Assessment of bone

Hx: Pain primarily localized. Consider sclerotomes. Boring, aching, or throbbing in nature.

I: Unremarkable in early stages; malalignment.

F: Aggravated by positions or activities that increase stress in the bone. In more severe cases, positions make no difference on the bone pain.

P: Tapping; vibrating bone. Local tenderness, deformity enlargements. (Some research indicates clinical ultrasound may be used to detect stress fractures.)

N: Negative in early stages.

S: Roentgenograms, bone scans, etc.

Assessment of joint capsules

Hx: Pain is usually localized but without strict boundaries. In cases of the back, it is usually unilateral to the midline of the back, but a specific level is often difficult to interpret. (There may be referred pain along dermatomal patterns.) Onset is often sudden, accompanying trauma, or gradual, such as with developing arthritis. If synovial membrane is irritated, there is usually an increase in synovial fluid volume, causing effusion of a joint without discoloration.

I: Patients avoid positions that stress the capsules involved, either stretching or compressing. There may be secondary muscle "guarding" (fluid accumulation).

F: Certain movements increase pain, and some decrease pain. Passive movements usually coincide with active movement patterns. There may be reflexogenic muscle guarding. Injurious movements that stress the capsule may be sudden or sustained. May be associated loss of coordinated trunk movements. May develop capsular pattern following periods of immobilization (Cyriax). Capsular end feel at extremes of motion.

P: Passive intervertebral movements as well as graded articulations help localize pain. Capsules of most peripheral joints and cervical joints can be palpated directly.

N: Negative.

S: Mobility roentgenograms, articular injection with local analgesic, and arthrograms.

Assessment of ligaments/fascia

Hx: Gradual or sudden onset. Aggravated by specific sudden or sustained movements that cause tension, stress. Pain gen-

erally localized. May complain of joint instability or of joint "giving way" reflexively.

I: May have accommodating loss of cervical or lumbar lordosis if central ligaments are stretched. May have secondary muscle splinting to guard against movement. Peripheral joints may become deformed if dysfunction not corrected; look for joint effusion.

F: Passive movements that stress the ligaments are painful and limited.

P: Superficial ligaments of the spine may be painful while performing passive intervertebral movements (PIVM). May have onset of pain at end of the available range of the joints(s) being tested; joint effusion may be present.

N: Negative. Sometimes tender trigger points in the back coincide with acupuncture points, which seem to occur where small cutaneous nerves perforate the dorsal fascia.

S: X-rays and injection of local analgesic.

Assessment of nerve roots

Hx: Onset of pain may be gradual or sudden. Symptoms may be intermittent or continuous, depending on type of lesion. Generally the pain is referred. Symptoms are aggravated by conditions that irritate or stress the nerve root.

I: Normal, or adopts a position that best avoids compromise of affected nerve root; spinal list shift.

F: Generally, extension or lateral bending on the side of the pain is limited and painful in the spine because of the reduced vertical dimension of the intervertebral foramen.

P: Variable. Paresthesia or hypoesthesia along specific dermatomes. Change in skin texture secondary to denervation of skin. Pain aggravated by segmental articulations (graded accessory movements), which may aggravate an irritated nerve root.

N: Besides paresthesia, in more advanced stages, motor weakness and reflex changes are noted. Straight leg raising and other tests that increase tension on irritated nerve roots aggravate symptoms.

S: EMG. Various tests on other conditions that may compromise nerve root, such as diskograms, CT-scans, venograms, and MRI.

Assessment of dura mater

Hx: Onset gradual or sudden, such as following spinal trauma. Pain is generally referred and extrasegmental.

Modified from D.A. Williams, MS, PT.

*Hx, History; I, inspection; F, function; P, palpation; N, neural exam; S, special tests.

etal disorders involves a determination of whether the patient has a primary arthrogenic or neuromuscular tissue involvement. Other abnormalities may involve the vascular system, the autonomic nervous system, and, in some cases, a component of the psychological system. The various joint-related structures tend to demonstrate their involvement in a particular pattern with each of the major areas of the exam demonstrating a rather classic clinical presentation. Consequently, the guidelines for assessing pain in the various

synovial joint structures outlined in the Box may be useful for both practicing clinicians and therapists who are in the early stages of developing their diagnostic acumen.

TRIAL TREATMENT

This chapter has presented an overview of evaluation procedures. However, clinicians should remember that their primary responsibility is to provide rehabilitation for the patient, which is dependent upon an accurate evaluation so

Guidelines for assessment of pain—cont'd

I: Usually patient adopts a list to avoid tension on the dura; appears apprehensive about moving.

F: Forward bending and contralateral bending aggravate pain. With adhesions, the patient continues to have some pathologically limited range on repeated movements.

P: Variable. Paresthesia extrasegmental. Often accompanied by trigger points.

N: Straight leg raise and other qualifying tests such as neck flexion, femoral internal rotation, adduction, and ankle dorsiflexion increase sciatica; positive Kernig's, Brudzinski's, and Valsalva.

S: Epidermal injection or qualifying tests for other tissues, which may compromise dura.

Assessment of muscle

Hx: May be gradual onset of pain following sustained or repeated contractions. Sudden onset of pain usually associated with lifting or a sudden jerk when the back or peripheral joints are unprepared. Pain is often continuous but worse in positions that apply tension. Pain is usually diffuse in paraspinal area.

I: Primary muscle guarding is common, along with occasional color changes, depending upon circulation and bleeding in the area.

F: Active movements painful and restricted and cause tension of the contractile unit. Static resisted movements painful. (Use Cyriax's interpretation when testing static resisted movements).

P: Local tenderness with guarding may have trigger points, palpable, visible gap in muscle, partial or complete rupture.

N: Negative.

S: Rule out other structures. Occasionally electromyography. Possible measure for muscle compartment pressures in the future.

Assessment of blood vessels

Hx: Onset gradual or sudden. Pain constant and pulsating or throbbing in nature. Sometimes intermittent claudication.

I: Generally negative. May see color changes in the skin.

F: Variable depending on which tissue may be damaged. Sometimes position makes no difference. Nocturnal pain common.

P: Secondary muscle guarding.

N: Negative, but may present like peripheral neuropathy.

S: Venograms, arteriograms, compartmental pressures, and so on.

Assessment of disks

Hx: Gradual or sudden onset. Usually sitting and lifting makes condition worse. Not always related to specific activity.

I: Variable, depending upon which pain-sensitive tissues are compromised.

F: Usually flexion, ipsilateral bending, and twisting increase pain. Again, it depends upon which pain sensitive tissues are compromised.

P: PIVM and graded articulation help locate involved segment.

N: Variable, depending upon compromises of neural tissue.

S: X-rays, diskograms, myelograms, CT-scan, MRI.

Assessment of articular cartilage

Hx: Most often a gradual onset of localized pain and discomfort. If systemic disorder, patient complains of similar problems in other joints. Because cartilage is not innervated, pain comes from either excessive loading on subchondral bone or from other excessive tissue tension secondary to mechanical dysfunction. The patient sometimes complains of grating, locking, or "giving out" of the joint.

I: Unremarkable initially. Look for genu varus, genu valgus at knee. In later stages, there may be secondary changes due to chronic biomechanical imbalances.

F: Active and passive movements may cause pain or minor locking in the joint. Joint distraction may ease any associated pain. In later stages, the active or passive movements are limited.

P: May sense grating, crepitus. Tissue pain where abnormal stresses have been experienced on other tissues. Note joint effusion; may palpate bony hypertrophy at joint margin.

N: Negative.

S: Radiography, arthroscopy, arthograms, and so on.

---

that the proper rehabilitation procedures will be directed at the involved tissue structures in a manner appropriate to the severity of involvement. The initial attempts at treatment actually lend themselves to the reevaluation process as the therapist moves from a provisional or preliminary diagnosis to a more definitive and confirmed diagnosis. The result of the initial treatment is really the first step in the process of continued reevaluation. Based on measurable changes and historical reports by the patient, the therapist notes that the provisional or prelimary diagnosis is either supported or refuted by the patient's response to treatment. The patient's response must be carefully evaluated so that verbal reports by the patient regarding symptom changes do not unduly influence information derived from measurement of the patient's progress. By evaluating both of these major

components (symptoms and signs), a more complete interpretation of the patient's response to treatment can be developed. At this point, therapists must be willing to modify their initial clinical impression as conflicting or contradictory information develops from the patient's response to trial treatment. Moreover, astute clinicians are patient during this time because the therapeutic benefit of many rehabilitation procedures is additive (cumulative over time) and does not necessarily occur following the initial treatment. As the patient's response to treatment is noted to change over time, the rehabilitation procedures similarly change in an effort to keep pace with the patient's progress. A commitment to constant reevaluation and measurement of the patient's improvements encourage healing with minimal delays or barriers.

INTERPRETATION OF TEST PROCEDURES

Physical therapy students and practicing clinicians who wish to be successful evaluators of patients with musculoskeletal conditions must commit themselves to developing the skill and accuracy necessary to perform the examination procedures. However, *interpreting* the results of the examination process in a clinically meaningful way requires more than the appropriate psychomotor performance of the various test procedures. Consideration should be given to four relevant issues with an impact on the nature of evaluation procedure interpretation:

1. Reliability of clinical measurements and tests
2. Validity of assumptions underlying standard measurement systems
3. Sensitivity of a given sign
4. Specificity of a given sign

The evaluation schemes of Cyriax and McKenzie are among the most commonly used methods for assessing patients complaining of low back pain. These schemes have contributed greatly to systematizing our examination approach to such patients. However, components of both systems of evaluation have been shown to have questionable reliability, especially when agreement in test interpretation between different therapists was studied.[17,24] Similarly, Hayes and associates recently examined the assumptions underlying Cyriax's evaluation format of selective tension and found their validity to be questionable.[10] Specifically, these investigators have reported that the pattern of restriction ("capsular pattern"), the pain-resistance sequence, and the end-feel descriptions for patients with known osteoarthritis of the knee are neither reliable nor valid. The reason for alerting the reader to these research findings is to point out the limitations in interpreting the information obtained from various examination procedures undertaken during the evaluation of patients with neuromusculoskeletal disorders. When possible, multiple measurements of the same basic anatomic structure should be attempted, as this strategy has been shown to dramatically improve the reliability of such measures.[5]

Interpretation and analysis of examination procedures depend not only on the reliability and validity of such measures but also upon the sensitivity and specificity of the "signs" elicited by the test procedures. The *sensitivity* (%) of a given sign is defined as the probability of its occurrence (e.g., positive straight leg raise) in the presence of the lesion that the sign is considered to indicate (in this example, nerve root compression).[28]

$$\frac{\text{TRUE } (+)}{\text{TRUE } (+) \text{ and FALSE } (-)} \times 100$$

By contrast, the *specificity* (%) of a given sign is defined as the probability of its absence (e.g., no straight leg raise pain) in the absence of the lesion that the sign is considered to indicate (in this example, no nerve root compression).[28]

$$\frac{\text{TRUE } (-)}{\text{FALSE } (+) \text{ and TRUE } (-)} \times 100$$

Although these concepts are useful for identifying clinical tests that are sensitive enough to detect anatomic and physiologic abnormalities and are sufficiently sophisticated that they do not incorrectly identify tissues as abnormal when they are not, they themselves are based upon underlying assumptions. The fact that the calculation of sensitivity and specificity are based on true-false positives and negatives assumes that we really know what a true or false positive or negative is; that is, a gold standard test is available against which others are evaluated to determine their relative merit or value. Such a gold standard test is often based on "direct" visualization (e.g., MRI results showing an extruded disk). Although we do not often think in such terms, even the gold standard, direct visualization is based on the assumptions that our senses are reliable and that they can be trusted to make the fine discriminatory assessments that are involved in analyzing what we see (or hear, feel, etc.).

CONCLUSION

The diagnostic process is a complex one about which our profession is learning more all the time.[7] Accurate diagnosis and sound clinical reasoning skills should lead to effective treatment of patients with musculoskeletal disorders. Skills of this nature are developed by students and clinicians who commit themselves to mastering the knowledge base and who gain clinical experience through constant practice of examination procedures. Our patients are the prime beneficiaries when careful, informed examination leads to appropriate rehabilitation procedures.

REVIEW QUESTIONS

1. What guidelines should be considered by the clinician when examining radiographs?
2. What steps should be used by the clinician when interpreting the results of the examination so that a musculoskeletal diagnosis can be developed?
3. What are the concepts of trial treatment and the interpretation of test procedures as they relate to musculoskeletal conditions?
4. What is the purpose of active, passive, and resistive tests in the diagnosis of musculoskeletal disorders?
5. What is the rationale for performing a clearing examination prior to proceeding with the clarifying examination of a musculoskeletal disorder?

REFERENCES

1. Beasley WC: Influence of method on estimates of normal knee extensor force among normal and postpolio children, *Phys Ther Rev* 36:21, 1956.
2. Bogduk N: The rationale for patterns of neck and back pain, *Pain Management* 13:17, 1984.

3. Bohannon RW, Gajdosik RL: Spinal nerve root compression: some clinical implications, *Phys Ther* 67:676, 1987.
4. Butler DS: *Mobilisation of the nervous system,* Melbourne, 1991, Churchill-Livingstone.
5. Cibulka MT, Delitto A, Koldehoff RM: Changes in innominate tilt after manipulation of the sacroiliac joint in patients with low back pain: an experimental study, *Phys Ther* 68:1359, 1988.
6. Cyriax J: *Textbook of orthopaedic medicine, vol 1, diagnosis of soft tissue lesions,* ed 8, London, 1982, Bailliere Tindall.
7. Delitto A, Snyder-Mackler L: The diagnostic process: examples in orthopedic physical therapy, *Phys Ther* 75:203, 1995.
8. Farrell JP, Jensen GM: Manual therapy: a critical assessment of role in the profession of physical therapy, *Phys Ther* 72:843, 1992.
9. Forrester DM, Brown JC: Radiographic evaluation of back pain, *Contemporary Diagnostic Radiology,* Baltimore, 1979, Williams & Wilkins.
10. Hayes KW, Petersen C, Falconer J: An examination of Cyriax's passive motion tests with patients having osteoarthritis of the knee, *Phys Ther* 74:697, 1994.
11. Hughston JC et al: Classification of knee ligament instabilities: part I, the medial compartment and cruciate ligaments, *J Bone Joint Surg Am* 58:159, 1976.
12. Jones MA: Clinical reasoning in manual therapy, *Phys Ther* 72:875, 1992.
13. Kaltenborn F: *Mobilization of the extremity joints,* ed 3, Oslo, 1980, Olaf Norlis Bokhandel.
14. Kessler RM, Hertling D: Assessment of musculoskeletal disorders. In Kessler RM, Hertling D, editors: *Management of common musculoskeletal disorders,* ed 2, Philadelphia, 1990, JB Lippincott.
15. Levine JD et al: Reflex neurogenic inflammation: I, contribution of the peripheral nervous system to spatially remote inflammatory responses that follow injury, *J Neurosciences* 5:1380, 1985.
16. Magee DJ: Principles and concepts. In Magee DJ, editor: *Orthopedic physical assessment,* ed 2, Philadelphia, 1992, WB Saunders.
17. Maher C, Adams R: Reliability of pain and stiffness assessments in clinical manual lumbar spine examination, *Phys Ther* 74:801, 1994.
18. Maitland GD: *Vertebral manipulation,* ed 5, London, 1986, Butterworth.
19. McKinnis LN: Fundamentals of radiology for physical therapists. In Richardson JK, Iglarsh ZA, editors: *Clinical orthopaedic physical therapy,* Philadelphia, 1994, WB Saunders.
20. Melzak R: The short-form McGill Pain Questionnaire, *Pain* 30:191, 1987.
21. Michaelis LS: Stenosis of carpal tunnel, compression of median nerve and flexor tendon sheaths, combined with rheumatoid arthritis elsewhere, *Proc R Soc Med* 43:414, 1950.
22. Nitz AJ: Limb denervation following anterior cruciate (ACL) reconstruction without tourniquet application, *Phys Ther* 68:822, 1988.
23. Price DD, McGrath PA, Rafii A: The validation of visual analogue scales as ration scale measures for chronic and experimental pain, *Pain* 17:45, 1983.
24. Riddle DL, Rothstein JM: Intertester reliability of McKenzie's classifications of the type of syndrome present in patients with low back pain, *Spine* (in press).
25. Rothstein JM: Manual therapy: a special issue and a special topic, *Phys Ther* 72:839, 1992 (editorial).
26. Sandover J: Dynamic loading as a possible source of low back disorders, *Spine* 8:652, 1983.
27. Saunders HD: *Evaluation, treatment and prevention of musculoskeletal disorders,* Minneapolis, 1985, Viking.
28. Uchihara T, Furukawa T, Tsukagoshi H: Compression of brachial plexus as a diagnostic test of cervical cord lesion, *Spine* 19:2170, 1994.
29. Upton ARM, McComas AJ: The double crush in nerve entrapment syndromes, *Lancet* 2:359, 1973.
30. Wells RM, Johnson EW: Study of conduction delay in median nerve of patients with rheumatoid arthritis, *Arch Phys Med Rehabil* 43:244, 1962.

CHAPTER 8

Basic Concepts of Orthopedic Manual Therapy

Robert C. Hall and Arthur J. Nitz

OUTLINE

History of manual therapy
Classification of synovial joints
Osteokinematics and arthrokinematics
    Osteokinematics
    Arthrokinematics
Concepts and rules of joint motion
    Convex-concave rule
    Positions of joint congruency
    Laws of vertebral motion
    Barriers to movement
Manual methods for assessing joint dysfunction
    Selective tissue assessment
    Contractile and noncontractile elements
    Systematic evaluation techniques
Palpation techniques
Traditional manual treatment techniques
    Manipulation/mobilization
Nontraditional manual techniques
    Myofascial release
    Muscle energy technique
    Craniosacral technique
    Strain counterstrain technique
Contraindications
Summary

LEARNING OBJECTIVES

After studying this chapter, the reader should be able to:

1. State the criteria used to classify synovial joints.
2. Define the terms *osteokinematics* and *arthrokinematics.*
3. State the convex-concave rule.
4. Describe the laws of vertebral motion.
5. Define and describe what is meant by the term *painful arc.*
6. Define and describe what is meant by the term *capsular pattern.*
7. Define and describe what is meant by the term *end feel.*
8. State the five possible responses to resisted movement testing.
9. List five gradations of oscillations used to objectively grade arthrokinematic (accessory) movement.
10. Describe the contraindications for the use of manual therapy techniques.

KEY TERMS

osteokinematics
arthrokinematics
vertebral motion
assessment

palpation
mobilization
manipulation

In the field of orthopedic physical therapy, manual therapy has rapidly evolved from a set of procedures that used passive mobilization movement techniques or manipulation. It is now a highly specialized yet eclectic system of both evaluation and treatment procedures of the neuromuscular skeletal system aimed primarily at relieving pain, increasing or decreasing mobility, and, in general, normalizing function. This approach to a patient with neuromuscular skeletal dysfunction requires not only clinical knowledge of a variety of philosophical approaches to evaluation and treatment but also skillful application of hands-on techniques in nonsurgical management of spinal and extremity dysfunction. This type of treatment requires continual reassessment and alteration of the techniques in order to optimize recovery to full function.

The actual practice of manual therapy has developed from the many techniques and concepts of numerous clinicians worldwide. Anatomy, biomechanics, and neurophysiology supply the supporting disciplines and theories for these approaches to manual therapy. Research of manual therapy, however, is complicated by a variety of factors:

1. The questionable etiology of musculoskeletal pain
2. Clinical findings rather than knowledge of musculoskeletal pathology often dictate the application of manual therapy techniques
3. The self-limiting nature of musculoskeletal conditions
4. The effect of human behavior and higher degree of bias with manual therapy

Nevertheless, as judged by the testimony of patients and clinicians and anecdotal observations, manual therapy continues to enjoy popularity among orthopedic physical therapists. This chapter is not meant as an instruction manual for specific techniques of any particular approach to manual therapy but rather as a comprehensive overview.

HISTORY OF MANUAL THERAPY

Manual therapy—or the manipulation of soft tissues—is certainly not new to the realm of physical therapy and, in fact, is mentioned quite frequently in ancient medical writings. As early as 460 BC, Hippocrates referred to a number of methods of mobilization in *Corpus Hippocrates* that are quite comparable to manual techniques used today.[1] He referred to the use of traction and immobilization, with the palm of the hand, as a technique for the reduction of fractures.[4] Hippocrates was also one of the first ancient medical practitioners to advocate exercise as a means of strengthening to retard muscle wasting as a result of inactivity.[3] In the second century AD, Galen even went so far as to recommend that an injured part undergo continuous but cautious movement after the application of heat.[2] Galen also gave a description of how to treat "outwardly dislocated" vertebrae. His theories remained unchallenged until the sixteenth century.[33] Movement in the form of graded mobilization, however, was first mentioned by Hippocrates for treatment of a shoulder dislocation. He advocated "rubbing" and gentle motion of the affected joint in order to enhance healing. Movement was also used to loosen a joint that had become stiff.[3,4] Treatment by manipulation and a form of traction using ropes tied to an individual who lay prone on a board were advocated by Ambrose Pare, a well-known physician of the Renaissance.[5] His description of the traction procedure involved stretching the patient from the arms and legs in order to reduce a spinal kyphosis.[33]

Families of bonesetters who practiced the art of manipulation of the limbs and spine in order to set or relocate bones that were out of place were popular in the seventeenth century in England. These bonesetters were especially successful at treating six common types of disorders[33]:

1. Stiff and painful joints that had been immobilized for prolonged periods after fractures, dislocation, or sprains
2. Stiffness and/or pain that resulted from disuse after soft tissue injuries
3. Internal derangements of soft tissues (menisci)
4. Luxation of the smaller bones of the hands and the feet
5. The development of ganglia around the wrist
6. A variety of neck and back disorders

Early medical literature often uses the term *massage* to indicate both soft tissue massage (as known today) and manipulation or mobilization of bone structure. Graham, in the 1800s, stated that massage meant any procedure that was done by the hands, including friction and manipulation.[33] Mennel, in the late eighteenth century, went as far as to define *massage* as a scientific method for treating disease and classified it as scientific manipulation.[2] The confusing multiple meanings of terms such as *massage, manipulation, mobilization,* and *passive range of motion* in the early course of medical history may be one of the factors that led many in orthodox medicine to reject manual therapy as a mainstream treatment approach to musculoskeletal dysfunction.[33]

In the United States, two main categories of manual practitioners developed almost simultaneously in the early eighteenth century. Unfortunately, the competition between these two schools of thought, as well as their advocation that all disease was treatable by manipulation, caused most physicians to disregard manipulation or mobilization as a viable treatment technique of any disorder.[33] Techniques referred to as the practice of osteopathy were introduced in the United States by Andrew Taylor Still in 1871. He maintained that the body as a unit has the inherent ability to fight off all disease. He also maintained that the cause of all disease could be traced to abnormal mechanical pressure upon both blood vessels and nerves that was produced by dislocated or subluxated bones, cartilage, and ligaments and by changes in muscle tension, primarily in the spine.[6,11,31-34] Osteopaths began to refer to the adverse mechanical pressure as an *osteopathic lesion,* and this became the focus of osteopathic manipulation.

In 1895, Daniel David Palmer founded the concept of chiropractic treatment. His concept, similar to that of the osteopaths, was based on malalignments of bones and the ability to realign the bones by using chiropractic manipulation. The chiropractic community basically remains split among two groups: the straights and the mixers. Those who hold to the straight view believe that the mechanical malalignment of bones produces adverse mechanical pressure, primarily on the nerves, and that dysfunction of nervous tissue is responsible for most illnesses. Their adjustments are aimed primarily at restoring nerve function and therefore restoring overall health.[31,33] Mixers view adjustments or manipulation as necessary for treating dysfunction of the spine as well as other structures. They also are amenable to the use of physiotherapeutic and nutritional measures in order to restore health.[31,33] Today the medical profession still reacts negatively to the concept of chiropractic medicine, whose practitioners are not recognized as physicians by the allopathic medical community. Osteopaths, by contrast, have diversified and upgraded their medical education to include pharmacology and even surgery. Osteopaths find themselves aligned with the allopathic medical profession and are recognized as physicians by the allopathic community in all states. Today, in fact, the majority of osteopaths do not practice manipulation on a routine basis but see it as a subspecialty within their own field.[8] Cyriax, a British orthopedist, advocated friction massage, fluid injection, and mobilization with traction, as well as exercise and modalities and patient education, as a system for treating dysfunction of contractile and noncontractile structures. His system of treatment was based largely upon the practitioner's ability to evaluate and differentiate contractile and noncontractile tissues in patients with musculoskeletal pain. The identification of the anatomical structure associated with a "lesion" is one of the key concepts in the evaluation and subsequent application of manual treatment, according to Cyriax.[8]

Mennel developed techniques of manipulation and mobilization utilizing specific joint play techniques to examine the synovial joints and treat joint dysfunction.[8,29,30] Mennel's manipulative techniques of extremities are the most specific to the joint with limited joint "play." The spinal techniques, however, are less specific than those of the extremities.[29] Maigne, a French physician, developed a system based on the two rules of "no pain" and "contrary movement." To relieve the stiffness of a joint and free the joint to have more mobility, he advocated moving it in the direction of the greatest amount of mobility available. He also believed that a painful procedure, such as moving in the direction of least mobility, should be avoided.[25,31]

Maitland developed and popularized the Australian approach to manual therapy, including graded oscillatory movements as a means of evaluation and treatment of joint stiffness in order to restore lost mobility. His approach relies heavily on a detailed subjective examination, using the S.I.N.S. algorithm to assess the severity, irritability, nature, and stage of the complaint associated with the pathology.[8,26,27] *Severity* is the term used to describe the clinician's assessment of the intensity of the patient's symptoms as they are related to a specific functional activity. Functional activities may include dressing, eating, and positions of particular posture. *Irritability* is a term used to describe the response to the clinician's assessment based on the amount of activity needed to bring on the patient's symptoms and the amount of time needed for the patient's symptoms to subside (duration).[8,26,27] The "nature of the complaint" represents the clinician's assessment of the patient's pain tolerance, including consideration of cultural differences, stability of the condition, type of pathology, and the physical therapist's hypothesis of the structures responsible for producing the pain complaint. The "stage of the pathology" describes the clinician's assessment of the patient's progression of symptoms, such as a patient who reports initially having had back pain and now having primarily lower extremity pain radiating into the foot, a different stage of pathology.[8] Maitland also maintains that successful treatment for restoring movement requires continual modification in order to meet the demands of the changing condition, based on the ongoing assessment of the condition with specific oscillatory techniques and utilizing the S.I.N.S. algorithm. Maitland graded his oscillatory techniques on a scale of 1 to 5; they vary in amplitude and frequency to affect the tissue's stability and joint stiffness at a variety of depths (see Fig. 8-6).[26,27]

Kaltenborn, of the Norwegian school of thought, approaches the assessment of joint movement from a more biomechanical model. A key concept to his treatment scheme involves the application of principles from the science of arthrokinematics (e.g., concave-convex, closed-loosely packed positions). He also uses graded oscillatory movements on a scale of 1 to 3, similar to those of Maitland, for the assessment and treatment of joint and soft tissue dysfunction.[17,31] Stanley B. Paris, a New Zealand physiotherapist, has greatly influenced American physical therapists with his teachings. His approach to manual therapy treatment of joint dysfunction is somewhat eclectic. He relies heavily upon Maitland and Kaltenborn. Paris contends that properly examining the spine from a mechanical standpoint for any signs of dysfunction leads to treatment in the early stages and reduces the likelihood of further deterioration, particularly in spinal dysfunction. He also contends that the facet joint is the primary source of pain and hence dysfunction in the spine.[31] Over the past two decades, Paris has probably been most responsible for popularizing manual therapy and creating a greater awareness of the various schools of manual medicine within the physical therapy community.

Paris, in his course notes, has summarized the principal goals shared by the various schools of thought in manual therapy:

1. The relief of nerve root pressure (primarily related to the spine)
   a. Specific action—chiropractic school of thought recommends the movement of one specific vertebrae on another
   b. Nonspecific—Cyriax recommends a more general manipulation with some form of manual traction
2. Relief of pain (further related to the spine but also the extremities)
   a. Graded oscillation—Maitland believes in graded oscillations but subthreshold to the level of pain
   b. Contrary movement—Maigne recommends therapeutic movement of the joint or extremity in the direction opposite to that which induces pain
3. Normalization and restoration of joint mobility (related to the spine or the extremities)
   a. Osteopathy—Those who advocate specific techniques for mobilization of the spine and extremities in order to restore or maintain normal structure and function
   b. Treatments of stiffness—Kaltenborn advocates kinematic principles to regain mobility without regard to pain[31]

CLASSIFICATION OF SYNOVIAL JOINTS

A sound knowledge of functional anatomy is critical to the student of orthopedic manual therapy. The primary structure affected by mobilization or manipulation is the synovial joint. Knowledge of the classification and characteristics of these joints enables visualizing the movement of the joint as various therapeutic techniques are applied to the tissues.

The anatomical synovial joint consists of two articular surfaces, the surrounding tissues (capsules, ligaments), and the interarticular structures. Grieve has suggested that the anatomical synovial joint can also be classified as a physiological joint by including the soft tissue that surrounds the joint (muscles, connective tissue, nerves, and blood vessels).[12,13] Anatomical synovial joints can be classified according to the number of articular surfaces or according to the type of articular surface. Joints that have only one space and two articulating surfaces and a single capsule are classified as *simple*. An example is the metacarpal phalangeal joint.[36] A joint that has a single capsule and two articulating surfaces is classified as *compound*. An example is the elbow.[36] *Complex* joints have a single capsule with meniscoid or intercapsular disk material interposed between two surfaces. An example is the knee.[36]

MacConaill and Basmajian have developed a classification of synovial joints according to their articular surfaces[24] (Fig. 8-1). Four classifications of joint articulating surfaces have been proposed:

1. Any modified ovoid ball and socket articulation in which the surfaces are spheroid, with three axes and 3 degrees of freedom (number of available movements

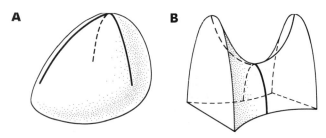

Fig. 8-1. Two basic types of articular surfaces: **A,** ovoid; **B,** sellar.

in cardinal planes). Examples of these articulations are the hip and shoulder joints.
2. Modified ovoid-ellipsoid and sellar articulation, in which the surfaces are convex or concave in all directions. The joints have two axes and allow 2 degrees of freedom. The best examples of a modified ovoid joint are the metacarpal phalangeal joints.
3. Unmodified sellar-saddle articulations, in which the surfaces are convex and concave at right angles to one another. These joints also have two axes and allow 2 degrees of freedom. Unlike the modified ovoid joints, they are usually accompanied by a loose capsule, which allows an easy directional change with movement. The best example of this type of joint is the first carpal-metacarpal joint.
4. Modified sellar ginglymus or trochoid joint, with one axis and 1 degree of freedom. Examples are the interphalangeal joints of the finger and the ulnar humeral joint.[14,36]

OSTEOKINEMATICS AND ARTHROKINEMATICS

Anatomical movements typically describe a gross movement of limbs by muscles through various cardinal planes. These traditional kinesiological terms serve anatomists and biomechanists well but offer little to therapists to describe the small movements in the practice of manual therapy. The term *kinematics* describes the subdivision and classification of movements into the independent movements of bones and joints. Osteokinematics is the study of the movement of bones, and arthrokinematics is the study of the movement of joints.[36]

Osteokinematics

Osteokinematics, or bone movement, involves two motions: spin and swing (Fig. 8-2). Spin is a pure motion, that of rotation around a mechanical axis. This rotation is either clockwise or counterclockwise and is not accompanied by any other type of movement. Such pure spin occurs in the human body only at the head of the femur, humerus, and radius.

Swing is any movement other than pure spin. It can be divided further into pure cardinal swing and impure or arcuate swing. Pure swing moves in a cardinal plane that is not necessarily simultaneous with the spin, and the move-

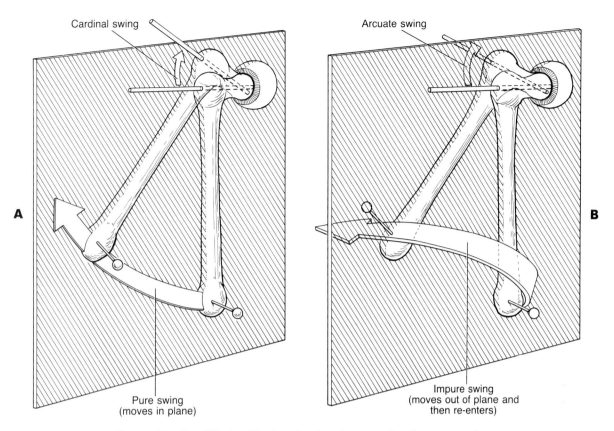

Fig. 8-2. MacConaill's classification of swing: **A,** pure swing; **B,** arcuate swing.

ment therefore traverses the shortest route between two points. Impure or arcuate swing involves swinging and rotation that occur simultaneously, and therefore the distance between two points is greater than in pure swing. Impure swing movement occurs within and outside the cardinal plane.[36]

Arthrokinematics

Accessory movements that take place at a joint are described as arthrokinematic movements. These movements include spin, glide, roll, rotation and translation[36] (Fig. 8-3). The accessory motion of spin involves rotation around a stationary mechanical axis and is similar to the term *spin* used in osteokinematics. Gliding occurs when a point on the resting surface comes in contact with two or more points on another surface. For pure gliding to occur, the two surfaces must be congruent and flat or congruent and curved. Gliding that occurs as an involuntary motion is referred to as *translation* or *translatory glide*.[14] During the anterior drawer test, the tibia is said to translate in an anterior direction or glide on the femur. Rolling occurs when new points on one surface come into contact with new points on a second surface. Unlike glide, this movement requires that the surfaces not be congruent and is most prevalent during joint movement when a convex surface moves on a concave surface.[17]

Rolling and gliding can occur simultaneously, but in the human body they do not necessarily occur in proportion to one another. In the knee, for example, the surfaces are incongruent, and the roll and glide movements that occur during flexion and extension of the knee are a result of both active and passive bone rotations. As the knee begins to flex from full extension, the first 15 degrees of motion involve pure rolling of the medial condyle. Beyond 15 degrees of flexion, the sliding component increases until the end of the range, where pure sliding occurs.[18] Direction of the roll-glide movement truly depends on the convex or concave shape of the surfaces that are moving.

CONCEPTS AND RULES OF JOINT MOTION
Convex-concave rule

All surfaces of a synovial joint have some degree of either convexity or concavity. Where surfaces appear flat, the addition of cartilage often alters the contour, as in the surface of the tibia at the knee joint. The tibia has the addition of the medial and lateral menisci cartilage that is thicker at the perimeters and serves to enhance the concavity of the joint surface as well as control and accommodate movement of medial and lateral condyles of the femur. In general terms, if both surfaces appear to be flat, the larger surface is considered to be the convex surface. In the combination of rolling and gliding movements, the gliding portion of the movement

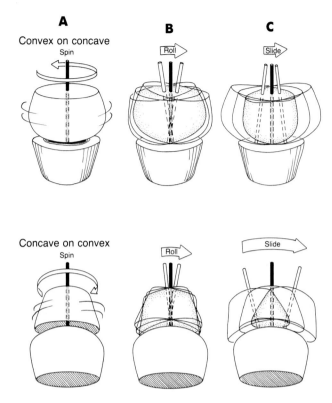

A
Convex on concave
Spin

B
Roll

C
Slide

Concave on convex
Spin

Roll

Slide

Fig. 8-3. MacConaill's classification of accessory movements: **A,** spin; **B,** roll; **C,** glide.

follows a set pattern, depending upon whether the moving surfaces are convex or concave. Kaltenborn has used these concepts to develop the convex-concave rule[17] (Fig. 8-4).

If the concave surface is stationary and the convex surface is moving, the gliding movement in the joint occurs in a direction opposite that of the bone movement. This difference is due to the axis of rotation always being maintained on the convex bone. For instance, during manual therapy techniques aimed at increasing the range of motion of flexion in a hypomobile glenohumeral joint, the therapist moves the head of the humerus in a caudal or downward direction against the fixed glenoid fossa while inducing flexion of the humerus. If the convex surface is to remain stationary and the concave surface becomes the moving surface, however, the gliding motion of the joint occurs in the same direction as the movement of the bone. Such is the case in the knee joint when the patient is sitting and the therapist is using manual techniques. To increase flexion, the therapist moves the proximal tibia in a posterior direction, while the distal tibia is also moving in a posterior direction.

Positions of joint congruency

In active physiological movement, often very little of the two joint surfaces is in complete contact, and the surrounding capsule of the joint is in a "loose state." Other instances of active movement show much greater congruence and more contact between the two surfaces of the joint, and the

capsule is in a "tighter state." Knowledge of positions of joint "looseness" or "tightness" is helpful to manual therapists for examining and treating pathology.

McConaill and Basmajian have described both the loose and tight positions of the joint in detail[24] (Fig. 8-5). A tight-joint is in the close-packed position; it occurs when the joint surfaces are at the maximum congruence. Close-packed positions minimize the intracapsular space, tighten major ligaments, and resist the pulling apart of the surfaces by nominal traction forces. The close-packed position restricts all degrees of freedom of movement in the joint during active movement. Therefore, the close-packed position is not the position of choice for mobilization or manual therapy techniques. However, the close-packed position does enable the examiner to assess pain and damage to the articular surfaces, ligament stability, and any internal derangement of cartilage or meniscus. An example of close-packed testing is the varus/valgus test for ligamentous instability with the knee held in extension. In most joints, including the knee joint, the interphalangeal joints, and the elbow joint with the forearm supinated, the closed-packed position is a position of full extension. Any other position of the joint that is not the close-packed position is a loose-packed position.

All joints have points of minimal tension or a maximal loose-packed position. The loose-packed position is the resting position of the joint. In the resting or loose-packed position of the joint, the surrounding tissues are as lax as possible, and the intracapsular space is at its greatest. Joint trauma and subsequent articular effusion of a joint most likely cause a patient to allow the joint to assume the loose-packed position, which allows for maximum fluid accumulation within the joint. For the manual therapist, the maximal loose-packed position or resting position is the optimal position for treatment utilizing joint mobilization techniques. Therapists may also utilize the loose-packed position to test the joint for roughness of articular surfaces and to assess the mobility or extensibility of the capsule by stretching the capsule in various directions. In the knee, the maximal loose-packed position is about 30 degrees of flexion with slight external rotation of the tibia. Kaltenborn has described all joint resting or loose-packed positions.[17] Understanding arthrokinematic and osteokinematic movements lays the framework for understanding the more complex active and passive joint movements that occur at isolated joints (as in the extremities) or at two or more joints (as in the spine).

Laws of vertebral motion

As a result of the nature of the anatomical relationships, as well as the relationship of the supporting structure (muscles, ligaments, vertebral disk, facet joints), movement of the spine does not normally occur between only two vertebrae. Rather, movement at the spine usually is described as movement of a basic functional unit, the spinal segment. The spinal segment is composed of typically three (but as

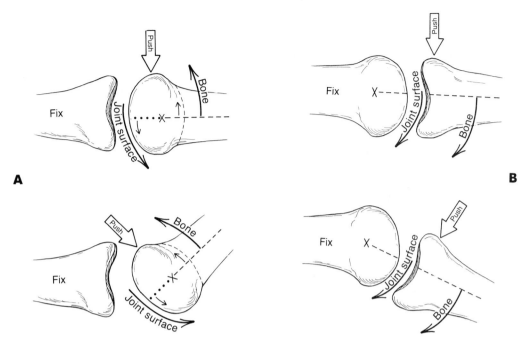

Fig. 8-4. A, Convex surface moving on concave surface. **B,** Concave surface moving on convex surface with a combination of roll, spin, and glide occurring in both simultaneously.

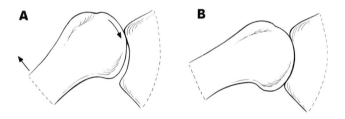

Fig. 8-5. The congruence of articular surfaces: **A,** loose-packed position; **B,** close-packed position.

many as five) sequential vertebrae.[31] A spinal segment typically acts as one moving unit, each vertebra contributing to the total motion, with varying degrees of movement occurring at each facet joint.

Within the spine, forward and backward bending in the sagittal plane is referred to as *pure* movement; that is, these two movements can take place without the imposition of any secondary movement (i.e., side bending).[31] However, in the spine the movements of rotation and side bending are referred to as combined or component movements because they cannot take place alone under normal circumstances and must always occur in combination. Hence, it is not possible to side-bend the spine without some degree of rotation within the spinal segment, nor is it possible to rotate the spine without having some degree of side bending occurring within the spinal segment.[31] Initial rotation of the head appears as pure rotation; as the patient actively moves into the range of rotation, however, close observation reveals

some degree of side bending in the same direction as the rotation of the head. These minor component motions in the spine occur because of the mechanical laws that affect spinal movement. These mechanical laws and the manner in which the combined movements take place are largely determined by the orientation of the facet joints in the spine.

Understanding the basic laws of spinal motion is critical for applying manual therapy techniques to spinal segments, for assessing pathology, and for grading dysfunction at individual or groups of spinal segments. As described by Paris, the rules of spinal motion are as follows:

1. Cervical spine: rotation and side bending of the vertebrae take place to the same side.
2. Thoracic and lumbar spine: rotation and side bending of the vertebrae take place to opposite sides.
3. Lumbar and thoracic spine: rotation and side bending of the vertebrae take place to the opposite side when the movements occur in the upright posture, but to the same side when the movement occurs in the flexed spine.
4. When any region of the spine is in neutral (neither flexed or extended), it must be side-bent before it can be rotated.
5. When any region of the spine is in extension, it must be rotated before it can be side-bent.[31]

The osteopathic physician Fryette developed three laws of spinal motion. He arrived at these laws from observations of patients with scoliosis and from Lovett's earlier biomechanical work.[11] These three laws are generally applicable to all areas of the spine and describe three types of vertebral motion.

Type I (Law I). When the spine is in neutral (no flexion or extension) and the facets are "idling" without the influence of ligamentous tension, rotation of the vertebrae always takes place opposite the direction of any side bending of the spine.

Type II (Law II). When the spine is in extension or nearly full flexion, the facets are in control; the vertebrae are under the influence of ligamentous tension and rotate toward the side to which side bending occurs.

Type III (Law III). If movement is introduced into a spinal segment in any one plane, the range of motion available in the other two planes is reduced. For instance, the patient who is sitting erect has more available range of motion in rotation than the patient who is sitting in the flexed position. In this instance, the flexion of the lumbar spine reduces the available range of motion for rotation to occur in the lumbar spine.

In the cervical spine, according to Fryette, the second law always applies in the typical cervical joint, where the facets are bearing the weight of the head and the facets are therefore always engaged. At the atlantoaxial joint, where the motion is almost all rotation and the facet orientation is quite different, however, the concepts of the second law of cervical motion do not apply. Likewise, at the occipitoatlanto joint, the facets are set at an angle to each other so that any little amount of side bending that takes place must always be accompanied by an even smaller amount of rotation of the atlas in the opposite direction. In the thoracic and lumbar spine, the first law applies. The second law has also been shown to apply to the thoracic region, but in the lumbar spine it has not been shown to apply with respect to the motion of full extension.[11] Rotation in positions of full extension of the spine does not always occur toward the side of the side bend in the lumbar spine.

Fryette's laws are key concepts to the application of the principles of osteopathic manipulative treatment, as specific facet dysfunctions are named according to the type of vertebral motion (type I, type II) that occurs as determined by palpation and motion testing throughout the spine. The types of dysfunction are named for the position of the vertebrae in question. For example, the dysfunction of a single vertebra in the lumbar spine may be said to be in a position of flexion, side bending, and rotation to the right, obeying Fryette's second law of vertebral motion and hence a type II lesion to the vertebrae[5,11] (Fig. 8-6 and 8-7).

Barriers to movement

Active movements of the joint, or movements produced by voluntary control, are the result of the activity of muscles surrounding the joint. Passive movement, or involuntary movement of a joint, is induced by an external force. Although most joints have more than one plane of motion, each plane of motion is constrained to movement within limits of motion. For efficient movement in a joint in any one plane of motion, there must be anatomical limits to motion provided by bone muscles, ligaments, or fascia. These limits

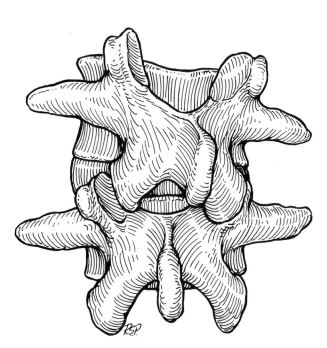

Fig. 8-6. Type II dysfunction (Fryette): Right facet is closed; superior vertebra is extended, rotated, and sidebent to the right.

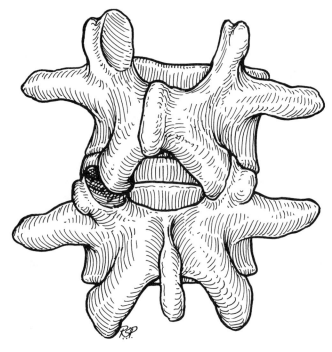

Fig. 8-7. Type II dysfunction (Fryette): Left facet is open; superior vertebra is flexed, rotated, and sidebent to the right.

to extreme motion provide stability and structure to the joint. When motion exceeds the boundaries of these anatomical barriers, injury occurs to the tissues in the form of fracture, dislocation, or the disruption of ligaments and other supporting tissue structures.

Between these boundaries of anatomical motion is the range of both active and passive available motion that is produced by muscles acting upon the joint (active) or by an external force (passive). The limits of passive motion can be described as a elastic barrier to motion. As the resting tension to soft tissue structures increases with passive movement, the potential space between the anatomical limits of motion and the end range of passive motion becomes an elastic barrier. Any further passive movement beyond the elastic barrier results in deformation of connective tissue. In normal tissues, the amount of available active movement is equal to or slightly less than the total amount of passive movement. Active motion is limited by physiologic barriers provided by the normal resilience and tension in the soft tissues

surrounding the joint. The space between the elastic and physiologic barriers is equal to the difference between the amount of passive and active motion available in the joint.

The amount of available range for active motion in a joint can be reduced by tightening of soft tissue fascia and an increase in connective tissue to form a restrictive barrier that limits the amount of active movement, usually in one direction of the plane of movement. The goal of manual therapy, therefore, is to attempt to restore the available active range of motion by removing this pathological restrictive barrier and reestablishing the amount of motion available in that particular plane of movement. Restrictive barriers may be in the form of myofascial shortening, muscle spasm, tissue fibrosis, or edema[11] (Fig. 8-8).

In physical therapy, restoring active range of movement to a joint that has lost movement in one or more planes typically involves using some form of passive range of motion. The method of applying the passive range of motion depends on what types of tissues are restricting normal active

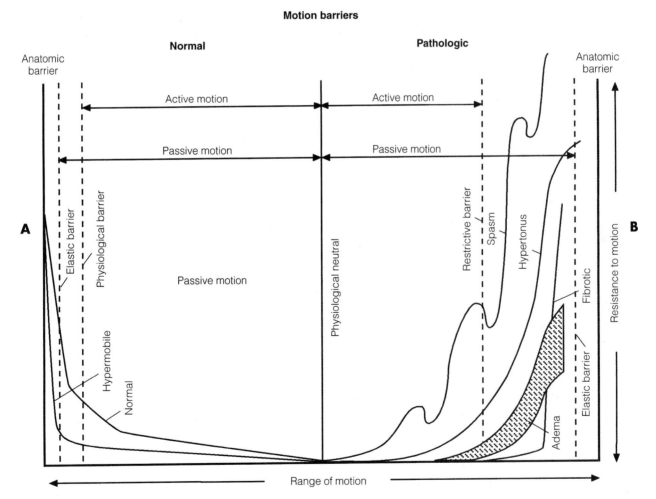

Fig. 8-8. A, Physiologic barrier limiting active motion and elastic barrier limiting passive motion in normal tissue. **B,** Restrictive barrier limiting active motion and elastic barrier limiting passive motion in tissue with underlying pathology. Note that tissue dysfunction has a decreasing effect on the available active range of movement.

motion. For example, if the tissue providing the barrier to normal active motion is muscular (in the form of muscle tightness), then muscle-stretching techniques would reduce the restrictive (muscular) barrier. If, as many contend, the barrier to joint motion results from a pathological abundance of connective tissue (e.g., frozen shoulder), however, then the use of a sustained stretch may not be indicated, as it may overstimulate the pain receptors and cause a reflexive contraction of muscles that is antagonistic to the desired increase in direction of range of motion. This contraction of muscles would not allow the therapist to restore full motion and would not reduce the connective tissue restrictive barrier in order to achieve full active motion.

MANUAL METHODS FOR ASSESSING JOINT DYSFUNCTION
Selective tissue assessment

Although manual therapy approaches are based on a variety of different philosophies, they all seem to share the common dimension of some form of systemic evaluation scheme that ultimately leads the manual therapy practitioner to a decision about the particular implementation of manual intervention in the treatment of musculoskeletal dysfunction.[8] The development of specific evaluation techniques that localize tissues or structures that require the use of manual therapy skills has been one of the greatest benefits of the increased interest in orthopedic manual therapy by physical therapists in North America. By adopting a systematic evaluation scheme and investigating dysfunction by way of clinical reasoning and decision making, the ultimate goal of understanding the cause of the dysfunction can be based on the interpretation of findings during the evaluation. Therapists involved in orthopedic manual physical therapy are continually challenged to develop the technical skills needed to perform manual therapy techniques. Manual therapists are further challenged to utilize the analytical skills needed to solve problems and ultimately arrive at a deliberate and specific intervention.

Contractile and noncontractile elements

The basis of the differentiation of tissue is division of soft tissue into contractile and noncontractile elements. As defined by Cyriax, contractile elements are tissues that originate in muscle, tendon, and tendon-bone interface at tendinous insertions.[6,7] Labeling dysfunctional tissue as a contractile element requires selective assessment of the structure involved through manual isometric testing. Isometric manual muscle testing that is normally used to identify weakened muscle tissue may also help to differentiate dysfunctional tissue by a response of pain, weakness, or both when the tissues are tested in the midrange position. When a structure is found to produce pain or weakness with isometric testing, the practitioner may further attempt to isolate the structure with specific palpation and special tests.

Noncontractile elements are tissues other than contractile

tissues that may also give rise to pain, including bone, nerve, ligaments, bursa, fascia, and dura. Dysfunctional noncontractile tissue may give rise to pain with stretching, tapping, or pinching. Contraction of muscle may also be a source of irritation to underlying noncontractile tissue if inflammation is present. The examiner must persist with specific tests and palpation, as well as consideration of all signs and symptoms, in order to differentiate contractile and noncontractile elements.

Systematic evaluation techniques

In general, the selective examination of specific tissues that may or may not be involved in musculoskeletal dysfunction can be broken down into testing for painful arcs, capsular patterns, end feels, and resisted movement.

Painful arcs. Active range of motion on a gross scale gives the therapist good indication of the quantity and quality of movement that the patient is able to produce with regard to the amount and limitation of pain that is a result of the dysfunction. As the patient performs specific active range of movement in specific planes of motion, the therapist can note the amount of pain that may occur at different points in the range of motion. Pain that occurs at one point in the range of motion but disappears at other points in the range of motion is said to occur in a "painful arc."[6] Cyriax contends that painful arcs occur because of the pinching of tissue, usually bone approximating bone with some tissue interposed. Painful pinching that occurs at a joint with normal joint motion is not considered normal; it may be the result of a biomechanical fault leading to abnormal osteokinetic movement, or it may be the result of hypertrophy of the tissue that is interposed between the two bony surfaces, for example, a rotator cuff injury. In the shoulder, the irritated rotator cuff muscle may be hypertrophied and becomes impinged between the head of the humerus and the acromion during an arc of motion as the arm undergoes abduction, flexion, or a combination of abduction, flexion, and rotation. Cyriax further claims he is a able to delineate the specific site where a structure may have a "lesion" by associating the specific site with a specific painful arc of motion. Painful arcs have also been noted to occur with passive movements.

Painful arcs may occur in both the extremities and the spine. McKenzie has proposed a classification of spinal derangement based on active movement examination and pain associated with different points during the movement, particularly spinal flexion and extension.[28] Pain at the extreme end range of a movement may be attributed to different causes, depending upon the specific movement pattern as well as the specific structure that is thought to be stressed during the movement. The structures include ligaments, tendons, and bursae. In the spine, however, pain that is associated with straightforward flexion may be rooted in stressing of a variety of tissues, including facet joint capsules, longitudinal ligaments, spinal musculature, posterior lateral protrusion of an intervertebral disk, or specific nerve roots. Pain may be localized to a specific area of the spine or may also be referred into the extremities with flexion movements. The movement of spinal extension may also produce pain that originates from a number of structures, including the anterior longitudinal ligament, bulging intervertebral disk, facet joints, and torn or irritated connective tissue anterior to the spine. The spine can also be stressed by the examiner with both side-bending and rotational movements in order to further delineate these specific structures that may be involved in producing the pain.[28]

Capsular patterns. According to Cyriax, passive range of motion is used to assess the amount of motion available, the amount and direction of any limitation of motion, and a sense of the quality of resistance to movement that the examiner feels when reaching the end point of a particular movement (the end feel).[6,8]

The sensation of a limitation of movement of a synovial joint when it is examined with active or passive movement can be helpful in determining the presence or absence of a capsular pattern. The capsular pattern is a joint-specific pattern of movement restriction that indicates involvement of the entire joint capsule. A noncapsular pattern deviates from the specific capsular pattern and can indicate the presence of a ligamentous or partial capsular adhesion, extraarticular tissue involvement, or internal derangements.[6] Cyriax contends that limitations in movement that follow a noncapsular pattern point to three possible extracapsular conditions that may be responsible for the dysfunction:

1. Ligamentous or partial capsular adhesions. Usually one movement is limited. Pain may or may not be present at the end of the range.
2. Extraarticular tissue involvement. Adhesions of structures outside the joint produce pain when stressed but do not produce pain with movements that do not stress that particular structure.
3. Internal derangement. Pain and limited motion caused by a loose structure within the joint. There is usually a history of recurrent sudden blocking of motion with localized joint pain.

End feels. The palpable sensation at the end of passive motion, known as *end feel,* is an assessment of the quality of resistance to movement that the examiner feels when reaching the end point of a particular passive movement. Cyriax proposes four "normal" end feels and four "abnormal" end feels.

Normal end feels

1. Capsular—"leathery" sensation of movement that occurs at the end of normal passive movement.
2. Bony—the abrupt stopping of normal movement that typically occurs without pain, such as extending the elbow to full extension. This may occur with a restriction before the end of movement, as in the case of heterotopic bone changes (e.g., degenerative joint disease or healing fractures).
3. Soft tissue approximation—a soft end feel produced by soft tissues approximating each other, as in elbow flexion or knee flexion.
4. Muscular—an elastic, reflexive sensation that occurs when muscular tightness limits normal full passive range of motion of a joint, as is the case with a straight leg raise and tightness of the hamstrings.

Abnormal end feels

1. Muscle spasm—when the movement stops abruptly with a rebound or muscle contraction to prevent further movement, usually accompanied with pain at the point of restriction.
2. Boggy—a soft, mushy type of end feel typically accompanies joint effusion and may even be present in the absence of significant synovial inflammation.
3. Internal derangement—a springy or rebound end feel. Typically it accompanies a noncapsular restriction produced by a cartilaginous or loose body blocking the motion of the joint, such as a torn meniscus in the knee.
4. Empty or loose—gives the examiner the sensation that the movement could continue without restriction, but the movement is typically stopped by the insistence of the patient because of severe pain. This end feel is rare but usually indicates significant pathology, such as rheumatoid arthritis or joint neoplasm.[6,19]

Resisted movements. Another significant aspect of Cyriax's selective tissue examination is assessment of the patient's ability to resist specific movements. He believes that this part of the examination gives the therapist information concerning the irritability or state of the inflammatory process in tissues, particularly the contractile elements of soft tissues, muscle, tendon, bone, and musculotendinous junctions. The tests require isometric contraction against manual resistance provided by the therapist, with the joint held in a midrange position. They are typically performed to gain selective information about one muscle or a very small group of muscles. Cyriax classifies responses to resisted movement testing in five categories:

1. Strong and painful. A minor lesion of the muscle or tendon is suspected; usually the tendon is involved (typically tendinitis or a mild first-degree strain.)
2. Strong and painless. No lesion or neurological deficit is noted in the muscle or tendon tested.
3. Weak and painful. This response indicates a partial rupture of the muscle or tendon with some fibers still intact. It may also indicate inhibition associated with severe pain produced by serious pathology, such as fracture, neoplasm, or a very acute inflammatory condition.

4. Weak and painless. This response may indicate a disruption of nerve supply to the muscle being tested. It often also indicates a complete rupture of a muscle or tendon with no fibers left intact from which pain can be elicited.

5. All muscles about a particular joint are painful. This response is not typical and may indicate an emotional or serious psychological problem. It may also be an ominous sign of serious underlying pathology.[6,19]

Until recently, the construct validity of this form of passive motion testing for selective tissues was not researched or questioned in orthopedic manual therapy. Recently, however, Hayes and colleagues examined the construct validity and test-retest reliability of the passive motion component of Cyriax's soft tissue diagnosis system. The subjects were 79 patients with a known history of osteoarthritis of the knee. Using four manual therapists as examiners, the investigators found poor reliability for end-feel and pain-resisted sequence testing among subjects. Also, very few subjects exhibited true capsular patterns as defined by Cyriax. The findings suggest that more investigation of selective tissue tension testing is needed to improve reliability and examine the validity of this type of evaluation scheme for orthopedic conditions.[15]

PALPATION TECHNIQUES

Critical to physical examination of patients in orthopedic medicine is the skill of palpation. In a gross sense, palpation reveals information about the integrity of skin, muscle, tendon, ligament, bone, and joint structures. In the realm of orthopedic manual physical therapy, palpation allows the examiner to assess the integrity of these structures in a more detailed manner and reveal subtle changes that gross palpation often overlooks. There is a direct relationship between the examiner's level of palpation skills and the ability to detect the following:

1. Changes in tissue texture
2. Asymmetry of position, in regard to joints or bony structure
3. Differences in mobility of structures throughout the total range of motion, the quality of the movement, and the end feel
4. A three-dimensional sense of position in space
5. Reassessment of improvement or lack of improvement in a patient's condition with respect to manual treatment intervention

The osteopathic school of thought has utilized the concept of establishing and utilizing eye dominance as a critical tool for accurate visual discrimination with palpation. Philip Greenman suggests the following technique for determining eye dominance:

1. Both arms are extended, and a small circle is formed with the thumb and index finger of each hand.
2. With both eyes open, the examiner sights through the circle formed, focusing on a fixed object across the room. The circle is made as small as possible but large enough to contain the object.
3. The examiner closes his or her left eye only. If the object seen remains contained within the circle, then the examiner is said to be right eye dominant. If the object is no longer seen contained within the circle, the examiner is said to be left eye dominant.
4. The procedure is repeated by closing the right eye first, and the differences are noted.[11]

Examining with the dominant eye is important in assessing symmetry between two anatomical structures. For example, to assess symmetry of the pelvis with the patient in the supine position, a right eye–dominant examiner should stand on the right side of the patient's body and face the patient. The examiner's right thumb should be on the patient's left anterior superior iliac spine (ASIS) and the left thumb on the patient's right ASIS. The examiner's dominant right eye is focused in the midline between the right and left thumbs. The examiner's eyes must be kept at the level of both ASISes, and in the same plane as the examiner's thumbs.

Different aspects of the hand can be utilized for palpating different structures. The palms of the hands are best suited for palpating extensive contour. The dorsal aspect of the hand is usually more sensitive to temperature variations. The finger pads of the hand are best utilized for palpation of textural differences. The tip of the thumb is particularly useful as a probe for assessing depth of structures. The pisiform bone can be utilized as an instrument for assessing "spring" and end feel, particularly at the vertebral joints.[11,31] Each therapist must develop the ability to utilize each of these points of manual contact in the hand.

As palpation and manual therapy involve the assessment of subtle changes in tissue, the manual therapist also has to be able to differentiate the relationship between various layers of tissue with palpation. Typically, differences in tissue layers are easiest to assess by palpating from the most superficial layer to the deepest structures. The integrity of the tissue at each layer can best be palpated in the following order:

1. Superficial skin. The examiner assesses warmth or coolness, roughness or smoothness, wetness or dryness, color, and thinness or thickness of the outermost layer.
2. Subcutaneous fascia. Here, gentle movement enables assessment of the mobility of the subcutaneous fascia, as well as thickness or thinness, and the integrity of vessels, arteries, veins, and even superficial nerves.

3. Deep fascia. Here the examiner looks for smoothness, firmness, and a continuous sense of the fascial layers by deeper pressure and gentle movements. A sense of the division of muscle tissue by fascial bundles is also obtained with palpation in this layer.
4. Underlying muscle. The examiner accesses the direction of the muscle fibers, the resting state of the muscle tissue, the presence or absence of hematoma, muscle integrity, and the ability of the muscle fiber to contract or relax with the active contraction and relaxation of the muscle by the patient.
5. Musculotendinous junction. Here the examiner palpates for the smoothness transition between muscle and tendon and for the integrity of the musculotendinous junction.
6. Tendon. The examiner palpates for smoothness, roundness, and integrity or firmness of the tendon. "Popping" and/or crepitation may be palpated with the patient's contraction and relaxation of the musculotendinous unit.
7. Ligamentous structure. The examiner may be able to palpate superficial ligamentous structures, especially at the peripheral joints. The examiner who palpates the entire length of the ligament for integrity may be able to appreciate the firmness and thickness of the ligament.
8. Bone. The examiner may be able to appreciate the smoothness of the surface of the bone as well as the general contours of the bone.
9. Joint space. The examiner palpates the joint space and is able to access increased tension in the joint capsule as well as possible displacement of cartilaginous tissues within the joint, such as the meniscus of the knee.

The best method for beginning manual therapists to improve their palpatory skills is repetitive palpation of all these tissue layers in asymptomatic subjects. In this way the therapist can develop a sense of what is normal for each structure. Only familiarity with the sensation of normal tissues enables appreciation of the subtle changes that reveal abnormal tissue changes in patients.

Another exercise in developing palpation skill requires having a friend hide a single human hair somewhere between two pieces of notebook paper. The examiner then palpates and attempts to locate the hair through the top layer of notebook paper. The skill of the examiner can be further challenged by repeating the exercise with more pages of notebook paper on top of the hair.

Manual therapists also use palpation to access normal and abnormal movement in tissue structures, particularly movement of joints. The examiner's ability to appreciate both the quality and quantity of movement and to correlate it to other palpatory findings is enhanced by the examiner's movement,

both active and passive, at the joint level. Abnormal movement at the joint level is classified as hypermobility or hypomobility. Hypermobility indicates excessive joint movement. The amount of increase in motion ranges from slight to unstable. Hypomobility refers to a loss of joint motion and therefore a limitation of mobility at the joint segment. Hypomobility may range from a minimal loss of joint motion, which may be normal for certain individuals, to a considerable or even complete loss of joint motion, which may be indicative of underlying pathology. Paris has developed the following grading scale of mobility with passive movement:

0—Ankylosis
1—Considerable limitation in movement
2—Slight limitation in movement
3—Normal or minimal limitation in movement
4—Slight increase in motion
5—Considerable increase in motion
6—Unstable[31]

The degree of joint hypermobility or hypomobility varies throughout the normal population, and the assessment of hypermobility or hypomobility alone may or may not correlate with other examination findings, including pain. Likewise, hypermobile joint segments rather than hypomobile joint segments may be the areas producing symptoms. The manual practitioner must take care to avoid utilizing manual therapy techniques that may increase the pathologic mobility of a hypermobile segment, especially in vertebral segments, where relatively hypermobile segments are next to hypomobile segments; the hypermobile segments compensate for the lack of mobility in the surrounding hypomobile segments. This condition is referred to as *compensatory hypermobility.*[11]

TRADITIONAL MANUAL TREATMENT TECHNIQUES

The specific treatment techniques manual therapy practitioners use vary greatly. One common underlying premise of nearly all traditional schools of manual therapy is that loss of mobility leads to dysfunction. On this base a framework of various manipulative and mobilization techniques is structured. In the realm of manual medicine, manipulation or mobilization of the skeletal system is aimed primarily at restoring lost mobility and relieving pain. Manual techniques aimed at affecting the skeletal system are seen as traditional, whereas soft tissue techniques are often referred to as nontraditional.

Manipulation/mobilization

One of the more "traditional" manipulative orthopedic practitioners was James Cyriax. His techniques are based largely on the identification of the exact contractile or noncontractile structure responsible for pain. He advocates heat and friction massage for contractile structures (such as strained tendon) and forceful manipulation with the application of manual distraction to treat intraarticular displacements. The object of his manipulation is restoration of full painless movement, and the treatments are discontinued once the maximum benefit has been achieved. He also advocates reexamination after each manipulation. The number of manipulative treatments varies according to the structure and the amount of dysfunction. However, he states that most intraarticular dysfunction requires no more than four treatment sessions.[6,7]

Kaltenborn believes that a joint restriction should be treated even if it is asymptomatic. He believes that over time a stiff and hypomobile joint leads to the hypermobility of other structures and places more strain on these structures, which eventually become symptomatic. He advocates the manipulation of hypomobile segments as a preventive measure.

Manipulative techniques may indeed provide for small increases in osteokinematic movements and a temporary reduction in pain. However, some practitioners believe that they may not achieve the desired effect of overcoming the restrictive barrier at the joint level. Accessory movement techniques are, by contrast, smaller passive techniques that are more controlled and measured in terms of millimeters of movement. These accessory techniques are aimed at creating increases in movement between the joint articular surfaces. The accessory movements these smaller and more controlled forces produce do not occur automatically with active motion, but they are components of joint motion that must occur to produce most active and passive motion at the joint. Accessory movements are often described in arthrokinematic terms such as *glide, spin,* and *roll,* which have been discussed previously (see Fig. 8-3). A manual therapist's application of accessory movements is a safer method of overcoming barriers to resistance to passive range of motion with less pain caused per degree of range of motion gained.[32] These techniques primarily address tight articular structures (Table 8-1). Maitland identified five gradations of oscillations that grade accessory movement more objectively (Fig. 8-9):

Grade I—small-amplitude movement conducted from the beginning to the available range of motion
Grade II—large-amplitude movement conducted within the range but not to the end of the range of the movement available
Grade III—large-amplitude movement that does reach the end of the available motion
Grade IV—movements of very small amplitude that are conducted at the very end of the range of motion
Grade V—the high-velocity thrust of very small amplitude at the end of the available range of motion but within the anatomical range—that is, beyond the physiological and elastic barrier but within the range of the anatomical barrier

Grade V mobilization (actually a manipulation) is typically referred to as a manipulation or high-velocity, low-amplitude manipulative thrust. This thrust technique is most often associated with the pop or crack sound that may

Table 8-1. Comparison of accessory and physiological movement

Accessory movement techniques	Physiological movement techniques
Used when primary resistance is encountered from the ligment and capsule of the joint and there is minimal muscular resistance	Used when primary resistance encountered is muscular
Can be done in any part of the physiological range of motion	Is effective only at the end of the physiological range of motion
Can be done in any direction (posteriorly, caudally, or anteriorly)	Is limited to one direction
Causes less pain per degree of range of motion gained	Causes more pain per degree of range of motion gained
Used for tight articular structures	Used for tight muscular structures
Is a safer method because it employs short lever-arm techniques	Is a less safe method because it employs long lever-arm techniques

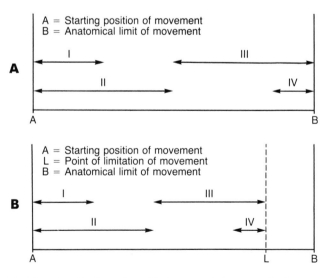

Fig. 8-9. A, Grades of oscillations used in manual therapy. **B,** Grades of oscillations used in manual therapy in relation to a joint with limited motion.

or may not occur during the manipulation.[31] The source of the sound that often occurs with a grade V manipulation is the subject of much debate among manual therapy practitioners of all disciplines. Hypotheses include actual movement of displaced bones or joint surfaces that are unlocking, a reduction in the vacuum seal that is produced by breaking the synovial fluid seal between two facet joint surfaces, and the actual tearing of connective tissue.[39] Maitland has advocated these graded oscillatory techniques for reducing both pain and stiffness.[26,27] He feels that Grades I and II oscillatory movements are more effective in reducing pain via stimulation of joint mechanoreceptors. Korr and Wyke performed research on joint mechanoreceptors and pain to support this theory.[28,32] Maitland believes that pain must be treated prior to stiffness. The pain is diminished with the application of Grades I and II oscillatory techniques; the manual therapist may apply grades III and IV techniques in order to correct problems of stiffness. Maitland also believes that asymptomatic stiffness should not be treated unless symptoms recur and these symptoms are correlated to the hypermobile area.[26] Paris has adopted a similar approach to oscillatory techniques and, in some instances, advocates classification of the disorder into one of five stages:

Stage I—Immediate (up to 30 minutes following the onset of the symptoms). Paris advocates self-mobilization in the grade III range or manual traction combined with skilled manipulation in the case of facet block.
Stage II—The acute stage (from 30 minutes to a few days). He advocates oscillations and manual traction in the grade I range, as well as positional distraction with the aim of eliminating muscle guarding and pain, while maintaining mobility and a goal of restoring function.
Stage III—The subacute stage (following the initial onset, when motion has improved and symptoms have decreased but return to the acute stage is probable without intervention). He advocates grade I and II oscillations, positional distraction, and rhythmic manual traction. The goal here is further removal of muscle guarding, maintaining range of motion with function, and hastening repair of damaged tissues.
Stage IV—The settled stage (relatively high tolerance to any residual pain with minimal or no muscle guarding). If blockage of movement remains, he advocates stretch or thrust procedures that may or may not be combined with oscillations. The aim is to restore full mobility and function and to prevent recurrences.
Stage V—The chronic stage may be after several years of suffering and the failure of sound conservative management. He advocates a more cautious approach with treatment techniques based on a meticulous assessment of a dysfunction. He adds that the prognosis is not good for most patients who are allowed to reach this stage.[31]

In contrast to Paris and Maitland, Robert Maigne believes in no pain and free movement.[25] His technique involves positioning joints in direct opposition to positions that increase pain or demonstrate restriction. This technique focuses on the interrelationship of structure and function in the body and the tendency toward "self-regulation." The practitioner using this technique is attempting to put the joint at ease by putting it in a position of less restriction. The hypothesis is that restoration of the proper afferent signals to the central nervous system returns the neurological traffic in the spinal cord segment to a more normal level and elicits a more normal neurological response. These techniques are based on a common neurological model in which the reduction of the flow of abnormal afferent impulses into the central nervous system reprograms the "central computer" to allow more normal function.[11] This type of approach is not without controversy; little research and few controlled clinical studies support such theories.

NONTRADITIONAL MANUAL TECHNIQUES

The majority of the nontraditional approaches to musculoskeletal dysfunction have been developed by osteopathic manual practitioners. Osteopathic manipulative treatment is based on the diagnosis of a structural dysfunction in the presence of—and associated with—significant somatic dysfunction. *Somatic dysfunction* is defined as impaired or altered function of related components of the somatic (body framework) system; skeletal, arthrodial, and myofascial structures; and related vascular, lymphatic, and neural elements. Somatic dysfunction is diagnosed by the presence of three criteria:

1. Asymmetry of the related parts of musculoskeletal system, either structurally or functionally
2. Range of motion abnormality, or alteration of joint range of motion, in the form of either increased or decreased mobility
3. Tissue texture abnormality, that is, an alteration in the characteristics of the soft tissues of the musculoskeletal system (skin, fascia, muscle, ligaments)[11]

The diagnosis of structural dysfunction is made from the presence of one or more of these criteria. The appropriate prescription for manual intervention is made with the goals of achieving postural balance and maximal painless movement of the musculoskeletal system. Osteopaths believe that achieving this goal results in overall balance of the somatic system.

Myofascial release

Soft tissue procedures, according to osteopaths, are those directed toward tissues other than the skeleton; the responses are monitored with diagnostic palpation skills. These procedures are described in relation to muscle fiber direction. They are aimed at affecting skin and the subcutaneous fascia, as well as the deep fascia surrounding the muscle. Often referred to as *myofascial release,* treatment is aimed at relieving barriers of soft tissue and fascia that may be the cause of abnormal dysfunction due to postural reflex and other changes. Osteopaths contend that myofascial barriers may have mechanical, circulatory, and neurological effects on the patient in both acute and chronic conditions. These procedures also encourage the circulation of fluid in and around the soft tissues to enhance venous and lymphatic systems and aid in decongesting areas of fluid stasis. Myofascial release techniques include lateral stretching, longitudinal stretching, separation of origin insertion, and deep pressure. Myofascial techniques are not without controversy, as research and clinical trials on the efficacy of such techniques are nearly nonexistent. Adding to the skepticism, some practitioners have sought to exploit and sensationalize their results. Others classify this approach as a form of emotional "healing," although this claim, too, has yet to be validated through research.

Muscle energy technique

Many physical therapists are familiar with "contract-relax" muscle-stretching techniques, which are typically used in conjunction with passive stretching of large muscle groups. On a much more specific and smaller scale, muscle energy technique relies upon postisometric agonist relaxation and reciprocal antagonist inhibition to aid the manual practitioner in overcoming restrictive barriers to joint movement. The term *muscle energy* is that of Fred L. Mitchell, who originally developed a series of contract-relax techniques to treat sacral and pelvis motion restrictions. He eventually developed a series of muscle energy techniques for treatment of the entire musculoskeletal system.[5] Using Fryette's laws of spinal motion, the practitioner of muscle energy technique first identifies the barriers to rotation, side bending, and flexion or extension. Assuming that a loss of joint motion may be concomitant with abnormal muscle tension on one side of the joint, muscle energy technique aims at restoring the normal muscle tension and allows the practitioner to overcome the restrictive barriers to joint movement. The practitioner seeks to take the joint manually to the barrier limits of motion in all three planes. At this point, the patient is instructed to perform a small isometric contraction while the practitioner provides resistance to the motion. The patient must attempt to move into the direction of the restricted motion. After about 3 to 5 seconds, the patient is instructed to relax and cease contraction, and the practitioner attempts to move the joint farther and overcome the restrictive barrier. The entire process is repeated 3 or 4 times, until a significant increase in joint motion is achieved. Osteopaths stress that the application of muscle energy techniques must be extremely specific in order to gain the desired effects.[11] The technique has gained popularity with orthopedic manual therapists, as it is relatively easy to learn and does not involve high-velocity forces.

Craniosacral technique

Originally developed around 1940 through the work of William G. Sutherland, an osteopath, craniosacral technique has been gaining favor with orthopedic manual physical therapists during the last decade.[13] As is the case with many manual medical procedures, craniosacral technique has not been wholeheartedly embraced by the mainstream medical community and has become increasingly controversial as it has become more popular among physical therapists. This approach to the treatment of craniosacral dysfunction is based on Andrew Taylor Still's principles on the articulations of the skull, the rhythmical motion of the coiling and uncoiling cerebral hemispheres, and the circulatory movement of cerebral spinal fluid (CSF) as it flows between the cranial vault and the spinal canal. The continuation of the intracranial membranes from the foramen magnum to the sacrum provides the basis for a theoretical rhythmical relationship between these structures.

The craniosacral rhythm (CSR) was initially thought to result from the rise and fall of CSF pressure that occurs with the contracting brain and ventricular system. The change in pressure was, in turn, believed to influence tension in the dura, with resultant motion within the cranium and at the sacrum.[13,35] Upledger and Vredevogd more recently proposed that the rhythm is a direct result of changes in CSF pressure secondary to the production and resultant reabsorption of CSF in the cranium. The changes in CSF pressure give rise to rhythmical movement that is transmitted through the dura to the sacrum.[35] No research exists to support either theory. The rate of CSR is said to be quite close to the patient's respiratory rate. Trauma, disease processes, psychological stress, exercise, and respiration are said to alter the craniosacral rate. The normal rate is said to be between 6 and 12 cycles per minute. Proponents of craniosacral therapy state that CSR changes can be palpated *anywhere* along the body, but especially on the skull.[37] Amplitude, symmetry, and quality of motion are other aspects of craniosacral motion that are said to be palpable. Craniosacral dysfunction assessment also includes an evaluation of the pattern of movement at the sphenobasilar junction and the flexion, extension, side bending, rotation, and torsional movements of the sphenoid bone. Motion of the sacrum between the fixed ilia is also assessed.

Treatment techniques are aimed at restoring the maximum mobility of the osseous cranium with a resultant balancing of membranous tension within the craniosacral system. Treatment involves "molding" techniques aimed at modifying the resiliency and contour of bones by the practitioner's application of external force in conjunction with the body's own internal activating force (respiratory motion).[13]

Even osteopathic practitioners of craniosacral technique attest to the highly specialized level of palpatory skill needed to assess CSR. One difficulty in measuring the reliability of such techniques is simply that very little has been done to verify the existence of craniosacral movement. Research fails to verify the existence of CSR and clearly questions the interrater reliability of CSR measurements by those who claim they can perceive such motions by palpation.[37]

Strain counterstrain technique

Developed by Lawrence H. Jones, another osteopath, the strain counterstrain technique is relatively new to manual therapy practitioners. The basis for this technique is the premise that musculoskeletal dysfunction is maintained by constant abnormal efferent signals from the spinal cord level. These signals are in response to abnormal afferent impulses from joint mechanoreceptors and nociceptors that occur with a disruption of the normal sensory input from the musculoskeletal system. Korr maintains that the muscle spindle is most likely the producer of the abnormal afferent signals for three reasons:

1. They are sensitive to musculoskeletal stress.
2. They are nonadapting receptors, able to sustain streams of impulses as long as they are mechanically stimulated.
3. Their influence is highly specific to the muscles acting on joints and the corresponding spinal segments.[21,22]

Jones believes that an overstretched muscle on one side of the joint (agonist) increases spindle firing from both its primary and secondary endings. At the same time, the muscle(s) on the opposite side of the joint (antagonist) become hypershortened and relaxed. If the body panics in an attempt to return the overstretched muscle to its normal state of tension, he contends, the shortened antagonist muscle(s) react reflexively with a contraction and prevent the joint from assuming a relaxed, nonstressed state. The antagonist, in effect, continues to be maintained in a state of abnormal shortening by the constant discharges of the gamma motor neurons of the corresponding spinal segment, keeping the spindle discharge frequencies at an exaggerated state, referred to as "high spindle gain." The resulting pathological state is such that the joint is unable to return completely from its overstretched position.[16,21]

Any attempts to return the joint to its normal resting state, either by moving it away from the direction of restricted motion or into the pathological barrier to motion, result in pain and increased resistance to movement. However, if a position of reduced pain is found that allows the muscle spindle to relax, that position is held involuntarily for at least 90 seconds, and the joint is slowly returned to the normal resting position, the normal spindle bias is restored and the pain alleviated.[13,16] A key concept of the strain counterstrain technique is the monitoring of tender points usually associated with the lengthened muscle (Fig. 8-10 a and b). These points, often corresponding to Travell's myofascial points or acupuncture points, are used to monitor the degree of therapeutic intervention by the practitioner. The practitioner continually monitors the amount of pain felt by the patient at a point always under the practitioner's finger. The patient is positioned to achieve the point of maximum pain relief for the 90-second hold treatment. No clinical research exists to support strain counterstrain treatment principles.

CONTRAINDICATIONS

Although the medical community often views manual therapy techniques as benign, manual practitioners are

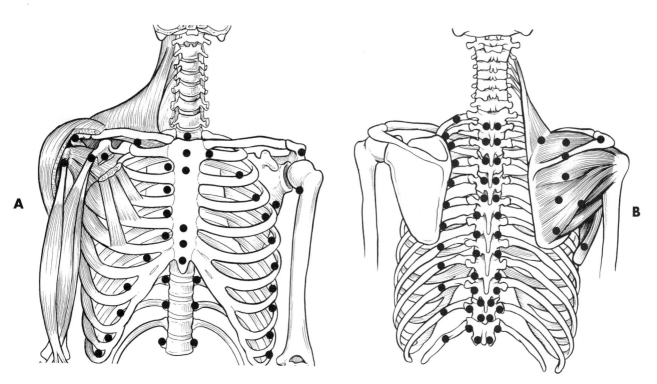

Fig. 8-10. Strain-counterstrain tender points of the trunk. **A,** Anterior. **B,** Posterior. (Modified from Jones LH: *Strain and counterstrain,* Colorado Springs, Colo, 1981, American Academy of Osteopathy.)

advised to avoid manipulation or mobilization for some conditions or to modify treatment techniques and proceed with caution[11,12] (Table 8-2). Absolute contraindications to manipulation or mobilization revolve around conditions that may lead to bone failure, spinal cord compromise, and circulatory damage. Relative precautions to manipulation or mobilization revolve around conditions for which treatment may result in increased pain, inflammation, and joint hypermobility.[5] Situations of relative precaution call for the practitioner to use the gentlest and most specific techniques available, with careful planning and perhaps consultation with other experienced practitioners.

The majority of circulatory accidents reported with manipulation were associated with high-velocity thrust techniques of the upper cervical spine with the head in a position of extension and rotation. The resulting insult is often a dissecting aneurysm of one of the vertebral arteries or a thrombosis of one of its branches. Krueger and Okazaki reviewed 10 cases of vertebral-basilar artery disruptions following chiropractic manipulation of the cervical spine. They reported one fatality and found that all of the patients manipulated had no previous history of neurological symptoms prior to chiropractic treatment. They suggest that cervical manipulation may be a factor in the pathogenesis of stroke in some patients but point out the difficulty in recognizing predisposing arterial abnormalities without the use of radiographic studies.[23] Fast and colleagues point out that the vertebral arteries are especially susceptible to damage where they penetrate the fibrous atlantooccipital ligament; however, the most frequent site of damage is the atlantoaxial junction, where compression or elongation may take place with sliding movement during head rotation and extension.[9] Greenman advocates testing for vertebral artery dysfunction during the cervical screening process by having patients actively move their heads into a position of maximum rotation and extension while in the seated position. The patient maintains this position for 5 minutes and is watched closely for anxiety, nystagmus, or dizziness, any of which indicates the need for extreme caution with manipulative treatment of the upper cervical spine.[13]

SUMMARY

This chapter is an overview of orthopedic manual therapy. Clinical practitioners of manual therapy must consider the scientific rationale for each approach, lest they blindly adopt one technique as their primary tool of practice. The understanding of the rationale supporting manual techniques is also critical to any future research in this area. An understanding of the foundation laid by osteokinematic and arthrokinematic principles, as well as the concepts and rules governing joint motion, allows the student of orthopedic manual therapy to begin building a set of manual evaluation and treatment skills. Only through the constant practice of basic palpatory skills and reassessment of bone and soft tissue response to manual interventions can novice manual practitioners become aware of their abilities to utilize manual interventions therapeutically in the treatment of musculoskeletal dysfunction. The development of adequate palpation skills is an ongoing and individualized process that requires the "laying on of hands" upon a multitude of patients; it should not frustrate or discourage beginning manual therapy practitioners. Most find that, with sufficient time and experience, their hands become their most valuable tools in assessing and treating musculoskeletal dysfunction.

Finally, research in the area of manual medicine is greatly needed to validate and substantiate the claimed successes of what many consider an art form. Although each of us, as rehabilitation specialists, strives to individualize a treatment

Table 8-2. Contraindications and precautions in mobilization and manipulation

Manipulation		Mobilization	
Absolute contraindications	**Relative precautions**	**Absolute contraindications**	**Relative precautions**
Bone disease	Hypermobility	Malignancy of area to be treated	Presence of neurological signs
Neoplastic disease of skeletal or soft tissue area to be treated	Joint irritability Severe pain	Presence of central nervous system signs	Rheumatoid arthritis Osteoporosis
Old bony deformities or anomalies of area to be treated	Protective muscle spasm	Active inflammatory arthritis	Spondylolisthesis
Inflammatory arthritis	Pregnancy	Infectious arthritis	Hypermobility
Presence of central nervous system signs		Bone disease of area to be treated	Pregnancy Previous malignant disease
Vascular disease related to area to be treated			
Advanced degenerative changes			

approach to a particular patient, as we struggle for recognition as scientific practitioners in the mainstream medical community, only the honest reporting and documentation of the clinical successes and failures of manual therapy will enable intelligent defense of any of the approaches discussed in this chapter. We can no longer expect to be able to hold forth the use of unsubstantiated manual interventions in a rapidly changing health care environment that demands "proof" rather than testimonials and weekend course certificates of "proficiency." The failure of manual practitioners to participate in the research process may very well in the future mean lack of recognition for a historically relevant and clinically significant method of treating musculoskeletal dysfunction.

REVIEW QUESTIONS

1. What are the differences and the similarities between the Australian and Norwegian approaches to the use of manual therapy?
2. How are the convex-concave rule and the positions of joint congruency used to determine the optimal articular position for extremity mobilization and manipulation procedures?
3. What methods or procedures are used to assess joint dysfunction and to determine whether the dysfunction is contractile or noncontractile in origin?
4. How does the clinician differentiate between a normal or typical end feel and an abnormal end feel?
5. How do the nontraditional manual therapy techniques, including myofascial release, muscle energy, craniosacral, and strain-counterstrain, differ from one another and from the traditional manual therapy techniques?

REFERENCES

1. Ackerknecht EH: *A short history of medicine,* New York, 1975, Ronald Press.
2. Beard G, Ward EC: *Massage principles and techniques,* Philadelphia, 1964, WB Saunders.
3. Bettman DL: *A pictorial history of medicine,* Springfield, Ill, 1962, Charles C Thomas.
4. Bick EM: *History of orthopedic surgery,* New York, 1933, The Hospital of Joint Disease.
5. Bourdillon JF: *Spinal Manipulation,* ed 5, Oxford, 1992, Butterworth-Heinemann.
6. Cyriax J: *Textbook of orthopedic medicine,* vol 1, *Diagnosis of soft tissue lesions,* London, 1969, Bailliere Tindall.
7. Cyriax J: *Textbook of orthopedic medicine,* vol 2, *Treatment by manipulation, massage and injection,* Baltimore, 1974, Williams & Wilkins.
8. Farrell J, Jensen G: Manual therapy: a critical assessment of role in the profession of physical therapy, *Phys Ther* 72(12):843, 1992.
9. Fast A, Zincola D, Marin E: Vertebral artery damage complicating cervical manipulation, *Spine* 12(9):840, 1987.
10. Glossary of osteopathic terminology, *J Am Osteopath Assoc* 80:552, 1981.
11. Greenman PE: *Principles of manual medicine,* Baltimore, 1989, Williams & Wilkins.
12. Grieve G: *Mobilization of the spine,* New York, 1965, Churchill Livingstone.
13. Grieve G: *Common vertebral joint problems,* New York, 1981, Churchill Livingstone.
14. Grimsby O: *Fundamentals of manual therapy: a course workbook,* Vagsbydgd, Norway, 1981, Sorlandets Fysikaiske Institute.
15. Hayes K, Peterson C, Falconer J: An examination of Cyriax's passive motion test with patients having osteoarthritis of the knee, *Phys Ther* 74(8):697, 1994.
16. Jones LH: *Strain and counterstrain,* Colorado Springs, Colo, 1981, American Academy of Osteopathy.
17. Kaltenborn F: *Mobilization of the extremity joints: examination and basic treatment techniques,* Universitetsgaten, 1980, Olaf Norlis Bokhandel.
18. Kapandjii IA: *Physiology of joints,* vol 2, *Lower limbs,* Edinburgh, 1970, Churchill Livingstone.
19. Kessler R, Hertling D: *Management of common musculoskeletal disorders,* Philadelphia, 1983, Harper & Row.
20. Kirkaldy-Willis WH: *Managing low back pain,* New York, 1983, Churchill Livingstone.
21. Korr IM: Proprioceptors and somatic dysfunction, *J Am Osteopath Assoc* 74:638, 1975.
22. Korr IM: *The neurobiologic mechanisms in manipulative therapy,* New York, 1977, Plenum.
23. Krueger BR, Okazaki H: Vertebral-basilar disruption infarction following chiropractic cervical manipulation, *Mayo Clin Proc* 55:322, 1980.
24. MacConaill MA, Basmajian JV: *Muscles and movements: a basis for human kinesiology,* Baltimore, 1969, Williams & Wilkins.
25. Maigne R: *Orthopedic medicine,* Springfield, Ill, 1976, Charles C Thomas.
26. Maitland GD: *Extremity manipulation,* London, 1977, Butterworth.
27. Maitland GD: *Vertebral manipulation,* London, 1978, Butterworth.
28. McKenzie RA: *Mechanical diagnosis and therapy,* Waikanae, New Zealand, 1981, Spinal Publications.
29. Mennell J: *The spinal column: the science and art,* New York, 1952, Little, Brown.
30. Mennell J: *Joint pain: diagnosis and treatment using manipulative techniques,* New York, 1964, Little, Brown.
31. Paris SV: *The spine: course notebook,* Atlanta, 1979, Institute Press.
32. Paris SV: *Extremity dysfunction and mobilization,* Atlanta, 1980, Prepublication Manual.
33. Schiotz EH, Cyriax J: *Manipulation: past and present,* London 1978, William Heinemann.
34. Stoddard A: *Manual of osteopathic practice,* London, 1969, Hutchinson Ross.
35. Upledger JE, Vredevogd JD: *Craniosacral therapy,* Chicago, 1983, Eastland.
36. Warwick R, Williams P: *Gray's anatomy,* ed 35, Philadelphia, 1973, WB Saunders.
37. Wirth-Patullo V, Hayes KW: Interrater reliability of craniosacral rate measurements and their relationship with subjects' and examiners' heart and respiratory rate measurements, *Phys Ther* 74:908, 1994.
38. Wyke B: Articular neurology: a review, *Physiotherapy* 58:94, 1972.
39. Zusman M: Spinal manipulative therapy: review of some proposed mechanisms, and a new hypothesis, *Aust J Physio* 33(2):89, 1986.

CHAPTER 9

Exercise and Rehabilitation Concepts

Barbara Sanders

OUTLINE

Limiting factors in exercise
    Physiologic limitations
Resistive and overload training
    Type of exercise
    Methods of overloading
    Principles of strength, power, and muscular endurance
      training
    Precautions and contraindications
Designing an exercise program
    General conditioning
    Body weight percentages for beginning conditioning
      programs
    Selecting various programs
Summary

KEY TERMS

exercise	closed kinetic chain
muscle	strength
resistance	power
open kinetic chain	endurance

LEARNING OBJECTIVES

After studying this chapter, the reader should be able to:
1. Define the concept of resistive exercise.
2. Describe the limitations and limiting factors in exercise prescription.
3. Describe the differences in isotonic, isometric, and isokinetic exercise.
4. State the difference between concentric and eccentric contractions.
5. State the difference between open kinetic and closed kinetic chain exercise.
6. Explain the various methods of overloading.
7. Describe the terms *strength, power,* and *endurance* in relation to muscle training.
8. List the precautions and contraindications for exercise.
9. Describe how the set and repetition system, light to heavy system, heavy to light system, and the circuit weight training system differ.
10. Design an exercise program incorporating concepts of overload, strength, power, and endurance.

Active-resistive exercise can be classified as having either a conditioning or a rehabilitative effect. The procedures followed in both areas to enhance one's muscular strength, power, and endurance are essentially the same. The major difference between the two areas exists in the intensity of the exercise regimens used. Exercise for conditioning purposes should be as intense as safely possible, thus eliciting optimal gains. The goal of rehabilitation, by contrast, is to restore the greatest possible function in the shortest possible time.

Mobility training, therefore, for whatever reason, must be restricted by individual limitations. An examination of specific physiological limitations can explain the complexity of exercise programs.

LIMITING FACTORS IN EXERCISE

A major concern of this chapter is to describe the factors involved in exercise. The effectiveness of exercise depends on the current physical performance levels of each individual, but analyzing the factors limiting exercise is a complex endeavor. To facilitate this task, an organizational paradigm (Fig. 9-1) was developed by Kearney.[16] The paradigm assumes that the core component of exercise is physical performance, which involves three primary factors: skill, cardiovascular conditioning, and neuromuscular coordination. Five modifying factors—genetic predisposition, anthropometric characteristics, psychological-sociological variables, ambient environment, and pain tolerance—are also important considerations that affect physical performance. To illustrate the primary factors, an activity performance profile (Fig. 9-2) should be used; that is, one end of the neuromuscular continuum should be designed to show strength and power as dominant, while the opposite end stresses muscular endurance. An athletic performance profile is then established for certain activities by subjectively assigning a grade for each primary factor. From these primary factors certain physiological, neurological, and histological elements are ultimately determined as being responsible for limiting performance and, consequently, limiting exercise.

In helping a client prepare to participate in a major sport, the main objectives the therapist should strive to achieve depend on the preceding elements. The amount of preparation time for activities varies according to the demands of the sport. Marathon runners and swimmers are continually practicing their activity as they train, but their performance is primarily determined by their physical conditioning. Discus throwers and golfers do not require the high degree of physical conditioning needed by distance runners and swimmers, but they do need to devote a greater percentage of prepara-

tion time to skill development. This diversity in sports preparation can be represented on the neuromuscular continuum and illustrates the basic differences in the training required for each sport. For example, a golfer needs to strengthen arms, wrists, and shoulders by performing specific strength-training exercises rather than relying on the weight of the club alone to increase strength. However, much of a golfer's training consists of complex skill movements, which are mastered by continual practice of the sport.

Fig. 9-3 identifies factors that determine skill limitations. The logical progression of the skill continuum is from simple (repetitive) tasks to highly complex tasks requiring modification by proprioceptive feedback or response to opponent actions.

The items listed in Fig. 9-4 represent limiting factors in cardiovascular conditioning, which in the *anaerobic* spectrum include (1) fuel sources, (2) enzymatic activity, (3) muscle fiber types, and (4) oxygen debt capacity. The respective limiting factors in the *aerobic* spectrum are (1) maximum oxygen uptake, (2) distribution of blood supply, (3) muscle fiber type, (4) fuel sources, and (5) fluid and ionic balances.

Within this cardiovascular framework, energy (capacity or ability to do work) represents the bottom line. The human body must be continuously supplied with its own form of energy to do work. Adenosine triphosphate (ATP) is used for the immediate (anaerobic) activities and is continuously resynthesized for long-duration (aerobic) energy activities. The key to successful enhancement of the cardiovascular elements is to identify the predominant means of energy

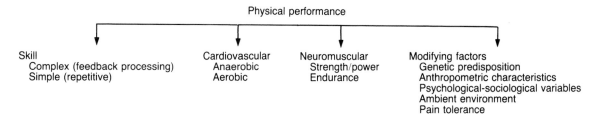

Fig. 9-1. Physical performance and its determining factors.

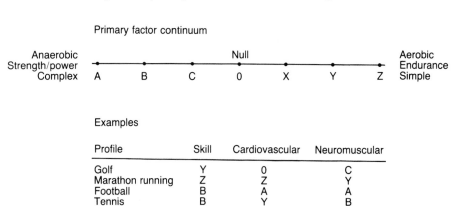

Fig. 9-2. Activity performance profile.

metabolism required for a desired area of performance and to train specifically to augment the capacity for that type of energy output.

Fig. 9-5 describes physiological factors limiting muscular strength and power, including (1) total cross-sectional area of a muscle, (2) cortical control factors, (3) muscle fiber type, and (4) ambient conditions influencing the rate of muscle fiber shortening. Factors limiting muscular endurance include (1) muscle fiber type, (2) state of training, (3) environmental factors, (4) circulatory conditions, and (5) type of activity involved.

Fig. 9-6 displays certain modifying factors that can enhance or restrict muscle performance. Of the factors cited, genetic predisposition is potentially the most significant.

To make clear the relative importance of certain limiting factors in the paradigm, one specific activity should be closely evaluated. Marathon running is the ultimate chal-

lenge of aerobic power training, involving cardiovascular ability, muscular endurance, neuromuscular coordination, and simple skill movements. Modifying factors, such as genetic predisposition (high percentage of slow-twitch red fibers), anthropometric characteristics, and psychologic and pain tolerance variables, also contribute to success in this activity.

With this information in mind, potential limitations that may occur in exercise can be demonstrated.

Physiologic limitations

In addition to the preceding factors, further specific physiological factors ultimately limit the ability of an individual to function at the maximal possible muscular efficiency as well as the minimal balanced bilateral muscular efficiency. Much of the evidence accumulated on muscular efficiency suggests that limitations exist within the muscle fibers themselves.* Muscles are composed of varying numbers of motor units that contribute to such contractile properties as speed, power, and resistance to fatigue. Consequently, muscle fibers can be classified accordingly:

1. Slow-twitch red (slow oxidative glycogenolytic)
2. Fast-twitch red (fast oxidative glycogenolytic)
3. Fast-twitch white (fast glycolytic)

There are two essential differences between the fiber types: (1) the dominant energy source may be either aerobic or anaerobic, and (2) the contraction time of the particular fiber may be fast-twitch or slow-twitch. However, the most important consideration in determining differences between fiber types is the tension that can be produced by a muscle fiber type. This force of contraction is ultimately dependent upon six variables:

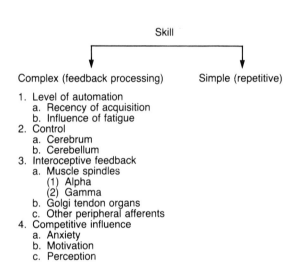

Fig. 9-3. Skill limiting factors.

* References 2, 5, 11, 15, 28, 29.

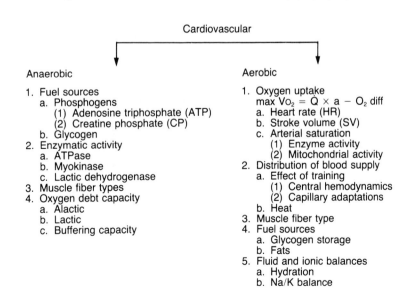

Fig. 9-4. Cardiovascular limiting factors.

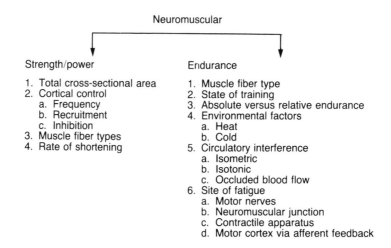

Fig. 9-5. Neuromuscular limiting factors.

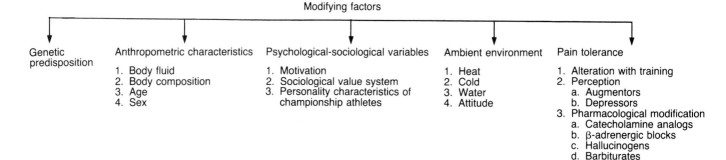

Fig. 9-6. Major modifying factors of physical performance.

1. Number of motor units firing
2. Size of motor units
3. Rate of firing of individual motor units
4. Velocity of muscle shortening
5. Length of muscle fiber
6. Condition of muscle fiber

Number of motor units firing. The number of motor units firing and thus contributing to muscular contraction depends on the integrity of the central nervous system and the motivational level of the individual. Coordination of movement is the responsibility of the central nervous system,* a fact that is important in understanding the development of strength. One theory is that with an intact central nervous system fewer inhibitory impulses are transmitted to different motor neurons, resulting in more motor units being activated at any one time.[2,3,14,22,27]

Size of motor units. Motor neurons may innervate less than 10 fibers or more than 1000 fibers. The size of such motor units varies between muscles and within an individual muscle. The initiation of muscle contraction is precipitated by small motor units. Recruitment of larger motor units is required as the demand for tension increases. The implications for exercise are obvious: Minimal contractions that elicit low muscle tension in effect activate tonic motor units. Consequently, a therapist who knows that a particular unit or fiber possesses a high resistance to fatigue could develop an exercise program requiring repeated submaximal contractions for long periods of time.

Rate of firing of individual motor units. A twitch contraction is initiated by a single action potential within a muscle fiber. Repetitive action potentials can produce a summation of twitch contractions to produce tetanus.[3,14]

Velocity of muscle shortening. The velocity of muscle shortening decreases as the load increases until the velocity is zero and an isometric contraction is produced. As velocity decreases, the tension that can be produced by a muscle increases. Consequently, a heavier load can be moved through space until the load creates zero velocity.†

Length of muscle fiber. The length of muscle fiber is determined not only by the type of muscle fiber involved but by each sarcomere as well. During actual muscle

---

*References 2, 3, 5, 10, 13, 28, 29.

†References 3, 14, 21, 23, 27, 28.

Table 9-1. Properties of the various fiber types

	Slow-twitch red	Fast-twitch red	Fast-twitch white
Histologic differences			
Size	Small	Intermediate	Large
Color	Red	Red	White
Myoglobin	High	High	Low
Sarcoplasmic reticulum and T tubules	Thin and sparse	Thin and sparse	Well developed
Nerve size (myelin)	Small	Medium	Large
Blood supply	High	High	Low
Mitochrondrial density	High	Medium	Low
Sarcoplasm	Less	Moderate	More
Fibrils	Few	Moderate	Many
Fibers per motor unit	Low	Medium	High
Physiologic differences			
Contraction time	Slow	Fast	Fast
Endurance	High	Medium	Low
Tension capacity	Low	Medium	High
Stretch sensitivity	Very sensitive	Moderately sensitive	Less sensitive
Biochemical differences			
K+ depletion	Slow	Moderate	Rapid
Metabolism	Oxidative	Both	Glycolytic
Myoglobin content	High	High	Low
Glycogen content	Similar	Similar	Similar
ATPase activity	Low	Moderate	High

contraction each cross-bridge elicits a constant amount of tension regardless of the distance between the two contractile proteins, actin and myosin. It is theorized that maximal tension occurs when the highest number of cross-bridges is interdigitated.[2-4,21,23,28,29]

Condition of muscle fiber. A number of physiological changes take place in a muscle when it is repeatedly subjected to overload training. Primary changes involve improvement of the neural pathways from brain to muscle and the tendinous attachment of the muscle to the bone, as well as the musculotendinous junction. Engaging in exercise will result in improved efficiency of the neural pathways and a more effective application of force.*

Although certain properties of muscle fiber function that determine contraction capability are shared by all fast-twitch red, fast-twitch white, and slow-twitch red fibers, a closer examination of histological, physiological, and biochemical properties can differentiate the fibers more clearly. Table 9-1 illustrates that slow-twitch red fibers have a high resistance to fatigue endurance and are adaptable to prolonged contractions because they rely on energy metabolism employing oxygen. The fast-twitch white fibers, by contrast, are capable of strong, rapid contractions essential for dynamic movements, but they have a low resistance to fatigue. These fibers rely on an adenosine triphosphate and creatine phosphate pool for their energy.

* References 2, 3, 14, 21, 27, 28, 30.

RESISTIVE AND OVERLOAD TRAINING

Use of the overload principle in conditioning and rehabilitation facilitates an increase in muscular strength, power, and endurance. Simply stated, workloads for both conditioning and rehabilitation have to impose a demand on the organism, and, as adaptation to increased loading occurs, more load needs to be added. Exercise of this type is called *progressive resistance exercise* (PRE).

Types of exercise

Isometric exercise. This type of exercise or muscle contraction occurs when a muscle attempts to shorten but is unable to overcome the resistance. Considerable muscular force is generated during an isometric contraction; however, there is no noticeable shortening of the muscle and no movement of the mass. Isometric or static resistance exercises normally are performed against an immovable object such as a wall, a barbell, or a weight machine that is loaded beyond the maximal concentric strength of the individual. Increases in strength from this type of exercise are related to the number of contractions, the duration of contractions, maximal versus submaximal effort, frequency of training, and joint angle specificity.[1] Submaximal, isometric actions are, in reality, the form used in most rehabilitation sequences.

Isotonic exercise. This exercise is dynamic and is traditionally defined as a muscular contraction in which the muscle exerts a constant tension. However, the tension is not usually constant but varies with the mechanical advantage of the joint during movement. Another way to think about isotonic exercise is that it is muscle movement with a constant load. Isotonic exercises normally are performed against some type of resistance, from handheld weights to equipment that can be used to perform dynamic constant resistance training.[12,26]

Concentric contraction. This type of muscular contraction occurs in dynamic rhythmical activities when the muscle fibers come together (shorten) as it develops tension, thus causing the "lifting" of the applied load.

Eccentric contraction. This type of contraction occurs when a weight is lowered through a range of motion (ROM) and a muscle lengthens at a controlled rate. It is also called *negative resistance exercise.* Eccentric exercise is a functional activity done every day. Walking down stairs requires the quadriceps to perform an eccentric exercise. Normal dynamic resistance training includes the eccentric component because lifting a resistance causes the muscle to shorten as it contracts (concentric contraction); lowering the resistance is a muscle-lengthening activity. Eccentric exercises can be performed with a variety of equipment from free weights to expensive weight machines.[19]

Isokinetic exercise. By defining isotonics as constant load and variable speed, isokinetic exercise can be defined as exercise with a constant maximal speed and variable load. In isokinetic exercise, the muscular contraction is performed at a constant maximal angular limb velocity, and the equipment varies the resistance. The reaction force mirrors the force applied to the equipment throughout the range of motion, which theoretically allows the muscle to exert a continual, maximal force over the full range. The advantages of isokinetic exercise are that it allows faster speeds of movement while minimizing muscle and joint soreness. Most isokinetic devices provide both concentric and eccentric exercise options. A disadvantage of this type of exercise is the cost of the equipment.[12]

Open kinetic chain exercise. Open kinetic chain activities are activities of the body in which the ends of limbs or parts of the body are free to move without causing motion at another joint. In the open chain, motion does not occur in a predictable fashion because the joints or limbs may function independently or in unison. An example of an open kinetic chain activity is that of the lower extremity in kicking a ball. The hip, knee, and ankle may flex to accelerate and then kick the ball, or just one joint may flex and propel the ball. Another example of an open chain exercise is a seated knee extension or a biceps curl.[20]

Closed kinetic chain exercise. Closed kinetic chain activities involve the integration of muscle joints acting in a predictable sequential order with combined weight-bearing and shear forces that are mediated by eccentric muscle action. This concept has become more popular in the literature and in professional seminars, although research on the effects of closed-chain principles is minimal. Empirical evidence in clinical trials shows apparent success in rehabilita-

tion and functional training for athletes, additional research into the clinical applications is warranted. An example of a closed kinetic chain exercise is a knee press or a squat lift. In the earlier kicking example, the support limb would be primarily eccentric in activation. Eccentric exercise, or closed kinetic chain activity, is normally incorporated into any exercise program, whether the equipment used is free weights, isokinetics, or weight machines.[20]

Methods of overloading

There are numerous ways to impose an overload on the muscular system. Most of the current therapeutic exercise equipment and many of the regimens employed use one or more of the following methods of overloading.

Increased weight/resistance. This is the most basic of all overloading techniques. The individual increases the resistance he or she is accustomed to, the muscular system is overloaded, and conditioning takes place. DeLorme popularized this approach in the mid-1940s by using a weight boot and increasing the resistance as individual adaptation occurred.[8,9]

Increased repetitions/sets. By increasing the number of times (repetitions) or group times (sets) an exercise is done, the individual can progressively overload the system. This regimen, also popularized by DeLorme, is usually coupled with increased resistance to enhance overloading.[8]

Increased frequency. This element of overloading is concerned with the number of times per week or per day that the individual trains. Studies of conditioning frequency indicate that significant levels of conditioning can be achieved if the frequency range is 2 to 4 times per week.*

Increased speed or rate of movement. The advent of speed training (isokinetic exercise) was popularized by use of Cybex† equipment. Isokinetic movements are muscular contractions that occur at a constant maximal speed through a full range of motion. The advantages of speed training are that the speed of contraction is fixed and a maximum of resistance is encountered through the full range of motion. No matter how much force is applied, the maximal velocity remains constant and the force accommodates[21,22] (Fig. 9-7).

Duration. Duration is the specific time element during which the individual is actually performing mobility exercises. The objective of the mobility training program determines the duration. Rehabilitation training may be conducted at lower intensities and for shorter time periods; the opposite is true for conditioning training.

Rest interval. Overloading can be intensified or decreased by adjusting the length of the rest interval between periods of intensity. An intense training session followed by a short rest interval before the next session causes a more extreme physical response:

---

* References 2, 4, 6, 9, 10, 29.
† Cybex, Ronkonkoma, NY.

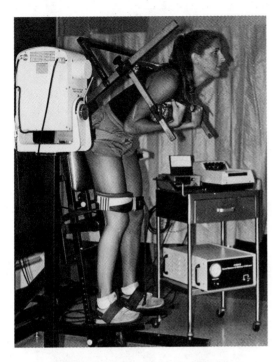

Fig. 9-7. Prototype Cybex back unit.

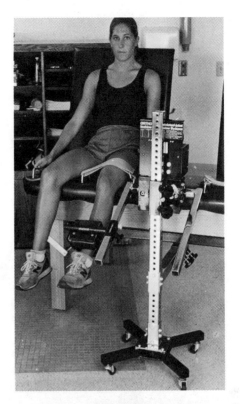

Fig. 9-8. Lumex Orthotron unit.

1. Heart rate is higher
2. Oxygen debt is incurred earlier
3. Respiration rate increases
4. Exhaustion occurs sooner

This response is desirable for mobility training in some conditioning programs, but for early stages of rehabilitation intense training is not recommended.

Isolation of the muscle. Some proponents of mobility training advocate isolation of a specific muscle group to elicit optimal development. Nautilus,* Cybex, and numerous other types of training equipment incorporate this principle in their machinery. Basically, this approach tries to avoid the incidence of *synergistic response* (i.e., when an injured and/or weak muscle group performs a dynamic movement, the action of other muscles assists in the movement). Use of this type of equipment theoretically isolates the specific area to be strengthened (Figs. 9-8 through 9-10).

Range of motion. Range of motion is determined by the relative distance a body part traverses during an exercise. While performing mobility exercises for conditioning, it is desirable to perform the exercise through the full range of motion. For example, a barbell curl should begin from a position where the elbow flexors are in complete extension and finish with the elbow flexors in complete flexion for proper overloading. Often, however, this is not possible immediately following an injury or surgery, but continued rehabilitation can gradually increase the range of motion so

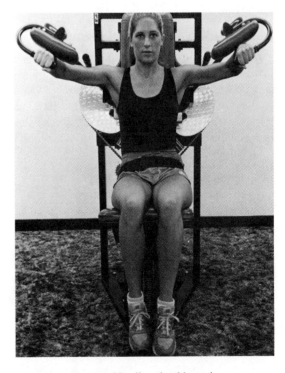

Fig. 9-9. Nautilus shoulder unit.

* Nautilus, Deland, Fla.

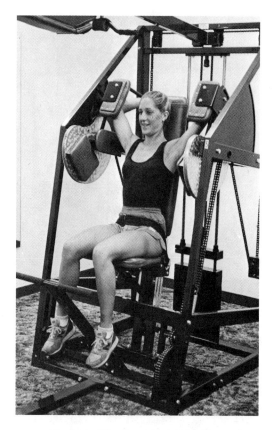

Fig. 9-10. Nautilus pullover machine.

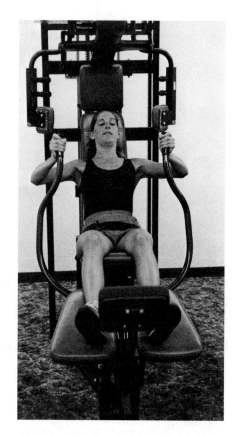

Fig. 9-11. Nautilus double chest machine.

that there will be an increase in the overload of affected muscles and a consequent restoration of function (Figs. 9-11 through 9-13).

Principles of strength, power, and muscular endurance training

Providing sufficiently descriptive semantic definitions for *strength, power,* and *muscular endurance* has been an ongoing problem in recent years, especially with the advent of isokinetics. *Strength* appears to be a pure component, but within the confines of the available training modalities, it can be defined in several ways*:

1. Strength is the maximum force that can be exerted against an immovable object (isometric strength).
2. Strength is the heaviest weight that can be lifted against gravity (isotonic strength).
3. Strength is the maximal torque that can be developed against a preset, prelimiting device at a specific contractile velocity (isokinetic strength).

Although absolute strength is an important component of exercise, *power* (force × distance) is dependent on the individual's level of strength. Time quantification of power

* References 2, 3, 10, 16, 17, 22.

has been achieved with the introduction of isokinetic equipment. Isokinetic devices, for instance, allow for an assessment of power from numerous muscle groups and joint motions by varying the speed at which the resistance moves. The implications for conditioning and rehabilitation are twofold: (1) isokinetic devices provide a diagnostic tool for assessing muscular imbalances and/or deficiencies, and (2) they enhance an individual's ability to improve general power development. For definitive purposes, muscular endurance can assume the same categories as strength.

Muscular endurance is the ability of a muscle to perform repeated contractions against an immovable object (isometric exercise), against gravity (isotonic exercise), and against a preset speed-limiting device (isokinetic exercise). Additionally, relative to dynamic or static movements, there can be a concentric contraction and/or an eccentric contraction (Fig. 9-14).

A *concentric contraction* is the most common type of muscular contraction and occurs in rhythmical activities when the muscle shortens as it develops tension (Fig. 9-15). An *eccentric activation,* by contrast, entails lengthening of the muscle. This is achieved when a weight is lowered through a range of motion. The muscle yields to the resistance, allowing itself to be stretched (Fig. 9-16).

The effect of exercise on the muscular system primarily centers on hypertrophy, although strength, power, and endur-

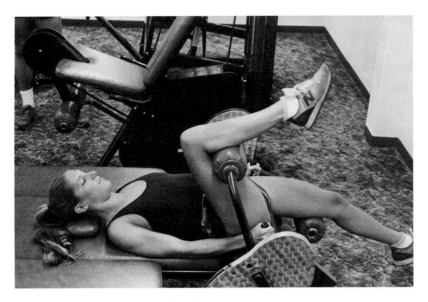

Fig. 9-12. Nautilus hip and leg machine.

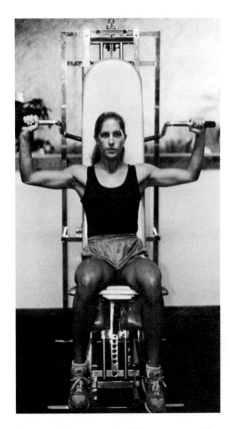

Fig. 9-13. Dynacam shoulder press machine.

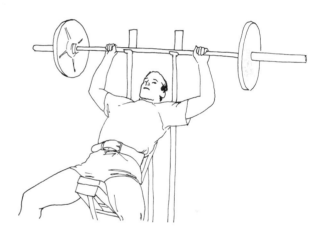

Fig. 9-14. Beginning phase.

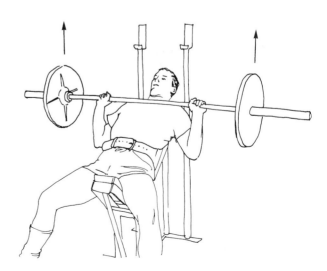

Fig. 9-15. Concentric phase.

ance gains can be achieved without increases in the size of muscle fibers.[2,7,27,29] Table 9-2 compares the biological changes that result in an individual who engages in exercise and one who engages in cardiovascular training. Certain chemical and histochemical similarities occur when various types of training are undertaken, and even cardiovascular training is a form of overloading.

Precautions and contraindications

Precautions. A major cardiovascular precaution is the Valsalva maneuver. Patients should be cautioned about holding their breath. In fact, instructions should include exhaling when performing a motion, and patients should be encouraged to talk, count, or breathe rhythmically while exercising. The Valsalva maneuver is most commonly seen when an individual is performing isometric or isotonic heavy resistance exercise. Individuals with cardiovascular problems should be carefully monitored during exercise.

Fatigue affects performance and should be a major

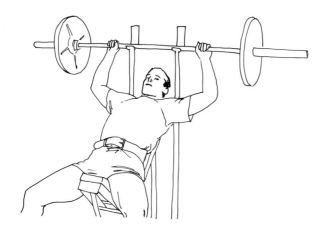

Fig. 9-16. Eccentric phase.

consideration during an exercise program. Fatigue can be either specific or general. Muscle fatigue is the diminished response of a muscle to a stimulus. It is a normal response that can occur during dynamic or static exercise programs and with high-intensity or low-intensity exercise bouts. When a muscle is fatigued, the response rate is slower and the range of motion is shortened. General fatigue (whole body) is the inability of the body to respond to prolonged exercise activity. It may be due to reduced blood glucose levels, a decrease in glycogen stores, and a depletion in potassium. These considerations are important in designing endurance and conditioning programs. Adequate recovery time should be built into any exercise program. Research indicates that performing light exercise during the recovery period facilitates recovery from fatigue more rapidly than total rest.

Overwork can be characterized as a temporary or permanent deterioration of strength as a result of exercise. Causes of overwork are not fully understood, and avoidance is the best solution. Overwork can be avoided if intensity, duration, and progression of exercise are appropriately monitored.

Osteoporosis is a loss of bone density or mass. It is often the result of inactivity, long-term immobilization, or prolonged bed rest. Postmenopausal women are also at high risk for the development of osteoporosis. The bone changes that occur in osteoporosis make the bone susceptible to fracture. Considerations in designing exercise programs should include the amount of resistance and the progression of exercise.

Immediate muscle soreness often develops as a result of strenuous exercise because of lack of adequate blood flow and oxygen and a temporary buildup of metabolites in the exercised muscle. This muscle soreness is transient and after exercise should resolve quickly with adequate blood flow and oxygen. Delayed-onset muscle soreness (DOMS) develops 24 to 48 hours after exercise and resolves within a week. Theories speculate that the soreness is caused by microtrauma to connective tissue and muscle fibrils. Eccen-

Table 9-2. Physiologic comparison between overload modalities in exercise and cardiovascular training

Biologic factors	Strength	Muscular endurance	Cardiovascular endurance
Collagen content	Increase	Increase	Increase
Connective tissue	Increase in density	Increase in density	Increase in density
Sarcolemma	Increase in density	Increase in density	Increase in density
Tendons and ligaments (volume)	Increase	Increase	Increase
Sarcoplasm	Increase	Increase	Increase
Contractile proteins (actin, myosin, troponin, tropomyosin)	Increase	Increase	Increase
Glycogen	Yes	Yes	Yes
Mitochondria (size and number)	Yes	Yes	Very high
Fiber type response	Fast-twitch white (FTW)	Fast-twitch white (FTW) and fast-twitch red (FTR)	Slow-twitch red (STR)
Succinic dehydrogenase	Little	Little	Very high
Phosphorylase activity	Little	Little	Very high

tric exercise seems to cause more DOMS than concentric exercise, perhaps because more damage occurs to muscle fibers and connective tissue with muscle lengthening against resistance. It can be reduced by having the client perform both warm-up exercises and stretching prior to the exercise program.

Contraindications. Inflammation is a contraindication for resistance exercise. Resistive exercises can lead to increased inflammation and swelling and further tissue damage.

Pain is another contraindication. If the client has severe joint or muscle pain that persists for more than 24 hours following exercise, resistance should be eliminated or drastically reduced. A thorough evaluation of the pain is indicated.

DESIGNING AN EXERCISE PROGRAM

Selection of the proper regimen for an exercise program is essential for optimal benefits. The core element, whether the program is for conditioning or for rehabilitation, is persistent reinforcement of effort to increase and improve muscle strength beyond prior limits. Resistive programs are varied and are designed for the cross-section of individuals who engage in resistive training for whatever purpose. They include the following types of individuals:

1. Athletes—individuals who are interested in developing strength/power specific to their sport
2. Olympic and power lifters—individuals interested mainly in acquiring strength/power necessary to achieve success in respective lifts, such as Olympic (the snatch and the clean-and-jerk) and power lifting (squat, bench press, and the deadlift)
3. Body builders—individuals wanting to attain massive muscular development and definition
4. Those in need of rehabilitation—individuals who work with resistive exercise for restoration of function in injured or affected structures
5. General physical fitness—individuals who desire general muscular toning

General conditioning

The following programs can be used to achieve optimal results in exercise: set and repetition system, light-to-heavy system, heavy-to-light system, and circuit weight training.[4,22,23]

Set and repetition system. This system was introduced by DeLorme in the mid-1940s and is, by far, the most widely used method of training.[8] *Repetition* refers to the number of complete and continuous executions of an exercise or the repetition maximum (RM) for a particular weight. A set constitutes the group number of repetitions of an exercise. If more than one set is performed, a short rest interval follows each set. This allows the person to quantify and objectively document the regimen.

EXAMPLE: EXERCISE

Bench press, 100 lb × 10 RM (100%) × 1 set
Rest
Bench press, 100 lb × 10 RM (100%) × 1 set
Rest
Bench press, 100 lb × 10 RM (100%) × 1 set

The DeLorme method is characterized by doing an initial set at 50% of 10 RM, a second set at 75% of 10 RM, and progressing to a third set at 100% of 10 RM.

EXAMPLE: EXERCISE

Bench press, 50 lb × 10 RM (50%) × 1 set
Rest
Bench press, 75 lb × 10 RM (75%) × 1 set
Rest
Bench press, 100 lb × 10 RM (100%) × 1 set

Light-to-heavy system. In this system[29] the individual starts with a lighter weight, does a certain number of repetitions, rests, adds more resistance, does fewer repetitions, rests, adds even more resistance but does fewer repetitions, and continues this process until a certain weight and repetition goal is achieved. The regimen of imposing increasingly greater amounts of resistance with fewer repetitions is used frequently by athletes seeking to acquire great mass and strength.

EXAMPLE: EXERCISE

Bench press, 100 lb × 10 RM × 1 set
Rest
Bench press, 120 lb × 8 RM × 1 set
Rest
Bench press, 140 lb × 6 RM × 1 set

Heavy-to-light system. Also called the *Oxford technique,* the heavy-to-light system retains the principle of heavy resistance and low repetitions but reverses the light-to-heavy pattern by starting with the heaviest weight first and progressively decreasing the load. Zinovieff believed that the DeLorme method was too fatiguing and that too great a strain was placed on the muscles.[31]

EXAMPLE: EXERCISE

Bench press, 100 lb × 10 RM (100%) × 1 set
Rest
Bench press, 75 lb × 10 RM (75%) × 1 set
Rest
Bench press, 50 pound × 10 RM (50%) × 1 set

Circuit weight training. Circuit weight training involves a sequential arrangement of weight training exercises resulting in a system of continuous activity that brings about improvement of strength, muscular endurance, body composition, and aerobic capacity.[13] Circuit weight training requires the trainee to exercise in short, all-out bursts, followed by short rest intervals. A circuit of eight or more exercise stations is established with a specific time allotment and/or a required number of repetitions performed at each station. Exercises are arranged in the circuit so that there is an alternation of arm, leg, shoulder, and back movements to prevent fatigue of one muscle group before the circuit is completed.

EXAMPLE:

Exercise	Repetitions	Rest
Bench press	10 RM (100%)	30 sec
Squat	10 RM (100%)	30 sec
Upright row	10 RM (100%)	30 sec
Sit-up	10 RM (100%)	30 sec
Curl	10 RM (100%)	30 sec
Dead lift	10 RM (100%)	30 sec
Dip	10 RM (100%)	30 sec
Leg raise	10 RM (100%)	30 sec

Exercises are done one after another until the circuit is completed. After a rest period, the circuit can be done two or three more times. To intensify the program the following can be done: (1) the rest interval can be decreased, (2) more repetitions can be added, and (3) more circuits can be completed. Regardless of the exercise systems or methods of overloading used, progressively overcoming increased resistance is necessary for the development of muscular strength, power, and endurance.

Overload and repetitions. Numerous studies* concerning the optimum amount of overloading and the proper number of repetitions for maximum conditioning gains (Table 9-3) have been conducted. However, no precise

* References 2, 4, 6, 9, 17, 23, 26-28.

amount of resistance or number of repetitions has been demonstrated conclusively as most effective. DeLorme advocated a system of heavy resistance and high repetition, beginning with a light weight for a specified number of repetitions and progressively increasing the load from 50% to 75% to 100% for that specific number of repetitions.[8,9] Zinovieff modified DeLorme's progression, called it the Oxford technique, and reversed the procedure, while still doing 10 repetitions.[31] MacQueen surveyed competitive weight lifters and bodybuilders and differentiated between a regimen for eliciting muscle hypertrophy and one for developing muscle power.[18] The study indicated that, generally, high repetitions and low resistance result in increased endurance while low repetitions and high resistance yield strength. The major practical implication that arose from this research was a definition of the effort required for muscular gains: RM, therefore, was defined as the maximum amount of weight a muscle can lift for that specific number of repetitions. Initially, determination of the RM was done on a trial-and-error basis.

Body weight percentages for beginning conditioning programs

Sanders implemented a formula to determine starting weights in resistive programs based on percentage of body weight.[24] These percentages represent median starting points for certain body parts and are used as a basic guideline in beginning programs. (Rehabilitative restoration of an injured area using exercise, however, necessitates a somewhat modified approach to body weight percentage. Determination of the RM is not easy, and, because of pain or fear of injury, the client may not understand the meaning of the maximum effort. It then becomes a problem of education and motivation on the part of the participant.)

The following percentages are recommended starting points for beginning lifters, doing three sets of 10 repetitions,

Table 9-3. Exercise programs

Programs	Rehabilitation	Conditioning
DeLorme[8]	B, I, A: 1st set × 10 repetitions × 50% of 10 RM 2nd set × 10 repetitions × 75% of 10 RM 3rd set × 10 repetitions × 100% of 10 RM	B, I, A: Same
Oxford technique (Zinovieff)[31]	B, I, A: 1st set × 10 repetitions × 100% of 10 RM 2nd set × 10 repetitions × 75% of 10 RM 3rd set × 10 repetitions × 50% of 10 RM	B, I, A: Same
MacQueen[18]	B, I, A: 3 sets × 10 repetitions × 100% of 10 RM A: 4-5 sets × 2-3 repetitions × 100% of 2-3 RM	B, I, A: Same A: Same
Sanders[24]	A: 4 sets × 5 repetitions × 100% of 5 RM (3 days/week) 1st day = 4 sets × 5 RM 2nd day = 4 sets × 3 RM 3rd day = 1 set × 5 RM 2 sets × 3 RM 2 sets × 2 RM	A: Same

B, Beginning (posttrauma); *I,* intermediate; *A,* advanced.

and should serve only as a guideline for starting a weight-lifting program:

1. Barbell squat—45% body weight
2. Universal leg press—50% body weight
3. Barbell bench press—30% body weight
4. Universal bench press—30% body weight
5. Universal leg extension—20% body weight
6. Leg extension (weight boot)—20% body weight
7. Universal leg curl—10 to 15% body weight
8. Upright rowing—20% body weight

Table 9-3 presents various progressive loading systems that are currently in use. The programs are arranged under conditioning and rehabilitation headings to illustrate the adaptability of various systems to both areas. In addition, further information is given as to whether the programs should be implemented in the beginning, intermediate, or advanced phase of rehabilitation using an exercise program.

The key to success in the various programs is always striving to increase resistance without sacrificing good mechanics. No matter what regimen is followed, progressively increasing the resistance results in increased strength, power, and endurance for conditioning as well as for restoration of the injured area. Knight[17] proposed a different technique of progressive resistance exercise (PRE) for postsurgical rehabilitation and provided another means to determine whether a client is working at maximum levels. Daily adjusted progressive resistance exercise (DAPRE) is a technique that allows for individual differences in the rate at which a person regains strength in the injured area. Tables 9-4 and 9-5 depict the DAPRE technique of weight adjustment and progressive resistance exercise.

The number of repetitions performed during the third set and the weight guidelines described in Table 9-5 are used for determination of the adjusted working weight for the fourth set. Additionally, Table 9-5 gives the number of repetitions performed during the third set, determines the weight used in the fourth set, and indicates that the number of repetitions done in the fourth set is used to determine weight for the next exercise session.

Selecting various programs

The selection of various progressive systems and modalities is ultimately determined by availability and the current status and desire of the individual. Pathological conditions require a more moderate approach both in equipment and in progressive system approaches. Rehabilitation following injury is better accomplished when an exercise can be applied selectively and when resistance can be employed where it is most needed.

Logically, a progressive increase in load with decrease in the repetitions would be the most efficient approach for optimal strength, power, and endurance gains. Not only is the loading system important but so is the selection of exercises. A marathon runner doing a barbell squat of 550 lb will find the exercise has little carry-over value for running 26.2 miles; a shotputter performing the same exercise will experience a needed conditioning effect.

Physical conditioning for any sport should correspond with the physiological demands of the activity. The fact that many physiological factors play a role in athletic performance dictates that many combinations of loading systems must be employed.

A sample regimen that combines a circuit routine employing three sets of 10 RM (3×10 RM) would be suitable for both conditioning and rehabilitation, as long as the selection of exercises was correct. The use of a combination of overloading systems with repetition and set schemes is endless and presents a unique opportunity for the therapist and/or trainer to maximize an individual's muscular gains. Shown here is a combination program of circuit training and 3×10 RM.

CONDITIONING (BASIC PROGRAM)

1. Barbell squat
2. Bench press
3. Barbell upright rowing
4. Barbell curl
5. Hamstring curls (Universal)

REHABILITATION (KNEE EXERCISES)

1. Straight-leg raise
2. Side-leg raise
3. Standing front-leg raise
4. Standing knee flexion

To complete the regimen for the conditioning program, the individual should perform the exercises in numerical sequence doing one set of 10 RM; then, after completing all five exercises, he or she should rest 2 minutes, repeat, rest, and repeat, consecutively, until three sets of 10 RM have been completed. The same procedure should be followed for

Table 9-4. DAPRE technique

Set	Weight	Repetitions
1	50% RM	10
2	75% RM	6
3	100% RM	Maximum
4	Adjusted working weight	Maximum

Table 9-5. Guidelines for adjusted working weight

Number of repetitions performed during set	Adjusted working weight (fourth set)	Next exercise session
0-2	−5-10 lb	−5-10 lb
3-4	−0-5 lb	Same weight
5-6	Same weight	+5-10 lb
7-10	+5-10 lb	+5-15 lb
11	+10-15 lb	+10-20 lb

the rehabilitation circuit. The intensity of the workouts could be increased by (1) increasing the number of exercises, (2) repeating the circuit more times, (3) increasing the resistance, and/or (4) reducing the rest intervals between or at the end of each cycle. It is clear, therefore, that no matter what the desired outcome or situation, multiple exercise programs can be designed and implemented.

SUMMARY

The basic underlying element in exercise that is responsible for optimal muscular strength, power, and endurance gains is the progressive reinforcement of efforts to extend beyond limits already reached. Overloading presents numerous possibilities to the therapist/facilitator. There is, of course, no definitive exercise regimen that is applicable to all conditioning and rehabilitation situations. However, research has demonstrated that a number of specific procedures can be followed, and, for practical purposes, the 3 × 10 RM exercise regimen or some modification thereof is usually sufficient. What is also important is understanding that there are individual physiological limitations that might restrict advancement. The selection of programs and/or equipment becomes a problem of time, money, space, and the current status of the individual. Several methods can and should be used with each individual to maximize muscular strength, power, and endurance gains.

REVIEW QUESTIONS

1. What physiological limitations limit the ability of an individual to function at a maximum level of muscular effiency?
2. What method of overload would you select to progress an exercise program? Explain your answer.
3. Why are the concepts of open kinetic chain and closed kinetic chain important in the formulation of an exercise program?
4. What criteria would you use to establish minimal expectations for a strength training program?
5. How would the lower extremity training program designed for an individual undergoing rehabilitation for postsurgical repair of their anterior cruciate ligament differ from that for the individual interested in developing strength and power specific to a sport?

REFERENCES

1. Albert M: *Eccentric muscle training in sports and orthopaedics,* New York, 1991, Churchill Livingstone.
2. Astrand PO, Rodahl K: *Textbook of work physiology,* New York, 1970, McGraw-Hill.
3. Basmajian JV: *Therapeutic exercise: student edition,* Baltimore, 1980, Williams & Wilkins.
4. Bjornaraa B: *Weight training systematized,* Stillwater, Minn, 1975, Croixside Press.
5. Burke EJ, editor: *Toward an understanding of human performance: readings in exercise physiology for the coach and the athlete,* Ithaca, NY, 1980, Movement Publications.
6. Capen EK: The effects of systematic weight training on power, strength, and endurance, *Res Q Exerc Sport* 21:83, 1950.
7. Clark DH: Adaptations in strength and muscular endurance resulting from exercise, *Exerc Sport Sci Rev* 1:73, 1973.
8. DeLorme TL: Restoration of muscle power by heavy resistance exercises, *J Bone Joint Surg Am* 27:645, 1945.
9. DeLorme TL, Watkins AL: Techniques of progressive resistance exercise, *Arch Phys Med Rehabil* 29:263, 1948.
10. de Vries HA: *Physiology of exercise for physical education and athletics,* ed 2, Dubuque, Iowa, 1974, William C Brown Group.
11. Dons B, Bollerup K: The effect of weightlifting exercise related to muscle fiber composition and muscle cross-sectional area in humans, *Eur J Applied Physiol* 40:95, 1979.
12. Fleck SJ, Kraemer WJ: *Designing resistance training programs,* Champaign, Ill, 1987, Human Kinetics Pub.
13. Gettman LR, Pollock ML: Circuit weight training: a critical review of its physiological benefits, *Physician Sports Med* 9:44, 1981.
14. Jaeger L: Course syllabus for therapeutic exercise, Physical Therapy Program, University of Kentucky, 1976.
15. Katch FI, McArdle WD: *Nutrition, weight control, and exercise,* Boston, 1977, Houghton Mifflin.
16. Kearney JT: Limiting factors in physical performance. Paper presented at physical therapy seminar, University of Kentucky, April 1976.
17. Knight KL: Knee rehabilitation by the daily adjustable progressive resistive exercise technique, *Am J Sports Med* 7:336, 1979.
18. MacQueen IJ: Recent advances in the technique of progressive resistance, *Br Med J* 11:1193, 1954.
19. Malone TR, Sanders B: Strength training and the athletic female. In Pearl AJ, editor: *The athletic female,* Champaign, Ill, 1993, Human Kinetics Pub.
20. Norkin CC, Levangie PK: *Joint structure and function, a comprehensive analysis,* Philadelphia, 1992, FA Davis.
21. O'Donoghue DH: *Treatment of injuries to athletes,* ed 3, Philadelphia, 1976, WB Saunders.
22. O'Shea JP: *Scientific principles and methods of strength fitness,* Reading, Mass, 1969, Addison-Wesley.
23. Ryan AJ, Allman FL Jr: *Sports medicine,* New York, 1974, Academic Press.
24. Sanders MT: *Weight training and conditioning.* In Sanders BR, editor: *Sports physical therapy,* Norwalk, Conn, 1990, Appleton & Lange.
25. Sanders MT: Resistive training, Unpublished study, 1978.
26. Sanders MT: A comparison of two methods of training on the development of muscular strength and endurance, *J Orthop Sports Phys Ther* 1:210, 1980.
27. Schram DA: Resistance exercise. In Basmajian JV, editor: *Therapeutic exercise,* Baltimore, 1980, Williams & Wilkins.
28. Stone MH: Considerations in gaining a strength-power training effect (machines vs. free weights), *Nat Strength Condition Assoc J* 4:22, 1982.
29. Stone WJ, Kroll WA: *Sports conditioning and weight training programs for athletic competition,* Boston, 1978, Allyn & Bacon.
30. Wilmore JH: *Athletic training and physical fitness: physiological principles and practices of the conditioning process,* Boston, 1976, Allyn & Bacon.
31. Zinovieff AN: Heavy resistance exercise, the Oxford technique, *Br J Physic Med* 14:129, 1951.

CHAPTER 10

Assessment of Strength

George J. Davies, Kevin Wilk, and Todd S. Ellenbecker

OUTLINE

SECTION I GENERAL PRINCIPLES
Purpose
Mode of muscle action
Terminology of resistance exercise
Isometric exercise
Isotonic exercise
Muscle strength assessment methods
    Manual muscle testing
    Handheld dynamometry
    Cable tensiometers
Isotonic muscle assessment
Computerized isokinetic dynamometer assessment
Computerized eccentric isokinetic dynamometer strength assessment
Computerized closed kinetic chain isokinetic dynamometer strength assessment
Open kinetic chain versus closed kinetic chain computerized isokinetic testing
Functional testing algorithm
Basic/fundamental measurements
Subjective examination
KT1000 testing
Digital balance evaluator
Closed kinetic chain isokinetic testing
Open kinetic chain testing
Closed kinetic chain squat isokinetic testing
Functional jump test
Functional hop test
Lower extremity functional test

SECTION 2 SPECIFIC ASSESSMENT FOR THE LOWER EXTREMITY
Isokinetic testing of the knee
Knee testing
Interpretation of test data
Functional testing
SECTION 3 SPECIFIC ASSESSMENT FOR THE UPPER EXTREMITY
Rationale for utilization of isokinetics in upper extremity strength assessment
Reliability of upper extremity isokinetics
Glenohumeral joint testing
Shoulder internal/external rotation strength testing
Interpretation of shoulder internal rotation/external rotation testing
    Bilateral differences
    Normative data utilization
    Unilateral strength ratios (agonist/antagonist)
Additional glenohumeral joint testing positions
    Shoulder abduction/adduction
Shoulder flexion/extension and horizontal abduction/adduction
Scapulothoracic testing (protraction/retraction)
Distal upper extremity testing
Concentric versus eccentric considerations
Relationship of isokinetic testing to functional performance

KEY TERMS

muscle strength
exercise types
muscle assessment

open kinetic chain testing
closed kinetic chain testing
functional testing

LEARNING OBJECTIVES

After studying this chapter, the reader should be able to:

1. State the purpose of a strength assessment.
2. State and describe the three primary types of exercise.
3. List the advantages and disadvantages of isometric, isotonic, and isokinetic exercise.
4. State the advantages and limitations of manual muscle testing.
5. Describe the differences in open kinetic chain versus closed kinetic chain isokinetic testing.
6. Describe the function testing algorithm (FTA) as a method of strength assessment.
7. Describe the components of the lower extremity functional test.
8. List 15 parameters of the standardized isokinetic knee testing protocol.
9. State 11 parameters used for the interpretation of an isokinetic test.
10. State a rationale for the utilization of isokinetics in upper extremity strength assessment.

Section I   GENERAL PRINCIPLES

Assessment of strength is performed ubiquitously in rehabilitation clinics and in sports performance and fitness centers. However, often strength is defined differently and consequently is measured in a variety of ways. A rehabilitation clinician may measure strength by determining whether a patient can independently sit to stand or by the use of manual muscle testing (MMT), handheld dynamometers, sophisticated computerized isokinetic dynamometers, or agility tests to measure functional strength. Therapists associated with sports performance centers will often use hand grip dynamometer tests, one-repetition maximum (RM) or 10 RM progressive resistive exercise (PRE) isotonic testing, computerized isometric or cable tensiometers, or agility tests to measure functional strength.

Because of the various methods that are frequently used to assess strength, it demonstrates the point that occasionally confusion results when assessing and evaluating strength. Therefore, when assessing and interpreting strength testing results, it is important for the clinician to remember the particular methods used. Moreover, for appropriate analysis, the proper terminology should be applied when describing the results such as torque, work, power, or force to have relative meaning. For example, if a rotary open kinetic chain (OKC) isokinetic test is performed, then the values should be reported as torque measurements (ft-pounds or NM). However, if the linear closed kinetic test is performed, the values are measured in pounds or newtons.

PURPOSE

The purpose of assessing strength is to try to quantify objectively the force production of the musculoskeletal system.

We are actually measuring muscle performance in an indirect manner via the selected method of analysis. These indirect measures are predicated not only on changes in muscle tension but also on changes dependent on many factors including mode of muscle contraction, position of patient relative to gravity, position of muscle relative to the length-tension ratio, the skeletal leverage biomechanics, and velocity of movement.

MODE OF MUSCLE ACTION

When assessing muscle strength, the mode of muscle contraction performed must be considered. The three primary modes of muscle action are isometric (static), concentric (shortening), and eccentric (lengthening). The assessment of the muscle's performance for a particular activity should be contraction-specific. However, most muscles actually function in all modes of muscle action with various activities. Therefore, using multiple assessment techniques is probably most appropriate.

There are advantages and disadvantages of assessing and using the particular modes of muscle actions in rehabilitation. The details of the specific application of the various modes of muscle actions in rehabilitation will be discussed throughout this text.

TERMINOLOGY OF RESISTANCE EXERCISE

Various forms of musculoskeletal exercise are available for the clinician to use when rehabilitating a patient.[13] Today three primary types of exercise are commonly employed in conditioning and rehabilitation: isometrics, isotonics, and isokinetics:

Isometrics: fixed speed (0°/sec); (immovable) fixed resistance

Isotonics: variable speed (approximately 60°/sec); fixed resistance

Isokinetics: fixed speed (1°/sec ≈ 1000°/sec – dynamic speed); accommodating resistance

ISOMETRIC EXERCISE

Isometric exercise is performed at 0°/sec speed, without observable joint movement (arthrokinematics) or osteokinematic movement.[13] The resultant observable action seen with isometric exercises is an increase in the size of the muscle belly as the muscle fibers contract and shorten, producing tension. The velocity is constant at zero, so the resistance varies to match the force applied, but no functional movement is possible. The application of isometrics in rehabilitation will be discussed in more detail in various chapters throughout the book. The advantages and disadvantages of isometric exercise are presented in the Boxes.

ISOTONIC EXERCISE

Isotonic exercise is also frequently referred to as progressive resistance exercise (PRE) or weight training.[13] Isotonic exercise has been performed through various modes including free weights (barbells, dumbbells, cuff weights), hydraulic systems (HYDRAGYM* and machine weights (Eagle,† Nautilus,‡ Universal,§ etc).

Isotonic exercise is divided into concentric and eccentric muscle loading. *Concentric muscle loading* involves a shortening muscle contraction where the muscle's origin and insertion approximate. The individual muscle fibers actually shorten with a concentric contraction. *Eccentric muscle loading* involves a lengthening muscle activation where the

* Hydra Fitness, Belton, Tex.
† Cybex, Ronkonkoma, N.Y.
‡ Nautilus, DeLand, Fla.
§ Universal, Cedar Rapids, Iowa.

Advantages of isometrics

Used early in rehabilitation without causing further joint irritation, because there is no joint motion
Increases static muscular strength
Helps retard atrophy
Assists in decreasing swelling (the muscles act as a muscular pump and assist in fluid removal)
Prevents neural dissociation through muscular contractions, which stimulate the mechanoreceptor system in the joint capsule and surrounding ligaments
Maintains neural association
Can be performed anywhere
No special equipment is needed
Can be performed in short periods of time
Has approximately a 20° physiological overflow through the range of motion (ROM)

Modified from Davies GJ: *A compendium of isokinetics in clinical usage,* Onalaska, Wis, 1992, S & S.

Disadvantages of isometrics

Muscular strength increases are fairly specific to the joint angle where the exercises are performed (≈20° physiological overflow)
Subject to physiological influences
Difficult to provide patient motivation
No contribution to muscular endurance
No improvement in functional force control accuracy
No eccentric work provided
Creates ischemic responses in muscle and subsequent pain

Modified from Davies GJ: *A compendium of isokinetics in clinical usage,* Onalaska, Wis, 1992, S & S.

muscle's origin and insertion separate. The individual muscle fibers actually go through a lengthening process with an eccentric action.

Fig. 10-1 compares the tension-developing capacity of various types of muscle actions.

MUSCLE STRENGTH ASSESSMENT METHODS

We have already mentioned numerous ways that strength can be assessed including MMT, handheld dynamometers, hand grip dynamometers, cable tensiometers, 1 RM or 10 RM PRE isotonic testing, computerized isokinetic dynamometers, and functional performance activities of daily living, ergonomic, agility, or sports performance testing.

Manual muscle testing

Manual muscle testing (MMT) is a commonly used method to assess muscle strength in a clinical environment. Dr. Robert Lovett was the originator of the gravity system of MMT.[24] Dr. Charles Lowman added a numerical system for grading muscle action using the gravity system but also incorporating ROM considerations.[25] Henry and Florence Kendall developed a percentage system that included ROM, gravity, resistance, and the element of fatigue.[22,23]

Signe Brunnstrum and Marjorie Dennen developed a system of grading movements rather than individual muscles.[11] Elizabeth Kenny introduced a system for recording the presence of function, spasm, and incoordination in muscle affected by poliomyelitis, which was called a muscle analysis.[12] There were other variations and refinements in MMT, but this brief overview has allowed an appreciation of its applications.

There are many advantages of using MMT. It is quick, readily available, inexpensive, and provides relatively reliable data, particularly with experienced clinicians. These data can be used for screening purposes, are relatively easy for the patient to understand, and clinicians can adapt the MMT for the many variables of the patient (age, sex, pathology, etc.). The significant limitations of MMT include subjective interpretation of the test by a clinician, poor reliability with inexperienced clinicians, numerous uncontrolled variables such as positioning, stabilization, amount of pressure exerted by examiner, patient's effort and motivation, leverage differences, sex differences, strength differences, age considerations, and biomechanical/muscle-length-tension related to specific ROM, compensations by patients, and lack of intertestor reliability and reproducibility in testing subjects who have greater than "normal" strength levels.

MMT is typically based on or evaluated on the interaction between the effects of gravity, movement through the ROM, and the presence/absence of a muscle contraction. MMT is often performed as an isometric "break" test, meaning the patient tries to hold or contract the muscle against the examiner's resistance. Another method of MMT is a "dynamic MMT" through the ROM. This has all the disadvantages described above in addition to trying to vary the resistance through the ROM based on the changing biomechanics, length-tension ratio and skeletal leverage of the muscle, and the particular pathology (pain inhibition, etc.). However, this can often be a valuable part of the total clinical examination to identify a "resisted painful arc syndrome" that may be present, although an active ROM painful arc was not present. Many times this clinically provides guidelines as to where to initiate rehabilitation or ROM to avoid.

Handheld dynamometry

To try to objectively quantify MMT, handheld dynamometers have become more popular recently.[1,5-9] Handheld dynamometers seem to be gaining in popularity and acceptance in clinical practice. Most of these units operate as pressure or strain gauges and are limited by the clinician's ability to overcome the musculature in question while not allowing uncontrolled movements.

One variation that has been used for many years is a hand grip dynamometer. This has often been used to specifically measure hand grip function or as an estimation of total arm strength.

Cable tensiometers

Cable tensiometers were used more frequently in the past and are rarely used in clinical practice today. The cable tensiometer testing is an isometric test and therefore has all the aforementioned described disadvantages. Furthermore, there is difficulty in performing specific types of tests often required for testing various pathologies.

ISOTONIC MUSCLE ASSESSMENT

The advantages and disadvantages of isotonics are outlined in the Boxes.

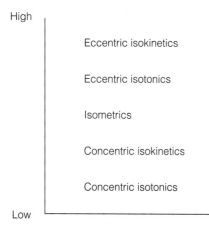

Fig. 10-1. Comparison of tension-developing capacities of various muscular contractions.

Advantages of isotonics

Some can be relatively inexpensive
Readily available
Provides motivation by achievement (lift more weight)
Can be progressively increased in varying increments for the overload principle
Work takes place through the ROM
Work occurs at speeds greater than 0°/sec
Has a concentric and eccentric component
Can improve muscular endurance (peripheral circulation) (greater than 10/15 reps)
Can affect neurophysiological system
Can be objectively documented
Various components of program can be manipulated to maintain workload (reps, sets, weight)
Increase muscular strength in few repetitions (1– ≈ 8/10)

Modified from Davies GJ: *A compendium of isokinetics in clinical usage,* Onalaska, Wis, 1992, S & S.

Generally, a 1 RM or 10 RM PRE isotonic strength assessment is used. Because isotonics use a fixed resistance throughout the ROM, one problem that occurs is that the "true maximal loading" only occurs at the weakest point in the ROM. Therefore, a 1 RM or 10 RM is really a repetition maximum only at one particular point (weakest) in the ROM. Furthermore, the velocity of the movement occurs at a variable speed depending on the patient's efforts. Most self-selected velocities of isotonics are performed at approximately 60°/sec. Although PREs are readily available, and they continue to be widely used, accurate and reliable isotonic strength assessment continues to be problematic.

COMPUTERIZED ISOKINETIC DYNAMOMETER STRENGTH ASSESSMENT

Isokinetics were developed in the 1960s and gained popularity through the 1980s and early 1990s. Most isokinetics have been performed in an open kinetic chain isolated joint pattern.

Isokinetics are defined as a fixed velocity with an accommodating resistance. The velocity is dependent on the technology but ranges from 1°/sec to approximately 500°/sec. Isokinetics have been used extensively for muscle performance evaluation and objective documentation and for rehabilitation.

The advantages and disadvantages of isokinetics are presented in the Boxes.

Extensive literature has been published in the area of concentric isokinetic testing and evaluation. Based on reliability, advantages previously described, and accuracy of human muscle testing, isokinetics probably represents the "gold standard" in assessment of OKC isolated muscle strength testing and rehabilitation today.

COMPUTERIZED ECCENTRIC ISOKINETIC DYNAMOMETER STRENGTH ASSESSMENT

Most of the research published in the area of isokinetics has been performed concentrically. Over the last decade, computerized isokinetic dynamometers with eccentric capabilities have been developed. Because of muscle performance using eccentric actions, it is important to also assess the eccentric capabilities of the muscle. The specificity of testing is important; however, most dynamometers have limited eccentric isokinetic velocities up to approximately 210°/sec. It is beyond the scope of this chapter to thoroughly discuss eccentric muscle assessment and rehabilitation. Consequently, the reader is referred to a comprehensive overview of eccentric isokinetics by Davies and Ellenbecker.[16]

Disadvantages of isotonics

Maximally loads a muscle only at its weakest point in the ROM

Is not safe if someone has pain during the ROM because the patient must still support the weight

If performed too soon ballistically, can cause a reactive traumatic synovitis

Once the weight starts moving, there is a momentum factor with the weight

Does not develop rapid force (quickness)

Does not develop accuracy at functional speeds

Difficult to exercise at fast functional velocities (without susceptibility for injury)

Does not provide reciprocal concentric exercise

Not usually performed in a diagonal or functional plane

Difficult to develop an aerobic training response

Muscular eccentric isotonics causes delayed onset muscle soreness (DOMS)

Unable to spread workload evenly over entire ROM

Modified from Davies GJ: *A compendium of isokinetics in clinical usage*, Onalaska, Wis, 1992, S & S.

Advantages of isokinetics

Accommodating resistance allows maximal dynamic loading of a muscle throughout the ROM

Provides maximal resistance through the velocity spectrum

Inherent safety factor, due to accommodating resistance; therefore minimal risk to patient

Minimal postexercise soreness with concentric isokinetic contractions

Validity of equipment

Reliability of equipment

Reproducibility of testing (reliability)

Isokinetic dynamometers and recording systems, computers, etc.

Exercise through velocity spectrum

Specificity of movements

Helps force development of quickness (time rate of torque development)

Develops force control accuracy

Decreases reciprocal innervation time of agonist/antagonist contractions

Efficiency of muscular contractions

Accommodation to pain

Accommodation to fatigue

Joint nourishment

Decreased joint compressive forces at high speed and length of time compression is placed on joint surface

Physiological overflow

Provides feedback to patient with recorders, computers, etc.

Neurophysiological "pattern" for functional speeds and movements

Objective supervision of submaximal and maximal programs and progression

Modified from Davies GJ: *A compendium of isokinetics in clinical usage*, Onalaska, Wis, 1992, S & S.

Disadvantages of isokinetics

Cost of some equipment

Eccentric loading stimulus to the muscles causes DOMS

Lack of personnel trained in use or interpretation of isokinetic testing and rehabilitation

The sensitivity of the equipment and recording devices in testing larger muscle masses such as hip, trunk

Availability of the equipment

Inconvenience of switching the equipment attachments for various joints and ease of various setups

Time-consuming if more than one joint is exercised/assessed

Some artificial parameters until the limb actually moves to reach the velocity of the dynamometer or decelerates

Modified from Davies GJ: *A compendium of isokinetics in clinical usage,* Onalaska, Wis, 1992, S & S.

COMPUTERIZED CLOSED KINETIC CHAIN ISOKINETIC DYNAMOMETER STRENGTH ASSESSMENT

With the increasing emphasis on closed kinetic chain (CKC) exercises being used in rehabilitation today, a very basic question arises as to how to assess CKC performance. Davies has recently completed a reliability study of the Linea Computerized Closed Kinetic Chain Isokinetic Dynamometer* providing intraclass correlation coefficients ranging from .85 to .94, which demonstrates good to excellent reliability.[15]

Open kinetic chain versus closed kinetic chain computerized isokinetic testing

Most isokinetic testing that has been published is open kinetic chain (OKC) or isolated joint testing. Recently, having the Linea available to do CKC or multiple joint testing has allowed us to compare the advantages and disadvantages of each type of testing for the lower extremities.

The Box demonstrates the forces produced by OKC isokinetic testing of the quadriceps compared with CKC isokinetic testing. CKC multiple joint/multiple muscle groups produce tremendous forces, approximately three times more than OKC at relatively slow speeds of testing, respectively.[14] Furthermore, after testing approximately 250 patients with a variety of knee injuries, the comparative results between OKC and CKC are presented in Table 10-1.[14]

This reinforces the need to perform both CKC and OKC testing. If only CKC testing is performed, then an isolated deficit may be missed as illustrated in Table 10–1.[14] The importance of doing isolated testing to identify specific weaknesses is often far from the actual injury site, as previously described by Nicholas et al,[27] Gleim et al,[20] and Boltz and Davies.[10]

* Loredan Biomedical, Inc., West Sacramento, Calif.

Comparison of OKC and CKC isokinetic testing with body weight

The peak torque to body weight for the quadriceps with OKC was:

(Slow speed)	60%s: $\approx 1 \times$ BW
(Medium speed)	180%s: $\approx 2/3 \times$ BW
(Fast speed)	300%s: $\approx 1/2 \times$ BW

The peak force to body weight for the leg extensors with CKC was:

(Slow speed)	10 inches/sec: $\approx 3 \times$ BW
(Medium speed)	20 inches/sec: $\approx 2^1/2 \times$ BW
(Fast speed)	30 inches/sec: $\approx 2 \times$ BW

Table 10-1. Lido linea closed kinetic chain: computerized isokinetic testing compared with Cybex open kinetic chain computerized isokinetic testing

$n = 250$ Patients (different knee injuries)			
Cybex		**Linea**	
	% Deficit		% Deficit
PT 60°/s Quads U - 142 ft-pounds I - 101 ft-pounds	29	PT 10 in/sec U - 462 pounds I - 420 pounds	9
PT BW 60°/s Quads U - 95% I - 66%	31	PT %BW 10 in/sec U - 298 pounds I - 266 pounds	11
PT 10°/s U - 99 ft-pounds I - 78 ft-pounds	21	PT 20 in/sec U - 374 pounds I - 331 pounds	11
PT BW 180°/s U - 64% I - 48%	25	PT% BW 5 in/sec U - 239 pounds I - 216 pounds	11
PT 300°/s U - 80 ft-pounds I - 64 ft-pounds	20	PT 30 in/sec U - 302 pounds I - 253 pounds	16
PT BW 300°/s U - 51% I - 41%	20	PT %BW 30 in/sec U - 193 pounds I - 171 pounds	11

The area of CKC objective muscle strength assessment is in its infancy. However, because so many clinicians are performing CKC exercises as part of their rehabilitation programs, without prospective randomized experimental studies to document their outcomes, there is a dire need for research to elucidate this process. Furthermore, long-term follow-up studies are necessary to evaluate the effectiveness of the CKC rehabilitation programs on selected parameters of performance, return to activity, injury recurrence, effects of early CKC compressive forces on the articular cartilage, and so forth.

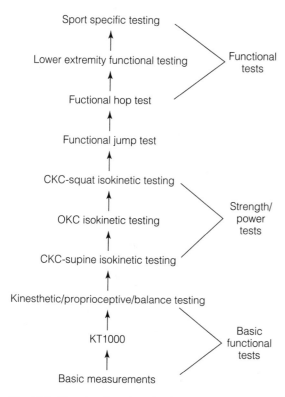

Fig. 10-2. Functional testing algorithm—lower extremity.

Table 10-2. Empirical guidelines for patient progression in the functional testing algorithm	
Tests	**Empirical guidelines**
Sport specific testing (SST)	
Lower extremity functional test (LEFT)	Female <2:00 min; Male <1:30 min
Functional Hop Test (FHT)	<15% bilateral comparison and norms
Functional jump test (FJT)	<20% compared to body height and norms
Closed kinetic chain (CKC) (standing)	<20% bilateral comparison
Open kinetic chain (OKC)	<25% bilateral comparison
Closed kinetic chain (CKC) (supine)	<30% bilateral comparison
Digital balance evaluation (DBE)	<.6
KT1000	<3 mm bilateral comparison
Basic measurements	<10% bilateral comparison
Subjective	Pain <3 (analog pain scale: 0-10)

FUNCTIONAL TESTING ALGORITHM

Davies has developed a functional testing algorithm (FTA) as one method to assess a patient in a systematic progressive manner.[17] We will describe the FTA and how it is used in the evaluation and progression of a patient through a rehabilitation program and back to a sporting activity. The FTA for the lower extremity is described in Fig. 10-2.

The FTA testing strategies are based on the principles of progression and "control." Each test in the progression testing sequence increases stresses to the athlete with less control. Progression to the next higher level of testing difficulty is predicated on passing each test in the FTA sequence. To pass from one level to the next in the FTA, the patient must meet a minimum level of performance to pass to the next higher stage in the FTA sequence. The criteria used for the progression through the FTA are presently based on our clinically based empirical guidelines. Correlation research is presently in progress; however, at the present time there is limited published research. Table 10-2 provides the empirical guidelines presently used for clinical decision making regarding patient progression.

The following information describes each stage of the FTA with emphasis on the integration of strength testing.

BASIC/FUNDAMENTAL MEASUREMENTS

The basic/fundamental measurements consist of the various components of the history and subjective examination of the patient and the physical objective examination of

the patient. The various components of the basic measurements are listed in the Box.

SUBJECTIVE EXAMINATION

Using an analog pain rating scale from 0 (no pain) to 10 (worst pain), preferably the patient's pain at rest and with activities will be less than 3 before they are progressed to more demanding testing. Part of the reason for this constraint is pain produces a reflex inhibition resulting in muscle "weakness," and the patient may not be ready to be progressed and tested through the FTA. As a general rule, criteria for progressing a patient to the next level of testing in the FTA include parameters within 10% in a bilateral comparison and clinical judgment.

KT1000 TESTING

Obviously this testing would be used for patients who have had ACL or PCL injuries. Ideally the difference of a bilateral comparison of the involved knee to the uninvolved side would be less than 3 mm. If greater than 3 mm difference is seen, then time from injury or surgery, bracing, and medical discretion is used to determine whether the patient is ready to be tested at that particular time in the next stage of the FTA. If the graft is more than 3 mm bilateral comparison in the early stages of rehabilitation, then we try to protect the graft by protected weight bearing, bracing, and modifying the rehabilitation program.

Functional testing algorithm (FTA) basic/fundamental measurements

History and Subjective Examination
Objective Examination
    Observation/posture
    Vital signs
    Gait evaluation
    Anthropometric measurements
    Leg length measurements
    Referral/related joints
    Palpation
Neurological Exam
    Sensation
    Reflexes
Balance/Proprioception/Kinesthesia
Manual Muscle Testing
Active Range of Motion
Passive Range of Motion
Flexibility Tests
Special Tests
Medical Tests

DIGITAL BALANCE EVALUATOR

Some method of measuring balance/proprioception/kinesthesia should be incorporated into the FTA. We use a digital balance evaluator (DBE), which is a single-plane balance board that has microswitches and counts the number of touches and time out of balance in a 30-second test protocol.[1] Our descriptive research over the last 20 years has produced clinical guidelines that we use to assess the patient's status. Criteria for progression is a score of less than .60. The average score is .50 with a range from .40 (good) to .50 (average) to .60 (worse) (% of Time in Balance). If the patient's score is greater than .60, then we emphasize kinesthetic exercise for neuromuscular control in his or her rehabilitation program for a period of time (variable based on the specific pathology) before we retest the patient.

CLOSED KINETIC CHAIN ISOKINETIC TESTING

With the increased emphasis on CKC exercise in rehabilitation protocols, the question certainly arises as to the need to also test in the CKC position. But the question still remains as to how we can test in the CKC position safely early in a rehabilitation program.

There are numerous reasons advocated for using CKC exercises. They are functional, the increased joint compressive forces increase knee stability, co-contractions of the quadriceps and hamstrings provide dynamic stability, and these exercises minimize translatory stresses to the ligaments, particularly the ACL.

The Linea is a lower extremity computerized isokinetic/isotonic testing and rehabilitation system. At this point in the FTA, we test the patient in a semi-sitting to supine position with CKC isokinetics. Davies[15] has performed a reliability study that demonstrates the ICCs to be .85 to .94, which demonstrates good to excellent results. We test the patient in this position because of the aforementioned reason for CKC. We think this is a safe position because of the CKC position, controlled speed, controlled ROM, and so forth. This position controls the stresses to the knee and prevents varus/valgus or rotational forces. Therefore, we feel this is an excellent way to test early in a rehabilitation program to get objective documentation of the patient's status to make changes to individualize the patient's rehabilitation program. Although there are various methods of testing, at the present time we are primarily using velocity spectrum isokinetic testing in a reciprocal lower extremity pattern. Other options include isokinetic testing (both concentric and eccentric) and a coupled/tandem symmetrical leg press pattern. Research is ongoing regarding the advantages and disadvantages of the modes and positions.

Our empirically based guidelines to progress a patient to the next higher level (increased stresses with less control) is a bilateral comparison of less than 30% in peak force, total work, (TW), TW/body weight (BW), average power (AP) and AP/BW. Because of research by Bandy et al,[3] we primarily focus on the peak force because there is a high correlation between peak force results and TW and AP. If the patient still has deficits in muscle performance greater than 30% bilateral comparison, then we continue integrated rehabilitation using both CKC and OKC techniques. The emphasis is on strength, power, and endurance training before we retest the patient's status to determine whether he or she is ready to progress to the next level of the FTA.

OPEN KINETIC CHAIN TESTING

Although many feel that OKC is a contraindication for testing certain knee pathologies, these authors think it is appropriate for most patients. Of course, there are always exceptions, and the clinical examination, soft-tissue healing times, and so forth may preclude this testing.

However, the safety factors that we feel do in fact allow OKC testing include the following: controls certain stresses to the knee including varus/valgus and rotational, a proximally placed tibial pad helps reduce anterior translation of the tibia (important for patients with ACL-deficient knees or ACL reconstructions), speeds are controlled (faster speeds can control anterior translation), decreased compressive forces, ROM can be precisely controlled, single or isolated joint testing is performed and prevents compensation so one really knows what they are assessing, and it allows assessment of the neural system's ability to "drive" the isolated muscle group.

Several authors[10,13,20,27] have already previously described and demonstrated the need for isolated joint testing. Furthermore, Nicholas et al,[27] Gleim et al,[20] and Boltz and Davies[10] have demonstrated the need for creating a composite score of total leg strength (TLS). Davies[14,17] has documented the importance of performing isolated joint testing (OKC) in conjunction with CKC testing for patients with various knee pathologies. We use many of the standard protocols previously published regarding indications, contraindications, guidelines, and protocols for testing various lower extremity injuries, surgeries, or both.

A clinically based empirical guideline we use for progressing the patient to the next level in the FTA is a bilateral comparison of less than 25%. If the patient still has a deficit in the quadriceps greater than 25%, we still have an isolated joint/muscle weakness (weak link of the kinetic chain), and we continue an integrated rehabilitation program to focus on the isolated deficit and to do total lower extremity patterns to facilitate the normal motor patterns.

Admittedly the patient does not perform in an isolated manner; however, there are studies that show that the OKC isolated testing does not correlate with functional performance,[2,21] whereas other studies do demonstrate a correlation between OKC testing and functional performance.[4,18,19,29-33]

CLOSED KINETIC CHAIN-SQUAT ISOKINETIC TESTING

In the process of progressing the patient from the previous tests to the actual weight-bearing (WB) position, we test the patient in the functional squat position using two legs and then to unilateral squat testing. The patient performs single-leg squats, and a bilateral comparison of the functional WB position is calculated. We expect the patients to have less than 20% bilateral deficit to progress them to the functional testing. If the patient has greater than a 20% deficit, then we emphasize single-legged concentrated training using integrated OKC and CKC rehabilitation techniques.

FUNCTIONAL JUMP TEST

This is a significant change during the FTA, because now there is no longer control superimposed on the patient; that is, when the patient jumps, there are varus/valgus and rotational forces that previously had been controlled with the various tests. The functional jump test (FJT) is a simultaneous two-legged jump. The purpose of the FJT is to measure functional simultaneous bilateral leg power. Therefore to prevent the segmental contributions of the arms, neck, and trunk,[13,18,19,26,28] we have the patient clasp the hands behind the back and minimize neck and trunk movements. We have the patient perform four gradient submaximal to maximal warmups (25%, 50%, 75%, 100%) followed by three maximal FJTs. The distance the patient jumps is averaged and then normalized to the patient's height. We expected healthy recreational or competitive athletes under 40 years of age to achieve the numbers listed in Table 10-3. Our criterion for the patient to progress to the next stage of the FTA is that the patient achieve less than a 15% deficit from the descriptive normative data. If the patient still has a greater than 15% deficit, we continue functional rehabilitation exercises until on retesting the patient performs at the

Table 10-3. Functional (relative/normalized) jump and hop test data for males and females

	Males	Females
Jump test (R + L)	90%-100%/Ht.	80%-90%/Ht.
Hop test (U)	80%-90%/Ht.	70%-80%/Ht.
Hop test (I)	80%-90%/Ht.	70%-80%/Ht.

minimum level of functional performance to progress to the next stage of the FTA.

FUNCTIONAL HOP TEST (FHT)

This is a major step in the FTA, because now uncontrolled stresses are placed exclusively on the involved extremity. This is also an important "psychological readiness test" on the part of the patient. Often, even though patients have passed all the previous tests in the FTA, they become hesitant or unable to perform a maximal hop test. The functional hop test is the test used as the functional test by the International Knee Documentation Committee (IKDC). However, the IKDC evaluates the FHT by just doing a bilateral comparison. We use similar guidelines for the FHT as described for the FJT. Patients hands are clasped behind their back, and head and trunk movements are minimized. The gradient submaximal warmups are used, and three maximal tests are performed. The data are analyzed in a bilateral comparison as described by the IKDC; however, the data are also normalized to body height similarly as the FJT (Table 10-3).

The patient must hop within 10% in bilateral comparison and be within 10% of the descriptive normative data in Table 10-3. If the patient has greater than a 10% deficit in either data analysis and interpretation, then functional rehabilitation exercises with single-leg activities are emphasized until the patient can perform and test to progress in the FTA.

LOWER EXTREMITY FUNCTIONAL TEST

When the patient/athlete reaches the terminal phases of the rehabilitation program, we use a lower extremity functional test (LEFT) test to evaluate various lower extremity patterns that are inherent to sporting activities. Furthermore, the specific dimensions of LEFT tests were designed based on in-clinic space constraints. Therefore, it makes it a practical functional test, and it does not require unrealistic space or equipment to perform the test. The dimensions of the floor layout are in a diamond shape with 30 feet in length and 10 feet in width (Fig. 10-3).

The test consists of a series of progressively more demanding functional movement patterns. The sequence of the LEFT test is described in the Box.

As the patient performs the LEFT, the quantity of performance (time) and the quality of performance (limping, hesitation, etc.) are also evaluated. The quality of performing the LEFT is evaluated empirically by the clinician to make a clinical judgment. The status of the "patient's readiness" to perform and the quality of his or her performance are

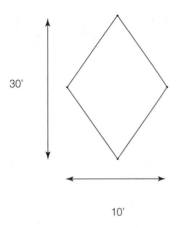

30'

10'

Fig. 10-3. Lower extremity functional test (LEFT) dimensions.

Sequence of the LEFT test
1. Sprint (frontwards)
2. Sprint (retro-run)
3. Side shuffles (both ways)
4. Cariocas (both ways)
5. Figure eights (both ways)
6. 45° angle cuts (outside foot) (both ways)
7. 90° angle cuts (outside foot) (both ways)
8. Crossover step (both ways)
9. Sprint (frontwards)
10. Sprint (retro-run)

Table 10-4. Lower extremity functional test (LEFT) descriptive normative data

Norms					
Males			Females		
90s	100s	125s	120s	135s	150s
	Avg			Avg	

critical interpretations of the test. The quantity of performance (time) for objective documentation is also measured. The descriptive normative data collected on more than 500 subjects and patients are illustrated in Table 10-4.

There are certainly many things to consider in the performance and interpretation of the LEFT. The patient's age, sex, somatotype, physical fitness level, sport position, and so on can influence the patient's performance. Therefore, there is a need to develop specific patient population norms. For example, if we are testing a 15-year-old 250-pound endomorphic male football player status post Grade 2, MCL

sprain, then the descriptive norms provided in Table 10-4 may have to be altered. Therefore, interpretation of test results relative to norms should be done carefully.

If the patient does not complete the test in the appropriate time (objective documentation) or does not perform in a qualitative manner that meets acceptable clinical guidelines, then the patient may not be ready to progress to the end stage, which is sport-specific testing. If the patient demonstrates a quantitative or a qualitative deficit in the LEFT test, then continued rehabilitation is necessary to "really" prepare the patient for the demands of his or her sport. Naturally, rehabilitation would be integrated with particular attention to the specific deficit. Goals for the patient are to be within the range of the descriptive normative data before progressing to the next level of the FTA. Table 10-4 lists the normative data. The final stage in the FTA is sport-specific testing, which often cannot adequately be evaluated in a clinical setting. Therefore, at this time the clinician must decide the appropriate testing methodology, location, and so forth. Fig. 10-4 summarizes the application of how the FTA provides the foundation of a progressive rehabilitation program done safely with an objective foundation to produce the final desired outcome. In summary, the FTA is a systematic progressive testing sequence that forms the scientific and clinical foundation for both testing a patient and for using the FTA results to guide the appropriate rehabilitation program. The following sections of this chapter present lower extremity and upper extremity strength assessment specifics. This introduction provides the overall framework of integration of strength into rehabilitation.

Section II SPECIFIC ASSESSMENT FOR THE LOWER EXTREMITY

The assessment of lower extremity muscular strength and functional capacity has significantly changed in recent years. Twenty years ago, lower extremity muscular strength was

assessed through manual muscle testing techniques. In addition, lower extremity function was often assessed through various functional activities such as the squatting,

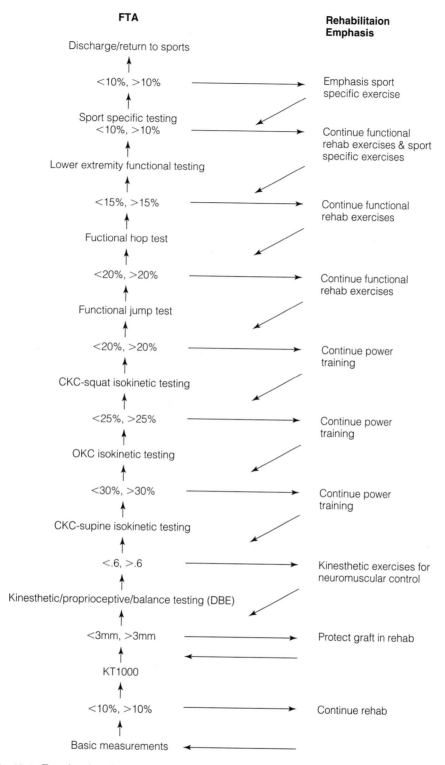

Fig. 10-4. Functional testing algorithm as the foundation for a progressive rehabilitation program.

vertical jumping, stair running, and duck waddle walk techniques. Since then, a metamorphosis occurred leading to today's specific and objective testing methods consisting of isokinetic muscular performance testing and specific functional test drills, which will be discussed in this chapter.

Tremendous demands are routinely placed on the knee joint with daily activities. These demands and stresses are accentuated with sporting activities, where the lower extremity is repetitiously loaded, such as with running, cutting, and jumping. During these strenuous and stressful sport activities, the tibiofemoral and patellofemoral joints are exposed to dramatic microtraumatic and macrotraumatic forces. This type of repetitive trauma can lead to deleterious effects on various noncontractile structures such as the articular cartilage, meniscus, and the ligamentous structures.

Knee joint stability is accomplished through three components: (1) the osseous structures, (2) ligamentous structures, and (3) the neuromuscular dynamic stabilizers. The dynamic stabilizers of the knee are the muscles surrounding the joint. The functions of these muscles are to provide movement (acceleration/deceleration) and dynamic joint stability and to control (absorption) of joint reaction stress. Thus, the musculature about the joint acts much like a shock absorber and therefore must be of appropriate integrity before demanding sport or work activities can be resumed or imposed. Hence, the documentation of muscular performance (strength) is critical in determining progression of the rehabilitation program and ultimate outcome.

The individuals' ability to activate muscles is critical to a successful rehabilitation outcome. In addition, positional sense (kinesthesia) and positional change (proprioception) are also extremely vital in the restoration of patient function. Therefore, the documentation of proprioception, kinesthesia, and reactive neuromuscular control is equally as important as muscular strength. This section of this chapter will discuss the objective documentation of muscular performance through isokinetic testing and through functional testing for the lower extremity.

When clinicians refer to the assessment of muscular performance, we often immediately consider manual muscle testing (MMT). Dr. Robert Lovett first described MMT in 1912 and discussed its application for neurologically involved patients.[132] Since its inception, there have been many revisions in the original technique. Two of the most popular versions of MMT have been developed by Kendall et al[59] and Daniels et al.[24] Between these two techniques there exists numerous inconsistencies in both the application and grading.[75,95,116] In addition, there are various inherent enigmas with MMT. Several authors have documented that the grading appears empirical,[49,83,129,131] it has poor inter-rater reliability,[49] and it appears as a relatively subjective test method.[81] In 176 postarthroscopy knee patients, Wilk et al[120] has demonstrated isokinetic knee extension deficits ranging from 23% to 31% in subjects who exhibited a "normal" MMT score bilaterally. Last, MMT does not allow the tester to document muscular performance parameters such as work, power, endurance, acceleration, and deceleration.[116] MMT determines the ability of the patient to exert tension or muscular force at a particular point in the range of motion. Consequently, the face validity of MMT for the orthopedic and athletic sports medicine patient may not be acceptable.[75,116,120]

Isokinetic testing experienced tremendous popularity during the 1980s and early 1990s but has recently come under considerable scrutiny. The efficacy of isokinetics has

Standardized isokinetic knee testing protocol

1. Patient education
2. Test uninvolved side first
3. Pretest warmup
4. Pad placement
5. Axis of rotation
6. Stabilization
7. Verbal commands
8. Visual feedback
9. Test repetitions
10. Rest interval between speeds
11. Gravity compensation
12. Calibration, system stability
13. Test environment
14. Firm end stop
15. Angular velocities

been questioned because of cost, necessity, lack of correlation to functional activities,[5] and possibly deleterious effects of open kinetic chain exercises.[58,86] Isokinetics is a dynamic, objective, and reproducible method of documenting muscular performance.[116] Therefore, it guides the clinician in determining treatment progression regarding muscular performance and assists the clinician in determining treatment progression such as return to work, sport, or functional activities. In addition, isokinetic testing provides the clinician with vital information regarding isolated muscular performance such as torque, work, power, and acceleration parameters.

ISOKINETIC TESTING OF THE KNEE

There have been numerous articles written regarding isokinetic testing of the knee. However, due to a lack of consistency in the method of testing and variations in testing protocol, often the existing literature is nonapplicable to the clinician. Recognizing these inconsistencies, Davies[27] and later Wilk et al[119] suggested a standardized isokinetic testing protocol. The purpose of the standardized testing protocol is to enhance test-retest reproducibility, and it would allow clinicians to share and compare test data. Fifteen "variables" should be standardized and controlled to ensure an objective, reliable, and reproducible isokinetic evaluation of the knee (see the Box and Fig. 10-5).

The first guideline is to ensure that the client is informed as to the purpose and intent of the isokinetic test. The client must be familiarized with the testing device, how it functions, and the results that will be provided. An informed knowledgeable client will be less apprehensive and will produce more reproducible tests. Wilk has shown (unpublished data) that subjects allowed one practice session prior to testing produced more consistent torque values in 83% to 88% of all test trials. Mawdsley[74] has reported significant

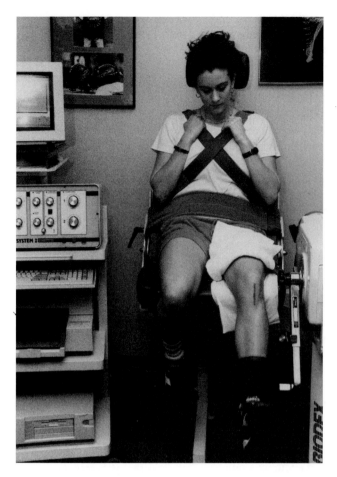

Fig. 10-5. Isokinetic testing of the knee joint musculature performed in the seated position utilizing a Biodex isokinetic dynamometer.

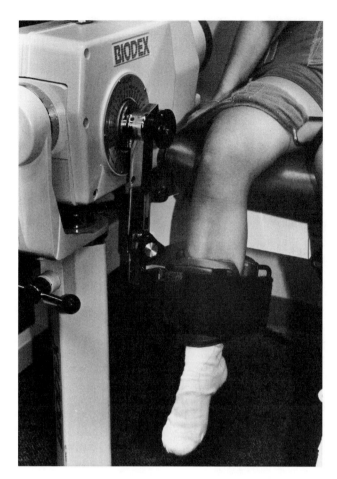

Fig. 10-6. The conventional resistance pad placement is 1 in. proximal to the medial malleolus. To minimize tibial displacement and more proximally placed pad is beneficial.

differences between the values demonstrated in the first testing session and those of all remaining sessions in a sequence of six trials. Therefore, it is recommended that whenever possible, clients undergo at least one isokinetic exposure prior to testing.

Testing the uninvolved side first is the next parameter to control. This serves three important functions: (1) it establishes a database for the involved knee, (2) it evaluates the client's willingness to be tested, and (3) it serves to decrease apprehension by allowing exposure to an isokinetic movement in the contralateral extremity first.[27,74,116]

The third testing guideline is the use of an active warmup prior to testing. Although three studies have documented no direct relationship between a warmup and enhanced isokinetic torque production,[25,27,114] definite physiologic rationale exists for performing an active warmup, as an active warmup should facilitate muscular performance by increasing blood flow, muscular/core temperature, oxygen utilization, and nervous system transmission and by decreasing muscular viscosity.[9,10,39,66,73] Based on these basic exercise physiology principles, a standardized warmup should be employed. The warmup includes a 5-minute lower body

cycling bout at a level of 90 repetitions per minute at a 600 kg/m workload, two sets of 10 repetitions of leg squats (0° to 60°) and five submaximal isokinetic repetitions, and at least one maximal repetition at each angular test velocity.[27]

The fourth parameter to standardize is the consistent placement of the resistance pad. Torque measurements are derived by multiplying force by its perpendicular distance from the axis of rotation.[75] However, when using an isokinetic device for torque acquisition, this calculation should be unnecessary, because the lever arm lengths of the machine and limb are equal and thus require no calculations. Three investigators have addressed the concern in changes in lever arm length related to torque production.[54,101,103] It has been determined that altering the pad placement greater than 25% of the total arm length (approximately 2 to 2½ in.) does significantly alter torque production.[54,103] We recommend documentation of arm length to ensure retest positioning and conventional placement of the resistance pad 1 in. proximal to the medial malleolus (Fig. 10-6).

The next guideline to consider is the alignment of the axis of rotation of the dynamometer with the knee joint. In the seated position, with the knee flexed to 90°, the axis of

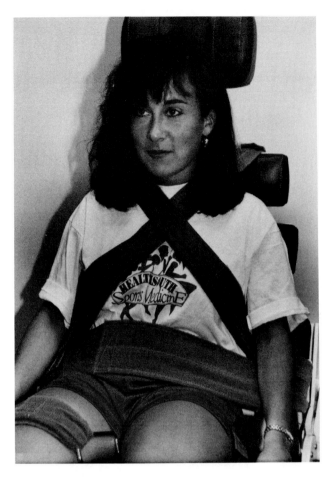

Fig. 10-7. When performing an isokinetic knee test, stabilization should be applied to the hips, thighs, and trunk to ensure isolation.

rotation of the tibiofemoral joint is .5 cm proximal to the joint line and through the lateral femoral condyle.[62] Accurate alignment of the axis of rotation will minimize translation of the resistance pad during testing.

The sixth parameter to control is proper positioning and stabilization of the subject to ensure test muscle isolation and enhance reproducibility (Fig. 10-7). Several studies have shown that changes in muscle length will produce significant differences in peak torque production.[18,43,65] Richard and Currier reported that back stabilization significantly improved knee extension peak torque production.[22,45,92] Currier documented that maintaining hip position at 110° to 130° resulted in maximum isometric torque production for the knee extensors.[22] Stabilization of the contralateral extremity has been shown not to have a significant effect on torque production,[88] whereas stabilization of the trunk and thigh results in enhanced consistency during isokinetic testing.[22]

The next guideline to standardize is the consistent use of verbal commands during testing. Johansson et al[53] demonstrated that loud verbal commands resulted in greater isometric torque values. It has been empirically stated[60,63] and it has been the author's clinical experience that aggressive verbal commands and encouragement, although enhancing torque values, results in the earlier occurrence of fatigue during both exercise and testing. Thus, it is recommended that verbal commands be consistent, encouraging, and moderate in intensity.

The eighth guideline is the utilization of visual feedback during testing. Numerous investigators have reported that knowledge of results during strength testing may enhance some parameters of performance.[36,44,72,91,111] Hence, visual feedback in the form of knowledge of results can significantly influence testing performance and must be consistently controlled during isokinetic testing. Because the use of visual feedback may lead to earlier muscular fatigue, it is not recommended.[36,116]

The number of test repetitions utilized during testing should also be standardized. Davies has reported that 10 isokinetic repetitions produce optimal training effects.[14] Johnson and Siegel[55] reported that at least three repetitions were required to establish a stable consistent isokinetic measurement. In addition, Croft[21] recommended eliminating the first test repetition from the data collection due to inconsistency. Arrigo and Wilk in a review of 500 isokinetic consecutive knee tests, have found that both peak torque and maximum work of the injured knee consistently occurred during the third repetition,[8] whereas for the uninjured knee the peak torque and maximum work repetition occurred during the second test repetition.[8] We recommend 10 to 15 repetitions at each test speed to establish work fatigue rates and endurance ratios.

The tenth parameter, controlling the rest interval during testing, is the next factor that must be standardized to ensure reproducibility. Ariki et al[7] have demonstrated that the optimal period of rest between each isokinetic test speed is 90 seconds. Based on these data, we recommended a 90-second rest between isokinetic test sets.

The limb that is undergoing testing should be gravity-compensated prior to testing. Significant differences have been demonstrated during isokinetic testing of muscle groups that were gravity-compensated when compared with those that were not.[37] When gravity compensation is not utilized, the muscles assisted by gravity will exhibit higher torque values, whereas the muscles that resist gravity will exhibit a lesser torque value. In addition, as the isokinetic angular velocity increases, so does the relative effect of gravity on torque values.[78,130] Therefore, we recommend that gravity compensation be performed prior to testing to ensure accuracy of performance.

The twelfth parameter to consider is the test system calibration. Although most manufacturers recommend calibration every 30 days, to ensure validity in test measures, the authors recommend calibration be performed every 2 weeks. In addition, the isokinetic system must be level and stabilized to the floor. A level, stable system will minimize artifact, overshoot, and oscillation interference during testing.[75]

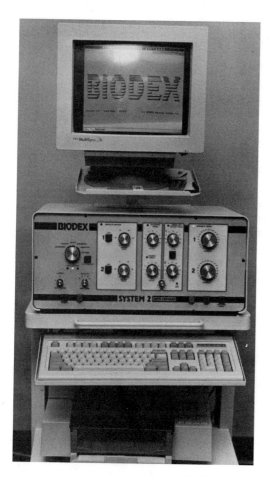

Fig. 10-8. The isokinetic dynamometer controller allows adjustment of the end range stop from soft stop (deceleration of limb applied) to hard stop (no deceleration effect).

Isokinetic angular velocity spectrum			
0-60°/sec Slow velocity	60-180°/sec Intermediate	180-300°/sec Fast	300-450°/sec Functional

The next guideline suggests that the test environment be conducive to human performance testing. A designated area should be available solely for testing and free from distractions. The skill and experience of the tester can greatly affect test reproducibility. An experienced tester can greatly allay client apprehension, ensure a reproducible standardized test from subject to subject, and maximize both the efficiency and the efficacy of isokinetic knee assessments.

The fourteenth parameter addresses the factor of the optimal amount of limb cushion at end range. Most isokinetic dynamometers allow the clinician to set the cushion of the end range stop from soft to hard abrupt stop. The cushion allows the patient enhanced comfort. Wilk et al have shown that altering the cushion during isokinetic testing of the shoulder abductors/adductors significantly affects peak torque.[122] This was observed with shoulder testing due to the long lever arm employed and end range torque spikes generated. This does not occur with knee testing. Thus, we recommend the use of a hard end stop to prevent the machine from assisting in limb deceleration during testing movements (Fig. 10-8).

The last parameter to standardize during isokinetic knee testing is the angular velocity to utilize. Significant debate persists regarding what angular velocities are most appropriate for knee testing. Davies has recommended testing throughout the velocity spectrum (60°/sec, 180°/sec, 300°/sec).[27] Conversely, Wilk has advocated fast-speed testing based on several factors. First, if we consider that the functional angular velocities of the tibiofemoral joint during walking range from approximately 230°/sec to 245°/sec[54] and approximately 1200°/sec during running,[33,87,109] then testing should be performed in a range related to function. Second, angular velocities in the intermediate and fast velocity spectrum (see the Box) minimize the amount of joint compressive, shear, and tibial displacement forces compared with slow-speed testing. Nisell et al[82] reported that during 30°/sec isokinetic knee extension movements, peak tibiofemoral compressive forces reached nine times body weight at 65° knee flexion. Kauffman et al[58] reported an anterior tibiofemoral shear force of 0.3 to 0.5 times body weight at 60°/sec and 0.2 times body weight during 180°/sec isokinetic knee extension (peak at 25° knee flexion). Kauffman et al[58] also reported a 1.8 and 1.4 times body weight posterior shear forces during isokinetic knee flexion at 60°/sec and 180°/sec, respectively. Wilk and Andrews[118] have reported increased anterior displacement of the tibia on the femur during slow-speed isokinetics when compared with fast-speed testing (Fig. 10-9). In addition, it has been my clinical experience that slow-speed testing (30°/sec, 60°/sec, 90°/sec) and training over a long period of time is detrimental to the patellofemoral joint and other knee extensor mechanism structures. Last, numerous studies have shown training at faster speeds results in physiologically based strength improvements at the slower speeds, and without the previously mentioned risks.[20,50,64] However, it should be noted that the optimal test velocity is based on the patient's functional demands and the clinician's preference.

Therefore, based on the information available, we suggest utilizing a velocity spectrum testing protocol that fits the specific functional requirements of the client. In the case of an elderly and relatively sedentary person whose goals are to return to ambulation only, our testing protocol would include testing at 180°/sec or 240°/sec, because these are the speeds at which this type of person will function most often. In the case of the athletic population, recreational or competitive, our testing velocity recommendations are 180°/sec, 300°/

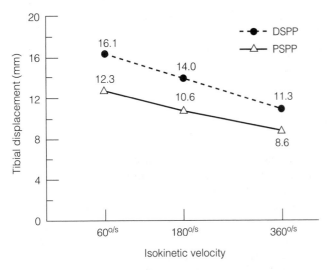

Fig. 10-9. The mean values of tibial displacements of both proximal and distal pad placement at three isokinetic speeds. (From Wilk KE, Andrews JR: The effects of pad placement and angular velocity on tibial displacement during isokinetic exercise, *J Orthop Sports Phys Ther* 17:24-30, 1993.)

sec, and 450°/sec. We test these clients at higher angular velocities because of the faster angular velocities achieved during sport movements. Wilhette et al have recommended the testing protocol progress from slower to faster angular velocities; this has been shown to improve reproducibility.[115] If the patient suffers from significant patellofemoral arthritis or chondrosis, then the application of an isometric test may be appropriate to minimize the patellofemoral and tibiofemoral shear force during testing.[69,70] Static testing of knee extensors/flexors has been advocated by Mangine and Mangine-Erfert[64,65]; however, there are limited published papers in this area. Mangine[64] suggests isometric testing of patellofemoral patients and with ACL reconstructed knees prior to dynamic testing. The authors recommended testing at 60° of knee flexion, and the patient performs three maximal effort repetitions for 10 seconds each.

KNEE TESTING

In the past, when isokinetic testing of the knee was discussed, the discussion was limited to isokinetic concentric testing only. Thus, the literature contains a tremendous number of articles relative to concentric isokinetic testing.* Presently, isokinetic dynamometers allow dynamic muscular performance testing with either concentric or eccentric muscular action. In addition, static muscle performance can be assessed through isometric muscular testing.[64,65] There have been only a limited number of studies performed on the knee musculature utilizing isokinetic eccentric activation.† This may be due to numerous factors such as delayed onset muscular soreness,[40,79] patient/clinician apprehension, and

* References 28, 29, 42, 67, 89, 96, 107, 133.
† References 15, 31, 41, 61, 77, 90, 99, 110, 112, 123.

Classification of test data

1. Torque

Peak torque
Mean torque
Mid range torque
Torque to body weight ratios
Unilateral muscle ratios

2. Muscular performance parameters

Total work
Average power
Work fatigue ratio
Work to body weight ratios
Power to body weight ratios

3. Neuromuscular performance parameters

Acceleration
Deceleration
Torque range
Force decay rate

4. Torque curve configuration

---

limited information pertaining to eccentric testing.[1] The authors believe that in time, additional information will be available to substantiate the application and efficacy of isokinetic eccentric testing.

We routinely assess knee extension/flexion in the seated position in a reciprocal fashion, based on the type of system we utilize (Biodex). One device (the Kin-Com) allows the clinician the ability to separately test knee flexors in the prone position and knee extensors in the seated position. Bohannom et al[19] have documented that reciprocal knee testing of agonist/antagonist muscles does not compromise reproducibility of isokinetic knee testing when a standardized testing protocol is utilized.

In addition, the measurement of muscular performance of tibial rotation may be important with selected knee disorders.[100] Several investigators have published data regarding tibial rotation muscular performance.[46,85,94] The positioning and stabilization described by Hester and Falkel[46] is what we presently utilize with a few modifications. The subject is seated in the accessary chair in a semi-reclined position (Fig. 10-10). This position affords excellent stabilization and isolation of the tibial musculature.

INTERPRETATION OF TEST DATA

Numerous publications are available to the reader that discuss the terminology of isokinetic test data. Rather than explain all isokinetic test parameters, we will classify the parameters and recommend ways to interpret the test data.

Test data can be divided into four interpretive classifications, as shown in the Box. These include torque

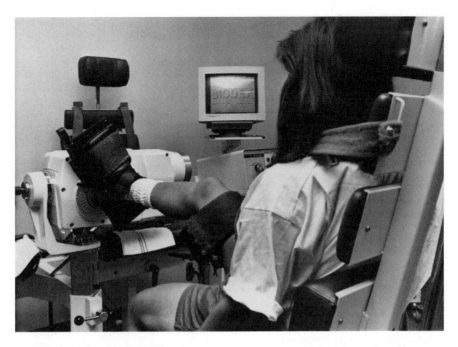

Fig. 10-10. Isokinetic testing/exercise for the tibial rotators in the seated position.

Table 10-5. Bilateral peak torque comparisons of patients following ACL reconstruction

	Extension		Flexion	
	180°	**300°**	**180°**	**300°**
12 weeks	69	76	94	98
26 weeks	73	81	97	100
52 weeks	91	95	110	112

Table 10-6. Quadriceps torque to body weight ratios

	Male	**Female**
60°/sec	100-115	80-95
180°/sec	65-75	50-60
300°/sec	45-55	35-45
450°/sec	35-45	20-30

*Biodex data.

parameters, muscular performance parameters, neuromuscular performance parameters, and torque curve shapes. We will briefly discuss several of these parameters and provide data for each.

The torque measurement most commonly utilized is peak torque, and it is most often used to compare the injured limb with the uninjured limb. Some authors have suggested a level of 80% to 85% of the opposite extremity be achieved prior to the return to sport activities.[67] This has come under some criticism of late.[75,95] We believe this parameter can be useful if carefully considered. Often the patient's opposite limb is not a sufficient standard of comparison due to gait abnormalities, leg preference, dominance, decreased activities, or underlying pathology. Therefore, we encourage a ratio as close to 1:1 as possible, usually within 10%. Active patients following ACL reconstruction exhibit a characteristic progression in quadriceps peak torque when compared with the opposite limb[117,121,126] (Table 10-5).

Another method for assessing peak torque is comparing it with body weight and establishing a ratio. This parameter,

torque to body weight ratios, are speed-, age-, and sex-dependent.[116] Davies[119] has recommended utilizing torque to body weight ratios for numerous years and has suggested this parameter is more appropriate than absolute torque measurements such as bilateral comparisons of peak torque. Table 10-6 represents quadriceps torque to body weight ratios utilized for males and females 18 to 29 years of age. For males and females these data decline 5% to 7% per decade of life. These data have been generated on the Biodex isokinetic dynamometer and may vary if another isokinetic device is utilized.[38,106,108,124,125]

Another method for interpreting torque measurements is unilateral muscle ratios. Several authors have published hamstring to quadriceps muscle ratios for various knee patients.[75,108,117,133] Table 10-7 presents the unilateral knee ratios we anticipate following various knee injuries.

The next group of parameters to interpret from the isokinetic test data are the muscular performance parameters, including work and power. We compare both these parameters relative to the opposite extremity and relative to

Table 10-7. Knee flexor/extensor unilateral ratios

Angular velocities	H/Q unilateral ratios
60°/sec	60-69%
180°/sec	70-79%
300°/sec	80-95%
450°/sec	95-105%

ACL clients add 10% to these values.
PCL clients subtract 10% from these values.

Table 10-8. Isokinetic torques to body weight ratio

	Extension	
	180°/sec	300°/sec
Total work/body weight	85-95	65-75
Total power body weight	160-175	155-170

body weight. When comparing bilateral data such as total work and average power, we attempt to establish a ratio as close to 1:1 as possible. Table 10-8 illustrates power and work to body weight ratios for athletic individuals. Work fatigue ratios are the amount of work performed during the first third of the test set compared with the last third of the test set. We strive for a ratio of 75% to 80% when evaluating this parameter.

The next area to consider when interpreting isokinetic test data is the neuromuscular performance parameter. This parameter assesses the acceleration/deceleration rate during the knee extension/flexion movement. The torque curve can be divided into three sections: the upslope or the acceleration range, the isokinetic load range, and the downslope or the deceleration range[127] (Fig. 10-11). The acceleration range is the portion of the motion it takes the individual to accelerate to the preset isokinetic speed. Our goal is for the patient to achieve at least 80% of his or her peak torque at 0.2 seconds before rapid sport movements are permitted. The deceleration range is the range of motion required for the patient to slow the limb prior to the end stop. This is represented as the force decay rate (FDR) of the torque curve.[27] Thus, the portion of the torque curve that the patient engages and maintains the preset isokinetic angular velocity is referred to as the "isokinetic load range."[127] We believe these neuromuscular performance parameters represent an important correlation to functional activities.[127] These parameters may also represent the status of the patient's "neurophysiologic system."

Another area to consider when interpreting the result of an isokinetic knee test is whether a consistent effort was performed by the test subject (patient). This has been a somewhat enigmatic area for many years. Was the patient or subject exerting a maximal effort for each repetition, or was he or she "holding back" for whatever reason? In the past, most clinicians assessed the isokinetic torque curves, and consistency of effort was measured by a gradual decrement in torque output. Today, most isokinetic systems determine the coefficient of variations among test repetitions. Several years ago, Arrigo and Wilk (unpublished data) assessed 500 consecutive knee tests to determine the normal range for the coefficient of variations. These data can be found in Table 10-9. Once again, these data were generated from a Biodex isokinetic system; values may vary if another isokinetic

device is utilized.[38,106,108,124,125] In addition, the data contained in Table 10-9 was based on 10 repetitions at 180°/sec and 15 repetitions at 300°/sec.

The last area to consider is torque curve shape. Numerous authors have investigated torque curve shapes as they relate to various pathologies.* This type of interpretation is difficult even for the most experienced of isokinetic testers. Most often, patients with patellofemoral chondrosis or arthritis will exhibit a torque curve with significant waviness and irregularities. These irregularities represent torque alterations secondary to pain inhibition (Fig. 10-12a). The reader is encouraged not to confuse the isokinetic angular velocity engagement with a torque curve irregularity. This type of torque curve is normal and represents no knee pathology (Fig. 10-12b). Wilk and Andrews have identified a characteristic torque curve with ACL deficient knees[118] (Fig. 10-12c). This type of torque curve represents a significant concavity in the force decay rate due to the mechanical subluxation of the tibia and is illustrated in an inability to sustain quadriceps torque in the last 30° of knee extension.[118] Thus, evaluating torque curves can be useful to the clinician; however, caution must be exercised not to "over-read" the curve. In addition, before any conclusions can be established from the torque curve, the data must be correlated to a careful and complete clinical examination. Most commonly, I perform analysis of the torque curve to determine the degree of smoothness of the curve and the presence of patellofemoral pain through waviness. For a thorough and concise summary of knee pathologies related to torque curves, the reader is referred to Davies.[27]

Anyone who has performed an isokinetic test or has attempted to interpret a test realizes that the amount of data generated is copious. One of the authors (Wilk) has recommended 11 parameters worthy of consistent evaluation when interpreting a test.[116] Interpretation of the same parameters each time has allowed the establishment of descriptive data more quickly and gained insight into data interpretation. The Box represents these parameters that are referred to as "The Bottom Line." The bottom line represents the order and isokinetic data evaluated routinely following each isokinetic test.

Isokinetic testing of the knee provides valuable information to the clinician regarding patient progression. It provides

---

* References 16, 27, 34, 35, 47, 48, 68, 76.

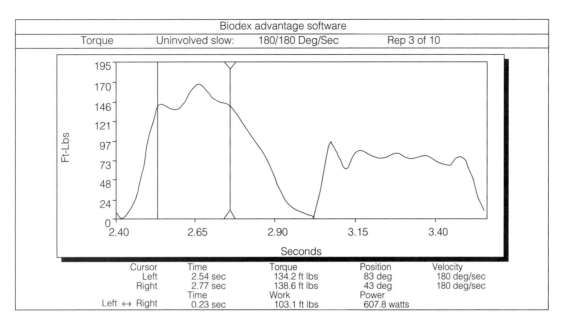

Fig. 10-11. The isokinetic torque curve can be divided into three compartments: acceleration range, isokinetic torque range, and deceleration range.

Table 10-9. Coefficient variations knee extension/flexion testing

	180°/sec	300°/sec
Extension (U)	5-9	7-12
(I)	5-9	8-13
Flexion (U)	5-9	8-13
(I)	5-10	8-13
$n = 500$		

U, Uninjured knee; *I*, injured knee.

Isokinetic interpretation "the bottom line"

Torque to body weight ratio
Torque curve analysis
Bilateral peak torque comparison
Total power to body weight ratio
Acceleration range
Torque range
Deceleration range
Unilateral muscle ratios
Bilateral comparison of total work
Work endurance ratio
Coefficient of variance analysis

objective reproducible data not obtainable in other forms of muscle testing. Several authors have advocated the use of handheld dynamometers to objectively assess muscular strength.[4,17] There are numerous types of handheld dynamometers such as spring-based, strain-gauge-based, hydraulic, load cells, and the traditional myometer types. For a thorough description of each including validity, reliability, and clinical application, the reader is referred to Amundsen.[2]

FUNCTIONAL TESTING

For numerous years, clinicians have attempted to objectively document lower extremity function and functional limitations through simulated activities. These simulated activities have been referred to as functional tests. Many investigators have included functional testing in their overall knee assessment and rating systems, but often the data collection procedures and analysis of test results have been relatively subjective in nature. In this section of the chapter, we will discuss the evolution of lower extremity functional assessment and discuss the current concepts in functional testing.

Marshall et al[71] in 1977 discussed the importance of a standardized knee evaluation method for determining knee function in surgical and nonsurgical patients. The authors indicated simulated functional activities should be a part of the knee evaluation. The functional tests included squatting, vertical jumping, and a duck waddle walk. The investigators observed the subjects performing the tasks and rated each subject on a scale of "can do" or "cannot do" basis. This is one of the first functional tests documented in the literature.

Later, Daniel et al[23] published results of three functional tests performed on ACL reconstructed knee patients and normal subjects. The three tests included a shuttle run, a one-legged hop for distance, and an isokinetic test performed at 60°/sec. The results of the normal population indicated that limb symmetry of 90% or greater was normal for males and 80% or greater was normal for females. In addition, 79%

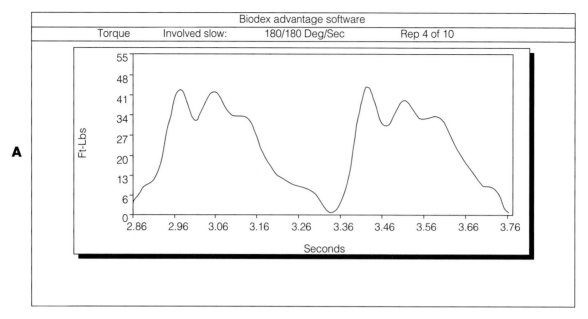

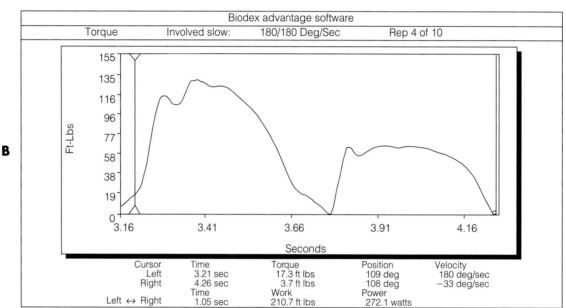

Fig. 10-12. Frequently seen isokinetic quadriceps (knee extension) torque curve shapes. **A** Illustrates significant pain inhibition of the quadriceps often secondary to patellofemoral chondrosis. **B,** A "normal" torque curve; the slight dip during the acceleration range is the engagement of isokinetic velocity.

of the ACL surgery treated patients had a normal functional test (hop test).

Jensen et al[51] observed several simulated sport type movements or functional activities; these included running in place, hopping, and the duck waddle walk. The examiners graded the activities as normal, asymmetrical, or unable to perform. Later, Jensen et al[52] modified the testing program to include stationary jogging, squatting, kneeling, duck waddle, and the leaning hop. The scoring consisted of yes (the patient was able to perform activity) or no (the patient was unable to perform the activity).

Tegner and Lysholm[104] performed four functional tests with two groups of patients; group one was ACL-deficient, and group two was ACL-reconstructed. The tests included a figure-eight running course, one-legged hop distance, a spiral staircase run, and an indoor slope run. The investiga-

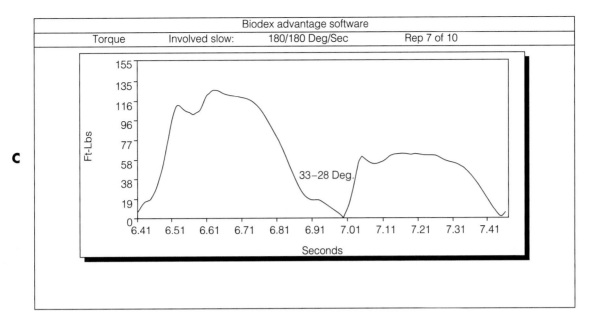

Fig. 10-12, cont'd.   C, An ACL-deficient knee torque curve; note the concavity during the deceleration portion of the curve.

tors compared the times and distances between subjects with and without a brace for all subjects. There was no statistical significance between the ACL-deficient knees and the patients who had surgery. Later, Tegner et al[105] reported results of functional tests of patients with an ACL-deficient knee compared with competitive soccer players. The tests included a figure-eight run, a one-legged hop for distance, a staircase run, and a slope run. Sixty-two percent of the ACL-deficient patients exhibited a normal one-legged hop for a distance test result. The authors concluded that the majority of patients with ACL-deficient knees will perform normally during hopping and straight running, which are more easily controlled motions, but will experience greater difficulty with turn-running and slope-running activities.

Barber et al[12] performed five hopping, jumping, and cutting functional activities with 35 ACL-deficient knee patients and 93 normal knee subjects. Specifically, the functional tests included a one-legged vertical jump, a shuttle without pivoting, and a shuttle run with pivoting. In addition, isokinetic testing at 60°/sec and 300°/sec was performed, and knee arthrometer testing was also performed. The results indicated no statistical significant differences between the right and left limbs related to sport activity level, gender, or dominant side. An 85% symmetry index score was reported for the normal population for the one-legged hop tests. In the ACL-deficient knee group, 50% of the patients exhibited an abnormal single-leg hop score. The investigators noted the cutting type tests and vertical jump, and did not detect functional limitations in a reliable manner. In addition, a statistically significant relationship was noted among abnormal hop scores and (1) self-assessed difficulty with cutting, and twisting, (2) quadriceps isokinetic weakness, and (3) patellofemoral compression pain. Specifically, patients with low quadriceps peak torque at 60°/sec did not perform the single-legged hop test (particularly distance hop) within the 85% limb symmetry index. The shuttle run and vertical jump test exhibited the lowest sensitivity rates in lower limb limitations. Based on these test trials, the investigators suggested performing at least two single-legged hop tests to accurately determine limb symmetry and using the opposite limb as a control.

Noyes et al[84] reported the lower limb function in 67 ACL-deficient knees. The investigators performed four one-legged tests: (1) single hop for distance, (2) timed hop, (3) triple hop for distance, and (4) crossover for distance. In addition, the subjects were isokinetically tested at 60°/sec and 300°/sec for knee extension/flexion, and knee arthrometer testing was performed to document anteroposterior knee laxity. The results indicated an abnormal limb symmetry score in 62% of the subjects when two hop tests were calculated. The crossover hop test rendered the same amount of abnormal scores as the single-hop tests and the timed hop test. In addition, a statistical correlation was reported between abnormal limb symmetry on the hop tests and low-velocity quadriceps isokinetic test results.

Several authors have documented a positive correlation between isolated isokinetic muscular performance test results and functional test maneuvers such as running, cutting, and hopping.* Others have reported no correlation between isokinetic results and athletic performance or functional simulation.[5,30,93] The investigators who have reported a positive correlation have noted this correlation for only the knee extension; none have reported a positive relationship between hamstring isokinetic performance and functional testing. In addition, the positive correlations were noted on isokinetic test systems, which allow reciprocal testing of knee extension and flexion functions. Conversely, the authors who reported no correlation performed with testing methods that employed concentric/eccentric muscle testing.

Recently, Wilk et al[127] assessed the subjective knee scores, isokinetic test results, and functional test scores in 50 ACL-reconstructed knees. Isokinetic testing was performed at 180°/sec, 300°/sec, and 450°/sec. Three functional test hops were performed: single leg for distance, single-leg timed hop, and crossover triple hop for distance. The results indicated a positive correlation between isokinetic quadriceps peak torque at 180°/sec and 300°/sec and all three functional hop tests. There was no positive correlation between hamstring function and functional hop testing. The subjective knee self-assessment scores compared favorably to the subject's ability to generate knee extension torque, accelerate the limb quickly during knee extension, and the timed hop and crossover triple hop. In addition, Wilk et al explored the concept of limb acceleration and deceleration range during knee extension/flexion movements. It was noted that individuals who required less acceleration range (thus accelerated quickly) and decelerated during a longer range scored higher on the hop tests. The authors discussed the role of the hamstrings as a critical decelerator in the last 25% of range during active knee extension. Wilk et al[127] reported a sequential doubling in deceleration range during knee extension from 180°/sec to 300°/sec and 300°/sec to 450°/sec. Basmajian[13] has reported that antagonist co-contraction is minimal except at high-velocity movements. This is the first study to document acceleration, deceleration, and torque range values for knee extension/flexion testing.[127]

Thus, based on the numerous articles published[102,105,127] there appears to be a positive correlation between quadriceps isokinetic muscular performance and functional hop test results. Recently, Bandy et al[11] examined the reliability and limb symmetry for five one-legged functional tests in normal subjects. The authors performed a horizontal hop test, vertical jump, timed hop test, triple hop for distance, and triple crossover hop test. The tests were performed on at least 16 subjects; all were tested three times across a 3-week period. The horizontal hop test, triple hop, and timed hop were shown to be the most reliable (.92 to .94). The vertical

jump test exhibited the poorest reliability (.85). Limb symmetry scores were within 1% for all tests.[11]

To date, our discussion of lower extremity functional assessment has been limited to higher functional level activities (sport-related) such as running, cutting, and single-leg hopping. Tests to document and quantify the strength of the knee extensors, knee flexors, ankle plantar flexors, and hip extensors during everyday functional activities may be beneficial in the general orthopedic lower extremity patient. For example, knee patients often complain of difficulty getting up from a chair or toilet seat and ascending or descending stairs; these functional movements should be tested with a logical and systematic functional strength test. Aniansson et al[6] have developed functional strength assessments for the elderly that measure the ability of an individual to ascend and descend a step of increasing heights (4, 8, 12, 16, or 20 in). The assessment includes whether assistance is required, level of pain, balance, and subjective exertion level.[3,6]

Wilk et al[128] have suggested three levels of functional testing based on the type of patient and phase of the rehabilitation program. Thus, level one functional tests are for low-demand patients, whose goals are independent and safe ambulation on level surfaces and stairs, and specific functions such as kneeling and squatting. The Box describes the various levels and functional tests that are utilized.

Level two includes patients who are moderately demanding of their knee joint. These individuals are involved in moderate-intensity recreational sports such as golf, tennis, walking, and bicycling. The tests for this group of patients are listed in the Box and are performed on a balance beam. For the aggressive athletic individual, level three functional testing should be utilized. Level three functions include running, jumping, and sharp cutting with deceleration. Individuals involved in sports such as basketball, volleyball and racquetball place high demands (level three) on their knee joint and require more challenging tests than level one or two individuals. The Box describes the various levels and functional tests that are utilized.

---

* References 12, 57, 84, 98, 102, 105, 113, 127.

Functional knee testing

Level one, low demand	Level two, moderate demand	Level three, high demand
• Single-leg step test	• Balance beam	• Single-leg hop test
• Squatting	–lateral step-up	–distance
• Level ambulation	–dip walk	–timed hop
• Ambulation/pivot	–walk-pivot	–triple crossover
• Sit to stand	–side shuffle	• 90° run/cut test
• Romberg test	–cariocas	• Shuttle run (yo-yo)
	–stance	

Section III SPECIFIC ASSESSMENT FOR THE UPPER EXTREMITY

Application of isokinetic exercise and testing for the upper extremity is imperative due to the demanding muscular work required in both ADL and sport-specific activities. The large unrestricted range of motion of the glenohumeral joint and limited inherent bony stability necessitates dynamic muscular stabilization to ensure normal joint arthrokinematics.[46] Objective information regarding the intricate balance of agonist/antagonist muscular strength surrounding the glenohumeral joint is a vital resource in rehabilitation and preventative evaluation of the shoulder. Utilization of therapeutic exercise and isolated joint testing for the entire upper extremity kinetic chain, including the scapulothoracic joint, is indicated for an overuse injury or postoperative rehabilitation of an isolated injury of the shoulder or elbow.[13]

RATIONALE FOR UTILIZATION OF ISOKINETICS IN UPPER EXTREMITY STRENGTH ASSESSMENT

Unlike the lower extremity, where most functional and sport-specific movements occur in a closed kinetic chain environment, the upper extremity almost exclusively functions in an open kinetic chain format.[51] The throwing motion, tennis serve, and ground strokes are all examples of open kinetic chain activities for the upper extremity. The use of open kinetic chain muscular strength assessment methodology allows for isolation of particular muscle groups, as opposed to closed chain methods, which utilize multiple joint axes, planes, and joint and muscle segments. Traditional isokinetic upper extremity test patterns are open chain, with respect to the shoulder, elbow, and wrist. The velocity spectrum (1°/sec to 500°/second) currently available on commercial isokinetic dynamometers provides specificity with regard to testing the upper extremity by allowing the clinician to assess muscular strength at faster, more functional speeds. Table 10-10 lists the angular velocities of sport-specific upper extremity movements.

The dynamic nature of upper extremity movements is a critical factor in directing the clinician to optimal testing methodology for the upper extremity. Manual muscle testing (MMT) provides a static alternative for the assessment of muscular strength using well-developed patient positions and stabilization.[10,41] Despite the detailed description of manual assessment techniques, reliability of MMT is compromised due to clinician size/strength differences and the subjective nature of the grading system (as discussed previously).[49,66]

Ellenbecker[20] compared isokinetic testing of the shoulder internal and external rotators with MMT in 54 subjects exhibiting manually assessed, symmetrical normal grade (5/5) strength. Isokinetic testing found relatively small mean differences between extremities in internal and external rotation. Of particular significance was the large variability in the size of this mean difference between extremities despite bilaterally symmetrical MMT. The use of MMT is an integral part of a musculoskeletal screening evaluation, because it provides a time-efficient, gross screening of muscular strength of multiple muscles using a static, isometric muscular contraction particularly in situations of neuromuscular disease or in patients with large muscular strength deficits.[49,66] The limitations of MMT appear to be most evident where only minor impairment of strength are present, and in the identification of subtle isolated strength deficits. Differentiation of agonist/antagonist muscular strength balance is also complicated using manual techniques as opposed to with isokinetic apparatus.[20]

RELIABILITY OF UPPER EXTREMITY ISOKINETICS

Several investigators have tested the reliability of isokinetic dynamometer systems on human subjects.[2,27,64] The vast majority of isokinetic reliability studies have utilized the knee extension/flexion movement pattern. Recently, isokinetic reliability studies have been published for the Cybex,[54]

Table 10-10. Upper extremity angular velocities of functional activities

Joint	Movement	Sport activity	Angular velocity	Source
Shoulder	IR	Baseball pitching	7000°/sec	Dillman[16]
Shoulder	IR	Tennis serve	1000°/sec-1500°/sec	Shapiro[60]
Shoulder	IR	Tennis serve	2300°/sec	Dillman[15]
Elbow extension		Baseball pitching	2500°/sec	Dillman[16]
Elbow extension		Tennis serve	1700°/sec	Dillman[15]
Wrist flexion		Tennis serve	315°/sec	Vangheluwe and Hebbelinck[65]

Biodex,[29,45] and KinCom[33] dynamometers using glenohumeral joint internal and external rotation with varying degrees of abduction. The findings of these studies report consistently these dynamometers as reliable devices for measurement of dynamic muscular strength. These studies also consistently report greater test-retest reliability for concentric as compared with eccentric modes of testing.[29,45] Despite the greater degree of inherent mobility and concerns regarding stabilization of the shoulder girdle, it appears that commercially available isokinetic dynamometers are capable of providing reliable upper extremity strength data.

GLENOHUMERAL JOINT TESTING

Dynamic strength assessment of the rotator cuff musculature is of primary importance in rehabilitation and preventative screening of the glenohumeral joint. The rotator cuff forms an integral component of the force couple in the shoulder described by Inman et al.[37] The approximating role of the supraspinatus for the glenohumeral joint and the inferior (caudal) glide component action provided by the infraspinatus, teres minor, and subscapularis must stabilize the humeral head within the glenoid against the superiorly directed forces exerted by the deltoid with humeral elevation.[43] Muscular imbalances, primarily in the posterior rotator cuff, have been objectively documented in patients with glenohumeral joint instability and impingement.[70]

SHOULDER INTERNAL/EXTERNAL ROTATION STRENGTH TESTING

Initial testing and training using isokinetics for rehabilitation of the shoulder typically involves the modified base position. The modified base position is obtained by tilting the dynamometer approximately 30° from horizontal base position.[11] This causes the shoulder to be placed in approximately 30° of abduction (Fig. 10-13). The modified base position places the shoulder in the scapular plane (30° anterior to the coronal plane).[58] The scapular plane is characterized by enhanced bony congruity and a neutral glenohumeral position that results in a mid-range position for the capsular ligaments and scapulohumeral musculature.[58] This position does not place the suprahumeral structures in an impingement situation and is well tolerated by patient populations.[11]

Isokinetic testing using the modified base position requires consistent application of the patient to the dynamometer. Studies have demonstrated significant differences in internal and external rotation strength with varying degrees of abduction, flexion, and horizontal abduction/adduction of the glenohumeral joint.[33,34,62,69] The modified base position utilizes a standing patient position that compromises both isolation and test-retest reliability. Despite these limitations, valuable data can be obtained early in the rehabilitative process using this neutral, modified base position.[11,24]

Isokinetic assessment of internal and external rotation

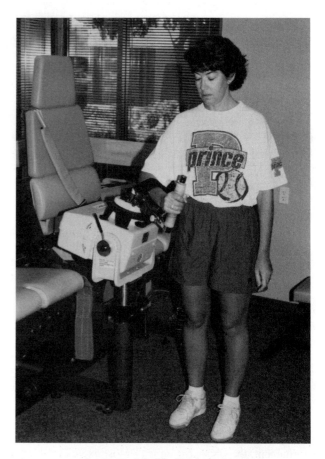

Fig. 10-13. Modified base position.

strength is also done with 90° of glenohumeral joint abduction. Specific advantages of this test position are greater stabilization in either a seated or supine test position on most dynamometers and placement of the shoulder in an abduction angle, corresponding to the overhead throwing position used in sport activities[26,16] (Fig. 10-14). Initial tolerance of the patient to the modified base position is required as a precursor to utilization of the 90° abducted position by these authors. Ninety-degree abducted isokinetic testing can be performed in either the coronal or scapular plane. Benefits of the scapular plane are similar to those discussed in the modified position and include protection of the anterior capsular glenohumeral ligaments and a theoretical length-tension enhancement of the posterior rotator cuff.[25,32,33] Changes in length-tension relationships and the line of action of scapulohumeral and axiohumeral musculature are reported in 90° of glenohumeral joint abduction, as compared with a more neutral adducted glenohumeral joint position.[4] Utilization of the 90° abducted position of isokinetic strength assessment will more specifically address muscular function required for overhead activities.

Heavy emphasis is placed on the assessment of internal and external rotation strength of the shoulder during rehabilitation. Rationale for this apparently narrow focus is provided by an isokinetic training study by Quincy and

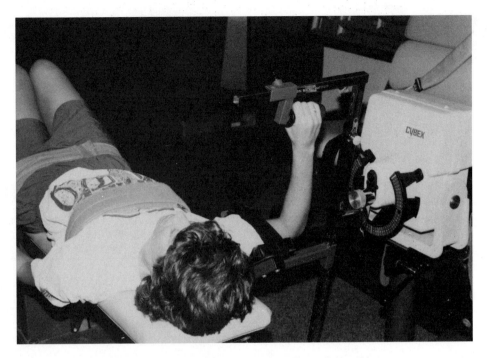

Fig. 10-14. Ninety-degree abducted IR/ER testing position.

Davies.[55] Six weeks of isokinetic training of the internal and external rotators produced statistically significant improvements not only in internal and external rotation strength but also in flexion/extension and abduction/adduction strength. Isokinetic training of flexion/extension and abduction/ adduction produced improvements only in the position of training. The overflow of strength caused by training the internal and external rotators provides rationale for the heavy emphasis on strength development and assessment in rehabilitation.

INTERPRETATION OF SHOULDER IR/ER TESTING
Bilateral differences

Similar to isokinetic testing of the lower extremity, assessment of an extremity's strength relative to the contralateral side forms the basis for standard data interpretation. This practice is more complicated in the upper extremity due to limb dominance, particularly in the unilaterally dominant sport athlete. In addition to the complexities added by limb dominance, isokinetic descriptive studies demonstrate disparities in the degree of limb dominance and the presence of strength dominance only in specified muscle groups.*

In general, a maximum limb dominance of the internal and external rotators of 5% to 10% is assumed in nonathletic and recreational level upper extremity sport athletes.[40] Significantly greater internal rotation strength has been identified in the dominant arm in professional,[7,23] collegiate,[9] and high school[36] baseball players and in elite level junior[8,18] and adult[17] tennis players. No difference between extremities has been demonstrated in concentric external rotation in professional[23,71] and collegiate[9] baseball pitchers and in elite junior[8,18] and adult[17] tennis players. This selective strength development in the internal rotators produces significant changes in agonist/antagonist muscular balance. The identification of this using isokinetic testing will be discussed in future sections of this chapter.

Normative data utilization

Utilization of normative or descriptive data can provide assistance to clinicians to further analyze isokinetic test data. Care must be taken to use normative data that is both population and apparatus specific.[28] Tables 10-11 and 10-12 present data from large samples of specific athletic populations on two dynamometer systems. Data are presented using body weight as the normalizing factor.

Unilateral strength ratios (agonist/antagonist)

The assessment of muscular strength balance of the internal and external rotators is of vital importance when interpreting upper extremity strength tests. Alteration of this external/internal (ER/IR) ratio has been reported in patients with glenohumeral joint instability and impingement.[70] The initial description of the ER/IR ratio on normal female subjects was published by Ivey et al[39] and confirmed by Davies[11] for both males and females. An ER/IR ratio of 66% is targeted in normal subjects. Biasing this ratio in favor of the external rotators has been advocated by clinicians[11,24,72]

* References 1, 8, 9, 17, 18, 23, 36.

Table 10-11. Isokinetic peak torque to body weight ratios from 150 professional baseball pitchers

Speed (°/sec)	Internal		External	
	Dominant	Nondominant	Dominant	Nondominant
180	27%	17%	18%	19%
300	25%	24%	15%	15%

Modified from Wilk KE, Andress JR, Arrigo CA, Kerins M, Erber DJ: The strength characteristics of internal and external rotator muscles in professional baseball pitchers, *Am J Sports Med* 61, 1993.

Table 10-12. Isokinetic peak torque and work to body weight ratios from 147 professional baseball pitchers

Speed (°/sec)	Internal		External	
	Dominant	Nondominant	Dominant	Nondominant
210 Torque	21%	19%	13%	14%
210 Work	41%	38%	25%	25%
300 Torque	20%	18%	13%	13%
300 Work	37%	33%	23%	23%

Modified from Ellenbecker TS, Dehart RL, Boeckmann R: Isokinetic shoulder strength of the rotator cuff in professional baseball pitchers (abstract), *Phys Ther* 72, 1992.

for both prevention of injury in throwing and racquet sport athletes and following insult or surgery to the glenohumeral joint.

Widespread reports of alteration of the ER/IR ratio due to selective muscular development of the internal rotators without concomitant external rotation strength are present in the literature.[9,17,18,23,36] This alteration has provided clinicians objective rationale for the global recommendation of preventative posterior rotator cuff (ER) strengthening programs for athletes in high-level overhead activities.[24,72] Examples of ER/IR ratios are presented in Table 10-13, with respect to population and apparatus specificity.

ADDITIONAL GLENOHUMERAL JOINT TESTING POSITIONS
Shoulder abduction/adduction

Isokinetic evaluation of shoulder abduction/adduction strength is an additional pattern frequently evaluated because of the abductor's key role in the Inman force couple[37] and the adductor's functional relationship to throwing velocity.[3,44] Specific factors important in this testing pattern are the limitation of range of motion to approximately 120° to avoid glenohumeral joint impingement and consistent utilization of gravity correction.[35]

Interpretation of abduction/adduction isokinetic tests follow traditional bilateral comparison, normative data comparison, and unilateral strength ratios. Ivey et al,[39] using normal adult females, reported abduction/adduction (AB/ADD) ratios of 50% bilaterally. Similar findings were reported by Alderink and Kluck[1] in high school and collegiate baseball pitchers. Wilk et al.,[73,74] reported dominant arm (AB/ADD) ratios of 85% to 95% using a Biodex

Table 10-13. Unilateral ER/IR ratios of professional baseball pitchers

Speed	Dominant arm	Nondominant arm
180 Torque	65	64
300 Torque	61	70
210 Torque	64	74
210 Work	61	66
300 Torque	65	72
300 Work	62	70

Modified from Ellenbecker TS, Dehart RL, Boeckmann R: Isokinetic shoulder strength of the rotator cuff in professional baseball pitchers (abstract), *Phys Ther* 72, 1992; and Wilk K, Andress JR, Arrigo CA, Keirns MA, Erber DJ: The strength characteristics of internal and external rotator muscles in professional baseball pitchers, *Am J Sports Med* 61, 1993.

dynamometer. His data utilized a windowing technique, which removed impact artifact following free limb acceleration and end stop impact from the data. Upper extremity testing, using long input adapters and fast isokinetic testing velocities, can produce torque artifact that significantly changes the isokinetic test result. Wilk et al recommends windowing the data by removing all data obtained at velocities outside 95% of the present angular testing velocity.[74]

Shoulder flexion/extension and horizontal abduction/adduction

Additional isokinetic patterns utilized to obtain a more detailed profile of shoulder function are flexion/extension and horizontal abduction/adduction. Both of these motions are generally tested in a less functional supine position to improve stabilization. Normative data are less prevalent in the literature on these positions. Flexion/extension ratios reported on normal subjects by Ivey et al[39] are 80% (4:5). Ratios on athletes with shoulder extension dominant activities are reported at 50% for baseball pitchers[1] and 75% to 80% for highly skilled adult tennis players.[17] Further development of normative data is needed to more clearly define strength in these upper extremity patterns. Body position and gravity compensation are, again, key factors affecting proper data interpretation.

Scapulothoracic testing (protraction/retraction)

In addition to the supraspinatus/deltoid force couple, the serratus anterior/trapezius force couple is of critical importance in a thorough evaluation of upper extremity strength. Gross manual muscle testing and screening attempting to identify scapular winging are commonly utilized in the clinical evaluation of the shoulder complex. Davies and Hoffman[14] have recently published normative data on 250 shoulders regarding isokinetic protraction/retraction testing. A nearly 1:1 relationship of protraction/retraction strength was reported. Testing and training the serratus anterior, trapezius, and rhomboid musculature enhances scapular stabilization and strengthens primary musculature involved in the scapulo-humeral rhythm. Emphasis on the promotion of proximal stability to enhance distal mobility is a concept used and recognized by nearly all disciplines of rehabilitative medicine.[63]

Distal upper extremity testing

Elbow extension/flexion. Despite the high velocity and maximal intensity muscular work by the muscles surrounding the elbow joint during sport activities, relatively few data have been published regarding dynamic strength assessment in this area. In addition to MMT,[10,41] which describes specific forearm positions to differentiate between forearm flexor muscle testing, similar positional relationships are reported with handheld dynamometers. Bohannon[6] reported significant differences in static muscular strength assessment with varying glenohumeral abduction and rotation angles. This, again, clearly demonstrates the need for standardization of patient application to the dynamometer to ensure reliable data acquisition.

Isokinetic elbow extension/flexion testing is performed in 45° of glenohumeral joint abduction on the Cybex and a seated adducted shoulder position on the Biodex. Concentric descriptive data generated on the Cybex show a 1:1 relationship between the elbow flexion and extension strength in normal subjects[59] and collegiate baseball players.[52]

Additional indications for isokinetic strength assessment of the elbow flexors and extensors is best explained by the important relationship of these muscles to the glenohumeral joint. The stabilizing role of the biceps long head has been described by several authors.[38,57] The forceful contractions

of the bicep musculature during the later portion of the acceleration phase of the throwing motion coupled with the intimate anatomic relationship of the bicep long head and the superior labrum,[57,61] make evaluation of the bicep musculature's integrity a valuable component in a thorough evaluation or rehabilitation program. The presence of increased bicep muscular activity has been reported in pitchers with glenohumeral joint instability as compared with a control population of pitchers.[30]

Wrist and forearm testing. The primary method for dynamic strength assessment of the forearm and wrist involves the use of isokinetic dynamometers. A gross estimate of wrist and finger strength can rapidly be generated using a hand grip dynamometer. The lack of isolation and static nature of this test proves limiting. Bechtol[5] has outlined a protocol for the Jamar hand grip dynamometer.

A dominance factor of 5% to 10% is reported in recreational athletes and in normal populations in isokinetic studies of distal strength.[50] Greater unilateral dominance of 15% to 30% has been measured distally in elite tennis players[17] and professional baseball pitchers.[21] Of particular importance in these studies is the presence of selective muscular development in these populations. Significantly greater dominant forearm pronation, wrist flexion, and extension strength were measured in elite tennis players without a dominance in supination.[17] Sport-specific activity patterns, requiring both concentric and eccentric muscle work in specific distal muscle groups measured with EMG, correspond to isokinetic strength profiles in these select populations.[48] Published test-retest reliability of distal upper extremity isokinetics is not currently available in the literature. Factors such as the standardization of elbow extension/flexion and forearm pronation/supination during testing are critical components of enhancing reliability in these areas.[19]

Concentric versus eccentric considerations

The availability of eccentric dynamic strength assessment has made a significant impact, primarily in research investigations. The extrapolation of research-oriented isokinetic principles to patient populations has been a gradual process. Use of eccentric testing in the upper extremity is clearly indicated, based on the prevalence of functionally specific eccentric work. Maximal eccentric functional contractions of the posterior rotator cuff during the follow-through phase of the throwing motion and tennis serve provide rationale for eccentric testing and training in rehabilitation and preventative conditioning.[40] Kennedy et al[42] found mode-specific differences between the concentric and eccentric strength characteristics of the rotator cuff. Further research regarding eccentric muscular training is necessary before widespread use of eccentric isokinetics can be applied to patient populations.

Basic characteristics of eccentric isokinetic testing, such as greater force production as compared with concentric contractions at the same velocity, are reported in the internal and external rotators.[12,22,47] This enhanced force generation is generally explained by the contribution of the series elastic (noncontractile) elements of the muscle-tendon unit to force generation in eccentric conditions. An increase in postexercise muscle soreness, particularly of latent onset, is a common occurrence following periods of eccentric work. Therefore, eccentric testing would not be the mode of choice during early inflammatory stages of an overuse injury.[12] Many clinicians recommend utilization of dynamic concentric testing prior to performance of an eccentric test. Both concentric and eccentric isokinetic training of the rotator cuff have produced objective concentric and eccentric strength improvements in elite tennis players.[22,47]

Relationship of isokinetic testing to functional performance

Dynamic muscular strength assessment is utilized to evaluate the underlying strength and balance of strength in specific muscle groups. This information is used to determine the specific anatomical structure that requires strengthening and to demonstrate the efficacy of treatment procedures. Isokinetic testing of the shoulder internal and external rotators has been used as one aspect in demonstrating the functional outcome following rotator cuff repair on select patient populations.[31,56,67,68]

An additional purpose for the utilization of isokinetic testing is to determine the relationship of muscular strength to functional performance. Several studies have tested upper extremity muscle groups and correlated their respective levels of strength to sport-specific functional tests. Pedegana et al[53] found a statistical relationship among elbow extension, wrist flexion, and shoulder extension, flexion and external rotation strength measured isokinetically, and throwing speed in professional pitchers. Bartlett et al,[3] in a similar study, found the shoulder adductors to correlate to throwing speed. These studies are in contrast to that of Pawlowski and Perrin,[52] who did not find a significant relationship in throwing velocity.

Ellenbecker et al[22] found 6 weeks of concentric isokinetic training of the rotator cuff resulted in a statistically significant improvement in serving velocity in collegiate tennis players. Mont et al,[47] in a similar study, found serving velocity improvements following both concentric and eccentric internal and external rotation training. A direct statistical relationship between isokinetically measured upper extremity strength and tennis serve velocity was not found by Ellenbecker[17] despite increases in earlier studies in serving velocity following isokinetic training. The complex biomechanical sequences of segmental velocities and the interrelationship between the kinetic chain link with the lower extremities and trunk make delineation and identification of a direct relationship between an isolated structure and a complex functional activity difficult. Isokinetic testing can provide a reliable dynamic measurement of isolated joint motions and muscular contributions to assist the clinician in

the assessment of underlying muscular strength and strength balance. The integration of isokinetic testing with a thorough, objectively oriented clinical evaluation allows the clinician to provide optimal rehabilitation for both overuse and postsurgical cases.

REVIEW QUESTIONS

1. What are the empirical guidelines for a patient progressing in the functional testing algorithm?
2. What factors must be considered by the clinician when evaluating the performance as well as interpreting the lower extremity functional test?
3. What is the function of the neuromuscular dynamic stabilizers of the knee joint?
4. What are four interpretive classifications used in the assessment of isokinetic test data?
5. How has functional assessment of the lower extremity developed over the past 20 years? What are the concepts currently used in lower extremity functional testing?

SECTION I REFERENCES

1. Agre JC, Magness JL et al: Strength testing with a portable dynamometer: reliability for upper and lower extremities, *Arch Phys Med Rehabil* 68:454, 1987.
2. Anderson MA, Gieck JH, Perrin D et al: The relationship among isometric, isotonic and isokinetic concentric and eccentric quadriceps and hamstring force and three components of athletic performance, *J Orthop Sports Phys Ther* 14:114, 1991.
3. Bandy WD, Lovelace-Chandler V: Relationship of peak torque to peak work and peak power of the quadriceps and hamstring muscles in a normal sample using an accommodating resistance measurement device, *Isok Exerc Sci* 1:87, 1991.
4. Barber SD, Noyes FR, Mangine RE et al: Quantitative assessment of functional limitations in normal and anterior cruciate ligament-deficient knees, *Clin Orthop Rel Res* 225:204, 1990.
5. Bohannon RW: Hand-held dynamometry: stability of muscle strength over multiple measurements, *Clin Biomech* 2:74, 1987.
6. Bohannon RW: The clinical measurement of strength, *Clin Rehabil* 1:5, 1987.
7. Bohannon RW: Make test and break test of elbow flexor muscle strength, *Phys Ther* 68:193, 1988.
8. Bohannon RW: Comparability of force measurements obtained with different strain gauge hand-held dynamometers, *J Orthop Sports Phys Ther* 18:564, 1993.
9. Bohannon RW, Andrews AW: Accuracy of spring and strain gauge handheld dynamometers, *J Orthop Sports Phys Ther* 10:323, 1989.
10. Boltz S, Davies GJ: Leg length differences and correlation with total leg strength, *J Orthop Sports Phys Ther* 6:123, 1984.
11. Brunnstrom S: Muscle group testing, *Physiotherapy Rev* 21:3, 1941.
12. Daniels L, Worthingham C: Muscle testing: techniques of manual examination, ed 5, Philadelphia, 1986, WB Saunders.
13. Davies GJ: *A compendium of isokinetics in clinical usage*, Onalaska, Wis, 1992, S & S.
14. Davies GJ. The need for critical thinking in rehabilitation, submitted to *J Sports Rehabil* 1993.
15. Davies GJ: Validity and reliability of the Lido Linea Closed Kinetic Chain Isokinetic Dynamometer, in review, *J Orthop Sports Phys Ther* 1996.

16. Davies GJ, Ellenbecker B: Eccentric isokinetic, *Orthop Phys Ther Clin North Am* 1:297, 1992.
17. Davies GJ, Malone TM: Proprioception, open and closed kinetic chain exercise: implications to rehabilitation and assessment, Proceedings of the Twentieth Annual Meeting of the American Orthopedic Society for Sports Medicine, Instructional Course 307, Palm Desert, Calif, June 1994.
18. Davies GJ, Romeyn R: Prospective, randomized single blind study comparing closed kinetic chain versus open and closed kinetic chain integrated rehabilitation programs of patients with ACL autograft infrapatellar tendon reconstructions. Research in progress, August 1992.
19. Davies GJ: Correlations between open kinetic chain isokinetic testing, closed kinetic chain isokinetic testing, functional jump test, functional hop test and lower extremity functional (agility) test. Research in progress, 1993.
20. Gleim GW, Nicholas JA, Webb JN: Isokinetic evaluation following leg injuries, *Phys Sports Med* 6:74, 1978.
21. Greenberger HB, Paterno MV: Comparison of an isokinetic strength test and a functional performance test in the assessment of lower extremity function (abstract), *J Orthop Sports Phys Ther* 19:61, 1994.
22. Kendall HO, Kendall FP: Care during the recovery period in paralytic poliomyelitis, U.S. Public Health Bull. No. 242, revised, 1939.
23. Kendall FP, McCreary EK: *Muscles: testing and function,* ed 3, Baltimore, 1983, Williams & Wilkins.
24. Lovette RW, Martin EG: Certain aspects of infantile paralysis and a description of a method of muscle testing, *J Am Med Assoc* 66:729, 1916.
25. Lowman CL: A method of recording muscle tests, *Am J Surg New Series* 3:588, 1927.
26. Luhtanen P, Komi PV: Segmental contribution to forces in vertical jump, *Eur J Appl Physiol* 38:181, 1978.
27. Nicholas JA, Strizak AM, Veras G: A study of thigh muscle weakness in different pathological states of the lower extremity, *Am J Sports Med* 4:241, 1976.
28. Robertson DGE, Fleming D: Kinetics of standing broad and vertical jumping, *Can J Sports Med* 12:19, 1987.
29. Sachs RA, Daniel DM, Stone ML, Garfein RF: Patellofemoral problems after anterior cruciate ligament reconstruction, *Am J Sports Med* 17:760, 1989.
30. Shaffer SW, Payne ED, Gabbard LR et al: Relationship between isokinetic and functional tests of the quadriceps (abstract), *J Orthop Sports Phys Ther* 19:55, 1994.
31. Tegner Y, Lysholm J, Lysholm M et al: A performance test to monitor rehabilitation and evaluate anterior cruciate ligament injuries, *Am J Sports Med* 14:156, 1986.
32. Timm KE: Post-surgical knee rehabilitation: a five year study of four methods and 5,381 patients, *Am J Sports Med* 16:463, 1988.
33. Wiklander J, Lysholm J: Simple tests for surveying muscle strength and muscle stiffness in sportsmen, *Intl J Sports Med* 8:50, 1987.

SECTION II REFERENCES

1. Albert MS: *Eccentric muscle training in sports and orthopaedics,* New York, 1991, Churchill Livingstone.
2. Amundsen LR: *Muscle strength testing: instrumental and non-instrumental systems,* New York, 1990, Churchill Livingstone.
3. Amundsen LR, DeVahl JM, Ellingham CT: Evaluation of a group exercise program for the elderly, *Phys Ther* 69:475, 1989.
4. An K, Chao E, Askew LJ: Hand strength measurements, *Arch Phys Med Rehabil* 61:366, 1980.
5. Anderson MA, Gieck JR, Perrin D et al: The relationships among isometric, isotonic and isokinetic concentric and eccentric quadriceps and hamstring force and three components of athletic performance, *J Orthop Sports Phys Ther* 14(3):114, 1991.
6. Aniansson A, Rundgren A, Sperling L: Evaluation of functional capacity in activities of daily living in 70 year old men and women, *Scand J Rehabil Med* 12:145, 1980.

7. Ariki PK, Davies GJ, Siewert MW et al: Optimum rest interval between isokinetic velocity spectrum rehabilitation speeds (abstract), *Phys Ther* 65(5):735, 1985.
8. Arrigo CA, Wilk KE: Peak torque and maximum work repetition during isokinetic testing of the knee. Submitted for publication, *Isokin Exerc Sci* 4(4):171, 1994.
9. Asmussen E, Boje O: Body temperature and capacity for work, *Acta Physiol Scand* 10:1, 1945.
10. Astrand PO, Rodahl K: *Textbook of work physiology: physiologic basis of exercise,* ed 2, New York, 1977, McGraw-Hill.
11. Bandy WD, Rusche KR, Tekulve FY: Reliability and limb symmetry for five unilateral functional tests of the lower extremity, *Isokin Exerc Sci* 4(3):108, 1994.
12. Barber SD, Noyes FR, Mangine RE: Quantitative assessment of functional limitations in normal and anterior cruciate ligament deficient knees, *Clin Orthop* 255:204, 1990.
13. Basmajian JV: *Muscles alive: their function revealed by electromyography,* ed 4, p. 93, Baltimore, 1978, Williams & Wilkins.
14. Bendle SR, Davies GJ, Wood KL: The optimal number of repetitions to be used with isokinetic training. In Davies GJ, editor: *The compendium of isokinetic,* ed 2, p. 522.
15. Bennett JG, Stauber WT: Evaluation and treatment of anterior knee pain using eccentric exercise, *Med Sci Sports Exerc* 18:256, 1986.
16. Blackburn TA, Eiland WG, Bandy WD: An introduction to plica, *J Orthop Sports Phys Ther* 3:171, 1982.
17. Bohannon RW: Manual muscle test scores and dynamometer test scores of knee extension strength, *Arch Phys Med Rehabil* 67:390, 1986.
18. Bohannon RW, Gajdosik RL, LeVeau BF: Isokinetic knee flexion and extension torque in the upright sitting and semi-reclined positions, *Phys Ther* 66:1083, 1986.
19. Bohannon RW, Gibson DF, Larkin P: Effect of resisted knee flexion torque, *Phys Ther* 66(8):1239, 1986.
20. Caiozzo VJ, Perrine JJ, Edgerton VR: Alterations in the in-vivo force velocity relationship (abstract), *Med Sci Sports Exer* 12:134, 1980.
21. Croft M: Isokinetic torque and test repetition. Master's thesis, University of Chicago, 1983.
22. Currier DP: Positioning for knee strengthening exercises, *Phys Ther* 57:148, 1977.
23. Daniel DM, Malcom L, Stone ML et al: Quantification of knee stability and function, *Contemp Orthop* 5:83, 1982.
24. Daniels L, Worthingham C: *Muscle testing: technique of manual examination,* ed 4, Philadelphia, 1980, WB Saunders.
25. Davies GJ: Cybex II isokinetic dynamometer measurements on the acute effects of direct active warm-ups and direct passive warm-ups on knee extension/flexion and power. Presented at Annual Conference of American Physical Therapy Association, June 1978.
26. Davies GJ: Isokinetic approach to the knee. In Mangine RE, editor: *Physical therapy of the knee,* p. 221, New York, 1988, Churchill Livingstone.
27. Davies GJ: *A compendium of isokinetics in clinical usage,* ed 4, Onalaska, Wis, 1992, S & S.
28. Davies GJ et al: A descriptive muscular strength and power analysis of the US cross country ski team (abstract), *Med Sci Sports Exerc* 12(2):441, 1980.
29. Davies GJ et al: Isokinetic characteristics of professional football players: narrative relationships between quadriceps and hamstrings muscle groups and relations to body weight (abstract), *Med Sci Sports Exerc* 13(2):76, 1981.
30. Delitto A, Irrgang JJ, Horner CD, Fu FH: Relationship of isokinetic quadriceps peak torque and work to one legged hop and vertical jump in ACL reconstructed knees (abstract), *Phys Ther* 73(6):585, 1993.
31. DeNuccio DK, Davies GJ, Rowinski MJ: Comparison of quadriceps isokinetic eccentric and isokinetic concentric data using a standardized fatigue protocol, *Isokinetic Exerc Sci* 1(2):81, 1991.
32. Dillman CJ, Ariel GB: The biomechanical aspects of Olympic sports medicine, *Clin Sports Med* 2:31, 1983.

33. Dillman DJ: A kinetic analysis of the recovery leg during sprint running. In Cooper JM, editor: *Biomechanics,* North Palm Beach, Fla, 1970, Athletic Institute.

34. Dohallow JH: Classification of patellofemoral disorders on the Cybex II isokinetic dynamometer, *Phys Ther* 60:738, 1981.

35. Dohallow JH, McIvor W, Lange D, Goheen D: A three year isokinetic knee evaluation study: diagnostic capabilities, *Phys Ther* 63:770, 1983.

36. Figoni SF, Morris AF: Effects of knowledge of results on reciprocal isokinetic strength and fatigue, *J Orthop Sports Phys Ther* 6:104, 1984.

37. Fillyaw M, Bevins T, Fernandez L: Importance of correcting isokinetic peak torque for the effect of gravity when calculating knee flexor to extensor muscle ratios, *Phys Ther* 66:23, 1986.

38. Francis KT, Hoobler T: Comparison of peak torque values of the knee flexor and extensor muscle groups using the Cybex II and Lido 2.0 isokinetic dynamometers, *J Orthop Sports Phys Ther* 8:480, 1987.

39. Franks DB: Physical warm-up. In Morgan WP, editor: *Ergogenic aids and muscular performance,* Orlando, 1972, Academic Press.

40. Friden J, Sjostrom M, Ekbrom B: A morphological study of delayed muscle soreness, *Expereita* 37:506, 1981.

41. Ghena DR, Durth AL, Thomas M et al: Torque characteristics of the quadriceps and hamstrings muscle during concentric and eccentric loading, *J Orthop Sport Phys Ther* 14(4):149, 1991.

42. Gleim GW: Isokinetic evaluation following leg injuries, *Phys Sports Med* 6:74, 1978.

43. Goslir BR, Charters J: Isokinetic dynamometry: normative data for clinical use in lower extremity cases, *Scand J Rehabil Med* 11:105, 1981.

44. Hald RD, Bottken EJ: Effects of visual feedback on maximal and submaximal isokinetic test measurements of normal quadriceps and hamstring, *J Orthop Sports Phys Ther* 9:86, 1987.

45. Hart DL, Stobbe TJ, Till CW et al: Effect of trunk stabilization on quadriceps femoris muscle torque, *Phys Ther* 64:1375, 1984.

46. Hester JT, Falkel JE: Isokinetic evaluation of tibial rotation, *J Orthop Sports Phys Ther* 6:46, 1984.

47. Hoke B: The relationship between isokinetic testing and dynamic patellofemoral compression, *J Orthop Sports Phys Ther* 4:150, 1983.

48. Hunter S: Preseason isokinetic knee evaluation in professional football athletes, *Athletic Training* 205:1979.

49. Iddings D, Smith L, Spencer W: Muscle testing, part 2: reliability in clinical use, *Phys Ther Rev* 41:249, 1961.

50. Jenkins WR, Thackaberry M, Killiam C: Speed-specific isokinetic training, *J Orthop Sports Phys Ther* 6:181, 1984.

51. Jensen JE, Conn R, Hazelrigg G, Hewett J: Systematic evaluation of acute knee injuries, *Clin Sports Med* 4:295, 1985.

52. Jensen JE, Slocum DB, Larson RL, James SL, Singer KM: Reconstruction procedures for anterior cruciate ligament insufficiency: a computer analysis of clinical results, *Am J Sports Med* 11:240, 1983.

53. Johansson CA, Kent BE, Shepard KF: Relationship between verbal command volume and magnitude of muscle contraction, *Phys Ther* 63(8):1260, 1983.

54. Johnson RJ, Wilk KE: The effect of lever arm pad placement upon the isokinetic torque during knee extension and flexion, *Phys Ther* 68:779, 1988.

55. Johnson J, Siegel D: Reliability of an isokinetic movement of the knee extensors, *Res Q* 49:88, 1978.

56. Jones HE: *Motor performance and growth: developmental study of static dynomometric strength,* Berkley, 1949, University of California Press.

57. Karlsson J, Lundin O, Lossing IW, Peterson L: Partial rupture of the patellar ligament: results after operative treatment, *Am J Sports Med* 19(4):403, 1991.

58. Kauffman KR, An KN, Litchy WJ, Morrey BF, Chao EY: Dynamic joint forces during knee isokinetic exercise, *Am J Sports Med* 19(3):305, 1991.

59. Kendall H, Kendall F, Wadsworth G: *Muscle testing and function,* ed 2, Baltimore, 1971, William & Wilkins.

60. Knott M, Voss D: *Proprioceptive neuromuscular facilitation,* p. 84, New York, 1968, Harper & Row, Hoeber Medical Division.

61. Kramer JF, Vaz MD, Hakansson D: Effect of activation force on knee extensor torques, *Med Sci Sports Exerc* 23(2):231, 1991.

62. Kreighblaum E, Barthels KM: *Biomechanics: a qualitative approach for studying human movement,* Minneapolis, 1985, Burgess.

63. Kryter KD: *The effects of noise on man,* p. 491, New York, 1970, Academic Press.

64. Lesmes GR, Costill DL et al: Muscle strength and power changes during maximal isokinetic training, *Med Sci Sports Exer* 10:266, 1978.

65. Lunner JD, Yack J, LeVeau BF: Relationship between muscle length, muscle activity and torque of the hamstring muscles, *Phys Ther* 57:148, 1977.

66. McArdle WD, Katch FL, Katch VU: *Exercise physiology: energy, nutrition and human performance,* ed 2, Philadelphia, 1986, Lee & Febiger.

67. Malone T, Blackburn TA, Wallace LA: Knee rehabilitation, *Phys Ther* 60:1602, 1980.

68. Malone TR, Mangine RE: Isokinetic testing of the ACL deficient knee. Presented at the APTA Annual Conference, 1983.

69. Mangine RE: *Isometric testing protocol of the knee Biodex clinical Advantage Program,* Shirley, N Y, 1991, Biodex Corporation.

70. Mangine RE, Mangine-Erfert MA: Isokinetic approach to selected knee pathologies. In Davies GJ, editor: *A comparison of isokinetics in clinical usage,* ed 4, p. 285, LaCrosse, Wis, 1992, S & S.

71. Marshall JL, Fetto JF, Botero PM: Knee ligament injuries: a standardized evaluation method, *Clin Orthop* 123:115, 1977.

72. Manzer CW: The effect of knowledge of output on muscle work, *J Exp Psychol* 18:80, 1935.

73. Martin BV, Robinson S, Wiogoma DC et al: Effect of warm-up on metabolic responses to strenuous exercise, *Med Sci Sports* 7:146, 1975.

74. Mawdsley RH, Knapik JJ: Comparison of isokinetic measurements with test repetitions, *Phys Ther* 62:169, 1982.

75. Mayhew T, Rothstein JM: Measurements of muscle performance with instruments, p. 57. In Rothstein JM, editor: *Measurement in physical therapy,* New York, 1985, Churchill Livingstone.

76. Mira AJ, Markley K, Greer RB: A critical analysis of quadriceps function after femoral shaft fracture in adults, *J Bone Joint Surg Am* 62A:61, 1980.

77. Mohtadi NGH, Kiefer GN, Tedford K: Concentric and eccentric quadriceps torque in pre-adolescent males, *Can J Sports Sci* 15(4):240, 1990.

78. Nelson SG, Duncan PW: Correction of isokinetic and isometric torque recordings for the effects of gravity, *Phys Ther* 63:674, 1983.

79. Newham DJ, Mills KR, Quigley BM: Pain and fatigue after concentric and eccentric muscle contractions, *Clin Sci* 64:55, 1983.

80. Newman LB: A new device for measuring muscle strength: the myometer, *Arch Phys Med Rehabil* 30:234, 1986.

81. Nicholas J, Sapega A, Kraus H, Webb J: Factors influencing manual muscle tests in physical therapy, *J Bone Joint Surg* 60:186, 1978.

82. Nisell R, Ericson MO, Nemeth G, Ekholm J: Tibiofemoral joint forces during isokinetic knee extension, *Am J Sports Med* 17(1):49, 1988.

83. Nitz M: Variations in current manual muscle testing, *Phys Ther Rev* 39:466, 1959.

84. Noyes FR, Barber SD, Mangine RE: Abnormal lower limb symmetry determined by function hop tests after anterior cruciate ligament rupture, *Am J Sports Med* 19(5):513, 1991.

85. Osterning LR, Bates BT, James SL et al: Patterns of tibial rotary torque in knees of healthy subjects, *Med Sci Sports Exerc* 12:195, 1980.

86. Palmitier RA, An KN, Scott SC, Chao EY: Kinetic chain exercise in knee rehabilitation, *Sports Med* 11(6):402, 1991.

87. Parker MG: Characteristics of skeletal muscle during rehabilitation: quadriceps femoris, *Athletic Training* 18:122, 1981.

88. Patteson ME, Nelson SG, Duncan PW: Effects of stabilizing the non

tested lower extremity during isokinetic evaluation of the quadriceps and hamstrings, *J Orthop Sports Phys Ther* 6:18, 1984.

89. Perrin DH: Reliability of isokinetic measures, *Athletic Training* 21:319, 1986.

90. Peterson SR, Bell GJ, Bagnell KM: The effects of concentric resistance training on eccentric peak torque and muscle cross-sectional area, *J Orthop Sports Phys Ther* 13(3):132, 1991.

91. Pierson WR, Rasch PJ: Effect of knowledge of results on isometric strength scores, *Res Q* 35:313, 1964.

92. Richard G, Currier DP: Back stabilization during knee strengthening exercises, *Phys Ther* 57:103, 1977.

93. Riezebos ML, Paterson DH, Hall CR, Yuhasz MS: Relationship of selected variables and performance in women's basketball, *Can J Appl Sport Sci* 8(1):34, 1987.

94. Robertson LD, Geeseman R, Nixon B: A device to strengthen and evaluate the medial rotator muscles of the leg, *Med Sci Sports Exerc* 6:277, 1974.

95. Rothstein JM: *Measurement in physical therapy,* New York, 1985, Churchill Livingstone.

96. Rothstein JM, Delitto A, Sinacore DR et al: Muscle function in rheumatic disease patients treated with corticosteroid, *Muscle Nerve* 6:128, 1983.

97. Rothstein JM, Delitto A, Sinacore DR et al: Electromyographic peak torque and power relationships during isokinetic movements, *Phys Ther* 63:926, 1983.

98. Sachs RA, Daniel DM, Stone ML, Garfein RF: Patellofemoral problems after anterior cruciate ligament reconstruction, *Am J Sports Med* 17:760, 1989.

99. Seliger V, Dolesjs L, Karas V: A dynamometric comparison of maximum eccentric, concentric and isometric contractions using EMG and energy expenditure measurements, *Eur J Appl Physiol* 45:235, 1980.

100. Shoemaker SC, Markolf KL: In vivo rotary knee stability. *J Bone Joint Surg Am* 64A:208, 1982.

101. Siewert WM, Ariki PK, Davies GJ et al: Isokinetic torque changes based on lever arm placement, *Phys Ther* 65:715, 1985.

102. Swarup M, Irrgang JJ, Lephart S: Relationship of isokinetic quadriceps peak torque and work to one legged hop vertical jump (abstract), *Phys Ther* 72(6):S88, 1992.

103. Taylor RC, Casey JJ: Quadriceps torque production on the Cybex II dynamiter as related to changes in lever arm length, *J Orthop Sports Phys Ther* 8:147, 1986.

104. Tegner Y, Lysholm J: Deterioration brace and knee function in patients with anterior cruciate ligament tears, *Arthroscopy* 4:264, 1985.

105. Tegner Y, Lysholm J, Lysholm M, Gillquist J: A performance test to monitor rehabilitation and for evaluation of anterior cruciate ligament injuries, *Am J Sports Med* 17:156, 1986.

106. Thompson MC, Shingleton LG, Kegerreis ST: Comparison of values generated during testing of the knee using the Cybex II+ and Biodex isokinetic dynamometers, *J Orthop Sports Phys Ther* 11(3):108, 1989.

107. Timm KE: Post-surgical knee rehabilitation: a five year study of four methods and 5,381 patients, *Am J Sports Med* 16(5):463, 1988.

108. Timm KE: Comparisons of knee extensor and flexor muscle group performance using the Cybex 340 and the Merac isokinetic dynamometers, *Phys Ther* 69:389, 1989.

109. Tolsma BC: Leg dynamics and maximum speed sprinting. Doctoral dissertation, Indiana University, Bloomington, 1979.

110. Tombenlin JP, Basford JR, Schwen EE: Comparative study of isokinetic eccentric and concentric quadriceps training, *J Orthop Sports Phys Ther* 14(1):31, 1991.

111. Ulrich C, Burke RK: Effect of motivational stress on physical performance, *Res Q* 28:403, 1957.

112. Vandervoort AV, Kramer JF, Wharran ER: Eccentric knee strength of elderly females, *J Gerontol* 45(4):125, 1991.

113. Wiklander J, Lysholm J: Simple tests for surveying muscle strength and muscle stiffness in sportsmen, *Int J Sports Med* 8:50, 1987.

114. Wiktorsson-Moller M, Oberg B, Edstrand V et al: Effects of warming up, massage and strengthening on range of motion and muscle strength in the lower extremity, *Am J Sports Med* 11:249, 1983.

115. Wilhette MR, Cohen ER, Wilhette SC: Reliability of concentric and eccentric measurements of quadriceps performance using the Kin-Com Dynamometer: the effect of testing order for three different speeds, *J Orthop Sports Phys Ther* 15(4):175, 1992.

116. Wilk KE: Dynamic muscle strength testing. In Amundsen LR, editor: *Muscle strength testing: instrumented and non-instrumented,* New York, 1990, Churchill Livingstone.

117. Wilk KE, Andrews JR: Current concepts in the treatment of anterior cruciate ligament disruptions, *J Orthop Sports Phys Ther* 15(6):279, 1992.

118. Wilk KE, Andrews JR: The effects of pad placement and angular velocity on tibial displacement during isokinetic exercise, *J Orthop Sports Phys Ther* 17(1):24, 1993.

119. Wilk KE, Arrigo CA, Andrews JR: A standardized isokinetic testing protocol: the throwers series, *Isokinetic Exercise Science* 1(2):63, 1991.

120. Wilk KE, Arrigo CA, Andrews JR: A comparison of individuals exhibiting normal grade manual muscle test and isokinetic testing of the knee extension/flexion, *Phys Ther* (abstract) 72(6):71, 1992.

121. Wilk KE, Arrigo CA, Andrews JR, Clancy WG et al: Anterior cruciate ligament reconstruction: a twelve week follow-up isokinetic testing, *Isokinetic Exerc Sci* 2(2):82, 1992.

122. Wilk KE, Arrigo CA, Keirns MA: Shoulder abduction/adduction isokinetic test results: window vs unwindow data collection, *J Orthop Sports Phys Ther* 15(2):107, 1992.

123. Wilk KE, Erber DJ, Pierce J, Gillespie C: The relationship between torque and speed during isokinetic eccentric exercise, *Phys Ther* 69(6):578, 1989.

124. Wilk KE, Johnson RJ, Levine B: A comparison of peak torque values of knee extensor and flexor muscle groups using Biodex, Cybex and Kin-Com isokinetic dynamometers, *Phys Ther* 67:789, 1987.

125. Wilk KE, Johnson RJ, Levine B: A comparison of peak torque values of knee extensor and flexor muscle groups using the Biodex, Cybex and Lido isokinetic dynamometers, *Phys Ther* 67:792, 1988.

126. Wilk KE, Keirns MA, Andrews JR et al: Anterior cruciate ligament reconstruction rehabilitation: a six month follow-up of isokinetic testing in recreational athletes, *Isokinetic Exerc Sci* 1(1):36, 1991.

127. Wilk KE, Rominello BR, Soscia S, Arrigo CA, Andrews JR: The correlation between subjective knee assessments, isokinetic muscle testing and functional hop testing in ACL reconstructed knees, *J Orthop Sports Phys* 20(2):60, 1994.

128. Wilk KE, Suarez K: Proprioceptible and neuromuscular training for the anterior cruciate ligament reconstructed knee patient. Submitted for publication, *J Orthop Sports Phys Ther,* 1995.

129. Williams M: Manual muscle testing, development and current use, *Phys Ther Rev* 36:717, 1956.

130. Winter DA, Wells RP, Orr GW: Errors in the use of isokinetic dynamometers, *Eur J Appl Physiol* 46:317, 1981.

131. Wintz M: Variations in current manual muscle testing, *Phys Ther Rev* 39:466, 1959.

132. Wright W: Muscle training in the treatment of infantile paralysis, *Boston Med Surg* 167:567, 1912.

133. Wyatt MP, Edwards AM: Comparison of quadriceps and hamstring torque values during isokinetic exercises, *J Orthop Sports Phys Ther* 3:48, 1981.

SECTION III REFERENCES

1. Alderink GJ, Kluck DJ: Isokinetic shoulder strength of high school and college aged pitchers, *J Orthop Sports Phys Ther* 7(4):163, 1986.

2. Bandy WD, McLaughlin S: Intramachine and intermachine reliability for selected dynamic muscle performance tests, *J Orthop Sports Phys Ther* 18(5):609, 1993.

3. Bartlett LR, Storey MD, Simons BD: Measurement of upper extremity torque production and its relationship to throwing speed in the competitive athlete, *Am J Sports Med* 17(1):89, 1989.

4. Basset RW, Browne AO, Morrey BF, An KN: Glenohumeral muscle force and moment mechanics in a position of shoulder instability, *J Biomech* 23(5):405, 1994.

5. Bechtol CO: The use of a dynamometer with adjustable handle spacings, *J Bone Joint Surg Am* 36A:820, 1954.

6. Bohannon RW: Shoulder position influences elbow extension force in healthy individuals, *J Orthop Sports Phys Ther* 12(3):111, 1990.

7. Brown LP, Neihues SL, Harrah A et al: Upper extremity range of motion and isokinetic strength of the internal and external shoulder rotators in major league baseball players, *Am J Sports Med* 16(6):577, 1988.

8. Chandler TJ, Kibler WB, Stracener EC et al: Shoulder strength, power, and endurance in college tennis players, *Am J Sports Med* 20:455, 1992.

9. Cook EE, Gray VL, Savinor-Nogue E et al: Shoulder antagonistic strength ratios: a comparison between college-level baseball pitchers, *J Orthop Sports Phys Ther* 8(9):451, 1987.

10. Daniels L, Worthingham C: *Muscle testing: techniques of manual examination,* ed 5, Philadelphia, 1986, WB Saunders.

11. Davies GJ: *A compendium of isokinetics in clinical usage and rehabilitation techniques,* ed 4, LaCrosse, 1992, S & S.

12. Davies GJ, Ellenbecker TS: Eccentric isokinetics, *Orthop Phys Ther Clin North Am* 1(2):297, 1992.

13. Davies GJ, Ellenbecker TS: Total arm strength rehabilitation for shoulder and elbow overuse injuries, *Orthop Phys Ther Home Study Course, Orthopaedic Section APTA,* 1993.

14. Davies GJ, Hoffman SD: Neuromuscular testing and rehabilitation of the shoulder complex, *J Orthop Sports Phys Ther* 18(2):449, 1993.

15. Dillman CJ: Presentation on the upper extremity in tennis and throwing. United States Tennis Association National Meeting, Tucson, March 1991.

16. Dillman CJ, Fleisig GS, Andrews JR: Biomechanics of pitching with emphasis upon shoulder kinematics, *J Orthop Sports Phys Ther* 18(2):402, 1993.

17. Ellenbecker TS: A total arm strength isokinetic profile of highly skilled tennis players, *Isokin Exerc Sci* 1(1):9, 1991.

18. Ellenbecker TS: Shoulder internal and external rotation strength and range of motion of highly skilled junior tennis players, *Isokin Exerc Sci* 2:1, 1992.

19. Ellenbecker TS: Elbow, forearm, and wrist testing and rehabilitation. In Davies GJ, editor: *A compendium of isokinetics in clinical usage,* ed 4, LaCrosse, 1992 S & S.

20. Ellenbecker TS: Muscular strength relationship between normal grade manual muscle testing and isokinetic measurement of the shoulder internal and external rotators, *J Orthop Sports Phys Ther* (abstract) 19(1): 72, 1994.

21. Ellenbecker TS: A distal upper extremity isokinetic profile of professional baseball pitchers. Submitted for publication, *Isokin Exerc Sci,* 1996.

22. Ellenbecker TS, Davies GJ, Rowinski MJ: Concentric vs eccentric isokinetic strengthening of the rotator cuff: objective data vs functional test, *Am J Sports Med* 16:64, 1988.

23. Ellenbecker TS, Dehart RL, Boeckmann R: Isokinetic shoulder strength of the rotator cuff in professional baseball pitchers (abstract), *Phys Ther* 72, 1992.

24. Ellenbecker TS, Derscheid GL: Rehabilitation of overuse injuries in the shoulder, *Clin Sports Med* 8:583, 1988.

25. Ellenbecker TS, Feiring DC, Dehart RL, Rich M: Isokinetic shoulder strength: coronal versus scapular plane testing in upper extremity unilaterally dominant athletes (abstract), *Phys Ther* 1992.

26. Elliot B, Marsh T, Blanksby B: A three dimensional cinematographic analysis of the tennis serve, *Int J Sport Biomech* 2:260, 1986.

27. Feiring DC, Ellenbecker TS, Derscheid GL: Test-retest reliability of the Biodex isokinetic dynamometer, *J Orthop Sports Phys Ther* 11(7):298, 1990.

28. Francis K, Hoobler T: Comparison of peak torque values of the knee flexor and extensor muscle groups using the Cybex II and Lido 2.0 isokinetic dynamometers, *J Orthop Sports Phys Ther* 8(10):480, 1987.

29. Frisiello S, Gazaille A, Ohalloran J, Palmer ML, Waugh D: Test retest reliability of eccentric peak torque values for shoulder medial and lateral rotation using the Biodex isokinetic dynamometer, *J Orthop Sports Phys Ther* 19(6):341, 1994.

30. Glousman R, Jobe FW, Tibone JE et al: Dynamic electromyographic analysis of the throwing shoulder with glenohumeral joint instability. *J Bone Joint Surg Am* 70A 220, 1988.

31. Gore DR, Murray MP, Sepic SB, Gardner GM: Shoulder muscle strength and range of motion following surgical repair of full thickness rotator cuff tears, *J Bone Joint Surg Am* 68A:266, 1986.

32. Greenfield BH, Donatelli R, Wooden MJ, Wilkes J: Isokinetic evaluation of shoulder rotational strength between the plane of the scapula and the frontal plane, *Am J Sports Med* 18(2):124, 1990.

33. Hageman PA, Mason DK, Rydlund KW et al: Effects of position and speed on eccentric and concentric isokinetic testing of the shoulder rotators, *J Orthop Sports Phys Ther* 11(2):64, 1989.

34. Hellwig EV, Perrin DH: A comparison of two positions for asessing shoulder rotator torque: the traditional frontal plane versus the plane of the scapula, *Isokin Exerc Sci* 1(4):202, 1991.

35. Hellwig EV, Perrin DH, Tis LL, Shenk BS: Effect of gravity correction on shoulder external/internal rotator reciprocal muscle group ratios (abstract), *Journal of the NATA* 26:154, 1991.

36. Hinton RY: Isokinetic evaluation of shoulder rotational strength in high school baseball pitchers, *Am J Sports Med* 16(3):274, 1988.

37. Inman VT, Saunders JB de CM, Abbot LC: Observations on the function of the shoulder joint, *J Bone Joint Surg Am* 26A 1, 1944.

38. Itoi E, Kuechle DK, Newman SR, et al: Stabilising function of the biceps in stable and unstable shoulders, *J Bone Joint Surg Br* 75B:546, 1993.

39. Ivey FM, Calhoun JH, Rusche K et al: Normal values for isokinetic testing of shoulder strength, *Med Sci Sports Exerc* 16:127, 1984.

40. Jobe FW, Tibone JE, Perry J et al: An EMG analysis of the shoulder in throwing and pitching. A preliminary report, *Am J Sports Med* 11(1): 3, 1983.

41. Kendall FD, McCreary EK: Muscle testing and function, ed 3, Baltimore, 1983, Williams & Wilkins.

42. Kennedy K, Altchek DW, Glick IV: Concentric and eccentric isokinetic rotator cuff ratios in skilled tennis players, *Isokin Exerc Sci* 3:155, 1993.

43. Kronberg M, Nemeth F, Brostrom LA: Muscle activity and coordination in the normal shoulder: an electromyographic study, *Clin Orthop Rel Res* 257:76, 1990.

44. Lace JE: *An isokinetic shoulder profile of collegiate baseball pitchers and its relation to throwing velocity* (unpublished masters thesis), Arizona State University, 1989.

45. Malerba JL, Adam ML, Harris BA, Krebs DE: Reliability of dynamic and isometric testing of shoulder external and internal rotators, *J Orthop Sports Phys Ther* 18(4):543, 1993.

46. Meister K, Andrews JR: Classification and treatment of rotator cuff injuries in the overhand athlete, *J Orthop Sports Phys Ther* 18(2):413, 1993.

47. Mont MA, Cohen DB, Campbell KR, Gravare K, Mathur S: Isokinetic concentric versus eccentric training of the shoulder rotators with functional evaluation of performance enhancement in elite tennis players, *Am J Sports Med* 22(4):513, 1994.

48. Morris M, Jobe FW, Perry J, Pink M, Healy BS: Electromyographic analysis of elbow function in tennis players, *Am J Sports Med* 17(2): 241, 1989.

49. Nicholas J, Sapega A, Kraus H, Webb J: Factors influencing manual muscle tests in physical therapy. *J Bone Joint Surg* 60:186, 1978.

50. Nirschl RP, Sobel J: Conservative treatment of tennis elbow, *Phys Sports Med* 9:43, 1981.

51. Palmitier RA, An K, Scott SG, Chao EYS: Kinetic chain exercise in knee rehabilitation. *Sports Med* 11(6):402, 1991.

52. Pawlowski D, Perrin DH: Relationship between shoulder and elbow isokinetic peak torque, torque acceleration energy, average power, and total work and throwing velocity in intercollegiate pitchers, *Athletic Training* 24(2):129, 1989.

53. Pedegana LR, Elsner RC, Roberts D, Lang J, Farewell V: The

relationship of upper extremity strength to throwing speed, *Am J Sports Med* 10(6):352, 1982.

54. Perrin DH: Reliability of isokinetic measures, *Athletic Training* 21: 319, 1986.

55. Quincy & Davies

56. Rabin SJ, Post MP: A comparative study of clinical muscle testing and Cybex evaluation after shoulder operations, *Clin Orthop Rel Res* 258: 147, 1990.

57. Rodosky MW, Harner CD, Fu FH: The role of the long head of the biceps muscle and superior glenoid labrum in anterior stability of the shoulder, *Am J Sports Med* 22:121, 1994.

58. Saha AK: Dynamic stability of the glenohumeral joint, *Acta Orthop Scand* 42:491, 1971.

59. Schexneider MA, Catlin PA, Davies GJ, Mattson PA: An isokinetic estimation of total arm strength, *Isokin Exerc Sci* 1(3):117, 1991.

60. Shapiro R, Stine RL: Shoulder rotation velocities. Technical report submitted to the Lexington Clinic, Lexington, Ky, 1992.

61. Snyder SJ, Karzel RP, Del Pizzo W et al: SLAP lesions of the shoulder, *Arthroscopy* 6:274, 1990.

62. Soderberg GJ, Blaschak MJ: Shoulder internal and external rotation peak torque production through a velocity spectrum in differing positions, *J Orthop Sports Phys Ther* 8(11):518, 1987.

63. Sullivan EP, Markos PD, Minor MD: *An integrated approach to therapeutic exercise theory and clinical application.* Reston, Va, 1982, Reston.

64. Timm KE, Genrich P, Burns R, Fyke D: The mechanical and physiological reliability of selected isokinetic dynamometers, *Isokin Exerc Sci* 2:182, 1992.

65. VanGheluwe B, Hebbelinck M: Muscle actions and ground reaction forces in tennis, *Int J Sport Biomech* 2:88, 1986.

66. Wakin KG: *Arch Phys Med Rehabil,* 1950.

67. Walker SW, Couch WH, Boester GA, Sprowl DW: Isokinetic strength of the shoulder after repair of a torn rotator cuff, *J Bone Joint Surg Am* 69A, 1941, 1987.

68. Walmsley RP, Szybbo C: A comparative study of the torque generated by the shoulder internal and external rotator muscles in different positions and at varying speeds, *J Orthop Sports Phys Ther* 9(6):217, 1987.

69. Walmsley RP, Hartsell H: Shoulder strength following surgical rotator cuff repair: a comparative analysis using isokinetic testing, *J Orthop Sports Phys Ther* 15(5):215, 1992.

70. Warner JP, Micheli LJ, Arslanian LE, Kennedy J, Kennedy R: Patterns of flexibility, laxity, and strength in normal shoulders and shoulders with instability and impingement, *Am J Sports Med* 18(4):366, 1990.

71. Wilk KE, Andrews JR, Arrigo CA, Keirns MA, Erber DJ: The strength characteristics of internal and external rotator muscles in professional baseball pitchers, *Am J Sports Med* 61, 1993.

72. Wilk KE, Arrigo CA, Andrews JR: Isokinetic testing of the shoulder abductors and adductors: windowed vs nonwindowed data collection, *J Orthop Sports Phys Ther* 15(2):107, 1992.

73. Wilk KE, Arrigo CA, Andrews JR: Standardized isokinetic testing protocol for the throwing shoulder: the throwers series, *Isokin Exerc Sci* 1(2):63, 1991.

74. Wilk KE, Arrigo CA: Current concepts in the rehabilitation of the athletic shoulder, *J Orthop Sports Phys Ther* 18(1):365, 1993.

PART THREE

Regional Considerations

CHAPTER 11

The Foot and Ankle

Thomas G. McPoil

OUTLINE

Anatomy
    Osseous components
    Ligamentous components
Joint mechanics
    Terminology
    Talocrural joint
    Subtalar joint
    Midtarsal articulations
    Intertarsal region
    The rays
    Windlass mechanism of the plantar fascia
    Closed chain movement of the foot articulations
    The functions of the foot
The typical pattern of rearfoot motion during walking
Examination of the foot and ankle
Physical examination procedures
Assessment and management
    Pronatory or excessive motion foot types
    Supinatory or limited motion foot types
Foot orthoses
    Fabrication methods
Common disorders of the foot and ankle
    Traumatic conditions
Case 1
    Chronic overuse conditions
Case 2

LEARNING OBJECTIVES

After studying this chapter, the reader will be able to:

1. Identify significant anatomic structures of the foot and ankle.
2. Describe the joint mechanics of the foot and ankle during walking.
3. Describe the typical pattern of rearfoot motion during walking.
4. Discuss the factors in the foot, ankle, and lower extremity responsible for causing or contributing to abnormal mechanical function of the foot.
5. Describe and list all the components of a physical examination of the foot and ankle.
6. Discuss those factors to consider when assessing the findings of the physical examination.
7. Discuss the use of footwear and foot orthoses for patients with foot problems caused by excessive foot pronation and supination.
8. Define *foot orthosis.*
9. List and describe the functions of foot orthoses.
10. Discuss fabrication techniques using premolded foot orthoses.

KEY TERMS

foot	foot orthoses
ankle	footwear
diagnosis	excessive pronation
examination	excess

The ability of the foot to function properly is essential for normal walking, as well as for other activities. During the stance phase of gait, the various foot articulations must work together to provide five important functions: supplying a dynamic base of support, transforming the foot into a supple accommodative structure, assisting the lower extremity in attenuating impact forces during early stance, providing a stable rigid structure during terminal stance, and allowing transverse plane rotation of the lower extremities when the foot is fixed to the supporting surface. The various foot articulations that are necessary for these functional movements are the talocrural joint, the subtalar joint, the articulations of the midtarsal and intertarsal regions, and the first through fifth rays. All of these articulations work in unison to provide the necessary motions. A traumatic or chronic overuse injury can prevent or delay any of these functions from occurring in their normal pattern of synchronization, thus leading to foot or lower extremity dysfunction. To treat clients with suspected foot dysfunction effectively, clinicians must understand the anatomy and mechanical function of these various articulations.

In planning treatment programs for individuals with foot dysfunction, clinicians must consider not only standard therapeutic procedures such as modalities, mobilization, and exercise but also the use of footwear, foot orthoses, and external devices attached to the shoe.

This chapter reviews the anatomy and normal mechanics of the principal articulations necessary for functional movement of the foot, clinical examination techniques for assessing both acute and chronic disorders of the foot and ankle, and common conditions that can cause dysfunction of the foot and ankle complex, with emphasis on management protocols using foot orthoses as well as footwear.

ANATOMY

The foot is composed of 26 bones and 30 major synovial joints.[43] Of these numerous articulations, 12 are essential for functional movements within the foot and ankle during activity:

1. The talocrural or upper ankle joint
2. The subtalar (talocalcaneal) or lower ankle joint
3. The two articulations of the midtarsal region, the talocalcaneonavicular and the calcaneocuboid
4. The three articulations of the intertarsal region, the cuneonavicular, cuboideonavicular, and intercuneiform joints
5. The first, second, third, fourth, and fifth rays

The osseous components of these articulations, as well as the significant ligamentous components that provide support to these articulations, are discussed here.

Osseous components

The talocrural joint is the articulation between the mortise, which includes the distal articulating surface and medial malleolus of the tibia as well as the lateral malleolus of the fibula, and the trochlea of the talus.

The subtalar (or talocalcaneal) joint is the articulation between the concave posterior facet on the inferior surface of the talus and the convex posterior facet on the superior surface of the calcaneus. Because the talus is an integral component of both the talocrural and subtalar joints, it is often referred to as the keystone of the ankle joint complex.[5]

The midtarsal region articulations are the talocalcaneo-

navicular and the calcaneocuboid. The talocalcaneonavicular joint is the articulation between the head of the talus and the posterior facet of the navicular bone, as well as the middle and anterior facets between the talus and calcaneus. The talocalcaneonavicular joint capsule is completely independent from the joint capsule of the subtalar joint. The calcaneocuboid joint is the articulation between the anterior facet of the calcaneus and the posterior facet of the cuboid. The literature refers to the fact that subtalar joint motion can directly influence the movements of the midtarsal articulations.[40,49] Because the posterior facets of both the calcaneus and talus form the subtalar joint and the two forward facts between talus and calcaneus are part of the talocalcaneonavicular, this concept has a strong anatomical basis. Subtalar joint movements directly affect the talocalcaneonavicular joint because both the talus and the calcaneus are components of both articulations.

The articulations of the intertarsal region include the cuneonavicular, cuboideonavicular, and intercuneiform joints. The cuneonavicular is composed of the articulations of the three cuneiforms (medial, intermediate, and lateral) as they articulate with the anterior facet of the navicular. The cuboideonavicular is the articulation between the cuboid and the navicular bone. The intercuneiform joints are the articulations between the medial and intermediate cuneiform bones, as well as between the medial and lateral cuneiform bones.

The rays are critical for normal foot function. The first ray is the functional unit between the first metatarsal and medial cuneiform bones. The second ray is the functional unit between the second metatarsal and the intermediate cuneiform bones. The third ray is the functional unit between the third metatarsal and the lateral cuneiform bones. The fourth and fifth rays are composed of only the fourth and fifth metatarsals, respectively, as they articulate with the anterior facet of the cuboid bone.

Ligamentous components

The talocrural joint is reinforced on both the medial and lateral aspects with a series of collateral ligaments. The lateral collateral ligaments of the ankle joint form three distinct structures: the anterior talofibular ligament, the calcaneofibular ligament, and the posterior talofibular ligament. A lateral view of the foot and ankle indicates that only the anterior talofibular ligament and the calcaneal fibular ligament are visible, the posterior talofibular ligament is not seen.[19] The posterior talofibular ligament travels directly behind the lateral malleolus to the posterior facet of the talus. Inman has reported that the average angle between the anterior talofibular and the calcaneal fibular ligaments is approximately 105 degrees in the sagittal plane.[19] Of all three ligaments on the lateral aspect of the ankle, only the calcaneofibular ligament provides support to both the talocrural and subtalar joints. On the medial aspect of the talocrural joint, several ligaments are consolidated into one large medial collateral ligament, the deltoid ligament. This triangular structure offers support to both the talocrural and subtalar joints. Turek notes that the strength of this ligament makes rupture rare; an injury to the medial ankle joint more commonly results in an avulsion of the medial malleolus.[50]

The subtalar joint is supported by two primary ligaments: the interosseous talocalcaneal and the cervical. The interosseous talocalcaneal ligament is a thick quadrilateral ligament that originates in the sulcus calcanei near the capsule of the posterior subtalar joint.[43] The fibers travel upward and medially to insert on the sulcus tali. The medial fibers are shorter than the lateral fibers, with the medial fibers becoming taut during subtalar joint pronation. The cervical ligament is the strongest of the ligaments connecting the talus and the calcaneus. The origin of the cervical ligament is the anterior medial aspect of the sinus tarsi near the insertion of the extensor digitorum brevis.[43] The fibers of this ligament travel upward and medially to attach on the inferior medial aspect of the neck of the talus. The cervical ligament becomes taut during supination of the subtalar joint.[43]

The articulations of the midtarsal and inner tarsal region, as well as the rays, are supported by small transverse and longitudinal ligaments, which reinforce the joint capsules of these various articulations. However, three important ligamentous structures on the plantar surface of the foot provide common support to all of these articulations. The long plantar ligament, the longest ligament in the foot, arises from the calcaneus, progresses anteriorly to attach to the cuboid bone, then continues forward to insert onto the bases of the third, fourth, and fifth metatarsals and, on occasion, the second metatarsal base.[43] The long plantar ligament forms a tunnel as it travels from the cuboid bone to the metatarsal bases for the peroneus longus tendon, which runs along the plantar aspect of the foot to insert into the first ray. Directly beneath the long plantar ligament is the short plantar ligament.[43] Both the short and long plantar ligaments are components of the plantar calcaneocuboid ligament. Located medially to the long plantar ligament is the plantar calcaneonavicular ligament or "spring" ligament. The spring ligament, by traveling from the calcaneus to the navicular, forms a ligamentous floor for the head of the talus to rest on.[43] These three ligaments are critical in providing support to not only the articulations in the midtarsal and intertarsal region but also in maintaining stability to both the medial and lateral longitudinal arches of the foot.

Another important structure that provides plantar stability to the various articulations of the foot is the plantar aponeurosis or fascia. There are three components or bands of the plantar aponeurosis: lateral, medial, and central.[43] The lateral band arises from the lateral tubercle on the plantar surface of the calcaneus, extends forward to cover the abductor digiti minimi muscle, and blends with the tendon of that muscle. The medial band, which often is not present, arises from the medial tubercle on the plantar surface of the

calcaneus, extends forward to cover the abductor hallucis muscle, and blends with the tendon of that muscle. The major component of the plantar fascia is the central band, which also originates from the medial tubercle on the plantar surface of the calcaneus. The central band extends forward and divides into five slips just before the metatarsal heads and continues to all five toes. Over the metatarsophalangeal joints, each slip further divides into a medial component and a lateral component, which wrap around both the medial and the lateral aspect of the proximal phalanx of the five digits.[43] Prior to dividing into medial and lateral components, the five slips of the plantar fascia have a superficial attachment to the plantar metatarsal fat pads.[43] This superficial attachment plays an important functional role in stabilizing the fat pads beneath the metatarsal heads to provide cushioning to these osseous structures during different types of activities, including walking. The functional significance of this unique insertion of the central band of the plantar fascia is reviewed with the windlass mechanism, which occurs during terminal stance phase.[14]

JOINT MECHANICS

The ability of the foot to provide the five functions that are necessary for walking, running, and other activities depends upon proper joint mechanics. Although common practice emphasizes subtalar joint function in any discussion of foot mechanics, it is important to realize that the movements of the foot articulations are initiated through the talocrural joint. Lower extremity rotation, caused by transverse plane pelvic rotation, initiates talocrural joint movement, which creates motion in the subtalar joint. Subtalar joint motion simultaneously causes movement in the other foot articulations, which are required to provide all five foot functions. Although the subtalar joint is an important component, it provides only one in a series of sequential movements involving numerous foot articulations, all of which are necessary to permit normal foot function. To discuss specific joint mechanics for each of the foot articulations, the terminology must be understood.

Terminology

Triplane motion. The term *triplane motion* refers to movement that occurs simultaneously in all three body planes, about a single axis.[40] The difference between triplane motion and triaxial motion, which occurs at the hip joint, is important. The hip joint has three distinct axes of motion, with one axis located in each of the three planes, the sagittal, the frontal, and the transverse. The hip joint is described as having 3 degrees freedom of motion. In addition, the three axes of the hip joint are positioned orthogonally or at a 90-degree angle to each other. The movements about the hip joint include flexion and extension in the sagittal plane, abduction and adduction in the frontal plane, and internal and external rotation in the transverse plane. A key point is that three specific axes are located orthogonally to one another and permit joint movement in a single plane. In the case of triplane motion, there is only one joint axis, but the axis is oriented in an oblique direction and thus positioned in all three body planes. When motion occurs about an articulation with a triplane axis, because the axis travels through all three planes, motion must occur simultaneously in each of the three planes.[39,40] This is one of the reasons why the early anatomical researchers developed the terms *pronation* and *supination*,[12,19] which describe the movement occurring in three planes simultaneously about a single axis. The articulations in the foot that exhibit triplane motion are the talocrural, the subtalar, the talocalcaneonavicular and calcaneocuboid articulations of the midtarsal region, and the first and fifth rays.[40] The remaining articulations discussed in this chapter are classified as plane joints, which indicates that they can have varying degrees of motion depending on the degree of capsular and ligamentous stability.

Closed chain movements. Closed chain movements of the foot articulations occur when the lower extremity has been loaded in a weight-bearing position, such as in the stance phase of walking. When the lower extremity has been fully loaded, frictional and ground reaction forces control movement of the foot because the plantar surface is held stationary to the supporting surface. Open chain movement occurs when the foot is not in contact with the ground, for example, when the foot is dangling off the edge of the examining table. The components and direction of joint movements can change as a result of going from an open to a closed chain. For example, the open chain description of subtalar joint pronation is calcaneal eversion with abduction and dorsiflexion of the forefoot.[45] In contrast, the closed chain description of subtalar joint pronation is calcaneal eversion with adduction and plantarflexion of the head of the talus.[45] Because most patients' foot problems are a result of repetitive daily stress during activities such as walking or running, movements of the various foot articulations are described as they occur in a closed chain situation.

Joint axis displacement during movement. Recent research has indicated that the axes of the different foot articulations, especially the joints in the subtalar and midtarsal regions, undergo displacement from their initial starting position during foot motion.[16] As a result of these findings, variation in the inclination of the axis during movements of the foot should be expected. Although various angles for the different joint axes are discussed here, during functional movements the angle of the axis changes secondary to displacements occurring in the foot articulations, especially in a closed chain situation.

Talocrural joint

The axis of the talocrural joint runs in an oblique direction between the tips of the malleoli. Anatomical investigations have demonstrated that the talocrural joint axis travels in an oblique direction and is positioned approximately 82 degrees from a vertical bisection of the tibia.[12,19] Although the talocrural joint has a triplane axis, Inman has demonstrated that the predominant motion of the talocrural joint is dorsiflexion and plantar flexion.[19] Inman further states that in approximately 80% of all cases, the talocrural articulation can be considered a uniplanar, single-axis joint with the primary motions of dorsiflexion and plantar flexion.[19] The degree of motion for the talocrural joint can range from 20 degrees of dorsiflexion to 50 degrees of plantar flexion. Although marked variations can occur in these ranges of motion for any given population, normal foot function during walking requires 20 degrees of plantar flexion and 10 degrees of dorsiflexion.[3] The 10 degrees of dorsiflexion should occur when the knee is extended and the foot is in a standing, relaxed posture. Because standing in a relaxed posture is often difficult to determine in a non–weight-bearing position, 10 degrees of dorsiflexion is often measured when the knee is extended and the subtalar joint is maintained in a neutral position. The assessment of dorsiflexion and plantar flexion is an important component of the examination. Individuals who lack dorsiflexion can compensate for this problem with early heel off or an increase in subtalar joint pronation.[48] A limitation in dorsiflexion range of motion and the resulting compensations can lead to dysfunction of the foot and ankle as a result of increased stress on the joint and surrounding soft tissues.

Subtalar joint

Several authors have described the average inclination angle of the subtalar joint axis as 42 degrees from the transverse plane and 16 degrees from the sagittal plane (Fig. 11-1).[11,27,39] The subtalar joint axis extends in an oblique direction from a posteriolateral, plantar position to a anteromedial, dorsal position in relation to the calcaneus. Because of the oblique placement of this single axis, the subtalar joint exhibits triplane motion. The two triplane motions of the subtalar joint are pronation and supination. Pronation of the subtalar joint in a closed chain is defined as the simultaneous movement of calcaneal eversion with adduction and plantar flexion of the head of the talus (Fig. 11-2, *C*).[45] Supination of the subtalar joint in a closed chain is defined as calcaneal inversion with abduction and dorsiflexion of the head of the talus (Fig. 11-2, *A*).[45] The motions of the talus are defined by describing the movement of the head of the talus. If the head of the talus from a neutral position moves superiorly or inferiorly, that motion is defined as dorsiflexion and plantarflexion, respectively. If the head of the talus from a neutral position rotates internally or externally, that motion is described as adduction and abduction, respectively. Because the subtalar joint demonstrates triplane motion, talar and calcaneal movements *occur simultaneously* during pronation and supination.

The prime function of the subtalar joint is to permit rotation of the leg in the transverse plane during the stance phase of walking.[17] A second function of the subtalar joint is to cause the lower leg (tibia) to internally rotate at a faster rate than the femur, thus permitting the knee joint to "unlock" during early stance. Knee joint flexion during the stance phase of walking is important in attenuating impact forces acting on the body. The subtalar joint, by pronating early in the walking cycle, can assist the popliteus muscle in causing the tibia to internally rotate at a faster rate and thus permitting the knee joint to flex during early stance. The average total range of motion for the subtalar joint ranges from 20 to 62 degrees.[19] In general, supination is approximately twice the value of pronation. The next section discusses the typical pattern of rearfoot motion and the degree of pronation and supination that occurs during a typical walking cycle.

Midtarsal articulations

The articulations of the midtarsal joint are the talocalcaneonavicular and the calcaneocuboid. The movement of these two articulations creates two axes in the midtarsal region: an oblique axis and a longitudinal axis. Although these two axes can move independently, the location of both axes during closed chain movement is dependent upon the position of the subtalar joint.[49] Thus, movements at the subtalar joint, when the foot is in a closed chain, help direct or guide the movements of the planes of the axes of the midtarsal articulations. Planes over the axes (Fig. 11-3, *B*) help to describe the relationship between subtalar movement and the two axes of the midtarsal joints. A sheet of plywood glued to the longitudinal axis and another to the oblique axis would enable observation of the movements of these planes of the axes (the sheets of plywood) during subtalar joint pronation and supination. The planes of the axes become more parallel to one another as the subtalar joint undergoes pronation. As can be observed in Fig. 11-3, *A*, which is a view of the anterior aspect of the subtalar joint, as the calcaneus everts, the talar head adducts, and plantar flexes, the planes of the midtarsal axes become parallel to each other. As the subtalar joint moves to a more neutral position, the planes of the axes tend to converge. The planes of the axes become increasingly more converged as the subtalar joint undergoes supination, as can be observed in Fig. 11-3, *C*. The functional result of this change in position of the axes is very important for general foot mobility during closed chain activities. The planes of the axes become parallel as a

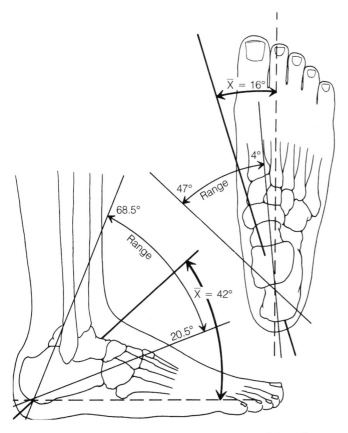

Fig. 11-1. Variations in the angle of the subtalar joint axis.

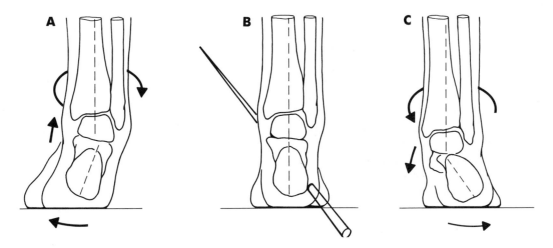

Fig. 11-2. Closed kinetic chain motion of the subtalar joint: **A,** supination; **B,** neutral position; **C,** pronation.

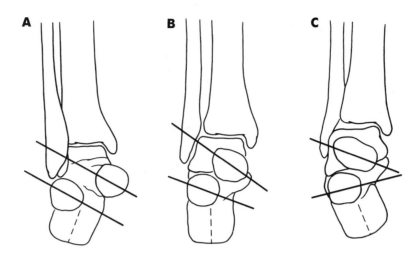

Fig. 11-3. Position of the planes of the axes of the midtarsal region during **A,** pronation; **B,** neutral position; **C,** supination.

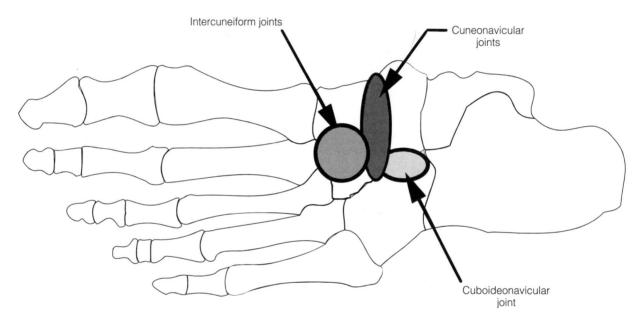

Fig. 11-4. Intertarsal region articulations.

result of subtalar pronation, which allows the articulations in the foot to become more flexible and mobile.[49] Using traditional orthopedic terminology, pronation of the subtalar joint and the resulting parallel position of the planes of the midtarsal region axes would cause the joints of the foot to assume a loose-packed position. As the subtalar joint undergoes supination, the planes of the axes of the midtarsal region become convergent. This convergence of the axial planes causes the articulations of the foot to become more stable.[49] Thus, convergence of the midtarsal axes, as a result of subtalar joint supination, would cause the foot articulations to assume a closed-pack position. The interaction between the position of the subtalar joint and the resulting change in the orientation of the midtarsal axial planes affects all of the joint articulations responsible for producing foot motion.

Intertarsal region

The cuneonavicular, cuboideonavicular, and intercuneiform articulations of the intertarsal region are primarily plane joints (Fig. 11-4). These joints' mobility is based on the ligamentous arrangement, as well as an individual's degree of soft tissue mobility. Thus, certain individuals may have more or less mobility in these joints, depending on these factors.

The rays

A marked variation exists in the amount of mobility of the first through fifth rays (Fig. 11-5).[40] The most mobile rays are the first and the fifth. Both the first and fifth rays exhibit triplane motion (Fig. 11-6). The most stable ray is the second, followed by the third ray (Fig. 11-7). The angle of

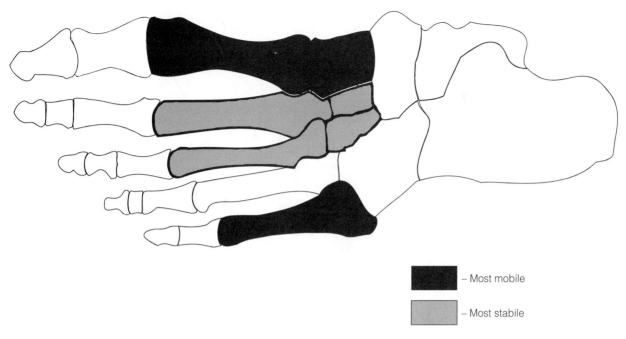

- Most mobile

- Most stabile

Fig. 11-5. The rays of the foot.

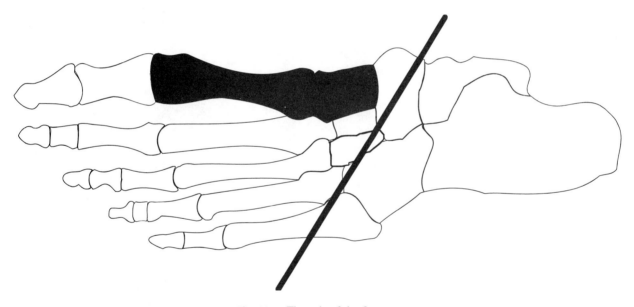

Fig. 11-6. The axis of the first ray.

the first ray is approximately 45 degrees in relation to the frontal and sagittal planes.[40] The first ray axis enters the transverse plane by only a few degrees. Thus, the predominant motions of the first ray occur in the frontal and sagittal planes.[40] The fifth ray axis is positioned at an angle of approximately 20 degrees from the transverse plane and 35 degrees from the sagittal plane.[40] Therefore, the predominant motions of the fifth ray are also in the frontal and sagittal planes.[40] The fact that the first ray and the fifth ray have their own axes and are the most mobile rays of the foot has important clinical implications. If the joints of the foot are permitted to be in a more mobile state during the terminal

portion of the stance phase of walking, the first and fifth ray may be unable to bear weight because of increased foot mobility. As a result, the second and third rays are forced to accept increased weight-bearing stresses because they are the most stable. This is one of the reasons why individuals with metatarsalgia often complain of pain under the second and third metatarsal heads.

Windlass mechanism of the plantar fascia

As previously discussed, the central band of the plantar fascia originates on the medial tubercle of the plantar fascia and travels toward the digits with a primary attachment to the

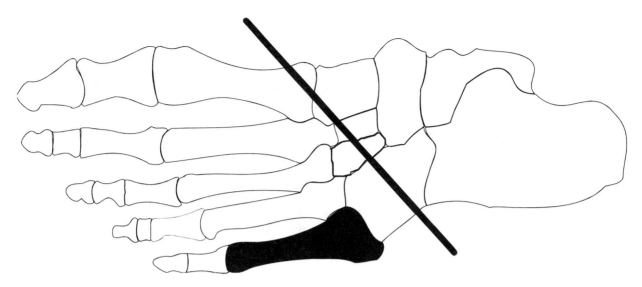

Fig. 11-7. The axis of the fifth ray.

medial and lateral aspects of the proximal phalanx of all five toes. This unique attachment permits the plantar fascia to affect the position of the foot when the toes are extended.[13] When an individual is standing in a relaxed posture with toes extended, the plantar fascia is wrapped around or pulled over the metatarsal heads of the five toes (Fig. 11-8).[41] This creates a functional shortening of the plantar fascia and an elevation of the medial longitudinal arch. Of course, the greatest effect of this windlass mechanism is at the first metatarsophalangeal joint because the first metatarsal head has the greatest radius. During the terminal portion of the stance phase of walking, as the calcaneus leaves the supporting surface and with the toes fixed to the floor, a functional shortening of the plantar fascia assists the foot in supinating. This functional shortening of the plantar fascia and the resulting increase in foot supination is termed the *windlass mechanism.*[14]

Closed chain movement of the foot articulations

Although the discussion of foot mechanics to this point has focused on each of the individual articulations or regions, all of the foot articulations work in unison to provide an overall movement pattern in the foot. For example, subtalar joint pronation and supination create a chain reaction in the midtarsal region, intertarsal region, and the rays to cause foot pronation and supination. A key question is how these movements in the various articulations of the foot are initiated.

Tibial rotation initiates movement in the articulations of the foot when the lower extremity is in a closed chain. Tibial rotation is caused by pelvic rotation in the transverse plane and is one of the six determinants for normal walking noted by Saunders and Inman when they investigated which factors were necessary for an energy-efficient walking pattern.[44] They found that during walking, in order to maintain the displacement of the body center of gravity to within a 2-inch square, six factors or determinants were

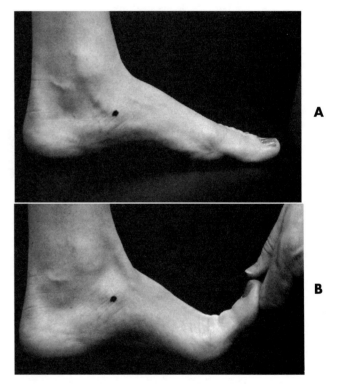

Fig. 11-8. The windlass mechanism: **A,** foot relaxed; **B,** elevation of medial longitudinal arch with toe extension.

necessary.[44] The first determinant was pelvic rotation in the transverse plane. The second determinant was transverse or pelvic rotation in the frontal plane. The third determinant was knee flexion during stance. The fourth and fifth determinants were classified as foot and ankle mechanisms. The sixth determinant was lateral displacement of the pelvis over the stance leg during the walking cycle. The first three determinants—pelvic rotation in the transverse and frontal planes, as well as knee flexion during stance—were identified as factors necessary to control vertical displacement of the center of gravity. These three components created a sinusoidal arc or pattern during the walking cycle. The fourth and fifth components create a smooth transition from arc to arc. The sixth determinant—lateral displacement of the pelvis over the stance limb—is critical in controlling the degree of lateral displacement of the center of gravity during walking.

The effect of transverse plane pelvic rotation in causing lower extremity and foot motion in a closed chain can be easily demonstrated by performing the following activity: Stand with your feet a shoulderwidth apart, place your hands on both hips, and then, while not moving your feet, begin rotating your pelvis forward and backward. If you consider that your left and right hands are on the left and right innominate bones, respectively, then the movement of each innominate and the resulting lower extremity motion can be observed. If you turn your pelvis toward the left, the left innominate bone moves posteriorly, causing the left lower extremity to undergo relative external rotation and the subtalar joint to supinate (Fig. 11-9). Simultaneously, the right innominate bone moves anteriorly, causing the right lower extremity to undergo relative internal rotation and the subtalar joint to pronate (Fig. 11-10). The opposite effect occurs if you turn your pelvis toward the right.

If these pelvic and lower extremity movements were applied to the walking cycle, the following sequence of motions for the right extremity would occur. From heel strike to foot flat (loading response) for the right lower extremity, the right innominate moves in an anterior direction and, with the foot fixed to the floor, causes relative internal rotation of both the femur and the tibia.[25] At the end of foot flat, the right innominate begins to move posteriorly as the left extremity begins its swing phase. As the right innominate bone moves posteriorly throughout the remainder of the stance phase, relative external rotation occurs in the femur and the tibia.[25] Thus, pelvic rotation in the transverse plane is the initiator of tibial rotation.[18] The key question to be asked is how tibial rotation can occur when the foot is fixed to the floor.

During the loading response phase of early stance, the tibia undergoes internal rotation,[25] which causes simultaneous internal rotation of the mortise. Internal rotation of the mortise causes the talus to adduct. Because the subtalar joint exhibits triplane motion, talar head adduction causes concurrent talar head plantar flexion and calcaneal eversion, resulting in subtalar joint pronation, which immediately causes the planes of the axes of the midtarsal region to become parallel, thus creating increased foot mobility in the midtarsal region as well as in the intertarsal region and the rays. At the end of loading response, the tibia begins to rotate externally.[25] External rotation of the tibia causes simultaneous external rotation of the mortise. External rotation of the mortise causes abduction of the talus. Because the subtalar joint exhibits triplane motion, talar head abduction causes concurrent talar head dorsiflexion and calcaneal inversion, resulting in subtalar joint supination. Supination of the subtalar joint immediately causes the planes of the axes of the midtarsal region to

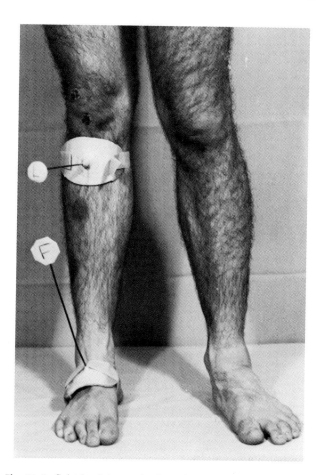

Fig. 11-9. Subtalar joint supination with tibial external rotation.

converge, thus restricting motion in the midtarsal and intertarsal regions, as well as in the rays.

Subtalar joint pronation and supination cause concurrent motion in the other articulations of the foot and thus create foot pronation and supination. Thus, the motions of foot supination and pronation are created by the movements of multiple joint articulations. Lundberg and colleagues investigated with three-dimensional stereoradiographic techniques which joints were the primary contributors to the overall motions of foot pronation and supination.[26] They concluded that the primary area of movement was in articulations of the midfoot region, followed by the subtalar joint. They further noted that the articulations both proximal and distal to the midtarsal region greatly added to the overall movement pattern of the foot as it underwent pronation and supination. The findings of Lundberg's study support the concept that the motions of foot pronation and supination are created by multiple foot articulations and not just the subtalar joint.[26]

The functions of the foot

The final aspect of the discussion of foot mechanics is how the various foot articulations work in concert to enable normal walking. The foot must provide the following five functions:

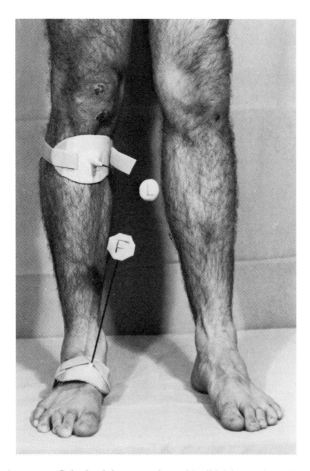

Fig. 11-10. Subtalar joint pronation with tibial internal rotation.

1. *Provide base of support during loading response.* The joints of the foot must allow the plantar surface of the foot to make contact with the supporting surface as soon as possible after heel strike to provide a stable base of support. Internal rotation of the tibia during loading response and the resulting subtalar joint pronation causes increased mobility in the midtarsal and intertarsal regions, as well as in the rays, as a result of foot pronation. This increased mobility, secondary to foot pronation, permits the plantar surface of the foot to contact the supporting surface as quickly as possible during the loading response phase of the walking cycle to provide a stable base of support. Patients with conditions such as hallux limitus or hallux valgus often have such severe pain in the first ray that they cannot effectively load the medial side of the forefoot during the loading response phase. Thus, they elevate the medial side of the forefoot in an attempt to decrease their level of pain. In doing so, however, the foot cannot satisfy this first foot function.

2. *Provide a supple accommodative structure at heel strike.* Foot pronation, as a result of subtalar joint pronation causing increased motion in the midtarsal and intertarsal regions as well as in the rays, increases mobility in all foot articulations. This increased mobility permits the plantar surface of the foot to adapt to the supporting surface during the contact phase of the walking cycle. Patients with limited foot mobility secondary to a high arch (pes cavus) foot type cannot satisfy this function and may require total-contact shoe inserts that increase the plantar surface area of the foot.

3. *Assist in attenuating impact forces during early stance.* The primary sources of shock attenuation during the early portion of the stance phase of walking are hip, knee, and ankle movements. These movements are controlled by eccentric contractions of the lower extremity musculature. The third determinant of normal walking is knee flexion during stance, which assists in controlling the vertical displacement of the center of gravity. Knee flexion, however, also causes a shortening of the lower extremity during the loading response. Because the lower extremity is in a closed chain, knee flexion would also result in motion at both the ankle (talocrural) and hip joints. The movements of the hip, knee, and ankle joints, which are controlled by eccentric muscular contraction, create a shortening of the lower extremity. The shock absorber of an automobile provides an excellent analogy to explain how the shortening of the lower extremity and the eccentric contraction of the muscles provide shock attenuation. The automobile shock absorber has two cylinders of different diameters that can move within one another. When going over a bump, the smaller-diameter cylinder moves into the larger-diameter cylinder to create shortening, and the spring positioned between the two cylinders compresses to absorb energy. The same principles of the automobile shock absorber—shortening and energy attenuation—are used by the lower extremity during the stance phase of walking. During the loading response, knee flexion causes simultaneous movement in the ankle and hip joints, which creates a shortening of the lower extremity, and eccentric muscle contraction acts as the spring in attenuating impact forces. The plantar heel pad also assists in attenuating early impact forces that occur 20 to 30 milliseconds after heel contact. Cavanagh has shown that these forces can be quite high (approximately 50% of body weight), especially during barefoot walking or during walking while wearing shoes with hard outsoles.[6]

4. *Provide a stable rigid base of support during terminal stance.* As a result of subtalar joint supination that causes increased stability in the midtarsal and intertarsal regions as well as in the rays, foot supination results in decreased mobility in all foot articulations. This increased foot stability provides a stable, rigid base of support to assist the lower extremity and trunk

during forward movement of the body at terminal stance. Factors that appear to initiate supination of the foot include the windlass mechanism of the plantar fascia, activity of the lower leg muscles, and external tibial rotation.

5. *Permit transverse plane rotation of the lower extremities with the foot fixed to a supporting surface.* The primary function of the subtalar joint, as previously mentioned, is to permit the lower extremity to undergo internal and external rotation during the stance phase of the walking cycle, when the foot is fixed to the supporting surface.[18]

THE TYPICAL PATTERN OF REARFOOT MOTION DURING WALKING

The majority of studies that have examined foot motion during walking have focused on the pattern of rearfoot motion that occurs during the stance phase. Root and colleagues proposed a specific pattern of motion for the subtalar joint during the stance phase of the walking cycle.[40] They noted that subtalar joint pronation occurred from heel strike to foot flat, with subtalar joint supination taking place from foot flat to toe off. An important point in Root and colleagues' description of the subtalar joint motion pattern was that the subtalar joint was in neutral position at either the instant of midstance or immediately after midstance during the walking cycle.[40] They based their description of subtalar joint movement on the research reported by Wright and colleagues, who studied the degree of subtalar joint motion using potentiometers on two male subjects.[52] Their results indicated that both subjects reached subtalar joint neutral position at 60% to 70% of the stance phase of walking. A critical issue is whether the Wright and Root groups use the same definition for neutral position of the subtalar joint. Wright and colleagues defined the neutral position of the subtalar joint for their investigation as the position when each subject was standing relaxed with the knees fully extended, arms at the sides, feet 6 inches apart, and a comfortable amount of toeing out.[52] They made no reference to placement of the subtalar joint in neutral in defining the "neutral" position for their study. Thus, Root and colleagues appear to have incorrectly interpreted the findings of the Wright group's study.

In an attempt to determine the relationship of subtalar joint neutral position to the pattern of rearfoot motion during walking, McPoil and Cornwall evaluated the pattern of rearfoot motion in 100 healthy, asymptomatic feet.[31] They used two-dimensional videography to record reflective markers placed on both the tibia and the calcaneus. Their results indicated that, just prior to heel strike, the rear foot was slightly inverted. From heel strike to foot flat, they found that the rear foot underwent the motion of pronation with the average time to maximum pronation approximately 40% of the stance phase. Rearfoot supination was initiated in all 100 feet by 50% of stance phase and continued until toe off. Their

findings were in agreement with the Wright group's results on their two subjects, except for the percent time to maximum pronation. The average amount of rearfoot pronation was approximately 4 degrees for both the Wright group study and the McPoil and Cornwall study. The average amount of rearfoot supination ranged from 4 to 8 degrees of supination. In addition to describing the pattern of rearfoot motion, McPoil and Cornwall also determined the relationship between the pattern of rearfoot motion and the static angles of the rear foot when each subject stood in a resting standing posture as well as with the subtalar joints positioned in neutral. They found that the mean pattern of dynamic rearfoot motion functioned around the static angle obtained with resting standing posture rather than the static angle obtained with the subtalar joint in its neutral position (Fig. 11-11).[31] They concluded that resting standing posture is the "functional" neutral position for typical rearfoot motion. These results refute the Root group's theory that the subtalar joint is in its neutral position at or just after midstance. Thus, the neutral position of the rear foot during walking is the position of the rear foot in relaxed standing posture.

In a second study, McPoil and Cornwall evaluated the relationship between the dynamic pattern of rearfoot motion and the static angle of the rear foot in resting standing posture and when standing on a single leg.[30] In this study, 62 feet were assessed with a similar research protocol. Their results indicated that the mean pattern of dynamic rearfoot motion functioned around the static angle of the rear foot in resting standing posture but did not cross the static angle of the rear foot in single-leg standing (Fig. 11-11).[30] These findings suggest that the typical pattern of rearfoot motion functions between the static angle of the rear foot in relaxed standing posture and single leg standing.

In summary, the typical pattern of rearfoot motion is as follows:

1. The rearfoot is slightly supinated prior to heel contact.
2. Pronation of the rear foot is initiated upon making contact with the ground and continues until approximately 40% of the stance phase.
3. Supination of the rear foot is initiated by 50% of the stance phase and continues until toe off.
4. The "functional" neutral position of the rear foot during walking is the angle of the rear foot in resting standing posture and *not* the subtalar joint neutral position.

EXAMINATION OF THE FOOT AND ANKLE

The procedures used for examination of the foot and ankle must include assessment techniques for both traumatic and chronic disorders. The theoretical basis for the evaluation procedures given here is the tissue stress model,[32] which is based on the load-deformation curve[7] and permits clinicians to adapt their evaluation and treatment protocols based on the tissues the client has stressed. The tissue stress model

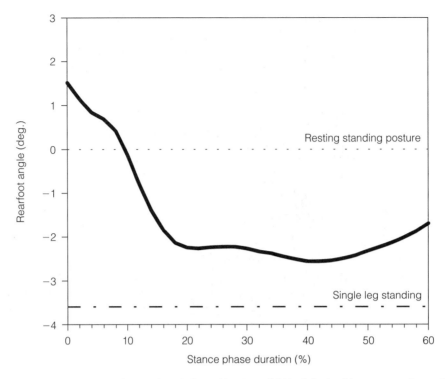

Fig. 11-11. Pattern of rearfoot motion (indicated by the solid black line) with respect to the angle of the rearfoot in resting standing posture and single leg standing.

can be applied to the examination of either a traumatic injury or a chronic overuse type of injury. Tissue stress in the foot and ankle can occur to both inert and contractile tissues. Inert tissues include joint capsule, ligaments, and plantar aponeurosis. Contractile tissues include the tendon, tenosynovial sheath, muscle fibers, and muscle origin. Tissue stress can be caused or intensified by excessive mechanical loading, frictional irritation, elevated tissue temperature, or nutritional imbalance.

Tissue stress can also be influenced by the speed at which the load is applied to the tissues as well as the ability of the lower leg muscles to provide dynamic stabilization during activity. To illustrate the influence of these two factors, consider an individual playing basketball. In attempting to shoot a layup, the player plants a foot and cuts toward the basket. As a result of the plantar flexion associated with this movement, the amount of foot surface area in contact with the gym floor is reduced because the player is bearing weight only on the forefoot. If the individual now loses balance, a moment is created causing their ankle to invert. The magnitude of the inversion moment as well as the speed of the moment could possibly cause a traumatic ankle sprain. The severity of the ankle sprain, including the extent of the ligamentous damage, is determined by the strength and response time of the peroneal muscles in attempting to arrest the inversion moment. Thus, both the strength and the response time of the dynamic stabilizers can significantly influence the amount of tissue stress.

The clinician must also remember that a major difference between upper extremity and lower extremity neuromusculoskeletal problems is the amount of force applied through the lower extremity during activities such as walking and running. This increased level of force results in significantly greater stresses being applied to the tissues of the lower limb and foot during normal walking. Thus, in the course of performing the physical examination, the examiner may not be able to apply enough force to provoke patients' pain or reproduce their symptoms.

The general examination scheme, using the tissue stress model for the patient with a foot or ankle disorder, is first to determine what tests are necessary in the physical examination. The selection of those tests should be based on the patient's symptomatic complaints and history. In a traumatic injury, the mechanism of injury usually directs the selection of the examination procedures. In a chronic overuse injury, however, the symptoms may be more obscure, and the patient may not have pain at the time of examination. In these cases, the examiner must obtain an adequate history in order to determine the tissues that are being overstressed and the direction of the applied forces that are causing the increased tissue stress. Regardless of whether the patient's injury is the result of trauma or of chronic overuse, the tissue stress model serves as the theoretical basis for examination and treatment. The goal of physical therapy intervention in clients with lower extremity traumatic or overuse injuries is to reduce tissue stress to a tolerable level.

The physical examination and management protocol for the tissue stress model includes the following steps:

1. Utilize the patient's history and subjective information to identify the involved tissues and attempt to determine the direction of force causing the excessive tissue stress.
2. Attempt to apply stress to the identified tissues through palpation and weight-bearing and non–weight-bearing tests to replicate the patient's symptoms. In addition, various factors identified as possible etiologies of overuse injuries are also assessed.
3. Based on the findings of the physical examination, determine if the patient's complaint is related to excessive mechanical loading or a nonmechanical problem. For example, a patient could be complaining of pain in the forefoot. Based on the results of the examination, if the diagnosis was metatarsalgia secondary to abnormal foot mechanics, the patient would be classified as having excessive mechanical loading. If the patient was determined to have a Morton's neuroma, however, it would be classified as a nonmechanical problem.
4. The management plan is then based on the following steps:
   a. Reduction of tissue stress to a tolerable level by utilizing footwear, arch strapping, or foot orthoses
   b. Healing the involved tissues through the use of pharmacological and physical agents.
   c. Restoration of soft tissue flexibility.
   d. Restoration of muscle strength.
   e. Use of an appropriate functional progression to allow the individual to resume desired daily activities.

The application of this tissue stress model to the individual with an acute injury requires less problem solving. If the patient reports a sprained ankle, then the examiner attempts to determine the direction of applied force that caused the sprain with specific special tests to stress the involved tissues. Thus, the patient's symptoms and the history guides the examiner in determining what specific tests are necessary as well as the organization of the physical examination.

With a chronic injury, however, the examiner must attempt to determine the region or specific tissues that are being overstressed and select the appropriate special tests to stress the involved tissues. In general, the two primary causes of chronic overuse injuries secondary to excessive mechanical loading are a pronatory foot type, causing excessive foot mobility, and a supinatory foot type, causing excessive foot stability.

The individual with excessive foot mobility associated with a pronatory foot type is subject to increased stress to osseous and soft tissues as well as overreliance on both intrinsic and extrinsic muscles to provide needed foot stability. Factors that can cause or contribute to a pronatory foot type include:

1. Excessive internal or external femoral rotation
2. Excessive internal or external malleolar torsion
3. Genu varum, genu valgum, or tibial varum
4. Limited flexibility of the calf muscle group, often referred to as a *functional equinus*
5. Excessive soft tissue mobility
6. Obesity
7. Severe intrinsic osseous deformities of the foot, including forefoot varus or valgus and rearfoot varus

The individual with excessive foot stability associated with a supinatory foot type is subject to decreased shock attenuation during loading response and increased forefoot plantar pressures secondary to decreased plantar surface area. Factors that can cause or contribute to a supinatory foot type include:

1. Neuromuscular disorders such as Charcot-Marie-Tooth disease
2. Traumatic injury secondary to industrial or motor vehicle accidents
3. Congenital foot deformities such as clubfoot
4. Idiopathic pes cavus
5. Severe intrinsic foot deformities such rigid forefoot valgus

In determining the necessary elements of the physical examination, an assessment of these factors should be included if the clinician suspects that the patient may have either a pronatory or supinatory foot type. The organizational scheme for the physical examination of the foot and ankle is listed in the Box on the following page.

Physical examination procedures

History and subjective exam. The goals of the history are to determine if the patient's symptom or problem is secondary to excessive mechanical loading and to delineate what foot region or tissues are being stressed. The following questions can guide the examiner in taking the history.

1. Does any position, movement, or activity either relieve or intensify the symptoms?
2. Are you awakened at night with pain?
3. What are your symptoms like when you first arise in the morning versus during the day with activity?
4. Do your symptoms increase with activity?
5. Have x-rays been taken? Were the x-rays weight bearing or not?
6. Have you had any recent injuries not related to the present symptoms?
7. What medications do you take? How do you rate your

general health? Have you had a significant recent weight loss?

8. If evaluating a child, determine if there has been a recent growth spurt.

9. What types of footwear do you most often use for work and recreational activities?

10. A family or personal history of any of the following problems should also be determined:

Rheumatoid arthritis	Lower extremity weakness
Diabetes mellitus	Flat feet or high arches
Ever worn special shoes	Sprain ankles frequently
Ever worn foot orthoses	Osteoarthritis
Neurological problems	Circulatory problems
Foot wounds or ulcers	Cold or burning feet
Sweaty feet	Toenail problems
Edema or swelling of feet	

Some of these questions may not be necessary for a patient with a recent traumatic injury, if the patient can describe how the injury happened and the likely mechanism of injury.

Objective examination

Patient observation. The examiner should observe the patient in an attempt to answer the following questions: Is the patient willing to move the foot? How does the patient position the foot and the medial longitudinal arch while standing? Can the patient bring the medial side of the forefoot, especially the first and second metatarsal heads, in full contact with the ground while standing? Is the patient standing on the lateral aspect of their foot, elevating the medial aspect of the foot so as to not load it?

Are any foot deformities obvious? Does the patient have a hallux valgus or bunion deformity? Is there clawing of one or more toes (Fig. 11-12)? Is there a hammer or mallet toe deformity (Fig. 11-12)? If a bunion is present, is the hallux compressing the second toe to create a hammer toe deformity? Does the patient have flatfoot (pes planus) or a high arch (pes cavus)?

Initial gait analysis. An initial gait analysis should be conducted to determine the presence of transverse or frontal plane deformities. For example, if the patient ambulates with a pigeon-toed walking pattern or if the patella is positioned medially during the last 50% of stance phase, a torsional deformity may be present. Based on these signs, an assessment of hip rotation and malleolar torsion should be included in the physical examination. A frontal plane deformity, such as genu varum or genu valgum, might be present if the patient demonstrates an excessively wide or narrow dynamic base of walking.

Screening. As noted with any other orthopedic assessment, the foot can be a possible area of referred pain. Pain can be referred to the foot from the lumbar spine, sacroiliac region, or the hip or knee joints. To rule out the possibility of referred pain from any of these anatomical regions, a range-of-motion assessment should be conducted for each

---

Physical examination scheme for the foot and ankle

I. History and subjective exam

II. Objective examination
  A. Patient observation
  B. Screening
  C. Functional tests
    1. Active and resistive motions of the ankle
    2. Passive motion
  D. Mobility testing
    1. Talocrural joint
    2. Subtalar joint
    3. Intertarsal joint
    4. Intermetatarsal joint
    5. Metatarso-phalangeal, proximal interphalangeal, and distal interphalangeal joints
  E. Palpation
    1. Bony and soft tissue
    2. Callus
    3. Peripheral arterial pulses
  F. Neurological examination
    1. Reflexes
    2. Sensory testing
  G. Special tests—acute injury
    1. Anterior drawer test
    2. Anterolateral drawer test
    3. Inversion stress test
    4. Thompson's test
    5. Compression test
    6. Homans' sign
    7. Tinel's sign
  H. Special tests—overuse injury
    1. First metatarsophalangeal joint range of motion (ROM)
    2. Ray mobility
    3. Malleolar torsion
    4. Hip joint ROM
    5. Talocrural joint ROM
    6. Resting standing foot posture (RSFP)
    7. Standing in subtalar joint neutral (SSJN) position
    8. Measurement of tibiofibular varum during single leg stand
  I. Final gait analysis

III. Assessment and treatment planning

---

possible referral area, with overpressure applied at the end of the available range. If, for example, the patient complains of a burning sensation over the lateral aspect of the foot, irritation of the sural nerve might be suspected, referred pain from the lumbosacral region.

Active, passive, and resistive tests. The patient is first asked to actively move the ankle in the directions of dorsiflexion, plantar flexion, inversion, and eversion. While the patient performs these active motions, the clinician should visually observe whether the movements are symmetrical or asymmetrical. If full range of motion is present bilaterally,

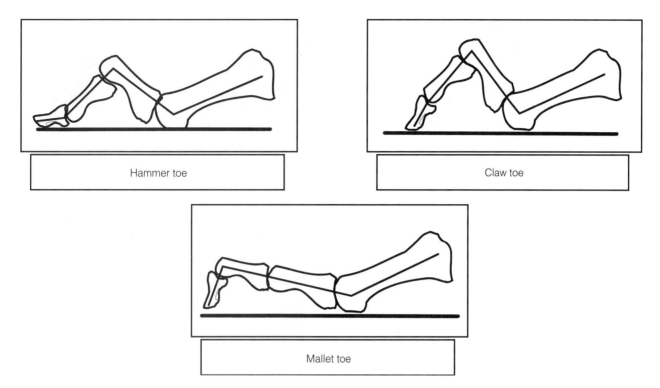

Hammer toe

Claw toe

Mallet toe

Fig. 11-12. The classifications of toe deformities.

the patient should be asked about any pain associated with active motions. Once active motion is completed, passive motion is assessed. Dorsiflexion of the ankle would be assessed with the knee first extended, then flexed, followed by plantar flexion, inversion, and eversion. Next, the passive motions of the midtarsal and intertarsal region are assessed with the patient long sitting. To assess motion in the oblique midtarsal and intertarsal region of the right foot, the examiner first grasps the calcaneus with the right hand to prevent subtalar movement (Fig. 11-13). The thumb and index fingers of the left hand then grasp the fourth and fifth metatarsals and then abduct and adduct the forefoot. While abducting and adducting the forefoot, the examiner should avoid dorsiflexing or plantar flexing the forefoot. To assess longitudinal motion of the midtarsal and intertarsal region, the examiner continues to stabilize the right calcaneus with the right hand. The examiner then grasps all five metatarsal heads between the index finger and thumb of the left hand and twists or rotates the metatarsal heads as a group internally and externally (Fig. 11-14). The passive motions of the midtarsal and intertarsal region are first done with the talocrural joint in the neutral position. If, however, the patient notes that most of the symptoms or pain occurs when the foot is plantar flexed, the examiner can place the ankle in various positions of plantar flexion and repeat the two tests. Passive range of motion of the first metatarsophalangeal joint (FMTPJ) is then assessed, with emphasis on extension. With the talocrural joint in slight plantar flexion, the FMTPJ is passively extended to the end of the range. The angle formed by the hallux and the shaft of the first metatar-

sal is observed for approximately 90 degrees of motion. Once the passive tests are completed, resistive tests are used to rule out involvement of contractile tissues. The motions of plantar flexion, dorsiflexion, eversion, and inversion are isometrically resisted in a position that does not replicate the patient's symptoms or pain. Active motion tests provide information on the patient's ability to move the joints of the foot through the range of motion. Pain or limited motion with passive tests, if conducted with the patient totally relaxed, can indicate inflammation or a restriction of inert tissues. Finally, pain or limited motion with resistive tests, especially if passive range of motion is normal, can indicate contractile tissue irritation.

Mobility testing. If passive range of motion is restricted or painful, then joint play or accessory motion is assessed with the use of various glides and distractions. Joint mobility testing for the talocrural joint includes distraction and anterior and posterior glides. Joint mobility testing for the subtalar joint is difficult in light of the articular anatomy previously discussed. A calcaneal distraction can be used to assess a limitation in joint mobility. In addition, the physiological motions of inversion and eversion are also assessed. Midtarsal mobility and intermetatarsal accessory mobility are evaluated by rolling or "sweeping" the metatarsal heads as well as performing dorsal and plantar glides for all the metatarsal heads. Finally, metatarsophalangeal, proximal interphalangeal, and distal interphalangeal joint mobility can be assessed with dorsal and plantar metatarsal glides and distraction.

Palpation. The following bony landmarks could be

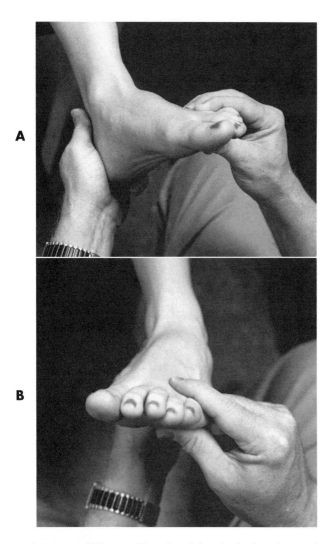

Fig. 11-13. Oblique midtarsal and longitudinal region motion: **A,** abduction; **B,** adduction.

palpated, based upon the patient's complaints: the medial and lateral malleolus, the head of the talus, navicular tuberosity, the first metatarsocuneiform joint, the medial aspect of the FMTPJ, the sustentaculum tali, the lateral aspect of the base of the fifth metatarsal, and the plantar aspect of all five metatarsal heads. In addition to bony palpation, appropriate soft tissue palpation should be performed, based on the patient's symptoms. Next, areas of callus on the plantar surface of the foot should be noted. Finally, the dorsalis pedis and posterior tibial arteries should be palpated to determine if a strong pulse is present.

Neurological tests. If the patient indicated possible signs of neurological involvement such as burning, tingling, or electrical shocks in the lower legs, then neurological tests, including an assessment of neural reflexes, joint proprioception, and cutaneous sensation, should be performed.

Special tests. The final aspect of the physical examination is specific tests, based on whether the person has a traumatic or chronic overuse injury.

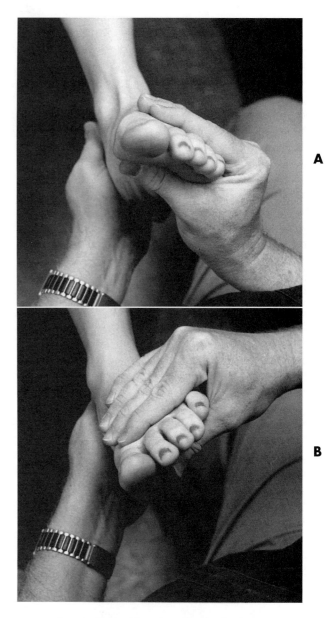

Fig. 11-14. Longitudinal midtarsal and longitudinal region motion: **A,** inversion; **B,** eversion.

Special tests for acute injuries

1. *Anterior drawer test.* The anterior drawer test is performed by having the patient sitting relaxed over the edge of the table.[42] The examiner grasps the calcaneus with one hand and stabilizes the tibia with the other hand. The hand on the tibia prevents forward movement of the mortise as the hand on the calcaneus attempts to pull the entire foot in an anterior direction. This action creates an anterior glide of the talus on the mortise (Fig. 11-15). The examiner should attempt to determine the degree of laxity in the ligaments of the ankle by judging the displacement of the talus in relation to the mortise. A positive test indicates involvement of the anterior talofibular ligament as well as the

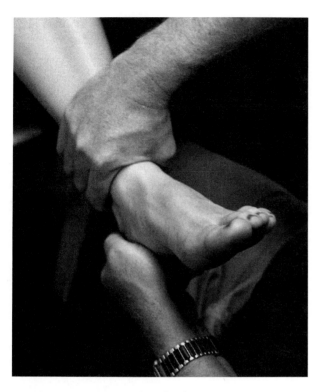

Fig. 11-15. Anterior drawer test.

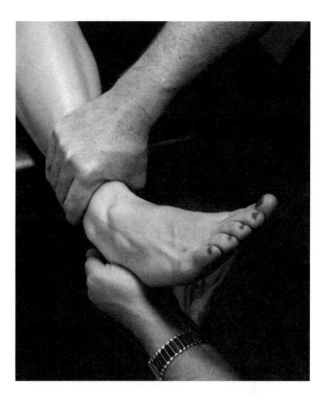

Fig. 11-16. Inversion stress test.

anterior capsule of the talocrural joint.[42] An *anteriolateral drawer test* is similar to an anterior drawer test, except that a rotational force is applied in addition to the anterior translation. As the clinician pulls the calcaneus forward, rather than doing just a pure anterior glide, the calcaneus is glided anteriorly as well as rotated in a medial direction to apply increased stresses to the anteriolateral tissues of the ankle.

2. *Inversion stress test.* To perform the inversion stress test, the examiner places one hand on the tibia, again to stabilize the lower leg.[42] The other hand is positioned on the lateral aspect of the calcaneus and forcefully inverts the calcaneus, as the tibia is prevented from moving. The clinician should observe for an increased degree of inversion on the involved ankle (Fig. 11-16). A positive inversion stress test would indicate possible involvement of the anterior talofibular ligament as well as the calcaneofibular ligament.

3. *Thompson's test.* Thompson's test determines if the Achilles tendon has ruptured.[2] The patient is prone on the table with knees flexed and feet handging off the edge. The clinician then squeezes the patient's calf. This maneuver normally causes plantar flexion of the ankle. If it does not, a rupture of the Achilles tendon should be suspected.

4. *Compression test.* The compression test is used to look for a possible stress fracture. To perform this test, the clinician compresses the involved bone proximally and distally to the site of the suspected fracture. Although the patient may complain of discomfort at the proximal and distal location of compression, a positive sign for a stress fracture is increased pain at the site of the possible stress fracture as a result of the compression. If a stress fracture is suspected, the patient should be immediately referred to a physician.

5. *Homans' sign.* Homans' sign indicates possible thrombophlebitis of the posterior tibial veins. For this test, the patient sits with legs off the edge of the examination table and both feet in a slight plantar flexed position. The clinician then compresses or squeezes the calf muscles and notes if the patient complains of pain or discomfort in the posterior leg. Pain in the calf muscles as a result of this test suggests thrombophlebitis. If thrombophlebitis is suspected, the patient should be immediately referred to a physician.

6. *Tinel's sign.* Tinel's sign determines whether a tarsal tunnel compression syndrome is present. For this test, the patient's foot is plantar flexed and everted. The examiner then taps over the flexor retinaculum, which is located between the medial malleolus and calcaneus (Fig. 11-17). A positive sign is replication of the symptoms or pain the patient reported previously.

Special tests for overuse injuries. Special tests for chronic overuse injuries assess factors that have been identified as causing or contributing to excessive mobility or limited mobility foot types.

1. *First metatarsophalangeal joint (FMTPJ) extension range of motion.* The measurement of FMTPJ extension is done to rule out a hallux limitus or hallux rigidus. To measure the FMTPJ extension, the stationary arm of a goniometer should be positioned parallel to the medial aspect of the shaft of the first metatarsal, with the moving arm on a medial bisection of the hallux (Fig. 11-18).[15] The axis of the goniometer should be placed medial to the FMTPJ axis. The typical value of FMTPJ extension required for walking is 65 degrees.[15]

2. *Ray mobility.* To assess the plantar and dorsal motion of all five rays, each metatarsal head is moved in a dorsal and plantar direction while the adjacent ray is stabilized (Fig. 11-19, *A, B*). For each ray, the clinician notes the amount of dorsal and plantar mobility. As previously discussed, the first and fifth rays should demonstrate the most mobility. The second should exhibit the least, followed by the third and fourth rays.

3. *Determination of malleolar torsion.* The patient sits over the edge of the table, and the femoral condyles are palpated and positioned so that they are parallel to the table edge (Fig. 11-20, *A*). The clinician then places one thumb on the anterior aspect of the lateral malleolus and the other thumb at the midpoint of the medial malleolus (Fig. 11-20, *B*). Once positioned, the alignment of the thumbs is assessed. If the thumbs form a line or plane parallel to the edge of the table, malleolar torsion is within normal limits. If the alignment of the thumbs creates a line or plane that is not parallel to the edge of the table, then a malleolar torsion deformity, either internal or external, is present.

4. *Hip joint range of motion.* The examiner should consider measuring hip joint range of motion if a rotational deformity is suspected. For the measurement, the patient can be either prone or sitting. The prone position should be avoided if the patient is also suspected of having a hip flexion contracture.

5. *Talocrural joint range of motion.* Talocrural joint dorsiflexion range of motion should be assessed to determine if the patient has approximately 8 to 10 degrees of dorsiflexion with the knee extended and flexed. Care should be taken not to pronate the foot during the assessment. For *dorsiflexion with knee extended,* the

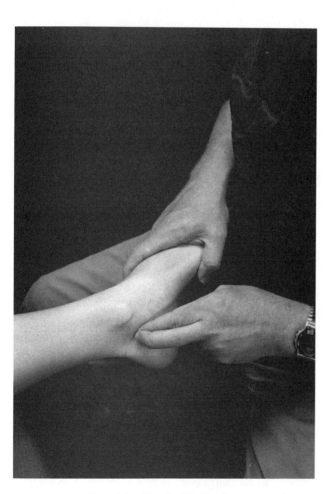

Fig. 11-17. Test for Tinel's sign.

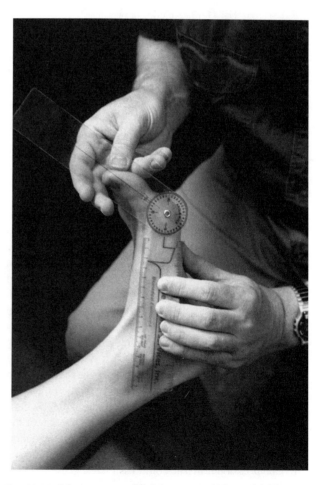

Fig. 11-18. Measurement of first metatarsophalangeal joint extension.

patient is prone. While the knee joint is maintained in an extended position, the foot is passively dorsiflexed to the end of the available range. The examiner should take care not to pronate the foot. At the end of the available passive range, the patient is asked to actively dorsiflex the foot. The stationary arm of the goniometer is then placed along the lateral aspect of the shaft

of the fifth metatarsal, while the moving arm is positioned along a line drawn from the lateral malleolus to the fibular head (Fig. 11-21, *A*). In addition to recording the range of motion measured, the joint end feel should also be noted. For *dorsiflexion with knee flexed,* the procedure described with the knee extended is repeated, except that the knee is flexed to 90 degrees prior to performing the measurement (Fig. 11-21, *B*). In general, a 5-degree increase in dorsiflexion range of motion is observed when the knee is flexed.

6. *Resting standing foot posture (RSFP).* RSFP allows the clinician to observe the patient's foot posture in standing as well as determine how the joints of the foot have adapted in static weight bearing. In addition, the amount of foot pronation and supination can be estimated by measuring the height of the navicular in RSFP and comparing it to the same measurement in the standing in subtalar joint neutral (SSJN) position. Prior to performing any measurements, a dynamic angle and base of gait template is made. The template serves as a permanent record of the foot position for that particular examination as well as for future examination sessions, thus increasing the repeatability of future measurements. Before being positioned on a piece of paper to have the feet traced, the patient is asked to walk so that the clinician can determine the dynamic angle and base of gait. As the patient is walking, the clinician observes the distance between the medial malleoli and the medial aspect of both knees to determine the dynamic base. As the patient continues to walk, the number of toes that are visible from the lateral aspect of the lower leg are noted, bilaterally. For example, if two toes are noted in rela-

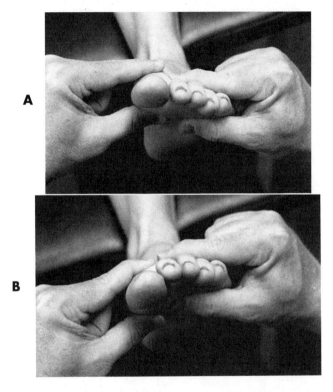

Fig. 11-19. Ray mobility: **A,** dorsal; **B,** plantar.

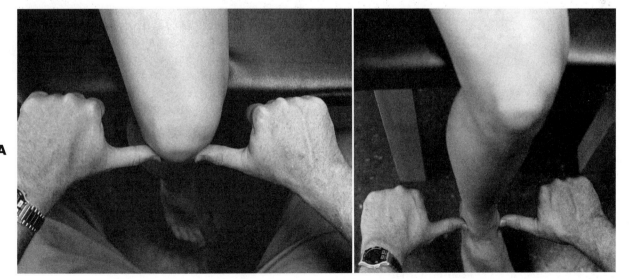

Fig. 11-20. Test for malleolar torsion: **A,** alignment of femoral condyles; **B,** alignment of the thumbs at the malleoli.

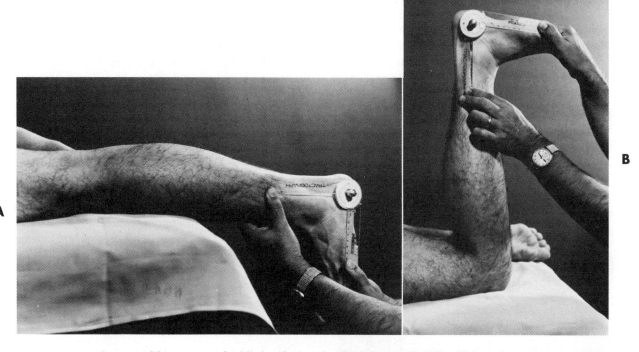

Fig. 11-21. Measurement of ankle dorsiflexion: **A,** with knee extended; **B,** with knee flexed.

tion to the lateral aspect of the lower leg while walk-ing, the patient would then be positioned with the same number of toes showing while standing on the paper used for the template. The patient is then placed on the paper in the patient's own dynamic angle and base of gait, and the feet are outlined (Fig. 11-22).

The entire foot, as well as the calcaneus, talus, and medial longitudinal arch, is then observed to deter-mine whether the foot is pronated or supinated. The patient is considered to have a pronatory foot type if the calcaneus is everted or vertical and if the head of the talus is displaced medially. Next, the tuberosity of the navicular is marked with a felt-tip pen. The height of the navicular tuberosity from the floor is then mea-sured and recorded in millimeters (Fig. 11-23). Finally, tibiofibular varum is measured. Previous research has indicated that tibial varum cannot be measured with-out a radiograph. Tibiofibular varum, however, can be measured clinically, and the best position for the as-sessment is RSFP.[34] To measure tibiofibular varum, the lower third of the lower leg is bisected with a felt-tip pen. The stationary arm of the goniometer is placed on the supporting surface, while the moving arm is aligned to the bisection line of the lower leg (Fig. 11-24). The angle measured represents the de-gree of tibiofibular varum.

7. *Standing in subtalar joint neutral (SSJN).* While the patient is still positioned on the angle and base template, the examiner individually places both sub-talar joints in the subtalar neutral position and

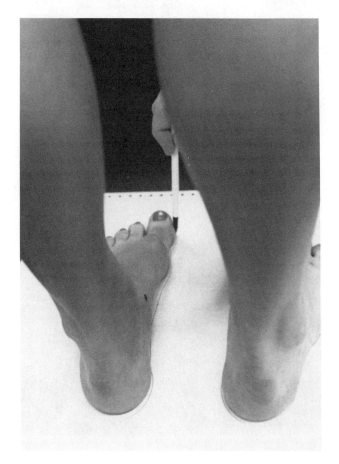

Fig. 11-22. Tracing feet to create a dynamic angle and base template.

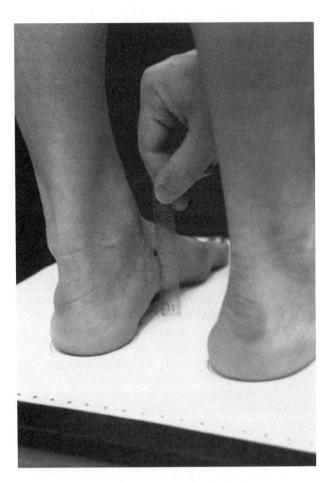

Fig. 11-23. Measurement of navicular height.

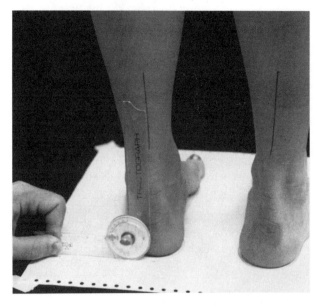

Fig. 11-24. Measurement of tibiofibular varum.

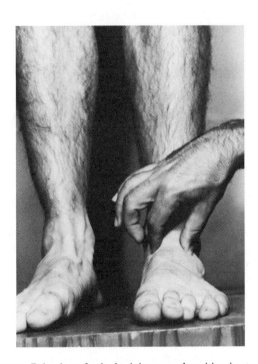

Fig. 11-25. Palpation of subtalar joint neutral position in standing.

maintains them there (Fig. 11-25). While in subtalar joint neutral position, the total foot, calcaneus, talus, and medial longitudinal arch are again observed to note alignment variations in comparison to RSFP. Finally, the measurement of the height of the navicular tuberosity from the floor is repeated and subtracted from the navicular height measurement obtained in RSFP. A difference of greater than 10 millimeters is considered significant and could be indicative of excessive foot pronation.[36] Although researchers have not established the criteria for a supinatory foot type, a difference in navicular height of less than 5 millimeters may indicate a limited motion foot type.

8. *Measurement of tibiofibular varum during single leg standing (SLS).* The patient is asked to practice standing on one leg, using only fingertips for the maintenance of balance. The examiner should observe the patient's weight shift during practice. Once the examiner is satisfied with the weight shift, the patient is then asked to stand on one leg. The measurement of tibiofibular varum is repeated with the technique previously described (Fig. 11-26). In general, a 5-degree change is usually observed when the tibiofibular varum angle obtained in SLS is subtracted from the angle in RSFP.

Final gait analysis. The last step of the examination is a final gait analysis to observe foot position as well as changes in foot posture that occur during walking. Although most video cameras have the capability of taking approximately 30 to 60 pictures per second, the human eye and brain can only take and process approximately 10 pictures per second. The examiner, therefore, can most likely observe the patient walking at only three locations during the walking cycle. The first point of observation should be just prior to and following heel strike. The rear foot should be in an inverted position prior to contacting the ground and immedi-

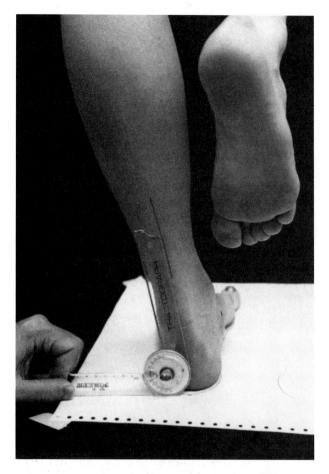

Fig. 11-26. Measurement of tibiofibular varum in one-leg stand.

ately undergo pronation after initial contact. As previously discussed, the average time to maximum pronation is approximately 40% of the stance phase with foot supination beginning just before or at midstance. The second point of observation should be at midstance. The easiest way to determine when the stance leg is at midstance is to note when the toes of the opposite foot leave the ground to begin their swing phase. At that point, the examiner switches his or her eyes back to the stance leg to observe if the foot is initiating supination. The third point of observation is when the heel of the stance leg begins to leave the ground. At this point in the walking cycle, the foot should be undergoing the motion of supination to enhance foot stability. If the foot is still pronated once heel off has occurred, excessive stresses are probably being applied to pedal soft tissue structures as a result of increased foot mobility.

In addition to these three specific points of observation, the examiner should also note the pattern of movement of the medial longitudinal arch during initial contact as the patient walks toward the examiner. Another important observation is whether the patient exhibits early heel off during the walking cycle. A patient whose heel leaves the ground too early may have limited calf muscle flexibility, also termed *functional equinus.*[48]

As the patient is walking toward the examiner, the position of the patella should be observed near midstance to determine if it is facing forward, inward, or outward. A patella facing inward could be indicative of a torsional problem or limited motion of the internal rotators of the hip. A patella facing outward could be indicative of excessive external torsion or limited motion of the external rotators of the hip. Finally, as the patient walks toward the examiner, the patient should be instructed to stop. The examiner should then place the patient in the dynamic angle and base of walking. In this position, the patient can then be maximally pronated and supinated, by passively internally or externally rotating the tibia bilaterally. The examiner is then able to observe the movement of the foot and medial longitudinal arch and the resulting effect on lower extremity movement.

ASSESSMENT AND MANAGEMENT

The assessment represents the analysis of the results that have been obtained from the physical examination of the foot and ankle. If the patient examined has had a traumatic injury, then an assessment must be made from the examination findings as to the presence of hypermobility or hypomobility of the involved joints. In addition, as a result of severe trauma, the patient may have had an ankylosis, or fusion, of one or more foot articulations. The management plan for this type of patient is based on the assessment of the examination findings. If the patient has joint hypermobility as a result of the trauma, then a major focus of the treatment program is a muscle-strengthening program to provide stabilization of the involved segment or joint. If the patient's primary problem is hypomobility, then the primary focus of the treatment program is articular and soft tissue mobilization techniques to the restricted area. If the patient has a joint fusion and cannot fully load the medial aspect of the forefoot because of restricted motion, then foot orthoses can be prescribed to "bring the supporting surface up to the foot" as well as increase total plantar surface area, resulting in decreased plantar pressures.

Remember that any patient who has had a prolonged antalgic walking pattern secondary to foot and ankle pain can develop weakness of proximal musculature as a result of limited use of the involved extremity. The proximal muscles that are often affected include the hip abductors as well as the internal and external rotators. Thus, an important goal of treatment should be to assist the patient in attaining a normal walking pattern as soon as possible to prevent proximal muscle weakness. In addition, the examiner should consider testing the strength of the proximal lower extremity musculature when evaluating patients who have a history of an antalgic walking pattern as a result of a foot and ankle injury.

In the assessment of the overuse injury, the clinician must first determine if the injury is mechanical or nonmechanical in origin. A mechanical problem is defined as symptoms or pain induced by increased activity causing excessive stress to osseous and soft tissue structures. An example of a nonmechanical problem is a patient who notes not having had any pain or discomfort in the right foot for 5 days while at work but severe pain in the right medial arch area while relaxing over the weekend. Individuals with this pattern of pain or symptoms should be sent to their referring physician for further examination. Patients with a mechanical problem present with pain or symptoms that are exacerbated with increased activity. If the patient's complaint is believed to be caused by a mechanical problem, then the examiner must determine whether the reported symptoms or the excessive stresses being applied to the tissues are related to an excessive pronation or excessive supination foot type. Once the foot type is determined, then an appropriate treatment program can be initiated. In both cases, the primary goal of treatment is to reduce tissue stress to a tolerable level.

Pronatory or excessive motion foot types

Patients with overuse injuries secondary to a pronatory foot type often lack the ability to convert the foot to a more stable structure during terminal stance and as a result have increased stress on soft tissues as well as overreliance on extrinsic and intrinsic muscles of the foot. In addition to pharmacological and physical agents and muscle-strengthening exercises, footwear and foot orthoses should also be considered to assist the patient in controlling excessive foot motion. Specific features that should be considered when prescribing footwear for pronatory foot types include (1) a rearfoot control system, (2) full or partial board lasting, and (3) five to six eyelets. If the patient has a severe pronation problem, then an all-leather shoe upper should also be considered.[28] A rearfoot control system in footwear consists of a snug-fitting, firm heel counter and a counter stabilizer, which is a separate plastic piece or a superior extension of the midsole that acts to reinforce and prevent distortion of the heel counter.[28] Board lasting, if available, provides a flat, firm surface within the shoe, which is desirable if foot orthoses are prescribed.[28] The high lacing pattern provided by five or six eyelets allows for proper stabilization of the midtarsal and intermetatarsal regions of the foot. Although researchers have shown that properly fitting shoes can aid in the control of excessive foot pronation,[20,35] the shoe also serves as the foundation for foot orthoses. Although foot orthoses may be prescribed to provide additional control of excessive pronation, proper footwear is always the first step in the treatment program. Additional measures to control foot pronation can include arch strapping with adhesive tape, custom-made foot orthoses, and premolded foot orthoses. Suggestions for the use of premolded foot orthoses are listed in the section on foot orthoses.

Supinatory or limited motion foot types

The problems associated with a supinatory or limited-motion foot type include decreased shock attenuation and increased plantar pressures, especially in the forefoot region.[28] Footwear for these patients should have a cushioned midsole. Total-contact foot orthoses to increase the area of contact between the shoe and the plantar surface of the foot should also be considered. Finally, if the patient stands and walks with the rear foot in a constantly inverted position or has a history of lateral instability of the ankle, then a lateral outflare should be prescribed for the shoe. Foot orthoses fabricated from rigid plastic materials should be avoided.[29]

FOOT ORTHOSES

Foot orthoses were originally used to support and statically control the medial longitudinal arch. The Schaffer and Whitman plates were fabricated from metal or leather and designed to control the medial longitudinal arch by preventing the navicular from dropping.[53] Arch supports, including navicular pads and cookies, were also utilized to control the position of the medial longitudinal arch. Arch supports were fabricated from different densities of materials and placed directly into the patient's shoes.[53] Although these early supportive devices were designed to statically support the medial longitudinal arch as well as prevent it from "falling," they all failed to permit dynamic foot movement during activity. As a result, patients complained of arch pain when they attempted dynamic activity with these devices. As previously discussed, foot pronation is required for normal walking. Thus, the key to an effective foot orthosis is to control excessive pronation but permit a normal amount of foot pronation.

In keeping with this principle, Root and colleagues described a functional foot orthosis for treating foot problems.[40] They defined what they believed was the normal foot alignment and classified deviations from it as intrinsic foot deformities[40]: forefoot varus, forefoot valgus, and rearfoot varus. The functional foot orthosis did not support the medial longitudinal arch, but rather used wedges and posts in either the rearfoot or forefoot regions.[45] Investigations of the Root approach measurement procedures have raised serious questions regarding the reliability and validity of these procedures.[10,24,46] Furthermore, although the concept of not using an arch support to control excessive foot pronation has merit, a key question is whether pronation in the midfoot and intertarsal regions can be adequately controlled through the use of wedges placed in the forefoot or rear foot. I believe that the only method to control excessive foot mobility in the midfoot and intertarsal regions is a total-contact foot orthosis. If the foot orthosis fully contacts the medial longitudinal arch, however, the materials used in the construction of the foot orthosis must be *dual density* in the region of the arch (Fig. 11-27). The concept of using dual-density materials in the fabrication of foot orthoses is described later in this section.

If foot orthoses are an important component of the management protocol, then the definition and functions should be delineated for the clinician. A foot orthosis is a device that improves foot function and supports as well as modifies the alignment of the foot.[53] Foot orthoses, in

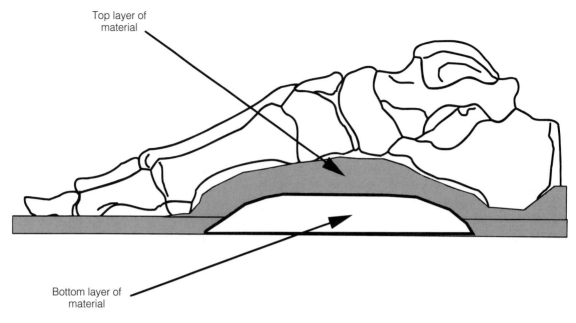

Top layer of
material

Bottom layer of
material

Fig. 11-27. The concept of dual-density materials in the medial longitudinal arch.

satisfying this definition, provide the following four functions:

1. Distribute the weight-bearing stresses and pressures acting on the plantar surface of the foot by using the principle of total contact
2. Reduce the stresses acting on the proximal structures of the lower extremity and spine secondary to excessive foot pronation or supination
3. Control excessive foot pronation by reducing both the magnitude and rate of foot pronation
4. If necessary, balance intrinsic deformities using appropriate posting

In addition to these four functions, foot orthoses should also have the following properties:

1. Have no harmful effects to other parts of the body
2. Be comfortable to wear
3. Be lightweight and durable
4. Be easy to fabricate and cost-effective
5. Be fabricated of breathable materials and able to absorb moisture

Commercially available premolded foot orthoses, made with thermoplastic materials, permit the fabrication of lightweight, comfortable, and durable foot orthoses that can control excessive foot pronation. A disadvantage of the thermoplastic premolded devices is their lack of breathability and inability to absorb moisture. The patient must thus always use cotton socks with the orthoses to assist in the absorption of moisture and enhance breathability. Even with this disadvantage, premolded foot orthoses permit the

clinician to fabricate an effective, inexpensive device in a relatively short period of time. In many cases, the premolded foot orthoses can be used directly from the package with minimal or no modification. As previously mentioned, the foot orthoses should be constructed to provide total contact over the entire plantar surface of the foot, including the medial longitudinal arch. To provide total contact in the area of the medial longitudinal arch, two densities of material must be used (Fig. 11-27). The top layer of the two materials should be moldable to provide total contact and also compressible. This top layer of material functions to permit foot pronation but decreases the speed of pronation as the material compresses. The bottom layer of material is firmer and less compressible, to control the magnitude of foot pronation. The concept of dual material density is critical for a total-contact foot orthosis. This type of foot orthosis allows the medial longitudinal arch (midtarsal and intertarsal regions) to be supported and, at the same time, permits the required amount of foot pronation.

Fabrication methods

Numerous techniques can be used to modify premolded foot orthoses, some of which require equipment such as a sander and oven. The different types of premolded devices and the materials that are used in the following fabrication procedures are listed in the Box, along with possible suppliers.

**Fabrication methods with no
equipment except a heat gun**

1. If the patient requires increased cushioning in footwear as a result of metatarsalgia, a full-length insole can be cut to replace the existing shoe sock liner. If the shoe sock liner is removable, then the old liner can be used to trace an

Supplies necessary to fabricate foot orthoses

Premolded foot orthoses

Accommodator (A) or AC (U)—Soft
BFO (A) or BF (U)—Medium
XPE (A) or XP (U)—Firm
MDT (U)—Flexible heel base with firm, plastic arch support

Insole materials

PPT ⅛ in. uncovered (A)
Ovafit 3 mm—medium (U)
Ovaflex 3 mm—soft (U)

Orthotic materials

UCOlite 2 mm (U)—excellent top covering
UCOlite 5 mm (U)—excellent reinforcement material
Plastizote #2 (¼ in.) (U) or (A)—compressible soft foam used to provide total-contact top layer with premolded orthoses
Quick Post Strips (U)—for wedging or posting (4 mm or 6 mm)
M/L Lifts—vinyl wedges (x-firm) (A)—for fabricating external metatarsal bars

Adhesives and lubricants

Hi-Performance Supertak (U)—spray adhesive
Silicone Lubricant USDA (U)—to reduce friction between orthotic top cover and foot
Superbond Adhesive (U)—for maximum adhesion
Master Adhesive (A)—for maximum adhesion

Equipment

Standing system   (U) or (A) $460.00–$1000
Steinel heat gun 3000 SLE (U) $ 180
Turbo convection oven   (U) or (A) $ 270
Heat protecting gloves $ 14

Suppliers

(U) indicates UCO International
16 East Piper Lane, Suite 120
Prospect Heights, IL 60070
(800) 541-4030

(A) indicates Alimed, Inc.
297 High Street
Dedham, MA 02026
(800) 225-2610

outline over one of the three insole materials listed in the Box. If the sock liner is not removable, then a paper tracing of the inside area of the shoe is used to trace an outline on the insole material.

2. To control excessive foot motion or to increase the surface area in contact with the plantar surface of the foot, a premolded foot orthosis (selected based on the desired density) could be placed under the existing removable shoe sock liner (Fig. 11-28). If the sock liner is not

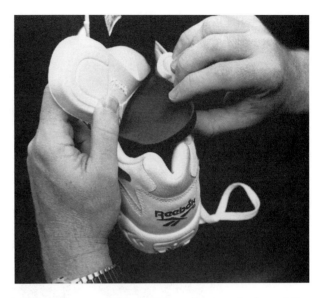

Fig. 11-28. Placement of premold foot orthoses under the sock liner of the shoe.

removable or if the liner is extremely worn, then a premolded foot orthoses could be placed in the shoe with a full-length piece of insole material glued to the top of the orthosis.

3. Finally, a premolded foot orthosis, selected on the basis of desired density, could just be placed within the shoe. Double-sided adhesive tape on the bottom of the orthoses can prevent sliding of the orthosis within the shoe.

Fabrication methods requiring a sander and oven

1. A selected premolded foot orthosis could be modified to provide both motion control and total-foot contact with the following fabrication procedure:
   a. Select one of the premolded devices based on appropriate density for the patient.
   b. Next, roughen the top surface of the foot orthosis with the sander to increase glue adhesion.
   c. Cut a full-length piece of Plastazote #2 ¼ in and apply glue to the top of the orthosis and the portion of the Plastazote that will cover the orthosis (Fig. 11-29).
   d. When the glue has dried, adhere the Plastazote to the foot orthosis. Trim the Plastazote so that approximately ¼ in overlaps the medial, lateral, and posterior edges of the foot orthoses (Fig. 11-30).
   e. Place the entire device into the oven for approximately 40 to 50 seconds at a temperature of 280° F.
   f. Remove the device from the oven, place it on the floor in front of the patient, and have the patient place a foot on the Plastazote (Fig. 11-31).
   g. Have the patient slightly elevate the medial longitudinal arch and stand while molding the material in the arch area with your hand and pushing down on the forefoot region, especially over the first and second metatarsals.

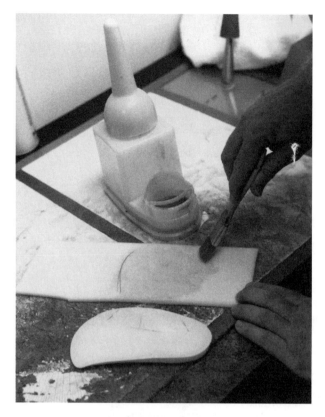

Fig. 11-29. Adhesive applied to the Plastazote II and the premolded foot orthoses.

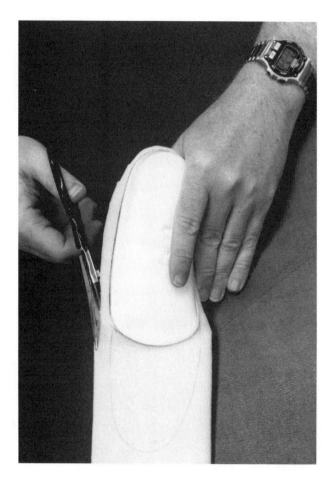

Fig. 11-30. Plastazote II trimmed to edges of the premolded foot orthoses.

h. After 2 minutes, the Plastazote is set and the device can be removed from the patient's foot.

i. After molding the other device, sand the Plastazote overlap on the sides of the orthoses by holding the bottom of the orthoses perpendicular to the sanding drum (Fig. 11-32).

j. To complete the orthoses, the Plastazote #2 is covered with either UCOlite 2 mm or one of the three insole materials (Fig. 11-33).

k. If after 3 to 4 weeks of wear, the Plastazote compresses excessively and the patient complains of decreased support, then a piece of UCOlite 5 mm material can be added to the entire length of the bottom of the orthoses. If the toe box region of the shoe is too tight, it may be necessary to remove 2 to 3 mm of the UCOlite 5 mm material from under the toe area.

2. To construct an extremely durable foot orthosis for an endurance runner or a patient requiring maximal pronation control, the following fabrication procedures could be used:

a. Select the appropriate size of multiple density thermoplastic (MDT) orthosis for the patient (NOTE: the plastic material should end just behind the metatarsal heads).

b. Modify the arch height of the MDT orthosis, if necessary, by using a heat gun.

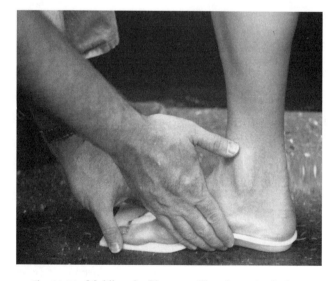

Fig. 11-31. Molding the Plastazote II to the patient's foot.

c. When satisfied with the fit of the MDT orthoses, cover it with a 5-mm piece of UCOlite, either full length or just to the end of the leather bottom cover of the MDT orthosis.

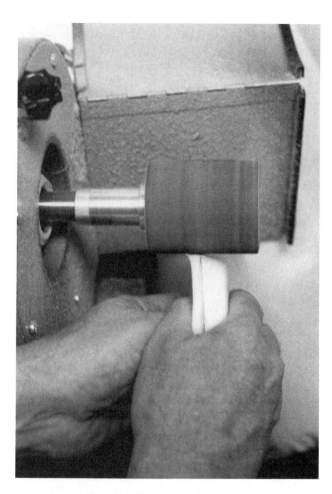

Fig. 11-32. Sanding the edges of the Plastazote II, keeping the bottom of the orthoses perpendicular to the sanding drum.

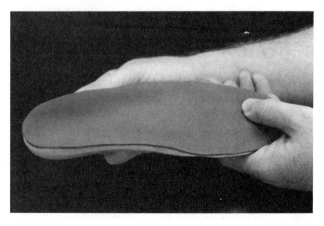

Fig. 11-33. Completed foot orthoses.

COMMON DISORDERS OF THE FOOT AND ANKLE
Traumatic conditions

Orthopedic trauma. The most common etiologies of orthopedic trauma are industrial accidents and motor vehicle collisions. These patients often have extensive fractures and bone-crushing injuries that result in marked limitation of joint mobility or ankylosis of one or more foot articulations. An important aspect of the examination of these patients is the determination of the available range of motion of the talocrural, subtalar, midtarsal, intertarsal, and first metatarsophalangeal articulations. Based on the results of the examination, the clinician must determine if the various joints of the foot will permit the plantar surface of the foot to fully contact the ground during both standing and walking. Inability to fully load the medial aspect of the forefoot as a result of restricted joint motion or ankylosis must be considered in planning the treatment program, which should include articular and soft tissue mobilization, exercises, and modalities to regain as much mobility as possible in the involved articulations. Footwear with both midsole cushioning and rearfoot stabilization should be prescribed. If the patient cannot fully load the medial aspect of the forefoot during closed chain activities, then foot orthoses should also be considered to bring the ground up to the foot. In addition, the foot orthoses should provide total contact and cushioning. In severe cases, surgical intervention, including joint arthrodesis, may be necessary.

Ankle joint sprains. Ankle sprains are one of the most common traumatic injuries affecting the ankle joint complex. Approximately 80% to 85% of all ankle sprains are inversion sprains with or without anterior translation of the talus.[23,37] The anterior talofibular ligament is most often involved, followed by the calcaneofibular ligament. Involvement of the anterior talofibular ligament causes increased anterior translation of the talus in relation to the mortise and is evaluated with the anterior drawer and anterolateral drawer tests. Involvement of the calcaneofibular ligament, caused by forceful ankle inversion, is evaluated with the inversion stress test. Inversion sprains usually occur when the ankle is positioned in plantar flexion. When the ankle joint is plantar flexed, the anterior talofibular ligament is in the best position to resist an inversion moment about the ankle.[19] As the ankle joint, however, becomes more dorsiflexed as the plantar surface of the foot comes down to the ground, the calcaneofibular ligament now assumes the best position to resist the inversion moment about the ankle.[19] Thus, depending on the speed and magnitude of the inversion moment about the ankle as well as the resistance to inversion provided by the peroneal muscles, either the anterior talofibular ligament, the calcaneofibular ligament, or both can be injured. Because the calcaneofibular ligament provides support to both the talocrural and subtalar joints, partial or complete disruption of this ligament can often result in severe instability, necessitating surgical repair.[47] Eversion ankle sprains occur less frequently because of ankle anatomy and the strength of the deltoid ligament. Often an eversion sprain results in an avulsion of the distal tip of the medial malleolus, rather than a disruption of the deltoid ligament.[50]

The treatment for ankle sprains is divided into an imme-

History

A 25-year-old female college student was referred to physical therapy for examination and treatment of right foot pain. She reported no previous history of lower extremity or spinal problems. She reported that yesterday, when walking down a flight of stairs after a snowstorm, she had lost her balance on the bottom step, fallen backward, and hyperextended her right first metatarsophalangeal joint (FMTPJ). The patient noted that she put an ice pack on her foot for approximately 20 minutes, about 2 hours after the injury occurred. She stated that today her "big toe joint" was very painful and that the only way she could walk was to limp, favoring her right foot. She was wearing a pair of cross-trainer athletic shoes that she said had the most room for her swollen right foot.

Examination Findings

Effusion was noted in the right FMTPJ. On palpation, the dorsal aspect of the right first metatarsal head was extremely painful to touch. Active extension range of motion without pain of the right FMTPJ was only 40 degrees. Passive range of motion without pain of the right FMTPJ was 45 degrees. Any attempt to passively extend the FMTPJ beyond 45 degrees caused immediate pain in the joint. Active and passive extension range of motion of the left FMTPJ was 95 degrees. The patient could tolerate a grade I distraction of the right FMTPJ, but any attempt to perform dorsal and plantar glides caused pain. When standing, the patient could not load the medial aspect of the right forefoot. She stated that it felt better to keep her forefoot elevated. She had an antalgic walking pattern, with a decreased stance period on the right.

Assessment

Based on the findings of the examination, the patient was diagnosed as having hallux limitus secondary to a traumatic injury to the right FMTPJ. The first step of the treatment program was to attempt to restore a normal walking pattern as soon as possible to prevent proximal problems caused by the antalgic walking pattern as well as to decrease the stresses applied to the right FMTPJ.

Treatment 1—Day 1 Postinjury

To assist the patient in attaining a more normal walking pattern, a ³/₈-in. external metatarsal bar was attached to the right shoe. Upon standing and walking, the patient's walking pattern immediately improved, and she no longer found it necessary to maintain the medial aspect of her right forefoot elevated. Because of the effusion in the FMTPJ, nothing was placed inside her shoe. The patient was instructed to apply an ice pack to the right medial forefoot for 20 to 25 minutes every 2 hours and to keep the right lower extremity in an elevated position whenever possible. After removing the ice pack and while maintaining the right lower extremity elevated, the patient was also instructed to actively extend her FMTPJ within the pain-free range. She was shown how to perform a gentle, nonpainful distraction to the right FMTPJ. The patient was instructed to perform these activities daily, always use the shoe with the external metatarsal bar, and report back to the clinic in 2 days. She was also told to call if her symptoms increased.

Treatment 2—Day 4 Postinjury

On returning to the clinic, the patient reported that the pain when she extended the right FMTPJ was decreased. The patient's walking pattern was normal and pain-free, as long as she used the shoe with the external metatarsal bar. The active and passive extension range of motion of the right FMTPJ was 55 degrees. The patient still noted pain when the right FMPTJ was extended beyond 55 degrees, both actively and passively. The patient was instructed to stop using ice packs but to continue using the shoe with the external metatarsal bar. In addition, the patient was instructed to perform the following movement activities 3 times a day: (1) actively extend and flex her right FMTPJ for 10 minutes, within the pain-free range of motion, 3 times a day, and (2) perform grade I and grade II distractions and dorsal-plantar glides on the right FMTPJ approximately 5 times in each direction. The patient was scheduled to return to the clinic in 6 days but was told to call if her symptoms increased.

Treatment 3—Day 10 Postinjury

On returning to the clinic, the patient reported no pain in the right FMTPJ with any of her movement activities. She was still using the shoe with the external metatarsal bar when walking; however, she had stopped wearing the shoe around her apartment. The active and passive extension range of motion of the right FMTPJ was 80 degrees with no pain. When passive motion was attempted past 80 degrees, she reported only mild discomfort until approximately 90 degrees. Upon palpation, the dorsal aspect of the right first metatarsal head was only slightly painful to touch. When asked to walk without using her shoes, the patient reported no pain or discomfort in the right FMTPJ and had a normal walking pattern, bilaterally. Based on these findings, the external metatarsal bar was removed from the shoe. The patient was instructed to continue the movement activities she had previously been doing and add active-assistive extension range of motion to the point of pain for the right FMTPJ. The patient was asked to return to the clinic in 1 week.

Treatment 4—Day 17 Postinjury

On reexamination, the patient had 90 degrees of active and passive extension range of motion of the right FMTPJ, without pain. The patient reported only slight discomfort with forceful palpation of the dorsal aspect of the right first metatarsal head. She reported that she has been walking without pain for the past week. Based on these findings, the patient was discharged from physical therapy but instructed to continue the active-assistive range of motion to the right FMTPJ for the next 2 weeks. The patient was also instructed to avoid any athletic activities for another 2 weeks and to call the clinic if she had a recurrence of her symptoms.

Follow-up at 2 Months

On examination 2 months after the injury, the patient had full active and passive range of motion of the FMTPJ, bilaterally without pain. The dorsal aspect of the first metatarsal head was also pain-free with forceful palpation. She demonstrated a normal walking pattern, fully loading the medial aspect of the forefoot during late stance bilaterally. She reported that she was jogging and taking an aerobics class 3 days per week, with no pain or symptoms in the right FMTPJ.

diate postinjury stage and a rehabilitation stage. The acronym *PRICE* is used to direct treatment during the immediate postinjury stage: (1) *p*rotected with a commercially available ankle brace, (2) *r*ested through the use of crutches depending on the initial extent of the injury, (3) *i*ce should be applied to the involved joint to prevent or reduce effusion, (4) *c*ompression to the involved joint with an elastic bandage to prevent effusion, and (5) the involved extremity should be *e*levated, to reduce joint effusion. The key to early treatment in the first 48 to 72 hours is to protect the involved joint from further injury and control the amount of joint effusion. As joint effusion and pain become stabilized, the rehabilitation stage can begin. The protective bracing can be removed and active movements within the pain-free range of motion can be initiated to the involved ankle. Grades I and II joint mobilizations can also be used for pain modulation, if necessary. For reduction of joint effusion, contrast baths can be initiated. The patient should continue wearing the ankle brace during walking and other activities. As the effusion and pain decrease further, resistive exercises in both an open and closed chain, balance activities, and flexibility exercises can be incorporated into the treatment program. To prepare the patient to return to the desired level of activity, a functional activity progression to apply controlled stresses to the injured joint should be implemented. The use of a commercial ankle brace as well as high-top athletic shoes, depending on the sport or work activity, should be prescribed to prevent a possible reinjury during functional progression activities. The criteria for return to activity should include the restoration of (1) normal accessory and physiological motion to the involved joint, (2) good muscle strength with balance between antagonistic muscle groups, and (3) functional use of the injured part in required activities.

Stress fractures. Stress fractures occur as the result of daily microfractures to the bones of the lower extremity and spine.[38] Although these microfractures occur with any stressful activity, they often do not produce symptoms or signs because of constant daily repair by the body. If, however, the microfractures occur at a rate too rapid for repair, the result can be a stress fracture. The most common sites for stress fractures in the foot and ankle are the second and third metatarsals (often referred to as a March fracture) and the proximal shaft of the fifth metatarsal (a Jones fracture).[1,4] Stress fractures are also quite common in the tibia and fibula, often presenting with the same symptoms as shin splints.

Differential diagnosis is difficult as roentgenograms are often negative 2 to 3 weeks after the initial diagnosis.[38] Even 4 weeks after diagnosis, all that is observed on the x-ray is a thin bony callus over the site of the suspected stress fracture. Subjectively, the patient complains of severe pain with activity; rest usually causes temporary relief.[38] If the examiner suspects a stress fracture, then compression test can be used in the evaluation. If the compression test is positive, the patient should be referred to the physician for further testing. The most common treatment plan is total rest from the aggravating activity for 5 to 6 weeks. At the end of 6 weeks, then the patient can begin a slow and gradual return to activity. These patients should be advised to use shoes with excellent midsole cushioning properties as well as cushioned, total-contact foot orthoses, if necessary. They should avoid using rigid or hard plastic foot orthoses.

Chronic overuse conditions

Plantar fasciitis. Although the term *plantar fasciitis* indicates inflammation of the plantar aponeurosis, three muscles have the same origin on the medial tubercle of the calcaneus as the plantar fascia.[21] These three muscles are the abductor hallucis, the flexor digitorum brevis, and the quadratus plantae. Thus, the management program for the patient diagnosed with plantar fasciitis must include treatment and rehabilitation of both connective and contractile tissue.

The four recognized types of plantar fasciitis are systemic, traumatic, degenerative, and mechanical (overuse).[22] Systemic plantar fasciitis is often seen in collagen tissue disorders, such as rheumatoid arthritis. The patient with this type complains of vague heel pain, but the history and symptoms are not typical for the mechanical or degenerative types of plantar fasciitis. The traumatic type of plantar fasciitis is usually a partial tear or complete rupture of the plantar aponeurosis secondary to the application of high forces, such as in an athletic activity. The degenerative type of plantar fasciitis is usually the result of continual trauma over many years. An important point to obtain from the history is that, while these patients have plantar fasciitis symptoms, they have no record of changing their level of activity or trauma to the foot over the past several years. In most cases, the mechanical or overuse type of plantar fasciitis is caused by excessive pronation, which results in microtears of the plantar fascia. The patients' histories almost always indicate a change in their level of activity, whether it be a dramatic increase in running mileage over a short period or a change in the level of activity at work.

The inflammation usually affects the central band of the plantar aponeurosis at the insertion on the medial tubercle of the calcaneus. The most common mechanical cause is excessive foot pronation, which increases the level of stress to the plantar fascia and surrounding intrinsic muscles. Increased stress is also placed on the calcaneal insertion of the plantar fascia, as a result of the excessive foot pronation. A bony hypertrophy of the medial plantar tubercle can occasionally occur at the site of the plantar fascia attachment, which is termed a *heel spur*.[9]

In general, the mechanical and degenerative forms of plantar fasciitis are most commonly referred for treatment. These two types of plantar fasciitis are often seen in patients participating in endurance sports, in occupations requiring prolonged standing or walking, or with increases in normal levels of physical activity. A common symptom for both the mechanical and degenerative types of plantar fasciitis is pain upon weight bearing after a period of inactivity. These patients often complain of severe heel pain first thing in the morning upon rising, followed by a slow reduction after an hour of activity.[22] This reduction in pain can last up to 3 hours, depending on the level of fascial irritability. When the patient sits down to rest their feet; however, heel pain will occur again when they assume a weight-bearing posture. Finally, patients do not usually have pain directly on the inferior aspect of the calcaneus, but slightly anterior and medial over the calcaneal insertion of the plantar fascia. To ensure that the origin of the plantar fascia is correctly palpated, the examiner should extend the first metatarsal phalangeal joint to place tension on the plantar fascia. The examiner can then palpate the fascia from the middle of the foot posteriorly to the region of the insertion on the plantar surface of the calcaneus.

Treatment for plantar fasciitis is divided into two stages:

CASE 2

History

A 62-year-old woman was referred to the physical therapy clinic for examination and treatment of left foot pain. The patient reported that she had had surgery on the left foot 10 years ago because of "extreme pain under the ball of my foot." Although she was not certain, the suture lines suggested that a resection of the second metatarsal head had been performed. She further noted that her current pain was similar to the pain she had before the surgery, except the location of the present pain was more on the lateral aspect of the ball of the left foot. The patient stated that she is retired but does volunteer work in which she must wear a pump shoe with a ½-inch heel. Otherwise, she usually wears walking shoes for her daily activities. The patient noted that the pain in the ball of her foot does not start until after she has been walking or standing for 2 hours. She further stated that she had seen the surgeon who did the original operation on her left foot but has decided not to have further surgery at this time.

Examination Findings

Active, passive, and resistive tests were within normal limits, bilaterally. Upon palpation, the patient had marked tenderness under the fourth metatarsal head of the left foot. A hallux valgus or bunion deformity was noted bilaterally, with the degree of deformity greater on the left than the right. As a result of the hallux valgus, first metatarsophalangeal joint (FMTPJ) extension was decreased on the left in comparison to the right. The range of motion measured for FMTPJ extension was 75 degrees for the left and 100 degrees for the right. In addition to the hallux valgus deformities, clawing was present in digits two through five, bilaterally. Although the toes were clawed, all the toes could be almost fully extended, bilaterally. When walking, the patient demonstrated excessive foot pronation bilaterally, with the amount of foot pronation greater on the left than on the right. Finally, the walking shoes were assessed for wear and fit. The walking shoes had been worn for less than 2 months and had a snug-fitting, firm-rearfoot stabilization system, as well as a leather upper.

Assessment

Based on the results of the examination, the patient was diagnosed as having metatarsalgia, with pain specific to the fourth metatarsal head. The primary objective of the treatment program was to decrease the stresses applied to the lateral aspect of the forefoot.

Treatment—Session 1

Although the patient had sufficient room in her walking shoes for a total-contact foot orthosis, the fit of the pump shoe was snug. Thus, to decrease the stresses acting on the ball of her foot while she was wearing her pump shoes, an external metatarsal bar was used. For her walking shoes, total-contact cushioned foot orthoses were fabricated from (1) BFO pre-molded foot orthoses, (2) a layer of Plastazote #2 (¼ in.) that was glued to the BFO and then molded to the patient's feet; and (3) a top cover of PPT insole material. Once the fabrication was completed, the patient walked in both shoes and reported no pain in either foot while walking. In addition, the patient was instructed to perform range of motion to the lesser digits of both feet after bathing each day to prevent the development of a fixed claw toe deformity. The patient was further instructed in how to perform foot intrinsic muscle exercises, bilaterally, using the towel rolling method. She was then scheduled to return in 3 weeks, unless her symptoms increased, at which time she was to call the clinic.

Treatment—Session 2

On return to the clinic after 3 weeks, the patient reported that her symptoms and pain under the ball of her left foot had not returned, as long as she used the pumps or the walking shoes. She also stated that she was doing the lesser toe stretching and intrinsic muscle exercises daily. At patient's request, an external metatarsal bar was placed on two other pairs of shoes that she also used for her volunteer work. Based on the progress report, the patient was discharged and instructed to call the clinic if any of her symptoms or pain recurred. In addition, she was instructed to call for an appointment to refurbish the foot orthoses, using UCOlite 5 mm, if she noted a decrease in the amount of foot support or cushioning.

Follow-up at 6 Months

The patient reported that she was doing very well and had no pain in the forefoot as long as she used either her walking shoes or the shoes with the external metatarsal bar. The patient further stated that she could perform all of her desired activities without forefoot pain.

short term and long term. Short-term treatment can include antiinflammatory medications often prescribed by the referring physician, modalities for symptom reduction as well as tissue healing, and premolded foot orthoses or arch strapping with adhesive tape to decrease the level of stress on the plantar fascia and related structures. Reducing the level of stress applied to the plantar fascia is critical prior to initiating treatments designed to decrease the degree of tissue inflammation. Thus, fitting premolded foot orthoses or arch strapping should be the first step in the short-term treatment program. The long-term treatment program is designed to prevent the recurrence of plantar fasciitis. It should include intrinsic and extrinsic muscle strengthening exercises and plantar fascia stretching activities. An effective exercise for intrinsic strengthening is towel rolling. For this exercise, the patient sits and places half of the heel on a linoleum or smooth floor and the other half on a towel. The rest of the towel is extended in front of the foot, and the patient uses the toes to pull the towel beneath the foot. For added resistance, cans or a weight can be placed at the end of the towel. Plantar fascia stretching can be accomplished with a simple rolling pin. For this exercise, performed while sitting, the patient places the plantar surface of the foot on the rolling pin and rolls it back and forth. The amount of pressure the patient applies depends on the irritability of the plantar fascia. If an increased stretch is desired, a piece of elastic exercise material or a towel can be used to extend the toes and place more tension on the plantar fascia during the rolling action. In severe cases of plantar fasciitis, night splints have been extremely effective.[51] They maintain tension on the plantar fascia and muscles while the patient is sleeping.

Metatarsalgia. *Metatarsalgia* is defined as pain or discomfort in the anterior segment of the foot.[5] The symptoms include pain and tenderness under the plantar surface of the metatarsal heads and the inability to progress from heel off to toe off during terminal stance (flat-footed walking pattern). The various etiologies of metatarsalgia include rheumatoid arthritis,[2] neurological disease,[5] Morton's toe,[5] Morton's neuroma or interdigital neuroma,[2] a pes cavus foot structure, and an alteration of normal foot mechanics of the forefoot.[33] The most common site of metatarsalgia caused by the alteration of normal foot mechanics is the second and third metatarsal heads. Excessive foot pronation can cause increased mobility in the foot articulations, including the first and fifth rays. During terminal stance, as a result of this increased foot mobility, the first ray may be unable to accept weight, and the load shifts to the second and third metatarsal heads. This increased load under the second and third metatarsal heads can eventually lead to the development of symptoms.[33]

Treatment for patients diagnosed with metatarsalgia can include modalities and medications to decrease symptoms, teardrop-shaped metatarsal pads placed inside the shoe, insole materials cut to fit the full length of the shoe, footwear with cushioned midsoles, and an external metatarsal bar. An external metatarsal bar functions to (1) decrease the load acting on the metatarsal heads during standing, (2) delay loading the metatarsal heads during walking, and (3) decrease the amount of first metatarsophalangeal joint extension during early terminal stance. To position the external metatarsal bar on the shoe properly, the patient should stand in full weight-bearing stance with shoes tied. The first and fifth metatarsal heads should be palpated and marks made just behind each metatarsal head (Fig. 11-34). The M/L Lift–Vinyl Wedge (see the Box) is then positioned on a line that would extend from the marks made for the first and fifth metatarsal heads (Fig. 11-35, *A* and *B*). The external metatarsal bar is an extremely effective treatment for metatarsalgia that should be considered for patients who cannot use a

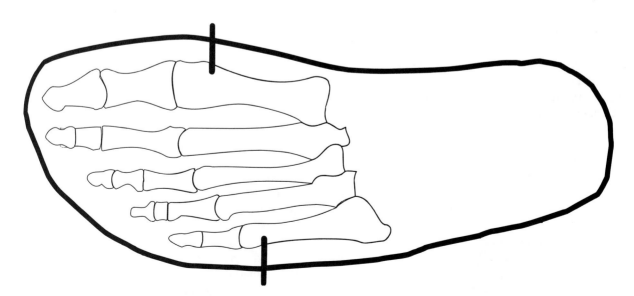

Fig. 11-34. Marking the placement of the external metatarsal bar on the plantar surface of the shoe.

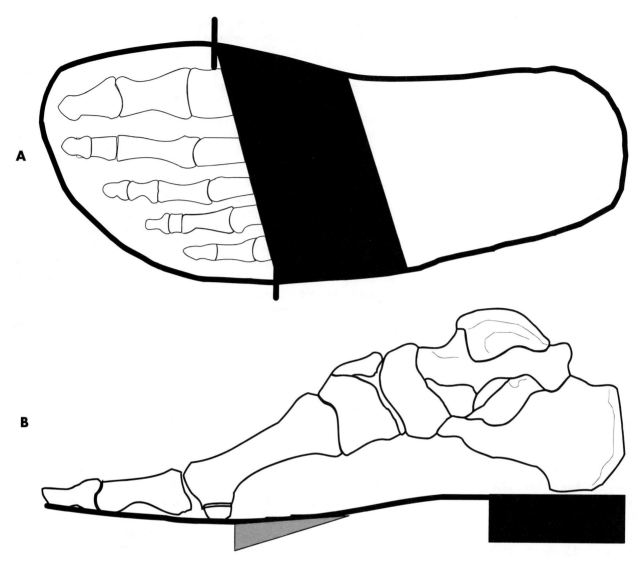

Fig. 11-35. Placement of the external metatarsal bar: **A,** view from the bottom of the shoe; **B,** view from the side of the shoe.

metatarsal pad or insole material because of limited room in their footwear.

Hallux limitus/rigidus. *Hallux limitus* is defined as a restriction in first metatarsophalangeal extension.[8] Because normal walking requires approximately 65 degrees of first metatarsophalangeal joint extension during the terminal stance period,[15] any limitation in this required amount of extension range of motion is classified as a hallux limitus. *Hallux rigidus* refers to an ankylosis or fusion of the first metatarsophalangeal joint.[5] Any condition that prevents the proximal phalanx of the hallux from gliding over the first metatarsal head during terminal stance would be considered an etiology of hallux limitus.[8] The various etiologies include (1) trauma to the forefoot region, (2) degenerative changes to the first metatarsophalangeal joint secondary to rheumatoid arthritis or a hallux valgus (bunion) deformity, (3) congenital variations in the shape of the first metatarsal head articular

surface, and (4) a dorsiflexed first ray deformity, which can also be termed a *metatarsus primus elevatus.*[39]

The symptoms of hallux limitus and/or hallux rigidus include (1) pain and restricted range of motion at the first metatarsophalangeal joint, (2) inability to progress from heel off to toe off during terminal stance (flat-footed walking pattern), and (3) walking on the lateral border of the foot or increased toe out on the involved side, in an attempt to limit first metatarsophalangeal joint extension while walking. Conservative management includes joint mobilization, especially in the case of recent trauma to the forefoot region. The patient should be advised to use stiff-soled shoes and avoid walking on inclines or stairs.[5] The external metatarsal bar should also be used, especially during the acute inflammatory stage; it can delay as well as decrease the amount of first metatarsophalangeal joint extension required during the early part of terminal stance.

REVIEW QUESTIONS

1. How does the windlass mechanism of the plantar fascia assist the foot in supinating during terminal stance?
2. What are the closed chain movements of the various foot articulations, and how do these movements permit the five functions of the foot to occur during gait?
3. What is the "functional" neutral position of the foot during walking, and how does it influence the placement of the foot for the fabrication of foot orthoses?
4. What steps are required for the physical examination and management of a foot disorder using the tissue stress model?
5. What special examination tests are used to assess acute injuries of the foot and ankle in comparison to chronic and overuse foot and ankle injuries?

REFERENCES

1. Acker JH, Drez D: Nonoperative treatment of stress fractures of the proximal shaft of the fifth metatarsal (Jone's fracture), *Foot Ankle* 7:152, 1986.
2. Alexander IJ: *The foot: examination and diagnosis,* New York, 1990, Churchill Livingstone.
3. American Academy of Orthopaedic Surgeons: *Joint motion: method of measuring and recording,* Chicago, 1965, author.
4. Anderson EG: Fatigue fractures of the foot, *Injury* 21:275, 1990.
5. Cailliet R: *Foot and ankle pain,* ed 2, Philadelphia, 1983, FA Davis.
6. Cavanagh PR: Forces and pressures between the foot and the floor during normal walking and running. In Cooper JM, Haven B, editors: *Proceedings of the Indiana University Biomechanics Symposium,* Indianapolis, 1980, Indiana State Board of Health.
7. Cornwall MW: Biomechanics of noncontractile tissue: a review, *Phys Ther* 64:1869, 1984.
8. Dananberg HJ: Functional hallux limitus and its relationship to gait efficiency, *J Am Podiatr Med Assoc* 76:648, 1986.
9. Doxey G: Calcaneal pain: a review of various disorders, *J Orthop Sports Phys Ther* 9:25, 1987.
10. Elveru RA et al: Goniometric reliability in a clinical setting; subtalar and ankle joint measurements, *Phys Ther* 88:672, 1988.
11. Green DR et al: Clinical biomechanical evaluation of the foot: a preliminary radiocinematographic study, *J Am Podiatr Med Assoc* 65:732, 1975.
12. Hicks JC: The mechanics of the foot: the joints, *J Anat* 87:345, 1953.
13. Hicks JC: The mechanics of the foot: the plantar aponeurosis and arch, *J Anat* 88:25, 1954.
14. Hicks JC: The foot as a support, *Acta Anat (Basel)* 25:34, 1955.
15. Hopson MM et al: Motion of the first metatarsophalangeal joint: reliability and validity of four measurement techniques, *J Am Podiatr Med Assoc* 85:198, 1995.
16. Huson A: Functional anatomy of the foot. In Jahss MH, editor: *Disorders of the foot and ankle: medical and surgical management,* ed 2, Philadelphia, 1991, WB Saunders.
17. Inman VT: The human foot, *Manitoba Med Rev* 46:513, 1966.
18. Inman VT: The influence of the foot-ankle complex on the proximal skeletal structures, *Artificial Limbs* 13:59, 1969.
19. Inman VT: *The joints of the ankle,* Baltimore, 1976, Williams & Wilkins.
20. Johanson MA et al: Effects of three different posting methods on controlling abnormal subtalar pronation, *Phys Ther* 74:149, 1994.
21. Kosmahl EM, Kosmahl HE: Painful plantar heel, plantar fasciitis, and calcaneal spur: etiology and management, *J Orthop Sports Phys Ther* 9:17, 1988.
22. Kwong PK et al: Plantar fasciitis, *Clin Sports Med* 7:119, 1988.
23. Landry ME: The common inversion sprain and its treatment in the athlete, *J Am Podiatr Med Assoc* 66:266, 1976.
24. Lattanza L et al: Closed versus open kinematic chain measurements of subtalar joint eversion: implications for clinical practice, *J Orthop Sports Phys Ther* 9:310, 1988.
25. Levens AS et al: Transverse rotation of the segments of the lower extremity in locomotion, *J Bone Joint Surg Am* 30:859, 1948.
26. Lundberg A et al: Kinematics of the foot and ankle: part 2, pronation and supination, *Foot Ankle* 9:248, 1989.
27. Manter JT: Movements of the subtalar and transverse tarsal joints, *Anat Rec* 80:397, 1941.
28. McPoil TG: Shoewear, *Phys Ther* 68:1857, 1988.
29. McPoil TG, Cornwall MW: Rigid versus soft foot orthoses, *J Am Podiatr Med Assoc* 81:638, 1991.
30. McPoil TG, Cornwall MW: The relationship between the rearfoot angle during one-leg stand and the pattern of rearfoot motion during walking, *Phys Ther* 73:S96, 1993 (abstract).
31. McPoil TG, Cornwall MW: Relationship between neutral subtalar joint position and the pattern of rearfoot motion during walking, *Foot Ankle* 15:141, 1994.
32. McPoil TG, Hunt GC: An evaluation and treatment paradigm for the future. In Hunt GC, McPoil TG, editors: *Physical therapy of the foot and ankle,* ed 2, New York, 1995, Churchill Livingstone.
33. McPoil TG, Schuit D: Management of metatarsalgia secondary to biomechanical disorders: a case report, *Phys Ther* 66:970, 1986.
34. McPoil TG, et al: A comparison of three positions used to evaluate tibial varum, *J Am Podiatr Med Assoc* 78:22, 1988.
35. McPoil TG, et al: Effects of foot orthoses on center-of-pressure patterns in women, *Phys Ther* 69:149, 1989.
36. Mueller MJ et al: Navicular drop as a composite measure of excessive pronation, *J Am Podiatr Med Assoc* 83:198, 1993.
37. Quillen WS: An alternative management protocol for lateral ankle sprains, *J Orthop Sports Phys Ther* 2:187, 1981.
38. Rankin EA, Baker GI: Stress fractures, *Annals of Family Practice* 13:71, 1976.
39. Root ML et al: Axis of motion of the subtalar joint, *J Am Podiatr Med Assoc* 56:149, 1966.
40. Root ML et al: *Clinical biomechanics: normal and abnormal function of the foot,* vol 2, Los Angeles, 1977, Clinical Biomechanics.
41. Rose GK: Pes planus. In Jahss MH, editor: *Disorders of the foot,* ed 1, Philadelphia, 1982, WB Saunders.
42. Roy S, Irwin R: *Sports medicine: prevention, evaluation, management, and rehabilitation,* Englewood Cliffs, NJ, 1983, Prentice Hall.
43. Sarrafian SK: *Anatomy of the foot and ankle,* ed 2, Philadelphia, 1993, JB Lippincott.
44. Saunders JBM et al: The major determinants in normal and pathological gait, *J Bone Joint Surg Am* 35:543, 1953.
45. Sgarlato TE: *A compendium of podiatric biomechanics,* San Francisco, 1971, California College of Podiatric Medicine Press.
46. Smith-Oricchio K, Harris BA: Interrater reliability of subtalar neutral, calcaneal inversion, and eversion, *J Orthop Sports Phys Ther* 12:10, 1990.
47. Staples OS: Ruptures of the fibular collateral ligaments of the ankle, *J Bone Joint Surg Am* 57:101, 1975.
48. Subotnick SI: Equinus deformity as it affects the forefoot, *J Am Podiatr Med Assoc* 61:423, 1971.
49. Subotnick SI: Biomechanics of the subtalar and midtarsal joints, *J Am Podiatr Med Assoc* 65:756, 1975.
50. Turek SL: *Orthopaedics: principles and applications,* ed 2, Philadelphia, 1967, JB Lippincott.
51. Wapner KL, Skarkey PF: The use of night splints for the treatment of recalcitrant plantar fasciitis, *Foot Ankle* 12:135, 1991.
52. Wright DG et al: Action of the subtalar and ankle joint complex during the stance phase of walking, *J Bone Joint Surg Am* 46:361, 1964.
53. Wu KK: *Foot orthoses: principles and clinical applications,* Baltimore, 1990, Williams & Wilkins.

CHAPTER 12

The Knee

Lynn A. Wallace, Robert E. Mangine, and Terry R. Malone

OUTLINE

Anatomy
    Osteology
    Menisci
    Knee capsule
    Bursae
    Musculature
Biomechanics/arthrokinematics
    Tibiofemoral joint
    Patellofemoral joint
    Kinetic chain
Knee injuries
    Mechanisms of injury
    Prevention of knee injuries
    Structural predisposition
    Functional predisposition
    Previous injury
    Muscular factors
    Proprioception
    Shoes
    Environmental factors
Physical examination of the knee
    Evaluation form
    Subjective examination
    Objective examination
    Reexamination
    Referral
    Specialized examination by physical therapists
Assessing and treating range-of-motion deficiencies
Treatment
    Passive joint mobilization for capsular problems
    Muscle-tendon techniques for noncapsular problems
Unacceptable results
    Rehabilitation
Case studies
Surgical management
    Specific pathologies
Summary

LEARNING OBJECTIVES

After studying this chapter, the reader should be able to:

1. List the articulations and identify the significant anatomic structures of the knee complex.
2. Describe the joint mechanics of the knee complex, including the tibiofemoral and patellofemoral articulations.
3. Describe the anterior, posterior, medial, and lateral musculature of the knee complex.
4. Discuss the mechanisms of injury to the knee complex.
5. List those factors resulting from a previous injury that can increase the risk of knee disorders.
6. Describe and list all the components of a physical examination of the knee complex.
7. Discuss factors to consider in assessing the findings of the physical examination.
8. Discuss parameters to consider in planning a rehabilitation program for the knee complex.
9. Discuss the use of surgical intervention for meniscal lesions and ligamentous repairs.
10. Describe the use of a functional progression in planning the sequence of rehabilitation for knee injuries.

KEY TERMS

knee complex
patellofemoral
biomechanics
examination

kinetic chain
treatment
surgical management

The frequency and severity of knee injuries in organized and recreational sports and in industry are well documented.[1,5,6] In American football, the knee is the most commonly injured joint.[6] Available data indicate that many of these injuries are preventable.[8,30,61] Many "overuse" knee injuries, which are common in noncontact sports, are also predictable and preventable.[56] Unfortunately, many of these macrotraumatic and microtraumatic knee injuries tend to recur, indicating that optimal treatment was not rendered.[5] This chapter, which is concerned with rehabilitating knee injuries, addresses both causes and symptomatology.

Current physical therapy involvement is primarily directed toward achieving long-term goals, such as restoration of range of motion and strength. Physical therapy has had minimal involvement in the areas of prevention, recognition, realizing short-term goals (such as controlling inflammatory response), immobilization, minimizing loss of motion and strength, and achieving terminal goals (such as identifying and correcting causative factors). We hope that graduate and postgraduate education programs will increasingly prepare physical therapists for involvement in the areas of prevention, recognition, and provision of both acute and terminal care. In addition, therapists must continue to educate the medical community and public at large about the availability of these services.

ANATOMY
Osteology

The osseous structures that form articulations at the knee are the femur, the tibia, and the patella. These three bony structures form two separate articulations: the patellofemoral and the tibiofemoral joints. Functionally, however, these two joints cannot always be considered separable, as there is a mechanical relationship between them. Evaluation of the client with an acute or chronic knee disorder demands thorough analysis of each articulation and its interrelated mechanics.

The proximal aspect of the knee consists of the distal femur, which is the longest bone in the body. It originates at the hip and courses in an inferior, medial, and distal direction as it descends distally. This combined direction of the shaft of the femur allows for the weight-bearing condyles of the bone to align with the axis of the lower extremity. In this alignment, a normal valgus angle is formed between the medially oriented femur and the slightly laterally oriented tibia as the two form the junction of the knee. Normal measurement of this angle is approximately 170 to 175 degrees. In women, generally, because of an increase in pelvic width, the angle tends to be less than 170 degrees, resulting in a tibia valga, or knock-kneed position. An angle greater than 175 degrees results in tibia vara, or a bowlegged position.

The distal aspect of the femur flares into a pair of large condyles presenting an articulation with both the patella and the tibia (Fig. 12-1). The articular condyles themselves are rather large and convex in both the sagittal and frontal planes. Anteriorly, the condyles are divided by a central sulcus, the trochlear groove, that forms the articular surface for the patella. Posteriorly, the condyles are divided and separated by the intercondylar notch, which is filled by the cruciate ligaments. When the femur is viewed in the frontal plane with the knee in a flexed position, the configuration resembles a large horseshoe. This formation presents an articular arrangement with a closed anterosuperior surface and an open posteroinferior area. The condyles are covered by smooth hyaline cartilage that is very thick in order to withstand the extreme forces placed on the articular surfaces during weight bearing.

Adjacent to the articular condyles are the large epicondyles, which are convex surfaces pitted with vascular foramina. These highly vascular areas are the site of attachment for the capsular structures, ligaments, and tendons that surround the knee. The medial epicondylar region is easily distinguished by the adductor tubercle, which serves as a site of insertion for the adductor tendon and also as the origin of the tibial collateral ligament. The lateral epicondylar region can be easily palpated because of the extremely thin tissue covering it.

The lateral femoral condyle is more in line with the shaft of the femur, given that structure's oblique medial direction. In its anterior-to-posterior direction, the lateral condyle is somewhat flattened in configuration when compared to the medial femoral condyle. In a medial-to-lateral direction, the lateral condyle is convex and slightly larger than the medial condyle in this plane. When viewed in a sagittal plane, the lateral condyle shows an increase in height in the region of the trochlear groove, which accommodates the large lateral facet of the patella and prevents subluxation or dislocation during normal function (Fig. 12-2).

The medial femoral condyle angles away from the shaft of the femur in comparison to the lateral side. This angle brings it into line with the mechanical axis of the lower limb. The medial femoral condyle's dimension is longer in its anterior-to-posterior direction and is convex in both the anterior-posterior and the medial-lateral orientation. This longer distance allows greater rolling on this condyle, resulting in rotation, particularly during the terminal extension phase.

The distal portion of the femur shows one epiphyseal growth center at birth that remains active until fusing occurs with the main shaft of the femur at approximately 18 years of age. This ossification center at the distal end of the femur transects the femur at the level of the adductor tubercle. The trabecular system of the distal femur shows a crisscrossing pattern within each condyle with long stress lines running up into the shaft. These lines of force run from the articular surface into the cortical bone. A second series of stress absorption lines forms in a transverse plane that serves to connect the two condyles.

The distal aspect of the knee consists of the proximal portion of the tibia, the tibial plateau (Fig. 12-3). The tibial plateau is composed of two flattened shelves that anteriorly

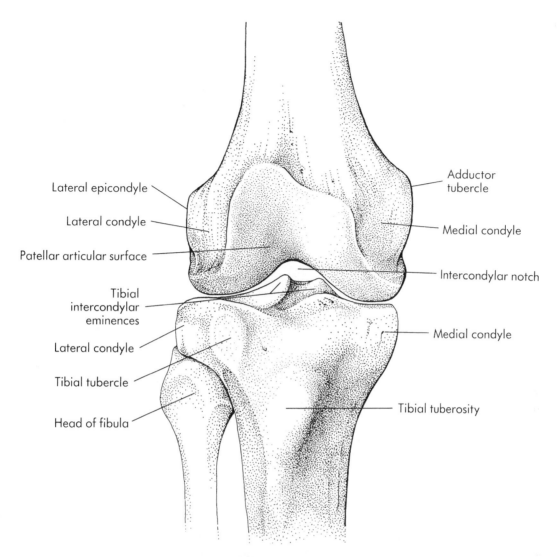

Fig. 12-1. The anterior view of the tibiofemoral joint in extension. (From Hughston JC: *Knee ligaments: injury and repair,* St Louis, 1993, Mosby.)

are even with the shaft of the tibia but posteriorly overhang the shaft. Viewed from the top, the tibial plateau resembles two round dishes that are, on first appearance, concave in both directions. The condylar surfaces are lined with hyaline cartilage, which drapes over the edge of the plateau by 2 or 3 mm. The capsule attachment falls along the edge of the periphery of the articular surface and also to the periphery of the menisci. The tibial plateau also has an epicondylar region that is adjacent to the condyles and is pitted with vascular foramina.

The medial tibial plateau is an oval dish that is seen to be concave in both the sagittal and frontal planes. This condylar region is the larger of the two plateaus in the anterior-to-posterior direction and accommodates the larger medial femoral condyle. Its lateral border is recognized as the intercondylar area. When the tibia is viewed from the lateral side, the posterior portion of the medial condyle does not overhang the shaft of the tibia as much as does the lateral

condyle. Posteriorly, however, the tibia, because of the attachment of the capsule, is heavily pitted with vascular foramina just below the articular surface.

The lateral tibial plateau is circular in shape and also descends posteriorly, thus overhanging the shaft. Further flaring occurs in the posterior lateral corner to accommodate articulation with the fibular head. In the medial-to-lateral aspect, it is easy to see the concavity that forms on the inner surface of the plateau. When viewed from the lateral aspect, however, the anterior-posterior direction of the plateau tends to be flat. This shape facilitates rotation of the femoral condyle during movement.

The medial and lateral tibial plateaus are divided by the intercondylar region. However, in a brief space anterior to this region, the medial and lateral tibial plateaus join and then follow the tibial shaft inferiorly to the tibial tubercle.

This intercondylar region is characterized by several features. The anterior region appears as a flattened depres-

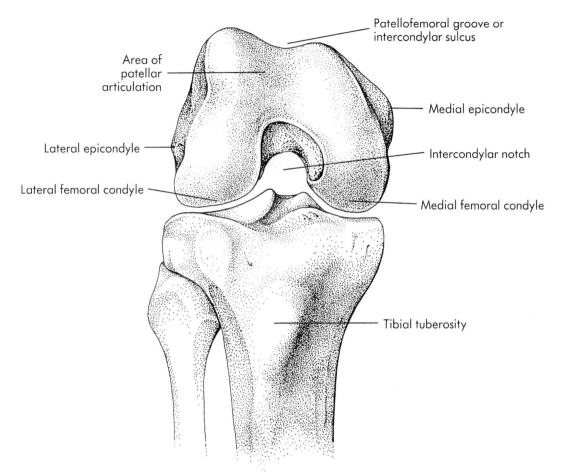

Area of
patellar
articulation

Patellofemoral groove or
intercondylar sulcus

Medial epicondyle

Lateral epicondyle

Intercondylar notch

Lateral femoral condyle

Medial femoral condyle

Tibial tuberosity

Fig. 12-2. The anterior view of the tibiofemoral joint with 90 degrees of flexion. (From Hughston JC: *Knee ligaments: injury and repair,* St Louis, 1993, Mosby.)

sion separating the medial and lateral intercondylar eminences or tibial spines. This depression serves as the site of attachment for the anterior cruciate ligament. The medial and lateral tibial spines are found in the midregion of the tibial plateaus and can be observed as little mountains projecting upward between the plateaus. The shape of these spines is compact and linear. They project into the femoral intercondylar notch with flexion, during which time the greatest amount of rotation can occur.

Anterior and inferior to the tibial plateau along the shaft border lies the tibial tuberosity. This serves as the attachment for the patellar ligament (quadriceps tendon) that is the extension of the quadriceps mechanism. It also serves as the lowest border for attachment of the capsule as it overflows the anterior tibial plateaus following the patellar ligament. The space occupying this region is filled with the inferior patellar bursa and fat pad.

At birth, the femur, like the tibia, displays an ossification center in its proximal portion. This center remains active until fusion at 16 to 18 years of age. The tibial tuberosity region has two possible ossification mechanisms: Ossification can occur as an extension of the proximal center itself, or it can occur as a separate ossification center that generally begins activity in about the twelfth year of life.

The trabecular systems of the tibia provide a similar model to those of the femur. Each condyle is represented as having crisscrossing stress lines that extend all the way from the articular surface to the underlying cortical bone. Overlying this system is a horizontal stress pattern that interconnects the two condyles for stress absorption in the transverse plane.

The patellofemoral articulation is formed by the anterior surface of the femur (trochlear groove) and the posterior facets of the patella. The patella is the largest sesamoid bone in the body and is interposed in the quadriceps mechanism. When viewed from a frontal plane, the patella appears as a large triangular bone with a broad superior border and a distal inferior apex. A transverse section of the patella also reveals a triangular pattern, with a broad superior border and a distal inferior apex, a broad superior apex (serving as the attachment site of the quadriceps extensor mechanism), and a posterior apex, which divides the articular surfaces into medial and lateral facets. The anterior surface of the patella is roughened and pitted with vascular foramina because of the extensive attachment of the femoral quadriceps muscle. Upon insertion over the broad superior border, the tendon continues inferiorly across the patellar surface, eventually narrowing into a tendinous band that extends into the inferior

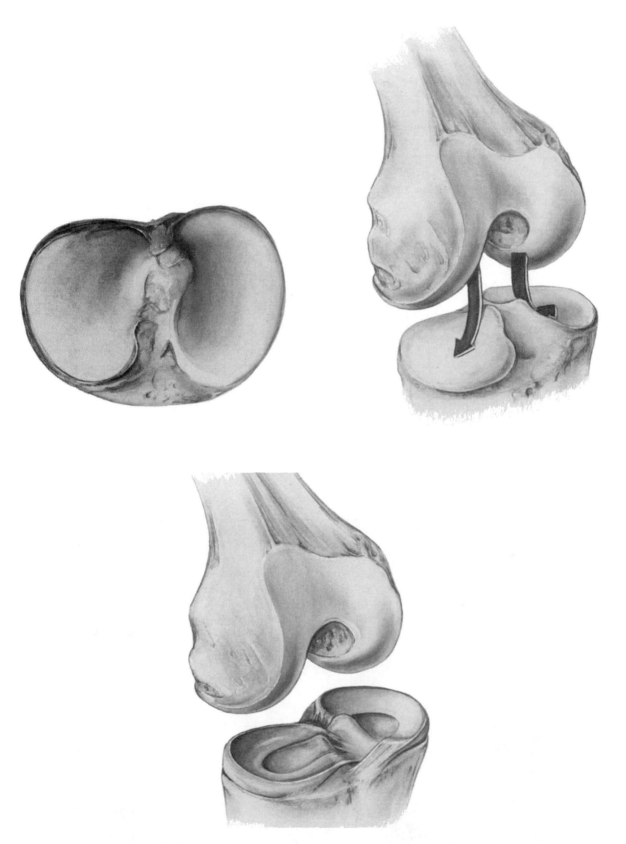

Fig. 12-3. The tibial plateau and its relationship to the femoral condyles. (From Hughston JC: *Knee ligaments: injury and repair,* St Louis, 1993, Mosby.)

insertion on the tibial tuberosity. The region from the inferior apex of the patella to the tibial tuberosity is called the *patellar tendon,* the *quadriceps tendon,* and/or the *patellar ligament.*

Posteriorly, the patella is divided by a vertical ridge into medial and lateral facet regions. Each side can further be subdivided into three facets: superior, middle, and inferior. These facets come into contact with the femur at various points in the range of motion. A seventh facet is also identified on the far medial aspect of the patella. This region, which comes into contact with the femur during extreme flexion, is identified as the flexion or "odd" facet. The

patellar facets are convex in shape in order to accommodate the concave femoral surface. The lateral patellar facet is correspondingly wider to accommodate the femoral condyle. The medial facet also is characterized by the aforementioned "odd" facet on the extreme medial border. The articular cartilage on the posterior surface of the patella is the thickest in the human body, approximately 5 mm in density.

At birth, the primary patella is composed of cartilage cells and is an easily palpable structure. Several separate ossification centers quickly fuse in about the sixth year of life. The trabecular system of the patella radiates in two directions: The first is parallel to the anterior surface, spanning in a

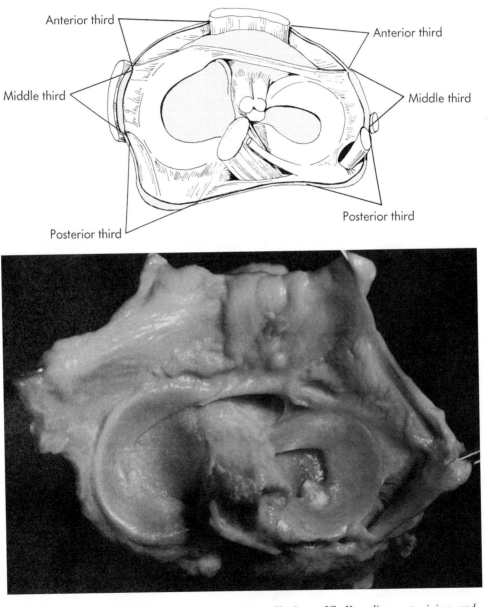

Fig. 12-4. The orientation of the knee menisci. (From Hughston JC: *Knee ligaments: injury and repair,* St Louis, 1993, Mosby.)

horizontal pattern. The second system runs in a perpendicular direction, radiating from the articular surface and moving superiorly to the anterior surface.

Menisci

The geometric shape of the knee is, from a bony standpoint, poorly designed for stability. To enhance stabilization, a fibroelastic meniscal system lies on the tibial shelf, thus deepening the tibial plateaus. Two intraarticular fibroelastic menisci are arranged along the peripheral border of the tibial shelf. The medial and lateral menisci are attached to the peripheral plateau of the tibia by the strong coronary ligaments (Fig. 12-4). Other functions of the menisci, in addition to increasing the integrity of the joint, are aiding in transmission of the weight-bearing forces, improving lubrication, and aiding in the rolling of the femoral condyles during motion. A sagittal view shows them to be wedge-shaped crescents with a rounded peripheral surface presenting a concave apex within the joint. The superior surfaces are concave to accept the shape of the femoral condyles but tend to be more flattened on the inferior or tibial surface. When viewed from above, the menisci follow the shape of the tibial surfaces on which they sit. The medial meniscus is semilunar in shape with a wide base of attachment at both the anterior and posterior regions, the "horns" of the meniscus. Furthermore, the body of the medial meniscus flares posteriorly and is wider in this portion than it is in the lateral meniscus. The lateral meniscus is more oval, with a narrow base of attachment at its anterior and posterior horns. This configuration results in a greater degree of mobility for the lateral meniscus than the medial meniscus during knee motion. The anterior horns of the menisci are connected by a transverse ligament.

The peripheral meniscal attachments are quite extensive and include both dynamic and static controlling features. As previously mentioned, the menisci receive a slip of the quadriceps expansion, thus allowing tension transfer, which results in an anterior translation of the menisci. Further attachment of the anterior horn of the medial meniscus occurs along the ridge of the anterior cruciate ligament, blending into the medial tibial eminence. This attachment flares anteriorly from the depression along the anterior crest

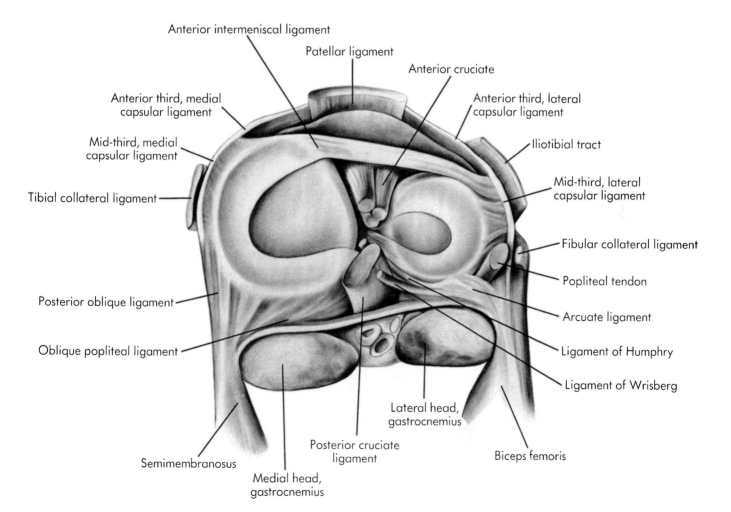

Fig. 12-4 cont'd.

of the plateau. The midportion of the medial meniscus is attached to the deep capsular layer of the tibial collateral ligament. The extensive capsular attachment also brings with it a vascular supply to the outer third of the meniscus. The inner portion of the meniscus is avascular. Posteriorly, the medial meniscus receives a slip of the semimembranous tendon by way of the capsule. This results in a posterior displacement during flexion. The extensive insertion of the medial meniscus in the capsule and aponeurotic slips result in a decreased movement in the anterior-posterior direction. The medial meniscus is thus allowed only approximately 6 mm of motion in this plane.

The lateral meniscus receives the same anterior attachment of the quadriceps expansion from the patella, which results in an anterior translation of this structure. Along its midportion, however, the insertion of the ligament in the capsule is not as extensive. On its posterior border, it receives a slip of the popliteal tendon through the capsule, which can be visualized during arthroscopy. The muscular attachment allows posterior displacement of the meniscus during knee flexion. The posterior horn of the lateral meniscus can receive an attachment from one of three possible structures: the posterior cruciate ligament, the ligament of Wrisberg, or the ligament of Humphrey. An important function of these structures is stabilization of the lateral meniscus during movement. The total movement of the meniscus in the anteroposterior direction is approximately 12 mm.

Knee capsule

The articular surfaces of the knee are encased in the most extensive capsule in the body. This capsule gains both static and dynamic support from the surrounding ligaments and musculotendinous structures. Attachment of the knee capsule follows the articular surface of the patellofemoral and tibiofemoral joints and inserts just peripherally to the articular margins. There are many distinguishable features about this capsule because of its immense size: It has a posterior recess that covers both the medial and lateral condyles, an indentation following the intercondylar notch of the femur, and a large superior patellar pouch. Further characteristics include capsular attachment of the menisci along the peripheral border of the tibia, thus holding the menisci to the articular surface. This peripheral attachment is referred to as the *coronary ligament.*

Anteriorly, the capsule descends in an inferior fashion over the crest of the tibia, following the patellar tendon and fanning outward to the medial and lateral areas in a **V** shape. This shape forms a small pocket that is filled by the inferior patellar fat pad and the infrapatellar bursa, thus reducing friction between the tendon and tibial crest. When the capsule dissects away from the patellar tendon either on the

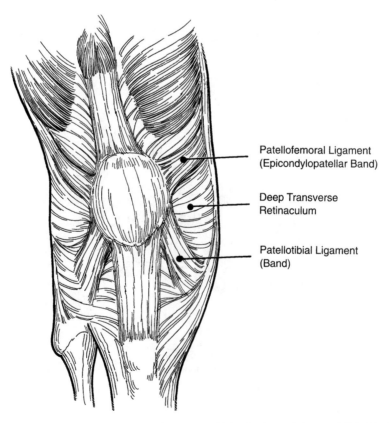

Patellofemoral Ligament (Epicondylopatellar Band)

Deep Transverse Retinaculum

Patellotibial Ligament (Band)

Fig. 12-5. The "patello" ligaments. (From Scott WN: *The knee,* St Louis, 1994, Mosby.)

medial or lateral side, it gains support from the aponeurotic expansion of the quadriceps mechanism. In the aponeurotic expansion, several thicknesses of ligament appear to help stabilize the patella and place tension on the menisci. These thickenings are the meniscopatellar ligaments and patellofemoral ligaments (Figs. 12-5 and 12-6). The meniscopatellar ligaments extend from the superior-inferior lateral and medial border of the patella to the anterior one third of the menisci. Tension is placed on the menisci by these ligaments when the quadriceps muscle contracts. The second expansion comes horizontally off the patella at about its midpoint and turns in a transverse direction, inserting into the lateral and medial epicondylar regions. These ligaments serve to provide stabilization of the patella as it glides through the trochlear groove. There is some question as to whether these bands form as a result of stress on the capsule or are evolutionary vestiges within it.

The midmedial portion of the capsule is reinforced by the tibial collateral ligament (Figs. 12-6 and 12-7). The deep portion of the capsule in this region, the short or deep collateral ligament, is divided into two segments. This first is a band-shaped superior portion running from the anterior surface of the femoral condyle to a midpoint above the superior border of the medial meniscus. The second portion runs from the peripheral border of the medial meniscus to the tibial crest just inferior to the articular surface. This deep layer is covered by a second outer superficial layer that is approximately 2.54 cm in width and originates from a fan-shaped attachment just below the adductor tubercle on the medial femoral epicondyle. A ligament descends past the joint line to a point approximately 3 or 4 cm below the tibial plateau, inserting beneath the pes anserinus tendon, and is separated from that tendon by the pes anserinus bursa. This superficial ligament is delta-shaped, going from a wide base of origin to a narrow base of attachment. The significance of this shape is that biomechanically a portion of the ligament remains taut throughout the range of motion, thus stabilizing the tibiofemoral joint against valgus stress. The greatest degree of tension, however, is seen in the extended position. Directly posterior to the tibial collateral ligament is the posteromedial corner of the capsule. This portion of the capsule inserts into the tibia along the roughened groove just inferior to the articular surface. It receives dynamic support from the tibial portion of the semimembranous muscle. Hughston and colleagues named this corner the *posterior oblique ligament* and emphasize its importance in stabilizing the knee against anteromedial instability.[22] This structure is very important in supporting the capsule and preventing excessive tibial rotation.

Posteriorly, the capsule forms two pouches that cover the articular surfaces of the femoral condyle superiorly and the tibial plateaus inferiorly. This aspect of the capsule also invaginates into the intercondylar notch, forming a large horseshoe shape and leaving the cruciate ligaments external to it. These ligaments are considered to be extracapsular, yet each is covered by a synovial sheath and is therefore intrasynovial. Superficial to the posterior cruciate, the two femoral condyles are bridged by the oblique popliteal

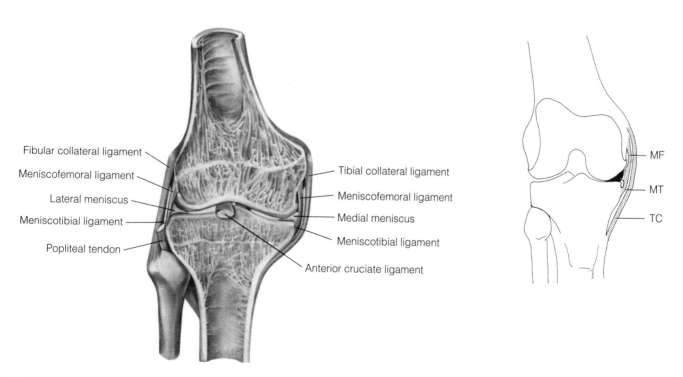

Fibular collateral ligament

Meniscofemoral ligament

Lateral meniscus

Meniscotibial ligament

Popliteal tendon

Tibial collateral ligament

Meniscofemoral ligament

Medial meniscus

Meniscotibial ligament

Anterior cruciate ligament

MF

MT

TC

Fig. 12-6. The medial capsular structures-anterior view. (From Hughston JC: *Knee ligaments: injury and repair*, St Louis, 1993, Mosby.)

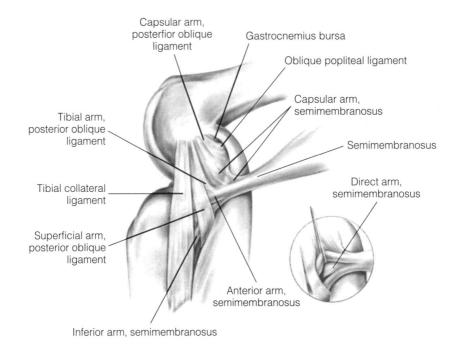

Fig. 12-7. The medial ligamentous and muscular orientation. (From Hughston JC: *Knee ligaments: injury and repair,* St Louis, 1993, Mosby.)

ligament. From a medial-to-lateral aspect, the popliteal ligament runs obliquely, superiorly, and transversely across the posterior cruciate, drawing dynamic support from the capsular arm of the semimembranous muscle. The semimembranous muscle, with its insertion in the oblique popliteal ligament as well as the posterior oblique ligament, can exert tension through the capsule to the medial meniscus. Contraction of that muscle during flexion results in a posterior glide of the corresponding meniscus, thus preventing impingement by the femoral condyle.

The posterior lateral aspect of the capsule is a complex of static and dynamic support structures. Capsular attachment follows the bulging lateral femoral condyle along its superior peripheral border. Support of this portion of the capsule is provided by the arcuate complex, the popliteal tendon, and the lateral head of the gastrocnemius muscle. The arcuate complex has an arching superior attachment originating on the oblique tendon, converging and inserting into the fibular head. The shape of the fibers upon cadaver dissection can be seen to be triangular with a broad superior border and an inferior apex. Further support of the capsule is provided by the popliteal tendon. Fibers of the tendon and muscle blend with the aponeurosis of the posterior lateral capsule, which has an attachment to the posterior portion of the lateral meniscus. As the popliteal tendon crosses posteriorly, it blends with the oblique popliteal ligament, thus preventing multidirectional fiber orientation. Further ligamentous support on the lateral and posterolateral aspects of the knee is provided by the fabellofibular ligament and the lateral collateral ligament. These three structures insert into the fibular styloid process and run in a superior (oblique)

direction to the lateral femoral condyle, with the fabellofibular ligament being the most posterior and the lateral collateral ligament being the most superficial. The combined result of these structures is a posterolateral pillar, similar in function to the posterior oblique ligament of the medial aspect, with the common goal being the prevention of excessive rotation of the tibia.

Two structures of the knee that have received wide attention are the anterior and posterior cruciate ligaments (Fig. 12-8, *A* and *B*). These structures lie in the intercondylar notch of the femur and are covered by their own synovial sheaths, separating them from the capsule of the knee joint. The term *cruciate* is descriptive in that the ligaments form a twisting pattern as the knee moves through a range of motion.

Girgis, Marshall, and Almonajem have further elucidated the anatomical shape and function of the cruciates.[16] The anterior cruciate lies most anteriorly in the intercondylar notch, originating in the depression anterior to the medial tibial eminence. From this origin it turns in a superior, oblique, posterior direction to insert on the lateral femoral condyle in a semicircular pattern, giving it a twisted configuration. At its tibial origin, the anterior cruciate is seen to have a slip that runs and attaches to the anterior horn of the lateral meniscus. Girgis and associates have not found an attachment to the medial meniscus to be common.[16] It is generally accepted that, by its mode of attachment, the anterior cruciate can be divided into two functional structures: the anteromedial and posterior bands. The anteromedial band is described as being taut in the flexed position because of its shortened anatomical dimension and its anterior position.

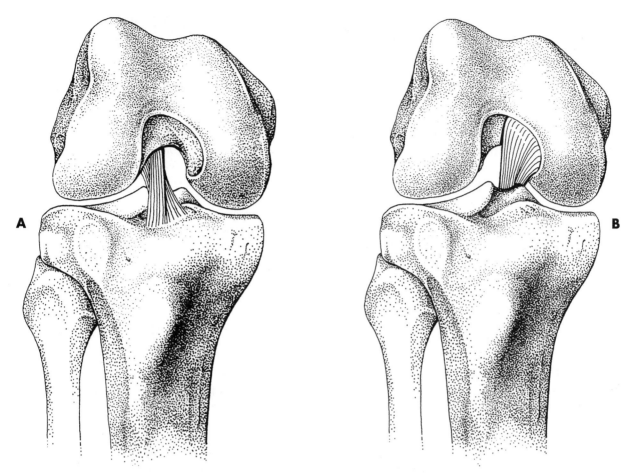

Fig. 12-8. The orientation of the ACL (**A**) and PCL (**B**) with the knee flexed 90 degrees. (From Hughston JC: *Knee ligaments: injury and repair,* St Louis, 1993, Mosby.)

The posterior cruciate lies in the posterior region of the intercondylar notch. The femoral attachment site is on the posterolateral aspect of the medial femoral condyle, forming a semicircular posterior pattern with the arch of the circle running adjacent to the femoral condylar articular surface. From this region, the posterior cruciate runs in a posterior, oblique, inferior direction to insert into the posterior depression between the tibial plateaus, continuing downward for approximately 1 cm, which gives it a very broad and convex configuration. Furthermore, the ligament sends a slip into the posterior horn of the lateral meniscus. The posterior ligament also can be divided into two functional structures: the anterolateral and posterior functional bands. Unlike the anterior cruciate, the posterior portion of the posterior cruciate ligament becomes taut in flexion, with the main bulk of the anterior portion being maximally stretched during extension. Both attachments in this ligament are posterior to the mechanical axis of the knee.

Two common but poorly understood posterior ligaments are the Wrisberg and Humphrey ligaments (see Fig. 12-4).[18] These ligaments are found in various combinations and are usually described as attaching on the posterior horn of the lateral meniscus and running in a medial direction to the medial femoral condyle. Gray describes these structures as giving support to the rotational movement of the tibia.[18]

Bursae

In excess of two dozen bursae are located in the area of the human knee.[18] Each of these bursae functions to reduce friction, between either muscle and tendon, tendon and tendon, or tendon and bone. Four of these bursae are routinely seen to be involved in inflammatory states: the prepatellar, infrapatellar, suprapatellar, and pes anserinus bursae. The suprapatellar, infrapatellar, and prepatellar bursae are generally injured as a result of direct trauma. Football, soccer, wrestling, and baseball are sports in which injuries to these bursae are common. These three bursae are located on the anterior aspect of the knee. The pes anserinus bursa, which is located just distal and medial to the medial joint space, is generally injured as a result of repetitive mechanical trauma. Such trauma might result if a long-distance runner participates in extremely long-duration running.[16] The mechanical cause of inflammation to this particular bursa may be the result of incorrect technique and/or a biomechanical dysfunction, such as foot pronation.

Clinically, it is important to distinguish between swelling

as a result of bursitis or swelling as a result of a primary joint effusion: Bursitis is localized and remains outside the knee capsule itself, whereas an effusion is an indication of a disordered status within the joint.

Musculature

The musculature about the knee plays an important role in both the normal functioning of the knee and in protection against injury.[3,52] The function of the musculature is to decrease the susceptibility of the knee to injury either directly (i.e., secondary to the ligamentous system) or indirectly (i.e., because of vastus medialis obliquus dysfunction causing patellar tracking problems).[31] A long list of references supports the importance of the thigh musculature in prevention of knee injuries, minimization of acute symptoms, and restoration of function to minimize future susceptibility.*

Anterior musculature. The anterior thigh musculature is dominated by the femoral quadriceps muscle group. The sartorius and the iliopsoas muscles are also included in the anterior group. The femoral quadriceps muscle group consists of the rectus femoris, vastus lateralis, vastus intermedius, and vastus medialis. Specifically, the vastus medialis obliquus must attach distally enough to allow for normal patellar tracking.[31] Much has been written in the literature regarding selective functions of different portions of the femoral quadriceps muscle group.[32] Visually observable atrophy of the vastus medialis is an indication of atrophy of the entire musculature.[33] Vastus medialis atrophy can occur because of the obliquity of its fibers, the distalness of its insertion, and its limited fascial covering.[33] Although attention in the literature primarily has been paid to weakness of the vastus medialis in relationship to the various patellar dysfunctions, there is some evidence that hypertonicity of the vastus lateralis muscle may also be a problem. We prefer to view the vastus medialis obliquus as a mirror of the femoral quadriceps musculature, meaning that the vastus medialis obliquus reflects the functional status of this structural group. The femoral quadriceps muscles can generate tremendous force in an athlete who through exercise has hypertrophied the group. It is not uncommon for athletic individuals to isotonically lift 40% of their body weight.

The iliopsoas muscles have also been identified as being related to certain lower extremity disorders. Weakness of this muscle group is a common finding following injury. It is not uncommon for someone with a previous knee injury to be evaluated years later with no apparent deficits in quadriceps and hamstring musculature, but with a significant difference in hip flexor strength. It should be remembered that the anterior muscle groups are only one portion of the four-part muscle system surrounding the knee. All of these groups

provide support for the knee, and proper attention to the posterior, lateral, and medial groups must be given for both prevention and rehabilitation of knee injuries.

Posterior musculature. The posterior thigh musculature includes the hamstrings group and the gastrocnemius and popliteal muscles. All three muscle groups provide posterior support for the knee; however, the hamstrings have an additional function. They have an indirect effect through their biarticular action upon the paired innominates. Weakness of this group can cause an anterior rotation of an innominate, and tightness can cause a posterior rotation of the innominate. The hamstrings also control rotatory movement of the tibia, whereas the semimembranous muscle, through its attachment to the posterior horn of the medial meniscus, functions to retract that structure during knee flexion. The femoral biceps muscle serves as an external rotator of the tibia; the semimembranous muscle functions as an internal rotator.

The hamstring muscles normally do not produce as much force as the quadriceps. However, during isokinetic testing at very high speeds, the force produced by the hamstrings approximate that of the quadriceps. The normal testing position for these muscle groups allows gravity to assist the hamstrings, thus possibly accounting for a portion of this increase and the consequent functioning of the muscles at a relatively enhanced level. The importance of the hamstrings as knee stabilizers is not commonly emphasized in the literature; however, the hamstring muscles certainly are important in protecting the knee. The function of each of these muscles must be considered in rehabilitating knee injuries, especially rotatory instabilities and their rehabilitative protocol.

Lateral and medial musculature. Rarely is either the lateral or medial musculature mentioned as important; however, one study indicates that both groups play an important role in stabilizing the knee as well as in affecting the knee indirectly through their influence on the pelvis. Weak lateral musculature can cause an upward movement of the innominate, resulting in a functional limb-length difference. Weakness of the medial musculature can cause pubic movement that can refer pain to the lower extremity as well as create a functional limb-length imbalance. The medial musculature also serves to stabilize the femur during activity, prevent rotation, and thereby allow normal function. Tightness of the iliotibial band, described as *excessive lateral compressive syndrome,* can be related to subluxation of the patella. All these possibilities emphasize that attention should be directed to the medial and lateral muscle groups rather than concentrate purely on the anterior and posterior structures.

BIOMECHANICS/ARTHROKINEMATICS
Tibiofemoral joint

The complex movements of the tibiofemoral and patellofemoral joints are coordinated and guided by the action of

---

* References 5, 8, 12, 30, 31, 41.

the musculature and the ligamentous structures previously described.

The tibiofemoral joint is best described as a rolling, gliding, rotating hinge joint. The contribution of each of these actions is required if the tibiofemoral joint is to function in its normal state. The key tibiofemoral joint movement is helicoid or spiral,[18] a description that allows visualizing the tibia as winding itself over the medial femoral condyle of the femur during flexion and extension. Studies of the movement of the tibia indicate that the axis of centroid allows the rotation or axis point to change during flexion to extension. This action distributes surface tension, thus allowing normal wear of the articular surfaces. Frankel and Nordin have done extensive research into this phenomenon.[15]

Patellofemoral joint

Mechanics of the patellofemoral joint are influenced significantly by the quadriceps muscle, the shape of the trochlear sulcus, the patellar shape, soft tissue restraints, and biomechanics at the hip and foot.[27] The patella's roles are to increase the distance from the joint axis, to provide a smooth articular surface (rather than allowing the quadriceps tendon to articulate), and to protect the anterior knee.[7] Normal function of the patella is to glide in the trochlear groove in a rhythmic pattern, which increases the leverage of the quadriceps muscle. However, to perform this activity, the patella must withstand shear and compressive forces placed on the articular surfaces.

In this extended position, the patella lies above the trochlear groove, resting on the suprapatellar fat pad and suprapatellar synovium. This position is slightly lateral because of the externally rotated end point of the tibia during extension and the physiologic valgus of the knee. Even in the extended position, the patella can be felt to slide superiorly approximately 1 cm with quadriceps contraction.[49] The patella is pulled distally during flexion into the trochlear groove. This distal movement allows the patella to pass over the medial femoral condyle because of the unlocking of the tibiofemoral joint as it internally rotates. According to Outerbridge,[49] occasionally a slight overgrowth of the osteochondral junction develops. Constant shearing of the patella over the ridge may lead to early medial-distal pull degeneration. At 20 to 30 degrees of flexion, the patella is well embedded in the trochlear groove and drifts to the lateral aspect, placing compressive forces across the medial and lateral facets. With further flexion, the pressure continues and the patellar articular surfaces segmentally come in contact with the trochlear groove, with the exception of the "odd" facet.[7] Continuation of flexion allows a smaller portion of the medial aspect of the patella to be contacted, with greater resultant pressure. With extreme flexion, the "odd" or flexion facet comes into contact with the inner margin of the medial femoral condyle in the region of the intercondylar groove. Lateral contact is of a similar nature and occurs in the extreme inner margin.

As flexion continues, the patella glides through the trochlear groove with increasing lateral pressure because of the tension of the lateral structures. Thus pressure is generated laterally during flexion; during extension, there is increasing medial pressure. Clinical observation of clients performing active progressive resistance exercises from a flexed to extended position shows that the medial facets are often the source of crepitus. Further observation demonstrates a slight lateral displacement of the patella as the knee nears terminal extension.

Arthrokinematically, the patella slides distally over the femoral trochlear groove, being pulled much like a glider being pulled through space. At the end of flexion, the patella tilts slightly laterally. This tilt can be observed in clients performing resistive movements. In extension, the patella glides proximally, being pulled upward by the quadriceps mechanism. At the end of extension, a lateral displacement of the patella is again observed.

Patellar stabilization is provided by static and dynamic mechanisms. Active stability is provided through traction of the vastus medialis with an emphasis on the oblique fibers of this muscle. This muscle also provides a degree of static stability through its insertion and acts with other soft tissue structures on the medial side of the knee to assist in providing a degree of static stability. Further static stability is provided by the trochlear groove in conjunction with patellar size and type of patellar vertical orientation. Thus the function of the patellofemoral joint is intricately linked to movement of the tibiofemoral joint, and total knee function includes a dynamic relationship among all functional components.

Kinetic chain

The kinetic chain concept allows viewing the action of the total lower extremity as a functional relationship. The open versus closed kinetic chain has a primary influence on knee injuries. The lower extremity is an open kinetic chain when the foot is off the ground and a closed kinetic chain when the foot is in contact with a supporting surface. The significance of this difference is that the closed kinetic chain is an encapsulated system prohibiting the function of one portion of the system (i.e., the foot) to the exclusion of the remaining parts (i.e., the knee and the hip). Forces, if abnormal, cannot be dispersed but must be absorbed into other tissues in the closed kinetic chain. The mandatory absorption of abnormal forces frequently leads to injury. Abnormal forces originating in the lower extremity, therefore, frequently have a profound effect upon the knee. Foot, pelvic, and soft tissue dysfunctions have the potential to produce these abnormal forces.

Abnormal foot function is not uncommon and causes a variety of knee ailments, including patellar tendinitis/tendinosis, lateral knee pain, and patellar pain.[54,56] For example, abnormal compensatory pronation causes excessive internal tibial rotation, forcing musculature to contract longer and out of phase.[56] The musculature may become glycogen-depleted and may cease to function in its shock-absorbing capacity.

With pelvic involvement (i.e., posterior innominate), the resulting change in limb length triggers a compensatory change in the foot (pronation, supination) or a change in the total extremity position (toe out, toe in).[40,49]

Soft tissue dynamics (flexibility, strength) also place stress on other tissues in the lower extremity kinetic chain. Abnormally tight hamstring muscles produce an increase in passive resistance to knee extension, causing an increased workload on the quadriceps muscles.[60] Weak muscles (i.e., hip extensor weakness causing an anterior innominate) can also trigger changes in lower extremity mechanical balance.[40,49]

KNEE INJURIES
Mechanisms of injury

Microtrauma includes a series of inflammatory reactions to submaximal loading that eventually produce clinical signs and symptoms. Microtraumatic injuries can occur as a result of several mechanisms, including excessive normal forces, abnormal forces, or excessive abnormal forces. Our bodies can absorb normal forces daily without causing inflammatory responses. A normal force is absorbed by an individual who walks several miles during a 15-hour day. However, if this same individual hiked 10 miles in a 5-hour period, an inflammatory condition would result from an excessive normal force. Excessive normal forces include either high-repetition activities with a low load or low-repetition activities with a high load.

Abnormal forces also cause microtraumatic injuries. A limb-length difference, pronatory problem, or a flexibility or strength deficit necessitates compensatory changes in lower extremity kinetic chain loading and a diminished ability to absorb or disperse such forces, which can lead to tissue breakdown.

However, some individuals get along well with abnormal forces until these forces become excessive. People with limb-length differences as great as ¾ inch, gross pronation, and very tight, weak muscles may never have problems until they change or increase their activity level. This mechanism, which produces microtrauma, is referred to as *excessive abnormal force*. Individuals unable to accommodate such forces increasingly find their way to physicians' offices and thus to physical therapy as the fitness boom continues. The microtraumatically induced inflammatory process that results from excessive abnormal forces can be located in the ligament, tendon, contractile unit, capsule, articular cartilage, and/or bone. It is not uncommon for several tissues to be involved and for the client to have previously had pain in other anatomic locations. When pain first appears, the client can either curtail activity or attempt to compensate, with compensation being the rule. Compensation, however, ultimately leads to pain in another area, and the process starts anew. The client who can no longer compensate seeks medical attention.

In treating the microtraumatic injury, the cause of the injury must be addressed. Frequently, if only the symptoms are treated, symptoms recur when the activity is resumed. The pathomechanical causes of lower extremity microtraumatic injuries are usually the big three and/or the little one: The big three are limb-length difference, foot dysfunction, and flexibility deficits; the little one is strength deficiency and/or imbalance.

Macrotrauma is trauma resulting from an injury of a magnitude that causes immediate clinical signs and symptoms. Macrotrauma can disrupt the ligaments, muscle-tendon units, joint capsules, bones, nerves, and/or blood vessels. Rarely does macrotrauma affect only one tissue. An individual can be predisposed to macrotraumatic injury. (Predisposing factors are discussed at the beginning of this chapter.) Macrotraumatic injuries can be a result of direct or indirect mechanisms. An example of direct injury to the knee joint occurs when varus force causes compression of the medial meniscus. An indirect injury occurs when a valgus force causes the medial joint space to open, thus applying traction forces to the medial collateral ligament and its attachment to the medial meniscus.

As with microtraumatic injury, in addition to treatment of the symptoms, the predisposing factors (causes) of the macrotraumatic injury must be identified and treated for successful management.

Prevention of knee injuries

The incidence and severity of knee injuries in sports mandate more attention paid to prevention. Abott and Kress[1] and Bender[5] have demonstrated that it is possible both to predict and to prevent knee injuries through appropriate intervention. Cahill and Griffin have demonstrated in high schools that some types of knee injuries can be prevented with appropriate exercise and preseason conditioning programs.[8] Nicholas has shown that muscle weakness as a consequence of knee injuries can persist, thus increasing the likelihood of reinjury, if the injury is not thoroughly rehabilitated.[40]

In addition, Cameron and Davis have discussed other factors, such as the type of foot gear worn, that are responsible for the incidence and severity of injuries.[9] Klein has pointed out that a limb-length difference can be responsible for both microtraumatic and macrotraumatic injuries of the knee,[29] and Blyth noted that the number and quality of coaches available in athletics have a direct effect upon the incidence and severity of injuries.[6]

These existing facts must be recognized and used in preseason screening and for treating past as well as present and future injuries. Neither the lack of a definite program of treatment nor the lack of thorough and aggressive rehabilitation, once an injury has occurred, can be tolerated. These facts supporting intervention to prevent knee injuries should not be ignored. Furthermore, these facts must be made available to the medical community and the general public.

Structural predisposition

An individual's biomechanical structure can be responsible for a predisposition to knee injuries. Abnormal positioning of the patella, hypermobile joints, hormonal influences in women, inherited or acquired biomechanical problems of the foot, and/or limb-length differences are all examples of structural predisposition. These factors should be identified as part of a screening examination, and the individual should be counseled as to beneficial types of sports and remedial exercise programs and/or supportive devices that might minimize the chances of injury.

Functional predisposition

An individual or athlete's gait pattern, such as a pronated or toed-out gait, can be a predisposing factor in many knee injuries. Additional factors include posture, genu recurvatum, an abnormally flexed knee, pes planus, and pes cavus.

Physical condition may also serve as a functional predisposition. Conditioning provides many benefits, such as increased tensile strength in the ligament when muscles around the joint are exercised.[57] Strength itself has been demonstrated to be a primary protective mechanism.[1,5,8] To be effective, this mechanism must have the ability to function repeatedly, thus emphasizing the need for endurance rather than just maximal muscular strength. Most epidemiologic data collected indicate that the majority of injuries in most sports take place at the end of the day (as in skiing) and/or in the final periods of play (as in football).[13]

Previous injury

Previous injury is also a predisposing factor to knee disorders. Variables resulting from previous injury that may predispose the athlete to injury include:

1. Decreased strength, power, and endurance
2. Instability
3. Insufficient collagen maturation
4. Decreased range of motion and flexibility
5. Delayed reaction time and decreased balance
6. Adhesions
7. Altered gait
8. Poor (or incorrect) diagnosis
9. Lack of (or insufficient) treatment

Muscular factors

Strength. The importance of muscular strength around joints for an athlete has been demonstrated many times. Exercising the muscles around the joint increases the tensile strength of the ligaments and also increases the strength of the ligament-bone interface. Exercise also increases the bone circumference, which provides further protection against bony injury.

Muscle groups that must be considered in relationship to knee injury include all of those of the lower extremity. Clinicians most frequently think only of the anterior compartment of the thigh because of the obvious importance of the quadriceps mechanism in maintaining the stability of the patella and in protection of the knee. The importance of this group in both prevention of injury and recurrence of injury cannot be denied, but the posterior muscular structures are equally important. The posterior muscle groups have a role to play in prevention of linear and rotatory instability. The medial and lateral structures of the knee also have been demonstrated to be of value in preventing knee injuries. Posteriorly and inferiorly the gastrocnemius muscle provides a support mechanism to the posterior aspect of the knee. Other muscle groups, such as the abdominals, hip rotators, and muscles of the leg that support the foot, indirectly influence the lower extremity kinetic chain and therefore can be responsible for applying abnormal stress to the knee if, in fact, they are not functioning optimally.

Evaluation of the strength of musculature around the knee demands the identification of parameters and normal values. Parameters that should be considered for these muscle groups include:

1. Strength of the group versus body weight
2. Right-versus-left ratio
3. Relationship of agonists and antagonists
4. Total leg strength (right to left)
5. Variations of these relationships with different speeds of testing

Power. Although the terms *strength* and *power* are often used synonymously, they are not interchangeable. *Strength* refers to the amount of force that a muscle-tendon unit can generate, whereas *power* refers to the amount of force that can be generated per unit of time. The importance of the ability to generate force in a short period of time cannot be overemphasized. If an athlete needs 100 foot-pounds of strength to stabilize or protect the knee joint in $\frac{1}{10}$ second, but that individual requires $\frac{1}{5}$ second to generate that much force, the joint has already been injured and the amount of force produced has been of no value. Therefore, power is a very significant aspect in both prevention and rehabilitation programs. Appropriate functional testing must be done to ensure that power requirements have been successfully met. We recommend a functional progressive program developed to fit the needs of each individual undergoing rehabilitation. This involves the delineation of performance tasks and the organization of these tasks in a continuum from the most easily accomplished through a return to the desired activity. The sequence includes open kinetic and closed kinetic chain exercise patterns.

Endurance. Endurance is another goal that must be considered and pursued vigorously. The ability of a muscle-tendon unit to produce strength and power is of no value if they cannot be successfully reproduced. Endurance must be adequately incorporated in a preventive program so that an athlete can avoid injury upon becoming fatigued. The development of adequate enzyme production, glycogen deposition, and oxygen utilization capabilities requires significant time and specific stimuli.

Flexibility. Lack of flexibility in muscle-tendon units around the knee can be responsible for either direct or indirect joint injury. Inflexible muscles are not as efficient and therefore may tire more quickly, causing opposing muscle groups likewise to tire more quickly because they must work to compensate for the passive resistance of a restricted or tight muscle. As muscle function increases, glycogen depletion takes place earlier, and the tired muscle is unable to complete the function of joint protection. Tight muscles may also cause abnormal stresses throughout the lower extremity kinetic chain, leading to knee disorders. For example, a tight gastrosoleus muscle group may cause an athlete to pronate the foot excessively, producing patellar tendinitis/tendinosis or chondromalacia of the knee.

Proprioception

Seldom are proprioceptive factors considered in a preventive program. However, through the work of Wyke,[63] the importance of this parameter has become increasingly clear. Obviously, an athlete with good balance and reaction time is less susceptible to injury. The athlete should be better able to avoid injury-producing situations and need to work less vigorously to restore body position after losing balance.

Balance can be tested with a modified Stork test timed with a stopwatch or, particularly for competitive athletes, with an objective testing mechanism, such as a mechanical balance evaluator or computerized assessment device. Testing protocols and normative data have been developed for this area, but a tremendous individual variation requires care in the application of such. We thus recommend norm creation on your specific group of subjects rather than using a nonspecific norm.

Shoes

Shoes can also be responsible for either microtraumatic or macrotraumatic knee injuries. Cameron and Davis have demonstrated that shoe design in football can make a difference in the incidence and severity of knee injuries.[9] Other clinicians have reported that shoes can be a primary cause of microtraumatic (overuse) types of injuries about the knee. Design, construction, fit, and wear (asymmetrical and excessive) are all possible factors.

Environmental factors

Environmental factors, such as uneven ground and slippery and sticky surfaces, are also primary considerations. Although environmental factors cannot always be controlled, they should be evaluated and minimized whenever possible.

PHYSICAL EXAMINATION OF THE KNEE
Evaluation form

We recommend the use of an evaluation form that establishes an encompassing, systematic format to be followed for each individual seen in the clinic. This type of form allows standardization of the evaluation process and enhances reliability. The International Knee Documentation Form is provided as an example. It is used in numerous "knee clinics" worldwide (Fig. 12-9).

Subjective examination

Physical examination of the knee begins with the examiner assuming the posture of an investigator and starting the investigation with a subjective assessment of the client's complaints. The following questions should be routinely included: How, when, and where did the injury take place? What was the immediate treatment? How rapidly did the knee swell (if swelling took place)? Has the knee "given way"? Does it catch or lock? Clarification of each of these questions and the importance assigned to them involves the length of time since the injury occurred. The client's description of how the injury occurred should include details such as the direction of forces, the position of the injured knee, whether the foot was planted, and the type of surface involved. Immediate treatment, including whether the individual continued with the activity or was unable to do so, is also extremely important to determine. Frequently, clients know more about their knees and their injuries than clinicians can assess by examination.

Intraarticular disorders of the tibiofemoral joint range from isolated entities to complex rotatory injuries. Surgeons such as O'Donoghue,[48] Slocum,[51] Hughston and colleagues,[23] Kennedy,[28] Noyes,[41-46] and Nicholas[40] have added new dimensions to injury recognition, surgical intervention, and time frames for healing. Furthermore, the advent and wide use of arthroscopy, which allows visualization of the injured structures, has helped advance surgical concepts.

Acute knee injuries, however, have created an aura of confusion among health care practitioners. Hughston and colleagues, for example, have attempted to classify injury mechanisms and resultant trauma.[22] Smillie,[53] Slocum,[51] and O'Donoghue[48] have contributed significantly to the delineation of mechanisms of injury.

Extracting subjective information in the orthopedic examination is crucial if the examiner did not see the injury occur. In clients with a chronic injury, the individual must attempt reenactment of the injury-producing situation—either verbally or by action—to help assess the direction of mechanical forces. Noyes stresses the importance of understanding joint mechanics in soft tissues that stabilize the joint.[46] This concept deals with primary and secondary restraints. The majority of clients' injuries occur in the loose-packed position, which provides only minimal stability of capsular and ligamentous structures.

1993-1994
THE IKDC KNEE LIGAMENT STANDARD EVALUATION FORM

Patient Name_____ Date_____ / _____ / _____ Medical Record#_____

Occupation_____ Sport: 1st Choice_____ 2nd Choice_____

Age_____ Sex_____ Ht_____ Wt_____ Involved Knee: ☐ Right ☐ Left Contralateral Normal: ☐ Yes ☐ No

Cause of Injury: Date of Injury:____ / ____ / ____   Procedure_____
☐ADL ☐ Traffic
☐ Contact ☐ Noncontact   Date of Index Operation:____ / ____ / ____   Postop Dx_____

ACTIVITY

	Pre-injury	Pre-Rx	Post-Rx
I. Strenuous Activity jumping, pivoting, hard cutting (football,soccer)			
II. Moderate Activity heavy manual work (skiing, tennis)			
III. Light Activity light manual work (jogging, running)			
IV. Sedentary Activity (housework, ADL)			

Eventual change knee related: ☐ Yes ☐ No

MENISCAL STATUS

	N1	1/3	2/3	Total
Med				
Lat				

Morphotype: Lax_____
Normal_____ Tight_____
Knee: Varus_____
Normal_____ Valgus_____

PREVIOUS SURGERY

Date: _____ Procedure: _____

Date: _____ Procedure: _____

Date: _____ Procedure: _____

EIGHT GROUPS	FOUR GRADES				* GROUP GRADE			
	A. Normal	B. Nearly Normal	C. Abnormal	D. Sev. Abnorm.	A	B	C	D
1. Patient Subjective Assessment								
How does your knee function?	☐ 0	☐ 1	☐ 2	☐ 3				
On a scale of 0 to 3, how does your knee affect your activity level?	☐ 0	☐ 1	☐ 2	☐ 3	☐	☐	☐	☐
2. SYMPTOMS	**I.** Strenuous Activity	**II.** Moderate Activity	**III.** Light Activity	**IV.** Sedentary Activity				
(Grade at highest activity level with no significant symptoms. Exclude 0 to slight symptoms.)								
Pain	☐	☐	☐	☐				
Swelling	☐	☐	☐	☐				
Partial Giving Way	☐	☐	☐	☐				
Full Giving Way	☐	☐	☐	☐	☐	☐	☐	☐
3. Range of Motion Ext/Flex: Index side:____ / ____ / ____ Opposite side:____ / ____ / ____								
Lack of extension (from 0°)	☐ <3°	☐ 3 to 5°	☐ 6 to 10°	☐ >10°				
△ Lack of flexion	☐ 0 to 5°	☐ 6 to 15°	☐ 16 to 25°	☐ >25°	☐	☐	☐	☐
4. Ligament Evaluation (manual, instrumented, x-ray)								
△ LACHMAN (25° flex)	☐ -1 to 2mm	☐ 3 to 5mm <-1 to -3 stiff	☐ 6 to 10mm <-3 stiff	☐ >10mm				
Endpoint: firm/soft	☐ firm		☐ soft					
△ Total A.P. Transl.(70° flex)	☐ 0 to 2mm	☐ 3 to 5mm	☐ 6 to 10mm	☐ >10mm				
△ Post. sag(70° flex)	☐ 0 to 2mm	☐ 3 to 5mm	☐ 6 to 10mm	☐ >10mm				
△ Med jt opening(20° flex)(valgus rot)	☐ 0 to 2mm	☐ 3 to 5mm	☐ 6 to 10mm	☐ >10mm				
△ Lat jt opening(20° flex)(varus rot)	☐ 0 to 2mm	☐ 3 to 5mm	☐ 6 to 10mm	☐ >10mm				
△ Pivot shift	☐ equal	☐ + (glide)	☐ ++(clunk)	☐ +++ (gross)				
△ Reverse pivot shift	☐ equal	☐ glide	☐ marked	☐ gross	☐	☐	☐	☐
5. Compartmental Findings			crepitation with	crepitation with				
△ Crepitus patellofemoral	☐ none	☐ moderate	☐ mild pain	☐ >mild pain				
△ Crepitus medial compartment	☐ none	☐ moderate	☐ mild pain	☐ >mild pain				
△ Crepitus lateral compartment	☐ none	☐ moderate	☐ mild pain	☐ >mild pain				
6. Harvest Site Pathology	☐ none	☐ mild	☐ moderate	☐ severe				
7. X-Ray Findings								
Med Joint space	☐ none	☐ mild	☐ moderate	☐ severe				
Lat Joint space	☐ none	☐ mild	☐ moderate	☐ severe				
Patellofemoral	☐ none	☐ mild	☐ moderate	☐ severe				
8. Functional Test								
One leg hop (% of opposite side)	☐ ≥90%	☐ 89% to 76%	☐ 75% to 50%	☐ <50%				
**FINAL EVALUATION					☐	☐	☐	☐

*Group Grade: The lowest grade within a group determines the group grade. **Final Evaluation: The worst group grade determines the final evaluation for acute and subacute patients. For chronic patients compare preoperative and postoperative evaluations. In a final evaluation, only the first 4 groups are evaluated but all groups must be documented.

△ Difference in involved knee compared to normal or what is assumed to be normal.

IKDC – INTERNATIONAL KNEE DOCUMENTATION COMMITTEE, Members of the Committee:
AOSSM: Anderson, AF, Clancy, WG, Daniel, D, DeHaven, KE, Fowler, PJ, Feagin, J, Grood, ES, Noyes, FR, Terry, GC, Torzilli, P, Warren, RF.
ESSKA: Chambat, P, Eriksson, E, Gillquist, J, Hefti, F, Huiskes, R, Jakob, RP, Moyen, B, Muller, W, Staeubli, H, vanKampen, A.

Fig. 12-9. The IKDC knee ligament standard evaluation form. (From the International Knee Documentation Committee.)

INSTRUCTIONS FOR THE IKDC FORM

The first part of the form establishes demographic information, history of prior surgery, findings of the index procedure, current status of the menisci (i.e., normal, 1/3 removed, 2/3 removed or complete removal), morphotype and knee alignment. For activity, the patient selects the highest activity level which he/she is able to perform; pre-injury, pre-treatment, and post treatment. This data is recorded but not graded.

The evaluation includes eight groups, each of which is assigned one of four grades. The eight groups are:

1. Patient Subjective Assessment:

How does your knee function? The patient is asked to rate the involved knee compared to the normal knee or what is perceived as normal.

2. Symptoms:

Grade at the highest activity level at which the patient thinks he/she would be able to function without significant symptoms, even if they were not actually performing activities at this level. Exclude 0 to slight symptoms. Performance at level I, strenuous activity, without symptoms is normal. Patients who are symptomatic at level I activity but not level II activities would be graded nearly normal.

3. Range of Motion:

Passive range of motion is measured with a gonimeter and recorded on the form for the index side and opposite or normal side. Record values for hyperextension/zero point/flexion, (e.g. 10 degrees of hyperextension, 150 degrees of flexion = 10/0/150). Hyperextension is recorded as a positive number and a flexion contracture as a negative number. Extension is graded from 0 degrees even if the patient has hyperextension of the normal knee.

4. Ligament Examination:

*The Lachman test, total AP translation at 70 degrees and medial and lateral joint opening may be assessed with manual, instrumented or stress x-ray examination. Only one should be graded, preferably a "measured displacement". A standard force of 30 lbs. (134N) is used in the instrumented examination. The numerical values for the side to side difference are rounded off, and the appropriate box is marked.

*The end point is assessed in the Lachman test. The end point affects the grading when the index knee has 3-5 mm. more anterior laxity than the normal knee. In this case, a soft end point results in an abnormal grade rather than a nearly normal grade.

*The 70 degree posterior sag is estimated by comparing the profile of the injured knee to the normal knee and palpating the femoral tibial stepoff. It may be confirmed by noting that contraction of the quadriceps pulls the tibia anteriorly.

The pivot shift and reverse pivot shift are performed with the patient supine, with the hip in 10-20 degrees of abduction and the tibia in neutral rotation using either the Losee, Noyes or Jakob techniques. The greatest subluxation should be recorded.

5. Compartment Findings:

Patellofemoral crepitation is elicited by extension against slight resistance. Medial and lateral compartment crepitation is elicited by extending the knee from a flexed position with a varus and then a valgus stress (i.e., McMurray test). Grading is based on intensity and pain.

6. Harvest Site Pathology:

Note tenderness, irritation or numbness at the autograft harvest site.

7. X-ray Findings:

A bilateral PA weightbearing roentgenogram at 35-45 degrees of flexion (tunnel view) is used to evaluate narrowing of the medial and lateral joint spaces. The Merchant view at 45 degrees is used to document patellofemoral narrowing. A mild grade indicates minimal changes (e.g., small osteophytes, slight scleorosis or flattening of the femoral condyle), but the joint space is wider than 4 mm. A moderate grade may have those changes and joint space narrowing (e.g., a joint space of 2-4 mm. wide). Severe changes include significant joint space narrowing (e.g., a joint space of less than 2 mm).

8. Functional Test:

The patient is asked to perform a one leg hop for distance on the index and normal side. Three trials for each leg are recorded and averaged. A ratio of the index to normal knee is calculated.

Fig. 12-9, cont'd.

However, injuries can also occur at the extremes of range of motion. For instance, an individual who attempts to stand from a squatting position may, with tibial rotation, pinch the meniscus. Significant ligamentous injuries occur in portions of the range of motion where ligament tension is required, hence sprains often occur in the last 30 degrees of extension.

In the loose-packed position, many injuries occur with application of a rotational force. The most common force applied is external rotation of the tibia, resulting in an injury described by O'Donoghue as the unhappy triad: damage to the medial collateral ligament, unstable medial meniscus, and damage to the anterior cruciate ligament.[48]

Other mechanisms of injury may include hyperextension, varus disorder, and internal rotation. Although none of these mechanisms is as common as those previously described, they can result in trauma equally significant to the anterior cruciate ligament, lateral collateral ligament, or lateral meniscus in the posterior lateral complex. With these mechanisms, the significance of the injury should not be underestimated.

In recording the client's subjective history, along with the mechanism of injury, the clinician should pay particular attention to the sequence of events following the injury. Many times the client complains of a popping or snapping sensation, which can be the result of a tearing of the intraarticular structures (such as the ligaments, menisci, or osteochondral structures) or dislocation of the patella. An associated acute hemarthrosis within 2 to 24 hours can occur with significant clinical findings.

In clients with an acute hemarthrosis, arthroscopy is becoming a routine diagnostic tool. Noyes found that 72% of acute hemarthroses show associated injury to the anterior cruciate ligament.[44] The overall correlation of clinical examination to arthroscopic evaluation has been well delineated by Oberlander and colleagues.[47] This knowledge has led to increased numbers of primary repairs to the anterior cruciate ligament. Today, such surgery is performed after the patient has regained a normal range of motion, thus minimizing surgical and rehabilitative complications.[19] Other associated disorders have been demonstrated through early arthroscopic examinations, including minimal involvement of associated ligamentous structures in 41% of treated cases and 62% of cases with meniscus lesions. Another condition that should be examined is a locked knee resulting either from meniscal displacement or hamstring muscle spasm. Locking can also be the result of effusion forcing the joint into a loose-packed position. The chief complaint then is inability to walk without a limp as the knee remains in a flexed position.

Clients with chronic knee disorders reveal a wide array of complaints. However, the clinician should not categorize complaints as always being evidence of a pathologic disorder. A client's complaint of the knee "giving way" must be treated specifically, as this problem can occur while walking down steps, twisting, or decelerating, and may be the result

of a wide range of problems. These problems can include subluxation of the patella, femoral quadriceps muscle weakness, meniscal pinching, ligamentous insufficiency, and effusion. Isokinetic documentation of quadriceps muscle weakness, in fact, has demonstrated that a significant decrease in strength occurs within weeks, and muscle output may be significantly decreased after 1 day. Often muscle weakness results in a sensation that the client's knee is going to "give way" or that the knee is too tired for continued walking.

A second common complaint in the client with chronic knee disorders is locking, which can result from hamstring muscle spasm, true meniscal locking with joint blockage, or inflammation of the fat pad as a result of an original injury. Some clients misinterpret the sensation of stiffness that often accompanies degenerative joint disease as a locking sensation. True locking, however, is the result of an injury associated with internal knee derangement, most commonly involving the meniscus.

Pain is one of the most common symptoms of clients with chronic or acute knee disorders. Careful attention should be paid to the client's description of the pain's location and intensity. The ability to reproduce this pain can assist the clinician in determining structural involvement and the extent of the injury. In a client with an acute knee injury, however, trauma or effusion pressing on capsular joint receptors may lead to inaccurate physical examination because of client apprehension. Remember that the location and intensity of the pain vary widely with the specific injury. In a subjective history the clinician must identify the different types of pain, such as dull, aching, local, radiating, intermittent, or constant. Ability to reproduce the pain over palpable sites also allows the clinician to effectively delineate the involved tissues. However, with chronic internal derangement, pain may be referred to other structures.

Objective examination

Observation of the lower extremities. The next sequence in the examination is objective inspection or observation of the lower extremities. For clients who complain of "giving way," stiffness, and an aching type of pain, a total lower extremity examination, including evaluation of tibia valgus, tibia vara, internal tibial torsion, patellar alignment, and tibial rotation with active extension and flexion, is important. In the client with acute knee injury, the primary emphasis should be on inspection for a locked-knee position, effusion, and the ability to ambulate, with or without a limp.

Examination of the tibiofemoral joint. Physical examination of the tibiofemoral joint is often difficult in a client with an acutely injured or inflamed knee. Although the role of arthroscopy in assisting the diagnosis and treatment of acute problems is increasing,[44,47] the physical portion of the examination should not be minimized. The importance and validity of the examination are enhanced if it is performed shortly after the injury. It is not unusual for a client to demonstrate significant instability initially, yet be unable to display instability 2 hours after the injury because of swelling, effusion, or both. Internal derangement of the knee as a result of acute injury may include meniscal lesions, ligamentous lesions, lesions in the articular cartilage, and lesions of the synovium and/or capsule. Thorough evaluation is necessary to determine whether a primary or secondary restraint is still functioning in the knee. As previously stated, the initial contact with the client should include a complete and accurate history, followed by a systematic physical examination.

Palpation. With an acute injury, pain location is usually local and can be reproduced through palpation. Thus palpation allows localization of involvement. A classic case of needing to determine local involvement occurs when a person receives a direct blow to the medial collateral ligament, whereupon palpation can delineate the site of the injury as a femoral attachment injury, tibial attachment injury, or midsubstance tear.

Careful palpation for acute injury should include examination of the following structures:

1. The medial collateral ligament should be palpated from its distal attachment just below the adductor tubercle of the femur to its insertion approximately 2 to 3 inches below the joint line on the tibia. (However, careful delineation from the pes anserinus bursa and tension at its tibial insertion is often difficult.)

2. The lateral collateral ligament should be palpated from the lateral femoral condyle to the fibular head. If pain and swelling permit, the examiner can accentuate the palpation of the lateral collateral ligament by flexing and crossing the affected leg over the unaffected leg, thus allowing the hip to fall into external rotation. This is often referred to as the *figure 4* position.

3. The entire length of the joint line should be palpated on both the medial and lateral aspects, starting at the tibial tubercle and palpating up the patellar tendon until the groove (the joint line), at which point the examiner should palpate medially and then laterally, pressing in an oblique inferior direction along the joint line. It is not uncommon in meniscal tears or coronary ligament involvement to have palpable tenderness at the joint line. Tenderness over the medial aspect of the joint line, however, is often compounded with meniscus or ligamentous injury.

4. Palpation of the patella and the surrounding capsule should be performed to assess capsular damage that may have occurred with acute subluxation or dislocation of the patella. Palpation should be done as low as the tibial tubercle because associated patellar tendon problems may also occur. Also, palpation from the medial border of the patella to the adductor tubercle must be accomplished to document the medial patellofemoral ligament.

5. Pes anserinus expansion palpation should be performed on the anteromedial aspect of the tibia where this tendon inserts superficially into the tibial attachment of the medial collateral ligaments and continues to the crest of the tibia. Palpating the tendon, bursa, and/or tibial attachment on the medial collateral ligament calls for caution. Pain in any of these structures may be the result of palpation in this area.

6. The lateral tibial crest is the site of the attachment of the iliotibial track. The lateral tubercle to which the iliotibial is attached is Gerdy's tubercle.

7. Soft tissue palpation of the posteromedial and posterolateral aspects of the proximal tibia is important. Rotational instabilities often create tenderness of tissues located in these areas.

8. Palpation of the hamstring musculature for insertional pain to determine excessive tension is important, as such tension can prevent full knee extension.

9. Palpation for joint effusion in an acute knee injury is usually simple. First, a simple ballottement examination should be used. The examiner places one hand on the suprapatellar pouch and exerts a caudal pressure, thereby pushing the synovial fluid beneath the patella. Meanwhile, the examiner's other hand palpates the middle of the patella. A posterior force is exerted on the patella to determine whether it has been raised off the femoral condyle by excessive fluid. In a second type of effusion test (commonly called *milking*), the examiner palpates the suprapatellar pouch on the medial and lateral sides with both hands. The hands are then moved in a caudal direction to squeeze the knee from a superior to inferior direction and force the fluid to move with the hands. Upon releasing the hands, an effusion can be seen returning in a rippling fashion into the suprapatellar pouch.

Accessory motion testing. The next section of the physical examination dealing with acute knee injury involves accessory motion testing, which is performed to establish the integrity of stabilizing structures about the joint.[17] The knee relies heavily on strong ligamentous and capsular expansions to provide the static stabilization necessary for normal motion. Stability examination, therefore, is important because primary repair of ligamentous injury is often thought to be crucial in successful return to full functional status. The extent of ligamentous injury has been classified many ways, including the classic orthopedic terminology of *grade I, grade II,* and *grade III* (depending upon the degree of mobility as compared to the noninvolved extremity) and Hughston's classification according to severity.[22] Manual therapy recommends the use of a 0 to 6 grading scale in which the involved knee is rated in comparison to the opposite or noninvolved extremity. According to this scale, a grade of 3 is normal, with the client serving as his or her own control. Regardless of the methodology of classification, adequate force must be used to provide relevant information. Noyes points out that frequently traditional joint-stability tests are performed in a rather low-force environment, thus leading to potentially false-negative results.[41] Anesthetization has been advocated for years for examination of clients with acute injuries to make possible a more accurate assessment of stability.

Assessment of both primary and secondary restraints available in the knee are important. Often, with injury to a primary restraint, the secondary static restraint or dynamic restraint may provide enough stability to cause a false-negative test result. Therefore, when performing joint-stability examinations, the clinician should follow four important rules:

1. Proper stabilization of both the proximal and distal segments is essential.
2. Proper clinician positioning is required for adequate palpation of the structure being tested.
3. In assessing accessory movement, not only the degree of opening but also the end feel achieved with testing is important.
4. The clinician should always start by testing the opposite extremity to allow the client to feel how the test is performed and to establish a baseline. Repeat or comparison testing is thus performed on the normal extremity.

Specific tests

Medial and lateral collateral ligament testing. Testing the stability of these ligaments involves the following steps:

1. The client should be supine to ensure total relaxation while the clinician secures the ankle between his or her elbow and the trunk so that the hand and the clinician's arm can extend up the medial aspect of the tibia, thus placing the index finger or (preferably) the middle finger on the medial joint line. The clinician's opposite hand should be placed on the lateral aspect of the client's knee joint in a secure manner.
2. At this time, the knee is flexed 30 degrees, and a valgus force is applied by pushing the hand on the outside of the knee and rotating the trunk in the opposite direction. This action results in a gapping of the medial aspect of the tibia on the femur that may be very obvious and palpable. As the clinician performs this task, a normal firm end point should be felt. If any end feel other than capsular is present, a disorder should be suspected. Upon relieving the pressure, the clinician may feel a reduction "clunk" of bony structures, which is often present in both normal and injured knees.
3. The test is then repeated with the knee in a more extended position but not into the fully locked-out position. Gapping in both the extended and flexed positions indicates involvement of the posterior cruciate ligament, posterior "corner" capsular structures, and the collateral ligament.
4. To test the lateral aspect of the knee, the reverse of the previous procedure is carried out, using a varus stress

at the knee. Again, this test must be performed in both 30-degree flexion and near extension to assess the stability of both primary and secondary restraints.

Anterior and posterior cruciate ligament testing. The anterior and posterior cruciate complexes provide stability for the knee to function in both planar and rotatory directions. These ligaments are found to be outside the joint capsule but within their own synovium. Classical testing of the anterior cruciate ligament (ACL) involves the following procedures:

1. The client should be supine, with hip flexed 45 degrees and knee flexed 90 degrees. (We suggest that one leg at a time be tested so as not to position the client where substitution will occur.)
2. The examiner's thumbs are placed on the anterior crest of the tibia along the joint line, with the index fingers placed posteriorly on the tibia to assess hamstring musculature. (A false-negative test is very common in clients who have dynamic hamstring support).
3. The test is performed simply by applying pressure in an anterior direction in an attempt to draw the tibia forward. In this position, an anterior displacement of 2 to 3 mm is considered normal. However, it is again necessary to check the opposite extremity as well as the end feel achieved. A ballistic movement may be necessary to assess the desired end feel.
4. The second and more sensitive and specific test for the ACL is Lachman's test, which is best described as performing an anterior drawer test at a 20- to 30-degree knee flexion position.
5. To check the posterior cruciate, the clinician simply applies the force in the opposite direction. It is sometimes better to move from 90 degrees of knee flexion to less flexion (60 to 80 degrees) for this assessment. Again, the amount and quality of movement and end feel should be compared to the opposite side. (Often a false-positive anterior drawer is assessed when in actuality the tibia has been posteriorly displaced). To assess this prior to performing the anterior and posterior drawer test, we advocate the use of the antigravity test. The client is placed in a supine position with the hips and knees flexed 90 degrees. The clinician holds the client's legs at the ankles, and a straight edge is applied across the crest of the tibia to allow assessment of a relative posterior displacement of the tibia. A positive antigravity test shows a valley appearance from the edge of the straight edge to the tibial tubercle.

Rotational examination. In association with drawer testing, Slocum and Larson advocate the use of internal-external rotation of the tibia to detect rotational instability.[52] External rotation of the tibia increases tension in the intact posterior medial structures, thereby reducing forward movement of the tibia, even with involvement of the anterior cruciate ligament. With internal rotation, there is an increase in tension of the posterior lateral structures, thereby reducing the anterior displacement. However, if in either instance the tibia continues to slide forward excessively, then an associated disorder is present in the structures. It is important to rotate the tibia only slightly on the femur because maximal rotation tightens whatever portion of the structure is still intact, thereby decreasing the displacement present.

Hughston and others have delineated the difference between straight and rotatory instabilities.[22] These rotatory instabilities have been classified as *anterolateral, anteromedial,* and *posterolateral.* They are usually the result of selective structural damage, which has caused a change in the rotatory pattern of the tibia on the femur. The anterolateral rotatory instability is the most common. Further assessment of this rotatory instability has been proposed by Hughston and others (the jerk test),[22] MacIntosh (the pivot-shift test), Noyes and colleagues (the flexion-rotation drawer test),[46] and Slocum (the anterior drawer test with an internally rotated tibia).[51] All of these tests are designed to detect subluxation of the tibia on the femur or reduction of the tibia on the femur.

It is important to assess throughout the range of motion the feeling perceived with the drawer test. Lachman advocates a test for the anterior drawer in which the leg is held externally rotated, and the test is performed in 15 degrees of knee flexion.[46] Torg and colleagues first described this positioning in 1976.[58] The purpose of this position is to allow the posterior horns of the menisci to clear the femoral condyles. These structures may block movement in the traditional 90-degree knee flexion anterior drawer test. In the client with acute knee injury and effusion, moreover, flexion beyond the 45-degree position also results in a decreased joint movement. Letting the client assume a loose-packed position of approximately 15 to 30 degrees with an externally rotated leg and then applying an anterior force on the tibia results in a much higher degree of accuracy in assessing the anterior cruciate ligament. However, the clinician should not forget the importance of clinical end feel and palpation of the relative joint movement.

The McMurray test was devised to detect posterior tears in the medial meniscus.[21] The medial meniscus, when damaged, may sublux in the intercondylar region of the knee joint. This examination combines the movement of flexion and extension with rotation of the knee. The examiner should palpate the joint lines in order to detect meniscal popping or snapping during the test if the test is positive. Occasionally, an audible clicking or popping can also be elicited with this maneuver. It should be recognized that this test is best used as a confirmation process as it has relatively poor specificity.

The McMurray test is performed with the client supine and the examiner grasping the bottom of the client's foot with one hand while palpating the joint line with the opposite hand. The knee is then flexed and placed into external rotation, after which the examiner applies a valgus force. The knee is then extended. A positive test elicits a popping or snapping sensation.

Appley's compression test for meniscal tearing is performed with the client in the prone position, knee flexed to 90 degrees.[21] The examiner grasps the plantar aspect of the client's foot and performs forceful compression through the foot to the knee joint. Simultaneously, the examiner performs internal-external rotation of the tibia, which may cause "catching" of the meniscus. A positive test again elicits clicking, snapping, or pain. (The client may need to have support under the thigh in order to prevent compression of the patella during this test maneuver. We also recommend that this test be done in different positions to duplicate function and test different portions of the meniscus.)

Spring test. The spring test for tearing of the collateral ligaments is performed like the preceding tests. With the client in the supine position, the examiner attempts to extend the client's knee. In a "locked" knee, forceful extension may be prohibited because of a displaced meniscus. This results in a springy end feel as the pressure is released from the inhibited range. The knee "springs back" to the loose-packed position if impingement on the meniscus is minimal.

Functional assessment. The last portion of the objective examination for acute knee injury involves functional assessment. A systematic functional examination requires, first, that a client perform activities such as ambulating, ascending and descending stairs, making sudden movements, squatting, and hopping. The next step is to ask the individual to actually perform the specific movements required by his or her daily activities to allow the clinician to determine the client's ability to function in the presence of pain, limited motion, crepitus, and excessive motion. Functional stability, not just static stability, needs to be assessed because functional assessment is much more important than static assessment.

Foot examination. Following the basic knee examination, other tests should be done for foot posture and gait. All three are closely related in evaluating macrotraumatic and microtraumatic injuries of the knee.

Foot dysfunction can be either intrinsic or extrinsic. Intrinsic foot dysfunction can include either rearfoot or forefoot varus or valgus.[20,55,56] Extrinsic problems include limb-length differences and flexibility deficiencies.[40,59] If the foot dysfunction is extrinsic in origin, orthotic management normally does not provide a satisfactory result. Similarly, if the foot dysfunction is intrinsic, flexibility and strengthening exercises yield poor results.

Static foot examination must include tests for both intrinsic and extrinsic problems. A quick test for intrinsic, biomechanical dysfunction of the foot is to place the client in a long-sitting position with the feet relaxed and passively hanging in a plantar-flexed position, which places the subtalar joint in a neutral position. An index card or business card is then held perpendicular to the rear foot, which allows identification of forefoot varus or valgus.[40] With the client in the same position, evaluation of dermatologic response to forces should also be initiated. Common findings are that the client has callus formation on the medial aspect of the first metatarsal joint and the medial aspect of the first distal interphalangeal joint. Callus formation in either location is indicative of a pronated foot.[4] Asymmetric pronation or supination can be evaluated in a functional (standing) position by measuring from the floor superiorly to the distal tip of the medial or lateral malleolus with a business or index card, making a corresponding mark on the card.[4] If there is a right-left difference in terms of vertical dimension in measuring from the floor to the medial malleolus, the side that is closer to the floor is probably in excessive pronation. The final portion of the preliminary foot examination should include analysis of shoe wear. Normal wear patterns are symmetric and occur in normal areas. Wear should be on the posterior lateral aspect of the heel, and toe off should not be at the metatarsal head but rather over the first toe.

An examination of the external forces affecting the foot should include flexibility and limb-length examinations. The flexibility examination should include assessment of the gastrocnemius and soleus muscles with the subtalar joint in a neutral position.[59] Hamstring muscles, hip rotators, the iliotibial band, and hip flexors should also be tested for flexibility. We believe that limb-length assessment should be done in a functional position with measurement from the anterior superior iliac spine (ASIS) to the distal tip of the lateral malleolus, accompanied by palpation of the iliac crest and the posterior superior iliac spine (PSIS). When assessing limb length, note whether dysfunction of the foot, recurvatum of the knee, or sacroiliac involvement affects limb length.

Posture. Client posture has a profound effect on forces affecting the knee. Clients should be evaluated for toeing in and toeing out, genu recurvatum, forward pelvis, forward shoulders, and excessive cervical flexion.[25] Many of these factors are interrelated, and all must be resolved to rule out their involvement with the client's knee problems.

Gait evaluation. Gait evaluation serves as a final dynamic assessment of the client's lower extremity function. Initially, this examination should be done while the client is walking normally; however, this can progress to jogging, jogging in place, or sprinting. Observation at fast speeds, of course, is very difficult, and a videotape and treadmill apparatus are desirable. Gait evaluation should follow a thorough static evaluation that can give clinicians an indication of likely problems.

Specifically, the clinician doing a gait evaluation should have the client do multiple circuits on the gait path while observation for only one dysfunction per circuit is made. We recommend that the first and last strides be ignored.[4] The following specifics should be viewed during gait evaluation: toe in and out, vertical calcaneus and heel position, patella alignment in relationship to the second toe, patella alignment in the frontal plane, the amount of knee extension, equality of

heel flexion during the gait cycle, genu recurvatum, excessive medial roll of the navicular bone, and early heel off.

Reexamination

Any tests that were suspiciously negative or that the clinician was unsure were conducted correctly should be repeated on future client visits. It is important to retest the knee because pain, swelling, and protective splinting can often lead to a false negative response. Repeating or expanding the examination process may be necessary if an initially minimum objective examination was performed on the client. It is not unusual to discover additional client problems at a later time during the treatment process. If a test is found to be positive once and then negative on recheck, it is reasonable to assume that a pathologic condition exists.

Referral

If at any time the clinician is less than 100% certain of what tissues are involved or how severely they are affected, the client should be referred to another practitioner. If there is any change that requires medical intervention, the sooner the client is referred, the better. The only error that can be made by the clinician is lack of prudence. Any errors should be on the side of caution.

Medical practitioners can perform tests that are not available to the physical therapist to further differentiate the client's problem. Included in this testing battery are stress radiographs, arthrograms, magnetic resonance imaging, arthroscopy, aspiration of joint fluid for culturing, and other blood and laboratory tests. Knee pain can often be of systemic origin or referred from other joints.

Specialized examination by physical therapists

In some situations, a minimal examination is all that is required. The rationale for a minimal examination is multifaceted. Frequently the clinician is faced with time constraints, originating either from the client in question or from other causes. In this case doing a portion of the examination to allow commencement of the treatment is acceptable. A minimal examination can be defined as that which is required for client convenience, comfort, and safety.

Subjective examination. The subjective examination may allow for simplification of the objective examination— that is, common overuse injury may be more easily handled by a subjective examination than a traumatic football injury. In a client with the overuse injury, the knee may have just been examined by an orthopedist who specializes in knee disorders. However, if important client information (such as type of surgery) is missing, extreme caution is required in the performance of stressful tests that may be indicated.

Minimal objective examination. A minimal objective examination may be acceptable if the clinician wants to save the most painful test until last and selects only those tests that provide necessary information.

The minimal objective examination that should be done

on a client referred to physical therapy for rehabilitation should include range-of-motion testing; effusion, strength, and pain determination; and joint "clearing." The range-of-motion testing should include tests for accessory, passive physiologic, and active physiologic movements.[10,26,35]

The presence of a joint effusion is critical to determination of the rehabilitation program as it affects range of motion and strength.[12] In its presence, forcing range of motion and active exercise through the range of motion may be contraindicated. Tests that should be included are those involving palpation and objective measurement. (The ballottement[21] and "milking" tests that involve palpation have both been described previously.) Objective measurements should be recorded in metric terms presented in the record as right-to-left difference. We suggest using a measurement from the joint space (which is thus reproducible) and using distances of 9 cm above the joint space, 20 cm above the joint space, and 15 cm below the joint space as reference points for objective testing.

Strength testing should be performed to determine the client's ability to contract the muscle, difficulty in maintaining the contraction, and/or any gross muscular deficiency. In the minimal examination, manual muscle testing is generally used as a timesaving measure. Other more objective tests can be used in the complete examination at a later time.

The assessment of pain is subjective, yet a measure of objectivity can be added by asking the client to place the degree of pain on a scale. The clinician can use either a 10- or 100-point scale, but in any case some type of continuum is necessary. The type of pain (burning, aching, shooting, constant, episodic) should be noted. Other key factors to note are whether there is pain with activity or only after activity and whether there is pain with active, passive, and/or resistive motions.

A "joint-clearing" examination should be performed on all joints that may refer pain or mechanically influence the knee. The foot, ankle, hip, sacroiliac complex, and lumbar spine should be "cleared." The joint clearing examination typically involves the use of overpressure at the extreme range of motion.[21] A quick knee-screening examination consists of the spring test (collateral ligaments), drawer test (cruciate ligaments), and Lachman's test (anterior cruciate).

This minimal objective examination for the knee can be completed in less than 10 minutes and provides the clinician with a data base from which to initiate treatment.

ASSESSING AND TREATING RANGE-OF-MOTION DEFICIENCIES

Range-of-motion deficiencies are a common clinical problem. Unfortunately, the usual clinical approach is to resort to a simplistic approach of whirlpool treatments, forcing motion, weight lifting, and hoping that the problem will resolve. A better approach is to systematically evaluate the deficiency and select specific treatment techniques. A four-part evaluation scheme and several specific treatment techniques are recommended.

The purpose of the evaluation scheme is to determine the tissue or tissues responsible for motion deficiency and their degree of involvement. After this has been done, selection of the appropriate treatment techniques can be clarified. The final portion of the scheme is designed to determine when it is appropriate to begin restoration of movement to the affected joint. The system consists of testing for capsular patterns, end feels, glides, and pain-resistant sequences.

Testing for capsular patterns, first described by Cyriax,[11] refers to the fact that any joint with a capsular involvement has a predictable loss of range of motion. The capsular pattern for a knee disorder is a slight limitation of extension and a gross limitation of flexion. The typical knee with a capsular involvement might exhibit a 15-degree loss of extension and a 60-degree loss of knee flexion.

End feel, also described by Cyriax,[11] refers to the feeling imparted to the examiner's hands at the end of the range of motion. There are six types of end feels (Table 12-1). However, only two indicate conditions treatable through physical therapy intervention. In particular, capsular and spasm end feels may be rectifiable with capsular and muscle-tendon techniques.

The evaluation of joint glides has been emphasized by

Table 12-1. Range-of-motion end feels

Name	Description
Capsular	Leathery Example: normal glenohumeral external rotation
Spasm	Firm, contracting muscle Example: cramping muscle
Springy	Bounces back Example: internal joint derangement, "loose" bodies, "bucket handle" meniscus tear
Bone-on-bone	Hard, solid, unmovable Example: normal elbow extension
Tissue approximation	Further range of motion (ROM) impeded by opposition of two tissues Example: maximum knee flexion (posterior leg touches posterior thigh)
Empty	Feels like more movement is there, but it is unobtainable Example: metastasis with referred pain

Modified from Cyriax J: *Textbook of orthopaedic medicine*, vol 1, Baltimore, 1975, Williams & Wilkins.

Kaltenborn.[26] *Physiologic movement* refers to the joint movement that is under the client's active control. *Accessory movements* are movements necessary for normal joint function that are not under the client's active control. An example would be the gliding movement of the tibia posteriorly on the femur with knee flexion. A tight posterior capsule would limit the ability of the tibia to glide posteriorly. A listing of accessory movements of the knee can be found in Table 12-2.

A pain-resistance sequence has been proposed by Cyriax to determine if the joint is ready to have range of motion restored.[11] The three possibilities of pain resistance are pain before resistance, pain with resistance, and resistance before pain. This system signals a red, yellow, or green light directing the therapist toward appropriate action. Table 12-3 provides additional information regarding this.

This four-part system for evaluating range-of-motion deficiencies can be completed in less than 1 minute and provides the therapist with the information necessary to proceed with a safe and efficient treatment approach.

TREATMENT

Treatment of knee injuries can be directed at either the capsule, the muscle-tendon unit, or, on occasion, both. Selection of proper treatment techniques optimizes results. Positive results can be measured as an increase in range of motion without a concomitant increase in pain or effusion.

Passive joint mobilization for capsular problems

Capsular restriction requires use of capsular treatment techniques—that is, passive joint mobilization. Joint mobilization is directed at restoring accessory joint motion by selectively stretching the shortened tissues. Three principles serve as a basis for joint mobilization: hypomobility, the convex-concave principle, and the graded application of mobilization techniques.

Hypomobility of a joint during an accessory movement is evaluated by comparison to the opposite unaffected side. This evaluation can be classified by using the Paris scale (Table 12-4). The theory of convex versus concave joints simplifies the process of mobilization.[26] The knee joint is a concave joint because the concave bone (tibia) moves on the convex bone (femur). Concave joints are mobilized in the same direction; therefore, if knee flexion is restricted, the tibia would be mobilized posteriorly on the femur.

Maitland's gradation of movement allows the therapist to carefully control the force applied to the client.[12] If the system is followed carefully, the client should experience no discomfort, and no damage should be done to a surgeon's work. Maitland's system consists of four movements (Table 12-5).

The therapist normally begins with a grade I movement and progresses according to client tolerance. At the end of the treatment, the therapist returns through the system, ending with a grade I. This reversal minimizes posttreatment discomfort.

Muscle-tendon techniques for noncapsular problems

The spasm end feel and noncapsular patterns require muscle-tendon techniques. Numerous treatment techniques are available. The wise clinician selects the best technique—that is, the technique that produces results and can be used most easily by the client. Heat, ice, spray and stretch,

Table 12-2. Accessory movements at the knee

	Flexion	Extension
Patellar movement	Cephalic	Caudal
Tibial movement	Posterior internal rotation	Anterior external rotation

Modified from Kaltenborn F: *Mobilization of the extremity joints*, Oslo, 1976, Olaf Norbis Bokhandel.

Table 12-4. Classification of accessory movement

Classification	Status
0	Ankylosed
1	Very hypomobile
2	Slightly hypomobile
3	Normal
4	Slightly hypermobile
5	Very hypermobile
6	Unstable

Modified from Paris S: *The spinal lesion*, Christchurch, New Zealand, 1965, Pegasus.

Table 12-3. Pain-resistance sequence

Reaction to movement*	Joint status	Physical therapy action
Pain before resistance	Acute	Red light—no attempt should be made to gain ROM
Pain with resistance	Subacute	Yellow light—gentle attempt can be made to regain ROM, but should be done cautiously (vigorous attempts may revert joint to acute state)
Resistance before pain	Chronic	Green light—vigorous intervention may be necessary to restore ROM

Modified from Cyriax J: *Textbook of orthopaedic medicine*, vol 1, Baltimore, 1975, Williams & Wilkins.
*Refers to passive movement through physiologic range.

Table 12-5. Maitland's grades of movement

Grade	Description*
I	Small-amplitude movement at the beginning of the accessory range
II	Large-amplitude movement within the available range but not to either limit
III	Large-amplitude movement beginning and extending up to the end of the accessory range
IV	Small-amplitude movement at the end of the accessory range
V	A manipulation (a high-velocity thrust)

Modified from Maitland GD: *Vertebral manipulation*, London, 1968, Butterworth Publishers.
*All movements take place within the accessory range.

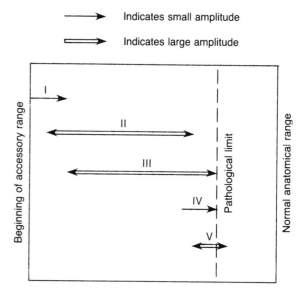

electricity, contract-relax, hold-relax, and active contractions are helpful techniques.

UNACCEPTABLE RESULTS

If treatment has not been initiated soon enough or if inappropriate techniques have been used, improvement may not result. There should be improvement during each treatment session, and the client at the next clinic visit should possess an equal—if not increased—range of motion.

If a knee will not move, transverse friction massage[10] and prolonged mechanical stretching may be used.[40] It should be remembered that some client's knees "can't move" because they are restricted by masses of adhesions. Two or three successive treatments without increase in range of movement should be considered a failure. Appropriate information should be conveyed to the referring physician, and consultation should be sought. We should not abuse but rather recognize our limitations of altering mature tissue.

Rehabilitation

Rehabilitation can best be viewed as a specified sequence of tasks performed to allow the accomplishment of desired activities. Therefore, rehabilitation must be individualized to fit the needs of each client by merging the goals and aspirations of the client, the physician, and the therapist.[38] Frequently this merger is neglected, and an unsuccessful outcome is the result. As stated previously, the sequence of activities should achieve functional progression, and this development is the responsibility of the physical therapist. Such an approach means that instead of following a "cookbook" system of rehabilitation, the physical therapist should follow a framework of parameters and phases of rehabilitation that can be used with a specific individual client.

Parameters of rehabilitation

Treating the total client. The client represents a complex entity that cannot be separated into distinct parts. Although it would be very convenient if a clinician could rehabilitate

a torn meniscus without dealing with the total client, it is doubtful that the rehabilitation process would be complete or fulfilling. Because each client possesses individual goals and aspirations, goal setting must involve examination and treatment of the total individual.

Psychologic and physiologic factors come together in this process to result in an acceptable social compromise. This compromise is an unwritten understanding of the intended outcome for treatment and rehabilitation. It is very effective to have a comprehensive plan of action outlining activities to allow accomplishment of the ultimate outcome. Monitoring intermediate accomplishments allows quantification of progress and a reorientation of activity when appropriate. Rehabilitation should be monitored much like an employee evaluation: results oriented rather than intention controlled.

Psychologic factors. Several psychologic factors must be addressed during rehabilitation. Client motivation is of primary importance and should be assessed through verbal and nonverbal means. It is not uncommon for an individual client to talk a good game while being frightened and apprehensive about returning to a stressful environment. This is particularly true when persons are involved in competitive activities that require a high degree of skill but also possess potential for injury or reinjury. Secondary gains are always a possibility in clients dealing with a specific injury. Each segment of society has determined a role model that the individual undergoing rehabilitation is expected to emulate. When an individual does not conform to the model, psychologic pressures may not allow successful rehabilitation.

Physiologic concerns. Physiologic concerns include the range of motion, accessory joint motions, inflammation, and effusion considerations discussed before. Additional factors, such as tissue damage and healing, immobilization, articular cartilage maintenance, and musculotendinous maintenance and strengthening, are also of primary importance and must be addressed in the rehabilitation process.[34]

CASE 1	Rehabilitation of an Athlete

A.E., a 21-year-old running back, sustained a significant (first to second degree) sprain of the medial collateral complex. As he was uncomfortable in full extension with weight bearing, he was provided with crutches and allowed to increase weight bearing as tolerated. Because he had a solid end point during examination but was quite tender with significant muscle inhibition, he wore an immobilizer when performing activities of daily living. He removed the immobilizer 4 or 5 times daily to permit ROM exercise. Once daily he performed isotonic strengthening (open and closed chain) in a protective ROM (20 to 70 degrees). He did hourly lower extremity isometrics. He was to maintain weight bearing to tolerance, and a general maintenance program for cardiovascular and other nonrelated muscle groups was followed. At 1 week, range-of-motion exercises, strengthening and endurance training, full weight bearing, and specific work to the active stabilizers were performed. This phase lasted for ap proximately 1 week and incorporated the early portions of a

functional progression. Two weeks of additional rehabilitation followed, involving a typical functional progression sequence including strengthening and endurance activities, specific activities of the sport, with an emphasis on the development of neuromuscular integrity.

A typical functional progression chart for this type of client would appear as follows:
1. Immobilization (when required)—primary healing
2. Range of motion (when required)—protected
3. Strengthening—endurance activities
4. Activities—progressive weight bearing, balance activities, proprioceptive redevelopment, functional strengthening, walk-jog sequence, jog-run sequence, hopping-jumping sequence, cutting sequence, sprinting sequence, agility drills, specific activities related to the sport of football
5. Return to sport

CASE 2	Rehabilitation of a Nonathlete

H.H., a 21-year-old mail carrier, slipped on wet pavement and sprained the medial collateral complex of her right knee. The mode of treatment was very similar to that used on the running back, but the functional progression was quite different. The initial stages of the progression were the same, but the advanced levels differed greatly. She was treated during the early phase exactly the same as the athlete. The early mobilization period saw emphasis placed on regaining range of motion and strength and on allowing progressive weight bearing.

In discussions with the client, the clinician should try to design a functional progression that involves balance activities, proprioception development, and functional strengthen-

ing, without placing emphasis on the advanced activities involved in a cutting sequence or sprinting. Thus the goals and aspirations of the client involve a return to the work environment, not to an athletic environment.

What follows is the functional progression outlined for the second client:
1. Immobilization (immobilizer)—primary healing
2. Range of motion—protected
3. Strengthening—endurance activities
4. Progressive weight bearing
5. Activities—proprioceptive redevelopment, functional strengthening, walk-jog sequence, hopping-jumping sequence, return to work environment

Phase concept. An effective method of integrating physiologic factors with physiologic parameters into a comprehensive rehabilitation protocol is to use a "phase" concept. Several different phase systems have been discussed in the literature.[24,36] We recommend a five-phase system that is comprehensive:

1. Phase 1 is termed the *maximum protection period* and includes treating inflammation, achieving primary tissue healing, and maintaining function.
2. Phase 2 is described as the *moderate protection period,* and its primary concerns are tissue maturation, strengthening, endurance, and protected development.
3. Phase 3 is known as the *minimum protection phase* and consists of determining the time segment needed to deal with tissue maturation/reorientation, basic light functional activity, and skill reacquisition/acquisition.

4. Phase 4 is the *advanced level of rehabilitation* and includes functional progression and a return to a skilled or demanding environment.
5. Phase 5 is referred to as the *maintenance period* and involves consistent effort to avoid the in-season/out-of-season trauma that is frequently seen with the "weekend warrior."

An interesting evolution of this process can be seen in the treatment of patients having undergone anterior cruciate ligament reconstruction.[2]

Exercise prescriptions. Exercise prescriptions must provide progressive stress on maturing tissues while also allowing a gradual increase in functional demands on noninvolved structures.[38] A common mistake in rehabilitation is to deal only with the injury and not provide adequate protection or attention to other related structures. The ability of the musculotendinous unit to generate tension and to function repeatedly is dictated by the complex interaction of functional demands. Inactivity not only affects the articular, bony, and ligamentous tissues but also greatly decreases the contractile element capabilities. A too-rapid increase in activity during rehabilitation often results in problems with a contractile-related element rather than the feared articular or ligamentous tissue involvement. In knee rehabilitation, patellar tendinitis is frequently observed in clients who are moved too quickly into too demanding an activity.

Rehabilitation protocols. Incorporating all the previously discussed features of the rehabilitation process, the development of functional progression allows the therapist to individualize the rehabilitation program to fit the needs of the individual client.[61] Functional progression is ideal because it not only outlines for the therapist what is expected but also dictates what is expected of the client. Monitoring the rehabilitation process is greatly facilitated by this process, as pain, swelling, and client apprehension are the parameters used to guide progression.

In order to describe the use of a functional progression in the rehabilitation of clients with different needs, two examples are presented.

The sequencing for these activities should involve an increase in speed from approximately half speed through full speed. The athlete should participate at four or five of the levels in a functional progression at any one time. This means performing at half speed a later portion of one phase of the sequence while performing at full speed at lower levels. The athlete should be able to perform the activity without an increase in symptoms with careful monitoring of pain and swelling. Client apprehension is another element that should always be monitored. It should be remembered that pain and swelling can be residual or acute.

Proprioceptive activities should commence as soon as weight bearing is permitted. These activities include weight bearing on both lower extremities, followed by individual extremity weight bearing. Weight shifting and the incorporation of proprioceptive boards (multiplanar and uniplanar) should begin as soon as permitted. Proprioception should be performed with the eyes open and closed to more accurately simulate the environment in which the athlete may be participating.

Of primary importance to the rehabilitation of a running back is the cutting sequence. The cutting sequence begins with general figure-eight running with an increase in speed and a decrease in the size of the figure eights. The cutting sequence proper involves the athlete running to a predetermined position, planting, and then cutting with a crossover or normal cut. These cuts should be at half to three-quarter speed and should increase until the individual is able to perform them at full speed. The final feature of these cutting sequences should involve the athlete cutting on command to either the right or the left, which much more closely simulates the environment to which the individual is attempting to return.

As the athlete proceeds through the sequence with increasing speed and effectiveness, protected activities can give way to a less protected environment. This less protected situation is typically termed the "dummy" activity and is often a portion of most football practice sessions. From the dummy activity, the athlete can proceed to a controlled scrimmage environment and finally to live scrimmage where teammates are the enemy! Although this is a game situation, there is still a degree of individual control. This sequencing allows the athlete to become acclimated to the competitive environment, thus gaining the confidence necessary to allow the final step in the process—safe return to the competitive sport.

Functional progression. The rehabilitative sequence for each and every client should be individualized to fulfill the needs of that client. As physical therapists attempt to develop rehabilitation protocols to meet specific pathologic conditions or surgical procedures, the functional progression outline can be easily modified to fit those conditions. By integrating healing constraints, phases of rehabilitation, and individual goals and aspirations, a well-defined rehabilitation progression emerges. Discussion of individual conditions and procedures is beyond the scope of this chapter. The following guidelines are presented only as basic tenets to be used in any rehabilitation program. Individual conditions and modes of exercise are presented to provide a general clinical framework for physical therapy management of knee problems.

Conservative management. Conservative management means noninvasive management of a particular condition. It typically involves monitoring of inflammation and determining range of motion, tissue reaction, swelling, and general response of the client to treatment. It is important not to neglect the overall maintenance of physiologic function in noninvolved structures during conservative management. The therapist should attempt to develop a balance between external forces and internal forces during this period to allow appropriate resolution of the condition. It is important to remember that many of the concepts of conservative management are incorporated into follow-up care for surgical management. Thus the application of proper procedures and consistent monitoring of client progress are necessary in both conservative and surgical management. Conservative management is an outgrowth or continuation of surgical treatment.

Exercise. Three basic forms of exercise are incorporated in the vast majority of rehabilitation programs. Isometric contractions are familiar to physical therapists as an early mode of intervention. Isometrics can be used at various points in the range of motion, thus giving much more effective functional results, and can be used throughout the rehabilitation process rather than only during the acute or immobilization phases. Isotonic weight lifting involves moving a weight through a range of motion at approximately 60 degrees per second. Its effectiveness has been well documented, and its uses are obvious. Isokinetic rehabilitation has received great attention in the recent past. It allows much higher speeds of exercise (several hundred degrees per second), thus more closely approaching functional speed. We recommend that all forms of muscular activity be used in a rehabilitation program to allow a true integration of function. We further recommend that weight lifting follow a progression very similar to that which is compatible with fibrous healing: The individual is not subjected to maximal stress but rather undertakes a sequence of lifting involving submaximal work. A limited range of motion is first used, progressing to full range of motion at submaximal levels, finally culminating in unrestricted range of motion with maximal effort. This sequence should obviously be modified according to the specific disorder treated, such as limiting terminal extension when dealing with patients presenting with certain cruciate instabilities or patellar subluxation and/or dislocation.

Flexibility. In all clients with knee instability, it is important to maintain flexibility in related muscle groups. The gastrocnemius-soleus complex, the femoral quadriceps (rectus femoris), the hamstring musculature, the tensor fascia latae (IT band), hip rotators, hip adductors, and hip abductors are examples of muscle groups that must be of appropriate length for normal mobility. Flexibility exercises are incorporated in the functional progression that involves both warm-up and cool-down processes. Static flexibility exercises are primarily used as a warm-up to involve affected muscle groups before heavy functional activity. Often an active ROM stretching progression is recommended.

SURGICAL MANAGEMENT

Surgical intervention is necessary for a condition that will not resolve through physiologic healing. Most orthopedic surgeons allow a conservative trial before surgical intervention in a large number of cases. If conservative management fails to resolve the condition, surgical treatment is indicated. One of the more exciting advances in surgical management of knee conditions has been the tremendous increase in the use of the arthroscope. The arthroscope allows a fairly benign comprehensive examination of the interior of the knee joint, in which some disorders can be arthroscopically corrected. The list of conditions treated by arthroscopic surgery continues to increase rapidly because of increasing surgeon awareness and skill acquisition.

Specific pathologies

Meniscus lesions. Meniscus lesions are typically corrected by surgery either arthroscopically or through an open arthrotomy. Initial care is dictated by the type of surgery and the specific details of the client's condition. The physical therapist should be aware of the client's general status before surgery, how much of the meniscus was removed or repaired, whether protection is needed or mobility is allowed, what levels of stress will be placed on the structure by the client, and the long-term goals for this particular individual. It is imperative for the therapist and surgeon to communicate

regarding the actual level and type of surgery as well as the precautions to be followed during rehabilitation.

As a therapist proceeds through a functional progression treating a client with a meniscus condition, it is important to minimize compressive loading of the tibia until adequate muscular protection and joint reorganization have been developed. This frequently means substituting more rapid running for shorter distances for jogging. We recommend mid-ROM (20 to 70 degrees) work to minimize rotational stress, or, early in the rehabilitation program, this type of loading can be minimized by substituting bicycling or swimming. It is important to make athletic individuals aware that the injured knee may develop a slight degree of swelling when heavy repetitive activities are performed. Typically, this is true for football players who practice 2 or 3 times a day. The athlete may complain of swelling toward the end of the day during summer practice, with resolution of the condition seen as practices become less frequent.

Ligamentous repairs. Ligamentous repairs require rapid surgical intervention to reposition or stabilize damaged tissues. Rehabilitative constraints should be based upon the actual procedure done and the structure involved. The therapist must be aware of what tissues have been violated in reaching the involved structure and what activities can be used to minimize stress or to increase stress on the damaged but healing tissues. A similar process should be followed for a ligamentous reconstruction. Reconstructions are usually performed later (usually after resolution of acute inflammation with a return of a complete ROM) and involve the substitution of a different tissue for a damaged structure. The rehabilitative protocol must be based on the structure used and what is going to be demanded of that tissue. The same rationale for stressing the tissue or minimizing stress to the tissue dictates the development of the program.

Key factors in rehabilitating ligamentous tissues involve biomechanically analyzing the stresses that will be placed on the joint and the developing tissues and designing a rehabilitation program to allow progressive stress. Progressive stresses allow normalization (reorganization) or maturation along lines of stress, thus providing the strongest tissue possible. An example of this process involves emphasizing exercise of the hamstring muscles in anterior cruciate–deficient knee disorders. Anterior cruciate repairs or reconstructions typically demand a rehabilitation protocol that minimizes open chain quadriceps muscle activity that attempts to anteriorly translate the tibia. This involves using closed-chain sequences, and mid-range open chain quadriceps muscle work, not using progressive resistance open chain terminal extension, and emphasizing hamstring muscle strengthening to provide active stabilization.[2]

Patellofemoral problems. Patellofemoral problems are often related to compressive syndromes of the articular surface of the patella. The overused term *chondromalacia patellae* has been used frequently to describe patellofemoral arthritis and patellofemoral compressive syndromes. To minimize compressive loading of the patella, it is recommended that terminal exercises, quadriceps-setting in extension, and straight-leg raises be used early in rehabilitation. As an individual improves, incorporation of weight loading (isometrics at specific points in the range of motion) and high-speed isokinetic exercises are often quite effective. An isokinetic progression should proceed from submaximal to maximal loading. It is important to recognize compression problems are not always the cause of anterior knee pain. Often these patients must be exercised lower in the ROM to maintain proper recruitment and stability (i.e., patients with subluxating patellas).

Tendinitis conditions. The tendon is a portion of the musculotendinous unit. Often the actual lesion is degenerative and is better described as tendinosis as inflammation is no longer primary. It is our experience that an eccentric emphasis is demanded of these patients, and recovery is somewhat slow, often requiring 12 weeks. We have frequently seen patellar tendonitis in clients who have been asked to perform high-speed or high-resistance work before the tissue is ready for such stresses. Thus it is very important not to ask clients to perform high-repetitive stress activities, such as high-speed isokinetics, with maximal effort until the individual is physiologically capable of handling such activities. These activities should progress as gradual overload stresses on the client, while clinical signs and symptoms are continually reassessed.

Articular conditions. Articular cartilage represents a unique tissue that requires mobility for nourishment, yet is frequently damaged by compressive/shear combination loading. Articular cartilage often responds quite positively to high-speed isokinetic exercise. This is typically performed at submaximal levels and probably is effective because of decreased compressive loading of a short duration and improved nutrition. However, this view is speculative and represents only initial clinical judgment.

SUMMARY

Our intention has been to present a concept of phased rehabilitation, which develops into an all-encompassing progression of activity termed *functional progression.* Rehabilitation is a multifaceted activity that involves the individual aspirations of all parties involved. The meshing of these goals is required if rehabilitation is to be successful. Rehabilitation can thus be viewed as a progression into function.

REVIEW QUESTIONS

1. What are the functions of the anterior cruciate and posterior cruciate ligaments?
2. When the lower extremity is in a closed chain, what factors influence the development of knee disorders, especially patellofemoral dysfunction?
3. What is the difference between structural and functional predispositions to knee injury?
4. What palpation procedures should be included in the physical examination to evaluate an *acute* knee injury?
5. State four important rules that should be observed in performing a joint stability examination of the knee complex.

REFERENCES

1. Abott HC, Kress JB: *Preconditioning in the prevention of knee injuries,* 1969, Physical Medicine and Rehabilitation Association.
2. ACL surgery and rehabilitation (special section), *J Orthop Sports Phys Ther* 15:256, 1992.
3. Basmajian J: *Muscles alive: their functions, revised by electromyography,* Baltimore, 1962, Williams & Wilkins.
4. Beckman S: Pronation syndrome. Paper presented at the Podiatric Physical Therapy Conference, La Crosse, Wis, 1980.
5. Bender JA: Factors affecting the occurrence of knee injuries, *J Am Phys Med Rehabil* 18:537, 1964.
6. Blyth CS: Football injury survey: I, *Phys Sports Med* 2, 1975.
7. Brattstrom H: Shape of the intercondylar groove normally and in recurrent dislocations of the patella, *Acta Orthop Scand* 8:226, 1964.
8. Cahill BR, Griffin EH: Effect of pre-season conditioning on the incidence and severity of high school football knee injuries, *Am J Sports Med* 6:372, 1978.
9. Cameron B, Davis O: The swivel football shoe: a controlled study, *Am J Sports Med* 1:2, 1973.
10. Cyriax J: *Textbook of orthopaedic medicine,* vol 2, ed 8, Baltimore, 1975, Williams & Wilkins.
11. Cyriax J: *Textbook of orthopaedic medicine,* vol 1, ed 8, Baltimore, 1975, Williams & Wilkins.
12. De Andrade JR, Grant C, Dixon SJ: Joint distension and reflex muscle inhibition in the knee, *J Bone Joint Surg Am* 47:313, 1965.
13. Ellison A, producer: Ski injuries, New Brunswick, NJ, 1972, Johnson & Johnson Co (film).
14. Evans PJ, Bell GD, Frank C: Prospective evaluation of the McMurray test, *Am J Sports Med* 21:604, 1993.
15. Frankel VH, Nordin M: *Basic biomechanics of the skeletal system,* Philadelphia, 1980, Lea & Febiger.
16. Girgis FG, Marshall JL, Almonajem RS: The cruciate ligaments of the knee joint: anatomical, functional, and experimental analysis, *Clin Orthop* 106:216, 1975.
17. Gould J: Spinal evaluation and treatment; course taught at Cleveland State University, March 1980.
18. Gray H: *Gray's anatomy,* Philadelphia, 1974, Lea & Febiger.
19. Harner CD et al: Loss of motion after anterior cruciate ligament reconstruction, *Am J Sports Med* 20:499, 1992.
20. Hlavek H: *The foot book,* Mountain View, Calif, 1977, World Publications.
21. Hoppenfeld S: *Physical examination of the spine and extremities,* New York, 1976, Appleton-Century-Crofts.
22. Hughston JC et al: Classification of knee ligament instabilities I and II, *J Bone Joint Surg Am* 58:159, 1976.
23. Hughston JC: *Knee ligaments,* St Louis, 1993, Mosby.
24. James A: Rehabilitation for anterior instability of the knee, *J Orthop Sports Phys Ther* 3:121, 1982.
25. James SC, Brubaker CE: Biomechanics of running, *Orthop Clin North Am* 4:3, 1973.
26. Kaltenborn F: *Mobilization of the extremity joints,* Oslo, 1976, Olaf Norlis Bokhandel.
27. Kaufer H: Mechanical function of the patella, *J Bone Joint Surg Am* 53:1153, 1971.

28. Kennedy JC, editor: *The injured adolescent knee,* Baltimore, 1979, Williams & Wilkins.

29. Klein K: Knee injuries. Paper presented at the Second Annual Physician-Therapist Conference, Chicago, December 1981.

30. Klein K, Allman FC: *The knee in sports,* Austin, Tex, 1969, Jenkins.

31. Larson RL: *Subluxation-dislocation of the patella.* In Kennedy J, editor: *The injured adolescent knee,* Baltimore, 1962, Williams & Wilkins.

32. Lieb FJ, Perry J: An anatomical and mechanical study using amputated limbs, *J Bone Joint Surg Am* 50:1535, 1968.

33. Lieb FJ, Perry J: Quadriceps function: an EMG study under isometric conditions, *J Bone Joint Surg Am* 53:749, 1971.

34. Light K, Kuzik S, Personius W: Low-load versus high-load brief stretch in treatment of knee contractures. Paper presented at the annual meeting of the American Physical Therapy Association, Anaheim, Calif, 1982.

35. Maitland GD: *Vertebral manipulation,* London, 1968, Butterworth Publishers.

36. Malek MM, Mangine RE: Patellofemoral pain syndromes: a comprehensive and conservative approach, *J Orthop Sports Phys Ther* 2:108, 1981.

37. McLaughlin R: Personal communication, March 1975.

38. Mennell J: *Joint pain,* Boston, 1974, Little, Brown.

39. Mitchell F, Moran P, Pruzzo N: *An evaluation and treatment manual of osteopathic muscle energy procedures,* Valley Park, Mo, 1979, American Osteopathic Medicine Association.

40. Nicholas JA: A study of thigh muscle weakness in different pathological states of the lower extremity, *Am J Sports Med* 4:241, 1976.

41. Noyes FR: Functional properties of knee ligaments and alterations induced by immobilization: a correlative biomechanical and histological study in primates, *Clin Orthop* 123:210, 1977.

42. Noyes FR, Delucas JL, Torvik PJ: Biomechanics of anterior cruciate ligament failure in primates. *J Bone Joint Surg Am* 56:236, 1974.

43. Noyes FR, Delucas JL, Torvik PJ: Biomechanics of ligament failure II: an analysis of immobilization, exercise, and reconditioning effects in primates, *J Bone Joint Surg Am* 56:1406, 1974.

44. Noyes FR et al: Effect of intra-articular corticosteroids on ligament properties: a biomechanical and histological study in rhesus knees, *Clin Orthop* 123:197, 1977.

45. Noyes FR et al: Arthroscopy in acute traumatic hemarthrosis of the knee: incidence of anterior cruciate tears and other injuries, *J Bone Joint Surg Am* 62:687, 1980.

46. Noyes FR et al: Clinical biomechanics of the knee: ligament restraints and functional stability. In Funk J, editor: *American Academy of Orthopaedic Surgeons: symposium on the athlete's knee,* St Louis, 1980, Mosby.

47. Oberlander MA, Shalvoy RM, Hughston JC: The accuracy of the clinical knee examination documented by arthroscopy: a prospective study, *Am J Sports Med* 21:773, 1993.

48. O'Donoghue DH: *Treatment of injuries to athletes,* Philadelphia, 1976, WB Saunders.

49. Outerbridge RE: The etiology of chondromalacia patellae, *J Bone Joint Surg Br* 44:752, 1961.

50. Paris S: *The spinal lesion,* Christchurch, New Zealand, 1965, Pegasus.

51. Slocum DB: Rotary instabilities of the knee. In Funk J, editor: *American Academy of Orthopaedic Surgeons: symposium on sports medicine,* St Louis, 1969, Mosby.

52. Slocum DB, Larson RF: Rotary instability of the knee, *J Bone Joint Surg Am* 50:211, 1968.

53. Smillie IS: *Injuries of the knee joint,* Edinburgh, 1970, Churchill Livingstone.

54. Spencer A: *Practical podiatric orthopaedic procedures,* Cleveland, 1978, Ohio College of Podiatric Medicine.

55. Subotnick SL: *Podiatric sports medicine,* Mt Kisco, NY, 1975, Futura.

56. Subotnick SL: Biomechanics of the ankle. Paper presented at the annual meeting of the American Physical Therapy Association, Phoenix, June 1980.

57. Tipton C, James SL, Mergner W: Influence of exercise on the strength of the medial collateral ligaments of dogs, *Am J Phys Med* 218:894, 1970.

58. Torg JS et al: Clinical diagnosis of anterior cruciate ligament instability in the athlete, *Am J Sports Med* 4:84, 1976.

59. Wallace L: Lower quarter pathomechanics. Paper presented at the Mississippi Sports Physical Therapy Association, Jackson, Miss, February 1982.

60. Wallace L: Rehabilitation of patellofemoral problems. Paper presented at the annual meeting of the American Physical Therapy Association, Anaheim, Calif, June 1982.

61. Wallace L, Davies GJ: Knee rehabilitation. In Davies GJ, editor: *Isokinetics in clinical usage,* ed 3, Onalaska, Wis, 1987, S & S.

62. Wallace L, McKitrick B: Balance testing as a prediction of knee injuries. Paper presented at the annual meeting of the American Physical Therapy Association, Anaheim, Calif, June 1982.

63. Wyke B: The neurology of joints, *Ann R Coll Surg Engl* 41:25, 1967.

SUGGESTED READING

Anatomy/Evaluation/Surgery

Hughston JC., *Knee ligaments: injury and repair,* St Louis, 1993, Mosby–Year Book.

Feagin JA, editor: *The crucial ligaments,* ed 2, New York, 1994, Churchill Livingstone.

Scott WN, editor: *The knee,* St Louis, 1994, Mosby.

Basic Science/Biomechanics

Daniel D, Akeson W, O'Connor J, editors: *Knee ligaments: structure, function, injury and repair,* New York, 1990, Raven.

Knee Rehabilitation

Greenfield BH, editor: *Rehabilitation of the knee: a problem solving approach,* Philadelphia, 1993, FA Davis.

Griffin LY, editor: *Rehabilitation of the injured knee,* ed 2, St Louis, 1995, Mosby.

Mangine RE, editor: *Physical therapy of the knee,* ed 2, New York, 1995, Churchill Livingstone.

CHAPTER 13

The Wrist and Hand

Carolyn Wadsworth

OUTLINE

Clinical anatomy and mechanics of the wrist and hand
  Osteology
  Arthrology
  Soft tissue relationships and mechanics
  Neurology
  Angiology
Examination procedures specific to the wrist and hand
  History
  Physical examination
Pathologic conditions and treatment guidelines
  The rheumatoid hand
  Insidious conditions and cumulative trauma disorders
  Acute hand injuries
  Work hardening
Joint mobilization techniques for the wrist and hand
Case study
Summary

KEY TERMS

wrist	examination
hand	rheumatoid hand
biomechanics	cumulative trauma disorders
distal radioulnar joint	

LEARNING OBJECTIVES

After studying this chapter, the reader should be able to:

1. Identify significant anatomical structures of the wrist and hand complex.
2. Describe the joint mechanics of the wrist and hand articulations.
3. State the functions of the arches of the hand.
4. Discuss the clinical ramifications of the "multi-joint" muscles crossing the wrist and hand.
5. List the extrinsic and intrinsic muscles of the hand.
6. Describe and list all of the components of a physical examination of the wrist and hand complex.
7. State four criteria that should be satisfied in order to conclude the physical examination.
8. Describe the pathomechanics and deformities associated with the rheumatoid hand.
9. List and describe the insidious conditions and cumulative trauma disorders that can affect the wrist and hand.
10. Discuss the role of physical therapy in the rehabilitation of acute and chronic injuries of the wrist and hand.

To evaluate and treat wrist and hand disorders competently, therapists must understand the anatomy, mechanics, pathokinesiology, and diseases of this precisely balanced part of the body. In addition, they should recognize the manifestations of injury, the healing process, and the patient's response to treatment. Therapists must also possess the technical skills needed to administer manual examination and treatment.

This chapter describes the fundamental functions of, and interactions between, the numerous structures that comprise the wrist and hand. It presents the etiology and clinical manifestations of common hand pathology. It also instructs the reader in applying the specific examination techniques and treatments necessary to restore this area to harmonious function.

CLINICAL ANATOMY AND MECHANICS OF THE WRIST AND HAND
Osteology

The radius, ulna, and 27 bones of the hand proper (excluding sesamoids) comprise the wrist and hand skeleton (Fig. 13-1). The distal radius displays a broad, concave, articular surface, marked by shallow depressions where it contacts the scaphoid and lunate bones. Laterally, the radial styloid process projects distally, where it limits radial deviation of the wrist to 15° to 20°. Medially, the ulnar notch indents the radius, providing a concave articular surface for junction with the ulnar head. Dorsally, Lister's tubercle protrudes near the center of the bone, forming a pulley around which the extensor pollicis longus (EPL) tendon passes.

The ulna expands slightly at its distal end, terminating in a convex ulnar head, and styloid process at its distal-most medial aspect. The ulnar styloid process is ½-in shorter than the radial styloid process, permitting ulnar deviation of 30° to 40°.

Anatomists commonly classify the bones of the hand into three parts: the phalanges, metacarpus, and carpus, according to similarities in structure and function (Fig. 13-1). The 14 *phalanges* resemble miniature long bones, with shafts and expanded ends. Their proximal ends, the bases, are concave. The bases of the middle and distal phalanges display two

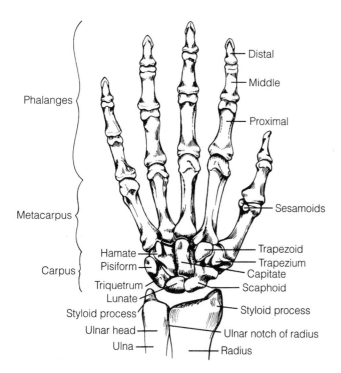

Fig. 13-1. Volar view of hand skeleton.

shallow depressions that fit the corresponding pulley-shaped heads of adjacent phalanges. The bases of the proximal phalanges differ in that they possess biconcave surfaces to articulate with the rounded metacarpal heads. The heads, at the distal ends of the proximal and middle phalanges, bear two small condyles and form the convex components of the interphalangeal (IP) joints. The heads of the distal phalanges taper into blunt points at the fingertips.

Five bones, also exhibiting elongated shafts and expanded ends, comprise the *metacarpus*. The bases of metacarpals 2 through 5 articulate with the distal row of carpal bones in the common carpometacarpal joint and with one another. Their convex distal heads are rounded rather than pulley-shaped like the phalanges. They articulate in the biaxial metacarpophalangeal (MP) joints, which possess more mobility but less bony stability than the IP joints. The first metacarpal, unlike the others, has a saddle-shaped base that articulates with the trapezium in the trapeziometacarpal (first carpometacarpal [CMC]) joint. The first metacarpal head is pulley-shaped, resembling the phalanges.

The bones of the *carpus* lie in two transverse rows, with four bones in each row. The distal row includes (lateral to medial) the trapezium, trapezoid, capitate, and hamate; the proximal row contains the scaphoid, lunate, triquetrum, and pisiform. The trapezium possesses a tubercle for the attachment of the flexor retinaculum, a groove for the flexor carpi radialis (FCR) tendon, and a saddle-shaped facet for articulation with the first metacarpal. The trapezoid, wedged between the trapezium and capitate, is the smallest bone in the distal row. The capitate, the largest and most centrally located carpal, articulates with seven other bones, and from it most of the intercarpal ligaments radiate. The hamate possesses an easily identifiable hooklike hamulus, which offers protection for the ulnar artery and nerve and a site of attachment of the flexor retinaculum. The scaphoid occupies the proximal row of carpals but actually bridges the midcarpal joint between the two rows. It receives forces transmitted through the radius when the arm supports the body weight and is thus commonly fractured in falls. Because of deficient circulation to the proximal pole of the scaphoid, a fracture through the waist or proximal pole of the bone often results in avascular necrosis, delayed union, or nonunion.[23,52] The scaphoid displays a prominent tubercle to which the flexor retinaculum attaches. The lunate, named for its semilunar shape, is the most commonly dislocated carpal, an injury that has potentially serious consequences if unreduced because of the bone's proximity to the median nerve. The triquetrum is three-sided and possesses a facet for articulation with the pisiform. The pea-shaped pisiform is the smallest carpal but has multiple attachments, including the flexor and extensor retinacula, pisohamate and pisometacarpal ligaments, and tendons of the flexor carpi ulnaris (FCU) and abductor digiti minimi (ADM) muscles.

Three volarly concave arches emerge from the arrangement of the wrist and hand bones to enhance prehensile function. The *longitudinal arch* spans the hand lengthwise, and two lateral arches run transversely, one at the level of the metacarpal heads and the other at the carpus. The flexible *metacarpal arch* is controlled by action of the intrinsic muscles, particularly the thenar and hypothenar muscles; it assists grasping and pinching functions. The relatively stable *carpal arch* forms a base for finger motion and the floor of the *carpal tunnel.* This tunnel serves as a conduit for the nine extrinsic flexor tendons of the fingers and thumb and the median nerve (Fig. 13-2).

When one views the hand from the radial side, the volar projections of the scaphoid and trapezium tubercles are prominent. They form the lateral boundary of the carpal tunnel and in addition provide a supporting base for the thumb in a plane that allows it to oppose the rest of the hand. The importance of thumb opposition to the grasping ability of the hand cannot be overemphasized. Disability compensation schemes attribute 50% of the value of the hand to the thumb.[15]

An ulnar view reveals the volar projections of the pisiform and hamulus, which form the medial boundary of the carpal tunnel. Another tunnel, the *distal ulnar tunnel,* conveys the ulnar artery and nerve. It lies between the hamate and pisiform, with the flexor retinaculum, pisohamate, and pisometacarpal ligaments forming its floor, and the palmar (volar) carpal ligament, palmaris brevis muscle, and the palmar aponeurosis forming its roof.

Arthrology

Distal radioulnar joint. The distal radioulnar joint contributes to both wrist and forearm function (Fig. 13-3). It is a double-pivot type of joint, connecting the distal ulna and radius and the ulna and articular disc. In an anatomical position, with the forearm supinated, the radius lies lateral and parallel to the ulna. During forearm pronation the concave ulnar notch of the radius sweeps around the convex ulnar head, bringing the distal radius into a medial position, while the proximal end remains lateral. During pronation and supination, the ulna also moves slightly, opposite to the direction of the radius (i.e., during pronation, the ulna moves

in a posterolateral and distal direction).[38] In conjunction with the proximal radioulnar joint, the distal radioulnar joint produces up to 170° of forearm rotation. Joint play movements include anterior and posterior glide of the radius and ulna on one another.

The articular disc unites the radius to the ulna. Fibrous bands that extend into the anterior and posterior radioulnar capsule reinforce the articulation. The base of the disc attaches to the medial radial margin, and its apex attaches to the ulnar styloid process. It is thicker peripherally but thins in its center, an area that is commonly perforated with injury or aging. The biconcave disc articulates proximally with the ulna and distally with the proximal carpal row, primarily the triquetrum, separating the ulna from the direct contact with the carpals. Anatomists refer to the components of the ulnomeniscotriquetral articulation as the triangular fibrocartilage complex (TFCC). The TFCC includes the capsular ligaments, the ulnar collateral ligament, the disc, and the ECU tendon sheath.

An articular capsule encloses the distal radioulnar joint, preventing its communication with the radiocarpal joint. The capsule is quite loose and does not provide support to the joint or limit its movement.[3] A synovial cavity extends from the ulnar head proximally between the bones, terminating in a pouchlike process, the *recessus sacciformis.*

Carpal joints. The carpus links the forearm and hand by a series of intercalated segments whose composite movement surpasses that of its individual parts. This innovative design produces extensive range of motion (ROM) but can lead to instability when injury or disease weakens supporting ligaments.

Short intercarpal ligaments bind the carpal bones firmly on their dorsal and volar surfaces, and deeper interosseous ligaments join the individual bones to one another. The carpals articulate in synovial joints and can be passively moved in relation to each other. The joint capsule and interosseus ligaments divide the synovial cavity of the wrist into the separate joints described in the following (Fig. 13-3).

The *radiocarpal joint* is the articulation between the

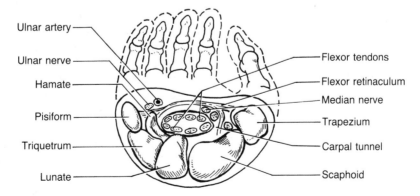

Fig. 13-2. The median nerve and extrinsic flexor tendons of the hand occupy the carpal tunnel bounded by the carpus dorsally and the flexor retinaculum volarly.

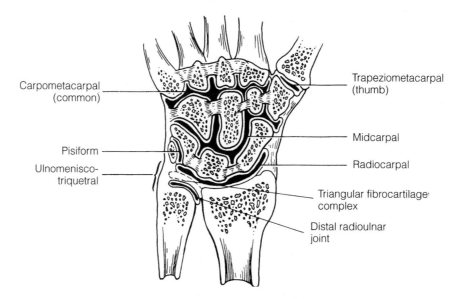

Fig. 13-3. Joints of the carpus.

convex proximal row of carpal bones and the concave radius and disc. The *midcarpal joint* lies between the distal and proximal rows of carpals; it is a *compound articulation* in which each row acts as a unit and each has both a convex and concave articulating portion. Together, the radiocarpal and midcarpal joints produce the movements that occur at the biaxial wrist joint: flexion, extension, radial deviation, and ulnar deviation.

The approximate ROM of the wrist is 80° of extension, 85° of flexion, 20° of radial deviation, and 35° of ulnar deviation. The position of the fingers, however, may influence this range because the length of the extrinsic tendons permits only a given amount of motion. For example, wrist flexion is less when the fingers are simultaneously flexed than when they are extended. Conversely, the wrist's position also affects finger ROM, that is, finger flexion is less when the wrist is simultaneously flexed than when it is extended. Because of this feature, a therapist should consider the importance of:

1. Maintaining a constant position of all other joints when measuring any one particular joint
2. Identifying hand position when measuring strength
3. Incorporating tenodesis into treatment planning, such as using wrist extension to enhance grasp in a C6 spinal cord injured patient, or wrist flexion to enhance finger extension in a patient with spastic cerebral palsy

The *common carpometacarpal joint* is an irregular combination of plane articulations between the distal row of carpals and the bases of the second through fifth metacarpals. It permits slight gliding and becomes more mobile toward the fifth metacarpal, allowing cupping of the palm.

The *trapeziometacarpal joint* is a saddle-shaped articulation between the trapezium and first metacarpal, which because of its exceptional mobility becomes the key joint of the hand. Its wide ROM includes pure movements of flexion, extension, abduction, adduction, and combinations of movements producing opposition and circumduction. During abduction and adduction the convex metacarpal surface moves on the concave trapezium, whereas in flexion and extension the concave metacarpal surface moves on the convex trapezium. By definition, motions of the thumb occur in a plane perpendicular to the plane of the same movement in the digits (i.e., thumb flexion occurs in a frontal plane, which is perpendicular to the sagittal plane in which finger flexion occurs). Average ROM of the thumb is 45° of abduction, 55° of extension, and 17° of axial rotation.[7]

The *pisiform-triquetral joint* is a small plane joint that has its own separate synovial cavity; it allows only a small amount of gliding. The *ulnomeniscotriquetral "joint"* unites the ulna, disc, and triquetrum; it is clinically significant because its gliding motion accompanies supination and pronation.[9] Joint play movements occur in all of these carpal joints in response to traction, gliding, and rotary forces.

The ligaments of the wrist form a complex system controlling force transmission and carpal stability.[35,47] The extrinsic ligaments include the radioscaphocapitate, radiolunate, radioscapholunate, ulnolunate, ulnotriquitral, dorsal radiocarpal, radial collateral, and ulnar collateral. The intrinsic ligaments include the short palmar, dorsal, and interosseous lunotriquetral, scapholunate, and scaphotrapezium ligaments and the long palmar (V or deltoid) and dorsal intercarpal ligaments.

Ligaments of the common carpometacarpal joint are the volar carpometacarpal ligaments, dorsal carpometacarpal ligaments, and intermetacarpal ligaments. At the trapeziometacarpal joint, the lateral ligaments, volar ligament, and dorsal oblique ligament provide support.

Metacarpophalangeal joints. The articulations be-

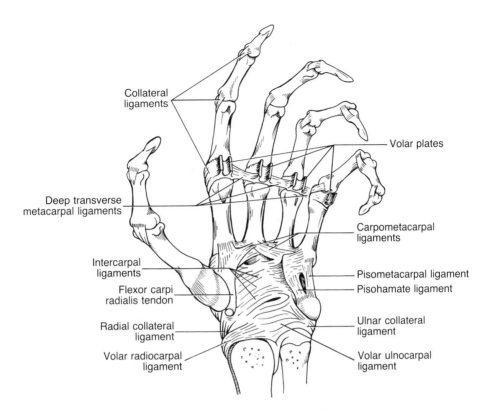

Fig. 13-4. Ligaments of the wrist and hand.

tween metacarpals two through five and the respective proximal phalanges are *biaxial joints*. Joint capsules enclose the individual MP joints. The dorsal hood apparatus reinforces (or replaces) the joint capsules. The volar plates reinforce the volar aspect of the capsules. The distal portion of the volar plate is cartilaginous and firmly fixed to the phalanx, whereas the proximal portion is membranous and loosely attached to the metacarpal. Adhesions may form between the membranous surfaces, which fold on themselves when immobilized in flexion. On their palmar surface the plates are grooved to receive and pad the flexor tendons of the finger (Fig. 13-4).

Laterally, collateral ligaments support the MP joints. They are strong cords that run obliquely from the dorsum of the metacarpals to the ventral aspect of the base of the phalanges (Fig. 13-4). Because of their eccentric placement and the camlike shape of the metacarpal head, which becomes larger palmarly and transversely, the collateral ligaments become taut as flexion increases.[15] Contractures of these ligaments contribute to loss of MP joint flexion. To prevent their shortening during immobilization, a therapist should splint the MP joints in 70° to 90° of flexion. Superficial and deep transverse metacarpal ligaments connect the metacarpal heads and offer indirect support for the joints. Active movement increases progressively from the second to the fifth MP joint but is approximately 90° flexion, 25° extension, and 20° abduction.

The articulation between the first metacarpal and the proximal phalanx of the thumb is a hinge joint. Bony stability is inherent in its configuration and is enhanced by volar and collateral ligamentous support (Fig. 13-4). Flexion occurs to approximately 50°. Traction, gliding, and rotatory joint play movements are also possible in all of the MP joints.

Interphalangeal joints. The articulations between adjacent phalanges are *hinge joints* because their pulley-like surfaces allow motion in only one plane. Proper and accessory collateral ligaments as well as volar plates maintain articular congruence (Fig. 13-4). The collateral ligaments differ from those of the MP joints in that they are most taut at 15° to 20° of flexion. This position, therefore, is ideal for splinting the fingers to prevent IP joint flexion contractures.[43] The accessory collateral ligaments suspend the volar plate and flexor sheath from the proximal phalangeal head at the proximal interphalangeal (PIP) joint and the volar plate from the middle phalangeal head at the distal interphalangeal (DIP) joint.[8] Active flexion at the PIP joints approximates 110°, at the DIP joints 90°, and at the thumb interphalangeal joint 90°. Traction, gliding, and joint play movements are also possible at the IP joints.

Soft-tissue relationships and mechanics

Disorders of the hand often involve soft-tissue pathology. This section presents the soft tissues as they are layered from superficial to deep and proximal to distal and investigates pathomechanics that may arise.

The subcutaneous tissue of the dorsum of the hand

structurally differs from the tissue of the palm. The dorsal areolar tissue is thin and elastic to permit stretching as one makes a fist. Its loose attachment and preponderance of lymphatic vessels and veins account for swelling that manifests predominantly on the dorsal surface, although the source of the problem often lies elsewhere in the hand. In the palm many strong, fibrous fasciculi connect the skin tightly to the adjacent palmar aponeurosis, permitting relatively little sliding of the skin and enhancing secure grasp. Dense fibrous tissue composes the palmar aponeurosis, just deep to the subcutaneous tissue. The palmar aponeurosis is continuous with the palmaris longus tendon and the fascia covering the thenar and hypothenar muscles and extends distally into the transverse metacarpal ligaments and flexor tendon sheaths. It provides protection for the ulnar artery and nerve and digital vessels and nerves and may transmit a weak flexion force from the palmaris longus tendon into the fingers (Fig. 13-5). Nodule formation or scarring in this structure produces the clinical entity known as *Dupuytren's disease,* which can produce flexion contractures of the digits.

The flexor retinaculum (transverse carpal ligament) deep to the palmar aponeurosis, spans the area between the pisiform, hamate, scaphoid, and trapezium (Fig. 13-5). It forms the roof of the carpal tunnel, which transmits the extrinsic flexor tendons and median nerve. The retinaculum offers attachment for the thenar and hypothenar muscles, helps maintain the transverse carpal arch, prevents bowstringing of the extrinsic flexor tendons, and protects the median nerve. The median nerve is subject to compression in this relatively unyielding space, a condition know as *carpal tunnel syndrome.*

Anatomists refer to muscles acting on the hand as extrinsic when their origin lies outside the hand and intrinsic when their origin is within the hand. The Box lists the extrinsic and intrinsic muscles. A thorough understanding of muscle origins, insertion, and actions is essential, but because of comprehensive coverage elsewhere, is not included in this text. The following paragraphs describe the kinesiology and pathomechanics of the soft tissues.

Operation of the hand requires a large number of muscles. The design of the extrinsics, with their muscle bellies lying in the forearm and tapering into tendons proximal to the wrist, allows the action of many muscles without inordinate bulkiness. In addition to powering the wrist and fingers, the extrinsic tendons also stabilize the wrist. The tendons of both the finger flexors and extensors compress the wrist joints by forcing the hand proximally into the concave radial surface during co-contraction (Fig. 13-5). The wrist muscles themselves enhance stability by achieving a balance of flexor and extensor forces through their attachment to the stable metacarpal bases.[28]

The extrinsic finger flexor tendons enter the hand deep to the flexor retinaculum. The flexor digitorum sublimis (FDS) muscle, which primarily flexes the PIP joints and secondarily assists MP joint flexion, divides into tendons that are capable of relatively independent action at each finger. The flexor

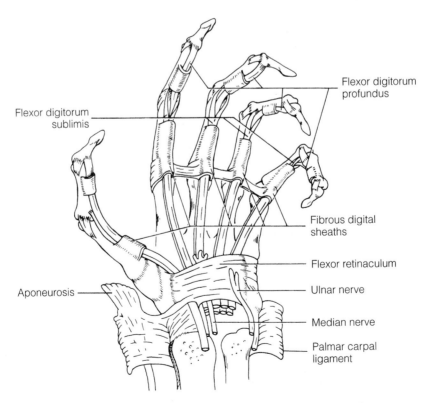

Fig. 13-5. Volar soft-tissue relationships in the wrist and hand.

digitorum profundus (FDP) muscle, which alone flexes the DIP joints and assists PIP and MP joint flexion, also supplies tendons for each finger. Unlike the FDS tendons, the FDP tendons of the middle, ring, and little fingers have a common muscle belly, so the tendons cannot operate independently in these fingers. When muscle testing, to isolate flexion of the PIP joint by the FDS muscle, one holds all of the fingers except the one being tested in extension to pull the common FDP muscle distally (Fig. 13-6). Because the FDP muscle cannot work independently in the finger being tested, only the FDS muscle can flex the PIP joint.[24]

Fibrous sheaths encase the flexor tendons between the distal palmar crease and the DIP joints.[44] Overlying these sheaths five annular and three cruciate pulleys stabilize the tendons. The first annular pulley, A1, produces a *trigger finger* when it impinges tendons that are inflamed.

The extensor retinaculum retains the extrinsic extensor tendons over the dorsal wrist (Fig. 13-7). Fasciculi of the retinaculum separate the tendons into compartments as follows:

I. abductor pollicis longus (APL) and extensor pollicis brevis (EPB)
II. extensor carpi radialis longus (ECRL) and extensor carpi radialis brevis (ECRB)
III. extensor pollicis longus (EPL)
IV. extensor indicis (EI) and extensor digitorum communis (EDC)
V. extensor digiti minimi (EDM)
VI. extensor carpi ulnaris (ECU)

Toward the distal ends of the metacarpals juncturae tendinae interconnect the four EDC tendons, limiting their independent motion (Fig. 13-7). For example, middle and little finger flexion hinder ring finger MP joint extension because the juncturae tendinae pull the ring finger EDC tendon distally, rendering it lax. Conversely, extension of the ring finger exerts an extensor force on its neighbors, so that the ring finger (EDC) can actively extend them, even if their tendons are severed proximal to the juncturae.[42]

As the EDC tendons cross the region of the MP joints, their main connection to the proximal phalanges is through the *sagittal bands,* which pass palmarward to attach to the volar plates (Fig. 13-8). The primary function of the sagittal bands is to transmit the extension force of the EDC tendons, thus extending the MP joints, but they also prevent bowstringing of the extensor tendons dorsally.[42] When one does not prevent hyperextension of the MP joints, contraction of the EDC muscles extends the proximal phalanges through the sagittal bands and simultaneously anchors the tendons, so that they are lax further distally; only the intrinsic muscles can then extend the PIP and DIP joints. Thus, to isolate intrinsic muscle action, a therapist instructs a patient to actively extend his or her MP joints and then attempt to extend the IP joints; this will only be possible if the intrinsics are functioning.

Between the MP and PIP joints, the EDC tendons divide into three parts: the central slip, which inserts into the base of the middle phalanx, and two lateral bands (Fig. 13-7). The lateral bands eventually rejoin into a terminal tendon, which inserts into the base of the distal phalanx. Rupture of this terminal tendon produces a *mallet finger,* in which the DIP joint drops into flexion. Fibers from the lumbrical and interosseous muscles join the EDC tendons over the proximal phalanx, forming the dorsal hood apparatus.

Extrinsic and intrinsic muscles of hand	
Extrinsic muscles	**Intrinsic muscles**
Extensor carpi radialis longus	Lumbricals
Extensor carpi brevis	Dorsal and palmar interossei
Extensor carpi ulnaris	Adductor pollicis
Flexor carpi radialis	Flexor pollicis brevis
Flexor carpi ulnaris	Abductor pollicis brevis
Palmaris longus	Opponens pollicis
Extensor pollicis longus and brevis	Flexor digiti minimi
Abductor pollicis longus	Abductor digiti minimi
Extensor indicis	Opponens digiti minimi
Extensor digiti minimi	Palmaris brevis
Extensor digitorum communis	
Flexor digitorum sublimis	
Flexor digitorum profundus	
Flexor pollicis longus	

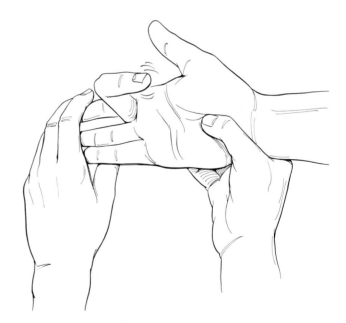

Fig. 13-6. An examiner tests the FDS muscle by holding the adjacent digits in extension to "tether" the FDP muscle distally, so that only the FDS muscle can flex the PIP joint. (Modified from Hoppenfeld S: *Physical examination of the spine and extremities,* New York, 1976, Appleton-Century-Crofts.)

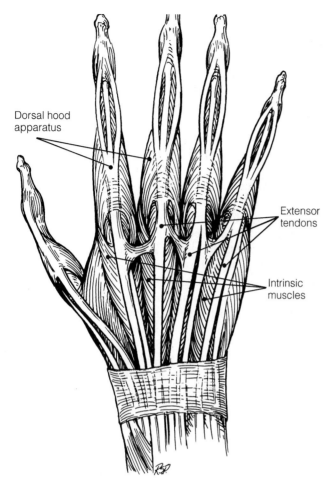

Fig. 13-7. Extensor tendons, dorsal hood apparatus, intrinsic muscles, and some ligaments of the fingers.

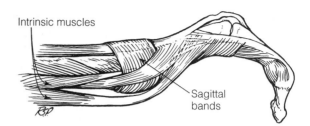

Fig. 13-8. An examiner tests the intrinsic muscles by having the patient actively extend his MP joint so that the sagittal bands transmit the extensor force of the EDC muscle to the proximal phalanx, rendering the distal end of the tendon "lax"; now only the intrinsic muscles will be able to extend the PIP and DIP joints.

Because the intrinsic muscles are volar to the MP joint axes, they can only flex the MP joints. The intrinsic tendons lie dorsal to the PIP and DIP joint axes and so exert an extension force on these joints.

The *transverse retinacular ligaments* link the lateral bands to the volar plates of the PIP joints and prevent them from dislocating dorsally (Fig. 13-7).[8] If these ligaments are stretched or lax, the lateral bands bowstring dorsal to the PIP joint. This produces excessive extension force at the PIP joint and contributes to hyperextension deformity. When the PIP joint hyperextends, it tightens the FDP tendon, which pulls the DIP joint into flexion through "passive tension," producing a *swan neck* deformity (Fig. 13-9).[42,43]

The *oblique retinacular ligaments* (Landsmeer's ligaments) also contribute to interdependence of IP joint movement. They attach between the PIP joint volar plate, where they are volar to the PIP joint axis, and the terminal tendon, where they are dorsal to the DIP joint axis (Fig. 13-7). When one extends his or her PIP joint, this tightens the oblique retinacular ligaments (ORL), which exert a passive extensor force on the DIP joint. When one flexes his or her

PIP joint, this relaxes the ORL so that they allow the DIP joint to flex. In the normal hand, the influence of the ORL is minimal. However, if they become contracted after burns or trauma, they produce a tenodesis effect; that is, when the PIP joint extends, the ligaments pull the DIP joint into extension.[30]

When the PIP joint flexes, the lateral bands slip volarly, decreasing the excursion required for full DIP joint flexion. Although PIP joint flexion passively enhances DIP joint flexion by relaxing the ORL and lateral bands, it weakens DIP joint extension. Full PIP joint flexion checkreins or anchors the extensor mechanism *distally* through attachment of the central slip to the middle phalanx. In this position the lateral bands are so lax that it becomes difficult to extend the DIP joint.[21] If, through injury or disease, the central slip ruptures from its insertion, the extensor mechanism migrates *proximally,* rendering the lateral bands taut. In this scenario, the combined forces of the intrinsic muscles and the EDC muscle act directly to extend the distal phalanx. Because the central slip rupture leaves the FDS muscle unopposed, it pulls the PIP joint into flexion, producing a *boutonniere deformity* (Fig. 13-10).[40,42]

The lumbrical muscles originate from the FDP tendons and insert into the dorsal hood apparatus. The only muscles in the body that originate from and insert into a tendon, the lumbricals coordinate the flexor and extensor systems.[25] During contraction, they exert a distally directed force on the FDP, along with a proximally directed force on the dorsal hood apparatus, thus possessing the unique ability to relax their own antagonist.[42] In instances of lumbrical muscle spasm or contracture, as in rheumatoid arthritis, attempts to flex the fingers via the FDP muscle result in force transmission through the lumbrical muscle into the extensor apparatus, contributing to IP joint extension rather than flexion. This may result in a *lumbrical plus* deformity, that is, MP joint flexion and IP joint extension. The lumbrical muscles serve as a primary feedback organ in the hand. They are ideally suited to link position and movement of the hand and finger joints, as Rabischong found that they contained more annulospiral endings per unit of length than any other muscle in the body.[51]

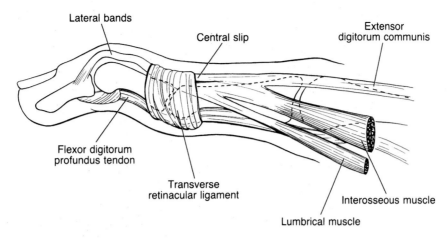

Fig. 13-9. Swan neck deformity, demonstrating transverse retinacular ligament laxity, with PIP joint hyperextension.

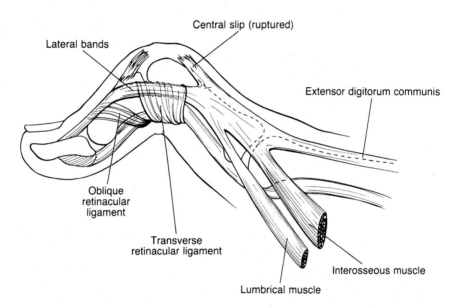

Fig. 13-10. Boutonniere deformity, demonstrating rupture of the central slip, with PIP joint flexion.

Neurology

Motor innervation. The median nerve supplies the following muscles in the forearm: pronator teres, FCR, palmaris longus, and FDS. Approximately 10 cm distal to the elbow, the anterior interosseous nerve branches off of the median nerve and supplies the flexor pollicis longus (FPL), pronator quadratus, and FDP muscles to the index and middle fingers. At the wrist the median nerve passes under the flexor retinaculum and enters the palm, splitting into a sensory branch and a motor branch. The latter supplies the abductor pollicis brevis (APB), opponens pollicis (OP), flexor pollicis brevis (FPB), and first and second lumbrical muscles.

Impairment resulting from median nerve dysfunction proximal to the wrist includes the inability to oppose the thumb, flex the IP joint of the thumb, and flex the first two fingers, resulting in a *benediction attitude* (Fig. 13-11a). Distal to the wrist, median nerve involvement, for example,

carpal tunnel syndrome, affects only the thenar and first two lumbrical muscles, which hinders one's ability to perform precision maneuvers.

The ulnar nerve supplies the following muscles in the forearm: FCU, and FDP to the ring and little fingers. In the hand, it innervates the flexor digiti minimi (FDM), ADM, opponens digiti minimi (ODM), adductor pollicis, palmaris brevis, third and fourth lumbricals, and the interosseus muscles.

Paralysis of the ulnar nerve produces loss of thumb adduction (lateral pinch), weakness in power grip and finger spreading, and inability to perform coordinated activities such as piano playing. An ulnar claw hand deformity, also known as an *intrinsic minus* hand, with MP joint extension and IP joint flexion, often results (Fig. 13-11b). This deformity is more severe in lesions distal to innervation of the FDP muscle.

The radial nerve supplies the brachioradialis, ECRL,

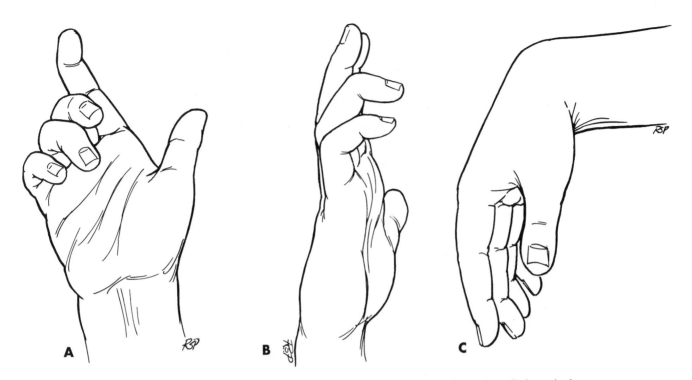

Fig. 13-11. Hand posturing after nerve injury. **A,** Median nerve injury produces a benediction attitude or ape hand with loss of thumb flexion and opposition, and index and middle finger flexion; **B,** ulnar nerve injury produces a claw hand with hyperextension of the ring and little finger MP joints; **C,** radial nerve injury produces loss of wrist, MP joint, and thumb extension.

ECRB, supinator, EDC, ECU, APL, EDM, EPB, EPL, and EI muscles. Radial nerve paralysis prevents wrist and finger MP joint extension (Fig. 13-11c). Because wrist extension is synergistic and stabilizing for finger flexion, radial nerve involvement can significantly hinder hand function. A patient with radial nerve injury also loses the ability to extend and abduct his thumb.

Sensory innervation. The hand serves as a "sensory organ" in some respects, because it contains a high percentage of sensory receptors. The hand's motor system depends on constant feedback from the sensory system. Branches of the three major peripheral nerves carry sensation from the hand in the following manner. The median nerve transmits sensation from the lateral portion of the palm and thenar surface, and the volar part of the thumb, index, middle, and lateral half of the ring fingers, extending over the dorsum of the terminal phalanges; innervation is purest at the tip of the index finger (Fig. 13-12a).

The ulnar nerve supplies the ulnar side of the hand, medial half of the ring finger, and little finger (both dorsal and volar surfaces); innervation is purest at the tip of the little finger.

The radial nerve innervates the dorsum of the hand lateral to the fourth metacarpal and the dorsal surfaces of the lateral three and one-half digits as far distal as the DIP joints; innervation is purest at the dorsal web space between the thumb and index finger (Fig. 13-12a).

Cervical nerve root pressure produces sensory changes in the most distal areas of the dermatomes, of which C-6, C-7, and C-8 extend into the hand. When a therapist evaluates the hand, knowledge of the dermatomal distribution helps differentiate between nerve root and peripheral nerve lesions. Root level representation includes C-6 to the lateral aspect of the hand and the thumb, C-7 to the middle of the hand and the index, middle, and ring fingers, and C-8 to the medial aspect of the hand and the little finger (Fig. 13-12b).[4] Because of the similar patterns of C-8 and ulnar nerve sensory distribution, a therapist often needs additional tests, such as muscle strength, to make a differential diagnosis.

Angiology

Arteries. The hand receives its blood from the radial and ulnar arteries. The radial artery courses along the lateral side of the forearm to the wrist, where its pulse is palpable just lateral to the FCR tendon. After giving off the superficial palmar branch, just proximal to the scaphoid, the radial artery winds laterally posterior to the first metacarpal; it gives off the dorsal carpal branch and the first dorsal metacarpal artery, then enters the palm between the first and second metacarpals, where it forms the deep palmar arch by uniting with the deep branch of the ulnar artery. The superficial palmar branch joins the corresponding ulnar branch, forming the superficial palmar arch. This arch is larger and more significant than the deep arch.

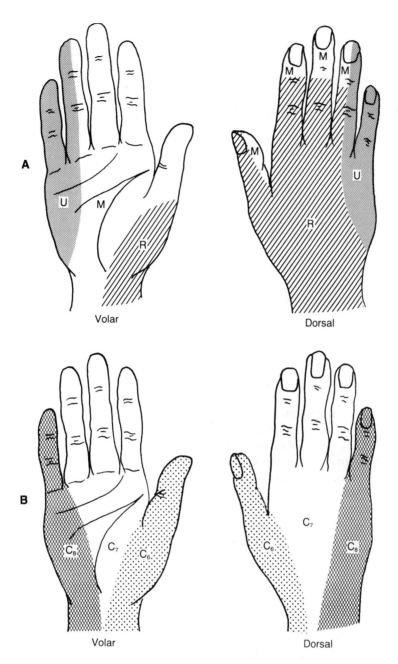

Fig. 13-12. Comparison of sensory innervation from peripheral nerves and cervical nerve roots. **A,** Peripheral nerves—radial *(R)*, median *(M)*, and ulnar *(U)*; **B,** cervical nerve roots—C6, C7, and C8. (Modified from Cailliet R: *Hand pain impairment,* ed 2, Philadelphia, 1975, FA Davis.)

The ulnar artery crosses the wrist medially, where it is superficial to the flexor retinaculum and palpable just lateral to the flexor carpi ulnaris tendon. Just distal to the pisiform, it divides into a superficial branch (which continues across the palm as the superficial palmar arch) and a deep branch (which joins the radial artery, completing the deep arch).

From the deep palmar arch arise the palmar metacarpal arteries, which join the common palmar digital arteries from the superficial arch. They extend into the fingers and divide into medial and lateral digital arteries.

Veins. A plexus of superficial and deep veins, of which the superficial is most significant, drain the hand. The superficial system is more extensive over the dorsal surface of the hand and becomes increasingly prominent with age. At the level of the wrist this system converges into the cephalic vein laterally and the basilic vein medially, both of which ascend superficially up the forearm. The deep veins of the hand travel in pairs with the arteries (vena comitantes). They ascend from the digits to the palmar arches to the radial and ulnar arteries.

Given an understanding of these anatomical and pathokinesiological concepts, the clinician has a sound foundation to proceed with the evaluation of the patient with hand dysfunction. Evaluation, in many respects, is the application of anatomy and kinesiology; by comparing the affected part with known norms, a clinician identifies aberrant structure and function.

EXAMINATION PROCEDURES SPECIFIC TO THE WRIST AND HAND

The rehabilitation goal of any patient with hand disability—whether it is caused by a birth defect, injury, or disease—is to obtain adequate hand and wrist function and cosmetic appearance and return to his or her former lifestyle in the shortest amount of time and at least expense possible. To accomplish this goal, teamwork is essential. Health professionals as well as the patient must join efforts in promoting the comprehensive care needed to achieve optimal results.

Accurate evaluation of the patient's condition is a critical element in the rehabilitative process and the responsibility of all members of the team. The evaluative results provide information for establishing a diagnosis, setting realistic goals, planning a program of treatment and management, and determining a baseline for measuring progress. Also, the evaluation establishes functional impairment and cosmetic defects and informs insurance companies and others of the patient's status. The rehabilitation team members may assume responsibility for different parts of the evaluation to accommodate their individual areas of expertise, but the overall process should yield a compilation of clear, precise, factual data that will be of subsequent use to multiple parties.

Chapter 7 presents the basic format for an examination. The following section elaborates only on tests and measurements that are unique to the wrist and hand. However, for the reader's convenience, the author has provided forms for a complete examination that one can adapt to most clinical settings. Because it is often difficult to visualize the relationship and extent of involvement of the numerous structures of the hand, a photographic record also helps to portray the condition.

The examination comprises two major areas: the patient's history and the physical examination (Fig. 13-13). The history gleans relevant information about the site, nature, and behavior of current symptoms as well as related background data. The content of the history, in conjunction with the provisional diagnosis, if available, dictates the scope of the physical examination that follows. The physical examination reveals abnormalities in structure and function, which an examiner documents objectively with measurements and test results. After obtaining both subjective and objective data, the therapist proceeds to develop a problem list and plan for further testing, treatment, and management.

To determine the extent of hand dysfunction, the therapist first performs a general assessment of the cervical spine and

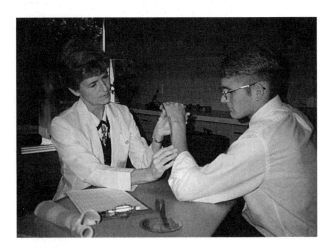

Fig. 13-13. History and physical examination, with involved part positioned for testing.

upper extremities. This ensures recognition of referred pain or multiple lesions and appreciation of their effect on the hand. The hand's location as the distal member of the extremity often makes it the recipient of pain that is commonly referred from a more proximal site. Therefore a therapist must "rule out" proximal disorders before concentrating on examination and treatment of the hand.

History

When obtaining the history, an examiner questions a patient to acquire identifying data and information pertinent to his or her present illness, past and family history, and lifestyle (Figs. 13-14 to 13-16).

In the event of trauma, an examiner requests details regarding the nature, mechanism, and ensuing results of the injury. For example, when a finger is forced beyond anatomical limits, knowing its position reveals the tissues most at risk for damage. In a fall, knowing the hand and arm position and the area of impact localizes involved structures. If the patient had an industrial accident, the examiner ascertains how the hand may have been trapped, for how long, and the type of moving parts that contacted the hand. He or she also notes the presence of thermal and chemical injuries, which can be more significant than mechanical trauma.[21]

An examiner should inquire whether there was deformity (i.e., interruption of bone, joint, or tendon continuity) and whether it was reduced. If the patient suffered disability following the incident, he or she should describe the type of disability (e.g., restricted motion), what he or she feels caused it (e.g., pain, bony block, weakness), and the time sequence of disability. For example, a fall on the dorsiflexed wrist may produce *immediate* pain, deformity, and restricted motion from lunate dislocation, then a day *later* produce symptoms of median nerve compression.

An examiner documents loss of motion and strength; in both instances he or she should describe the type of motion

WRIST AND HAND EXAMINATION FORM

A.   HISTORY

      1.   Identifying data

Name _____   Age _____   Sex _____   Date _____

Provisional diagnosis _____   Precautions _____

Chief complaint _____

Dominant hand   R _____   L _____   Prior conditions _____

      2.   Present Illness or episode

Date of injury/onset _____   Insidious _____   Abrupt _____

Dates of hospitalization _____   Duration of incapacity_____

  Nature and mechanism of injury _____

_____

Audible sounds at time of injury _____

Results of injury _____

Deformity _____   If and how corrected _____

Disability: Type _____   Reason _____

Time sequence _____

Loss of motion (specify) _____   Time sequence _____

Loss of strength (specify) _____   Time sequence _____

Swelling: Immediate _____   After 24 hours _____

Bleeding: Location _____   Amount _____

Treatments, dates and results _____

_____

_____

Fig. 13-14. Wrist and hand examination form: history, including identifying data and present illness through treatments.

(e.g., MP joint flexion) or strength (lateral pinch) and the sequence of involvement. The loss may be immediate, such as in rupture of a contractile structure, or slowly progressive, such as increasing effusion within an unyielding space occupied by nerves and vessels susceptible to compression.

An examiner is particularly attentive to the patient's description of the present status of his or her condition (Fig. 13-15). A body chart and scales for rating severity and impairment play important roles in this section. "Behavior" of the patient's symptoms, including when they occur and what worsens or lessens them, may provide valuable diagnostic information. For example, morning stiffness lasting more than 2 hours characterizes rheumatoid arthritis. In contrast, stiffness after awakening or periods of rest that resolves with stretching and exercise is a common sequela of hand trauma. Many musculoskeletal disorders, such as tendinitis, are aggravated by activity but relieved by rest. An examiner ascertains exactly which motion or posture reproduces the chief complaint to isolate the affected structure.

WRIST AND HAND EXAMINATION FORM cont.

Present status of   acute _____   chronic _____   intermittent _____   static _____   better _____
condition: worse _____

Musculoskeletal structure behavior

Joint: catches _____   locks _____   grates _____   clicks _____   dislocates _____

Muscle: spasm _____   weak _____   inc. tone _____   dec. tone _____

Other: _____

Description of symptoms:
    Location (code)
    Key: ////   =   pain
                ====   =   paresthesia
                oooo   =   numbness
                xxxx   =   pain

    Severity
    Scale: 1   =   best
             10   =   worst
    0————————————————10

    Impairment:
    Scale: 0% - 25%   =   annoying
             25% - 50%   =   interferes with activity
             50% - 75%   =   prevents activity
             75% - 100%   =   prevents activity and causes distress
    0————————————————10

    Nature

Ache _____   Stab _____

Throb _____   Twinge _____

Burn _____   Tingle _____

Other _____

    Constancy

Constant _____   Varies in intensity _____

When _____   What elicits _____

What worsens _____

What improves _____

How long lasting _____

Morning stiffness _____   Duration _____

Fig. 13-15. Wrist and hand examination form: history, including present illness from present status through description of symptoms.

WRIST AND HAND EXAMINATION FORM cont.

3.   Relevant past history

History of similar condition   Dates _____   Nature _____

_____

Treatment _____

Other body parts affected _____

Other relevant illnesses _____

General health status _____

4.   Family history

Health problems of immediate family _____

Familial diseases _____

5.   Life-style

Occupation _____   Habits _____

Living conditions _____

Regular (3 times/week) physical activities requiring:

Strength _____   Agility _____

Endurance _____   Flexibility _____

Other _____

What patient does to promote wellness _____

Patient's concept of cause of condition _____

Patient's concept of functional deficit _____

Patient's concept of cosmetic deficit _____

Anticipated life-style and goals _____

6.   Other considerations

Current medications _____

Imaging studies _____

Fig. 13-16. Wrist and hand examination form: history, including relevant past history, family history, lifestyle, and other considerations.

After determining the condition of the involved wrist and hand *prior* to the present illness or episode (identifying data) an examiner asks about the relevant past history. An examiner notes previous injury or preexisting pain that may alter a patient's ability or willingness to perform particular exercises (Fig. 13-16). If other areas of the body are affected in addition to the hand, it is feasible to investigate for the presence of congenital anomalies or systemic disorders. A family history may reveal the presence of any familial diseases. A lifestyle summary should include the occupation, habits, living conditions, and physical activities of the patient. What the patient does to promote wellness may give some indication of the responsibility he or she will be likely to assume in a rehabilitation program. Also, the patient's description of functional and cosmetic deficits produced by the condition and anticipated lifestyle, goals, and treatment expectations are important in assessing the overall severity of the case and in planning for future management. Other considerations, including a listing of current medications and the interpretation of imaging studies, complete the patient's history.

Physical examination

A therapist analyzes the data from a patient's history to determine the scope and focus of the physical examination. The following paragraphs describe all sections of the physical examination, but professional judgment may dictate that certain parts be abbreviated or deleted.

The physical examination begins with inspection, during which an examiner observes the appearance of the hands, resting posture, hand use, protective mechanisms, and the relationship of the hands to the rest of the body. Normally, the hand resting supine demonstrates moderate finger flexion that increases in a cascade fashion from the index to the little finger. The thumb MP and IP joints are slightly flexed, and the CMC joint is in mid-position between abduction and adduction.

The attitude of the hand at rest may portray deformities, such as ulnar deviation, volar subluxation of the MP joints, swan neck, and boutonniere deformities common in rheumatoid arthritis (Fig. 13-17). The hand might also demonstrate collapse of the normal longitudinal or transverse arch framework—invariably affecting function—which can result from skeletal malalignment, muscle imbalance, or joint instability.

Next an examiner describes the shape of the hand (Fig. 13-18). He or she notes visible changes in contour that may result from protuberances or nodules (such as ganglia or Heberden's nodes), loss of arches, absence of digits, narrowed web spaces, deviations in length and alignment, and swelling or atrophy. An examiner may objectively document subtle increases or decreases in hand size by circumfer-

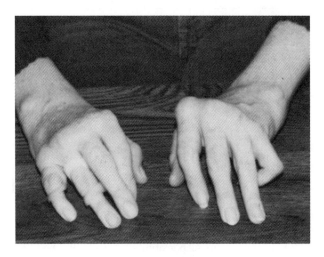

Fig. 13-17. Inspection of rheumatoid hands.

ential measurements at a specific site. Volumetric measurements of water displacement from a standardized volumeter provide another objective procedure. Conditions that affect hand size include peripheral neuropathies that typically produce widespread atrophy of thenar and hypothenar eminences and guttering over the area of the interossei. Median nerve damage occurring in carpal tunnel syndrome produces selective thenar atrophy. Ulnar nerve loss causes hypothenar and intrinsic muscle atrophy. Immobilization can produce generalized atrophy, but edema can mask this atrophy, possibly misleading an examiner during cursory inspection. Bilateral comparison helps identify subtle abnormalities.

An examiner observes how a patient uses the hand as he or she moves about and prepares for examination (e.g., when removing necessary clothing) (Fig. 13-19). Does he or she use it in an effortless, coordinated manner, or are movements labored, jerky, stiff, or protected? How does the patient compensate for hypermobility or hypomobility? Is he or she unwilling to put weight on the wrist when pushing up from a chair? If so, this may indicate a painful arthritic condition or sprain of the carpal ligaments. Reflex sympathetic dystrophy often produces a painful edematous hand that the patient protects and uses reluctantly, if at all. Jerky, uncoordinated movements may stem from a neurological disorder.

An examiner next inspects the hand for scars, skin lesions, color, quality, hair patterns, and nail changes. Trophic changes of the skin are common in peripheral vascular disease, diabetes mellitus, reflex sympathetic dystrophy, and Raynaud's disease. Pulmonary dysfunction may produce clubbing and cyanosis of the nails. A hand diagram facilitates localization of skin defects (Fig. 13-19).

Inspection ends with review and description of the patient's splints and adaptive devices. The examiner notes their intended purpose (e.g., a cock-up wrist splint worn to alleviate symptoms of carpal tunnel syndrome or a dynamic flexor splint worn to protect a healing flexor tendon repair) and whether they are effective.

The next part of the physical examination deals with the assessment of movement. Because of the detail this area encompasses, it is one of the therapist's most important contributions to the overall evaluation process. A clinician divides movements into two groups, functional and physiologic, for testing purposes. Functional active movements include various types of grips, grasps, and pinches. One may assess these functions according to the ease with which the patient completes tasks and handles common objects (Fig. 13-20). Standardized tests, such as the Minnesota Manual Dexterity, Jebsen-Taylor Hand Function, Crawford Small Parts Dexterity, and Purdue Pegboard, provide objective documentation of functional capability.[21,50] The BTE Work Simulator* is a computerized device that offers objective data on functional performance.

---

* Baltimore Therapeutic Equipment, Colo.

WRIST AND HAND EXAMINATION FORM cont.

B.   PHYSICAL EXAMINATION

1.   Inspection

a. Posture

General appearance of extremity

Joints affected: shoulder _____   elbow _____   wrist _____   thumb _____

fingers   I _____   M _____   R _____   L _____

Hand posture/attitude at rest _____

Integrity of arches _____

b. Shape

Key: X   =   missing digit

At   =   atrophy

S   =   swelling

D   =   deviation

⊖   =   lacks web

An   =   ankylosis

SN   =   swan neck

B   =   boutonniere

D/S   =   dislocation/subluxation

M   =   mallet finger

Z   =   collapse deformity

N   =   nodule

Circumferential measurements: arm _____   forearm _____   wrist _____   hand _____

Volumetric measurement: involved hand _____ ml displaced

uninvolved hand _____ ml displaced

Symmetry of extremities: yes _____   no _____   (explain) _____

_____

_____

Fig. 13-18. Wrist and hand examination form: physical examination, including inspection of posture through shape.

Composite range of motion involves measurement of total motion with the individual joints either simultaneously flexed or extended. One does this simply by measuring the distance (in inches or centimeters) the fingertip lacks from reaching the proximal palmar crease (Fig. 13-21, *A*) or the dorsal plane (Fig. 13-21, *B*). To determine composite motion of only the PIP and DIP joints, measure the distance from the fingertip to the MP joint crease.

WRIST AND HAND EXAMINATION FORM cont.

c. Use

Hand protected/use restricted

Handles clothing: independently minimum assistance maximum assistance

Movement: jerky stiff uncoordinated limited by pain

Compensates for hypermobility hypomobility

d. Skin

Key:	C	=	cyanotic
	R	=	reddened
	W	=	whitened
	S	=	scar
	L	=	lesion
	F	=	fixation
	Na	=	nail deformity
	T	=	texture changed
	Ne	=	necrosis
	H	=	abnormal hair pattern

e. Splints & adaptive devices   sling _____   splint _____   orthosis _____   other _____

Description _____

Purpose _____

Fig. 13-19. Wrist and hand examination form: physical examination, including inspection of use, skin, and splints.

A Jamar* dynamometer provides objective determination of grip strength. One performs this test with the patient seated, the arm at the side, the elbow flexed 90°, the forearm in neutral rotation, and the wrist slightly extended and ulnarly deviated (Fig. 13-22).[32] The patient squeezes the dynamometer, alternating right and left hands, performing three trials in each of the handle positions. The graphed values should fall into a bell-shaped curve, peaking at the second or third handle position.[21,27,37] Subjects attempting to fake strength measurements produce a flatter curve.[37] Table 13-1 contains normal values.

To test pinch strength, the patient assumes the same position as for grip strength, and the examiner hands him or her a B & L pinch gauge† (Fig. 13-23).[32] The patient performs

three trials of three-point (thumb, index, and middle finger pulp opposition), lateral (key), and tip (thumb and index tip opposition) pinches, alternating between right and left hands. Table 13-2 contains normal values.

Special tests include the Finkelstein test for tenosynovitis of the EPB and APL tendons in the first dorsal compartment. The patients flexes the thumb and ulnarly deviates the wrist to produce maximal tension in the involved musculotendinous structures (Fig. 13-24). A positive test occurs when there is sharp pain over the radial aspect of the wrist and is indicative of deQuervain's syndrome.

An examiner performs the Bunnell-Littler test to ascertain intrinsic muscle tightness. If the PIP joint lacks flexion, the problem could result from tightness of either the intrinsic muscles, the extrinsic extensor muscles, or the joint capsule. To distinguish which it is, an examiner passively

* Asmow Engineering, Los Angeles, Calif.
† B & L Engineering, Santa Fe Springs, Calif.

2. Movement

a. Functional active movements

Power grip _____ (hammer)

Precision grip _____ (writing)

Hook grip _____ (suitcase)

Lateral pinch _____ (key)

Cylinder grasp _____ (2.5 cm cylinder)

Key: C = completes task

D = completes task with difficulty/discomfort

N = not able to complete task

Spherical grasp _____ (5 cm ball)

Standardized tests _____

_____

_____

Composite range of motion:

Distance (cm)	I	M	R	L
Fingertips to PP crease				
Fingertips to MP crease				
Fingertip to dorsal plane				

Grip strength

Jamar handle position	#1	#2	#3	#4	#5
Trial 1	_____	_____	_____	_____	_____
Trial 2	_____	_____	_____	_____	_____
Trial 3	_____	_____	_____	_____	_____
MEANS	_____	_____	_____		

Pinch strength

B & L pinch gauge	lateral pinch	3-point pinch	tip pinch
Trial 1	_____	_____	_____
Trial 2	_____	_____	_____
Trial 3	_____	_____	_____
MEANS	_____	_____	_____

Special tests	+	−	Comments
Finklestein			
Bunnell - Littler			
Oblique retinacular ligament			
Froment's sign			
Weight bearing on extended wrist			

Fig. 13-20. Wrist and hand examination form: physical examination, including functional active movements and special tests.

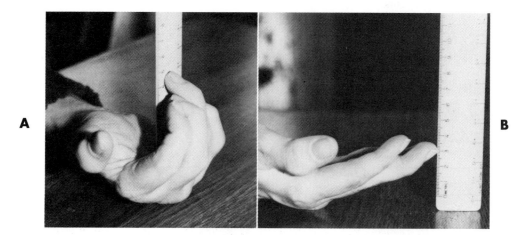

Fig. 13-21. Gross measurements of composite motion. **A,** Flexion is the distance between the fingertip and the proximal palmar crease; **B,** extension is the distance between the fingertip and dorsal plane.

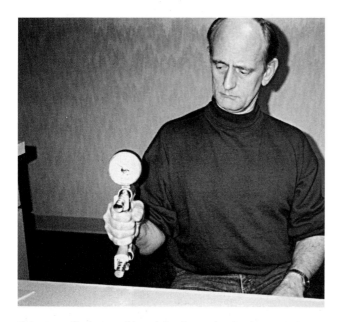

Fig. 13-22. Patient positioned for Jamar hand grip strength test.

extends the MP joint to tense the intrinsics, then measures PIP joint flexion; he or she then passively flexes the MP joint to relax the intrinsics and again measures PIP joint flexion; if PIP joint motion has increased, the intrinsic muscles are tight (Fig. 13-25, *A*). A test for oblique retinacular ligament tightness follows the same principle; if the DIP joint lacks flexion, the problem could result from either tightness of the ligament, the extensor tendons, or the joint capsule. To distinguish which, the examiner passively extends the PIP joint to tense the ligament, then measures DIP joint flexion; he or she then passively flexes the PIP joint to relax the ligament and again measures DIP joint flexion; if DIP joint motion has increased, the ligament is tight (Fig. 13-25, *B*).

An examiner elicits Froment's sign by requesting a patient to hold a thin object with a lateral pinch. If the thumb "collapses" into flexion at the IP joint, then the FPL muscle has overpowered the thumb extensor mechanism. This usually indicates ulnar nerve involvement, with weakness in the adductor pollicis and deep head of the FPB muscles, which contribute to the dorsal hood of the thumb and assist extension.

The final special test involves bearing weight on an extended wrist, such as when pushing up from a chair. If this maneuver produces pain, this is a positive indication for injury or inflammation of the carpal joint ligaments, capsule, or synovium.

Physiological movement testing involves measuring a large number of individual joints and muscles. One can record values in a chart format (Fig. 13-26). A therapist uses appropriate goniometric procedures to obtain precise measurements of active and passive ROM. The type of joint dictates the size and type of instrument to use (Fig. 13-27). The American Academy of Orthopaedic Surgeons recommends use of the neutral zero method (measure all motions from zero, starting in anatomical position). One should also position the proximal joints in a neutral position when measuring the distal joints to standardize the influence of multijoint muscles.

In the hand it is important to distinguish between the *active* and *passive* ROM of a joint. Active ROM is normally 5° to 10° less than passive; if the difference is greater than this, a musculotendinous or neurologic problem may be decreasing active motion. One of the most common causes of decreased AROM is adhesion formation in the hand. This will limit tendon gliding, or "pull through," but does not affect PROM.

A therapist must also consider the effects of *active* and *passive insufficiency* in the hand. Active insufficiency implies the inability of a musculotendinous unit, crossing two or more joints, to shorten sufficiently to move all of the

Table 13-1. Grip strength norms in pounds

Age		16-19	20-29	30-39	40-49	50-59	60-69	70+
Male	Right	101	121	121	113	107	90	71
	Left	86	108	112	107	93	77	60
Female	Right	70	72	76	66	62	52	46
	Left	59	62	67	59	52	43	41

(Adapted from Mathiowetz V: Grip and pinch strength measurements. In Admundsen LR, editor: *Muscle strength testing,* New York, 1990, Churchill Livingstone.)

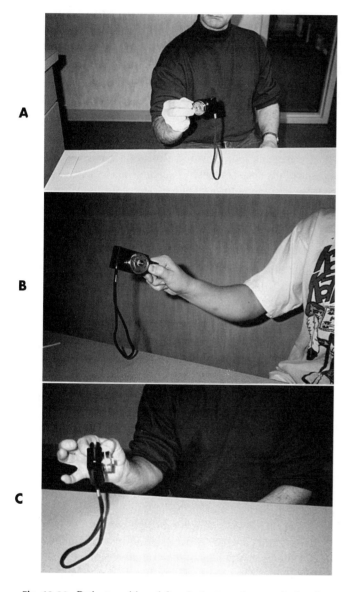

Fig. 13-23. Patient positioned for pinch strength tests. **A,** 3-point; **B,** lateral; **C,** tip.

joints it crosses through their full excursion simultaneously. For instance, due to active insufficiency, the FDP muscle loses mechanical efficiency when actively flexing the wrist and all finger joints simultaneously, so consequently grip strength is weaker when the wrist is flexed than when the wrist is extended. Passive insufficiency is the lack of enough extensibility of a musculotendinous unit, crossing two or more joints, to passively allow all of the joints it crosses to reach their full excursion simultaneously. For instance, when the EDC muscle is stretched maximally by simultaneous passive wrist and finger flexion, passive finger joint flexion is less than when the wrist is extended.

Standardized manual muscle testing procedures provide reliable and valid data on muscle strength. The grading scale uses a numerical or descriptive system in which 5 = normal, 4 = good, 3 = fair, 2 = poor, 1 = trace, and 0 = zero. It is necessary to isolate specific muscles when testing strength in the hand. Because either the FDS or the FDP muscle can flex the PIP joint, if one wants to isolate only the FDS muscle function he must anchor the FDP muscle distally by holding all fingers except the one being tested in extension, the patient then attempts to flex the PIP joint, which only the EDC muscle can affect (Fig. 13-6). Similarly, because either the EDC muscle or intrinsic muscles can extend the PIP joint, if one wants to isolate only the intrinsic muscle function, he or she instructs the patient to extend the MP joint, thus anchoring the EDC muscle proximally; the patient then attempts to extend the PIP joint, which only the intrinsic muscles can affect (Fig. 13-8).

An examiner may gain additional information for differential diagnosis by application of the concepts of selective tissue tension testing and end feel (Chapter 8).[9] Through understanding of the function of the different contractile and inert structures that may produce or restrict movement, one can selectively apply tension to each. By reproducing the patient's symptoms, an examiner can identify structures at fault. An examiner notes the structure responsible for limiting motion or reproducing symptoms (e.g., "intrinsic muscle contracture limits PIP joint flexion" or "collateral ligament contracture limits MP joint flexion") under the "passive movement" section of the examination form (Fig. 13-26). The examiner records symptoms produced by contractile structures under the "resistive movement" section of the examination form (Fig. 13-26).

To conclude the assessment of movement, an examiner applies joint play movements to the wrist and hand joints (Fig. 13-28). He or she grades joint mobility based on the following scale: 0 = ankylosis, 1 = extremely hypomobile,

Table 13-2. Pinch strength norms in pounds

Age		16-19	20-29	30-39	40-49	50-59	60-69
Male							
Right	3 Pt.	23	26	26	24	24	22
	Lateral	23	21	26	26	25	23
	Tip	16	18	18	18	17	16
Left	3 Pt.	22	26	26	24	23	21
	Lateral	22	25	26	25	25	22
	Tip	15	17	18	18	16	15
Female							
Right	3 Pt.	19	18	18	18	17	15
	Lateral	18	18	18	17	16	15
	Tip	13	12	12	12	12	10
Left	3 Pt.	18	17	18	17	16	14
	Lateral	17	16	17	16	15	14
	Tip	12	11	12	12	11	10

(Adapted from Mathiowetz V: Grip and pinch strength measurements. In Admundsen LR, editor: *Muscle strength testing,* New York, 1990, Churchill Livingstone.)

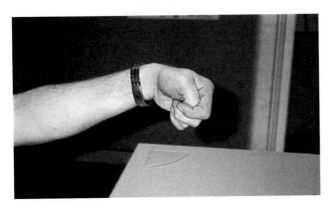

Fig. 13-24. Finklestein test for DeQuervain's syndrome: patient flexes his thumb, then ulnarly deviates his wrist; pain occurring at the radial styloid process indicates a positive test.

2 = slightly hypomobile, 3 = normal, 4 = slightly hypermobile; 5 = extremely hypermobile; 6 = unstable.

Palpation follows in the examination sequence. Most tissues in the hand are superficial and readily palpable, making it easy to detect structural and physiologic changes (Fig. 13-29). Progressing from superficial to deep, the examiner first palpates the skin and subcutaneous tissues for tenderness, temperature change, swelling, moisture, or decreased mobility. The dorsal tissues are normally thin and loose, allowing for a 30% increase in length from the wrist to fingertips during hand flexion. The lack of dorsal fascial attachments may permit the collection of edematous fluid over the dorsum of the hand when the source of inflammation could be in the palm or elsewhere. By contrast, the palmar tissue should feel thick to palpation and have relative lack of mobility. The signs of inflammation readily detectable on palpation include heat and swelling. Sympathetic changes that occur after nerve injury include vasomotor alterations (i.e., skin is warm initially but later becomes cool) and

sudomotor = sympathetic sweating response alterations (i.e., usually there is less sweating, but occasionally excessive moisture occurs). Profuse sweating may also suggest neurosis or vasomotor instability. Decreased tissue extensibility may signify scar adhesions or a contracted skin graft.

Palpating muscles and tendons may reveal tenderness, loss of continuity, loss of mobility, or changes in resting length, tone, or bulk. An examiner identifies the intrinsic muscle bellies and extrinsic muscle tendons, resisting movement when necessary to make them more prominent. He or she determines whether a tendon is severed, adherent, or not gliding smoothly within its sheath. The EPL tendon is especially subject to irritation at the dorsal radial (Listner's) tubercle, around which it makes a 45° turn. Tendon sheaths and bursae may be tender or swollen.

An examiner palpates bones and joints for the presence of tenderness, swelling, mechanical alterations, hypomobility, or hypermobility. He or she may palpate the carpus systematically, beginning with the styloid processes as landmarks. The ulnar styloid marks the level of the radiocarpal joint. Just distal to it lies the triquetrum, which becomes prominent with radial deviation. The pisiform is quite superficial, resting on the triquetrum at the ulnar edge of the distal skin crease of the wrist. To locate the hamate, the examiner places his or her thumb in the direction of the patient's web space with the IP joint over the patient's pisiform; the hamulus will lie directly under the pulp of the examiner's thumb.

Radially, the *anatomical snuffbox* lies just dorsal and distal to the radial styloid process, bordered by the EPL and EPB tendons. A scaphoid fracture produces tenderness in this area. The tubercle of the scaphoid is prominent volarly under the distal wrist skin crease. Just distal to the scaphoid but proximal to the thenar eminence is the trapezium, and one may locate its articulation with the first metacarpal by moving the thumb. Adjacent to the ulnar border of the trapezium is the trapezoid. One best palpates the adjacent

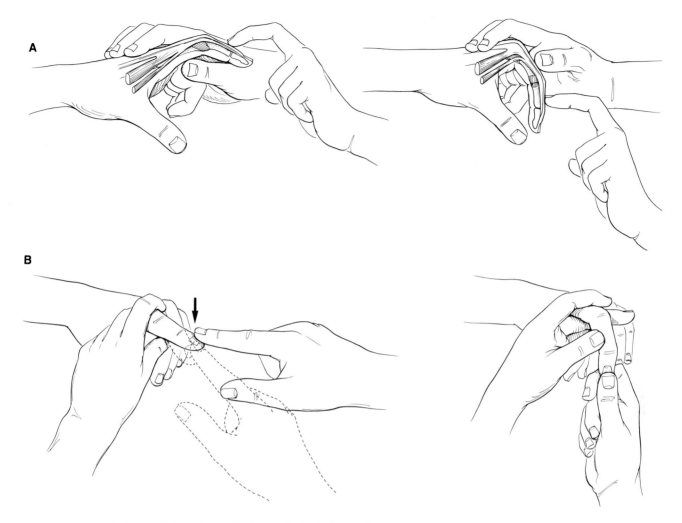

Fig. 13-25. A, The Bunnell-Littler test for intrinsic muscle tightness is positive when PIP joint flexion increases as the MP joint is flexed; **B,** the oblique retinacular ligament test is positive when DIP joint flexion increases as the PIP joint is flexed.

lunate and capitate dorsally on a line connecting the dorsal radial tubercle and base of the third metacarpal. With the wrist at 0° of extension, one palpates the prominence of the capitate, whereas the lunate lies in a depression. Flexing the wrist moves the lunate out from underneath the capitate, filling out the depression.

At the onset of the examination, the therapist identifies visible deformities or changes in joint shape. At this point in the examination the therapist acquires additional information regarding the site of tenderness and instability of the joints through palpation. Ligaments are normally not sensitive to pressure or stretch, so pain elicited by palpation may be indicative of injury or disease. One cannot feel a normal joint capsule; however, synovial proliferation can render it accessible, and perhaps painful, to palpation.

Palpation may also reveal certain qualities of arteries and nerves. One locates the pulse of the ulnar artery just proximal to the pisiform and lateral to the FCU tendon by pressing the artery against the ulna. A therapist palpates the radial pulse

lateral to the FCR tendon and medial to the radial styloid process. An examiner performs an Allen test to determine the patency of the radial, ulnar, and digital arteries. He or she asks the patient to exsanguinate the hand by clenching a fist several times; the patient then maintains a fist while the examiner occludes both arteries at the wrist; the patient next opens the hand, which appears white. The examiner notes arterial filing on the respective side as he or she releases pressure from one artery at a time. An examiner applies the same maneuver to the digital arteries by applying pressure to occlude flow at the base of the fingers.

In 1915 Tinel described a tingling sensation produced by pressure on an injured nerve. This phenomenon, now referred to as *Tinel's sign,* provides a test to identify the level of regeneration following repair of a nerve, by tapping along the course of the nerve from distal to proximal toward the site of injury. Resulting paresthesias in the nerve's distribution are an indication of regeneration at the point where it was tapped. Paresthesias may also result from tapping at the

WRIST AND HAND EXAMINATION FORM cont.

b/c/d. Physiological movements: active / passive / resistive			Active			Passive				Resistive	
			Degrees	Symptoms	Quality	Degrees	Symptoms	End-feel	Limiting structures	Strength	Symptoms
Forearm		supination									
		pronation									
Wrist		extension									
		flexion									
		abduction									
		adduction									
Thumb	CM	extension									
		flexion									
		abduction									
		adduction									
	MP	extension									
		flexion									
	IP	extension									
		flexion									
Index	MP	extension									
		flexion									
		abduction									
		adduction									
	PIP	extension									
		flexion									
	DIP	extension									
		flexion									
Middle	MP	extension									

Fig. 13-26. Wrist and hand examination form: physical examination, including physiological movements.

WRIST AND HAND EXAMINATION FORM cont.

b/c/d. Physiological movements: active / passive / resistive			Active			Passive				Resistive	
			Degrees	Symptoms	Quality	Degrees	Symptoms	End-feel	Limiting structures	Strength	Symptoms
Middle	MP	flexion									
		abduction									
		adduction									
	PIP	extension									
		flexion									
	DIP	extension									
		flexion									
Ring	MP	extension									
		flexion									
		abduction									
		adduction									
	PIP	extension									
		flexion									
	DIP	extension									
		flexion									
Little	MP	extension									
		flexion									
		abduction									
		adduction									
	PIP	extension									
		flexion									
	DIP	extension									
		flexion									

Fig. 13-26, Cont'd.

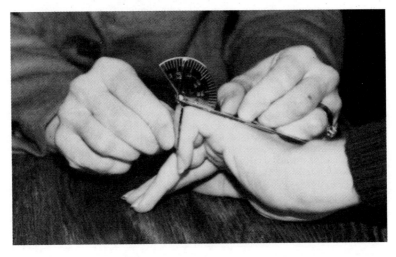

Fig. 13-27. Therapist using a finger goniometer to measure PIP joint ROM.

WRIST AND HAND EXAMINATION FORM cont.

e.   Joint play movements

		Mobility (grade 0 - 6)	Symptoms
Radiocarpal and midcarpal joints	dorsal glide		
	volar glide		
	ulnar glide		
	radial glide		
Ulnomeniscotriquetral "joint"			
Intercarpal joints	scaphoid		
	lunate		
	triquetrum		
	pisiform		
	trapezium		
	trapezoid		
	capitate		
	hamate		
Carpometacarpal joints	1st		
	4th		
	5th		
Intermetacarpal joints	2 - 3		

Fig. 13-28. Wrist and hand examination form: physical examination, including joint play movements.

WRIST AND HAND EXAMINATION FORM cont.

		Mobility (grade 0 - 6)	Symptoms
Intermetacarpal joints	3 - 4		
	4 - 5		
Metacarpophalangeal joints	1		
	2		
	3		
	4		
	5		
Proximal interphalangeal joints	1		
	2		
	3		
	4		
	5		
Distal interphalangeal joints	2		
	3		
	4		
	5		

Fig. 13-28, cont'd.

site of a *peripheral nerve entrapment.* Common areas of entrapment include the cubital tunnel, which is posterior-lateral to the medial humeral epicondyle, the carpal tunnel, which lies deep to the flexor retinaculum, and the distal ulnar tunnel, between the pisiform and hamate bones.

One performs Phalen's test to detect signs of median nerve compression within the carpal tunnel. A positive test occurs when wrist flexion, maintained for 60 seconds, reproduces sensory changes in a median nerve distribution (Fig. 13-30).

The neurological portion of the examination reveals abnormalities in the conduction of neurological impulses that may be responsible for a patient's signs and symptoms (Fig. 13-31). Sensory disturbance, aberrant deep tendon reflexes, weakness, or loss of motor control and coordination reveal neurological dysfunction. An examiner attempts to localize the source of the problem to a nerve root, peripheral nerve, or central nervous system lesion, remembering that

there may be overlaps and anomalies in innervation patterns. Making a definitive diagnosis may therefore require a combination of results of several tests.

Involvement of either the cervical nerve roots and peripheral nerves may affect both muscle strength and sensation in the upper extremity. One determines the level of root involvement, if present, without testing every muscle by identifying a *key muscle* or joint action that is representative of a given root level. The key muscles acting on the hand include the ECRL and ECRB (representing C-6), EDC (representing C-7), FDS and FDP (representing C-8), and the interossei (representing T-1) (Fig. 13-31).[24]

One determines peripheral nerve involvement by testing representative muscles as well. The opponens pollicis muscle (median nerve), the palmar interossei (ulnar nerve), and the EPL muscle (radial nerve) may reveal weakness, leading the examiner to further testing.

An examiner next performs sensibility evaluation to

WRIST AND HAND EXAMINATION FORM cont.

3.   Palpation (note location and nature of abnormality)

a.   Skin and subcutaneous tissues: tenderness _____   temperature _____   swelling _____

moisture _____   decreased mobility _____

b.   Muscles and tendons: tenderness _____   loss of continuity _____   loss of mobility _____

other _____

c.   Tendon sheaths and bursae: tenderness _____   swelling _____

d.   Bones and joints: tenderness _____   swelling _____   prominences

e.   Arteries and nerves: radial artery pulse _____   ulnar artery pulse _____   Allen test _____

Tinel's sign _____   Phalen's test _____

Fig. 13-29. Wrist and hand examination form: physical examination, including palpation.

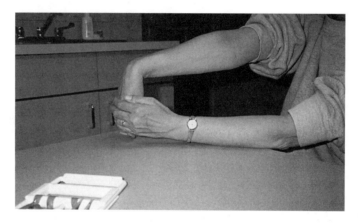

Fig. 13-30. Phalen's test for carpal tunnel syndrome is positive when sustained wrist flexion for 60 seconds reproduces median nerve symptoms.

identify the area of a nerve lesion and its associated functional disability. He or she must localize the area of involvement and distinguish dermatomal versus peripheral patterns of aberrant sensation, just as when testing the motor system. In a case involving nerve regeneration; he or she also determines the most distal level of return. A hand diagram assists in mapping the results of various sensory tests.

Numerous tests are available to evaluate the various sensory modalities. An examiner may utilize light touch and discrimination of sharp and dull, or hot and cold, sensation to initially distinguish a *pattern* of involvement. These tests, however, do not necessarily predict functional recovery. Objective tests are available, which eliminate the subjectivity of a patient's response but also may not correlate with the return of sensibility.[14] These include a sudomotor test in which ninhydrin applied to the palm reacts with sweat if the sympathetic system is functional, and a "wrinkle" test in

which a hand immersed in warm water (104°F) for 5 minutes wrinkles when sympathetic nerves are intact. Objective tests also include measurement of nerve conduction velocity and muscle response to electric stimulation.

Two-point discrimination (2PD) tests the ability to discriminate whether one or two blunt points are applied to the skin. It assesses *innervation density* and is useful in charting nerve regeneration. An examiner applies a caliper or discrimination device marked in millimeter increments to the volar surface of the patient's supported finger, while his or her vision is occluded (Fig. 13-32). Although some conditions may require testing the entire palm, usually a therapist only applies the stimulus to the volar digital pulp, which is the most concentrated area of receptor density.[36]

Static 2PD assesses the slowly adapting fiber receptor system. An examiner applies the prongs of the testing device parallel to the long axis of the finger, randomly alternating

WRIST AND HAND EXAMINATION FORM cont.

4.   Neurological evaluation

Key muscles (grades 0 - 5)

a. Nerve roots

C_6:   ECRL and ECRB _____

C_7:   EDC _____

C_8:   FDS and FDP _____

T_1:   Dorsal interossei _____

b. Peripheral nerves

Median: opponens pollicis _____

Ulnar: palmar interossei _____

Radial: extensor pollicis longus _____

Sensibility

Key: A =   monofilament

B =   sharp vs. dull

C =   temperature discrimination

D =   sweating (ninhydrin test)

E =   two-point discrimination (static)

F =   two-point discrimination (moving)

G =   30 cps vibratory perception

H =   256 cps vibratory perception (moving)

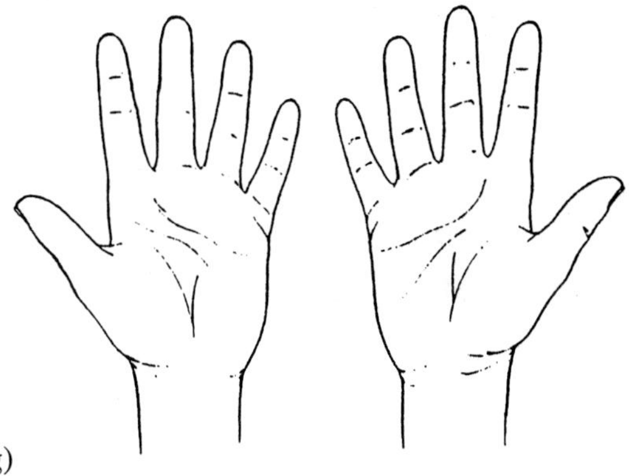

c. Motor function: spastic _____   flaccid _____   rigid _____   clonic _____

d. Coordination

Trace a diagram _____

Button a button _____

Tie a bow _____

Key: N =   completes with normal speed and coordination

CD =   completes slowly with minimal coordination difficulty

SM =   completes with searching movements

U =   unable to complete

5.   Other tests recommended

Imaging studies

Laboratory

Electrodiagnostic

Other

Fig. 13-31. Wrist and hand examination form: physical examination including neurological evaluation and other tests.

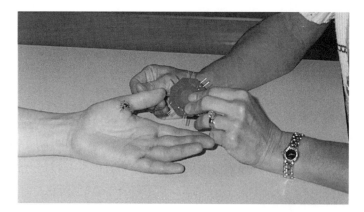

Fig. 13-32. Two-point discrimination test: randomly apply one or two points to the fingertip.

Table 13-3. Sensory norms

	Two-point distance in millimeters		Monofilament number
Normal	3-5 mm	Normal light tough	1.65-2.83
Fair	6-10 mm	Diminished light touch	3.22-3.61
Poor	11-15 mm	Diminished protective sensation	3.84-4.31
Protective	One point perceived	Loss of protective sensation	4.56-6.65
Anesthetic	Nothing perceived	Untreatable	>6.65

between one and two points. He or she narrows the interprong distance until the patient perceives only one point; 7 out of 10 correct responses are required to document a discrimination distance (see Table 13-3 for standard values).

Moving 2PD assesses the quickly adapting receptor system, which correlates best with tactile diagnosis and function. An examiner applies the prongs in a manner similar to static tests, except he or she *moves* the instruments in a stroking fashion, from proximal to distal. The examiner aligns the points transverse to the long axis of the finger and moves them parallel to the finger. The capacity to detect M2PD returns before S2PD, following the repair of a nerve laceration.

Semmes-Weinstein monofilaments constitute a threshold test that measures *stimulus intensity.* It is useful for assessing sensory loss associated with nerve compression. Calibrated sets of monofilaments are commercially available, ranging from very fine to very thick fibers. An examiner applies the thinnest monofilament perpendicular to the fingertip until it bends, while occluding a patient's vision (Fig. 13-33). The patient indicates with a response such as "touch" whenever he or she perceives a stimulus. If he or she does not perceive it after three applications, then the examiner applies the next thicker monofilament, repeating this progression until the patient feels the stimulus. (See Table 13-3 for standard values.)

Vibratory testing evaluates the threshold of stimulus needed to elicit vibration perception. It is useful in monitoring nerve compression and correlates with functional ability. Vibration is administered via 30 cps or 256 cps tuning forks or vibrometers and is a noninvasive type of test. Meissner receptors perceive 30 cps vibration and Pacinian receptors 256 cps. An examiner applies the vibratory instrument to a patient's fingertip and asks him or her to discern differences between involved and noninvolved parts (Fig. 13-34). With use of a vibrometer a patient reports when vibration is detected as the therapist gradually increases the amplitude.

An examiner describes the status of the motor system in terms of spasticity, flaccidity, rigidity, and clonicity. The presence of any of these abnormal patterns characterizes a central nervous system disorder. Conversely, a peripheral nerve lesion produces only localized muscle spasm or paralysis. One tests coordination by asking a patient to trace a diagram, button a shirt, or tie a bow. A code on the examination form relates to the patient's competence in carrying out the designated activities (Fig. 13-31).

A therapist may request other tests to clarify the results of the examination. Imaging studies, laboratory work, electrodiagnostic studies, etc., may provide additional information if the clinical examination is not conclusive.

After a therapist completes the examination and obtains all of the necessary data, he or she faces the task of

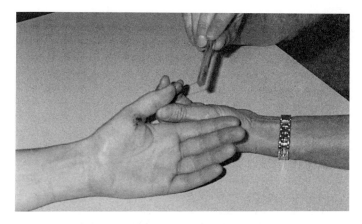

Fig. 13-33. Semes-Weinstein monofilament test: apply light pressure until the filament bends.

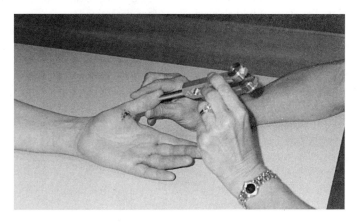

Fig. 13-34. Vibratory sensation test: apply the tip of a 256 cps tuning fork to the fingertip.

interpretation. He or she must recognize and dismiss irrelevant data. He or she must identify patterns and trends among the information that lead to defining the patient's status in terms of specific problems, structure(s) at fault, and baseline functional impairment (including rate and direction of change relative to the predicted course of similar types of impairment).

One may successfully conclude an examination when he or she can satisfy the following standards: (1) ascertain the consistency of the patient's status with the provisional diagnosis, (2) provide data for making a definitive diagnosis, (3) provide data for recommending patient disposition (including physical therapy intervention), and (4) determine the need for additional data. If the examination determines that the patient requires physical therapy treatment, the therapist can then proceed with program planning and implementation.

PATHOLOGIC CONDITIONS AND TREATMENT GUIDELINES
The rheumatoid hand

Rheumatoid arthritis is a chronic systemic disease that produces inflammatory changes in synovial joints and other connective tissues. Rheumatoid disease often affects the hand, causing pain, joint disorganization, and deformity. Because of the disease's chronicity and potentially devastating effects, it is prudent to institute proper management as early as possible.

The pathological elements that lead to deformity include microvascular injury, edema, and synovial inflammation and proliferation. The diseased synovium exuberates granulation tissue that extends across the joint surface as pannus. The pannus contains hydrolytic enzymes capable of eroding articular cartilage, subchondral bone, ligaments, and tendons. Joint capsules and supporting structures, weakened and distended by the inflamed tissue, yield under external forces, rendering the joints susceptible to the development of laxity and instability. Tendons, likewise, undergo fibrous dissolution, lengthening, and eventual rupture. Atrophy and shortening occur in both intrinsic and extrinsic muscles, which authorities propose result from disuse secondary to inhibition by pain stimuli.[15] These events act in combination to destroy the delicate balance among the muscles, tendons, and bones of the hand. The following paragraphs describe the mechanisms that deform specific joints in the rheumatoid hand.

Rheumatoid arthritis often afflicts the distal radioulnar and wrist joints. Because these joints comprise a link system between the forearm and hand, their dysfunction severely compromises hand function in several ways. Involvement of these more proximal joints may make the hand unstable, from lack of a supportive base. It also limits positioning of the hand, which affects the force the extrinsic finger muscles can generate because they depend on the wrist's position for mechanical leverage. When the rheumatoid process deforms the digital joints as well, this loss of extrinsic muscle power is especially devastating.

Wrist deformity usually involves flexion, radial deviation, and palmar subluxation of the carpal bones. Spontaneous fusion may occur with the wrist in flexion. The digital flexor muscles then become slack and lose much of their power. Another deformity involves dorsal subluxation of the ulnar head at the distal radioulnar joint. The deformity displaces the ECU tendon palmarly so that it no longer affords ulnar stability during wrist extension, thumb abduction, and finger flexion. Ankylosis occurs within the intercarpal and carpometacarpal joints as well, destroying the transverse arch framework and the cupping ability of the hand.

Rheumatoid arthritis frequently produces MP joint deformity, namely, ulnar deviation and palmar subluxation of the proximal phalanges. This particular configuration is partially related to the normal anatomy of the MP joints. Ulnar deviation and rotation normally accompany MP joint flexion in most hand activities because of the asymmetry of the collateral ligaments and the ulnar slope of the metacarpal heads.

The disease process accentuates this normal ulnar deviation by weakening the supporting structures. This leaves the MP joints vulnerable to the propagation of the deformity by ordinary forces generated in using the hand.[15] During pinch and grasp activities the extrinsic flexor tendons produce a force having ulnar and palmar components (Fig. 13-35). The bases of the proximal phalanges shift ulnarly and palmarly, causing the flexor tendons to bowstring away from the joint axis, which increases the dislocating forces.

Likewise, the disease weakens the dorsal fibers that stabilize the extensor tendons. The tendons shift from the dorsum to the ulnar sulci adjacent to the MP joints. In this position they lie volar to the joint axes and no longer function as extensors. Thus the aberrant forces become self-perpetuating, because the extensor tendons now contribute to flexion as well as ulnar deviation.

The intrinsic muscles also become deforming elements as they develop contractures, producing MP joint flexion and ulnar deviation.

Last, ulnar deviation at the MP joints occurs as part of a collapse deformity. With the wrist in radial deviation, the fingers move in the opposite direction, attempting to remain in alignment with the forearm.

The *swan neck* deformity, represented by hyperextension of the PIP joint and flexion of the DIP joint, results from imbalance of flexor and extensor forces in the presence of PIP joint laxity. Synovitis may restrict PIP joint flexion, concentrating flexor force at the MP joint. Intrinsic muscle contracture contributes to PIP joint extension. Laxity of the transverse retinacular ligaments allows the lateral bands to bowstring over the PIP joint, and the deformity progresses (Fig. 13-9). Hyperextension of the PIP joint increases tension in the FDP tendon, which then exerts more flexion force at the DIP joint.

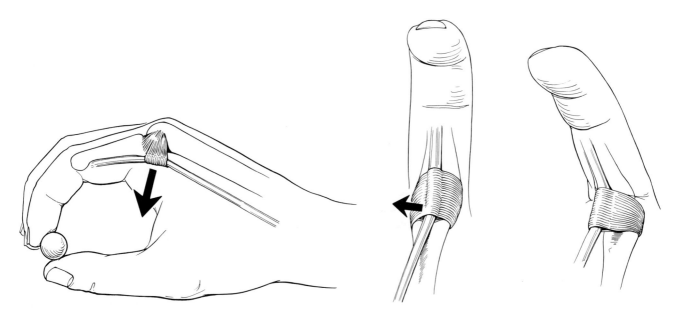

Fig. 13-35. Normal flexor tendon forces contribute to ulnar deviation and volar subluxation of the MP joint when rheumatoid arthritis weakens the supporting structures. (Modified from Flatt AE: *Care of the arthritic hand,* ed 4, St Louis, 1983, Mosby.)

The *boutonniere* deformity, characterized by PIP joint flexion and DIP joint extension, commonly results when the disease process weakens or ruptures the central slip of the EDC tendon. Proximal IP joint flexion is then essentially unopposed. The lateral bands accentuate this flexion, because they dislocate and slip volar to the joint axis, becoming PIP joint flexors (Fig. 13-10). The flexed PIP joint relaxes the FDP tendon so that it becomes mechanically weaker. The DIP joint hyperextends because the FDP muscle cannot oppose the extensor force of the terminal tendon.

Thumb dysfunction occurs commonly in rheumatoid arthritis. The thumb is the most important digit of the hand, and its impairment can impose severe restriction on prehension and grip strength. The most common deformity is the boutonniere, in which the MP joint flexes and the IP joint extends (Fig. 13-36, *A*). Synovitis at the MP joint initiates this condition, stretching the capsule and dorsal hood. Laxity of the supporting tissues displaces the EPL tendon and the adductor pollicis muscle ulnarly. The EPB tendon is stretched and weakened and cannot extend the MP joint (*extrinsic minus* thumb). The power of the extensor mechanism concentrates distally, producing hyperextension of the distal phalanx (*intrinsic plus* thumb). Attempts to use the thumb in pinch activities aggravate the deformity by exaggerating the collapse of the MP and IP joints.

A swan neck thumb deformity, in which the MP joint extends and the IP joint flexes, may also occur. Destructive changes at the trapeziometacarpal joint produce radial subluxation of the first metacarpal and contracture of the adductor pollicis muscle. The MP joint hyperextends in response to the stretch forces present during pinch. Tension in the FPL tendon passively flexes the IP joint (Fig. 13-36, *B*).

Treatment and management of the rheumatoid hand involve close interaction of all members of the rehabilitation team. In the acute phase of the disease and during subsequent exacerbations, a clinician's primary goal is protection of the inflamed hand. A physician may prescribe medications, and a therapist may use modalities to control pain and inflammation. Splinting helps relieve pain and edema, maintain proper joint alignment, and aid in prevention of deformity during the early stages of the disease. Examples of splints are a cock-up wrist splint, which positions the wrist functionally while allowing movement of the thumb and fingers, and a resting hand shell, which immobilizes the wrist and hand (Fig. 13-37).

During acute flare-ups a therapist limits exercise to isometric muscle contraction and gentle ROM activities. One should avoid excessive stretching, which only increases pain and the potential for tissue damage. Local heat application through use of paraffin, whirlpool, or ultrasound helps stimulate circulation, reduce pain, and increase mobility. Cryotherapy, if tolerated by the patient, also may alleviate inflammation, pain, and edema.

As acute inflammation and spasm subside, joint movement is less painful to the patient. A therapist intersperses controlled activity with periods of immobilization. Active

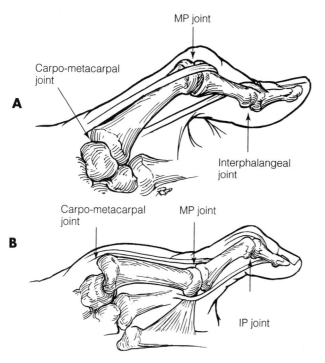

Fig. 13-36. Thumb deformities. **A,** Boutonniere, demonstrating loss of MP joint extension; **B,** swan neck, demonstrating subluxation of the base of the metacarpal with adduction and hyperextension of the MP joint. (Modified from Swanson AB: *Reconstructive surgery in the arthritic hand and foot,* CIBA Clinical Symposia, 31(6), 1979.)

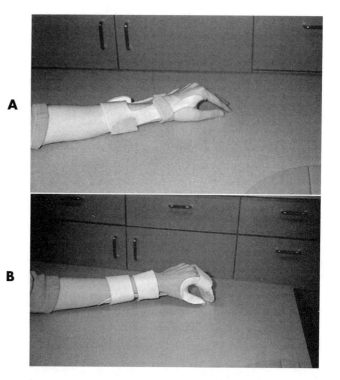

Fig. 13-37. Resting splints used for acute rheumatoid arthritis. **A,** Cock-up; **B,** hand shell.

assistive exercise reduces joint stiffness and tendon adhesions. Isotonic exercise enhances both strength and joint mobility. A therapist should emphasize exercises to strengthen finger extension, which becomes weaker as the EDC tendons sublux into the sulci between the fingers. A therapist builds functional activities into a patient's rehabilitation program to make the transition back to self-care and performance of daily tasks easier. He or she usually discourages resistive exercises because of the excessive force they impart to weakened and mechanically deranged tissues.

One should consider the effects of fatigue when planning the treatment program. Inflammation and other factors in the disease may cause a patient to tire easily. To prevent undue strain on the joints, a therapist incorporates rest periods as part of the overall program. Shorter, more frequent exercise sessions throughout the day are better than one prolonged period. Dynamic splints replace protective splints as the patient resumes more active function. A therapist should educate the patient regarding ADL and should provide appropriate adaptive devices.

In the chronic phase of the disease a vicious cycle of increasing malfunction develops; contractures and deformities decrease hand use, which leads to stiffness and further contractures.[15] A therapist deals with the problem by encouraging activity and fabricating splints that control joint position and direct muscle action. Examples of appropriate splints include knuckle-benders and dynamic wrist and MP joint splints.

Surgery may be necessary to alleviate symptoms, correct deformities, and restore function. One should recognize, however, that surgical techniques will not completely restore normal anatomical function, nor will they provide permanent correction. Surgery is not used in isolation but requires therapeutic management, both in preoperative and postoperative phases. Preoperatively, physical therapy helps decrease the extent of surgery necessary by increasing mobility and muscle strength and by altering alignment through splinting. Postoperatively, the therapist attempts to restore as much function as possible. A combination of modalities, exercise, splinting, patient education, environmental adaptation, and possible vocational rehabilitation assist in reaching this goal.

A patient shoud not postpone surgery until total joint destruction has occurred. Prophylactic synovectomies help protect the adjacent joint structures from the destructive effect of the diseased synovium. Intrinsic muscle contracture releases may prevent the development of MP joint subluxation, ulnar deviation, and swan-neck deformities. A surgeon can excise portions of diseased tendons and repair them by end-to-end apposition in small areas or use free tendon grafts in larger areas of involvement. Extensive tendon damage may require tendon transfers followed by a thorough program of muscle reeducation to ensure the patient makes optimal use of the new motor ability.

Joint reconstruction procedures generally fall into three categories: arthrodesis, arthroplasty, and prosthetic replacement. A surgeon selects joints for arthrodesis if their stability is necessary for function based on the overall condition of the rest of the hand. Examples of joints chosen for fusion include the wrist, the thumb trapeziometacarpal, the MP and IP joints, and the finger PIP joints.

Arthroplasty involves realigning joint surfaces and rebalancing soft tissues. This procedure improves function in the MP and PIP joints. Following the immobilization period, a therapist closely supervises an exercise program so that the patient learns to perform the desired movements and avoid deforming stresses.

Implant resection arthroplasty involves replacing diseased articular components with flexible silicone implants.[48] The implants serve as dynamic spacers and maintain alignment during healing as the body *encapsulates* the new joints. Finger and thumb MP and IP joints, intercarpal joints, and wrist joints are all candidates for implant resection arthroplasty. This procedure enhances stability, mobility, and durability while alleviating pain. Following surgery, a therapist initiates early motion to reduce edema, prevent soft-tissue contractures and adhesions between gliding surfaces, and maintain strength.

It is important to carefully control movement to prevent excessive stress on healing tissues. A dynamic splint serves as an adjunct to the exercise program to control motion in the desired plane and range and to assist flexor and extensor power following MP joint arthroplasty. As healing progresses, a therapist instructs the patient in joint protection principles, such as prevention of deforming positions, substituting pulp-to-pulp pinch for lateral pinch, building up small-handled utensils, employing proper body mechanics in all activities, and using adaptive and assistive devices to meet specific needs.

Joint replacement arthroplasty also restores motion and reduces pain. It is often functionally superior to fusion, but there are limits to the life of the prosthesis and its ability to remain seated within bone. Following prosthetic replacement, a therapist should recognize the restraints inherent in the prosthetic design, so that he or she does not attempt to force movement beyond what the prosthesis allows.

Home programs for continuation of therapeutic measures benefit patients with rheumatoid arthritis, whether they are undergoing conservative management or surgical treatment. A therapist should thoroughly educate a patient regarding the nature and course of his or her disease, signs and symptoms warning of impending flare-ups, and techniques of treatment and joint protection that he or she can use at home. A paraffin bath is a good modality for applying local heat to the small joints of the hand and one that a patient can easily utilize at home. A patient can perform passive, active, and resistive exercises but must continuously monitor the changing status of his or her musculoskeletal structures. The patient should also consider energy-saving devices whenever feasible.

Insidious conditions and cumulative trauma disorders

Carpal tunnel syndrome. Carpal tunnel syndrome is the most common peripheral compression neuropathy.[49] Any condition that decreases the area of the carpal tunnel or increases the volume of its contents may contribute to median nerve compression. Examples include synovial hypertrophy, tenosynovitis, ganglia, fracture callus, and tumors. Compression of the perineural vasculature leads to localized metabolic disturbance in the nerve.[11,22,29]

A typical history reveals a gradual onset of numbness, pain, and paresthesias in the median nerve distribution distal to the wrist, but sparing the thenar eminence. Symptoms often awaken the patient at night or occur during driving. Vigorous use of the hand, which may produce venous engorgement or flexor tendon synovitis within an unyielding space, aggravates a patient's symptoms. In advanced cases, weakness, clumsiness, and thenar atrophy may occur.

The clinician bases diagnosis of carpal tunnel syndrome on clinical history and provocative, sensory, and electrophysiologic tests. Studies reveal that a decrease in 256 cps vibratory perception is one of the earliest detectable changes, followed by decreased sensation in a Semmes-Weinstein monofilament test; loss of two-point discrimination occurs in later stages of the syndrome.[18,49]

Nerve conduction velocity reveals first an increase in distal sensory latency (greater than 3.5 mm/sec), then distal motor latency (greater than 4.5 mm/sec). Electromyography reveals the presence of fibrillation (or denervation) potentials in the median innervated intrinsic muscles. Of the provocative tests, Phalen's is more sensitive than Tinel's.[20,49]

Treatment of carpal tunnel syndrome involves eliminating the aggravating cause, if possible, such as repetitive movement, particularly with the wrist flexed and ulnarly deviated. Conservative management is often beneficial and may simply require restriction of activity and use of resting splints at night. Oral nonsteroidal anti-inflammatory drugs (NSAIDS) or steroid injection around the flexor tendons within the carpal tunnel may also afford relief.

Surgery is indicated for cases with intolerable sensory changes and progressive loss of function. After surgical division of the flexor retinaculum (transverse carpal ligament), the physician applies a compression dressing incorporating a wrist cock-up plaster slab. He or she instructs the patient to elevate the hand for the first 3 days and to actively move the fingers that are left free of the dressing. After dressing removal on the fourth day, the therapist instructs the patient in active exercises according to a written home program. The patient may also perform functional activities but must avoid lifting more than 2 pounds. At 2 weeks, following suture removal, the therapist instructs in light resistive exercises using theraputty (Fig. 13-38). Patients generally resume all activities, including full duty at work, approximately 4 weeks after an endoscopic release and 6 weeks after an open release.

Distal ulnar tunnel (Guyon's canal) syndrome. Nu-

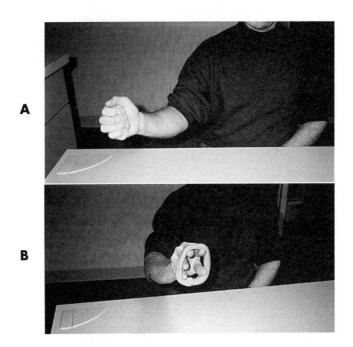

Fig. 13-38. Theraputty exercises for light resistance after carpal tunnel release. **A,** Flexion; **B,** extension.

merous etiologies that include ulnar artery thrombosis or aneurysm, fractures of the triquetrum or hamate, deep carpal ganglia, occupational compression, and blunt trauma can decrease the space within the distal ulnar tunnel.

A patient's history involves the insidious development of numbness, pain, and paresthesias over the palmar aspect of the medial side of the hand and medial 1½ digits. A patient occasionally experiences an acute onset of symptoms following blunt trauma or sustained compression (e.g., long-distance bicycling). Weakness occurs in the third and fourth lumbrical muscles, the interosseous muscles, and the adductor pollicis muscle. The syndrome also affects the hypothenar muscles unless compression occurs distal to the branch that supplies them, in which case the patient displays unopposed abduction of the little finger, known as *Wartenberg's sign.*

To manage this condition, eliminate the cause, such as repetitive trauma to the base of the hand, if possible. Administer NSAIDS and immobilize or rest the hand as necessary. If symptoms progress, surgical release of the distal ulnar tunnel is indicated. The rehabilitation protocol is similar to the one described for carpal tunnel syndrome.

De Quervain's syndrome. De Quervain's syndrome is inflammation of the synovial sheath surrounding the APL and EPB tendons at the wrist. Direct trauma to the tendon sheath or, more commonly, repetitive irritation, may elicit this condition. It produces tenderness over the radial styloid process, aggravated by active abduction of the thumb. A passive stretch produced by thumb adduction and wrist ulnar deviation is also painful (Finklestein's test). Treatment involves cold application and immobilization of the thumb in a forearm-based splint during the acute phase. When the condition becomes subacute, apply heat, phonophoresis, and active exercise. In recalcitrant cases, steroid injection or surgical incision of the first extensor compartment is necessary. After surgery, active exercise is initiated in 2 to 3 days upon dressing removal.

Dupuytren's disease. Dupuytren's disease is a progressive fibrosis of the palmar aponeurosis of unknown cause. It primarily affects men older than 40 years of Northern European ancestry; an increased incidence occurs in persons with alcoholism, epilepsy, or gout.[41] This painless condition may be limited to nodule formation in the area of the proximal palmar crease or may involve collagenous bands that produce a fixed flexion contracture of one or more digits. Moderate to severe cases require surgical excision of the diseased tissue. Following fasciectomy, a therapist initiates active ROM exercises on the third postoperative day. A patient performs all thumb, finger, and wrist movements regularly and progresses until he or she obtains full ROM. A hand-based extension splint for the involved finger(s) may be necessary until healing is complete (Fig. 13-39).

Trigger finger/thumb. Trigger finger/thumb involves thickening within the fibrous tendon sheath in the area of the A-1 pulley (Fig. 13-40). This condition usually results from repetitive trauma, such as gripping or utilizing a hand tool with a sharp edge. A patient complains of progressive pain, swelling and stiffness in his or her palm, with localized tenderness over the involved aspect of the flexor tendon sheath. An annoying momentary locking (triggering) occurs upon attempts to actively flex or extend the finger/thumb. A mobile nodular enlargement is often palpable in the palm.

Conservative treatment involves localized rest with a hand-based splint that maintains the MP joint at 0° but ends proximal to the PIP joint, leaving the rest of the digit free to move. Surgical treatment involves incision of the A-1 pulley, freeing the fibrous sheath. Postoperative rehabilitation begins on the third day with active digit movement and decongestive massage. Light resistive exercises utilizing foam or putty may begin on the fourteenth day. The patient may expect full recovery in approximately 8 weeks.

Acute hand injuries

Crush injury. A crush injury is the most devastating of all hand injuries. It typically produces widespread damage to numerous tissues, including skin or nail loss, vascular compromise, tendon or nerve laceration, ligamentous damage, and fractures. Posttraumatic edema complicates recovery and contributes to fibrosis and adhesions. After surgical repair of the skin and soft tissues and fracture reduction and fixation, a therapist begins edema control measures and early motion of as many joints as possible.[6] The patient often requires a customized splint to meet his or her unique needs.

An extensive rehabilitation program follows, emphasizing selective tendon gliding exercises, isolated and compos-

A

B

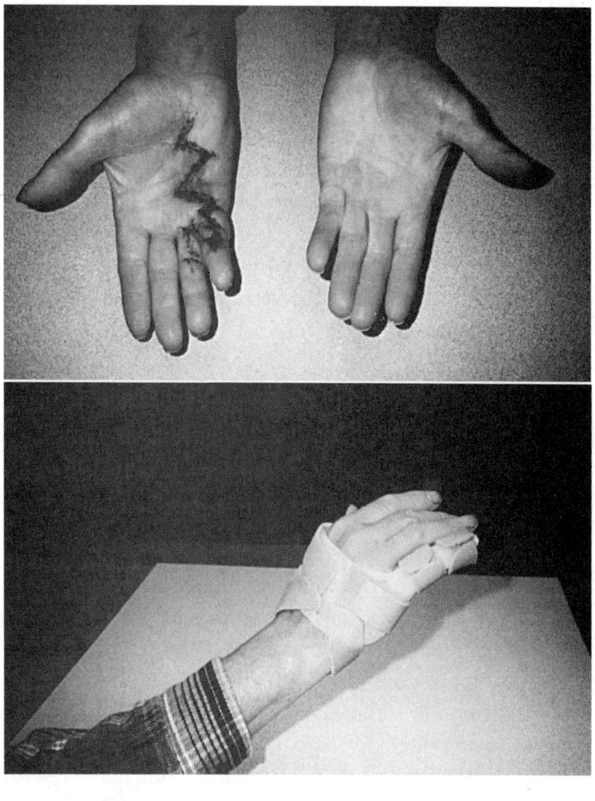

Fig. 13-39. Dupuytren's disease. **A,** Incision following surgical release; **B,** dorsal splint, maintaining extension following release.

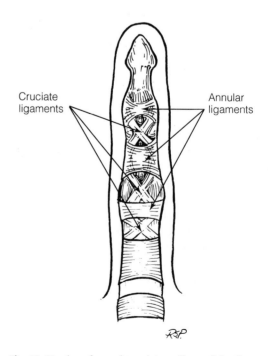

Fig. 13-40. Annular and cruciate pulleys of the finger.

ite joint motion, passive stretching, and joint mobilization. The program progresses to functional activities, strengthening, and endurance exercises. A therapist must be keenly aware of the healing status of the different tissues, as it may be appropriate to start exercise of a phalangeal fracture in 3 weeks, but the tendon repair in that digit will not withstand active contraction until 4 weeks. Please refer to the case study for additional details.

Sprains and dislocations

Lunate. A fall on the outstretched hand is the mechanism that produces most wrist injuries. This forces the wrist into its close-packed position of extension, with a potential for ligamentous damage, dislocation, fracture, or combinations of these injuries. The most common type of wrist dislocation involves an anterior dislocation of the lunate or a dorsal dislocation of the rest of the carpus relative to the lunate (perilunate dislocation).

Clinically, the volar projection of the lunate disrupts the normal surface configuration of the wrist and helps confirm the diagnosis. Because of the proximity of the median nerve, either lunate or perilunate dislocation can produce an acute compression syndrome if not reduced. These injuries may restrict flexor tendon gliding within the carpal tunnel as well. The volar radiocarpal ligament remains intact and theoretically preserves the lunate's blood supply.[33] Sometimes following trauma avascular necrosis occurs in the lunate (Keinbock's disease), producing wrist pain and lunate collapse.[1]

The treatment of choice for lunate dislocation is closed reduction followed by cast immobilization. However, if the dislocation is not diagnosed and treated within 2 weeks, it usually requires open reduction. A therapist initiates an exercise program during the period of casting to maintain shoulder, elbow, and finger function. After removal of the cast, the patient begins active thumb and wrist exercises. Attempts to restore motion lost because of immobilization must not stress the ligaments damaged by the initial injury. One must treat any complications, such as median nerve palsy, accordingly.

First MP joint. Forceful hyperextension or abduction of the thumb can rupture the ulnar collateral ligament of the thumb (Fig. 13-41). This is a common sports injury sustained from a fall on an abducted thumb. In cases of complete rupture or dislocation, gross clinical instability and pain, along with the mechanism of injury, make diagnosis relatively straightforward. If the dislocation can be reduced without interposition of soft tissue, it is accomplished through closed means; otherwise, open reduction is necessary. Treatment requires 4 to 6 weeks of immobilization to restore stability.[33] Thereafter, a therapist initiates protected range of motion and strengthening exercises, with stability taking precedence over mobility.

Second through fifth MP joints. A hyperextension injury of the second through fifth MP joints produces a sprain or dislocation and, in extreme cases, forces the metacarpal volarly between the lumbrical muscle and extrinsic flexor tendons. Severe twisting or lateral stress may also produce MP joint dislocation. A surgeon usually performs open reduction to ensure appropriate exposure when treating MP joint dislocation. After successful reduction, the joint is relatively stable and the patient can initiate early motion in a dorsal block splint. The splint maintains the MP joint at 60°, permitting active flexion from 60° to 90° (Fig. 13-42). A patient wears the splint for 5 weeks, then progresses to full ROM.[33]

Proximal interphalangeal joints. The small hinged PIP joints are the most commonly injured joints in the hand and rank second to the wrist in incidence of all upper extremity

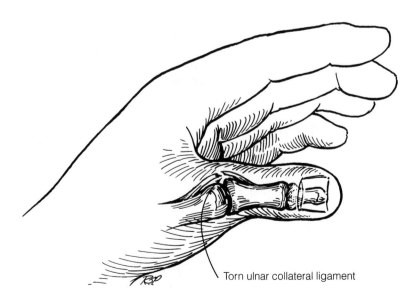

Torn ulnar collateral ligament

Fig. 13-41. Thumb ulnar collateral ligament injury.

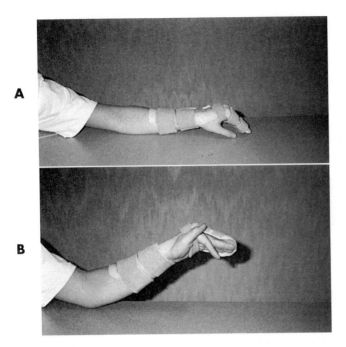

Fig. 13-42. Dorsal block splint. **A,** Maintaining the MP joint at 60°. **B,** Finger may be exercised from 60° to 90°.

trauma.[43] They are particularly vulnerable to injury because they have only one plane of motion, and the distal and middle phalanges serve as a relatively long lever arm in transmitting bending and rotatory forces from the fingertip. The most common injury is a hyperextension sprain, which usually occurs when a person catches a ball or when the finger is jammed into a solid surface. Hyperextension may damage the capsule, transverse retinacular ligaments, or collateral ligaments. A more forceful injury may produce subluxation or dislocation with disruption of the volar plate. Lateral angulation is less common but does occur during forceful grasping of an object that is jerked sideways.

Clinical characteristics of PIP joint injury include acute pain, localized swelling, and aberrant motion. The degree of instability will give the examiner an indication of the severity of the injury. If reduction is necessary, closed manipulation is usually satisfactory. Proximal IP joint immobilization follows a strict protocol with regard to position and duration. Because the PIP joint is more vulnerable to a flexion than an extensor contracture, one should splint it in no more than 20° of flexion to avoid shortening of the collateral ligaments, capsule, and the volar supporting structures, which become redundant as flexion increases.[43] A dorsal block splint, allowing flexion from 20° to 110°, helps prevent adhesions between the gliding tissue planes surrounding the flexor and extensor tendons. After 3 weeks, the splint is discontinued and the patient starts full active exercise. He or she buddy-tapes the injured finger to an adjacent finger for additional protection for 3 more weeks. Coban wrap assists in edema control. Restoration of full painfree motion may take as long as 6 to 9 months.[33]

Fractures

Radius. The distal radius sustains fractures more than any other bone in the body. As one attempts to break a fall with the outstretched arm, the hand fixed on the ground transmits force up through the forearm. The pronator quadratus and the brachioradialis muscles create a supination moment, producing maximal stress at the junction of cortical and cancellous bone in the distal radial metaphysis.

Abraham Colles, an Irish surgeon, first described a fracture of the distal radius 1 to 2 in. above the carpal extremity. The term *Colles' fracture* applies to most dorsally angulated fractures of the distal 2 in. of the radius, with or without accompanying ulnar fracture (Fig. 13-43). A similar fracture with a volarly angulated distal fragment is a Smith's fracture. A fracture through the dorsal articular area of the radius with dorsal and proximal displacement is termed *Barton's fracture.*

Treatment of a Colles' fracture consists of closed reduction, which may require anesthesia, followed by immobilization in an above-elbow plaster cast or an external fixator. During immobilization it is extremely important to stress full ROM of noninvolved joints and muscle-strengthening exercises. When the physician removes the cast or fixator in 6 to 8 weeks, a therapist initiates active and passive forearm, wrist, and thumb movements. He or she may also use other modalities to reduce pain and enhance mobility. Complications may include malunion, subluxation of the distal radioulnar joint, joint stiffness anywhere in the upper extremity, and rupture of the EPL tendon where it contacts Lister's tubercle near the roughened fracture site. One treats each complication as indicated. Rehabilitation of Smith's and Barton's fractures is similar to the Colles' fracture protocol.

Scaphoid. When a young athletic individual falls on his or her outstretched, supinated hand, he or she is more likely to fracture the scaphoid than the radius. Several unique features of this type of fracture make diagnosis difficult and yet necessitate adequate treatment to minimize serious late complications. The fracture, which is often transverse through the waist of the bone, may be difficult to recognize on initial radiographs. Scintigraphy and CT scans may assist diagnosis. Pain and swelling, localized in the "anatomical snuffbox," are good indications of a fracture even if there is no immediate radiographic evidence of such.

Treatment of scaphoid fractures requires immobilization in a thumb spica cast extending to the IP joint of the thumb. Displaced fractures may require ORIF. Even when the diagnosis is uncertain, the area should be immobilized until a physician can rule out or confirm a fracture. If one inaccurately diagnoses a scaphoid fracture as a wrist sprain and does not immobilize it, this increases the risk for nonunion. Because the blood supply only enters the distal pole of the scaphoid in many cases, healing is slower, and the incidence of nonunion, avascular necrosis, and degenerative changes over time increases. This fracture typically requires

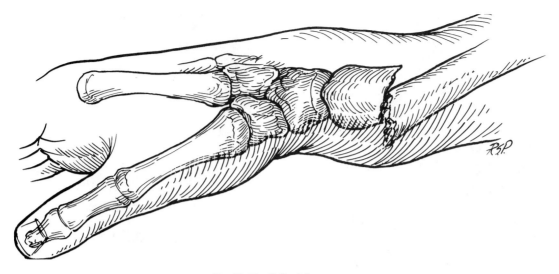

Fig. 13-43. Colles' fracture.

9 to 12 weeks to heal. When healing does not occur following prolonged immobilization, the fracture may require a bone graft. Prosthetic scaphoid implants are another option in cases of nonunion and avascular necrosis. A young client is usually able to regain hand function by activity alone, so extensive rehabilitation is not necessary.

Metacarpals and phalanges. A direct blow, crush, or twisting force may fracture the metacarpals or phalanges. Pain, instability, and possible angulation are the chief clinical features. A physician performs closed reduction if feasible; otherwise, he or she uses ORIF with bone plating or Kirschner wire (K-wire) fixation. If a patient requires immobilization, one applies a splint or cast. A physician usually discontinues immobilization in 2 to 4 weeks; then a therapist may begin exercises.

Tendon injury

Avulsions. Terminal extensor tendon avulsion from the base of the distal phalanx is the most common closed tendon injury affecting athletes. A forceful impact upon the tip of the extended finger, such as being struck by a ball that one is attempting to catch, is the usual mechanism that produces this injury. The patient experiences pain, swelling, and immediate loss of active DIP joint extension. The resultant drooping of the distal phalanx is a mallet finger deformity.

Treatment consists of simply splinting the DIP joint in slight hyperextension for a minimum of 6 to 8 weeks. One may use a commercially available stax splint or fabricate a custom splint to immobilize only the DIP joint. The patient starts AROM exercise in 8 weeks but continues to wear the splint at night for 4 more weeks. If the injury avulses a bone fragment with the tendon, surgical repair with K-wire fixation is indicated.

Extensor tendon central slip avulsion from the base of the middle phalanx is the second most common closed-tendon injury sustained in sports. The mechanism involves a forceful impact or "jamming" of the extended finger. The patient loses active PIP joint extension, and if the injury is left untreated, a chronic boutonniere deformity develops.

Conservative treatment involves splinting the PIP joint in extension while leaving the DIP free to move for 4 weeks. Surgical treatment incorporates reattachment of the tendon and K-wire stabilization for 5 to 6 weeks. Then the patient begins exercises to restore motion while guarding against PIP joint extension lag.

Flexor digitorum profundus avulsions from the distal phalanx occur when a sudden extension force is imparted to the actively flexed finger. This injury can occur when an athlete attempts to grab an opposing player's jersey that is forcefully pulled from his or her hand. After avulsion, a patient may experience a painful "snap," then be unable to actively flex the DIP joint.

This injury requires surgical tendon repair, and if a bony fragment is avulsed, it must be wired back into place. The therapist fabricates a dorsal block forearm-based dynamic splint, placing the wrist in slight flexion, the MP joints at 70° flexion, and the IP joints in 20° flexion. Rubber band traction flexes the finger to touch the palm, and the patient performs active extension within the limits of the splint. The splint is discontinued after 4 weeks, and the patient starts AROM exercise. At 6 weeks he or she starts progressive resistive exercise and resumes normal function at 10 weeks.

Flexor tendon lacerations. Sharp trauma may produce a partial or complete tendon laceration. Lacerations involving more than 25% to 50% of the tendon, depending on the tendon's condition, require surgical repair.[26,44] Surgeons divide the hand into zones that indicate the area of injury and the specific treatment required (Fig. 13-44).[45] The goal of flexor tendon repair is to achieve full painfree excursion without loss of power.

The unique characteristics of flexor tendon healing, which involve both intrinsic and extrinsic sources of blood supply, may impede optimal results.[44] A fibrous sheath

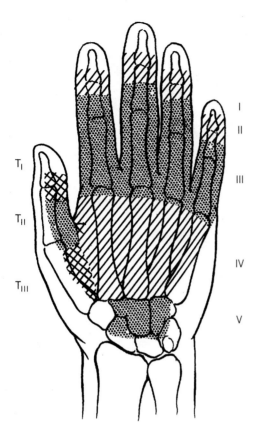

Fig. 13-44. Zones of flexor tendon injury: I—distal to the FDS insertion; II—between the A1 pulley and the FDS insertion; III—area between the distal carpal tunnel border and the A1 pulley; IV—within the carpal tunnel; V—proximal to the carpal tunnel; T I—from the thumb IP joint distally; T II—between the thumb A1 pulley and the IP joint; T III—area of the first metacarpal bone.

encases the flexor tendons between the DIP joint and the A1 pulley and contributes a substantial part of the tendon's extrinsic vascular supply. Continuity with the sheath facilitates tendon healing but also is the culprit in adhesion formation. Trauma to the tendon and surrounding tissues creates a fibroblastic response, and adhesions form between the tendon and adjacent structures, including the FDS and FDP tendons themselves. Differential wound healing is critical to a successful outcome; following tendon repair, the severed tendon ends must remodel with strength sufficient to transmit muscular forces, whereas the collagen between the tendon and adjacent tissues must remain randomly oriented and elastic to permit tendon gliding. To accomplish this, one performs passive gliding of the repaired tendon while protecting it from active forces until healing has progressed.[17,19,46] Passive motion enhances tendon healing by stimulating wound maturation, increasing tensile strength and linear excursion, and decreasing adhesions at the tenorrhaphy site.

A surgeon initially immobilizes the hand in dressings for 48 hours to decrease excessive bleeding and tissue reaction. Then a therapist fabricates a dorsal block forearm-based

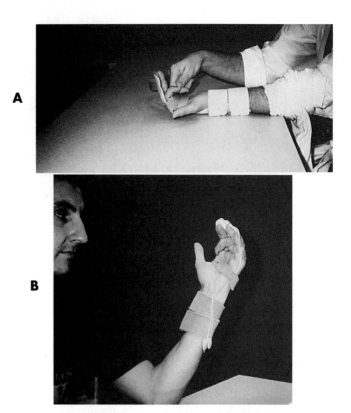

Fig. 13-45. Dorsal forearm-based splints after flexor tendon repair. **A,** Controlled passive motion; **B,** dynamic traction.

splint to maintain the wrist in 20° to 45° of flexion, the MP joints in 70° to 90° of flexion, and the IP joints in 0° to 20° of flexion. The fingers are passively flexed either manually (Duran protocol) or by dynamic traction (Kleinert protocol); the patient then actively extends his or her fingers within the confines of the splint (Fig. 13-45).[5,26,46]

When utilizing the Duran protocol of "controlled passive movement," 10 repetitions of full flexion are performed individually for the DIP and PIP joints. Then both joints are moved together in 10 repetitions of full composite flexion, every 2 hours.[5,45] With the Kleinert protocol, the patient performs active finger composite extension, then relaxes and allows the rubber band traction to flex the fingers 10 repetitions, every 2 hours. Modifications to the original Kleinert splint now incorporate a palmar pulley to ensure full flexion of all finger joints.[26,45]

Four weeks after repair a therapist replaces the splint with a wrist cuff incorporating dynamic traction; the cuff serves as a reminder for the patient not to perform forceful finger flexion while allowing full wrist ROM. The patient begins gentle active finger flexion and finger extension out of the cuff with the wrist extended only to a neutral position. (Full wrist extension in combination with finger extension is not permitted, because it would place excessive stress on the healing repairs at this time.)

Six weeks after repair, the therapist instructs the patient to discard the wrist cuff and initiate blocking exercise to

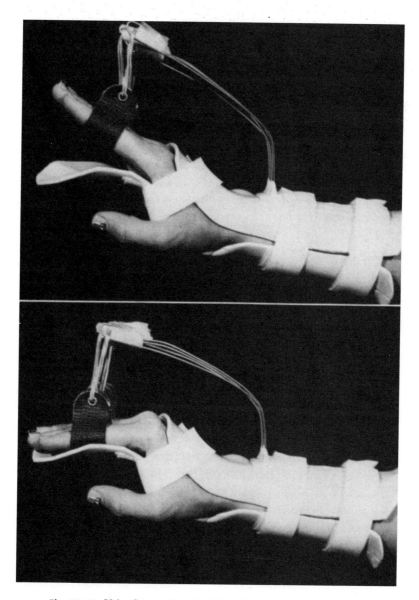

Fig. 13-46. Volar forearm-based splint after extensor tendon repair.

isolate individual joint motion and differential tendon gliding, taking care not to apply full force through the flexor tendons. A therapist may administer scar management and contracture control measures, if indicated. At the ninth week the patient may progress gradually to resistive exercises, returning to full function after the twelfth week.

Extensor tendon lacerations. Sharp trauma, crush injuries, and burns are mechanisms that produce extensor tendon injury. Following surgical repair, a therapist fabricates a volar block forearm-based splint to maintain the wrist in the 30° extension, the MP joints in 60° flexion, and the IP joints extended (Fig. 13-46). Although most utilize a static protocol, a forearm-based dynamic extension splint in which the patient performs active flexion while rubber bands produce passive extension is an alternative reported to be effective by Evans and Burkhalter.[13]

As with flexor tendon injuries, zones indicate the area of damage, but because of anatomical differences, these dorsal zones differ from the palmar zones (Fig. 13-47). As one moves distally into the hand, the extensor tendons become thinner and weaker, so immobilization is progressively maintained longer, and active exercise is started later than with proximal injuries. Please see Fig. 13-48 for the general treatment protocol.[2,12]

The burned hand. The hands are frequently involved with burns, because they are usually exposed and used for extinguishing a fire or handling hot objects. Hand burns produce cosmetic concerns, severe pain, deformity, and loss of function. A therapist directs therapeutic management toward restoring appearance, mobility, and function.

In the emergent phase, up to 72 hours after injury, burn shock threatens a patient's life. He or she usually requires

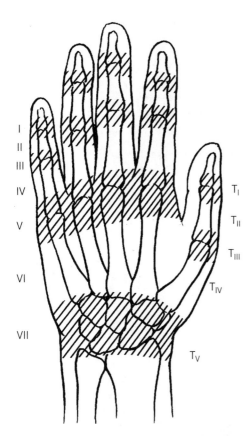

Fig. 13-47. Zones of extensor tendon injury: I—DIP joint and distal phalanx; II—middle phalanx; III—PIP joint; IV—proximal phalanx, V—MP joint; VI—metacarpal bone; VII—wrist; T I—IP joint and distal phalanx of the thumb; T II—proximal phalanx of the thumb; T III—thumb MP joint; T IV—metacarpal bone of the thumb; T V—wrist.

intensive fluid replacement. The added fluid in combination with the inflammatory response at the burn site contributes to massive edema, which reaches its peak approximately 2 days after a burn. Escharotomy and fasciotomy may relieve pressure and restore circulation. To combat edema the hands must remain elevated. A soft sling cradling the arm proximal to the elbow will assist in positioning the arm overhead, but caretakers must ensure that it does not place excessive tension on the brachial plexus or compression on the ulnar nerve at the elbow.[39]

Dorsal swelling and a position of comfort sought by the patient contribute to wrist flexion and clawing deformities. These contractures develop because wrist flexion produces extension of the MP joints through tenodesis of the EDC muscle; the MP joint collateral ligaments are lax and shorten to produce a fixed MP joint extension contracture. The action of the central slip may be lost at the PIP joint either by fixation of the sagittal bands at the MP joint by burn scar, or by direct disruption of the dorsal hood by the burn. A PIP joint flexion contracture then develops from constant tension of the unopposed FDS muscle.

A therapist splints the hands at the onset of treatment in an antideformity position, which is 0° to 30° of wrist extension, 70° to 90° of MP joint flexion, and IP joint extension. Extra compression or padding helps maintain the web spaces. As the edema subsides, a therapist revises the splints to maintain optimal position. One should carefully position and secure the splints, or they may contribute to, rather than alleviate, the deformity. A patient wears his or her splints at all times, except during periods of exercise and when they interfere with functional use of the hands.

After the emergent phase, the acute phase begins and lasts up until wound closure. A therapist initiates passive, active-assistive, and active exercise with the goal of reducing edema, maintaining muscle tone and ROM, and preventing capsular and ligamentous contractures and tendon adherence. Tendon adherence is common because the abundance of protein-rich exudate in the burned hand renders it susceptible to fibrotic changes, especially when immobilized.[34] Specific hand exercises include wrist circumduction, finger extension and abduction, thumb opposition, and cupping of the palm. Because dorsal burns are likely to involve the dorsal hood apparatus, a therapist should avoid composite flexion, that is, when attempting to increase flexion of one particular joint, he or she should block the other joints of the same digit in extension. The patient should perform self-care and ADL as soon as possible. These tasks exercise the hands and contribute to independence.

In addition to maintaining hand position and mobility, the therapist provides other aspects of burn care, such as preventing infection and achieving healing. Most burns require daily whirlpool treatments to assist wound cleansing and debridement, increase eschar pliability, and facilitate exercise. A therapist applies topical antibacterial agents or dressings after hydrotherapy to reduce the incidence of infection and pain. Synthetic dressings maintain wound hydration and enhance epithelialization.

Rapid wound closure is a major goal when treating the acutely burned hand. Many partial-thickness burns will heal eventually, but grafting may be preferred for functional and cosmetic purposes. If one chooses tangential excision and grafting, ideally a surgeon will do this procedure between the third and fourth days after injury.[16] Full-thickness burns always require grafting. The skin graft phase involves immobilizing the immediate area of the graft for 5 to 7 days. During this time the immobilized parts can perform isometric exercises, while other areas of the body may continue their regular program.

The rehabilitation phase extends from wound closure until scar maturation (up to 2 years). A therapist works with the patient to maintain scar pliability and decrease hypertrophy through massage, custom-fit pressure garments, and contact with silicone gel sheets.

After discharge the patient must also continue with exercise and splinting, if indicated, to ensure maximal recovery. Regular physical therapy follow-up is extremely important for the therapist to objectively reassess progress,

Days 0 through 3:   elevation in post surgical dressing:

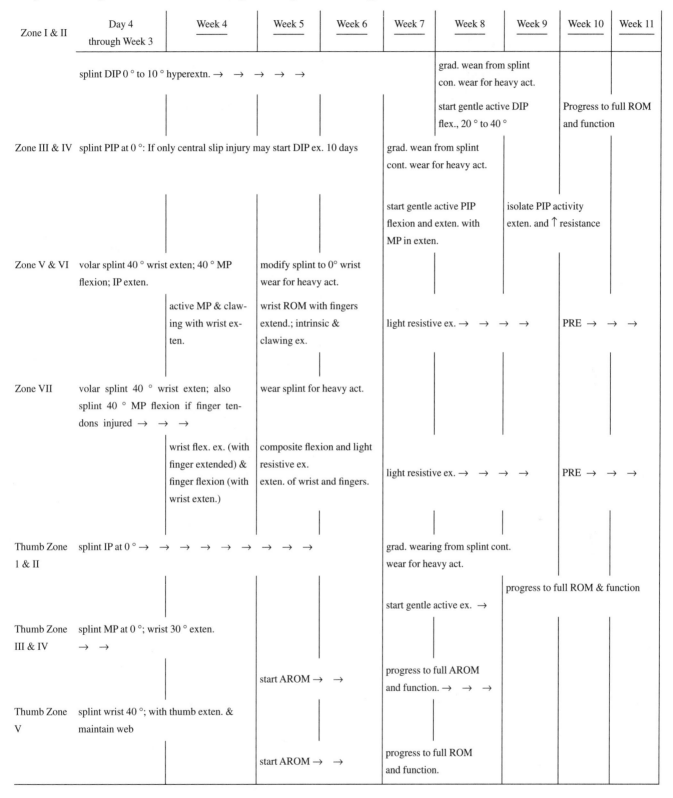

	Day 4 through Week 3	Week 4	Week 5	Week 6	Week 7	Week 8	Week 9	Week 10	Week 11
Zone I & II	splint DIP 0 ° to 10 ° hyperextn. → → → → →					grad. wean from splint con. wear for heavy act. start gentle active DIP flex., 20 ° to 40 °		Progress to full ROM and function	
Zone III & IV	splint PIP at 0 °: If only central slip injury may start DIP ex. 10 days					grad. wean from splint cont. wear for heavy act. start gentle active PIP flexion and exten. with MP in exten.	isolate PIP activity exten. and ↑ resistance		
Zone V & VI	volar splint 40 ° wrist exten; 40 ° MP flexion; IP exten.	active MP & clawing with wrist exten.	modify splint to 0° wrist wear for heavy act. wrist ROM with fingers extend.; intrinsic & clawing ex.			light resistive ex. → → → →		PRE → → →	
Zone VII	volar splint 40 ° wrist exten; also splint 40 ° MP flexion if finger tendons injured → → →	wrist flex. ex. (with finger extended) & finger flexion (with wrist exten.)	wear splint for heavy act. composite flexion and light resistive ex. exten. of wrist and fingers.			light resistive ex. → → → →		PRE → → →	
Thumb Zone I & II	splint IP at 0 ° → → → → → → → → →					grad. wearing from splint cont. wear for heavy act. start gentle active ex. →		progress to full ROM & function	
Thumb Zone III & IV	splint MP at 0 °; wrist 30 ° exten. → →		start AROM → →			progress to full AROM and function. → → →			
Thumb Zone V	splint wrist 40 °; with thumb exten. & maintain web		start AROM → →			progress to full ROM and function.			

Fig. 13-48. The general protocol for extensor tendon repair progression.

to revise exercises, splints, and garments as needed, and to encourage the patient toward maximal function.

Peripheral nerve injuries. Following an injury, the status of motor and sensory innervation is the single most important factor determining the recovery of hand function. A client's age, type and extent of injury, precision of surgical repair, and rehabilitation program influence the extent of recovery from nerve injury.

Seddon classifies peripheral nerve injuries as follows:

Neuropraxia—contusion that does not cause degeneration; the nerve will completely recover in 6 weeks.
Axontomesis—axonal disruption from blunt trauma or stretch without disruption of the Schwann tubes, allowing Wallerian regeneration to be completed through the original tube in approximately 6 months.
Neurotomesis—laceration or traction that completely disrupts the nerve, requiring precise surgical approximation with unpredictable recovery.

Two different factors influence the reinnervation process. One is the size of the nerve fibers. As axons sprout into regenerating endoneurial sheaths, the nerve cell bodies in the dorsal ganglia must produce axoplasm to replenish the nerves. Because the smaller fibers do not require as much axoplasm, they regenerate fastest; B & C afferent fibers, which are only from .2 to 3 μm in diameter, will be filled before A fibers, which are 12 to 20 μm in diameter.[10]

The other factor that affects reinnervation is the ratio of the axons to the cutaneous receptors. If there is only one axon to supply many receptors (axon:receptor = 1:>1 = <1), the chances and speed of recovery are less than if there are many axons relative to each receptor (axon:receptor = >1:1 = >1). Because Meissner corpuscles receive many axons, they will reestablish continuity first. Meissner corpuscles convey moving touch, flutter, and 30 cps vibration, so these sensory modalities return first. The Merkel cell-neurite complex recovers next, transmitting constant touch, deep pressure, and static 2PD. Pacinian corpuscles are the last to return; they convey moving touch and 256 cps vibration. It is interesting to note that the axon:receptor ratio for the Merkel cell-neurite complex is <1, whereas the ratio for the Pacinian corpuscles is 1:1; authorities hypothesize the delay in return of the Pacinian receptors is because of a "mechanical barrier" across which the regenerating fibers have to grow.

Ideally, a surgeon will repair a nerve within a few weeks of injury. This procedure takes advantage of the increase in metabolic activity of the nerve cell body in preparation for producing new axoplasm. Precise surgical alignment of fascicles enhances the prognosis, although functional recovery is never complete. It is essential to protect the nerve repair from tension for 2 to 4 weeks. A therapist fabricates a splint to immobilize the involved part with the joints positioned to maintain the nerve on slack.[29]

The examination section of this chapter describes numerous sensory, functional, motor, and sympathetic tests that can determine the status of nerve injury, regeneration, or both. A therapist uses these test results to plan and progress the rehabilitation process. A therapist usually initiates treatment with efforts to reduce edema and fibrosis. He or she accomplishes this through elevation, massage, and movement through a range of motion that does not traumatize the repair. Strengthening exercises for noninvolved muscles should continue throughout the course of treatment. When tissue healing is sufficient, the patient begins passive ROM exercises for the involved part(s). He or she attempts to use the extremity for goal-directed functions, utilizing adaptive devices as necessary. He or she must be aware of potential complications caused by insensitivity and trophic changes.

Functional splinting following nerve loss maintains functional hand position and prevents deformities resulting from muscle imbalance.[14] Although splint requirements differ according to individual needs, there are some common factors. Median nerve involvement requires a splint that at least maintains thumb abduction. Ulnar nerve loss typically produces clawing from loss of the intrinsic muscles in the fourth and fifth digits (Fig. 13-11); a therapist fabricates a splint that counteracts hyperextension of the MP joints. A radial nerve lesion precludes active wrist extension, so a cock-up wrist splint is necessary to position the hand in a functional position.

A therapist employs reeducation to enhance recovery of sensory modalities. This technique requires cortical correlation of sensory impulses with known stimuli. The sequence of sensory modality recovery usually occurs in the following pattern: pain, 30 cps vibration, moving touch, constant touch, and 256 vibration.[10] When the patient can perceive 30 cps, he or she attempts to relearn moving touch by heavy tracing of objects from proximal to distal areas. As recognition improves, the patient may gradually replace the heavy stimulus with lighter materials. Direction of movement is acquired by tracing numerals on the involved surface. Next, the patient learns constant touch by feeling or handling objects until he or she can recognize them without visual input (tactile gnosis).

Static two-point discrimination returns after light constant touch. Most young adults do not acquire better than 15 mm two-point discrimination following repair of nerve injury. Motor function, such as picking up and handling objects, accompanies sensory reeducation and is a useful training tool for developing movement patterns. Therapy sessions continue for a period of months, with the goal of gradually turning the program over to the responsible patient.

Work hardening

A majority of hand injuries occur in individuals who plan to return to the work force. A work capacity evaluation and a work hardening program improve the transition to gainful employment for many. An individualized program can assist a patient in developing sufficient strength, endurance, and coordination to return to his or her former occupation or a satisfactory alternate occupation. Use of a work-oriented treatment program with a productivity-based outcome is a cost-effective and time-saving link between medical rehabilitation and returning to work.[31]

A therapist plans graded activities according to a patient's specific job demands. For example, at the lowest level of resistance (0 to 1 pounds) he or she may begin with sorting objects (e.g., varied sizes of nuts and bolts), picking up and placing blocks or items in designated spaces, or macrame. Progressing to more resistance (2 to 3 pounds), he or she may perform activities such as exercise putty, assembling plumbing parts with or without tools (Fig. 13-49), leather work, and weight-resisted or mechanically resisted exercise. At a higher level (greater than 3 pounds) he or she can train at prehension tasks requiring speed, accuracy, strength, and sustained grip, such as woodworking, lifting and carrying boxes, progressive resistive exercise, and actual job-stimulated activity. Equipment such as the BTE Work Simulator* helps by reproducing job tasks and daily functions in a controlled clinical setting and provides feedback on the amount of torque generated and work performed (Fig. 13-50).

Advancing through these levels of activities allows a patient to improve work tolerance, speed, and proficiency. Through instruction and supervision he or she learns

appropriate techniques of pain mastery, body mechanics, and use of assistive or adaptive devices. Working toward an eventual goal of maximizing employability, a patient should ultimately reach his or her work tolerance level or plateau. The therapist discharges the patient from the program and advises him or her regarding acceptable levels of performance. In the event that he or she demonstrates inability to return to work, the program helps resolve the client's status in an unequivocal manner that may lead to justified pursuit of disability awards.[31]

JOINT MOBILIZATION TECHNIQUES FOR THE WRIST AND HAND

A therapist applies joint mobilization as a form of passive exercise in many cases of hand dysfunction to relieve pain

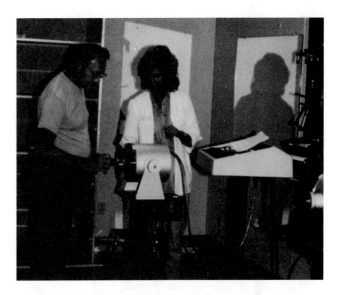

Fig. 13-50. The BTE Work Simulator records objective data for evaluating upper extremity function and offers a variety of attachments for simulating job tasks.

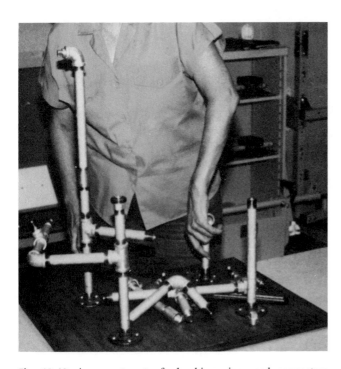

Fig. 13-49. An assortment of plumbing pipes and connectors provides functional hand exercise for increasing strength, endurance, ROM, and manipulative skills.

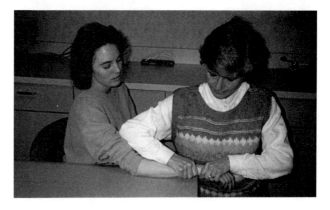

Fig. 13-51. Distal traction of carpus. Therapist stabilizes patient's arm, holding close to the joints; mobilization force is parallel to the long axis of the extremity, moving the carpus distally.

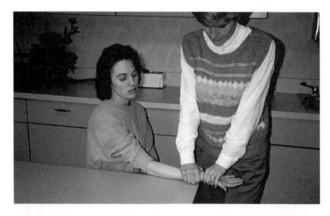

Fig. 13-52. Dorsal glide of the carpus. Therapist stabilizes the dorsal surface of the patient's forearm against the table, places distal traction on the carpus, and mobilizes the carpus volarly, perpendicular to the long axis of the extremity.

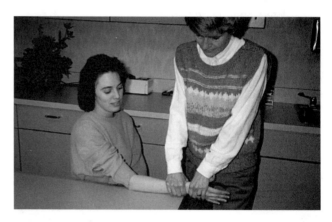

Fig. 13-54. Ulnar glide of the carpus. Therapist stabilizes the ulnar surface of the patient's forearm against the table, places distal traction on the carpus, and mobilizes the carpus volarly, perpendicular to the long axis of the extremity.

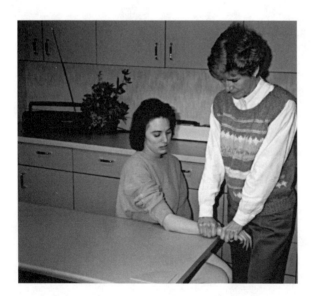

Fig. 13-53. Volar glide of the carpus. Therapist stabilizes the volar surface of the patient's forearm against the table, places distal traction on the carpus, and mobilizes the carpus volarly, perpendicular to the long axis of the extremity.

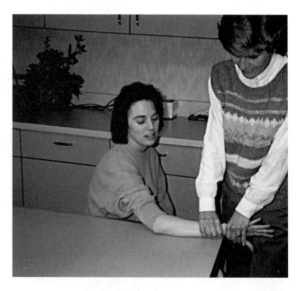

Fig. 13-55. Radial glide of the carpus. Therapist stabilizes the radial surface of the patient's forearm against the table, places distal traction on the carpus, and mobilizes the carpus volarly, perpendicular to the long axis of the extremity.

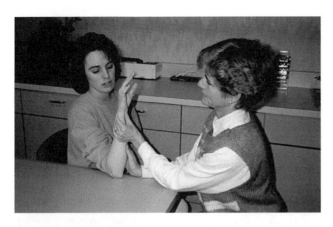

Fig. 13-56. Dorsal-volar glide of the meniscus and triquetrum on the ulna. Therapist stabilizes the patient's elbow on the table; with thumb over the pisiform and index finger over the dorsal ulnar styloid, a pinching force mobilizes the triquetrum dorsally and the ulna volarly.

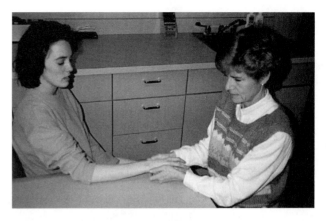

Fig. 13-57. Dorsal-volar glide of the metacarpals. Therapist stabilizes the patient's forearm on the table, grasps the metacarpals, and mobilizes the metacarpals one upon another or in combination to promote cupping of the palm.

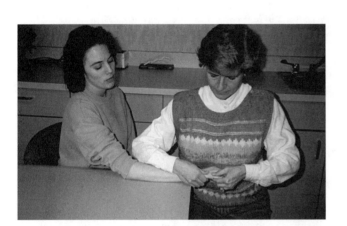

Fig. 13-58. Traction or glide of the MP or PIP joints. Therapist stabilizes the patient's hand on the table and grasps the adjacent metacarpal and phalanx close to the joint surfaces; mobilization force is parallel to the long axis of the finger; for glide or rotation techniques, he places distal traction on the phalanx and mobilizes in the appropriate direction.

and increase mobility. The therapist should perform a given technique in a controlled, reproducible manner with the appropriate grade and position to treat stiffness, pain, or spasm. Chapter 8 (Basic Concepts of Orthopedic Manual Therapy) discusses the indications for and the desired results of administering joint mobilization. The following paragraphs describe joint mobilization techniques for the wrist and hand.

Traction of the radiocarpal and midcarpal joints serves as a trial treatment (to determine a patient's response to joint mobilization) or as a technique for treating hypomobility in any direction (Fig. 13-51). Dorsal glide is the technique a therapist uses to increase wrist flexion. He or she moves the

convex carpus dorsally on the concave surface of the radius and disc (Fig. 13-52). A volar glide technique increases wrist extension. A therapist glides the carpus volarly on the radius and disc (Fig. 13-53). An ulnar glide technique increases radial deviation (Fig. 13-54), and a radial glide technique increases ulnar deviation (Fig. 13-55).

A therapist mobilizes the ulnomeniscotriquetral joint to increase forearm supination and pronation (Fig. 13-56). A dorsal-volar glide of the metacarpals, either individually or as a unit, improves metacarpal mobility and the carpal arch (Fig. 13-57).

Mobilization of the finger joints involves moving a concave surface on a convex surface (the opposite of articular surfaces at the wrist). Traction at the MP, PIP, or DIP joints provides a trial treatment or an exercise to increase any hypomobility (Fig. 13-58). Dorsal glide increases extension, whereas volar glide increases flexion. Medial/lateral and rotational motions also increase joint play.

SUMMARY

A patient with hand dysfunction desires the fullest recovery in the shortest time possible. This demands a fully coordinated team effort, with the patient being prepared to take responsibility for lasting results. Appropriate therapy requires an in-depth understanding and working knowledge of the clinical anatomy, mechanics, and pathology of the hand, as well as skill in evaluation, interpretation, and treatment techniques. This chapter correlates anatomical structure and function and pathological conditions that are commonly seen. Also, it presents a detailed format for evaluation and interpretation of results. Treatment considerations include appropriate timing and application of exercises, modalities, splinting, and joint mobilization.

CASE 1   Case Study

History

The patient is a 55-year-old male factory worker. He suffered a crush injury of his right (dominant) hand in a press. His diagnosis included fractures of the third metacarpal and proximal phalanx of the ring finger, and severe soft-tissue injury to the dorsum of the hand, palm, and the index finger (including avulsion of the MP joint volar plate), and the ring finger (including A4 pulley) (Fig. 13-59). He underwent surgical exploration and debridement of his hand wounds, ORIF of the fractures (K-wires in the metacarpal and a bone plate in the phalanx), and repair of the soft tissues. All digital neurovascular bundles and tendons were reportedly intact. He was referred to physical therapy on the fourth postoperative day for splint immobilization. He had no complications but was experiencing moderate pain.

Physical Examination

Inspection revealed a moderately edematous hand. Sutures were intact in numerous incisions, including the lateral aspect of the index finger and palm, the volar and dorsal surfaces over the third metacarpal, and the medial aspect of the ring finger, extending into the palm. Two K-wires protruded from the distal aspect of the third metacarpal (Fig. 13-60). A volar forearm-based splint was fabricated to maintain the wrist in 20° of extension, the MP joints in 70° of flexion, and the IP joints in 0° of extension. It was necessary to compromise the middle finger MP flexion to 60° due to the fracture fixation. The patient was instructed in splint care and was to wear it continuously except for removal briefly every 2 hours for skin inspection and cleansing. He was to maintain hand elevation at all times. He was to perform active motion of his thumb, which was uninjured and left free of the splint.

Problems

1. Healing status of fractures and soft-tissue injuries, requiring splint immobilization
2. Edema
3. Pain
4. Loss of hand motion and function

Treatment Goals

The goals of treatment were to initially provide immobilization during bone and soft-tissue healing and then to initiate motion and strengthening as soon as feasible. Edema and pain control were additional goals of therapy.

Treatment

The patient returned in 5 days for splint revision, including increasing MP joint flexion to 75° in all fingers. He also started A and PROM of the IP joints of all fingers except the ring, in which he was to perform only AROM. He was issued a written home program and instructions to exercise every 2 hours. He was to continue to maintain hand elevation.

Two weeks following injury the hand appeared moderately edematous. The patient complained of pain with joint movement but was compliant with his exercise program.

Three weeks following injury the sutures were removed and the splint discontinued. The patient was experiencing stiffness throughout his hand and was encouraged to strive for increased motion with his exercises. The patient was in-

structed in retrograde massage and Coban wrapping for edema control. He began MP joint motion in the index and ring fingers.

Four weeks following injury the pins were removed from the third metacarpal, and active motion of the MP joint was begun, in addition to other exercises. The patient was issued a foam gripper for light resistive exercise and an isotoner glove for edema control. He received physical therapy three times weekly and continued his home program.

Five weeks following injury the patient was experiencing less tenderness, but joint stiffness persisted throughout the hand. All incisions appeared well healed, and the edema had resolved. The patient was attempting to use his hand for functional activities and was performing his home exercises for an hour, three times daily. Physical therapy treatment included whirlpool, scar tissue massage, aggressive stretching exercise, and progressive resistive activities.

Six weeks following injury the patient's chief concern was lack of full active flexion. He was performing farm duties and using his hand for woodworking activities, in addition to structured exercises. Passive ROM was as shown in Table 13-4.

A volar forearm-based splint with static-progressive components was fabricated to enhance MP joint flexion (Fig. 13-61). The patient wore the splint at night and for periods during the day when he was not exercising his hand. His exercise program was advanced to include intrinsic muscle stretching and aggressive joint mobilization.

Three months following injury the patient returned to his factory job. He had complete passive composite extension in his fingers and sufficient passive flexion to allow the fingertips to touch the proximal palmar crease (PPC). However, he had a significant lag in AROM, lacking $1\frac{1}{2}$ in (index), $1\frac{3}{4}$ in (middle), and $1\frac{1}{2}$ in (ring) from touching the PPC. He continued to receive physical therapy three times weekly for an hour per session.

Six months following injury the patient underwent surgical tenolysis to free the index, middle, and ring finger flexor tendons from dense scar tissue. He was immediately placed on a continuous passive motion machine, which he continued to use at home for 2 weeks. He also performed active and passive ROM exercises and selective tendon gliding.

Eight months following injury the patient again returned to full duty. He continued to experience joint stiffness, but through diligent, aggressive exercise, he maintained full PROM and almost achieved full active extension (Fig. 13-62). He was unable to obtain full active flexion, however, lacking $1\frac{1}{4}$ in (index), 1 in (middle), and 1 in (ring) from touching the PPC in composite flexion (Fig. 13-63). His grip strength was 61% of age-matched norms in his right hand, compared with 105% age-matched norms in his left, uninvolved, hand.

In conclusion, fibrosis and residual flexor tendon adhesions prevented full return of active flexion. The patient's strong motivation, and aggressive therapeutic management did produce remarkable recovery from the devastating injury and allowed the patient to return to his former employment. He was to continue his home exercise program and return for medical and physical therapy reevaluation at 3-month intervals.

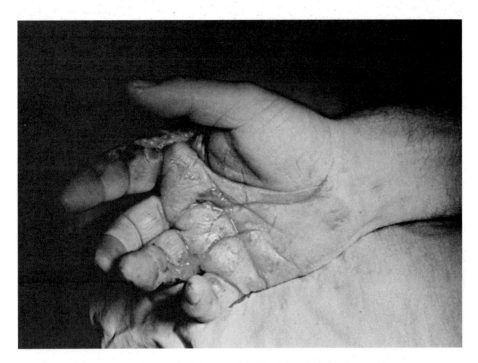

Fig. 13-59. Acute crush injury with "burst" soft-tissue lacerations.

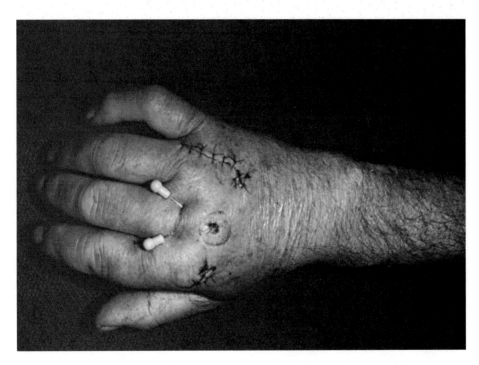

Fig. 13-60. Crush injury postoperatively, with pin fixation of the metacarpal fracture.

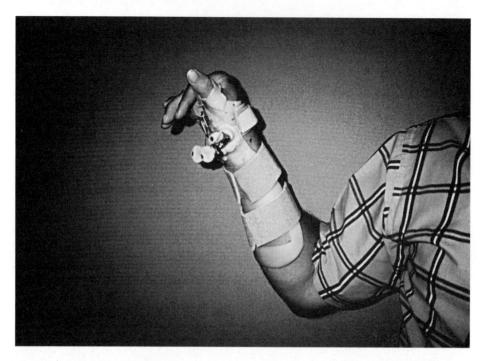

Fig. 13-61. Volar, forearm-based splint with static progressive components for increasing MP joint flexion.

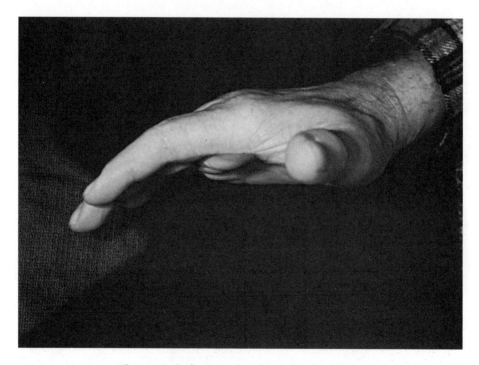

Fig. 13-62. Active extension, 8 months after injury.

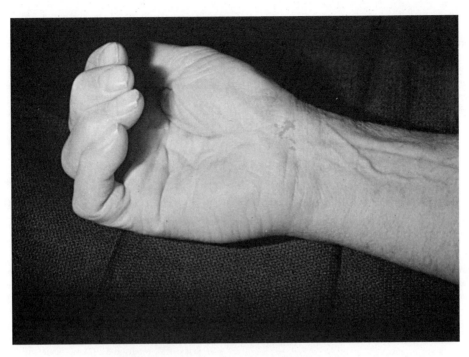

Fig. 13-63. Active flexion, 8 months after injury.

Table 13-4. Case study: passive ROM

	Index	Middle	Ring	Little
MP Joint	10-80	17-70	0-55	Not measured because of deformity from old injury; not involved in this injury.
PIP Joint	10-85	5-85	20-94	
DIP Joint	0-56	0-67	0-50	

REVIEW QUESTIONS

1. What are the "pure" spots for testing median, ulnar, and radial nerve sensation?
2. What is the normal configuration of the values in the five handle positions derived from a grip strength test?
3. What does a positive Bunnell-Littler test indicate? A positive Froment's sign?
4. What are the most common symptoms of carpal tunnel syndrome? Specifically where are they located?
5. What is the correct position for splinting an acutely burned hand?

REFERENCES

1. Alexander AH, Litchman DM: Kienbock's disease. In Lichtman DM, editor: *The wrist and its disorders*. Philadelphia, 1988, WB Saunders.
2. Blair WF, Steyers CM: Extensor tendon injuries, *Orthop Clin North Am*, 23(1):141, 1992.
3. Bogumill GP: Anatomy of the wrist. In Lichtman DM, editor: *The wrist and its disorders*, Philadelphia, 1988, WB Saunders.
4. Cailliet R: *Hand pain and impairment*, ed 2, Philadelphia, 1975, FA Davis.
5. Cannon NM, Strickland JW: Therapy following flexor tendon surgery, *Hand Clin*, 1(1):147, 1985.
6. Carter PR: Crush injury of the upper limb, *Orthop Clin North Am*, 14(4):719, 1984.
7. Cooney, WP III, Lucca MJ, Chao EYS, Linscheid RL: The kinesiology of the thumb trapeziometacarpal joint, *J Bone Joint Surg Am*, 63A(9):1371, 1981.
8. Craig SM: Anatomy of the joints of the fingers, *Hand Clin*, 8(4):693, 1992.
9. Cyriax J: *Textbook of orthopaedic medicine*, ed 6, vol 1, Baltimore, 1975, Williams & Wilkins.
10. Dellon AL: *Evaluation of sensibility and re-education of sensation in the hand*, Baltimore, 1981, Williams & Wilkins.
11. Ditmars DM Jr, Houin HP: Carpal tunnel syndrome, *Hand Clin* 2(3):525, 1986.
12. Evans RB: Therapeutic management of extensor tendon injuries. In Hunter JM, Schneider LH, Mackin EJ et al, editors: *Rehabilitation of the hand*, ed 3, St Louis, 1990, Mosby.
13. Evans RB, Burkhalter WE: A study of the dynamic anatomy of extensor tendons and implications for treatment, *J Hand Surg* 11A(5):774, 1986.
14. Fess EE: Rehabilitation of the patient with peripheral nerve injury, *Hand Clin* 2(1):207, 1986.
15. Flatt AE: *Care of the arthritic hand*, ed 4, St Louis, 1983, Mosby.
16. Fleegler EJ, Yetman RJ: Rehabilitation after upper extremity burns, *Orthop Clin North Am* 14(4):699, 1983.
17. Gelberman RH, Manske PR: Factors influencing flexor tendon adhesions, *Hand Clin* 1(1):35, 1985.
18. Gelberman RH, Szabo RM, Williamson RV, Dimick MP: Sensibility testing in peripheral-nerve compression syndromes, *J Bone Joint Surg Am* 65A(5):632, 1983.
19. Gelberman RH, Woo SL-Y: The physiological basis for application of controlled stress in the rehabilitation of flexor tendon injuries, *J Hand Ther* 2(2):66, 1989.

20. Gellman H, Gelberman RH, Tan AM, Botte MJ: Carpal tunnel syndrome, *J Bone Joint Surg Am* 68A(5):735, 1986.

21. Gupta A, Kleinert HE: Evaluating the injured hand, *Hand Clin* 9(2):195, 1993.

22. Hecker FR, Jabaley ME: Evolving concepts of median nerve decompression in the carpal tunnel, *Hand Clin* 2(4):23, 1986.

23. Hill NA: Complications of acute injuries of the wrist and reconstruction. In Sandzen SC Jr, editor: *The hand and wrist,* Baltimore, 1985, Williams & Wilkins.

24. Hoppenfield S: *Physical examination of the spine and extremities,* New York, 1976, Appleton-Century-Crofts.

25. Idler RS: Anatomy and biomechanics of the digital flexor tendons, *Hand Clin* 1(1):3, 1985.

26. Jaeger SH, Mackin EJ: Primary care of flexor tendon injuries. In Hunter JM, Schneider LH, Mackin EJ et al, editors: *Rehabilitation of the hand,* ed 2, St Louis, 1984, Mosby.

27. Janda DH, Geiringer SR, Hankin FM, Barry DT: Objective evaluation of grip strength, *Occup Med* 26(7):569, 1987.

28. Kapandji IA: *The physiology of the joints,* vol 1, Baltimore, 1970, Williams & Wilkins.

29. Lovett WL, McCalla MA: Nerve injuries: management and rehabilitation, *Orthop Clin North Am* 14(4):767, 1983.

30. Massengil JB. The boutonniere deformity, *Hand Clin* 8(4):787, 1992.

31. Matheson LN, Ogden LD, Violette K et al: Work hardening: occupational therapy in industrial rehabilitation, *Am J Occup Ther* 39(5):314, 1985.

32. Mathiowetz V: Grip and pinch strength measurements. In Amundsen LR, editor: *Muscle strength testing,* New York, 1990, Churchill Livingstone.

33. McCue FC III, Baugher WH, Kulund DN, Gleck JH: Hand and wrist injuries in the athlete, *Am J Sports Med* 7(5):275, 1979.

34. Miles W: Soft tissue trauma, *Hand Clin* 2(1):33, 1986.

35. Mooney JF III, Siegel DB, Koman LA: Ligamentous injuries of the wrist in athletes, *Clin Sports Med* 11(1):129, 1992.

36. Moran CA, Callahan AD: Sensibility measurement and management. In Moran CA, editor: *Hand rehabilitation,* New York, 1986, Churchill Livingstone.

37. Niebuhr BR, Marion R: Detecting sincerity of effort when measuring grip strength, *Am J Phys Med* 66(1):16, 1987.

38. Palmer AK, Werner FM: Biomechanics of the distal radioulnar joint, *Clin Orthop* 187:26, 1984.

39. Puddicombe BE, Nardone MA: Rehabilitation of the burned hand, *Hand Clin* 6(2):281, 1992.

40. Rettig AC: Closed tendon injuries of the hand and wrist in the athlete, *Clin Sports Med* 11(1):77, 1992.

41. Rowland E: Dupuytren's disease, *First Hand News* 4(2):1, 1994.

42. Smith RJ: Balance and kinetics of the fingers under normal and pathological conditions, *Clin Orthop* 104:92, 1974.

43. Sprague BL: Proximal interphalangeal joint injuries and their initial treatment, *J Trauma* 15(5):180, 1975.

44. Steinberg DR: Acute flexor tendon injuries, *Orthop Clin North Am* 23(1):125, 1992.

45. Stewart KM: Review and comparison of current trends in the postoperative management of tendon repair, *Hand Clin* 7(3):447, 1991.

46. Strickland JW: Biologic rationale, clinical application and results of early motion following flexor tendon repair, *J Hand Ther* 2(2):71, 1989.

47. Stuchin SA: Wrist anatomy, *Hand Clin* 8(4):603, 1992.

48. Swanson AB, Swanson GdG: Flexible implant resection arthroplasty of the proximal interphalangeal joint, *Hand Clin* 10(2):261, 1994.

49. Szabo RM, Madison M: Carpal tunnel syndrome, *Orthop Clin North Am* 23(1):103, 1992.

50. Totten PA, Flinn-Wagner S: Functional evaluation of the hand. In Stanley BG, Tribuzi SML, editors: *Concepts in hand rehabilitation,* Philadelphia, 1992, FA Davis.

51. Wynn Parry CB: *Rehabilitation of the hand,* ed 3, Sussex, 1973, Butterworth.

52. Zemel NP, Stark HH: Fractures and dislocations of the carpal bones, *Clin Sports Med* 5(4):709, 1986.

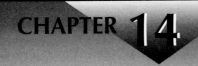

CHAPTER 14

The Elbow Complex

Richard W. Bowling and Paul A. Rockar, Jr.

OUTLINE

Anatomy
    Osteology
    Arthrology
Examination of the elbow complex
    Functional examination
Treatment of the cubital complex
    Dysfunction of noncontractile tissues
    Dysfunction of the capsule and accessory ligaments
    Treatment of hypomobility associated with connective tissue dysfunction
    Accompanying dysfunction of the capsule and accessory ligaments (hypermobility)
    Hypomobility as a result of dysfunction of the noncontractile component of the muscle
    Hypomobility as a result of articular surface dysfunction (springy motion barrier)
    Hypomobility as a result of articular surface dysfunction (bone-on-bone motion barrier and capsular barriers resistant to treatment)
    Noncontractile lesions (nerves and bursae)
    Dysfunction of contractile tissues
Case 1 Patient A
Case 2 Patient B
Summary

LEARNING OBJECTIVES

After studying this chapter, the reader should be able to:

1. List the articulations and identify the significant anatomic structures of the cubital complex.
2. Describe the joint mechanics of the cubital complex.
3. Discuss those factors that restrain elbow movements in the sagittal and frontal planes.
4. Describe the mechanics of the proximal and distal articulations of the forearm.
5. Describe those factors that limit pronation and supination of the forearm.
6. Describe and list all the components of a physical examination of the elbow complex.
7. Discuss those factors that must be considered when assessing the findings of the physical examination.
8. Describe the treatment of elbow complex hypomobility associated with connective tissue dysfunction.
9. Describe the treatment of elbow complex dysfunction associated with hypermobility of noncontractile structures.
10. Discuss the treatment program for contractile lesions affecting the elbow complex.

KEY TERMS

elbow	treatment
forearm	hypermobility
functional examination	hypomobility
cubital complex	

The cubital articulation is formed by the joints between the radius and humerus, the ulna and humerus, and the radius and ulna. All these joints share a common articular cavity. The first two are collectively known as the elbow and function as a hinge to allow flexion and extension of the forearm. The superior radioulnar joint belongs functionally to the joints of the forearm and participates in the movements of supination and pronation of the forearm along with the distal radioulnar joint.

The most common problem encountered by physical therapists in management of clients with dysfunction of the elbow complex is loss of motion as a result of trauma or immobilization. The goal of treatment in such cases is the restoration of a full and pain-free range of motion. The manner in which this goal should be accomplished, however, is controversial. On the one hand, most textbooks of orthopedic surgery advocate early active motion and state unequivocally that passive movement is contraindicated.[19,21] On the other hand, physical therapists who are experienced in the application of passive movement techniques are aware that properly selected and applied passive movement can supplement the effects of active exercise.[11,17]

The ability of the physical therapist to manage the problems encountered at the cubital complex hinges on understanding functional anatomy, pathokinesiology, principles of examination, and the principles of treatment of the musculoskeletal system used in therapeutic exercise. Selection of the appropriate treatment modality is no different at the cubital complex than at any other region of the musculoskeletal system. It involves the ability to perform a clinical examination to determine the nature and state of the pathologic condition present, as well as the ability to select and apply therapeutic techniques that can influence the problem identified in a positive manner.

ANATOMY
Osteology

Distal humerus. The distal end of the humerus is flattened in the frontal plane and projects anteriorly from the shaft of the humerus at an angle of approximately 45 degrees.[13] It bears two articular condyles, a medial or trochlear surface, providing articulation with the trochlear notch of the ulna and a lateral surface, or capitellum, for articulation with the proximal surface of the radial head.[22]

Three concavities, or fossae, are situated on the distal humerus. Anteriorly, the coronoid fossa is located just superior to the trochlear surface. It receives the coronoid process of the ulna during flexion of the forearm. Similarly, the radial fossa lies on the anterior surface just proximal to the capitellum, and during flexion of the forearm it accommodates the radial head.[7] Both of these anterior fossae increase the potential for flexion of the forearm.[13]

On the posterior aspect of the humerus, the olecranon fossa is located just superior to the trochlea, and it receives the olecranon process of the ulna during extension of the forearm, thus augmenting the range of extension.[13]

The trochlea covers the anterior, inferior, and posterior aspects of the medial humeral condyle.[22] It is a sellar articular surface that is concave in the frontal plane and convex in the sagittal plane. The trochlea is marked centrally by a deep groove that dictates the path that the ulna must follow during flexion and extension of the forearm.[15] The axis of motion of the elbow joint lies perpendicular to this groove. Laterally, the trochlea is separated from the capitellum by the capi/totrochlear groove.[22] Medially, the trochlea projects prominently downward below the rest of the bone.[22]

The capitellum is a roughly hemispheric body located on the anterior aspect of the distal humerus. Kapandji has described this articular condyle as lying entirely in front of the distal end of the humerus.[13] Thus, the radial head does not fit congruently with the capitellum when the elbow is extended. The capitellum has an ovoid articular surface that is convex in all planes.

The medial epicondyle is a blunt projection on the medial side of the medial condyle of the humerus.[22] The flexor muscles of the forearm (flexor carpi radialis, flexor carpi ulnaris, flexor digitorum superficialis, palmaris longus, and part of the pronator teres) take their origin from the anterior aspect of the medial epicondyle.[22] This structure also serves as the proximal attachment of the medial collateral ligament of the elbow joint.[22] The ulnar nerve runs in a groove on the posterior aspect of the medial epicondyle and is easily palpable in this location. The nerve is susceptible to trauma at this site because of its superficial position.

The lateral epicondyle is the lateral portion of the nonarticular region of the lateral condyle of the humerus. It gives origin to the superficial extensor muscles of the forearm (extensor carpi ulnaris, extensor digiti minimi, and supinator), as well as the lateral collateral ligament of the elbow joint.[22]

Proximal radius. The proximal end of the radius includes the head, neck, and bicipital tuberosity. The radial head is shaped somewhat like a disk, and its superior surface bears a shallow, cuplike articular surface for articulation with the capitellum of the humerus.[13,22]

The circumference of the radial head also bears an articular surface. This convex surface articulates with the radial notch of the ulna.[13] Just distal to the head of the shaft of the radius is a constricted region, the neck of the radius. It bears a roughened tuberosity on its medial aspect for attachment of the biceps brachii.

Proximal ulna. The upper end of the ulna presents two prominent processes: the olecranon and the coronoid. It also contains two articular surfaces, the trochlear notch and the radial notch, which articulate, respectively, with the trochlea of the humerus and the circumference of the radial head.

The olecranon process is the most proximal portion of the ulna. It projects upward and bends anteriorly to form a prominent beak that enters the olecranon fossa of the humerus when the elbow is extended.[22] The anterior aspect of the olecranon forms the upper part of the trochlear notch of the ulna.

The coronoid process is a small projection on the anterior aspect of the bone. Its superior surface forms the lower part of the trochlear notch.[22]

The trochlear notch, like the trochlea of the humerus with which it articulates, is a sellar surface. It is concave in the sagittal plane and convex in the frontal plane. Centrally, it is marked by a prominent ridge that corresponds to the groove found on the trochlear surface of the humerus.[15]

The radial notch is a concave articular depression located on the upper portion of the lateral aspect of the coronoid process of the ulna. It articulates with the circumference of the radial head to form the proximal radioulnar joints.[13]

Arthrology

MacConaill and Basmajian have classified the cubital complex as a paracondylar joint because one bone (the humerus) articulates with two others (the radius and ulna) by way of two facets.[16] This enables one of the latter two bones to undergo a movement independent of the other (e.g., rotation of the radius during pronation and supination of the forearm). The complex has two degrees of freedom. Flexion and extension of the forearm occur in the sagittal plane, and supination and pronation of the forearm are permitted in the transverse plane.

Kinematic analysis of the cubital complex can be simplified if the joint is divided functionally into the following components: (1) the elbow, which permits the movements of flexion and extension, and (2) the joints of the forearm, which permit supination and pronation.

Elbow. The elbow is composed of the humeroulnar and the humeroradial joints. The former possesses sellar articular surfaces, whereas the latter is ovoid in configuration. For practical purposes, these two joints can be considered to function as a uniaxial hinge joint.

Conflicting reports of elbow kinematics have been presented in the literature.[6,14,15,18] In a recent review, London discussed some of the major contributions in this area and noted some deficiencies in analytical techniques that were employed.[15] With what he considered an improved methodology, he determined that the instantaneous axes of rotation (IAR) for flexion and the IARs for extension of the humeroulnar joint were tightly clustered around the center of the arc formed by the trochlear sulcus of the humerus. Exceptions occurred during the last 10 degrees of extension when the IAR moved proximally and posteriorly toward the olecranon fossa.[15]

The IARs of the humeroradial joint demonstrated a similar distribution around the center of the arc formed by the capitellum.[15] During terminal flexion, the IAR moved proximally and anteriorly toward the radial fossa, and on terminal extension the IAR moved toward the posterior aspect of the capitellum.

The axis of motion of the elbow can be approximated by a line that connects the center of the arc of the trochlear sulcus with the center of the arc of the capitellum. This axis makes an angle of 94 to 98 degrees with the humeral shaft that declines from lateral to medial.[15] The position of the axis is also internally rotated with respect to the plane of the humeral epicondyles by 3 to 8 degrees (Fig. 14-1).[15]

In the plane of flexion and extension of the elbow, both of the moving surfaces (trochlear notch and radial head) are concave articular surfaces. Thus, the swing of the two bones is accompanied by gliding of the articular surfaces in the same direction.[16,22]

At the extremes of flexion and extension, the gliding movement of the articular surfaces is augmented by rolling.

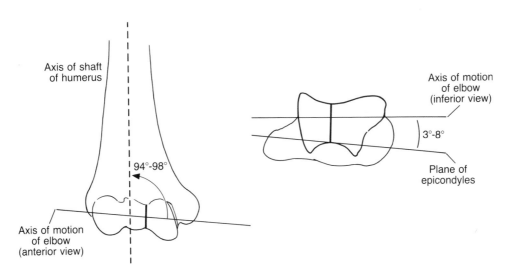

Fig. 14-1. Axis of motion of elbow joint.

The rolling movement also occurs in the same direction as the swing of the bones.[16,22] This rolling movement accounts for the displacements of the IARs that London has reported.[15]

The range of motion of elbow flexion and extension depends on whether the movement is produced actively or passively.[13] From the anatomic position, the elbow can flex through a range of 145 degrees actively and 160 degrees passively. Movement from the position of full flexion back to the anatomic position is termed *extension*. In some individuals, movement is permitted beyond the anatomic position. This motion is termed *hyperextension* and may reach a range of 5 to 10 degrees (Fig. 14-2).[13]

When the elbow is in the anatomic position (extended), a valgus angulation is evident between the arm and forearm. This angle is termed the *carrying angle* and usually ranges between 10 and 15 degrees.[13] The angle is generally larger in women than in men. There is some controversy over whether the valgus angulation remains constant or alters as the forearm is carried into flexion. Morrey and Chao state that the carrying angle varies in a linear manner from a valgus angle in extension to a varus angle in flexion,[18] but Grant[7] and London[15] state that the carrying angle is relatively constant throughout the range of flexion and extension. On careful clinical observation, the carrying angle does appear to remain constant if care is taken to prevent medial rotation of the humerus at the glenohumeral joint as the elbow is flexed.

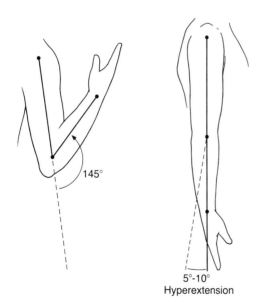

145°

5°-10°
Hyperextension

Fig. 14-2. Range of motion of elbow. From the anatomic position, the elbow can move through a range of 145 degrees of flexion actively. The joint is capable of 160 degrees of flexion passively. A range of 5 to 10 degrees of hyperextension is possible in some individuals. (Modified from Kapandji IA: *The physiology of the joints,* vol 1, *The upper limb,* London, 1970, E & S Livingstone, Inc.)

Supporting structures of the elbow. The elbow is supported by static and dynamic structures. The static structures include the fibrous capsule, the collateral ligaments, the osseous structures, and the dynamic supporting structures include the muscles that cross the joint. The static supports of the elbow region are described here; the reader is referred to any standard anatomic text for a review of dynamic supporting structures.[22]

Static supporting structures

Fibrous capsule. The anterior portion of the fibrous capsule is thin and broad. It is attached to the anterior surface of the humerus just above the radial and coronoid fossa. Inferiorly, it attaches to the anterior surface of the coronoid process and to the annular ligament of the superior radioulnar joint. On either side, it blends with the collateral ligaments.[22]

The posterior portion of the capsule is also thin and loose. Superiorly, it attaches to the humerus directly behind the capitellum and the lateral margin of the trochlea. It extends around the rim of the olecranon fossa and on to the posterior aspect of the medial epicondyle. Inferiorly, the posterior capsule is attached to the superior and lateral margins of the olecranon process. Laterally, it is continuous with the capsule of the superior radioulnar joint deep to the annular ligament.[22]

The synovial membrane extends from the margin of the articular surfaces of the humerus, lines the coronoid, radial, and olecranon fossa, and covers the flattened, medial, nonarticular surface of the trochlea. It is then reflected over the deep surface of the fibrous capsule and attaches inferiorly to the margins of the trochlear notch of the ulna and to the radial neck. It forms a saclike pouch below the radial head that permits rotation of the radius without tearing of the membrane.[22]

Between the fibrous capsule and the synovial membrane are three pads of fat. The largest of these is situated over the olecranon fossa. During flexion of the elbow, it is pressed into the fossa by the tendon of the triceps. On extension, it is displaced from the fossa.[22]

Anteriorly, two smaller fat pads are situated over the radial and coronoid fossae. These fat pads are pressed into their respective fossae during extension and are displaced during flexion.[22]

Normally, the fat pads are not visible on a lateral radiograph of the elbow. If they are displaced from the fossae by an effusion or a hemarthrosis, they are visible as radiolucent zones. This fat pad sign may be the only radiographic evidence of an occult fracture of the elbow.[6]

Ulnar collateral ligament. The ulnar collateral ligament provides a major contribution to stability of the elbow.[20] It is composed of two functional bands, both of which emanate from the medial epicondyle. The most anterior portion, the anterior oblique ligament, passes downward and anteriorly to insert into the medial aspect of the coronoid process of the ulna. This band is further subdivided into two functional components, one of which is taut in all positions of flexion or extension of the joint.[20]

The posterior portion of the ulnar collateral ligament is weaker than the anterior oblique portion. It is shaped like a fan and attaches to the medial and posterior aspects of the olecranon process. This portion of the ligament is taut only when the joint is in full extension.[20]

Radial collateral ligament. The radial or lateral collateral ligament is not as strong as the ulnar collateral ligament. It passes from its origin on the lateral humeral epicondyle downward to insert into the annular ligament of the superior radioulnar joint.[20] A few fibers may pass over that ligament to insert into the superior portion of the supinator crest of the ulna.[22] The radial collateral ligament is not capable of providing much protection against varus stress to the elbow joint.[20]

Restraint to motion in the sagittal plane. The capsule of the elbow is designed to permit free movement in the sagittal plane and does not offer much resistance to movement under normal circumstances.

Extension is limited primarily by impact of the olecranon process with the olecranon fossa. In this position the humeroulnar joint is in its most stable state, the close-packed position.[11] Interestingly, while the humeroulnar joint is in its close-packed position, the humeroradial joint is in its least stable position, the maximal loose-packed position (resting position).[11] Therefore, when in full extension, the ulna would appear to be the primary weight-bearing bone of the forearm. A joint that is stressed abnormally while in its close-packed position is prone to fracture of one of its bony members, whereas a joint that is stressed while in its resting position is prone to dislocation.[16] This phenomenon may explain the mechanism of Monteggia's fractures, in which the proximal ulna is fractured concomitant with dislocation of the radial head.

Extension is also limited, but to a lesser degree, by the anterior capsule and by the flexor musculature of the joint.[13] Under pathologic conditions, either of these structures may become the primary limiting factor to elbow extension.

Flexion of the elbow is limited primarily by contact and compression of the soft tissue masses of the anterior aspects of the arm and forearm.[2] When the movement is performed actively, the block to movement occurs at approximately 145 degrees because of the relative incompressibility of actively contracting muscle tissue.[13]

Passive flexion may also be limited by soft tissue compression in mesomorphic individuals (at 160 degrees) but is just as often brought to a halt by impact of the radial head and coronoid process into their respective fossae. As was the case with elbow extension, flexion may be limited by the posterior capsule and by the extensor musculature, although the role played by these structures under normal circumstances is relatively insignificant.

It was noted that the humeroulnar joint reaches its close-packed position in full extension. The close-packed

position of the humeroradial joint occurs at approximately 80 degrees of flexion with the forearm in the midposition between full pronation and full supination.[11] This position also corresponds to the resting position of the humeroulnar joint.[11] It might be expected that trauma in this position would produce a fracture of the humeroradial joint and dislocation of the humeroulnar joint.

Restraint to motion in the frontal plane. The collateral ligaments of hinge joints are typically designed to prevent motion outside the normal plane of movement of the joint. The capsule of the elbow permits free movement in the sagittal plane, whereas the ulnar and radial collateral ligaments limit movement in the frontal plane. From a clinical standpoint, the only restraint required is resistance to valgus stresses, in that varus stresses at the elbow are rarely encountered in functional activities.

The principal restraint to valgus angulation is provided by the ulnar collateral ligament, a portion of which is taut in all positions of the joint.[20] Tearing of this ligament results in instability of the joint with a tendency to recurrent dislocation. A further buttress to valgus angulation is provided by the bony configuration of the humeroradial joint.[20] This joint is capable of resisting compressive stresses that occur on the lateral side of the joint with a valgus stress, particularly when the joint is in a semiflexed attitude.

Joints of the forearm. The joints of the forearm include the proximal radioulnar joint and the distal radioulnar joint, both of which are ovoid synovial joints. The middle radioulnar syndesmosis must also be included. Movement of the joints of the forearm depends on movement at the humeroradial joint, which permits the joints to function in any position of flexion or extension of the elbow.

The joints of the forearm permit rotation of the radius in medial and lateral directions. Medial rotation of the radius is termed *pronation,* whereas lateral rotation is known as *supination.* Supination is usually permitted through a range of 90 degrees. Pronation is permitted through a somewhat smaller excursion of 85 degrees.[13]

On a cursory analysis, supination and pronation appear to be simple rotations of the radius about a fixed or stationary ulna. However, closer observation reveals the movements to be more complex. In fact, the axis of rotation of the radius appears to move in a manner that depends on the required functional activity; that is to say, the axis of rotation appears to shift to the radial side of the forearm, the ulnar side of the forearm, or to any position between these two extremes.[13]

An analysis of these movements must begin with the joints that participate. First, at the superior radioulnar joint, the convex peripheral rim of the radial head articulates with a concave surface formed by the annular ligament and the radial notch of the ulna. The radial head is capable of rotating within this fibroosseous ring in a clockwise or a counter-clockwise direction. The axis of rotation is at the center of curvature of the ring. Because the major portion of the ring is fibrous tissue, the axis may shift somewhat if the configuration of the ring is distorted. However, the axis does not displace to a significant degree because of this mechanism.

At the distal radioulnar joint, the convex articular surface of the head of the ulna articulates with a concave facet on the medial aspect of the distal radius. The axis of rotation of this joint must lie at the center of curvature of the head of the ulna. This position is near the point of attachment of the articular disk to the base of the styloid process of the ulna.[13,14]

Because the shafts of the radius and the ulna are united at each end by a joint and are relatively inflexible, the radius must rotate in relation to the ulna about an axis that passes through the axes of both the proximal and distal radioulnar joints. Motion can occur about any other axis only if one of the bones or one of the joints fails (Fig. 14-3).

The apparent shift in the axis motion must occur through a concomitant movement of the ulna. The distal end of the ulna may be observed to move in a lateral direction (abduction) during pronation and in a medial direction (adduction) during supination. This movement of the ulna in the frontal plane carries the distal pole of the axis of rotation of the forearm with it.[13,22]

When the frontal plane movement of the ulna is minimal, the functional axis of motion is near the ulnar side of the forearm. When ulnar movement is maximal, the axis shifts to the radial side of the forearm.

Ulnar motion in the frontal plane may occur at the humeroulnar joint because of the sellar configuration of the joint.[22] Because this is the case, the humeroulnar joint should be included in the detailed examination of motion disturbances of the joints of the forearm.

Thus far, the motion of the radius in space (osteokinematics) has been described. Also important are the articular movements (arthrokinematics) that occur when the radius moves in supination and pronation. Rotation of the radius depends on movement in the proximal radioulnar joint, the distal radioulnar joint, the middle radioulnar syndesmosis, and the humeroradial joint.

It is somewhat confusing to consider the long axis of the radius as the mechanical axis of the bone. For the sake of a better understanding of the arthrokinematics of these joints, it is helpful to construct a mechanical axis that is perpendicular to the plane of the concave joint surfaces.

The mechanical axis of the bone can be arbitrarily established as perpendicular to the plane of the distal articular surface of the radius. Supination, or lateral rotation, is a swing of the axis in a lateral direction, and pronation, or medial rotation, is a swing in a medial direction.

At the superior radioulnar joint, the moving articular surface is the convex radial head. Thus, the circumference of the radial head rolls in the same directions as the swing of the axis. It glides in the opposite direction of the swing. Motion of the radial head at this articulation appears to be mostly gliding, with little rolling.

The inferior radioulnar joint is formed by the articulation of the concave facet on the medial surface of the distal radius with the convex ulnar head. The concave radial surface is the moving surface. It rolls and glides in the same direction as the swing of the mechanical axis of the bone.

The shafts of the radius and ulna are connected by the oblique cord and by the interosseous membrane of the forearm. The latter is the most important structure functionally. Its fibers slant downward and medially from the interosseous border of the radius to that of the ulna. The fibers of the membrane are supposedly directed to transmit force from the radius to the ulna and hence to the humerus. However, the fibers of the membrane are taut only when the forearm is midway between full supination and full pronation and are relaxed at the extremes of these positions.[22] Primarily, the membrane appears to increase the surface area for muscle attachment, but, as will be seen, it can limit the range of motion under certain pathologic conditions.

Factors limiting supination. Supination is limited by the quadrate ligament at the proximal radioulnar joint and by the anterior ligament and capsule at the distal radioulnar joint. The pronating muscles, however, provide the greatest restraint to supination.[13,14]

Factors limiting pronation. Pronation is also limited by the quadrate ligament at the proximal joint. Movement is regulated by the posterior capsule and triangular ligament of the distal radioulnar joint. The primary restraint to pronation, however, is compression of the soft tissues covering the shafts of the radius and ulna as the two bones are crossed.[13,14]

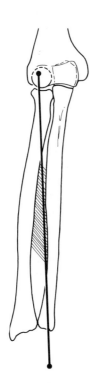

Fig. 14-3. Axis of joints of forearm.

As previously stated, the interosseous membrane is slack at the extremes of both supination and pronation. Thus, it cannot be a factor in restricting either of these movements under normal circumstances. It becomes taut midway between full supination and full pronation and appears to play a role in providing stability to the joints in this close-packed position of the forearm. The joints of the forearm reach the close-packed position in approximately 5 degrees of supination.[11] The joints of the forearm cannot be placed in their resting positions simultaneously. The distal radioulnar joint reaches the resting position at 10 degrees of supination, whereas the proximal radioulnar joint is in the resting position at 35 degrees of supination, when the elbow is flexed to approximately 70 degrees.[11]

The complex bowing of the radius also appears to be an important factor that influences range of motion in pronation and supination. The radius is bowed in the opposite direction (laterally) in relation to the ulna when the forearm is in the close-packed position. This factor appears to produce tension in the interosseous membrane. Following fractures of the forearm, if the bones are allowed to unite with an angular malunion, a significant reduction in the range of motion of pronation and supination occurs.[1]

EXAMINATION OF THE ELBOW COMPLEX

The objective of the examination of a part of the musculoskeletal system is to provide data from which decisions regarding management can be made. All too often a diagnosis or naming of a disease process is overemphasized. In many cases, a traditional diagnosis is impossible to obtain. In other cases, clients with the same diagnosis should be managed differently. This is one reason, in fact, for the disrepute of passive movement exercises at the elbow joint.

The objectives of a physical therapist's examination may be different from those of the physician. The physician is concerned with identification of major disease processes that may produce disorders of the musculoskeletal system, whereas the primary concern of the physical therapist is the determination of the client's reaction to movement of the joint. Of course, the physical therapist must also be alert for signs of pathologic conditions of a more serious nature.

Often, a diagnosis can be stated only in terms of altered motion. At other times, when a traditional diagnosis can be made, an understanding of the altered motion state that results from the pathologic condition present is of more use. It can be stated in terms of an abnormal response to active motion, passive motion, or both.

Once the movement disorder has been identified through a thorough examination of the effects of movement on the symptoms, management is directed toward improving the dysfunction. The methods of management are derived from a continual, dynamic process that involves the selection and application of treatment technique, reevaluation of the dysfunction, and maintenance or alteration of the treatment program, depending on the outcome; that is to say, if one

movement in the examination scheme appears to have the most effect on the client's symptoms, that movement may be selected as a treatment technique. After the movement has been applied as a mode of therapeutic intervention, its effects on the symptoms are assessed during the reevaluation. If the dysfunction has improved, the treatment may be continued with no changes. If the dysfunction has not changed or has become worse, a different treatment technique may be selected.

In this chapter only those portions of the subjective and objective examination that are most important to the physical therapist (see the Box) are stressed. A thorough discussion of the numerous pathologic conditions that affect the elbow has already been given in a number of standard orthopedic texts, and the reader is referred to them for further information.[8,9] However, certain aspects related to pathologic conditions at the elbow that are important to understanding the examination and treatment of movement disorders of this joint complex are discussed here.

Functional examination

The functional examination is that portion of the objective examination scheme (see Box) from which the physical therapist derives the most useful information regarding movement dysfunction. The functional examination includes an assessment of (1) active movements, (2) passive movements, (3) accessory movements, and (4) resisted tests.[11]

Active movement. The examination of active movement serves the following purposes: (1) The willingness of the client to move the joint may be assessed, and (2) if the range of motion is abnormal or painful, a baseline may be established to measure the effects of treatment.[2]

Active movement, in and of itself, is not diagnostic because it stresses both contractile and noncontractile tissue.[2] The findings must be interpreted along with those of subsequent portions of the examination. The client's response to active movement may provide a valuable gauge in determining how to proceed with the remainder of the examination. For example, if a client complains of a considerable increase in pain while performing an active movement or if the discomfort provoked by movement takes a considerable length of time to subside, the examiner must be alerted to the fact that caution should be employed in the performance of passive and resisted tests. If no pain is reported by the client and the range of motion is full, however, a more vigorous application of the remaining examination techniques may be appropriate.

The client is instructed to perform the following active movements: flexion, extension, supination, and pronation. The last two movements should be performed with the elbow held in varying degrees of flexion. As stated previously, the examiner should note any abnormality, including pain, decreased range of motion, or increased range of motion, compared to the uninvolved limb.

Passive movement. Passive movements are intended to

Examination of the elbow complex

Subjective

What caused the client to consult a physician?
- If pain
  - Where is the pain felt?
  - Is it constant or intermittent?
- If constant
  - Does it vary in intensity?
  - What makes it worse?
  - What eases it?
- If intermittent
  - What brings it on?
  - How long does it last?
- If loss of motion
  - What are the functional limitations?
  - How did this problem begin?
  - Any history of the same or a similar problem in the past?
  - Any related problems?

Objective

Inspection
- Functional movements
- Posture
- Shape
- Skin
- Aids

Function
- Active movements
- Passive movements
- Accessory movements
- Resisted tests

Palpation
- Skin and subcutaneous tissue
- Muscle and tendon
- Tendon sheaths and bursae
- Joints
- Nerves and blood vessels

Neurologic tests
- Nerve trunk
- Reflexes and key muscles
- Sensory examination
- Motor examination
- Coordination

Additional examinations
- Radiography
- Laboratory tests
- Electrodiagnosis
- Punctures (e.g., biopsy, aspiration)
- Special examination (referral to other practitioner)

Objective examination modified from Kaltenborn FM: *Manual therapy for the extremity joints, specialized techniques: tests and joint mobilization,* ed 2, Oslo, 1976, Olaf Norlis Bokhandel.

stress noncontractile tissues.[2] This portion of the examination may be the most valuable tool for the physical therapist. Much can be learned about the state of the tissues in and around the joint from a careful analysis of the passive range of motion permitted at the joint. While the movements are performed, the examiner must focus on three phenomena that follow: (1) the range of motion possible, (2) the nature of the motion barrier, and (3) the relationship of pain to the motion barrier.[2]

Range of motion. The passive movements included in the examination of the elbow joint are flexion, extension, pronation, and supination. On completion of these test movements, one of three possibilities will have been found: The range of motion will be normal, restricted, or excessive.

Excessive motion usually implies damage of the supporting connective tissues or muscles surrounding the joint. In an adolescent, this finding may warrant the inclusion of stress radiographs to rule out the possibility of epiphyseal fracture near the joint.

If the range of motion is limited, it will be limited in one of two patterns. Cyriax has termed these the *capsular* pattern and the *noncapsular* pattern.[2]

The capsular pattern has been defined as a proportional limitation of the movements available at a particular joint. The capsular pattern of the elbow is usually such that a greater limitation of flexion is found as opposed to extension. Generally, supination and pronation are not affected significantly. At times, the restrictions of flexion and extension may be nearly equal, and, in advanced cases of arthritis, movement of the forearm may also be limited.[2] At the elbow, as at other joints of the musculoskeletal system, a capsular pattern signifies a total joint reaction; that is, an inflammation of the joint is likely.[2]

The mechanism behind the proportional limitation of movement is not understood clearly. The joint may be splinted (by muscles surrounding the joint) in the position where the joint capsule can accommodate the greatest volume of fluid.[6] There is also some preliminary evidence that suggests an imbalance between the preaxial and postaxial musculature associated with a withdrawal reflex.[3,4] This area requires further investigation.

Although the finding of a capsular pattern does provide a diagnosis (a joint inflammation or arthritis), it does not provide enough information for decisions regarding treatment. These data are provided in subsequent portions of the examination.

If the restriction of motion does not fit the proportional requirements of the capsular pattern, a noncapsular pattern of restricted motion is present. Noncapsular patterns may be caused by lesions that are capable of restricting range of motion but that do not involve the entire joint. The following categories of pathologic conditions fit these requirements: (1) adhesions of ligaments (uncommon at the elbow), (2) internal derangements, and (3) extraarticular lesions.[2]

Noncapsular patterns of restriction at the elbow are usually caused by internal derangement, which results from a loose body of bone or cartilage within the joint.[2] Depending on which aspect of the joint is affected, movement is limited in one direction and free in the other. For example, if a loose body lies in the anterior aspect of the joint cavity, flexion is limited and extension unaffected; conversely, if the loose body lies posteriorly, extension is blocked and flexion is free.

At times, a confusing picture may appear with regard to the pattern of restriction. It occurs in the joint with a loose body that develops a simultaneous inflammation. The joint inflammation produces the characteristic proportional limitation of movement or capsular pattern. However, the loose body may block movement to a greater degree than expected in one direction. The identification of these cases is facilitated once the motion barrier is examined.[2]

Appraisal of the motion barrier. When a joint is moved passively, movement is brought to a halt when a barrier to motion is met. Under normal circumstances, the motion barrier prevents excessive movement. This may be termed an *anatomic motion barrier* and may be provided by (1) apposition of bony surfaces, (2) the development of tension in the connective tissues, or (3) approximation and compression of the soft tissues.

In each of these situations, as the movement is brought to a halt at the anatomic motion barrier, a distinctly different sensation is imparted to the hands of the examiner. Cyriax has termed this sensation *end feel.*[2]

When the barrier is provided by bony apposition of the members of the joint, the movement comes to an abrupt stop, and no further movement is possible, regardless of how hard the movement is forced. If the motion is restrained by tension in the connective tissues, the movement also comes to an abrupt stop, but continued forcing of the joint yields a small increase in the range of motion. Cyriax has termed this sensation a *capsular end feel.*[2] The sensation is much the same as that obtained from stretching a piece of leather.

Contact and compression of the soft tissues overlying the moving members of a joint provide yet another sensation to the examiner. The movement is felt to slow down as contact occurs, but continued forcing yields considerably more motion as the soft tissues are compressed.

Before an account of pathologic motion barriers can be given, the normal barriers to movement at the elbow and forearm need to be discussed. When the elbow is extended, movement is stopped as the olecranon process engages the olecranon fossa. In thin individuals, flexion is stopped in a similar manner when the radial head and coronoid process are received, respectively, into the radial and coronoid fossae. The motion barrier in these situations is one of bony approximation.

In mesomorphic individuals, when the elbow is flexed, the anterior surface of the arm comes into contact with the anterior surface of the forearm before bony approximation can occur. The motion barrier to flexion in these individuals is soft tissue compression.

Supination of the forearm is limited by connective tissues and by the pronator muscles. It usually has a capsular end feel. Pronation is limited by the soft tissues, which are interposed between the radius and ulna, thus producing a soft tissue approximation end feel.

When motion of the joint is restricted, a pathologic motion barrier impedes movement of the joint before the anatomic barrier is reached. The same factors that create an anatomic barrier may also constitute a pathologic barrier; that is, movement can be limited by bony approximation, soft tissue compression, or tension in the connective tissues before the anatomic range of motion is attained. In order to make appropriate decisions regarding treatment, determining the quality of the motion barrier is of the utmost importance.

If the pathologic motion barrier is one of bony approximation, no form of movement—active or passive—increases motion in the direction of the barrier. If the motion barrier is soft tissue compression, which may occur prematurely if the arm or forearm is edematous, the initial objective may be to reduce the edema. If the movement is limited by contracture of connective tissues, however, a combination of active and passive movements may be used to improve the range of motion. The motion may be limited by a loss of flexibility in either the joint capsule or the accessory ligaments of the joint. Alternatively, the movement may be limited by shortening of the connective tissues of antagonistic musculature, which gives rise to a similar motion barrier.

The length of these tissues can be modified with the application of appropriate stresses. The appropriate stress to induce lengthening of connective tissue is tension, which is produced by stretching. Although tension can also be induced with active movement, in many cases the optimal manner of providing the appropriate stress is with passive movement.

Two other types of motion barriers are encountered when passive movements are examined, and both springy block and muscle guarding are common at the elbow joint. If either type of barrier is encountered, forceful passive stretching in the direction of the barrier is clearly contraindicated. The failure of physical therapists to observe this contraindication is undoubtedly one of the reasons for the disrepute of passive movement treatment at this joint.

A springy motion barrier is usually found at the elbow when motion is limited by a loose body.[2] A loose body produces a noncapsular pattern of restriction, and either flexion or extension may be limited. As the joint is moved into the barrier, a sensation of resistance develops. The block to motion is not abrupt, and, if the examiner persists in the movement, more range can be obtained. If the joint is moved toward the barrier to the position where resistance is first met and then suddenly moved into the barrier (through a small amplitude), the joint springs back in the opposite direction when the force is released.

Motion may also be limited by spasm of the antagonistic muscles to the movement. The muscles may arrest the movement by contracting involuntarily when passive movement is produced. The muscle guarding may be termed low guarding or fast guarding. Both types of muscle guarding indicate an acute inflammation of the joint or the extraarticular tissues. Motion should never be forced in the presence of muscle guarding. If this rule is not observed, the good intentions of the physical therapist have the opposite effect: The joint loses even more motion.

The physical therapist must also keep in mind that the motion barrier may change. For example, if elbow extension is found to have a restriction of 30 degrees with a capsular barrier, appropriate treatment may include passive mobilization. If the restriction has been reduced to 20 degrees following the treatment, the motion barrier must be assessed at this point. If the barrier is still capsular, treatment may be continued with passive movement. If a bone-on-bone barrier occurs at the new position, however, this treatment is contraindicated.

Relationship of pain to the motion barrier. As the joint is moved passively, the client is instructed to inform the examiner when any sensation of pain is experienced. The pain may be related to the motion barrier in several ways. First, it may occur before the barrier is met, in which case it indicates an acute lesion. It may also occur simultaneously with engagement of the motion barrier. This, too, represents an acute lesion but differs from the former situation.[2] In both of these cases, treatment must progress with caution, with the initial objective of treatment being relief of pain.

Finally, pain may be experienced after the barrier to motion is met.[2] In this case, the pain is usually caused by stretching of contracted connective tissues (if the barrier has this quality), and the pain is typically not intense. The treatment goal in this instance should be directed toward improving the range of motion by increasing the flexibility of the connective tissues.

Accessory movement. Accessory movements or joint play movements are involuntarily passive movements in a joint.[22] Two types of accessory movements are found at the elbow. The first type is characterized by abduction and adduction of the ulna at the humeroulnar joint. Performing these motions voluntarily in isolated fashion is not possible, although they do occur when the forearm is supinated and pronated.[22]

The second type of accessory movement depends on the laxity of the supporting connective tissues. This type of accessory movement includes distraction of the articular surfaces and gliding movements of the surfaces. Through an examination of these accessory movements, the examiner can determine whether isolated portions of the capsule and accessory ligaments are contractured or excessively lax. Thus, treatment decisions are based on these findings. If an accessory movement reveals a limited range of motion and the corresponding passive movement is also limited, for example, the treatment of choice is to restore the lost range of motion through passive stretching. Restoration of movement is best accomplished by using the accessory movement rather than the physiologic movement. This eliminates problems associated with compression of the articular surfaces.

Alternatively, if the accessory movement is excessive in range and the corresponding passive movement is limited, passive stretching is not the treatment of choice. The limita-

Table 14-1. Accessory movements at the elbow

Joint	Movement
Humeroulnar joint	Abduction of the ulna
	Adduction of the ulna
	Medial glide of the ulna
	Lateral glide of the ulna
	Distraction of the ulna
Humeroradial joint	Distraction of the radius
	Compression of the radius
	Ventral glide of the radius
	Dorsal glide of the radius
Proximal radioulnar joint	Ventromedial glide of the radius
	Dorsolateral glide of the radius

tion of passive motion is not caused by contracture of the capsule and accessory ligaments because the accessory movement is excessive. The limitation of motion may be caused by an extraarticular lesion.

The accessory movements performed in the examination of the elbow complex are listed in Table 14-1.

Resisted tests. The primary objective of resisted testing is identification of painful lesions on the contractile elements of the musculoskeletal system.[2] Examples of these types of lesions include tendinitis and tears of the elements of the contractile units. Disorders that result in weakness of the muscles tested may also be identified, although this may be better accomplished with a conventional manual muscle test.

The resisted tests are performed by placing the joint in its resting position. This step is included so that the tension on the noncontractile tissues is at a minimum.[2] The client is then asked to hold the joint in a static position while the examiner attempts to move the joint in a direction that activates the muscle or group being tested. In this manner, as much movement as possible is prevented in the joint while the stress or tension in the contractile unit is increased.

The theoretic basis of resisted testing rests on the following assumptions: (1) No movement occurs that stresses the noncontractile tissues, and (2) increasing the tension in the contractile unit increases the client's complaint of pain by stressing a painful lesion.[2] In theory, these assumptions may appear valid, but enough false-positive and false-negative results are found with this type of examination to warrant further discussion.

In general, the purpose of muscle force is to produce torque or movement across the joint. This force results in a torque that resists or does work against an external load. In addition, there are large compressive forces created at the joint between the two bones; if the joint is not permitted to move, large shear stresses may also be created that tend to displace one bone with respect to the other. Therefore, it may be concluded that eliminating stress on noncontractile tissue during a resisted test is impossible. When a muscle contracts, it has the capacity to compress a joint or to produce gliding movement in a joint without visible motion of the joint. If the joint is acutely painful, the resisted test may produce an increase in the client's pain that may be attributed wrongly to a lesion of contractile tissue.

In this situation, although pain may have been elicited by a resisted test, the pain produced by examination of passive movement is usually worse. Correlation of the results of the entire functional examination is essential to eliminate this source of false-positive resisted testing.

A similar situation may exist at locations where a contracting muscle can compress a painful, noncontractile structure. This situation may be observed in cases of acute bursitis, but, again, passive movements generally elicit a more intense pain.[2]

Another type of problem may appear as a simple contractile lesion with pain on one or more resisted tests. Such pain may be caused by a fracture near the insertion of the muscle being tested (avulsion fracture). Contraction of the muscle produces pain that may be mistakenly diagnosed as tendinitis. If it is followed by treatment with deep friction massage, the therapist may exacerbate rather than alleviate the condition. To prevent this possibility, therefore, an adequate radiographic examination must be carried out if there is any history of trauma.

False-negative results of resisted tests are usually not a factor at the elbow, although they may be encountered in athletes. The lesion may be aggravated by stresses encountered in competition that are impossible to duplicate with clinical testing. In these situations, it may be helpful to have the client engage in the activity that precipitates the symptoms before examination. This activity may produce sufficient irritation of the painful structure to permit localization of the lesion with resisted testing.

The resisted tests that are performed at the elbow complex usually include elbow flexion, elbow extension, supination of the forearm, pronation of the forearm, extension of the wrist, and flexion of the wrist.[2]

After completion of these examination procedures, the examiner must correlate the results. (Table 14-2 lists test movements and the muscles that may be involved with each test.) For example, a client may complain of an increase in pain with resisted flexion of the elbow, which may be caused by a contractile lesion located in the biceps brachii, the brachialis, or the brachioradialis. If the problem lies within the biceps, the client also complains of increased pain with resisted supination. If the lesion is in the brachioradialis, pain may be exacerbated by resisted pronation in full supination and resisted supination in full pronation. If the lesion is in the brachialis, no pain is elicited with resisted supination or pronation.

A similar process of elimination should be used for the remaining resisted tests. Once the lesioned muscle has been identified, the examiner may palpate the muscle to locate the lesion.

Table 14-2. Interpretation of resisted tests at the elbow

Test	Affected muscle
Flexion	Biceps brachii
	Brachialis
	Brachioradialis
Extension	Triceps brachii
	Anconeus
Supination	Supinator
	Biceps brachii
	Brachioradialis (full pronation to neutral)
Pronation	Pronator teres
	Pronator quadratus
	Brachioradialis (full supination to neutral)
Wrist extension	Extensor carpi radialis longus
	Extensor carpi radialis brevis
	Extensor carpi ulnaris
	Extensor digitorum
Wrist flexion	Flexor carpi radialis
	Flexor carpi ulnaris
	Flexor digitorum superficialis
	Palmaris longus

TREATMENT OF THE CUBITAL COMPLEX

After the examination of the cubital complex, the physical therapist should have sufficient data to formulate a plan of care. Client problems that require physical therapy will have been identified. At this point, the therapist must establish a goal or objective of treatment for each problem and design a plan of care that responds to each problem.

Four primary goals become evident through a detailed assessment of the elbow region: (1) reducing pain, (2) reducing mobility, (3) increasing mobility, and (4) preventing recurrence of the problem, if possible.[11]

Musculoskeletal dysfunction can be divided into the broad categories of lesions of the noncontractile tissues and lesions of the contractile tissues.[2] The former is identified by an abnormal response to passive movement, whereas the latter is identified by an abnormal response to resisted testing.

Dysfunction of noncontractile tissues

The following noncontractile tissues may be involved in a pathologic process at the cubital complex: (1) the bones or their articular surfaces; (2) the articular capsule, synovial membrane, synovial bursae, or the accessory ligaments of the joint; (3) the passive component of the muscles that cross the joint; and (4) nerves that are located in a position that subjects them to trauma near the joint.

Client problems that may result from lesions of the noncontractile structures include one or more of the following: pain, limited movement (hypomobility), excessive movement (hypermobility), and paresthesias.

Dysfunction of the capsule and accessory ligaments

The articular capsule and accessory ligaments of the elbow are connective tissues. Connective tissue dysfunction is characterized by an abnormal response to passive movement. The motion may be abnormal in that it may be restricted or excessive. Either type of dysfunction may be accompanied by pain. If pain is the predominant feature, determining the type of dysfunction that is present may, in fact, be difficult because of muscle guarding. Occasionally, the physician must examine the joint with the client under anesthesia to determine whether the joint is hypomobile or hypermobile.

Because pain and muscle guarding may obscure the nature of the problem, the initial objective in the acutely painful joint is pain relief. Once it has been obtained, a more thorough examination of movement is permitted, and the type of dysfunction may be identified.

Regardless of the type of connective tissue dysfunction present—hypomobility or hypermobility—the goal of treatment is to return the joint to the best possible function in the shortest possible time. Obviously, the methods used to achieve this goal vary, depending on the pathologic condition identified in the examination and on the stage of the pathologic process. The physical therapist should be aware that the client's primary problem may change during the course of treatment. When this occurs, the treatment plan should be modified accordingly.

When the connective tissues are traumatized (or affected by a systemic disease), an inflammatory reaction occurs. The inflammatory reaction typically produces a capsular pattern of limitation at the joint. As noted previously, the presence of a capsular pattern of limitation of passive movement must be correlated with the results of other examination procedures in order to select the appropriate treatment modality. Treatment effectiveness is enhanced if the stage of the inflammatory process is identified.

Early stage of inflammation. *Inflammation* is a term used in reference to a large group of normal processes provoked by injury or alien material. Acute inflammation as a response to trauma is caused by the function of collagen in the activation of molecular systems (chemical mediators) that set off the inflammatory process.[10,12]

When collagen is exposed by injury, the chemical mediators of inflammation produce vascular changes in the area of tissue injury that result in exudation.[10] Cells and solutes that are normally intravascular pour out into the injured area to neutralize the noxious stimuli (damaged tissue). Dead or dying tissue must be disposed of in preparation for the repair process.

The local vasodilation, leakage of fluid into the extravascular space, and interruption of lymphatic drainage produce the classic signs of inflammation (i.e., redness, swelling, and heat). Pressure and chemical stimulation of nociceptors produce the fourth sign (i.e., pain).

In most uncontaminated injuries, the early inflammatory period subsides in 3 to 5 days.[10] During this period, an examination of the joint may reveal pain at rest or pain on movement that occurs before any barrier to movement is felt. If a motion barrier is reached, it is usually one of fast muscle guarding.

Although a capsular pattern of motion restriction is found during this period, restoration of motion is not the primary goal of treatment. The goal is the reduction of pain and limitation of the inflammatory process. Toward this end, ice and other modalities, such as transcutaneous electrical nerve stimulation (TENS) or high-voltage galvanic stimulation, may be used.

The joint is usually immobilized with a sling or with a sling and splint to prevent further tissue damage. Immobilization should be maintained only long enough for adequate tissue healing. Complications of management may arise if the joint must be immobilized for a prolonged period following an unstable fracture, dislocation, or a similar injury. A dense scar may form in the area of tissue injury, along with adhesions between adjacent tissue planes and generalized shortening of the connective tissue structures.

Intermediate stage of inflammation. As the damaged tissues are neutralized in the area of injury, the intermediate stage of inflammation—early repair—can begin. There is no sharp line of demarcation between the early and intermediate stages of inflammation. Both may exist simultaneously in different regions of the injured tissues.[10] For this reason, distinguishing between these two stages of inflammation on a clinical basis is sometimes difficult.

The intermediate stage is an early repair process that is characterized by an ingrowth of capillary buds into the injured region to reestablish circulation. As the circulation is being reestablished, fibroblasts appear in the injured region and begin to manufacture collagen and ground substance. Collagen may be found in the healing region as early as the first day after injury, but peak production occurs 5 to 7 days after injury.[10]

The early collagen is a gel-like substance that serves as a support for the new, fragile capillary system.[10] The tissue formed during this stage is termed *granulation tissue*. It is a highly vascularized connective tissue that is very fragile and easily torn by the application of tensile stress.

During the intermediate stage of inflammation, the motion barrier to passive movement is usually muscle guarding, and a capsular pattern of restriction is found. The sequence of pain to the motion barrier is variable. Generally, the client experiences pain at the same time the examiner feels the motion barrier. However, the pain may be felt slightly before or slightly after the barrier to motion.

Treatment during this phase of inflammation is important and has considerable bearing on the final outcome of the problem. It requires the coordinated efforts of the physician and the physical therapist.

Conceptually, treatment during this period is a balance between the immobilization that was required during the early stage of inflammation and the vigorous mobilization that is required, in some cases, in the late stage of repair. In fact, the objective of treatment at this time is preventing the formation of dense, inflexible scar tissue that can create problems that require vigorous mobilization later.

The referring physician is responsible for determining when to allow movement of the joint. The physical therapist is responsible for supervision of the client during this period, and must ensure that movement is sufficient to produce desirable results without disruption of the healing tissues.

Movement during the intermediate stage is intended to provide an adequate stimulus for the functional orientation of collagen fibers. If movement is not sufficient, the fiber orientation is such that free movement of the joint may be impeded. If movement is excessive, the fragile connective tissues are torn, and the joint may develop a chronic inflammatory reaction with an even greater loss of motion. Alternatively, if the initial trauma involved a significant disruption of the capsule and ligaments, excessive movement may result in permanent lengthening of these tissues with resultant instability of the joint.

Active and passive movement of the joint may be used in the management of the joint during this stage. Both should be guided by the same treatment principle. Pain should not be experienced as the joint is moved, and no muscle spasm should be provoked. Between periods of exercise, the joint should be protected with a sling.

Late stage of inflammation. The late stage of inflammation involves the maturation and remodeling of the young connective tissues that were formed during the intermediate stage. Again, there is no sharp line of demarcation between the intermediate and the late stages of inflammation.[10]

Maturation occurs through the formation of chemical crosslinks between adjacent collagen fibers. If appropriate stresses are not provided during the repair process, excessive crosslinking may occur, and the organization of the collagen fibers is at random.[10] The tissues formed are dense, inflexible, and ill suited to the needs of a freely movable joint such as the elbow.

Examination of the joint during this stage reveals a problem that is primarily lost motion, not pain. Motion is restricted in a capsular pattern and limited by contracture of connective tissues. The motion barrier thus has a capsular end feel. The accessory movements of the joint are also limited.

Pain that is produced on passive movement occurs only after the motion barrier is met and the pressure is maintained in a manner that forces movement into the barrier. The pain is usually not severe, and it generally abates once the force is released.

The goal of treatment at this stage is to increase the range of motion, which is accomplished by increasing the flexibility of the connective tissues. The most advantageous method of achieving this end is the application of tensile stress to the tissue.

Treatment of hypomobility associated with connective tissue dysfunction

Various forms of passive movement that can be used in the treatment of hypomobility of the elbow complex that is caused by contracture of the connective tissues have been well described in the literature.[2,11,17] Detailed discussion of all passive movement techniques that can be used in the management of these problems is beyond the scope of this chapter. Furthermore, the intention of this chapter is not to teach the reader how to perform passive movement techniques, which can be accomplished only through supervised practical experience. For the sake of illustrating the most important aspects of passive movement, however, selected techniques are described here in some detail.

Passive movement can be divided into accessory joint movement and physiologic joint movement.[17]

Accessory movements. The accessory movements used in the treatment of the elbow complex are identical to those used in the examination of the joints (see Table 14-1). During the examination, the purpose of performing accessory movement is to assess the range of motion, which is restricted in cases of hypomobility caused by connective tissue contracture. The purpose of accessory movement in treatment is to restore the range of motion. When the range of motion of the accessory movement has been regained, that of the associated physiologic movement is also restored.[11]

Accessory movements are used in the treatment of joints during either the intermediate stage or the later stage of the inflammatory process. Because the demands of treatment in each of these stages vary, the application of the treatment movement must be modified accordingly by altering the position of the joint, varying the amplitude of the movement, varying the rate of movement, and varying the number of movements performed.

First, the factor of joint position must be addressed for performing accessory movement. Joint position has a definite effect on the accessory movement of distraction of the humeroulnar joint. During the intermediate stage of the inflammatory process (when pain is the predominant feature) the joint should be positioned in its resting position.[11,17] This position minimizes the tension on all portions of the fibrous capsule and on the ligaments of the joint. Theoretically, distraction performed in this position increases the tensile stresses in all portions of the connective tissues, but the increase in stress is not great in any area. Thus, distraction of the humeroulnar joint in the resting position has the capacity to improve motion in flexion and extension and is relatively safe in that it does not produce significant increases in stress within the capsule (Fig. 14-4).

If distraction is used to treat the humeroulnar joint in the late stage of the inflammatory process (when loss of motion is the predominant feature), the joint is usually positioned at a motion barrier. When the joints move to the flexion motion

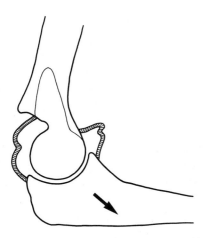

Fig. 14-4. Distraction of humeroulnar joint with joint in resting position. When the physical therapist performs distraction movement of humeroulnar joint in resting position, stress created in all portions of capsule is small. This is so because the capsule is relaxed in all regions. Note that direction of distraction force is perpendicular to the plane of concave joint surface (trochlear notch of ulna).

barrier, the posterior aspect of the capsule becomes taut while the anterior portion of the capsule relaxes. A distraction movement applied to the joint in this position produces a significant increase in the tension within the posterior capsule and has little or no effect on the anterior capsule. Although treatment in this position is usually more effective because tensile stress can be increased more readily, it also carries more inherent danger. If the joint is not capable of tolerating the stress, the condition may be exacerbated.

Distraction can also be performed with the joint positioned at the extension barrier. In this situation, the stress is applied selectively to the anterior portion of the capsule (Fig. 14-5).

A second factor that can be used to modify the effects of accessory movement is the amplitude of the movement. Kaltenborn[11] and Maitland[17] have developed systems for describing the amplitude of passive movement. Maitland's grading system is used to describe both accessory and physiologic movement because he uses both of these in treatment. He has classified movement into four grades, which are based on how far the movement is carried into the available range of motion and also on the amplitude of the movement.

A grade I movement is a small-amplitude movement performed at the beginning of the range. A grade II movement is a large-amplitude movement performed within the range but not reaching the limit. A grade III movement is also a large-amplitude movement performed up to the limit of the range. A grade IV movement is a small-amplitude movement that is performed at the end of the range (Fig. 14-6).[17]

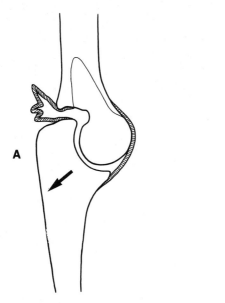
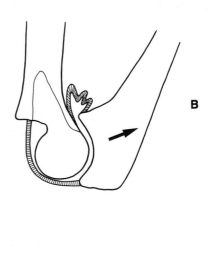

Fig. 14-5. **A,** Distraction of humeroulnar joint with joint positioned at motion barrier. When the joint is moved to motion barrier before application of distraction force, a portion of the capsule becomes taut while another portion becomes relaxed. Extension relaxes posterior capsule and tightens anterior capsule. **B,** The converse is true on flexion. Posterior portion of capsule becomes taut while anterior aspect is relaxed. When distraction force is applied in either of these positions, it has greater influence on the area of capsule that is prestressed. Thus, when movement is performed at flexion barrier, flexion is improved. When movement is performed at extension barrier, extension is improved.

Kaltenborn describes three grades of movement. The first movement is always performed in the direction of distraction. In fact, this movement may not actually move the joint surfaces apart but neutralizes the compressive forces that tend to bind them together. Kaltenborn's remaining two types of movement are based on the feel of the connective tissues rather than on the range of motion. The first is performed in the selected direction of motion but only until the slack is taken out of the connective tissues. The final grade is performed in such a manner that movement is carried beyond the slack in an attempt to stretch the connective tissues that restrain the joint movement (Fig. 14-7).

In treating a joint in which pain is the predominant feature, the physical therapist can perform accessory movements starting with Maitland's grade I and progressing to grade II as the inflammatory process subsides. Similarly, if the therapist uses Kaltenborn's system of grading accessory movement, the treatment may begin with a grade I, or small-distraction movement, and progress to taking up the slack in the direction of the movement selected.

When the predominant feature of the dysfunction is loss of motion, as occurs in the late stage of repair, the therapist may select Maitland's grade III and progress to grade IV. If Kaltenborn's system is used, the accessory motion is taken to stretch.

The rate of movement can also be varied in treatment with accessory movements. Maitland performs these movements as a series of oscillations,[17] whereas Kaltenborn performs the movement in a slower, rhythmical manner, with the joint held at the terminal point in the movement for several (5 to 8) seconds.[11] Table 14-3 gives a comparison of Maitland's and Kaltenborn's grades of movement.

Of course, the intensity of treatment is also affected by the number of treatment movements that are performed. Generally, acutely painful joints are treated with a much smaller number of movements before the joint is reexamined, whereas the stiff joint can tolerate more treatment movements before reexamination.

Physiologic movement. Physiologic movements can also be used in the treatment of dysfunction at the elbow complex. Maitland has provided a detailed description of the use of these movements in the treatment of the elbow.[17] He also has provided a description of the use of physiologic movements in combination with accessory movements.

Physiologic movements used in the treatment of hypomobility can also be graded. Maitland's grading system is well suited for describing physiologic movement. In general, grade I and grade II movements are used in the treatment of painful conditions, whereas grade III and grade IV movements are used in the treatment of stiff joints.

Although passive movement is useful in the management of dysfunction caused by connective tissue contracture, the ultimate success of the treatment program hinges on the physical therapist's ability to instruct the client in the performance of active exercises. Often, considerable time and effort are spent in the performance of passive movement and little attention is paid to instruction in a home exercise program.

Active exercises should be governed by the same factors that guide passive movement. In the intermediate stage of the inflammatory process, the client must be instructed to perform active range of motion within the pain-free range. During this stage of the inflammatory process, the fragile granulation tissue may just as easily be damaged by improper application of active movement as by excessive passive motion. The client must be carefully instructed as to which motions can be performed and the frequency with which the movement should be done. The client has to realize that pain and muscle guarding should not be provoked by the exercises.

With a dysfunction in the later stage of repair, the exercises are further modified by increasing the frequency of the movement rather than the intensity of active effort. Again, the exercises should not provoke pain.

Accompanying dysfunction of the capsule and accessory ligaments (hypermobility)

The most common form of instability at the elbow complex is medial laxity,[20] which is evidenced by excessive motion on valgus stress testing. The major contribution to stability in this direction is provided by the anterior oblique portion of the medial collateral ligament. This ligament is also instrumental in providing stability in the anteroposterior direction. Secondary restraints to motion in the valgus direction are provided by the flexor muscles of the forearm and by the humeroradial joint, which is able to resist compressive forces that occur on the lateral side of the joint complex with this motion.[20]

Although it is important for the physical therapist to recognize the existence of stability, treatment of this problem is within the realm of the orthopedic surgeon. If the surgeon does not feel that the client is a candidate for surgical

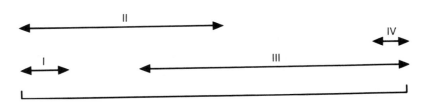

Fig. 14-6. Maitland's grades of movement.

Table 14-3. Grades of movement

	Kaltenborn	Maitland
Grade I	A small movement in the direction of distraction that is done before the performance of a gliding movement (only enough movement to neutralize the joint compression forces)	Small-amplitude movement performed at the beginning of the range
Grade II	A movement that takes up the slack in the soft tissues	Large-amplitude movement performed within the range but not reaching the limit of the range
Grade III	A movement that is taken beyond the slack (an attempt to stretch the soft tissues)	Large-amplitude movement performed up to the limit of the range
Grade IV		Small-amplitude movement performed at the limit of the range

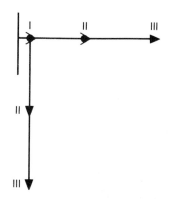

Fig. 14-7. Kaltenborn's grades of movement.

stabilization, the client may be referred to physical therapy for strengthening of the flexor muscles. The exercises performed should not cause engagement of the motion barrier, which may result in further stretching of the already compromised or lengthened connective tissues.

Hypomobility as a result of dysfunction of the noncontractile component of the muscle

If the joints of the elbow complex demonstrate a limited range of motion of physiologic movement but a normal or slightly hypermobile range of accessory movements, the limitation of motion may be caused by insufficient length of the antagonistic muscles to the movement being tested. The pattern of motion restriction may be noncapsular because the problem is extraarticular.

In this situation, the muscles may be lengthened with a contract-relax procedure. The joint is positioned at the motion barrier, which is provided by the shortened muscle, and the client is instructed to contract the muscle to be treated against the unyielding force of the therapist. This contraction is maintained for 5 to 10 seconds; then, the client is instructed to relax. After relaxation, the joint is moved into the motion barrier again. At this point, the client performs another isometric contraction and then relaxes, and the joint is again moved into the motion barrier. A series of 5 to 10 procedures is generally required.

When contract-relax techniques are used, the therapist must follow the same guidelines for repositioning the joint at the motion barrier as those described for the use of any passive movement. Pain and protective muscle guarding should not be provoked.

These techniques must be used with particular caution when elbow extension is limited. Extension may be limited by myositis ossificans, in which case the use of contract-relax procedures or any form of passive stretching is contraindicated.

Hypomobility as a result of articular surface dysfunction (springy motion barrier)

If a springy motion barrier is present on either flexion or extension of the elbow, a loose body of cartilage or bone may be lodged between the articular surfaces. Cyriax has described the passive techniques that may be used to reduce the displacement (move the loose body from its position between the articular surfaces).[2] However, he stresses that recurrence of the block is common and advocates surgical removal of the fragment.

Hypomobility as a result of articular surface dysfunction (bone-on-bone motion barrier and capsular barriers resistant to treatment)

Perhaps the most important consideration in the treatment of limited passive movement that results from trauma at the elbow joint is the establishment of realistic goals of treatment.

Following a fracture in the elbow region, a full range of motion is unlikely if the fracture fragments cannot be anatomically reduced. This is also true if the fracture is complicated by significant soft tissue injury.

During the course of treatment, the physical therapist must constantly reassess the nature of the motion barrier. When a barrier to motion changes, the goals of treatment often need to be changed accordingly.

If, at any time, a bone-on-bone barrier is encountered, continued efforts to regain motion in the direction of the barrier are futile and contraindicated. Several situations in

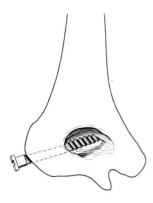

Fig. 14-8. Compression screw used to stabilize humerus, causing motion barrier.

the management of fractures of the bones around the elbow require special consideration.

If a compression screw has been used to stabilize the fragments of a fracture of the distal humerus and the screw passes through or projects into the olecranon fossa, motion in extension is blocked.[5] The motion barrier is most likely bone on bone—a hard, abrupt end feel. Obviously, efforts to regain extension in this situation exacerbate the condition (Fig. 14-8).

If an intercondylar fracture of the humerus is reduced with a residual rotary deformity or malalignment of one of the humeral condyles, the biomechanics of the joint are disturbed.[5] Motion of the elbow in the sagittal plane is limited as a result of malalignment of the axes of the humeroulnar and the humeroradial joints. If, for example, the lateral condyle (capitellum) is tilted ventrally with respect to the humeral shaft, bone-on-bone contact may occur prematurely as the forearm is flexed at the elbow. During extension, the humeroradial portion of the joint reaches the limit of its excursion prematurely. In this situation a bone-on-bone end feel is present in extension. Neither barrier responds to treatment with active or passive movement (Fig. 14-9).

Fractures of the forearm that are permitted to unite with malalignment also permanently limit the range of motion of pronation and supination of the forearm. If the radius is fractured and unites with the proximal fragment in supination and the distal fragment in pronation, forearm rotation is restricted. The loss of motion is in a one-to-one proportion to the rotational malalignment.[1] During supination, the proximal radioulnar joint reaches its anatomic motion barrier prematurely, and on pronation the same occurs at the distal radioulnar joint. Limitation of the range of motion may be present with no pathologic condition at either the proximal or distal radioulnar joints. This condition may be suspected when the physiologic range of motion is limited and the range of motion of the accessory movements is normal.

Treatment of a problem of this nature with active or passive movement may convert a painless limitation of motion into a painful condition (Fig. 14-10).

The complications of angular malunion of the forearm have already been mentioned. When normal curvature of the radius is disturbed, the range of motion in pronation and supination is limited (Fig. 14-11).[1] This probably occurs because of the development of abnormal or premature tension within the interosseous membrane.

When the joint in question presents a bone-on-bone motion barrier or fails to respond to an adequate program of treatment, one of the previous problems may be the cause. If the range of motion present is sufficient to allow reasonable function, further attempts to regain motion should be terminated. If the range of motion is nonfunctional, the client should be sent back to the physician for further care.

Noncontractile lesions (nerves and bursae)

Lesions of the nerves that traverse the cubital region are discussed in the chapter on the wrist and hand.

The most common type of bursitis seen at the elbow is olecranon bursitis. Pain at the elbow exists and is usually not aggravated by motion or by resisted testing.[2] The diagnosis is usually based on palpable thickening or tenderness over the olecranon bursa.

Dysfunction of contractile tissues

Dysfunction of contractile tissues is identified by an abnormal response to resisted testing.[2] An abnormal response may include weakness of the muscle or muscles being tested, pain that occurs as the muscle contracts isometrically, or a combination of the two. Pain combined with weakness is often associated with serious pathologic conditions in the region and thus requires further investigation.[2]

If weakness is detected, further investigation is also indicated to uncover the cause. The treatment for weakness is described in the chapter on the wrist and hand.

Pain on resisted testing in the presence of a strong contraction indicates the presence of a contractile lesion.[2] A *contractile lesion* is defined as a macroscopic or microscopic tear of the substance of the musculotendinous unit, which includes (1) the muscle belly, (2) the musculotendinous junction, (3) the tendon, and (4) the tenoperiosteal junction.

The unit may have been injured or torn by a single violent contraction of the muscle or, as is more often the case, by repeated submaximal overuse. Regardless of the mechanism of injury, an inflammatory reaction identical to that previously described occurs. Inflammatory reactions that involve the contractile units can be divided into two broad categories: acute and chronic. These categories are based more on the irritability of the tissues (severity of pain) than on the longevity of the symptoms. For example, a client with a long history of a contractile lesion may have an acute problem because of a recent exacerbation of the condition.

Treatment of contractile lesions. The objectives of treatment for contractile lesions vary, depending on the phase of the inflammatory process and the severity of the tear. In the acute phase, the goals of treatment are to

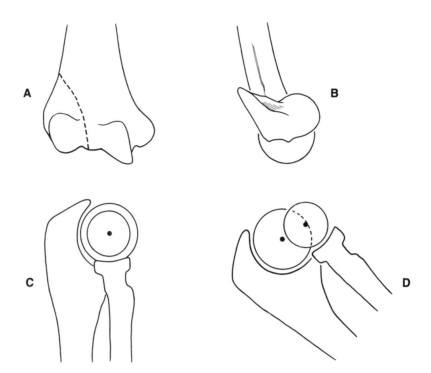

Fig. 14-9. Effects of condylar malalignment. Centers of articular arc of separate condyles are located on same horizontal line through distal humerus (**A, C**). When there is malalignment of one condyle with another (**B, D**), flexion and extension of elbow are blocked. (Redrawn from Magnuson PB and Stack JK: *Fractures,* ed 5, Philadelphia, 1949, JB Lippincott Co.)

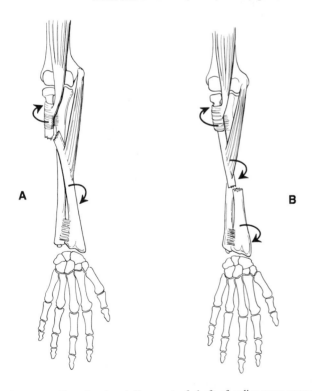

Fig. 14-10. Rotational malalignment of shaft of radius may occur following fracture of radial shaft. **A,** In fracture of upper shaft of radius between insertion of supinator and pronator teres, proximal fragment is supinated and lower fragment pronated. **B,** In fracture of middle or lower shaft between insertions of pronator teres and pronator quadratus, proximal fragment is in midposition.

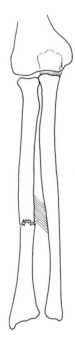

Fig. 14-11. Angular malalignment of radial shaft. When normal lateral bow of radius is lost, length of interosseous membrane is not maintained. Shortening of membrane impedes rotation of forearm.

CASE 1 ▼ Patient A

The patient is a 42-year-old female. She reports the onset of right lateral elbow pain during the rehabilitation of her right shoulder following a subacromial decompression. She recalls no specific injury but feels it was caused by repetitive exercise she performed to increase the strength in her right shoulder. She describes the pain as a dull ache to a stabbing pain that occurs with use of her right arm, such as driving and pitching a softball to her children. She states the pain has been present for the past 15 months. The patient reports slight decrease in pain with antiinflammatories and an injection approximately 6 weeks ago. The patient is able to perform all active movements of the elbow complex. Passive range-of-motion (ROM) testing reveals full flexion, extension, pronation, and supination with motion barriers comparable to the uninvolved side. The passive ROM of wrist flexion is mildly limited with a

muscle insufficiency motion barrier and pain after resistance. Resisted testing reveals wrist extension to be strong and painful. The remaining resisted tests of the elbow complex are strong and painless. Mobility testing revealed the right elbow to have increased medial gap of the humeroulnar joint. The physical therapy diagnosis was lateral epicondylitis syndrome. The patient was started on a program of ultrasound, moist heat, iontophoresis with a 2% dexamethasone solution, forearm flexibility, and cryotherapy. Progression was made to a forearm-strengthening program with light resistance in an attempt to stabilize the elbow complex and to increase endurance. The patient was instructed in a home program of moist heat/cryotherapy and exercise (including an eccentric emphasis). The patient was also to continue to wear the forearm band issued by the orthopedist.

CASE 2 ▼ Patient B

The patient is a 45-year-old male laborer in a steel mill. He suffered a fracture and dislocation of the left elbow complex during a fall at work. The surgical report indicates the presence of an intraarticular fracture of the distal humerus (two part), as well as a fracture of the proximal aspect of the olecranon process. An open-reduction internal fixation was performed, and there is good alignment of the fragments. However, a review of the standard x-rays reveals the screw fixation of the humeral fragments traverses the coronoid fossa. The fractures are well healed. A discussion of the case with the attending orthopedic surgeon revealed that this fracture was difficult to stabilize, this was the only option available, and it is not anticipated that this fixation will be removed. The patient is now 6 weeks postsurgery and immobilized in full arm cast. This cast permitted the patient to perform active motion of the digits. The patient is referred for progressive ROM and strengthening. The patient reports no pain with rest and moderate pain with movement. He states the pain worsens with repeated movement. He voices concern over the fact that he may never regain full movement of his left elbow. The patient can perform all active movements of the elbow and wrist-hand complex but exhibits severe restriction. Passive

ROM reveals: flexion to 100 degrees with capsular motion barrier, 35 degrees from full extension with slow muscle guarding, pronation to 45 degrees with slow muscle guarding, and supination to 45 degrees with slow muscle guarding. There are 10-degree limitations of wrist flexion and extension and a minimal loss of finger flexion. These motion barriers are capsular. Muscle testing revealed the elbow and wrist musculature in the 3/5 range. The patient was started on a program of whirlpool, active/active assistive ROM, mobilization at grades I and II, and cryotherapy. The patient's progress was slow. As the slow muscle-guarding motion barriers became more capsular in nature, the mobilization grades were progressed to grades III and IV. In addition, progressive strengthening was initiated. After 10 weeks of treatment, the ROM increased to flexion of 135 degrees, extension lacked 8 degrees from full, pronation was 80 degrees, supination was 80 degrees, and the wrist-hand movements were all normal. The extension motion barrier was hard, and it became evident there would be no further progress in this area. The strength increased to 4+/5 in all areas, and the patient was able to return to full employment.

reduce pain and to prevent the formation of adhesions between tissue planes. While these goals are being accomplished, care must be taken to ensure that no further tissue damage occurs. In chronic cases with existing adhesions, the objectives of treatment include improvement of the gliding function between tissue planes by stretching of adhesions with transverse friction massage.[2]

Ultimately, the client should be provided with a treatment program designed to prevent recurrence of the problem. It may include an exercise program designed to develop strength, power, and endurance in the musculotendinous unit, if deficiencies are identified, and a stretching program to promote flexibility. The total program should include instruction in activities of daily living to prevent overload of the structures involved. The athlete may require instruction in technique or alterations in equipment.

Contractile lesions in the elbow region may involve the flexors and extensors of the elbow joint as well as the pronators and supinators of the forearm.[2] These lesions are not encountered frequently. The precise identification of these lesions and their treatment has been described by Cyriax.[2]

By far the most common contractile lesions in the elbow region involve the proximal attachments of the wrist extensors and wrist flexors. If the wrist extensors are involved, the condition is known as *lateral epicondylitis,* or *lateral tennis elbow.* This syndrome is identified by pain produced by isometric contraction of the wrist extensors with the elbow in the extended position. The lesion is usually caused by overload of these muscles by repetitive use. It is common in tennis players but also occurs frequently in those whose occupation demands repeated use of the muscles in question.

When the wrist flexors are involved, the condition is termed *medial epicondylitis* or *golfer's elbow.* Medial epicondylitis is not seen as commonly as lateral epicondylitis. It, too, results from repeated overuse of the musculotendinous units and is often found in athletes who engage in the action of throwing.

A treatment program for contractile lesions has been outlined here. The plan can be modified for any contractile lesion found in this region.

I.   Acute stage
  A. Ice
  B. Aspirin
  C. Oral or injected antiinflammatory agents
  D. Electrical stimulation (muscle placed in shortened position to prevent excessive tension)
  E. Gentle transverse friction massage (to minimize formation of adhesions)
II. Chronic stage
  A. Heat applications before periods of activity
  B. Ice following periods of activity
  C. Deep transverse friction massage to mobilize adhesions
  D. Ultrasound (may be used before transverse friction massage)
  E. Orthosis (tennis elbow splint)
III. Prevention of recurrence
  A. Exercise for strength, power, and endurance of involved muscle (often eccentric emphasis)
  B. Exercise to promote flexibility
  C. Activities of daily living to improve technique, avoid stressful situations, and/or modify equipment

SUMMARY

This chapter provides a description of the functional anatomy of the elbow complex, which is essential for understanding the examination and treatment of this region of the musculoskeletal system.

An outline of the examination protocol has been provided, with an emphasis on the functional examination and its interpretation. Attention to the details of this examination should enable the physical therapist to identify movement dysfunctions of the elbow, which can be divided into dysfunctions of the noncontractile tissues and dysfunctions of the contractile tissues.

Interpretation of the results of the examination is most important. The physical therapist must determine which tissues are involved and the states of the pathologic process. From this information, rational goals or objectives of treatment can be set.

If the physical therapist follows these examination and treatment principles, the client may benefit from a more rapid return to optimal function. This is not to say that all clients attain a full and pain-free range of motion; in many situations, this is not possible. However, the client should not be made worse as a result of treatment. When treatment is directed toward unattainable goals, the final outcome of the process is usually unfavorable. Improper goal setting and failure to heed the principles of treatment of the musculoskeletal system have both contributed to the disrepute of physical therapy in the management of movement dysfunction of the elbow complex.

Before attempting to treat movement dysfunctions of the elbow complex, the physical therapist should receive supervised instruction in the examination and treatment of the musculoskeletal system, particularly if passive movement is used in the management of problems found in this joint.

REVIEW QUESTIONS

1. What is the difference between capsular and noncapsular patterns of the elbow complex?
2. Define the term *motion barrier,* and state those factors that limit motion under normal circumstances.
3. What is the theoretical basis for the use of resisted testing in the physical examination of the elbow complex?
4. How do the three stages of tissue inflammation influence the treatment of noncontractile structures?
5. What factors in the physical examination differentiate between contractile and noncontractile tissues as the cause of elbow complex dysfunction?

REFERENCES

1. Anderson LD: Fractures of the shafts of the radius and ulna. In Rockwood CA and Green DP, editors: *Fractures,* vol 2, Philadelphia, 1975, JB Lippincott.
2. Cyriax J: *Textbook of orthopaedic medicine,* vol 1, *Diagnosis of soft tissue lesions,* ed 5, Baltimore, 1969, Williams & Wilkins.
3. DeAndrade JR et al: Joint distension and reflex muscle inhibition in the knee, *J Bone Joint Surg Am* 47:313, 1965.

4. Dunn JS: Personal communication, 1981.

5. Eppright RH, Wilkins KE: Fractures and dislocations of the elbow. In Rockwood CA and Green DP, editors: *Fractures,* vol 2, Philadelphia, 1975, JB Lippincott.

6. Eyring EJ, Murray WR: The effect of joint position on the pressure of intra-articular effusion, *J Bone Joint Surg Am* 46:1235, 1964.

7. Grant JCB: *A method of anatomy,* Baltimore, 1937, William Wood & Co.

8. Heppenstall RB: Fractures of the forearm. In Heppenstall RB, editor: *Fracture treatment and healing,* Philadelphia, 1980, WB Saunders.

9. Heppenstall RB: Injuries of the elbow. In Heppenstall RB, editor: *Fracture treatment and healing,* Philadelphia, 1980, WB Saunders.

10. Hunt TK, VanWinkle W: Wound healing. In Heppenstall RB, editor: *Fracture treatment and healing,* Philadelphia, 1980, WB Saunders.

11. Kaltenborn FM: *Manual therapy for the extremity joints: specialized techniques: tests and joint mobilization,* ed 2, Oslo, 1976, Olaf Norlis Bokhandel.

12. Kang AH: Connective tissue: collagen and elastin. In Kelly WN et al, editors: *Textbook of rheumatology,* vol 1, Philadelphia, 1981, WB Saunders.

13. Kapandji IA: *The physiology of joints,* vol 1, *The upper limb,* London, 1970, E & S Livingstone.

14. Kapandji IA: The inferior radioulnar joint and pronosupination. In Tubiana R, editor: *The hand,* vol 1, Philadelphia, 1981, WB Saunders.

15. London JT: Kinematics of the elbow, *J Bone Joint Surg Am* 63:529, 1981.

16. MacConaill MA, Basmajian JJ: *Muscles and movements: a basis for human kinesiology,* Baltimore, 1969, Williams & Wilkins.

17. Maitland GD: *Peripheral manipulation,* New York, 1970, Appleton-Century-Crofts.

18. Morrey BF, Chao YS: Passive motion of the elbow joint: a biomechanical analysis, *J Bone Joint Surg Am* 58:501, 1976.

19. Muller ME et al: *Manual of internal fixation: techniques recommended by the AO-Group,* ed 2, New York, 1979, Springer-Verlag.

20. Schwab GH et al: Biomechanics of elbow instability: the role of the medial collateral ligament, *Clin Orthop* 146:42, 1980.

21. Sisk TD: Fractures. In Edmonson AS and Crenshaw AH, editors: *Campbell's operative orthopaedics,* vol 1, ed 6, St Louis, 1980, Mosby.

22. Williams PL, Warwick R, editors: *Gray's Anatomy,* ed 36, Philadelphia, 1980, WB Saunders.

ADDITIONAL READINGS

Tennis elbow

Baumgard SH, Schwartz DR: Percutaneous release of the epicondylar muscles for humeral epicondylitis, *Am J Sports Med* 10:233-235, 1982.

Brattberg G: Acupuncture therapy for tennis elbow, *Pain* 16:285-288, 1983.

Burton AK: Grip strength and forearm straps in tennis elbow, *Br J Sports Med* 19(1):37-38, 1985.

Dimberg L: The prevalence and causation of tennis elbow (lateral humeral epicondylitis) in a population of workers in an engineering industry, *Ergonomics* 30:573-580, 1987.

Gieck JH, Saliba E: Application of modalities in overuse syndromes, *Clin Sports Med* 6:427-466, 1987.

Groppel JH, Nirschl RP: A mechanical and electromyographical analysis of the effects of various joint counterforce braces on the tennis player, *Am J Sports Med* 14(3):195-200, 1986.

Halle JS, Franklin RJ, Karalfa BL: Comparison of four treatment approaches for lateral epicondylitis of the elbow, *J Orthop Sports Phys Ther* 8:62-67, 1986.

Heyse-Moore GH: Resistant tennis elbow, *J Hand Surg* 9B:64-66, 1983.

Leach RE, Miller JK: Lateral and medial epicondylitis of the elbow, *Clin Sports Med* 6:259-272, 1987.

Lee DG: Tennis elbow: a manual therapist's perspective, *J Orthop Sports Phys Ther* 8:134-141, 1986.

Lehman RC: Surface and equipment variables in tennis injuries, *Clin Sports Med* 7:229-232, 1988.

Morrey BF, editor: *Elbow and its disorders,* ed 2, Philadelphia, 1993, WB Saunders.

Morrey BF, editor: *The elbow,* New York, 1994, Raven Press.

Moss SH, Switzer HE: Radial tunnel syndrome: a spectrum of clinical presentations, *J Hand Surg* 8:414-419, 1983.

Nirschl RP: Prevention and treatment of elbow and shoulder injuries in the tennis player, *Clin Sports Med* 7:289-308, 1988.

Noteboom T, Cruver R, Keller J, Kellogg B, Nitz AJ: Tennis elbow: a review, *J Orthop Sports Phys Ther* 19(6):357-366, 1994.

Snijders CJ, Volkers ACW, Melchelse K, Vleeming AK: Provocation of epicondylalgia lateralis (tennis elbow) by power grip or pinching, *Med Sci Sports Exerc* 19(5):518-523, 1987.

Stoeckart R, Vleeming A, Snijders CJ: Anatomy of the extensor carpi radialis brevis muscle related to tennis elbow, *Clin Biomech* 4(4):210-212, 1989.

Stonecipher DR, Catlin PA: The effect of a forearm strap on wrist extensor strength, *J Orthop Sports Phys Ther* 6:184-189, 1984.

Stratford P, Levy DR, Gauldie S, Levy K, Miseferi D: Extensor carpi radialis tendonitis: a validation of selected outcome measures, *Physiother Can* 39(4):250-255, 1987.

Stratford P, Levy DR, Gauldie S, Miseferi D, Levy K: The evaluation of phonophoresis and friction massage as treatments for extensor carpi radialis tendinitis: a randomized controlled trial, *Physiother Can* 41(2):93–99, 1989.

Wadsworth TG: Tennis elbow: conservative, surgical, and manipulative treatment, *Br Med J* 294:621-623, 1987.

Wadsworth CT, Nielsen DH, Burns LT, Krull JD, Thompson CG: Effect of the counterforce armband on wrist extension and grip strength and pain in subjects with tennis elbow, *J Orthop Sports Phys Ther* 11(5):192-201, 1989.

CHAPTER 15

The Shoulder

Kevin E. Wilk

OUTLINE

Anatomy
  Glenohumeral joint
  Acromioclavicular joint
  Sternoclavicular joint
  Scapulothoracic joint
Biomechanics
Joint stabilization
  Dynamic stabilizers
  Static stabilizers
  Basic muscle function
Evaluation
  Physical examination
Observation
Inspection
  Cervical spine screening
Motion assessment
Inferior stability assessment
Anterior stability assessment
Posterior stability assessment
  Impingement sign
Biceps brachii assessment
Vascular examination
Neurological assessment
Resisted movements
Palpation
  Muscular performance testing
  Functional performance testing
  Summary of the examination process

The scapulothoracic joint
Acromioclavicular joint injuries
Instability
  Surgical approach to instability
  Historical overview
  Bankart procedure
  Overview-Bankart procedure
  Bristow
  Magnuson-Stack procedure
  Putti-Platt procedure
  Capsular shift
Rehabilitation following shoulder stabilization
  Rehabilitation following Bankart procedure
  Rehabilitation following capsular shift procedures
Rotator cuff pathologies
Surgical repair of the rotator cuff
Rehabilitation following rotator cuff repair
Glenoid labrum lesions
Neurovascular compression syndromes
Adhesive capsulitis
The shoulder joint in sports
  Overhead throwing
  Tennis strokes
  Golf swing
  Swimming
  Prevention

KEY TERMS

glenohumeral
scapulothoracic
scapulohumeral rhythm
instability

rotator cuff
neurovascular compression
adhesive capsulitis

After studying this chapter, the reader should be able to:

1. Identify significant anatomical structures of the shoulder complex.
2. Describe the joint mechanics of the glenohumeral, scapulothoracic, sternoclavicular, and acromioclavicular articulations.
3. State three components contributing to dynamic stability of the glenohumeral joint.
4. Describe and list the components of a physical examination of the shoulder complex.
5. State most common mechanism of injury to the acromioclavicular joint.
6. List five factors that form the basis of shoulder instability classification.
7. Describe what is meant by a capsular shift procedure.
8. State three functions of the rotator cuff.
9. List those factors that determine the type of rehabilitation program following a rotator cuff repair.
10. Describe the four stages of the adhesive capsulitis disease process.

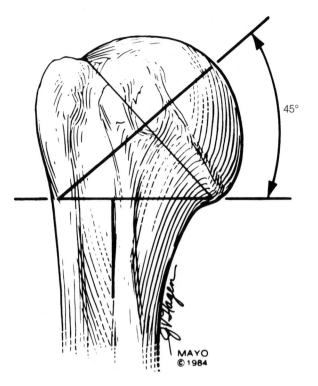

Fig. 15-1. The orientation of the humeral head. (From Morrey BF, An KW: Biomechanics of the shoulder. In Rockwood CA, Matsen FA, editors: *The shoulder,* Philadelphia, 1990, WB Saunders. Reproduced with permission.)

The shoulder joint complex is an intriguing region of the human body because of its complexity, integration of multiple joints, and susceptibility to injury. The shoulder joint complex is composed of the glenohumeral, acromioclavicular, sternoclavicular, and scapulothoracic joints and truly represents a functional kinetic chain movement pattern in all activities. The shoulder joint exhibits the greatest amount of motion of any joint in the human body.[377] However, it is also the most commonly dislocated joint of the human body.[75,186,336] Thus the glenohumeral joint sacrifices stability for the sake of mobility. Additionally, the shoulder joint is frequently injured as a result of both microtraumatic insults and macrotraumatic forces; consequently, a wide variety of injuries from fractures, dislocations, ligamentous lesions, to rotator cuff failures can be present throughout this joint complex.

In this chapter we will discuss the structure and function of the shoulder complex. Additionally, a review of the physical examination with attention to special tests will be discussed. And last, a thorough description of various injuries will be conducted, including both surgical and nonsurgical treatment suggestions.

ANATOMY

The anatomical discussion of the shoulder joint must include the entire upper quadrant. There are four articulations vital to normal shoulder joint function. These include the glenohumeral, sternoclavicular, acromioclavicular, and scapulothoracic joints. In addition, the cervical, thoracic, and lumbar spine also function in concert with the upper quadrant, enabling full unrestricted function. When discuss-

ing anatomy we can divide the anatomic structure into three components: the osseous structures, the ligamentous structures, and the neuromuscular system. All three components contribute to the functional stability of the joint.

Glenohumeral joint

The glenohumeral articulation is a diarthrodial joint and is often considered a spheroidal or multiaxial ball-and-socket joint.[377] This type of articular configuration allows tremendous mobility but is inherently unstable. The articular surfaces are formed by a large humeral head that articulates with the relatively small and flat glenoid cavity of the scapula. The head of the humerus is two to three times larger than the glenoid fossa. The articulation is often likened to the relationship between a golf ball and a golf tee.[318] Thus the glenohumeral joint relies greatly on the capsuloligamentous structures and neuromuscular system for functional stability, placing it at risk for injury.

The joint geometry (osseous structures) of the glenohumeral joint is conducive to excessive mobility but sacrifices static osseous stability. The humeral head articular surface is shaped somewhat as a sphere, but not a perfect sphere.[324,325] The head of the humerus is directed in a posterior, medial, and superior direction (Fig. 15-1). In contrast, the glenoid cavity is directed in an anterior, lateral, and superior direction.

The humeral head is covered with articular cartilage that

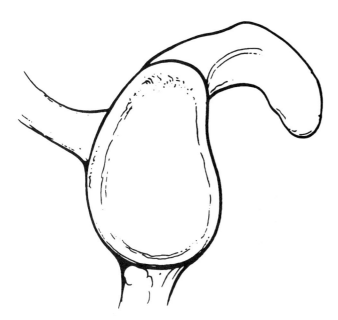

Fig. 15-2. Lateral view of glenoid fossa illustrating the pear-shaped appearance.

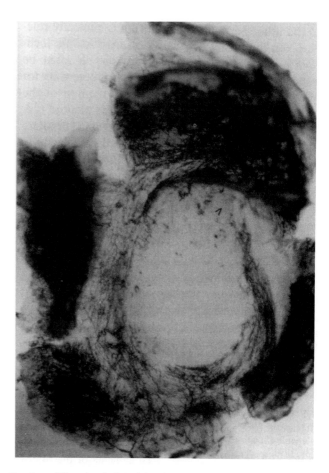

Fig. 15-3. The vascularity of the glenoid labrum. (From Cooper DE, Arnoczky SP, O'Brien SJ et al: Anatomy, histology and vascularity of the glenoid labrum: an anatomical study, *J Bone Joint Surg* 74A:46-52, 1992. Reproduced with permission.)

is thickest in the center and thinnest at its peripheral margin.[377] The articular surface represents approximately one third of an irregular sphere with a radius of curvature of about 2.25 cm.[327] The humeral head is inclined approximately 130° to 150° and is retroverted approximately 20° to 30°.[180,324,325,327]

The glenoid's articular surface is pear-shaped, with the inferior half being 20% larger than the superior half[277] (Fig. 15-2). The glenoid's articular surface is much smaller than that of the humeral head, and the surface area of the humeral head is approximately three to four times that of the glenoid.[340] The surface area ratio between the humeral head and glenoid has been referred to as the glenohumeral index (maximum diameter of the glenoid/maximum diameter of the humeral head). This ratio is approximately 0.75 in the sagittal plane and approximately 0.60 in the transverse plane.[324] Additionally, at any given point during normal motion only 25% to 30% of the humeral head is actually in contact with the glenoid.[55,83,345] This lack of articular contact contributes to the inherent instability of the glenohumeral joint. The articular cartilage of the glenoid is thicker at its peripheral margins and is thinner in its central area.[377] The peripheral margin of the glenoid is slightly raised and forms a rim that serves as an attachment point for the glenoid labrum. The glenoid fossa faces superiorly, laterally, and anteriorly. Thus the glenoid is tilted superiorly. Basmajian and Bazart[37] have reported this superior tilt limits the inferior translation of the humerus on the glenoid. There is a wide variation of the actual size, shape, tilt, and version of the glenoid fossa, which may or may not contribute to shoulder stability.[63,163,323]

The glenoid labrum is a fibrous rim that serves to slightly deepen the glenoid fossa and allows for the attachment of the

glenohumeral capsule to the glenoid rim. Several investigations have reported that a small amount of fibrocartilage exists at the junction of the glenoid and the fibrous capsule.[240,358] The superior labrum and the long head of the biceps brachii blend together at their attachment to the supraglenoid tubercle. This labrum-biceps tendon complex is often a site of lesion or injury. The superior aspect of the labrum is loose and "meniscal-like," whereas the inferior attachment is firm and relatively unmovable.[269] Additionally, the labrum does receive blood supply to its periphery. Cooper et al.[89] recently examined the vascular supply of the labrum and found that the superior and anterosuperior positions of the labrum were less vascular than the posterosuperior and inferior portions (Fig. 15-3). Additionally, Prodromos et al.[286] have reported that the vascularity of the labrum decreases with age.

The role of labrum as a stabilizing structure has been debated in the literature.[160,211,383] The labrum functions to deepen the glenoid from 2.5 mm to approximately 5.0 mm.[160] The labrum appears to assist in contributing to joint stability with the glenohumeral capsule and may serve a role as a "chock block" in controlling glenohumeral translation.

The capsule of the glenohumeral joint completely encircles the articulation. It is attached to the entire circumference of the glenoid cavity just medial to the glenoid rim and extends across the joint, attaching onto the anatomical neck of the humerus. The capsule is a loose and redundant structure that is approximately twice the surface area of the humeral head normally.[38] The inferior portion of this capsule extends inferiorly, exhibiting a redundant fold often referred to as the infraglenoid recess, or axillary fold. Obliteration of this fold in the capsule is considered a major cause of adhesive capsulitis.[259] Additionally, the capsule is lined throughout by a synovial membrane that is reflected inferiorly along the anatomical neck of the humerus. The synovial membrane also lines the bicipital groove and reflects over the biceps tendon.

The shoulder joint capsule is large, loose, and redundant, thereby allowing for the large range of motion naturally available at this articulation. The shoulder joint capsule is composed of multilayered collagen fiber bundles of differing orientation and strength. Gohlke et al.[135] have reported that the joint capsule collagen fiber orientation is composed of radial fibers that are linked to each other by circular elements. Thus rotational movements produce tension within the fibers, which leads to compression of the joint surfaces centering the humeral head within the glenoid. The antero-inferior capsule is the thickest and strongest portion of the capsule due to the presence of densely organized collagen fibers, evident by the reinforcing ligaments of the inferior glenohumeral ligament complex (IGHLC). The capsule is reinforced with capsular ligaments, which contribute greatly to joint stability. However, there is a wide variation in the size, strength, and orientation of these capsular ligaments.[103,240,271] These ligaments function when the joint is placed in extremes of motion to protect against excessive translation or instability of the humeral head on the glenoid.

The anterior aspect of the capsule is reinforced by three collagen thickenings referred to as the glenohumeral ligaments: the superior glenohumeral ligament (SGHL), middle glenohumeral ligament (MGHL) and IGHLC[103,271,362] (Fig. 15-4). The SGHL arises from the fovea capitis of the humerus adjacent and just superior to the lesser tuberosity and transverses in a superior and medial direction to the superior rim of the glenoid near the upper pole of the glenoid fossa, blending with the glenoid labrum and biceps tendon. This ligament has been found to be present in 90% to 96% of all specimens.[103,271] The MGHL, when present, usually arises from the labrum just inferior to the attachment of the SGHL. The ligament then transverses downward and laterally to insert just medial to the lesser tuberosity. Near its insertion, the ligament lies beneath or adherent to the subscapularis muscle. This ligament is present in approximately 68% to 73% of specimens studied and is considered to have the greatest amount of variation in size and presence.[103,121,271] Thus the ligament may be thick and robust or thin and ill-defined (when present). The IGHLC is

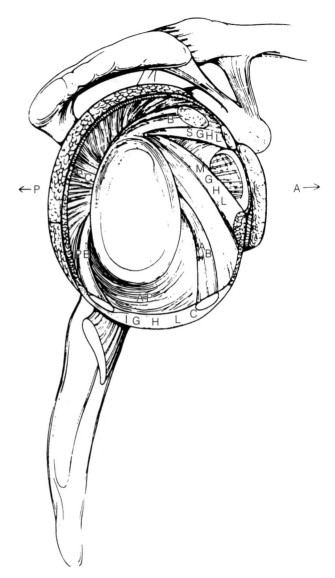

Fig. 15-4. The glenohumeral ligaments: the long head of the biceps (B), the superior glenohumeral ligament (SGHL), the middle glenohumeral ligament (MGHL), and the inferior glenohumeral ligament complex (IGHLC) consisting of the anterior band (AB), axillary pouch (AP), and posterior band (PB). (From O'Brien SJ, Neves MC, Arnoczky SP et al: The anatomy and histology of the anterior glenohumeral ligament complex of the shoulder, *Am J Sports Med* 18:449-456, 1990. Reproduced with permission.)

composed of three functional portions: an anterior band, a posterior band, and an axillary pouch[270] (Fig. 15-5). The anterior band of the IGHLC attaches to the glenoid between the 2 and 4 o'clock position. The IGHLC attaches to the humerus just inferior to the articular cartilage. The anterior and posterior bands of the IGHLC have been shown to exhibit great variations in thickness but are present in most specimens. This structure, when distinct in configuration, has been shown to be the strongest of the three distinct glenohumeral ligaments.

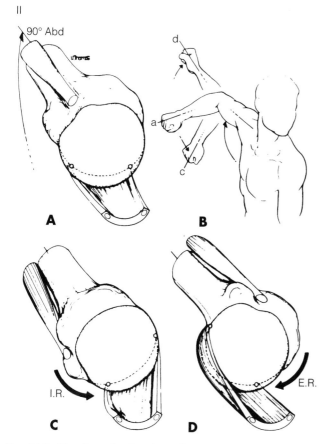

Fig. 15-5. The dynamic function of the inferior glenohumeral ligament complex. (D) during abduction to 90° and external rotation the (AB) anterior band fans out and supports the humeral head against anterior humeral head displacement. (C) the reverse is true during abduction and internal rotation.

a large rotator interval. Harryman et al.[145] reported that this portion of the capsule plays a significant role in preventing inferior subluxation in the adducted shoulder.

The posterior capsule of the glenohumeral joint does not exhibit the functional ligamentous bands present in the anterior capsule, other than the posterior band of the IGHLC. The posterior capsule is rather thin and provides only moderate joint stability at best. Although the entire shoulder capsule blends with the rotator cuff musculature, this is especially true with the posterior capsule. The supraspinatus, infraspinatus, and teres minor musculotendinous units blend intimately with the shoulder capsule and play a vital role in stabilizing the joint.

There are numerous bursae about the shoulder joint. Codman[83] has identified 13 surrounding the shoulder. Bursae are believed to assist in reducing friction between two surfaces or structures. The bursae normally are the thickness of a sheet of paper. The most commonly discussed bursae are the subacromial, subdeltoid, and coracobrachialis bursae, which are essential for normal function of the shoulder complex.

The muscles surrounding the glenohumeral joint provide dynamic stabilization to the inherently unstable joint and play a significant role in normal shoulder function. The anatomical description of each muscle can be found in several textbooks.[170,188,377] The primary dynamic stabilizers of the glenohumeral joint include the rotator cuff muscles (subscapularis, supraspinatus, infraspinatus, teres minor), the deltoid, and the long head of the biceps brachii. The secondary stabilizers include the teres major, latissimus dorsi, pectoralis major, and triceps brachii. The actual mechanics of dynamic stability will be discussed later in this chapter under biomechanics.

Acromioclavicular joint

The acromioclavicular (AC) joint is classified as a diarthrodial joint and is formed by the distal end of the clavicle and the inner margin of the acromion. The AC joint can be considered a plane joint because the articulating surfaces are relatively flat. The distal end of the clavicle is positioned higher than the acromion, and the acromion is angled or slanted downward (Fig. 15-6). The two articulating surfaces do not produce a congruent joint; consequently the AC joint is frequently injured. The articular surfaces are covered with hyaline cartilage.[308] Tyurina[363] reported that the articular cartilage of the distal clavicle is hyaline cartilage until approximately 17 years of age. It then acquires the structure and properties of fibrocartilage. The articular surface of the acromion changes slower and does not become fibrocartilaginous until about 23 to 24 years of age. There is a significant amount of variation in the shape and inclination of the AC joint, which may contribute to various injuries. A small articular disk projects into the joint from above. The disk has great variation in size and shape and in some cases is either complete or partial, which resembles more of a

The coracohumeral ligament (CHL) extends from the base and lateral border of the coracoid process, just below the coracoacromial ligament, and attaches to the greater tuberosity. The ligament is often described as two bands (anterior and posterior),[182] but on dissection usually the anterior portion is more distinct than the posterior position.[89] The fibers of the coracohumeral ligament intermingle with the superior glenohumeral ligament.[403] The cross-sectional size of the CHL at mid-position is 52 mm^2.[403] This is compared with a cross-sectional size of the SGHL of approximately 11 to 22 mm^2. [403]

The transverse humeral ligament crosses the intertubercular groove and provides static stability to the long head of the biceps brachii tendon. The ligament transverses from the greater to lesser tuberosities. The size of this ligament varies from individual to individual.[89]

The rotator interval is the space located between the superior border of the subscapularis and the anterior margin of the supraspinatus muscles. The SGHL and CHL are located in this region of the capsule. Nobuhara and Ikeeda[265] have reported an association between inferior instability and

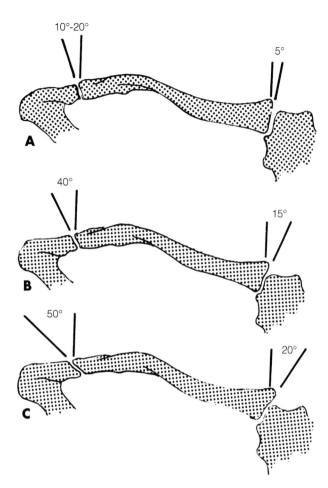

Fig. 15-6. Variations in the orientation of the acromioclavicular and sternoclavicular joints. (From Rockwood CA, Young DC: Disorders of the acromioclavicular joint. In Rockwood CA, Matsen FA, editors: *The shoulder,* Philadelphia, 1990, WB Saunders. Reproduced with permission.)

meniscoid pattern. Several investigators have reported that the meniscus or disk undergoes rapid degeneration until approximately 40 years of age, when it is no longer functional.[101,136,284] The articular disk serves to distribute forces evenly within the joint. The nerve supply to the acromioclavicular joint is from branches of the axillary, suprascapular, and lateral pectoral nerves.[308]

The joint is surrounded by a thin capsule that is reinforced above and below by the superior, inferior, anterior, and posterior acromioclavicular ligaments.[308] The fibers with the deltoid and upper trapezius muscles, which attach to the superior aspect of the clavicle and acromion process, serve to strengthen the acromioclavicular ligaments and stabilize the acromioclavicular joint.

The coracoclavicular ligaments are very strong, thick ligaments that run from the coracoid process of the scapula to the outer inferior surface of the clavicle. There are two distinct ligaments—the conoid and the trapezoid ligaments. The conoid ligament is cone-shaped and is more medial and posterior than the trapezoid ligament. The trapezoid liga-

ment is quadrilateral and broad and thin. The primary function of the coracoclavicular ligaments is vertical stability of the acromioclavicular joint. In addition, these ligaments (especially the conoid) guide motion occurring between the clavicle and the acromion.

Sternoclavicular joint

The sternoclavicular joint is a diarthrodial type of joint. This joint is the only true articulation between the upper extremity and the axial skeleton. The articular surface of the clavicle is much larger than that of the sternum, and both are covered with fibrocartilage. The medial end of the clavicle is concave front to back and convex vertically, thus creating a saddle-like joint articulation with the sternum (clavicular notch).[136,137] The articular surface area on the sternum is the clavicular notch, which is curved, making the joint noncongruent. Thus less than half of the medial clavicle articulates with the sternum, making the sternoclavicular joint the least stable from an osseous standpoint.[306]

Because the sternoclavicular joint lacks congruency, stability must be provided by the ligamentous structures. The capsular ligaments cover the anterosuperior and posterior aspects of the joint and represent thickenings of the joint capsule. The anterior sternoclavicular ligament is stronger than its posterior counterpart. The anterior sternoclavicular ligament is covered anteriorly by the sternocleidomastoid tendon and blends posteriorly with the intraarticular disk. The posterior sternoclavicular ligament blends with the tendons of the sternothyroid and sternohyoid muscles posteriorly. The interclavicular ligament is a flat ligament that extends from one clavicle to the other and binds to the upper margin of the sternum. The costoclavicular ligament is a strong rhomboid-shaped structure that runs from the superior aspect of the first rib to the inferior surface of the medial clavicle. This ligament has a somewhat twisted appearance.[137] The costoclavicular ligament assists in resisting displacement of the medial clavicle and guides clavicular motion. The intraarticular disk ligament is a very dense fibrous structure that arises from the synchondral junction of the first rib and runs to the sternum. This ligament passes through the joint, dividing it into two separate joint spaces. The intraarticular disk blends into the capsular ligaments both anteriorly and posteriorly, acting as a checkrein against medial clavicular displacement.

Scapulothoracic joint

The scapulothoracic joint is not a true anatomical joint but rather is considered a physiological joint that relies on soft tissue to maintain its relationship to the thoracic wall. The scapula is vital to normal arm and upper extremity function. It has a slightly concave ventral surface that glides on the convex thoracic wall. This positioning places the scapula in an orientation ranging between 30° to 45° anterior to the coronal plane. This position is referred to as the plane of the scapula[83,180,325] (Fig. 15-7).

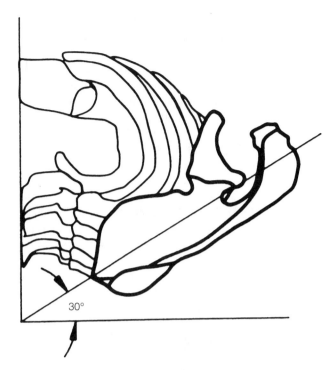

Fig. 15-7. The scapular plane; approximately 30 degrees anterior to the coronal plane. (From Morrey BF, An KN: Biomechanics of the shoulder. In Rockwood CA, Matsen FA, editors: *The shoulder,* Philadelphia, 1990, WB Saunders. Reproduced with permission.)

Typically, the resting position of the scapula is usually the following: the superior angle is level with the spinous process of T_2, with the inferior angle level with spinous process of T_7. The medial border of the scapula is approximately 5 to 6 cm from the spinous processes of the thoracic spine. The scapula is usually slightly upwardly rotated, although the literature offers some controversy.[128,288] Frequently, individuals involved in unilateral sporting activities or heavy work exhibit a depressed scapula on the dominant side. Also, the glenoid fossa is retroverted 7°[323] and inclined 3° to 5°,[37] which serves to enhance static stability inferiorly and posteriorly.

The scapulothoracic joint relies on muscular support to position the scapula on the thoracic wall. Muscular control also serves to provide mobility, allowing the humeral head to follow the scapula and maintain normal scapulohumeral rhythm. Thus if the scapular stabilizers are weak, injured, or ineffective, scapular posture and scapulohumeral rhythm will be affected. This may lead to or contribute to glenohumeral joint pathologies.

BIOMECHANICS

The study of biomechanics refers to the movement of structure through space and attempts to explain both the quantity and quality of joint movements. The movement of the arm and hand through space is greatly dependent upon the glenohumeral joint and the delicate interaction of the various joints that compose the upper extremity kinetic chain.

When the biomechanics of the shoulder joint complex is being discussed, an area of frequent discussion is the normal acceptable range of motion present at the glenohumeral joint. Numerous studies have published values described as "normal shoulder range of motion." Numerous factors such as age, gender, arm dominance, activity level, and body type may influence shoulder motion.[54,132,149,247]

Osteokinematics refers to the movement of the bone in space (i.e., shoulder flexion or external rotation), whereas arthrokinematics refers to the movement between two adjacent joint surfaces (i.e., posterior glide and anterior roll).

Scapulohumeral rhythm is a vital element allowing normal shoulder function. This concept refers to the synchronous motion of the humerus and scapula during arm elevation. It is generally accepted that scapulohumeral rhythm occurs in a 2:1 ratio, with the humerus moving 2° for every 1° of scapulae motion. This overall ratio is correct, but the scapulohumeral rhythm varies depending on numerous factors such as arm position, gender, unresisted or resisted motion, and glenohumeral capsule mobility.

During the first 30° of arm elevation (flexion in the scapular plane), the scapula is attempting to stabilize itself on the thoracic wall. This is referred to as the setting phase.[168] After this phase, the scapulohumeral rhythm is relatively consistent. Inman et al.[168] noted a 2:1 ratio from 30° to 170° of arm elevation. However, for the same range of motion Saha[325] has reported a ratio of 2.3:1; whereas Freedman[128] reported a ratio of 3.2:1. Doody et al.[111] stated the overall scapulohumeral rhythm as 1.74:1. Poppen and Walker[288] noted a ratio of 1.25:1 from 30° to 180° of motion.

Therefore scapulohumeral rhythm should be based on arm position during elevation. The setting phase takes place during the first 20° to 30° of elevation, and during this phase scapula motion is very inconsistent in that it may elevate, depress, or rotate on the thoracic wall. From 30° to 90° of arm elevation the humerus moves 2° to 2.75° to every 1° of scapular motion. From 90° to 160° of motion the scapula moves 1° of every 1° of humeral motion. Adding resistance in the hand causes the setting phase to occur more rapidly and increases the scapular rotation component in the early phases of elevation. Additionally, the scapulohumeral rhythm is also significantly affected by the type of motion, whether active or passive.

Additionally, during arm elevation the clavicle must elevate to allow the scapula to upwardly rotate. The clavicle rotates approximately 70° in an upward fashion during arm elevation.[168] This motion occurs at approximately 90° and continues as the arm elevates. The sternoclavicular and acromioclavicular joints allow for unrestricted clavicular motion to occur. This motion is guided by the costoclavicular, coracoclavicular, and conoid ligaments.

The sternoclavicular joint is a saddle-type joint that allows 6° of freedom. Elevation occurs up to 45°, and depression occurs approximately 5° in the sagittal plane.[236] Elevation is limited and guided by the costoclavicular ligament.[42,75,100] Approximately 15° of clavicular protraction and retraction occurs in the frontal plane. The anterior sternoclavicular ligament restricts retraction, and the posterior sternoclavicular ligament prevents excessive protraction.[42,236,345] Rotation occurs through the longitudinal axis, accounting for approximately 40° of upward rotation and 10° of downward rotation.[168,236]

The acromioclavicular joint is a plane-type of joint that allows 3° of freedom. Motion at the acromioclavicular joint is significantly less than at the sternoclavicular joint, but it does play a critical role in allowing full arm motion. Inman et al.[168] suggested that the total range of motion of the acromioclavicular joint is approximately 20°. The first motion occurs through the vertical axis and allows the acromion to glide forward and backward. In the scapular plane the scapula abducts and adducts. In the coronal plane the clavicle tilts slightly both anteriorly and posteriorly. The acromioclavicular joint is stabilized by the acromioclavicular and coracoclavicular ligaments. Rockwood and Matsen[308] summarize the stabilizing effects of these ligaments by stating that horizontal stability is controlled by the acromioclavicular ligament and vertical stability by the coracoclavicular ligament. When the acromioclavicular joint is irritated, inflamed, or degenerated, motion is restricted and active movements often become extremely painful.

The glenohumeral joint is a multiaxial ball-and-socket joint that exhibits tremendous mobility but sacrifices static stability. The arthrokinematic motions that occur at the glenohumeral joint include a rotation or spin, a roll, and a glide or translation. Rotation or spin is defined as multiple points on the humerus contacting sequentially with only one point on the glenoid surface. Rolling occurs when multiple contact points on the humerus articulate with multiple points on the glenoid. Gliding or translation is defined as one humeral contact translating over multiple glenoid points.

MacConail and Basmajian[214] in 1969 developed the term roll-gliding to describe joint motion. The roll and glide component is dependent on whether the concave or convex surface is moving. The convex/concave theory of arthrokinematics states that if the convex surface is moving on the concave surface, then the glide occurs in the direction opposite of the roll. Thus during shoulder elevation, glenohumeral arthrokinematics would suggest that there is an anterior-superior roll and a posterior-inferior glide. Poppen and Walker[288] reported through radiographic analysis that during the first 30° to 60° of arm elevation the humeral head glides upward within the glenoid fossa approximately 3 mm. After this initial 3 mm rise of the humerus, the center of rotation remains constant, moving only 1 to 2 mm relative to the glenoid during the remainder of arm elevation. The authors stated that after the superior glide occurs, the humeral head will rotate or spin on a relatively fixed center with little, if any, excursion. Howell

et al.[161] also reported that the humeral head glides superiorly 3 mm during the first 30° to 45° of shoulder elevation. Harryman et al.[144,145] found an average superior displacement of the humeral head of 0.8 mm during shoulder flexion. Kelkar et al.,[187] using three-dimensional steriophotogrammetry on cadaveric shoulders, noted an average superior migration of the humeral head of 1.29 mm and approximately 1 mm of superior glide during the first 30° of motion. These authors all concluded that the initial rise (superior translation) of the humeral head was due to the starting position of the humeral head within the glenoid, which when unloaded is approximately 1 to 3 mm below the center of the glenoid (Fig. 15-8). The authors noted that initially there is a glide to center the humeral head within the glenoid, but after 30° of elevation pure rotation (spin) occurs within the glenohumeral joint.

Howell et al.[161] examined both anterior and posterior humeral head translations on normal shoulder subjects and patients with known anterior instability. They concluded that with the arm positioned in 90° of abduction, full external rotation, and maximum horizontal abduction, the humeral head translates 4 mm posteriorly in the normal shoulders. Conversely, patients with anterior instability demonstrated an anterior translation of 3 to 4 mm when placed in this position. Harryman et al.[144] also noted a posterior glide of the humerus within the glenoid during external rotation with the arm positioned at the side.

It would appear that the direction of the translation is based on the capsuloligamentous integrity. Thus in the presence of a normal shoulder capsule there appears to be an initial translation of a few millimeters to center the humeral head within the glenoid, and then a rotation or spin takes place to facilitate complete motion. To further demonstrate

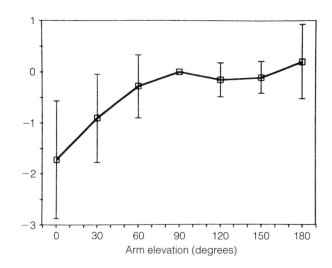

Fig. 15-8. During arm elevation in the scapular plane the humeral head glides superiorly. (From Kelkar R, Flatow EL, Biglianni LU et al: A stereophotogrammetric method to determine the kinematics of the glenohumeral joint, *Adv Bioeng* 19:143, 1992. Reproduced with permission.)

this point, Harryman et al.[144] analyzed the amount of translation of the humeral head in cadaveric shoulders. The researchers noted that the humeral head translated 3.8 mm anteriorly during shoulder flexion. The authors then tightened the posterior capsule, which significantly increased the anterior translation between 8 to 12 mm.[144] Therefore in the presence of a significantly tight capsule in one or more areas, excessive translation will result in the direction opposite that of the tightness. Hence, joint mobilization techniques can play an essential role in reestablishing full motion by improving capsuloligamentous extensibility. We would suggest the mobilization techniques and the direction of the glides are determined through the evaluation and assessment of the capsular tightness and must not be based solely on the convex-concave rule.

JOINT STABILIZATION

As previously mentioned, the humeral head maintains contact within the glenoid throughout the arc of motion and most likely translates only a few millimeters during any motion within a normal joint.[6,144,161,288] Maintenance of the humeral head within the glenoid is through a complex interaction of the active and passive stabilizers of the glenohumeral joint.

Dynamic stabilizers

There are several mechanisms in which the active or dynamic stabilizers act to improve the stability of the glenohumeral joint. We have discussed previously the muscles considered dynamic glenohumeral stabilizers, which act together in an agonist/antagonist relationship and function as components of two vital force couples to dynamically stabilize the glenohumeral joint. Force couples, by definition, are two parallel forces of equal magnitude but opposite direction applied to a structure at equal distances from the center of the mass, producing a rotation.[168] The force couples of the glenohumeral joint are the subscapularis counterbalanced by the infraspinatus/teres minor muscles acting in the transverse plane, and in the coronal plane the deltoid counterpoised by the infraspinatus/teres minor. The action of these force couples is a cocontraction that produces compression of the humeral head within the glenoid. Joint compression forces can significantly enhance joint stability. Lippett et al.[209] reported that joint compression resisted up to 60% of the transglenoid force. Bowen et al.[59] also noted joint compression significantly diminished joint displacement. It appears that the compression forces generated by the surrounding musculature appear to "center" the humeral head within the glenoid and subsequently reduce the magnitude of aberrant translations.

The second method of dynamic joint stability is provided through the blending or interlacing of the rotator cuff tendons into the shoulder capsule. Thus as the cuff muscles contract, tension is produced within the capsular ligaments, thus centering the humeral head and producing slight tension within the capsule. This concept has been referred to as dynamic ligament tension.[79] McKernan et al.[224] and Cain,[73] in cadaveric experiments, have illustrated that maximal contraction of the posterior cuff muscles reduced strain of the anterior capsule.

The third component contributing to dynamic glenohumeral stability is termed neuromuscular control.[388,392] This concept refers to the continuous interplay of afferent input and efferent output. Thus it is the individual's awareness of joint position (proprioception) and force (kinesthesia) and the ability to produce a voluntary muscular contraction that also contribute to joint stability. Recently, several investigators[351,369] have demonstrated the presence of mechanoreceptors within the capsulolabral structure, especially the inferior aspect of the capsule, which may contribute to this component of glenohumeral proprioception.

Numerous other structures such as the biceps brachii[13,276] and the scapulothoracic joint[276,373,388] also contribute to dynamic glenohumeral joint stability.

The active dynamic stabilizers play a vital role in stabilizing the glenohumeral joint. The dynamic stabilizers most likely have the greatest stabilization in mid ranges of glenohumeral joint motion, and the static stabilizers contribute most significantly at the end ranges of this motion.

Static stabilizers

Numerous structures are directly or indirectly related to static shoulder stability.

The bony geometry of the glenohumeral joint is conducive to excessive joint mobility but sacrifices static osseous stability seen at many other joints. Though the glenohumeral joint may appear grossly unstable from an osseous standpoint, the thick articular cartilage along the glenoid rim and the glenoid labrum may improve the stability somewhat. The glenoid labrum functions with the dynamic joint compression forces and the glenohumeral capsule to stabilize the humeral head within the glenoid by deepening the glenoid fossa. Additionally, the labrum serves as a "chock block" in controlling mild to moderate translation forces at the glenohumeral joint.

The glenohumeral joint capsule is relatively thin and redundant, and, to some degree, contribution to the overall stability of the glenohumeral joint is questionable.[234] The ligaments of the glenohumeral joint reinforce the capsule and significantly improve static stability.[234,272,275,353,358] The ligaments of the glenohumeral joint function to guide proper motion and act in conjunction with other structures to refrain excessive motion.

The three major ligaments of the glenohumeral joint are the anterior superior, anterior middle, and anterior inferior glenohumeral ligaments. The role the glenohumeral capsule and the ligaments play in stabilizing the glenohumeral joint is complex. The "circle stability concept" was formulated by Warren et al.[376] to pathomechanically describe the degree of tissue damage necessary for shoulder instability to occur.

Warren et al.[376] examined in the cadaveric shoulder the constraints to posterior instability. They noted that damage to both the anterior and posterior capsular structures was necessary to allow complete posterior dislocation. Recently, several investigations have validated this circle stability concept in the pathomechanics of anterior instability.[53,358] Therefore the stabilizing structures preventing the humeral head from subluxing or dislocating are located on both sides of joint, and insult to both sides must be present for complete dislocation.

The SGHL functions with the CHL, preventing inferior humeral head subluxation with the arm at the side in 0° of adduction.[372] It has also been reported that the SGHL limits external rotation at 0° of abduction.[272,353,362] Additionally, the SGHL functions with the anterior MGHL in preventing anterior humeral head subluxation with the arm at the side.[60]

The anterior MGHL has been found to prevent anterior humeral head subluxation with the arm abducted to 45° or in the mid-range of shoulder motion.[60,121,275] As mentioned previously, the MGHL assists in preventing anterior humeral head translation with the arm at the side.

The IGHLC is the thickest and possibly the most important ligament about the glenohumeral joint. O'Brien et al.[270] have demonstrated that the IGHLC is composed of three functional bands: the anterior band, axillary pouch, and posterior band. The anterior band attaches between the 2 and 4 o'clock position on the glenoid. The posterior band was found to attach between the 7 to 9 o'clock position. The axillary pouch is the redundant area of the capsule that lies between these two bands. Recently, the functional relationships between the static ligamentous structures and arm motions have been better defined. With abduction and external rotation the anterior band of the IGHLC fans out and surrounds the anteroinferior aspect of the humeral head, much as a hammock, preventing anterior subluxation. The posterior band shifts and fans out inferiorly to prevent the humeral head from subluxing inferiorly. With internal rotation and elevation, the anterior band of the IGHLC moves inferiorly to resist inferior subluxation while the posterior band shifts posterosuperiorly to prevent posterior translation. The anterior band of the IGHLC restrains anterior humeral head subluxation with the arm in 90° of abduction.[270] The tensile properties of the IGHL complex have been studied by Biglianni et al.[48] The investigators noted the anterior band of IGHLC to be consistently the thickest portion (approximately 2.79 mm).

As a general rule, the superior capsular structures play a significant role in joint stability when the arm is adducted. Conversely, the inferior structures are preeminent in joint stability from 90° abduction to full elevation. Additionally, the primary stabilizing structure of the glenohumeral joint is dependent on joint position. The ligaments of the glenohumeral joint guide motion but at end range act to prevent excessive humeral head displacement.

The CHL is located in the superior aspect of the capsule and runs from the coracoid process to the greater and lesser tuberosity. This ligament is intimately related to the supraspinatus muscle.[77] Tension placed on the CHL through arm positions such as adducted with external rotation result in strain being placed on the supraspinatus muscle. This is important to realize when rehabilitating a patient who has undergone rotator cuff repair. It has been shown that the CHL also acts with the SGHL to restrict inferior humeral head subluxation at 0° abduction while also resisting external rotation and extension.[144,272,353]

In the anatomically normal glenohumeral joint the capsule is sealed in an airtight fashion, enhancing stability. Normally, there is very little fluid present within the capsule (less than 1 ml).[222] Additionally, the normal intraarticular pressure is negative, creating a relative vacuum effect that resists glenohumeral joint translation.[67,133,198] If these properties are disrupted by a puncture or tear in the capsule that introduces air or fluid, humeral head subluxation tends to occur. Kumar et al.[198] noted that when the capsule was punctured, the humeral head tended to sublux regardless of the location of the puncture in the capsule. Several investigators have noted that venting the capsule increases humeral head translation between 45% to 65%.[133,372,404] Additionally, the synovial fluid produces an adhesion/cohesion mechanism that also enhances stability. Adhesion is described as fluid holding to a surface. Cohesion, on the other hand, is the joining of two surfaces by fluid. This adhesion/cohesion is best described by Matsen et al.[222] through the analogy of two wet microscope slides that are able to slide easily on each other but are difficult to pull apart. The glenohumeral joint mimics this concept at the contact area between the humerus and glenoid.

Basic muscle function

The deltoid muscle consists of three large heads, anterior, middle, and posterior, which act to move the arm and provide contour to the shoulder. Contraction of the deltoid muscle predominately produces arm elevation. Specifically, the middle deltoid is active in all planes of elevation,[267,287,332] whereas the anterior head produces flexion, and the posterior head assists in shoulder extension. The deltoid, functioning with the supraspinatus, has always been thought of as the force couple responsible for arm elevation. Although this motion is initiated by these two muscles, which are prime movers for arm elevation, total normal arm elevation is made possible by the stabilizing effects of the surrounding rotator cuff muscles. Both the deltoid and supraspinatus are active with arm elevation. Their specific roles, however, have been debated in the literature. Bechtol[43] has found that the absence of the deltoid causes a uniform decrease in abduction strength by approximately 50%, regardless of joint motion. Conversely, supraspinatus absence and/or rotator cuff absence allows nearly normal abduction initiation strength with a rapid dropoff in strength at elevation angles greater than 30°. Colachis et al.[85,86] have reported a 35% to 80% isometric torque deficit in shoulder flexion when the deltoid muscle is paralyzed. The deltoid, due to its line of insertion and pull on the humerus with the arm at the side, tends to cause the humeral head to migrate superiorly, producing a superior shear force. At rest, the middle and anterior deltoid angle of pull is approximately 24° to 27°; this results in a superior shear force, which the rotator cuff must attempt to negate.[287] Conversely, at 90° of abduction the line of pull of all three deltoid heads is approximately 60°, therefore changing the role of the deltoid to more of a compressive muscle than one that produces a superior shear force.[287] Hence, the deltoid functions to elevate the arm and acts as a prime mover but must work in concert with the other muscles about the glenohumeral joint for normal function. Therefore the deltoid produces significant superior shear forces at the lower angles of arm elevation but at the higher angles works as a glenohumeral joint compressor.

The supraspinatus muscle is active throughout the entire arc of elevation motion. This muscle should not be thought of as an isolated initiator of shoulder abduction.[168,169] It appears that the supraspinatus assists in elevating the arm but also acts as a stabilizing muscle to the glenohumeral joint. Colachis and Strohm,[85] after inducing a suprascapular nerve palsy, demonstrated a 30% abduction torque deficit at 0°, increasing to 65% at 30° and reducing to 35% at 150° of abduction. Thus the deltoid muscle was considered the prime abductor and the supraspinatus muscle a stabilizer and secondary abductor. In our laboratory we have noted increased electromyographic activity as the arm is abducted when performing external rotation/internal rotation movements.

The infraspinatus and teres minor muscles blend with the posterior shoulder capsule and are active throughout active elevation.[168,267] These posterior cuff muscles function as part of two vital force couples of the glenohumeral joint. Additionally, these muscles act as a barrier to posterior translation, with the combined cross-sectional area being approximately 1.74 cm².[38] Electromyographic activity of the posterior cuff muscles is greatest during scapular plane movements.[168] The author (KEW) believes that the infraspinatus is of paramount importance in rotator cuff patients, and reestablishing adequate strength is critical to dynamic humeral head stability and thus the ability to actively elevate the arm above shoulder level.

The subscapularis is a large triangular muscle that blends with the anterior shoulder capsule and has a cross-sectional area of 16.3 cm².[38] The subscapularis acts synergistically with the posterior cuff to stabilize the humeral head. It has been reported that the subscapularis is more active during abduction than in flexion, with peak activity between approximately 90° to 120°. The subscapularis is not an isolated stabilizer to anterior subluxation but rather works in concert with the other muscles about the glenohumeral joint to provide anterior stability.

The biceps brachii muscle, although predominantly an elbow flexor and forearm supinator, can assist in shoulder flexion. It also acts as a glenohumeral stabilizer.[13] Pagnani et al.[276] recently examined the stabilizing capability of the biceps brachii long head. They concluded that the biceps can reduce anterior translation when the arm is internally rotated and reduces posterior translation when the arm is externally rotated. The stabilization capability of the biceps brachii is most effective in mid-elevation ranges of motion. The biceps tendon is of notable strength, approximately four times stronger than the subscapularis tendon.[403] There is a wide variation in the size of the biceps tendon depending on the individual and location of the tendon.

The muscles of the scapulothoracic joint will be discussed later in this chapter.

EVALUATION

A thorough and systematic approach to the clinical evaluation of the shoulder complex is vital to the successful recognition of specific pathologies, their subsequent diagnosis, and effective treatment. A consistent evaluation routine ensures completeness, thoroughness, and a standardized systematic approach to the evaluation sequence. The clinical evaluation sequence utilized by the authors is illustrated in Table 5.

Before any clinical physical examination can be performed, a thorough and meticulous subjective history must be obtained. Several key facts can significantly assist in making a diagnosis. One of the first questions asked should be the patient's age and activity level. Age is important because it may suggest the type of pathology present. Most patients who are exhibiting shoulder instability will be younger than 30 years of age. Traumatic glenohumeral dislocations may occur at any age, but several studies have indicated that individuals younger than 20 and older than 50 years of age are most susceptible.[186,227,317] Conversely, rotator cuff pathologies usually occur in individuals older than 40 years of age, and rotator cuff tendinitis is commonly seen in individuals from 30 to 40 years of age.[237] Second, the patients should be asked their current and previous activity level and how their condition has affected their daily activities, work, and sports participation. Also establishing the patient's level of irritability can be helpful when designing the rehabilitation program. We routinely ask the patient how sore his or her shoulder region is and to grade the subjective response mild, moderate, or severe. This can also be performed using an analog (0 to 10) pain scale. In addition, the patient's general health, occupation, hand dominance, sports, and leisure activities should be documented. Next, we establish the patient's chief complaint (i.e., Why are you here today? When and how did the problem begin? Was the onset insidious in nature, or was there a specific traumatic event?) If a traumatic event is the cause, a thorough description of the injury mechanism should be established, with particular attention paid to the position of the arm at the time of injury. A common injury mechanism producing anterior instability occurs when the shoulder is abducted and externally rotated and is forced beyond its normal motion, producing capsular failure and resulting in an anterior dislocation. In contrast, posterior instability occurs from a force driving the humerus posteriorly, such as a fall onto an outstretched arm or while pushing an object. Often patients will convey that their symptoms are worse when a specific movement takes place, such as reaching above the head to grasp something. A thorough understanding of shoulder biomechanics can provide extremely valuable information regarding the possible pathology present.

If instability is suspected, the subjective questioning should attempt to establish the degree of instability (subluxation vs dislocation), the onset (traumatic vs atraumatic), the severity, and the primary direction of the instability (anterior, posterior, inferior, or multidirectional).

The patient should be asked what movements or activities aggravate the condition or reproduce the symptoms. Additionally, what positions alleviate the condition should also be obtained. The patient should be asked if he or she is able to sleep at night. This renders information about the degree of irritability of the shoulder but also sleeping positions tolerated.

The patient should be asked to verbalize the pain he or she is experiencing at the shoulder. This should include the location, type, intensity, and frequency of the pain. Often pain patterns at the shoulder can be misleading due to cervical spine involvement, motion compensations, secondary tendinitis, and referred pain. Commonly the levator scapulae and trapezius muscles can develop a painful trigger point or spasm. This can be related to cervical pathology such as facet or nerve root irritation, disk pathologies, or motion compensation of the scapulae to elevate the entire arm. The physical examination should differentiate these findings. Pain about the deltoid, typically laterally near the deltoid insertion, is commonly seen with several soft tissue lesions. Patients with rotator cuff tears often complain of pain in this region, within the C_5 dermatome. This referred pain pattern, explained by the cerebral and limb embryologic development, thus produces diffuse pain over the lateral aspect of the upper arm. Frequently, patients with capsular restrictions (i.e., capsular hypomobility) complain of pain over the lateral arm near the deltoid insertion. Patients exhibiting "impingement" often complain of pain over the anterolateral aspect of the shoulder directly over the biceps and supraspinatus muscles radiating inferiorly. Patients with instability often complain of pain on the opposite side of the instability. For example, patients with anterior unstable shoulders frequently complain of pain posteriorly, whereas multidirectional unstable patients frequently note diffuse muscular soreness.

The patient's pain intensity should be documented; an analog pain scale may be useful for this.[291] Pain frequency is also important to note. Night pain is quite common with shoulder dysfunctions. Patients with rotator cuff pathology often find it difficult to lie on the involved shoulder due to pain. The ability to sleep on the involved shoulder is often a sign of mild symptoms or a gradual recovery.

The ability to ascertain a meaningful subjective history should be thought of as a blend of art and science. Through a properly sequenced history the clinician should be able to formulate the pathology present, or at least begin to suspect a type of pathology. The physical examination should then be used to confirm this suspicion. The subjective history taking should be practiced thoroughly by the clinician with the goal to master the process in a meaningful, sequential, and uniform manner.

Physical examination

The physical examination is a clinical skill used to diagnose and design a rehabilitation program. During the examination the clinician's goals should be to determine a differential diagnosis, identify all involved structures, and determine the level of irritability within the shoulder complex. The sequence and proper format of a physical examination has been thoroughly discussed in Chapter 7, but the unique elements and tests specific to the shoulder will be discussed in this chapter.

The clinician should always perform a consistent evaluation to ensure completeness. Additionally, the clinician should always examine the uninvolved side first to establish a baseline or what is normal for that patient, but as the clinician's skill and experience grow, the clinician can better appreciate what is "normal" for a shoulder. The evaluation process may be frequently reordered due to patient complaints. The evaluation process must proceed from least to most provocative activity or test.

OBSERVATION

The observation of the patient must begin when the patient is walking into the evaluation area. General observation regarding upper extremity swing during gait, side-to-side shoulder height, ability to remove clothing, and in general normal movement patterns can all provide vital information regarding irritability and functional limitations of the shoulder.

INSPECTION

The inspection of the entire upper quadrant is performed next. Determining asymmetries in soft tissues and/or bony deformities is critical. The patient's shoulder complex, with scapulae and spine included, should be properly exposed. Bony prominences such as the acromioclavicular joint, sternoclavicular joint, scapulae, spine, and humeral head should be viewed for symmetry and alignment. Inspection of the soft tissues about the shoulder complex may provide valuable information and should include at a minimum the deltoid, pectoralis major, posterior rotator cuff, scapulae and arm muscles, and paraspinal musculature. The patient's posture is also extremely important to note, both in sitting and standing. Spinal alignment (such as thoracic kyphosis and forward head) directly influences shoulder girdle orientation and function.

Cervical spine screening

The cervical spine should be routinely screened with any upper quadrant involvement to rule out any primary or secondary associated pathology.[343] Active cervical motions are assessed for symmetry, amount of motion, and reproduction of symptoms. These active motions include flexion and extension, as well as both side bending and rotations. Frequently patients will report neck pain with specific motions such as extension or side bending (particularly older patients), which may be due to cervical facet degeneration. Additionally, a patient may note tightness, or a pulling with specific motions, due to soft tissue restriction. These types of symptoms must always be correlated with the patient's chief complaint. Cervical compression and traction with the head in a neutral position also may be useful in determining cervical involvement.

MOTION ASSESSMENT

The assessment of motion should include the evaluation of both physiological and accessory joint motions. The motion should be assessed to determine quantity, quality, and end feel.

Active range of motion is assessed first. This can render valuable information about the patient's condition. Active motion is utilized to determine not only quality and quantity of motion but also the patient's willingness to move the shoulder, apprehension of specific joint positions, presence of a painful arc, the location of symptoms, irritability, and scapulohumeral rhythm. We routinely ask the patient to perform four active motions: arm elevation, horizontal abduction/adduction, external rotation behind the head, and internal rotation behind the back. It should be noted the American Academy of Orthopaedic Surgeons (AAOS) no longer differentiates flexion from abduction and instead has adopted the term elevation.[9] We ask the patient whether he or she is experiencing any pain or discomfort during these movements. The location of any pain should be documented. If the patient notes pain over the acromioclavicular joint, a careful examination of that particular joint is necessary. Acromioclavicular joint degeneration is present commonly with rotator cuff pathologies. Additionally, patients with anterior instability will exhibit apprehension of movement during horizontal abduction and/or external rotation. This should be carefully noted and explored later.

Rotator cuff patients frequently describe a painful arc with active range of motion. A painful arc is pain noted during arm elevation usually between 60° to 120° of elevation.[83,96,97,102,249,253] Neer describes the painful arc as occurring during flexion when the greater tuberosity passes underneath the anterior acromion, causing impingement of the subacromial bursae and supraspinatus tendon on the acromion. Numerous factors can contribute to and produce a painful arc. These will be discussed in the rotator cuff portion of this chapter.

In addition, during active arm motion, scapulohumeral rhythm should be assessed. The scapulohumeral rhythm should be smooth and symmetrical, and the scapula should maintain congruency with the thoracic wall at all times.

Next, passive range of motion is assessed. Typically, the assessment includes forward flexion, external rotation in the place of the scapulae, as well as internal and external rotation in 90° of abduction. During passive range-of-motion assessment the clinician should attempt to determine: (1) quantity of motion, (2) type of end feel, (3) pain-resistance sequence, and (4) overall quality of motion. Cyriax[96] has described a capsular pattern as a proportionate restriction of motion due to a lesion of the capsule or synovial membrane. Cyriax[96] reported the capsular pattern of the shoulder to be "so much limitation of abduction, more limitation of lateral rotation, less limitation of medial rotation." Commonly a capsular pattern is noted in patients exhibiting adhesive capsulitis, stiff and painful shoulders, or any capsular hypomobility. Wilk and Andrews[388] have reported a characteristic pattern referred to as a "reverse capsular pattern" for patients with shoulder impingement. The reverse capsular pattern is characterized by internal rotation being restricted more than elevation and external rotation exhibiting only a mild limitation.

The end feel assessment of the shoulder joint can provide the clinician extremely vital information about the patient's condition. The "end feel" is the sensation perceived by the examiner at the end range of available motion. Cyriax[96] very eloquently describes the end feel as:

"When the examiner tests passive movements at a joint, different sensations are imparted to his hand at the extreme of the possible range. They possess great diagnostic importance."

Cyriax has noted six end feels in the human body:

1. Bone to bone
2. Spasm
3. Capsular feel
4. Springy block
5. Tissue approximation
6. Empty feel

The "normal" end feel perceived at the shoulder joint is one of a capsular feel. This consists of a "hardish" arrest of movement, with some give to it, as if you were stretching a thick piece of leather. End feels such as a spasm (muscle guarding) or empty feel can be elicited when the patient has extreme pain. A springy block may suggest intraarticular derangement such as a labral lesion. However, it should be noted that there appears to be several normal end feels with various shoulder movements. The end feel that is perceived with external rotation is different than that of shoulder flexion or the end feel of internal rotation.

The sequence of pain and end range resistance can also provide valuable patient information. Cyriax[96] states:

"the experienced physiotherapist faced with stretching a painful tissue is guided—often unconsciously—by what she feels the joint will accept."

Cyriax has noted three pain-resistance sequences:

1. Pain before resistance: suggests active lesion unsuitable for stretching
2. Pain synchronous with resistance: (capsular feel) gentle stretching may be cautiously attempted (hard feel) postpone stretching
3. Resistance before pain: strong stretching is acceptable

This sequence provides information dictating the aggressiveness of the treatment approach and should be carefully assessed.

Last, the overall quality of motion should be assessed, frequently with palpation during passive motion. We suggest palpating the SC, AC, and GH joints during passive motion to determine the degree of crepitation, ease of motion, and presence of abnormal arthrokinematics.

The assessment of accessory motions or joint play is performed next to determine the status of the noncontractile glenohumeral joint capsule. The evaluation of accessory motions assesses capsular pliability. The assessment of joint play for the glenohumeral joint is performed in the loose pack position, which is defined as 55° of abduction, and 30° forward flexion (neutral rotation).[181] In this loose pack position, the capsular structures are relaxed or placed on slack, thus allowing the greatest amount of passive joint play excursion. The glenohumeral joint accessory motions routinely assessed are anterior, posterior, inferior, and lateral (nonspecific) glides. The SC, AC, and ST joints should also be assessed for accessory motion. The SC joint accessory motion is assessed with the patient supine and relaxed. The accessory motions assessed are the dorsal, ventral, cranial, and caudal glides of the clavicle on the sternum. The same accessory motions are assessed for the acromioclavicular joint. Last, the scapulothoracic joint is assessed with the patient sidelying and the arm positioned at approximately 60° of elevation. The medial border of the scapula is grasped with both hands and glided in a lateral, medial, superior, and inferior manner. The purpose for assessing these accessory motions is to determine each joint capsule's mobility (hypomobility, normal, hypermobility) and joint play.

The author (KEW) recommends performing special tests prior to assessing resisted movements to determine the degree of joint stability prior to resisting specific motions.

The special tests included in this chapter are stability tests, impingement maneuvers, and tissue tension signs.

The assessment of glenohumeral joint stability requires the examiner to appreciate several interrelated objective components. First, the examiner must document the amount of passive translation present between the humeral head and the glenoid fossa during the examination. Second, the examiner should attempt to assess the end point to each directional stress applied. Last, the clinician should attempt to reproduce any symptoms of subluxation and/or apprehension subjectively described by placing and stressing the shoulder in provocative positions. Through an objective static stability assessment the examiner attempts to classify the type of shoulder instability according to the direction of the laxity demonstrated.

INFERIOR STABILITY ASSESSMENT

The first direction that should be assessed for instability in the shoulder patient is the inferior direction. This can be assessed through a sulcus test. This test is performed with the patient in a relaxed, seated position with arms at the side resting on the thighs, head facing forward. Next the elbow is grasped at the bicondylar axis of the humerus, and an inferior traction force is applied through the long axis of the humerus (Fig. 15-9). The space underneath the acromion is palpated to provide an impression concerning the amount of inferior humeral head translation present. If the amount of translation is greater than the contralateral shoulder, then the patient is believed to exhibit a positive "sulcus sign."[256,257] With the arm positioned at the side the primary restraint to inferior translation is the superior glenohumeral ligament and the coracohumeral ligament.[362,372] Inferior stability can also be assessed at 45° and 90° of abduction, with neutral rotation (Figs. 15-10 & 15-11). With the arm positioned at 45° of abduction the primary stabilizing structure to inferior translation is the anterior band of the IGHLC.[271] At

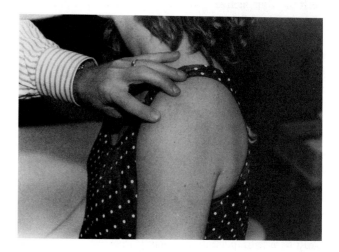

Fig. 15-9. The sulcus sign or test performed at 0° of arm abduction.

90°abduction, the primary restraint to inferior translation is the posterior band of the IGHLC.[270]

ANTERIOR STABILITY ASSESSMENT

Anterior glenohumeral joint instability is the most common instability pattern noted at the shoulder joint. The load and shift test or anterior drawer test is a commonly performed test to assess anterior stability.[54,149,150] The patient is seated with the arms relaxed and resting on his or her thigh. The examiner is behind and to the side of the patient. The examiner stabilizes the scapula with one hand while the other hand grasps the proximal humeral head (Fig. 15-12). The humeral head is then gently compressed into the glenoid to center it within the glenoid fossa, ensuring a neutral starting position. From this neutral starting position, the humerus is then pushed forward to determine the amount of anterior glenohumeral displacement. A "normal" shoulder reaches a firm end point with only slight anterior

displacement. In this position, the primary anterior restraints are the superior and middle glenohumeral ligaments.[59]

The drawer test is performed with the patient supine. In this position, the patient may be more relaxed, and the scapula is fixed by the examination table. The examiner grasps the arm at the bicondylar axis of the distal humerus and holds it in neutral humeral rotation. The patient's arm is placed in the scapular plane. The examiner's other hand grasps the humeral head, which is gently compressed, then anteriorly translated. The anterior drawer test may be performed at 0°, 45°, and 90° of abduction to individually assess the integrity of specific capsular ligaments (Fig. 15-13). The middle GHL plays a major role in limiting anterior translation in mid-range abduction.[59,121,275] As the arm is abducted to 90°, the stabilizing structures shift inferiorly and the inferior GHLC becomes the primary restraint.[270,271]

The fulcrum test is performed with the patient supine at the edge of the examination table and the arm abducted to 90°. The examiner places one hand on the posterior aspect of the glenohumeral joint to act as a fulcrum while the other hand grasps the elbow and gently extends and externally

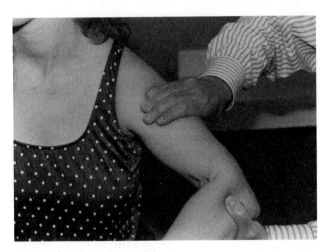

Fig. 15-10. Inferior displacement test performed at 45° of arm abduction.

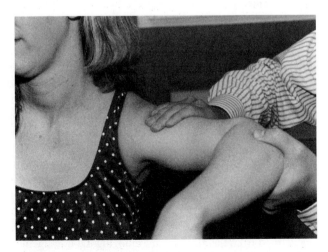

Fig. 15-11. Inferior displacement test performed at 90° of arm abduction.

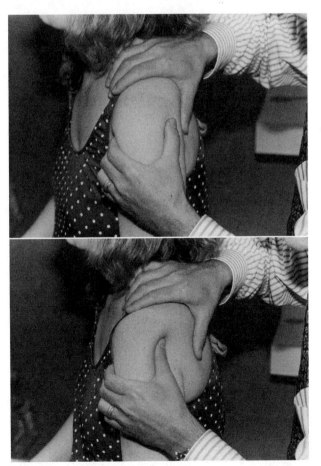

A

B

Fig. 15-12. (A) The load and shift test, starting position, **(B)** and as the humeral head is gently translated anteriorly and slightly medially.

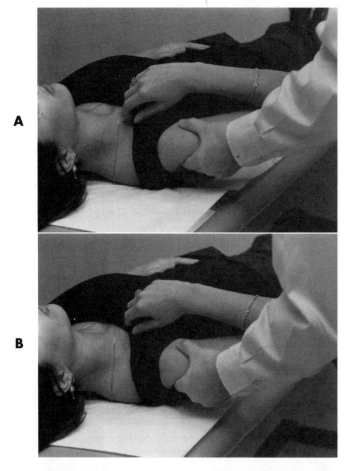

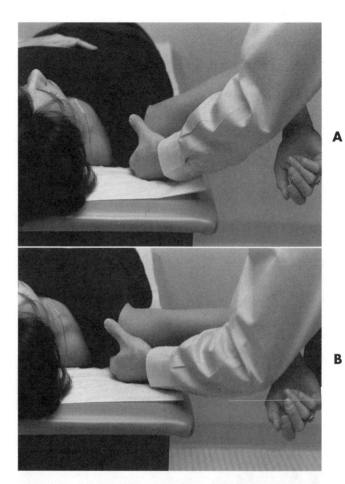

Fig. 15-13. The anterior drawer test: (**A**) starting position with the arm placed in the scapular plane (**B**) and as the humeral head is gently translated anteriorly.

Fig. 15-14. The anterior fulcrum test: (**A**) the starting position (**B**) and as the humeral head is fulcrummed over the proximal examiner's hand.

rotates the arm over this fulcrum (Fig. 15-14). In this position the anterior band of the IGHLC wraps around the anteroinferior aspect of the humeral head and acts as a hammock to prevent anterior humeral head displacement.[270] The examiner should expect to feel minimal displacement and an abrupt and hard end point in the normal shoulder. In the patient with anterior instability there will be excessive anterior displacement and a soft end feel. Additionally, the patient may become apprehensive as this test is performed.

An apprehension sign is used to reproduce the symptoms of anterior instability. The test can be performed in the seated or supine position[54,149,150] but is most commonly performed with the patient supine. The patient is positioned supine, and the examiner grasps the elbow and hand, gently abducting and externally rotating the arm. The examiner may place one hand on the posterior aspect of the humerus, pushing anteriorly for leverage. With increasing external rotation, an impending feeling of anterior instability may be produced, and an apprehensive look or protective muscular contraction may occur.

The diagnosis of anterior shoulder instability in an overhead athlete is often difficult because of the normal excessive hypermobility exhibited by these athletes. Fowler[342] and later Jobe[172,174] have advocated the use of the relocation test to determine pathological laxity in the overhead athlete. The patient is positioned supine, and the arm is abducted and externally rotated, hence in the apprehensive position, while the examiner gently pushes anteriorly on the humeral head (Fig. 15-15). If the test is positive, the patient complains of pain (not apprehension) as anterior subluxation occurs. The test is then repeated with a posteriorly directed force on the anterior aspect of the humeral head while the arm is externally rotated. This force reduces and maintains the humeral head in its normal position within the center of the glenoid fossa. If this maneuver relieves the patient's pain complaint, it is suggestive of anterior shoulder subluxation. By manually relocating the humeral head posteriorly, the supraspinatus is lifted from the glenoid rim, relieving the impingement and thus relieving all complaints of pain. It is often difficult to separate pain from true apprehension; but it can best be

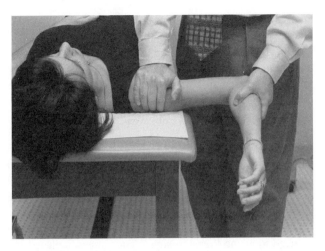

Fig. 15-15. The relocation test for anterior instability.

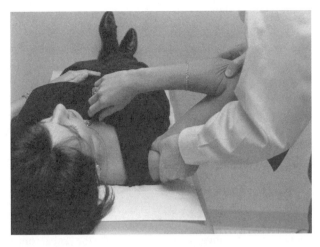

Fig. 15-16. The posterior drawer test.

recognized as pain occurs at the end of expected range as capsular tissues become maximally tense, and it may be appreciated bilaterally.

POSTERIOR STABILITY ASSESSMENT

The incidence of posterior instability is estimated at approximately 2% to 5%.[154,321] Additionally, it has been noted that the diagnosis of posterior instability is missed in approximately 60% to 79% of all cases.[281,321]

The clinical tests used to determine posterior stability are similar to those used to assess anterior stability. The posterior load and shift test is performed in the identical fashion as the anterior tests, except the translation should be redirected posteriorly (Fig. 15-12). The posterior drawer test is also performed in a similar manner, with the patient supine and the humeral head gently displaced posteriorly. The test is routinely performed at both 45° and 90° of abduction (Fig. 15-16). The primary restraints are the posterior capsule (at 45°) and the posterior band of the IGHLC at 90° of abduction.

The posterior fulcrum test is another useful test maneuver to assess posterior stability. The patient lies supine near the edge of the table. The examiner places one hand on the anterior glenohumeral joint to act as a fulcrum while the other hand grasps the elbow and gently horizontally adducts the arm (Fig. 15-17). As the arm is brought across the patient's body, the examiner gently pushes posteriorly on the anterior humerus. The test is performed in both 45° and 90° of abduction. Several other tests can be performed to determine posterior stability, including the jerk test and the push-pull test.[149,222,390]

The quantification of both the anterior and posterior translation test can be difficult to assess accurately by the clinician due to the significant joint play seen routinely at the glenohumeral joint. Grading of these tests is usually determined through a bilateral comparison. The examiner should always

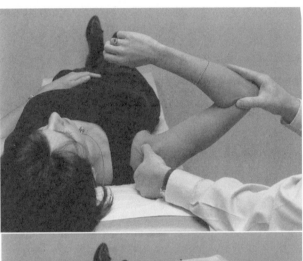

A

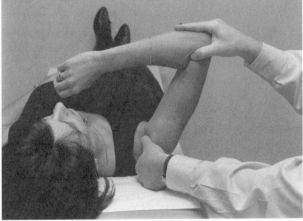

B

Fig. 15-17. The posterior fulcrum test: (A) the starting position and (B) as the arm is horizontally adducted.

assess the uninvolved shoulder first to provide a baseline assessment for that particular patient. Additionally, the examiner should assess joint end feel and symptom reproduction when performing stability tests.

Impingement sign

The impingement sign maneuver was popularized by Neer and Welsh[257] to assist in the diagnosis of rotator cuff pathologies related to impingement. The test is performed with passive arm elevation while the scapula is stabilized to minimize the upward rotation of the scapula, thus causing the supraspinatus tendon to impinge against the acromion. The test is positive if pain is elicited. Hawkins[149] has modified this test for eliciting impingement of the supraspinatus tendon against the coracoacromial ligament. In this impingement maneuver the arm is flexed to 90° and then forcibly internally rotated (Fig. 15-18). This test can be performed with the arm at various degrees of horizontal adduction. This may provide information regarding the degree of inflammation present within the subacromial bursae and supraspinatus tendon.

The "impingement test" is the patient's response to an injection of lidocaine or Marcaine (10 ml of 1%) into the subacromial bursae. Following the injection, which anesthetizes the tissues, the impingement sign is repeated. If there is a significant reduction or abolition of the patient's pain, this is a positive impingement test.[54]

BICEPS BRACHII ASSESSMENT

The biceps brachii is frequently involved with various shoulder pathologies. Palpation of the biceps brachii is possible in the bicipital groove; it often elicits a painful response. In most instances the diagnosis of biceps brachii involvement is made through palpation and the use of two or three provocative stress tests to confirm localized pathology.

The Yergason test is an extremely popular test performed for this purpose. The elbow is flexed to 90°, and the forearm is pronated. The examiner holds the patient's wrist while the patient is directed to actively supinate against the examiner's resistance. If pain is localized within the bicipital groove

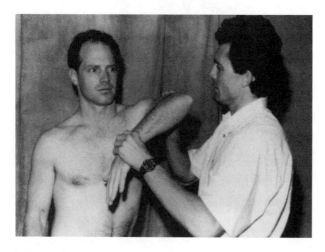

Fig. 15-18. Impingement sign; forced internal rotation at 90 degrees of arm elevation.

area, this suggests pathology of the long head of the biceps tendon within the tendon sheath.[405]

The Speed's test is performed with the elbow extended and forearm supinated. Forward flexion of the humerus is thus resisted at approximately 60°. A positive test provokes localized pain in the area of the bicipital groove.

The Ludington test is performed with the patient placing both palms on the top of the head with fingers interlocked. The patient then contracts and relaxes the biceps muscles. If pain occurs, the patient may have a biceps lesion. The examiner should palpate the biceps muscle belly during the test to determine the degree of contraction or rupture of the tendon.[212]

Another test the author (KEW) performs routinely is referred to as the "tension sign." The patient is placed in a similar position as the Speed's test, but the elbow is flexed between 30° and 45°, and full forearm supination and forward shoulder flexion is resisted from 30° to 90°. This test maneuver places significant demands on the long head of the biceps to elevate the arm. The test is positive if the action is significantly weak and painful, suggesting primary or secondary biceps tendinitis and/or a glenoid labrum lesion.

VASCULAR EXAMINATION

The vascular evaluation involves the assessment of a wide variety of clinical manifestations such as skin color, temperature, hair growth, and alterations in sensation. The assessment should include checking the radial, ulnar, brachial, axillary, and subclavian pulses. The examiner must remember that vascular compression from a thoracic outlet syndrome can result in pain at the shoulder.

The Adson maneuver is a frequently employed test to assess the vascular status of shoulder patients. The test is performed with the patient seated; the patient takes a long breath, elevates his or her chin and turns his or her head to the affected side. The examiner palpates the radial pulse for any change or obliteration. In this maneuver the subclavian artery is compressed within the interscalene space.[2] A common variation of this test is to turn the chin to the opposite side while placing the arm at 90° of abduction and externally rotating it.[54]

The Halstead's test is performed with the patient extending the neck and turning the head to the opposite shoulder, and then downward traction is placed on the involved arm.[54]

The hyperabduction test maneuver is performed with the patient seated, elbow flexed to 45°, and shoulders flexed to 90°. The arms are brought back into abduction. During this maneuver the neurovascular bundles are brought tightly under the pectoralis major muscle and the clavipectoral fascia. The examiner should be looking for any asymmetry during this test.

Another vascular test commonly performed is the provocative elevation test or overhead exertion test. The patient elevates both arms above his or her shoulders and is instructed to rapidly open and close his or her hands approximately 15 times. If fatigue, cramping, or tingling occurs in the hands or forearm, this may be suggestive of vascular insufficiency.[54]

These maneuvers previously discussed to determine neurovascular integrity when thoracic outlet syndrome is suspected are somewhat unreliable. Thus caution must be exercised when interpreting these test maneuvers. Numerous sites may cause impingement or compression of the vascular and/or neurological bundles supplying the upper extremity. These include the scalene muscles, pectoralis minor, first rib, fascia, and numerous other structures. When thoracic outlet syndrome is suspected, these tests should be performed, but assessment of each of these suspected structures should also be carried out in isolation to confirm the suspicion and identify the involved structure(s) so that proper treatment can be carried out. The validity of these clinical tests will be discussed in the thoracic outlet syndrome section of this chapter.

NEUROLOGICAL ASSESSMENT

The documentation of the patient's sensation and reflexes should be performed routinely. Sensation testing should include light touch, sharp touch, deep pressure, and thermal discrimination for all dermatome segments. In addition, reflexes must be tested for C_5 through C_7.

RESISTED MOVEMENTS

The examiner should assess the musculotendinous unit of various muscle groups about the shoulder joint to determine the integrity of the musculotendinous unit and its neurologic status and to grade overall muscle strength. The elements of performing a manual muscle test have been previously discussed in this text. Manual muscle testing should include motions to appropriately assess both the glenohumeral and scapulothoracic joints. In addition, specific muscles should be tested in isolation when possible.[98,155,189]

PALPATION

The use of skillful palpation can lend significantly to the physical examination process. Palpation of shoulder structures can be performed earlier in the evaluation, if desired; however, the authors prefer to perform the palpation late in the evaluation process so as not to provoke excessive tenderness or pain, which alters the findings of other tests. Palpation is useful only if the clinician has a thorough understanding of anatomy and biomechanics.

During palpation several elements are being assessed: (1) tenderness or pain, (2) swelling, (3) deformities, (4) muscle deformities, (5) contour changes, (6) temperature, (7) overall irritability, and (8) relationships to various structures. The assessment of various structures related to these elements is typically provided through palpation.

The sternoclavicular joint can be palpated easily. We assess clavicular motion at the SC joint routinely by palpating the joint when the patient elevates the arm completely and/or depresses the shoulder girdle.

The acromioclavicular joint is palpated during passive horizontal abduction/adduction. During these motions the distal clavicle translates slightly and places tension within the acromioclavicular capsule and may elicit pain. Acromioclavicular joint pathology is common in the rotator cuff patient.[283]

The glenohumeral joint can be assessed by the examiner placing the hand over the anterior then the posterior aspect of the shoulder as the arm is passively internally and externally rotated.

All three of these joints should be palpated during active and/or passive motions to document ease of joint movement, crepitus, pain, and arthrokinematics. In addition, increased local temperature may be present, which may suggest an inflammatory process (infection, RA, OA).

The supraspinatus tendon insertion is frequently palpated by clinicians. There are several techniques to assess this structure. One popularly utilized technique is placing the patient's arm in extension, adduction, and internal rotation. This position has been stated to completely expose the tendon.[96,361] In this position the supraspinatus tendon is located approximately 2 cm inferiorly to the anterolateral acromion. Frequently, this position is painful for some shoulder patients. Another technique to palpate the supraspinatus tendon is performed with the patient supine and the arm placed onto the table and internally rotated, so that the hand rests on the anterior superior iliac spine. In this position the clinician can palpate the supraspinatus tendon comfortably.

The biceps brachii (long head) can also be palpated in the supine or seated position. In the supine position, the patient's arm is abducted 45°, forearm supinated, and arm internally rotated 10° to 15° (this places the bicipital groove anteriorly). The biceps brachii is then palpated in the groove. To confirm the location the elbow is flexed to 90° and the arm passively internally and externally rotated; the tendon should slide underneath the examiner's fingers. The same technique can be performed with the patient seated.

Additionally, other muscles such as the infraspinatus, teres minor, teres major, pectoralis major, trapezius/rhomboids, and triceps brachii should be routinely palpated. When palpating muscle tissue, assess contour, temperature, and tone. Denervation of a muscle causes a flabby, atonic consistency. Significant atrophy may suggest chronicity of a shoulder problem.

Muscular performance testing

In some shoulder patients, a more detailed and objective muscular assessment may be necessary to document subtle bilateral deficits. This is especially true with athletes. Frequently, when assessing muscular strength through the conventional MMT technique, the involved shoulder muscles appear equal to the uninvolved. But upon iso-

Table 15-1. Isokinetic performance values in baseball pitchers

Bilateral comparisons				
Velocity degree/sec	ER	IR	ABD	ADD
180	98-105	110-120	98-105	110-125
300	85-95	105-113	96-102	110-125

Unilateral muscle ratios		
Velocity degree/sec	ER/IR	ABD/ADD
180	65-75	78-84
300	61-71	66-75

Torque to body weight ratios				
Velocity degree/sec	ER	IR	ABD	ADD
180	18-23	27-33	26-32	32-38
300	15-20	25-30	19-25	28-34

kinetic testing we have noted, as have others,[115,394] bilateral differences from 18% to 26%. Thus we routinely use isokinetic testing for our athletic patients with shoulder pathology to document muscular strength. Wilk et al.[389,393,396] have published several articles documenting the isokinetic characteristics of baseball pitchers. A summary of these data can be found in Table 15-1.

Functional performance testing

In the 1990s there has been an increasing need to document the functional status of the patient at various times in the rehabilitation process such as initial evaluation, during rehabilitation, and at discharge. By documenting functional performance the clinician can document that rehabilitation has a positive effect on the recovery. Several authors have documented various evaluation forms that can be used for documenting shoulder function.[36,120,143,318] Utilizing the information from these collective works we have modified the evaluation to include six areas to evaluate and document listed in the Box. These areas include (1) subjective pain level, (2) motion/flexibility, (3) strength, (4) static stability, (5) functional abilities, and (6) patient-perceived functional ability. Points are accumulated for each evaluation technique, with a maximum of 100 points possible. We have utilized these forms for several years and have found them extremely useful in the general orthopedic patient population in documenting outcome measurement.[385]

Summary of the examination process

The evaluation of the shoulder complex is an acquired skill that takes time and experience to master. It is the combination of art and science. The clinician must attempt to develop a sense about the patient and the shoulder they are evaluating. But the clinician must first understand the science of the shoulder, which includes the anatomy, biomechanics, and what specific tests are assessing directly or indirectly. The evaluation process should be more than location of the pain but more important, the cause of the pain and dysfunction. Therefore the treatment can be planned to treat the cause of the pain and/or dysfunction and not the symptom.

THE SCAPULOTHORACIC JOINT

The scapula plays a vital role in arm function. The scapula is positioned against the thoracic rib cage and serves to stabilize the upper extremity against the thorax. The scapulothoracic joint is a physiologic joint in that there is no true articulation; rather, the scapula is suspended on the thoracic wall by the surrounding musculature and soft tissue. Therefore the scapula must be mobile, but it also must exhibit a stabilizing role so that the glenohumeral joint has a stable base from which to function. Frequently, if not always, scapula pathology leads to glenohumeral dysfunction.

The primary functions of the scapula are to (1) provide a site of muscular attachment for scapular and glenohumeral musculature, (2) serve as an anchor or stable base from which the humerus can function, and (3) maintain a consistent and efficient length-tension relationship for the glenohumeral joint. This is accomplished through the interaction of the scapulohumeral rhythm, thus enabling the glenohumeral muscles to work efficiently.

Scapulohumeral rhythm has been discussed previously in this chapter, describing the many muscles responsible for rhythm control. The scapular muscles include the trapezius fibers (upper, middle, lower), levator scapula, rhomboids, pectoralis minor, and serratus anterior (upper and lower digitations). These muscles work in a synergistic fashion to provide a stable yet mobile base (from which the arm can function). Loss or significant weakness of any of these muscles can significantly affect scapula mobility and shoulder function.

Mobility of the scapula is produced and controlled by the scapular muscles working synergistically in a force couple relationship. One of the most significant force couples acting at the scapulothoracic joint is the trapezius counterbalance by the serratus anterior. Electromyographic activity demonstrated that during the setting phase and early shoulder elevation, the upper trapezius and levator scapulae are counterbalanced by the lower digitations of the serratus anterior. With the initiation of scapular rotation, upper trapezius continues to increase in a linear fashion as the

Functional shoulder assessment

Patient Name: _____ Chart # _____ Date: _____

Diagnosis: _____ Duration Days/Weeks Post Injury or Surgery: _____

Age: _____ Occupation: _____ Injured Shoulder: R L   Dominant Shoulder: R L

1. Subjective Pain Level (10 points)   _____

0	1	2	3	4	5	6	7	8	9	10

Emergency Room Pain	Constant Pain	Moderate Pain	Mild Pain	No Pain

2. Motion/Flexibility (20 points)   _____

Arm Elevation	170°-180°
External Rotation @ 90° Abduction	80°-90°
Internal Rotation @ 90° Abduction	75°-85°
External Rotation Scapular Plane	35°-45°
Shoulder Extension	30°-40°

Passive ROM (Maximum 10 points)   Active ROM (Maximum 10 points)

Motion Scoring
100% Motion	=	10 points
90% Motion	=	9 points
80% Motion	=	8 points
70% Motion	=	7 points
60% Motion	=	6 points
50% Motion	=	5 points
40% Motion	=	4 points

3. Strength (Maximum 21 points)   _____

Shoulder Flexion
Shoulder Abduction
External Rotation
Internal Rotation
Supraspinatus (Empty Can)
Biceps Brachii (Elbow Flexion)
Shoulder Extension

Muscle Scoring
5/5	=	3 points
4/5	=	2 points
3/5	=	1 point
2/5	=	0 points

4. Stability Testing (Maximum 9 points)   _____

• Sulcus Sign (Inferior)
• Anterior Drawer
• Posterior Drawer
• Apprehension Sign

Stability Scoring
0	=	Severe instability
1	=	Moderate instability
2	=	Mild instability
3	=	Normal

5. Functional Abilities (Maximum 30 points)   _____

• Reaching into back pocket
• Reaching to opposite axilla
• Reaching behind head and neck
• Reaching overhead
• Dressing
• Lying on involved side
• Use in perineal care
• Reach out at shoulder level
• Ability to lift 1-2 lbs to shoulder height and out
• Carrying object (10-15 lbs)

Scoring
3	=	Normal
2	=	Mild compromise
1	=	Difficulty
0	=	Unable

6. Perceived Functional Ability (maximum 10 points)   _____

0 ←————————————————→ 100
Unable to use   Perfect
arm and shoulder   Shoulder

Perceived Functional Ability Scoring:	Place decimal point one place to left; example 75 score = 7.5 points

Total Score: _____

scapula rotates superiorly.[168] The axis of rotation is located near the superior medial scapular angle. As the arm elevates and the scapula upwardly rotates, the muscular activity of the lower trapezius increases significantly. The electromyographic activity of the lower trapezius doubles from 70° to 120° of abduction and increases significantly from 120° to 150° of abduction. As elevation progresses past approximately 70°, the primary scapular force couple moves inferiorly to the lower trapezius counterposed by the upper serratus anterior. The axis of rotation now occurs near the acromioclavicular joint. The rhomboids/middle trapezius act with the serratus anterior to also stabilize the scapula on the thoracic cage. The middle trapezius and rhomboids serve to fix the scapula within the plane of motion during abduction but are not as active during flexion.[168] Recognition of scapula dyskinesias is vital to normal shoulder function.

Therefore the scapula rotates approximately 30° about its first axis; thus the inferior angle of the scapula moves outward along the thoracic wall, and the glenoid is positioned slightly superiorly. From about 30° to 45° of upward rotation, tension is generated within the costoclavicular and coracoacromial ligaments, which produces conjunct posterior rotation of the clavicle. This clavicular rotation allows the scapula to upwardly rotate, transferring the center of rotation superiorly.

When evaluating the scapula, the clinician should evaluate the scapulohumeral rhythm during both active and passive arm motions. The clinician is evaluating for asymetries, abnormal scapulohumeral rhythms, the inability to stabilize the scapula, and lack of motion. In an attempt to objectively measure and document scapula dynamic stability, Kibler[193] advocated the use of a lateral scapulae slide test. In this test the patient's T_7 spinous process is located and marked, and the inferior angle of scapula is also marked. The subject is then asked to place his or her arms at his or her side, followed by hands on hips in full internal rotation, and last, abduction to 90° and internally rotated. In each of these three positions the distance from the T_7 spinous process to the inferior angle of the scapula is measured. Kibler[193] reported that subjects with an asymmetry of more than 1 cm demonstrated a positive correlation to impingement complaints. Davies and Hoffman-Dickoff[99] have also advocated a similar test, except these authors suggested documenting the lateral scapular slide in five different arm positions (0°, 45°, 90°, 120°, 150° of abduction).

The evaluation of the scapulothoracic joint should include both active and resistive motion assessments. The scapulohumeral rhythm should be assessed with the patient actively elevating the arm. Additionally, scapulohumeral rhythm should be assessed with resistance applied to the arm during elevation. This can be done with manual resistance, a light hand weight, or with exercise tubing. By applying resistance, the scapula should stabilize more rapidly during the motion so that the contribution to humeral head elevation occurs earlier in the range.[111] This is a valuable clinical tool to illustrate insufficient scapular stabilization. Also, the clinician should be aware that there are differences in scapulohumeral rhythms between genders, morphologic compositions, and various pathologic conditions.

As previously discussed, the scapular muscles contribute greatly to the overall function of the shoulder complex. Paralysis of the serratus anterior results in significant functional impairment, with significant weakness and an altered movement pattern when attempting to flex or abduct the arm.

A rehabilitation program to restore or enhance the scapular stabilizers is critical to the total success of all shoulder patients. Recently, Mosely et al.[241] performed an electromyographic study analyzing specific exercises used for strengthening the scapular muscles. In this study the investigators analyzed the rhomboids, serratus anterior, pectoralis minor, levator scapulae, and upper, middle, and lower trapezius muscles. Each subject performed 16 different exercises.

In addition to these exercises, we have noted several exercise movements that are extremely beneficial in enhancing scapular stabilization. If scapular passive mobility is limited, soft tissue mobilization, scapular mobilization, and stretching may be utilized in appropriate combination to restore full, unrestricted mobility.

Scapular injuries and pathologies occur but are somewhat unusual. Fractures of the scapula occur infrequently, accounting for approximately 3% of all shoulder girdle injuries.[142,316] Scapular fractures are classified and described by anatomical area and can occur at the glenoid neck, scapular body, acromion, and coracoid. Butters[70] has thoroughly described and discussed these fractures, and the reader is encouraged to read this chapter for further information.

Another scapular pathology occasionally seen is a condition known as os acromiale. This condition represents a failure of the adjacent ossification centers of the acromion to coalesce and clinically appears as an acromial fracture. The unfused apophysis is present in 2.7% of patients and when present has a bilateral incidence of 60%.[206] Several investigators have noted an association between os acromiale and rotator cuff tears.[47,242,250,266] For further information regarding os acromiale the reader is recommended to the following resources.[47,70,242,250,266]

Two other conditions, closely related, are snapping scapula and scapulothoracic bursitis. Snapping scapula is a condition that presents when an osseous or osteocartilaginous lesion, arising from either the anterior scapula or posterior thorax, moves against the opposite surface.[229,230] Thus, instead of a smooth gliding of the scapula on the thorax, coarse crepitus and pain occurs in the periscapular region. Although scapular noises are not uncommon in the normal population, in snapping scapula the noise is louder, coarse, painful, and restricts function. Published articles discussing this condition are limited; however, several are listed as references for further information.[223,229-231]

Scapulothoracic bursitis is closely related to snapping scapula and is often misleading. Milch[229] differentiated between patients of these conditions as the following: scapular snapping is the result of an osseous or osteocartilaginous lesion involving the scapulothoracic interval; conversely, scapular crepitus occurs secondary to bursa inflammation due to overuse or local trauma. There are three bursae located in the periscapular region. These include the bursa mucosa angulae superiosis scapulae, located in the superior lateral scapula, second is the bursa mucosa serrata, which is located between the serratus anterior and lateral chest wall, and the third is located at the inferior scapular angle.[223] Treatment for scapulothoracic bursitis includes local injections, nonsteroidal antiinflammatories, modification of activities, light strengthening exercise, and motion. If nonoperative treatment fails, surgical removal of the bursae may be necessary but is considered rare. For additional literature regarding scapulothoracic bursitis, several authors describe the pathology and its treatment at length.[21,74,223,302]

Other scapula-related conditions such as serratus anterior paralysis,[156,202] trapezius paralysis,[112,347] and levator scapulae tendinitis[40] were not discussed due to length restrictions. The reader is encouraged to review the references listed for additional information concerning these pathologies.

ACROMIOCLAVICULAR JOINT INJURIES

The acromioclavicular (AC) joint is a frequent site of injury and/or pain in the shoulder patient. Injuries to the AC joint may occur indirectly due to degeneration or as the result of a direct traumatic injury. The AC joint is a joint that commonly exhibits rapid degeneration and is a site of osteoarthritis, which may retard the progress of the rotator cuff patient. The most common mechanism of injury is due to a direct force to the AC joint and is caused by a direct fall onto the point of the shoulder (the lateral acromion) with the arm at the side in an adducted position. This mechanism of injury is common in specific sports such as football and wrestling. Additionally, this type of macrotraumatic injury may also occur at the work place. The result of the downward force on the acromion is a driving of the acromion downward behind the clavicle.[308] In this scenario the clavicle may fracture, or the AC joint may become injured. As the force is imparted onto the joint, the acromioclavicular ligaments are first stretched (mild sprain); then as the force continues, the acromioclavicular ligaments tear, and the coracoclavicular ligaments are stretched (moderate sprain). As the downward force continues, the coracoclavicular ligaments tear along with the muscle attachments of the deltoid and trapezius muscles, resulting in a severe AC joint sprain (complete dislocation).[308]

Injuries to the acromioclavicular joint are classified according to the amount of tissue involvement created by the applied force. Several classification systems have been published.[5,309,357] Rockwood and Matsen[308] have identified six types of AC joint sprains.

Dislocations of the AC joint account for approximately 12% of all shoulder dislocations.[308] Incomplete injuries to the AC joint are two to three times more common than complete dislocations, and males tend to be injured at a 5:1 to 10:1 ratio when compared with females.

Patients presenting with AC sprains commonly complain of pain, tenderness, swelling, and possible deformity. Swelling, although minimal in a type I sprain, is more prominent in a type II or III sprain, often making palpation of the clavicle difficult. In type III AC joint injuries, significant pain and swelling are evident with a significant prominence of the distal clavicle. The patient typically presents with the upper extremity adducted close to the body and held upward by the other arm to relieve the traction discomfort at the AC joint. Type II injuries may be associated with an increase in anterior-posterior instability. This may be demonstrated by grasping the distal clavicle and gently displacing it anteriorly and posteriorly. In type III to IV injuries, the coracoclavicular ligaments are injured in addition to the acromioclavicular ligaments. This results in additional vertical instability (superior-inferior). This may be demonstrated by applying a superiorly directed force at the distal humerus (through the elbow joint), which reduces the acromion to the clavicle. Injury to the coracoclavicular ligaments causes an inferior displacement of the arm and shoulder rather than a superior displacement of the clavicle.

The diagnosis of AC joint sprains is usually made through the subjective history (description of injury), physical examination, and routine radiographs. Routine bilateral anteroposterior views are utilized with the patient's arms hanging unsupported. A comparison is made between the involved side and the uninvolved side, inspecting the amount of acromioclavicular joint separation. An axillary view may be used to demonstrate any posterior displacement of the injured clavicle, as seen in a type IV sprain. In patients in whom it is difficult to differentiate a type II from a type III injury, stress films of both shoulders may be helpful. These AP views are taken with 10- to 15-pound weights suspended from each wrist.[308] These stress films test the integrity of the coracoclavicular ligaments. A difference of 25% or greater, when comparing injured with uninjured shoulder, confirms the diagnosis of a complete separation.

Management of acute AC joint injuries depends greatly on the severity of the injury and type of patient (activity level) injured. Most authors agree on nonoperative treatment of type I and II sprains. Type IV, V, and VI injuries often require open reduction and internal fixation. Treatment of type III AC separations is extremely controversial.[56,290] In most cases nonoperative treatment will yield a good functional result.[167] Operative repair for type III separations may be indicated in patients who are involved in heavy manual labor[310,311] or in select contact sports athletes.[11]

The treatment for type I AC separations consists of a sling for comfort for several days, modalities such as ice to control pain and inflammation, and active assisted range-of-motion exercises. Additionally, the patient is initiated on isometric strengthening and progresses to isotonics and normal activities when the symptoms allow.

The nonoperative treatment of type II injuries includes some type of additional support to the AC joint. Many authors have advocated the use of a sling[147]; others have recommended adhesive tape strappings,[296] harnesses,[44] or even a sling harness immobilizing device.[5] The use of these types of immobilization devices has been advocated for 3 to 6 weeks. Heavy weightlifting activities and contact sports should be avoided for approximately 8 to 12 weeks, until the ligaments have healed. Although nonoperative treatment of type I and II injuries has been recommended, reports from Bergfeld et al.[44] and Cox[94] suggest that these injuries may lead to symptomatic problems later.

The management of type III injuries has created much controversy in the orthopedic literature. Numerous authors have recommended a nonoperative approach.* Many experts agree a simple sling is adequate for rest and comfort for approximately 7 to 21 days following the injury. The use of a harness to reduce the dislocation may be beneficial, but it must be worn continuously for approximately 6 weeks. Gentle active assisted range-of-motion exercises and isometric strengthening are performed once the symptoms begin to abate. Isotonic strengthening exercises can usually be initiated at 4 weeks, and from this point a gradual strengthening program is advanced as tolerated. Numerous investigators have documented 90% to 100% satisfactory results with nonoperative treatment of type III AC joint injuries.[51,107] In addition, studies comparing operative and nonoperative treatment of these type III injuries have also supported the nonoperative treatment approach.[32,129,201]

The surgical treatment for acute complete AC joint injuries include these options: acromioclavicular repair, coracoclavicular repair, or dynamic muscle transfer. A distal clavicle resection (Mumford procedure) is usually confined to chronic AC joint dysfunction.[243,308]

Primary acromioclavicular joint repair is a commonly performed procedure that utilizes a small, smooth, or threaded Steinmann pin. With the pin in place most authors recommend motion below 40° of elevation and gentle isometrics.[308] Once the pins have been removed (6 to 8 weeks), the rehabilitation program may be accelerated and advanced as tolerated.

Primary coracoclavicular ligament fixation can be performed using screw fixation. Several authors have reported successful results with this type of surgery.† The use of stainless steel wires[4,41] and Dacron grafts[183,279] has been advocated by several authors. In these techniques the wire or graft is looped around the coracoid process and the distal clavicle. The rehabilitation program following the stainless steel wires and synthetic grafts is much more accelerated. A sling may be used for comfort during the first several days

*References 32, 107, 129, 134, 147, 201.
†References 33, 56, 190, 192, 310, 311, 367.

following surgery. Immediate motion is utilized; full range of motion should be present in 10 to 21 days. Isometric strengthening is employed immediately and progressed to isotonics as motion and symptoms permit. Usually, the patient can return to heavy lifting or sports approximately 8 to 12 weeks after surgery. Comparisons of the acromioclavicular and coracoclavicular operative repairs have been reported in the literature and can be reviewed in the references.[34,200,349]

The use of a dynamic muscle transfer has also been advocated in the literature.[25,45,106] In this technique the coracoid process is osteomized with its muscular attachments of the biceps and coracobrachialis and is fixated to the clavicle with a screw.

The acromioclavicular joint is one joint that demonstrates early degenerative changes; thus osteoarthritis of the AC joint is not uncommon. Osteophyte proliferation is often present with spur development along the inferior aspect of the joint.[285] This may compromise the supraspinatus outlet, causing impingement. Often the degenerative changes seen are due, in part, to a previous traumatic injury. Patients can complain of localized pain at the AC joint, pain with motion, and pain upon direct palpation. Radiographs will often demonstrate AC joint narrowing and degenerative changes. Treatment of this pathology depends on the patient's symptoms. Nonoperative treatment consisting of physical therapy, activity modification, and antiinflammatory medications is the treatment of choice. A long-acting corticosteroid injection into the joint can significantly reduce the pain and inflammation. If conservative treatment fails, the surgeon may choose to excise the distal 2 cm of the clavicle either arthroscopically or through an open incision.[243] In athletes, the Mumford procedure has been shown to be extremely successful in returning full painless function for those with type I and II injuries.[88]

Acromioclavicular joint pathology is common in the general orthopedic and sports medicine shoulder patient. The acromioclavicular joint should always be carefully examined as part of a routine shoulder examination.

INSTABILITY

Instability of the glenohumeral joint is an extremely common condition encountered by clinicians in an orthopedic and sports medicine setting. The glenohumeral joint is the most commonly dislocated joint in the human body.[75] The glenohumeral joint exhibits the greatest amount of motion of any joint in the human body. Because the joint capsule must be loose enough to allow this motion, it is often difficult to determine the normal amount of capsular and physiologic laxity. This paradox contributes to the wide variety of "instabilities" seen at the shoulder joint.

The term "shoulder instability" is a vague and nonspecific term that represents a wide spectrum of shoulder joint conditions. This spectrum ranges from gross instability to subtle subluxation. To further understand shoulder instability, we must first understand the definitions of some common terms. A shoulder dislocation is a complete separation of the articular surfaces that do not spontaneously reduce. Thus someone else, or a special movement, must be utilized to reduce the dislocated joint. Shoulder subluxation is a condition where there is a complete separation of the articular surfaces with a spontaneous reduction; thus the subluxation is transient. Subluxation may or may not be associated with pain, apprehension, or disability.[375] The force required to dislocate the shoulder depends on previous injuries, patients' ligamentous laxity, and the forces involved in injury.[271]

The concept of shoulder joint laxity and shoulder instability is also important to fully understand. Matsen[218] describes shoulder laxity as the ability of the humeral head to be passively translated on the glenoid fossa. Conversely, shoulder instability is a clinical condition in which unwanted translation of the humeral head on the glenoid compromises the *comfort* and *function* of the shoulder.[218] Thus laxity is what is felt on clinical examination and instability is a condition the patient experiences that restricts normal function.

The classification of shoulder instability attempts to explain the type of instability the patient is experiencing. The classification may be based on five factors: onset, degree, frequency, volition, and direction.

The onset of the instability can be extremely important to document. Traumatic onsets, either dislocations or subluxations, usually cause tissue trauma and damage. The shoulder can be dislocated by direct trauma, such as a force directed to the proximal humerus or due to an indirect force. When the arm is forced into extreme external rotation, the shoulder is abducted and extended, commonly resulting in anterior dislocation. The mechanism of injury is important to document and should include arm position, amount of force applied, and the point of force application. Thus the amount of trauma is important to note. A violent injury such as a fall onto an arm that is fixed in abduction and external rotation and is forced in greater external rotation, often results in a Bankart lesion.[282] A Bankart lesion is the detachment of the capsulolabral complex from the glenoid. The incidence of Bankart lesions in traumatic anterior dislocations is *approximately* 87% in the *average population* and is a common cause for recurrent instability.[29,315] However, a recent study by Wheeler et al.[380] and Arciero et al.[19] has reported an incidence of Bankart lesions of 97% in young active cadet-athletes at the U.S. Military Academy. Conversely, an atraumatic onset can occur with everyday activities such as work or activities of daily living, during which the patient feels shoulder discomfort and dysfunction due to the shoulder slipping in and out of the joint. An onset contributed to overuse is common in sports medicine. As the athletic patient participates in strenuous shoulder activities and the shoulder muscles fatigue, a temporary loss of dynamic stability results in the patient experiencing transient shoulder instability. Several authors[87,103,310] have documented the

importance of distinguishing between traumatic and atraumatic instability of the shoulder. This distinction is critical in the treatment approach, whether nonoperative or operative.

The degree of instability is also important and includes the difference between dislocations and subluxations. The rate of recurrent dislocations is extremely high (80% to 95%) in younger patients, especially young athletic patients.[153,228,314] The term "silent subluxators" was originally described by Jobe[173] to describe the pathophysiology of shoulder pain in the overhead athlete. The subtle subluxation experienced by the overhead thrower leads to the shoulder capsule becoming sore and inflamed, related to the increased humeral head displacement during activity.

The frequency of the instability renders information about the nature of the instability. Acute instability usually presents with a recent episode of either a subluxation or dislocation. Acute usually refers to the first couple of days following the injury occurrence. Following an acute episode, most patients exhibit significant muscular spasm, guarded motion, and their arm is held "splinted" at the side. Recurrent instability is used to describe instability on multiple occasions. Recurrent instability may consist of repeated glenohumeral dislocations, subluxations, or both. Unfortunately, the rate of recurrent dislocations is extremely high and approaches 80% to 95% in younger patients, especially young athletic patients.[19,29,153,228,314,380] The rate of recurrent dislocation in patients older than 40 years of age is 10% to 15%. With recurrent anterior instability a Hill-Sachs lesion may develop. This is an impaction fracture of the posterolateral aspect of the humeral head and develops as the humeral head compresses against the anterior glenoid rim as it subluxates anteriorly. A dislocation is locked (or fixed) if the humeral head has been locked on an edge of the glenoid, making reduction of the dislocation difficult.

The clinician should routinely ask the patient whether he or she can subluxate the shoulder voluntarily. If the patient can subluxate the shoulder voluntarily, the classification of voluntary instability can be easily determined. The patient with voluntary instability usually has no history of injury (atraumatic history), unstable in multiple directions, and surgical stabilization is often difficult. Patients unable to voluntarily sublux the shoulder are considered to have involuntary instability.

One of the most common classifications of shoulder instability is based on the direction of the instability. Anterior instability is the most common type of instability, accounting for approximately 95% of all shoulder instabilities. The most common type of anterior dislocation is a subcoracoid dislocation, when the humeral head is anterior to the glenoid and inferior to the coracoid process. The second most common instability is the subglenoid dislocation, when the humeral head is below and anterior to the glenoid fossa.[219] Other types of instabilities are more rare. Posterior dislocations may occur but are infrequent, accounting for approximately 4% to 5% of shoulder dislocations.[52,328] Multidirectional instability (MDI) can be defined as shoulder instability occurring in more than one plane of motion. Neer and Foster[256] first described MDI in 1980. They described and classified patients into one of three MDI groups: anteroinferior with posterior subluxation, anteroinferior with anterior subluxation, or global (equally loose in all three directions). Patients with MDI are generally atraumatic in nature and exhibit excessive ligamentous laxity, which results in recurrent subluxations.

Thus patients are often classified as either traumatic or atraumatic in the onset of their instability. Matsen[219] has classified instability based on several factors. He has described the classification with two acronyms, TUBS (traumatic, unidirectional, Bankart lesion, requiring surgery) and AMBRI (atraumatic, multidirectional instability, bilateral shoulders, rehabilitation, inferior capsular shift).[219] This classification scheme may be beneficial to the clinician when designing an appropriate treatment approach.

What is the importance of classifying the shoulder instability and the relevance to rehabilitation? Burkhead and Rockwood[69] have documented the rate of success of nonoperative treatment for traumatic and atraumatic shoulder instability. The success in the atraumatic shoulder patients was noted as 80% or better, whereas the traumatic shoulder patients had a 16% success rate for a full unrestricted return to symptom-free activity.

Following shoulder dislocation, the patient presents to the clinician in obvious painful distress. Following the typical anterior dislocation, the shoulder is held in an adducted and internally rotated position. By holding the arm close to the side the patient feels more comfortable. Immediately following an acute dislocation, the patient experiences significant pain, muscular spasms, and acute inflammation.

Acute dislocations should be reduced as quickly and safely as possible to prevent injury to the neurovascular structures, minimize muscular spasms, and improve patient comfort. Plain radiographs should be taken prior to the reduction to ensure that a fracture has not occurred. Additionally, plain radiographs are required following the reduction to confirm the relocation of the joint and to rule out any possible fractures.

The patient usually exhibits a marked loss of motion, especially abduction and external rotation in the case of the anterior dislocation. Horizontal adduction is often painful and limited in the case of the posterior dislocation. The patient exhibits apprehension to specific motions and exhibits muscular spasms, significant weakness, and diffuse soreness. A thorough neurologic examination should be performed to clear the axillary nerve and/or humeral circumflex artery. Specific stability tests such as the load and shift, drawer tests, and sulcus sign should be gently performed to document the degree of instability. Plain radiographs may be beneficial in assessing the direction of the instability, glenoid rim, humeral head defects, and/or fractures. The use of computed tomography (CT) scans and magnetic resonance imaging (MRI) may be helpful in documenting glenoid labrum and/or capsular integrity (Bankart lesion).

The nonoperative treatment of a patient following a shoulder dislocation is to be immobilized in adduction and internal rotation. The ideal period of immobilization is somewhat controversial. A longer period of immobilization is advocated for younger patients (younger than 20 years) compared with older patients (older than 40 years) because of the higher rate of dislocation recurrence in the younger individual. Thus some physicians recommend that the younger patient be immobilized for a period of 4 to 6 weeks and that the older patient be immobilized only 2 to 3 weeks. The theory behind immobilization following dislocation is to allow capsular healing. This concept has come under serious scrutiny in the past several years. Several authors have reported that the length and type of immobilization has little to no effect on the incidence of recurrent instability.[114,158,227,320] Thus for the past several years we have advocated a sling for immobilization during functional activities but the use of immediate guarded motion to minimize the patient's pain and discomfort.

The type and length of the rehabilitation program employed is dependent upon several factors: (1) severity of injury, (2) stage of condition, (3) patient's age, (4) type of instability, (5) status of dynamic stabilizers, and (6) the level of activity to which the patient plans to return. The program is based on a four-phased approach.

In the first phase, the acute phase, the goals are to reestablish full motion, retard muscular atrophy, diminish pain/inflammation, and allow capsular healing. Emphasis is directed toward the gradual restoration of motion. The performance of AAROM exercises using an L-bar can be beneficial in gradually reestablishing full motion. Initially, the internal rotation/external rotation exercises are performed in the scapular plane, then gradually progressed to 60° and then 90° of abduction as pain subsides. Submaximal, pain-free, multiangle isometrics are also immediately initiated for all major shoulder muscle groups. The author believes that early initiation of isometrics is critical in reestablishing humeral head dynamic stability and preventing/minimizing rotator cuff shutdown/inhibition and atrophy. In addition, joint mobilization, ice, and high-voltage galvanic stimulation can all be beneficial in diminishing inflammation and pain.

In the second phase the program emphasis is placed on dynamic stabilization exercise drills to enhance the dynamic stability of the glenohumeral joint. Exercises that produce a cocontraction such as rhythmic stabilization PNF (proprioaptive neuromuscular facilitation) drills are extremely beneficial. Isotonic strengthening for the rotator cuff, scapular muscles, and surrounding shoulder muscles is also valuable in the rehabilitation process.

The third phase, the advanced strengthening phase, is

geared toward improving the neuromuscular control of the shoulder joint, especially in the apprehension position. In athletes, the patient will exercise internal rotation/external rotation at 90° of abduction. In addition, plyometric contractions are performed to teach dynamic control of the glenohumeral joint.[397] The progression of these drills is from an adducted position gradually progressing to 45° and then 90° of abduction. In the general orthopedic patient, these exercise drills are not emphasized; rather, the patient is placed on a gradual progressive exercise program.

The final phase of the rehabilitation program is the return to activity phase. It is designed to gradually and progressively return the athlete to unrestricted symptom-free work or sport participation. The patient must continue a strengthening program to maintain dynamic stability. Occasionally, the athletic patient involved in contact sports may be required to wear a brace that restricts abduction and external rotation, which may prevent recurrent instability.[197]

The conservative treatment of a patient with atraumatic multidirectional instability is somewhat different from that of traumatic unidirectional instability. The initial treatment is focused on improving the efficiency and effectiveness of the force couples about the glenohumeral joint. Exercises that have been proven beneficial are rhythmic stabilization techniques, cocontraction exercise drills, closed kinetic chain exercises, and neuromuscular control drills. The primary and essential goal of this program is the dynamic stabilization of the humeral head due to collagen elasticity of the glenohumeral joint capsule.

Surgical approach to instability

There are and have been numerous shoulder surgical stabilization procedures throughout the years. The type of surgical stabilization procedure performed is based on the type of instability exhibited by the patient.

Historical overview

Documentation of early treatments of shoulder dislocations dates back to the time of Hippocrates, who first described a burning treatment to the anterior aspect of the shoulder, followed by prolonged immobilization. Although treatment of shoulder instability has evolved considerably, the basic principle of creating scar tissue anteriorly to prevent further dislocations may hold true for many current treatment options. The most common type of shoulder instability is an anterior dislocation of the shoulder joint. In 1923 Bankart[30] introduced the concept that the essential lesion in a glenohumeral dislocation was a detachment or rupture of the capsule from the glenoid ligament. A few years later, Bankart[31] went on to describe the essential lesion as a detachment of the glenoid ligament from the anterior margin of the glenoid cavity, and he recommended repair of the lateral capsule back down to the bone of the anterior glenoid with sutures placed through the glenoid rim.

Surgical stabilization of the glenohumeral joint is indi-cated in patients who experience recurrent instability despite a trial of rehabilitation. Many different surgical procedures have been described for the treatment of recurrent instability. These include tightening of the subscapularis tendon, directly reattaching the capsule and glenoid labrum to the glenoid, augmentation of the bony anterior glenoid rim with a bone transfer, or treatment of a posterolateral humeral head defect by either rotational osteotomy or filling of the defect.

More recently, the advantages of anatomical repair or restoration of the normal anatomical structures of the shoulder joint have been recognized. With an anatomic repair the subscapularis tendon is not shortened, and it is easier for the patient to regain external rotation. Surgical stabilization of the shoulder joint involves a balance between correcting the instability and maintaining a functional range of motion.

Bankart procedure

Although this repair is called the Bankart procedure, it was apparently first introduced by Perthes[282] in 1906. He recommended repair of the anterior capsule to the anterior glenoid rim. The procedure, however, was first described by Bankart[31] in 1939, as mentioned previously. He reported on 27 consecutive cases and noted that there had been no recurrence of dislocation and that a full movement of the joint had been achieved following surgery.[31] In 1979 Hovelius et al.[159] compared the results between performing a Bankart and Putti-Platt operation. They found a 19% redislocation rate after the Putti-Platt compared with a 2% redislocation rate after the Bankart procedure. More than one third of the patients who were younger than 25 years of age were unhappy with the results of the Putti-Platt procedure. This was followed 2 years later by a report from Rowe and Zarins[322] that reported on a series of 15 subluxating shoulders with 94% good or excellent results after Bankart repair. In 1978 Rowe et al.[319] reported on a series of 145 patients who underwent a Bankart repair with only a 3.5% recurrence rate of instability, and 69% of the patients had regained their full range of motion.

The primary advantage of the Bankart procedure is that it restores the normal anatomy of the shoulder joint. By repairing the detached labrum, a potential pocket of tissue for the humeral head to slip into is removed. The size of the labrum in patients varies greatly, and it may be simply a detachment of the capsule off the anterior glenoid versus detachment of a discrete labral structure. Arthroscopic examination of the shoulder has resulted in better definition in the difference in the size and type of Bankart lesions.

The disadvantage of the Bankart procedure is that if a Bankart lesion is present, a capsular-shift procedure may be indicated. The incision that is made for a Bankart procedure may limit the approaches to a capsular shift, if it is not carefully planned. This can be avoided by determining the presence of a Bankart lesion prior to opening the capsule with an initial arthroscopic examination of the shoulder.

When a Bankart lesion is present, the Bankart-type repair is the procedure of choice to correct anterior instability of the shoulder. If the labrum is not detached from the glenoid and the anterior instability is a result of anterior capsule laxity, then a capsular shift procedure is indicated, and the anterior capsular incision is planned accordingly.

Overview-Bankart procedure

An anterior approach to the shoulder is typically used. This consists of approximately a 3-in incision made in the skin fold just above the axilla. In some cases an incision can be made in the axial crease and then the skin mobilized superiorly to create a more cosmetic incision. Careful layer-by-layer dissection occurs with some muscular and tendon splitting or releasing depending on the surgeon's preference. Care is then taken to protect nerve tissue as exposure to the Bankart lesion is obtained. In order to gain access to the glenohumeral joint, the subscapularis tendon and capsule need to be incised. The upper border of the subscapularis tendon can be defined as the rotator cuff interval, which is the potential opening of the joint between the supraspinatus and the subscapularis tendons. A defect in this interval itself has also been cited as a potential source of anterior instability.[122] Multiple techniques of accessing the actual joint through the subscapularis tendon have been described.[171,211,219] More recently, Andrews and Satterwhite[17] have reported on an approach to the Bankart lesion in which the rotator cuff interval is used, and the subscapularis is left intact or only detached partially at its lateral insertion on the humerus. This avoids cutting across the anterior capsular structure and, in theory, preserves the important glenohumeral ligaments anteriorly.

Once the capsule is exposed, it can either be taken off the humerus laterally or transversely incised across its midportion. A recent study has shown that imbrication of the capsule in the inferior-superior plane is better than tightening the capsule in the mediolateral plane. Because of this, the surgical technique is moving from the standard vertical incision as described by Rowe[319] to either a detachment laterally or a more transverse incision as described by Jobe.[171]

Once the capsule has been incised, the underlying Bankart lesion is then exposed. This consists of the labrum detached along the anterior rim of the glenoid. In order for the soft tissues to heal back down to bone, it is necessary to create bleeding bone by decorticating the surface of the glenoid. Once this is done, the labrum can be attached to the glenoid either by use of sutures through small holes made in the rim of the glenoid or by suture anchor-type devices that are placed into drill holes in the anterior glenoid. It is very important to repair the inferior portion of the detached labrum in order to reestablish to inferior glenohumeral ligament. The suture placed in the 6 o'clock position on the glenoid rim is very important for shoulder stability. A common cause of recurrent anterior instability after Bankart repair is inaccuracy of repairing the inferior portion of the labrum. Surgically it can be difficult to expose the labrum in this area, and surgeons may be hesitant to be aggressive with the proximity of the axial nerve. Typically sutures or suture anchors are placed at the 6 o'clock, 4 o'clock, and 2 o'clock positions on a right shoulder in order to repair the labrum back down to the glenoid. Once this is done, the capsular defect is repaired, and the superior rotator cuff interval is closed. Depending on the amount of laxity that the patient had before the operation, the capsule may be imbricated slightly in order to decrease the residual laxity. The subscapularis is then repaired anatomically, and the interval between the deltoid and pectoralis muscle is loosely approximated. The skin is then closed, and a dressing is applied.

With the increasing popularity of outpatient surgery, this procedure can either be done on a same-day basis or with an overnight stay in the hospital. After the operation the patient may have a significant level of pain for the first 24 to 48 hours; this can usually be managed with oral narcotics. Either a general anesthetic or an interscalene block is utilized during this procedure.

Bristow

This procedure is commonly referred to as the Bristow procedure, although it was developed, used, and reported on by Helfet,[152] who named this after his former chief, Dr. Bristow. In this procedure the tip of the coracoid process is detached, leaving the conjoined tendons attached. The bony block is then placed directly down onto the anterior glenoid in order to reinforce the defective part at the anterior joint. The bony block can either be passed directly through the subscapularis or over the superior border of the subscapularis.[356]

The advantages of the Bristow procedure is that it is a relatively simple operation that has bone-to-bone healing in order to repair the defect anteriorly. Unfortunately, the disadvantage of the Bristow procedure far outweighs any advantages it may offer. This procedure fails to address the anterior-inferior capsulolabral insufficiency, and the instability itself may not be corrected. Recurrent instability rates are as high as 13%.[157] In addition, this procedure tends to limit external rotation of the shoulder, and in one large series only 16% of the athletes were able to return to their preinjury level of throwing.[356] The use of a metal screw to fix the bone block is associated with a high risk of complications from either loosening of the screw or penetration of the joint by the screw.[407] A revision stabilization procedure is especially difficult after a Bristow procedure due to the extensive scarring of the anterior capsule and subscapularis tendon. Despite these limitations, the Bristow is still used occasionally in either nonthrowing athletes or a nondominant arm, where limitation in range of motion is not as detrimental. It may also be indicated if there is indeed a bony defect anteriorly, for example, that may occur after a fracture of the anterior glenoid. However, overall, the Bristow recently has been viewed with increasing disfavor.

Magnuson-Stack procedure

This was originally described by Magnuson[215] in 1940. It involved the transfer of the subscapularis tendon from the lesser tuberosity across the bicipital groove to the greater tuberosity. In 1955 the procedure was modified slightly in that the tendon was transferred across the bicipital groove and distally into an area between the greater tuberosity and the upper shaft of the humerus, allowing the subscapularis muscle tendon unit to create a plane to support the head of the humerus as the arm is abducted.[294] In the past the Magnuson-Stack procedure was popular, but as the advantages of anatomical surgical repairs have become more apparent, this procedure is now primarily of historical interest. If indeed isolated laxity of the subscapularis muscle contributed recurrent instability, it should be addressed by the rehabilitation exercises in strengthening the rotator cuff. Complications of this procedure include excessive anterior tightening, posterior subluxation and dislocation of the joint, damage to the biceps tendon, and recurrent instability.[219] The edge of the subscapularis is often fixated with a staple, and the staple can cause impingement on the long head of the biceps tendon and pain from the staple itself.

Putti-Platt procedure

This procedure was first described in 1948 by Osmond-Clark,[274] although neither Putti or Platt ever described the techniques themselves in the literature. In this procedure the subscapularis tendon is divided 2.5 cm from its insertion, and the capsule is also opened in the same plane as the tendon so the joint can be visualized. The lateral stump of the tendon is then attached to soft tissues along the anterior rim of the glenoid cavity. If the labrum is stripped from this area, it is attached directly to the anterior glenoid. Once the lateral tendon stump is secure, the medial muscle stump is then overlapped anteriorly, producing a shortening of the capsule and subscapularis muscle. Although short-term follow-up for this procedure results in increased stability of the shoulder, this is usually accompanied by a significant loss of motion. Reagan et al.[298] noted limitation and weakness of external rotation in all patients after Bristow, Magnuson-Stack, and Putti-Platt procedures. Of these three procedures, the Putti-Platt affected external rotation to the greatest degree. This procedure is also associated with osteoarthritis from overtightening (joint constraint).[148] The Putti-Platt procedure is contraindicated in patients with multidirectional instability, because tightening the front of the shoulder will only increase the likelihood of posterior instability. With the development of successful anatomical repairs, the Putti-Platt procedure is also basically of historical interest alone.

Capsular shift

The capsular shift procedure is used to remove the redundancy of the capsule of the glenohumeral joint. Anterior capsular redundancy can be seen rarely after an isolated anterior shoulder dislocation, usually as associated with multidirectional instability. The most common multidirectional instability that is seen is in the anterior-inferior direction. Multidirectional instability is usually atraumatic and can be secondary related to inherent tissue laxity, aplasia of the shoulder joint, nerve injury to the shoulder, or after a stroke (CVA). In addition, a traumatic dislocation can be superimposed on a shoulder with preexisting inherent capsular laxity, resulting in a multidirectional instability of the shoulder that is very difficult to treat with rehabilitation alone. Atraumatic instability is treated with a specific rehabilitation program emphasizing strengthening the deltoid, the rotator cuff, and the scapular stabilizers. The patient is given at least 6 months of rehabilitation and is carefully observed for signs of voluntary habitual subluxation or dislocation. The patient with voluntary subluxation or dislocation must be approached cautiously regarding possible surgical stabilization.

The surgical approach for a capsular shift is essentially the same as that used for Bankart-type operations. Once the capsule is isolated, there are several different techniques described to incise and tighten the capsule.[7,17,171,219,256] The balance between restoring the stability of the glenohumeral joint while allowing functional motion is even more difficult in a capsular shift procedure compared with a Bankart procedure. The position of the arm while the capsule is tensioned is very important, especially in throwing athletes. The tendency to overtighten the capsule to prevent recurrent instability must be tempered by the importance of allowing required residual shoulder motion. A position of 45° of abduction of the humerus with 45° of external rotation is frequently used to provide adequate postoperative motion.

REHABILITATION FOLLOWING SHOULDER STABILIZATION

The rehabilitation program following shoulder stabilization surgical procedures is based on six specific factors. These include (1) the type of surgical procedure performed, (2) the type of instability, (3) open versus arthroscopic technique, (4) tissue fixation method, (5) patient variables (tissue quality, activity level, dynamic stabilizers), and (6) the patient's rehabilitation ability. The rehabilitation sequence following shoulder stabilization uses a multiple phase approach, with each phase addressing specific goals and criteria.

In the first phase, the immediate postoperative period, the goals are to protect the surgical procedure while minimizing the negative effects of immobilization. Thus during this phase early protected and guarded motion is essential for collagen tissue synthesis and organization. In addition, submaximal isometrics are initiated to minimize muscular atrophy and improve dynamic shoulder stability. It is also important to diminish the patient's postoperative pain and inflammation. Modalities such as cryotherapy, mobilization, motion, and TENS, may be useful in diminishing the patient's pain, which may have an inhibitory effect on muscular action.

The second phase emphasizes the advancement of shoulder mobility. During this phase motion is gradually increased, the shoulder complex arthrokinematics are normalized, and improvement of the patient's strength and endurance is emphasized. Techniques to improve motion such as joint mobilization, physiological stretching, active assisted motion, and proprioceptive neuromuscular facilitation techniques may all be beneficial. Strengthening exercises to enhance dynamic shoulder strength such as manual resistance PNF, isotonics, and neuromuscular control drills should be utilized.

In the third phase, the advanced strengthening period, the goals are to enhance the patient's strength, power, and endurance, but also to maximize the effect of the dynamic stabilizers. Specific exercises based on the demands of the patient should be emphasized during this phase. For the athletic patient, exercises such as plyometrics, eccentrics,

PNF, isotonics, and functional drills should be employed.

The final phase, the return to activity, utilizes specific and progressive functional drills to prepare the patient and/or athlete for his or her return to work and/or sports. During this phase a comprehensive strengthening and stretching program should be performed to maximize the surgical outcome.

With these guidelines in mind, we now discuss the specific rehabilitation programs for the Bankart and capsular shift procedures to serve as models.

Rehabilitation following Bankart procedure

The rehabilitation process following a Bankart procedure is dependent on the type of surgical procedure performed (open versus arthroscopy). In the case of the open procedure, gentle active assisted motion may be initiated a few days following the surgery (see the Box). The capsule may be moderately stressed into abduction and external rotation at 3 to 4 weeks after surgery. At 5 to 6 weeks the shoulder may

---

Anterior capsulolabral reconstruction in throwers (open procedure)

Phase I: immediate motion phase

Week 0-2
- Sling for comfort (1 week)
- Immobilization brace for 4 weeks (sleeping only)
- Gentle AAROM exercises with T-bar
  • Flexion to tolerance (0°-120°)
  • ER at 20° abduction to tolerance (maximum 15°-20°)
  • IR at 20° abduction to tolerance (maximum 45°)
- Rope and Pulley
- Elbow/hand ROM
- Isometrics; ER, IR, Abd, Biceps
- Squeeze ball
- Elbow flexion/extension
- Ice

Week 3-4
- AAROM exercises with T-bar
  • Flexion to tolerance (maximum 120°-140°)
  • ER to 45° abduction (acceptable 20°-30°)
  • IR at 45° abduction (acceptable 45°-60°)
- Initiate light isotonics for shoulder musculature abduction, supraspinatus, ER, IR, biceps
- Initiate scapular strengthening exercises emphasis-rhomboids, trapezius, serratus anterior

Week 5-6
- Progress all ROM with AAROM T-bar
  • Flexion (maximum 160°)
  • ER/IR at 90° abduction
    ER to 45°-60°
    IR to 65°-95°
- UBE arm at 90° abduction
- Diagonal patterns, manual resistance
- Progress all strengthening exercises

Phase II: intermediate phase (week 8-14)

Week 8-10
- Progress to full range of motion (week 8-10)
  Flexion to 180°
  ER to 90°
  IR to 85°
- Isokinetic strengthening exercises (neutral position)
- Program all strengthening exercises
- Scapular strengthening exercises

Week 10-14
- Continue all flexibility exercises, self capsular stretches
- Throwers Ten Program (see Box, p. 434)
- UBE 90° abduction
- Diagonal pattern (manual resistance)

Phase III: advanced stage (month 4-6)

- Continue all flexibility exercises
  ER stretch
  IR stretch
  Flex stretch
  Self capsular stretches
- Continue Throwers Ten Program
- Isokinetics ER/IR (90/90 position)
- Isokinetics test (throwers series)
- Plyometrics exercises
- Initiate interval throwers throwing (physician approval necessary)

Phase IV: return to activity phase (month 6-9)

- Continue all strengthening exercises
- Throwers Ten Program
- Continue all stretching exercises

be gradually stretched at 90° of abduction while performing external and internal rotation stretching. Full passive range of motion is obtained at approximately 8 weeks after surgery. Strengthening exercises are initiated immediately after surgery, and more aggressive strengthening drills are permitted at 10 to 12 weeks and plyometrics exercise drills at 14 to 16 weeks. The throwing patient may progress to interval throwing at approximately 4 months and a return to overhead sports at approximately 6 months.

The rehabilitation program following an arthroscopic Bankart procedure is slightly slower than following an open procedure due to slightly poorer fixation methods. The program is particularly slower initially (see the Box), with the goal of full passive motion at approximately 10 weeks. An aggressive strengthening program is allowed at approximately 12 to 13 weeks, and a throwing program is permitted at 4 to 4½ months.

Rehabilitation following capsular shift procedures

The rehabilitation program following a capsular shift procedure is based on four key factors: (1) type of shift procedure performed (anterior vs posterior), (2) tissue integrity of the patient (capsular and muscular integrity), (3) type of patient (athletic vs nonathletic), and (4) the patient's

Arthroscopic anterior capsulolabral reconstruction in the overhead athlete

Phase I: "restricted motion" - maximal protection phase

Week 0-2
- Sling for comfort (2 weeks)
- Immobilization brace for 4 weeks (sleeping only)
- Gentle AAROM with T-Bar
  Forward flexion 0°-60°
  ER at 20° abduction (maximal motion 0°)
  IR at 20° abduction (maximal motion 45°)

- DO NOT abduct and ext rot shoulder during first 4 wks

- Elbow/hand ROM
- Isometrics, submaximal subpainful contraction ER, IR, abduction, biceps with arm at side (0° abduction)
- Squeeze ball
- Ice, modalities to shoulder to control pain

Week 3-4
- Discontinue use of sling
- Continue use of immobilization for sleep
- Continue gentle AAROM with T-Bar
  Flexion 0°-90°
  ER at 20° abduction (maximal motion 15°)
  IR at 20° abduction (maximal motion 65°)
- Continue isometrics
- Continue elbow/hand motion exercises

Week 5-6
- Discontinue use of immobilization for sleep
- Gradually progress all ROM exercises with T-bar
  Flexion (0°-135°)
  ER at 45° abduction (maximal motion 30°)
  IR at 45° abduction (maximal motion 60°)
- Initiate *light weight* isotonic shoulder exercises IR, ER, abduction, supraspinatus, biceps, triceps
- Initiate light weight isotonic scapular strengthening retraction, protraction, elevation, depression
- Initiate UBE at 70° abduction

Phase II: moderate protection phase (week 7-14)

Week 7-9
- Progress all motion exercises
  Flexion (0°-180°)

ER at 90° abduction (maximal motion 75°)
IR at 90° abduction (maximal motion 85°)
- Continue isotonic strengthening program
- Initiate diagonal strengthening program
- Continue all scapular strengthening
- Initiate isokinetic exercises (neutral position)
- Initiate exercise tubing ER/IR (at 0° abduction)

Week 10-14
- Goal full range of motion (week 12-14)
- Continue and progress all exercises as stated above
- Initiate manual resistance exercise programs

Phase III: minimal protection phase (week 15-21)

Week 15-18
- Continue all flexibility exercises, capsular stretches to maintain full ROM
- Initiate throwers ten program (see Box, p. 434)
- Initiate *light* swimming
- Initiate exercises in the 90° position

Week 18-21
- Continue flexibility exercises
- Begin interval throwing program when:
  1. Full non-painful ROM
  2. Strength 90° of contralateral side
  3. No pain or tenderness
  4. Satisfactory clinical exam
- Continue Throwers Ten Exercise Program
- Initiate Plyometric Exercise Program

Phase IV: advanced strengthening phase (week 22-26)

- Aggressive strengthening program for shoulder and scapular musculature.
- Continue Throwers Ten Program
- Continue Plyometric Program
- Progress to Phase II of interval throwing

Phase V: return to activity phase (month 7-9)

- Continue all strengthening exercises
- Continue all stretching exercises
- Begin unrestricted throwing

desired activity level. All four of these factors must be considered to determine the rate and aggressiveness of the program. The rate of progression is slower for a posterior capsular shift compared with an anterior capsular shift. This is because of the inherently poor capsular tissue posteriorly compared with anteriorly. The rehabilitation of an overhead athlete is generally much more aggressive than that of a nonathletic patient. Most commonly the overhead athlete has gradually stretched his or her capsule out over time; thus the capsular structures are usually strong. In contrast, the MDI patient has poor capsular structures, and the rehabilitation must be slower so as not to overstress the capsular restraints. Also, the athletic patient generally exhibits more efficient dynamic stabilizers. Therefore we advocate the clinical usage of two rehabilitation approaches following a capsular shift. The first approach, the accelerated approach, is applicable to the overhead athletic patients with emphasis on motion, dynamic stability, and an early return to functional activities (see the Box). Conversely, the general orthopedic patient progresses more slowly related to inadequate capsular and muscular stabilization.

The accelerated rehabilitation program is based on immediate protected motion, which assists in pain control, capsular healing, collagen alignment, and early functional activities. Active assisted range-of-motion stretching exercises for external rotation/internal rotation are initially performed with the arm at 30° abduction, then progressed to 45°, and then to 90° of abduction. The goal of full passive range of motion should be obtained at 8 weeks after surgery. The patient does utilize a sling for protection for approximately 10 to 14 days after anterior capsular shift following the accelerated program. Strengthening exercises are initiated immediately following surgery in the form of isometrics; isotonics are initiated at approximately 2 weeks, with aggressive strengthening drills permitted at 10 to 12 weeks and plyometrics initiated at 12 weeks. A progressive interval throwing program may be initiated at 20 to 22 weeks with pitching (from the mound) beginning between 23 to 26 weeks after surgery.

The rehabilitation program following an anterior capsular shift procedure in the general orthopedic patient who exhibited MDI prior to surgery is generally slower and more conservative than the previously discussed program. Several authors have advocated the use of an immobilization brace or sling for 3 to 6 weeks.[175,219,271] The patient performs daily range-of-motion exercises gently with no stretching of the capsule allowed. In addition, active and active assisted exercises are delayed until after the initial immobilization period. Our program is slightly more aggressive and allows *gentle* immediate motion, which is gradually increased. During the program the clinician must assess the patient's shoulder capsule integrity periodically to determine the patient's response to surgery and the exercise program. Thus, based on these assessments, the program may be more aggressive or slower. The general orthopedic patient should

exhibit full passive range of motion at approximately 10 to 12 weeks after surgery.

The goal of both rehabilitation programs is complete restoration of full unrestricted function, full painfree motion, and strength that provides dynamic stability. It is important for the clinician to realize that the postsurgical anterior capsular shift patient should be expected to obtain full range of motion, unless the static stabilizers are grossly inadequate.

The rehabilitation program following a posterior capsular shift procedure is generally slower than for an anterior shift procedure. Frequently a brace is utilized to immobilize the shoulder in abduction, external rotation, and slight extension. After a short period of immobilization a gentle range-of-motion program as well as gentle strengthening may be initiated. Limiting movements such as horizontal adduction and internal rotation may be beneficial during the early phases of rehabilitation. The expectations following this type of repair are less positive than that of an anterior repair; therefore this procedure is less frequently utilized in the athletic population. A return to full unrestricted activities is usually permitted at approximately 7 to 9 months after surgery.

In general, patients who exhibit ligamentous laxity and have a preoperative diagnosis of atraumatic multidirectional instability should undergo a more conservative rehabilitative program slightly slower related to congenital laxity. The excessive laxity presented by these patients generally allows them to obtain motion more rapidly and have little to no difficulty achieving full motion. Therefore the goal is to gradually restore motion and dynamic stability while maintaining static stability. Neer[252] reported the ideal motion for these patients may actually be a slight loss of motion (i.e., 10° flexion and 20° less of rotation) than the contralateral shoulder.

In summary, when rehabilitating a patient following a shoulder stabilization surgery, the clinician must consider numerous factors, previously discussed, before initiating any treatment program. The rehabilitation program must match the surgical procedure as well as the skill and philosophy of the surgeon. During the rehabilitation process the goal should be restoring full physiologic motion and enhancing dynamic stabilization. Functionally, the patient should strive for a complete return to function.

ROTATOR CUFF PATHOLOGIES

Rotator cuff pathologies are among the most common shoulder injuries seen by the clinician treating orthopedic problems. The rotator cuff musculature serves a vital role in normal shoulder function. The functions of the rotator cuff are (1) dynamic glenohumeral joint stability, (2) controlling humeral head translation, and (3) movement such as external or internal rotation.

The tendons of the rotator cuff interlace with each other and are interwoven with the adjacent muscles. The interdigitation of these tendinous fibers assists in controlling

Anterior capsular shift rehabilitation protocol (accelerated)

This rehabilitation program's goal is to return the patient/athlete to their activity/sport as quickly and safely as possible while maintaining a *stable shoulder*. The program is based on muscle physiology, biomechanics, anatomy, and the healing process following surgery for a capsular shift.

The capsular shift procedure is one where the orthopedic surgeon makes an incision into the ligamentous capsule of the shoulder and pulls the capsule tighter and then sutures the capsule together.

The ultimate goal is a functional stable shoulder and a return to a presurgery functional level.

Phase I - protection phase (week 0-6)

Goals: Allow healing of sutured capsule
  Begin early protected range of motion
  Retard muscular atrophy
  Decrease pain/inflammation

A. Week 0-2
  Precautions:
  1. Sleep in immobilizer for 4 weeks
  2. No overhead activities for 4-6 weeks
  3. Wean from immobilizer and into sling as soon as possible (orthopedist or therapist will tell you when)
  Exercises:
  Gripping exercises with putty
  Elbow flex/extension and pronation/supination
  Pendulum exercises (nonweighted)
  Rope & Pulley active assisted exercises
    shoulder flexion to 90°
    shoulder abduction to 60°
  T-Bar Exercises
    external rotation to 15° with arm abducted at 30°
    shoulder flexion/extension to tolerance
  AROM cervical spine
  Isometrics
    flexors, extensors, ER, IR, ABD
  Criteria for Hospital Discharge:
  1. Shoulder range of motion (AAROM) flexion 90°, abduction 45°, external rotation 25°
  2. Minimal pain and swelling
  3. "Good" proximal and distal muscle power

B. Week 2-4
  Goals: Gradual increase in ROM
    Normalize arthrokinematics
    Improve strength
    Decrease pain/inflammation
  1. Range of Motion Exercises
    T-Bar active assisted exercises
    ER @ 30° ABD to 45°
    IR @ 30° ABD to 45°
    Shoulder flex/ext to tolerance
    Shoulder abduction to tolerance
    Shoulder horizontal ABD/ADD
    Rope & Pulley flex/ext
    • All exercises performed to tolerance
      - take to point of pain and/or resistance and hold
      - *gentle* self capsular stretches

2. Gentle joint mobilization to reestablish normal arthrokinematics to:
  - scapulothoracic joint
  - glenohumeral joint
  - sternoclavicular joint
3. Strengthening exercises
  - isometrics
  - may initiate tubing for ER/IR at 0°
4. Conditioning program for:
  - trunk
  - lower extremities
  - cardiovascular
5. Decrease pain/inflammation
  - ice, NSAID, modalities

C. Week 5-6
  AAROM flexion to tolerance
  IR/ER @ 45° ABD to tolerance
  Initiate IR/ER at 90° ABD to tolerance
  Initiate isotonic (light wt.) strengthening
  Gentle joint mobilization (Grade III)

Phase II - intermediate phase (week 7-12)

Goals: Full nonpainful ROM at week 8-10
    Normalize arthrokinematics
    Increase strength
    Improve neuromuscular control

A. Week 7-10
  1. Range-of-motion Exercise T-Bar active assisted exercises
    Continue all exercises listed above
    Gradually increase ROM to full ROM week 8-10
    Continue self capsular stretches
    Continue joint mobilization
  2. Strengthening Exercises
    Initiate isotonic dumbbell program
    - sidelying ER
    - sidelying IR
    - shoulder abduction
    - supraspinatus
    - latissimus dorsi
    - rhomboids
    - biceps curls
    - triceps curls
    - shoulder shrugs
    - push-ups into chair (serratus anterior)
    Continue tubing at 0° for ER/IR
  3. Initiate Neuromuscular Control Exercises for Scapulothoracic Joint

B. Week 10-12
  1. Continue all exercises listed above
  2. Initiate tubing exercises for rhomboids, latissimus dorsi, biceps, and triceps
  3. Initiate aggressive stretching and joint mobilization, if needed

Phase III - dynamic strengthening phase (week 12-20) advanced strengthening phase

A. Week 12-17
Goals: Improve strength/power/endurance

Anterior capsular shift rehabilitation protocol (accelerated)—Cont'd

Improve neuromuscular control
Prepare athlete to begin to throw
1. *Criteria to Enter Phase III:*
   a. Full nonpainful ROM
   b. No pain or tenderness
   c. Strength 70% or better compared to contralateral side
Emphasis of Phase III:
   - high speed; high energy strengthening exercises
   - eccentric exercises
   - diagonal patterns
Exercises:
Throwers Ten Exercises:
   - Initiate tubing exercises in 90/90 position for IR and ER (slow sets, fast sets)
   - Tubing for rhomboids
   - Tubing for latissimus dorsi
   - Tubing for biceps
   - Tubing for diagonal patterns D2 extension
   - Tubing for diagonal patterns D2 flexion
   - Continue dumbbell exercises for supraspinatus and deltoid
   - Continue serratus anterior strengthening exercises push-ups floor
2. Continue trunk/LE strengthening exercises
3. Continue neuromuscular exercises
4. Continue self capsular stretches

B. Week 17-20
   - Continue all exercises above
   - Initiate plyometrics for shoulder:
     - ER at 90° ABD
     - IR at 90° ABD
     - D2 extension plyometrics
     - Biceps plyometrics
     - Serratus anterior plyometrics

Phase IV - throwing phase (week 21-26)

Goals: Progressively increase activities to prepare patient for full functional return
Criteria to Progress to Phase IV:
1. Full ROM
2. No pain or tenderness
3. Isokinetic test that fulfills criteria to throw
4. Satisfactory clinical exam
Exercise:
   - Initiate interval throwing program
   - Continue throwers ten exercises
   - Continue plyometric five exercises
A. Interval Throwing Program at 20th Week
   1. Interval Throwing Program Phase II - 24th week
B. Return to Sports: 26-30 weeks

---

stresses, maintaining humeral-glenoid compression, distributing forces, and resisting failure.

The vascularity of the rotator cuff has been a controversial subject for numerous years. Lindblom[208] proposed that the rotator cuff was hypovascular or avascular near the supraspinatus attachment to the greater tuberosity. Codman[81,82] referred to this avascular area as the "critical zone" where many lesions occur. Several others[62,295,313] have reported undervascularity in this zone. Moseley and Goldie,[239] using microradiography and histology to study the vascular supply of the cuff, concluded that this area is not less vascular than the remainder of the cuff, but rather that this area represents the anastomoses between the osseous and tendinous vessels. Recent studies utilizing laser Doppler technique have revealed substantial blood flow in the critical area.[165,253,348] Some authors have proposed compromise of supraspinatus blood flow based on arm movements. Rathbun and Macnab[295] noted when the arm is adducted, it puts the tendon under tension and in effect causes a "wringing out" of the vessels. Sigholm et al.[333] reported a significant increase (increase by fivefold) in subacromial pressure when the arm is elevated from 0° to 45°. If sustained, these pressures are sufficiently high to substantially reduce the tendon microcirculation.

There are numerous types of pathologies and injuries observed at the rotator cuff musculotendinous junction.

Subacromial impingement appears to be one of the most common pathologies discussed. Impingement is defined as the "encroachment" of the rotator cuff (usually the supraspinatus) on the acromion, coracoacromial ligament, coracoid process, and/or acromioclavicular joint as the shoulder is moved, particularly elevation and internal rotation. in 1972 Neer popularized the term "impingement," but the condition was recognized by many other clinicians such as Codman[80] in 1927 and Armstrong,[20] McLaughlin,[225] and Smith-Petersen et al.[338] in the 1940s. Neer et al.[254] has described impingement as a progressive pattern involving a distinct three-stage process. In stage one, the lesions are described as a condition of cuff inflammation, edema, and hemorrhage, reversible with conservative treatment. In stage two, the lesion involves fibrosis and cuff tendinitis and may be treated conservatively. Stage three lesions involve bony changes (spurs) and cuff failure, necessitating surgical intervention.

Recently, Flatow et al.[124] studied the contact patterns of the rotator cuff on the undersurface of the acromion. The investigators used stereophotogrammetry to determine contact areas while applying forces along the rotator cuff and deltoid muscular force lines. It was noted that contact and proximity was located at the anterolateral edge of the acromion at 0° elevation and shifted medially to the anteromedial edge with increasing arm elevation. In all cases (nine) and all test positions, contact involved only the anterior portion of the acromion. On the humeral side, contact was located at the proximal biceps region and supraspinatus tendon at 0° of elevation and shifted distally along these tendons with increasing arm elevation. In the range from 60° to 120° of arm elevation, the authors noted contact was focused at the supraspinatus insertion. Furthermore contact and proximity were consistently more pronounced in shoulders with a type III acromion or diminished external rotation. Thus in the normal shoulder, the rotator cuff, particularly the supraspinatus and biceps, contacts the acromion with arm elevation. And it is when the forces are concentrated in one region such as on the supraspinatus tendon when failure may occur.

It is important for the rehabilitation specialist to realize numerous factors may contribute to subacromial impingement. These factors have been classified as either structural or functional (see the Box).[221,388] Often these two factors are referred to as primary or secondary. In structural impingement there is a structure that is responsible for the encroachment. The acromion is a commonly discussed site of impingement. If the acromion fails to ossify or unite, a condition referred to as os acromiale occurs. This results in a downward hanging acromion, which has been demonstrated to cause subacromial impingement.[47,242,266] Variations of acromial shape are commonly observed in patients with impingement and cuff tears. Bigliani et al.[47] have identified three types of acromion: type I (flat), type II (curved), and type III (hooked) (Fig. 15-19). Other structural factors such as degeneration or spurring off the acromioclavicular joint or the anterolateral acromion may cause impingement. Bursal inflammation or thickening, or rotator cuff abnormalities may contribute as well.

Function or secondary impingement occurs as a result of an underlying condition that causes the encroachment. Numerous examples of functional impingement are listed in the Box. There are three common mechanisms that we will describe. Patients with subacromial impingement appear to exhibit a characteristic loss of motion pattern, described by Wilk and Andrews[388] as a "reverse capsular pattern." Internal rotation is restricted the most and elevation second, with a slight loss of external rotation. In this loss of motion pattern, usually the posterior capsule appears tight. Normal posterior capsular laxity allows the humeral head to stay centralized within the glenoid. Posterior capsular tightness results in an anterosuperior migration of the humeral head causing encroachment of the humerus on the coracoacromial ligament and/or acromion. Thus this impingement is secondary to capsular tightness; the treatment must be directed at normalizing the capsular flexibility.

In contrast, capsular hypermobility can also cause secondary impingement. If the capsule is excessively lax and/or the dynamic stabilizers are inadequate, the humeral head will displace excessively, which may cause secondary impingement. The author (KEW) believes this may be one

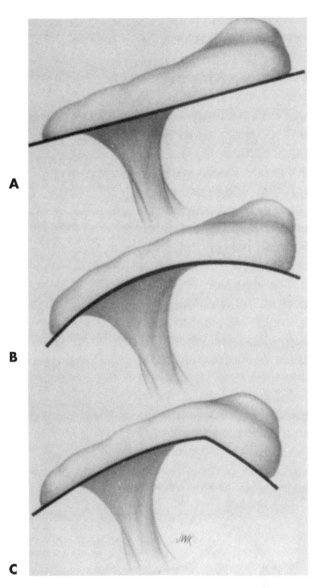

Fig. 15-19. Three types of acromion (A) Type I, flat, (B) Type II, curved, (C) Type III, hooked. (From Biglianni LU, Ticker JB: Impingement pathology of the rotator cuff. In Andrews JR, Wilk KE, editors: *The athlete's shoulder,* New York, 1994, Churchill Livingstone. Reproduced with permission.)

of the causes for the painful arc. The treatment must be directed at improving joint stability. Muscular weakness of the rotator cuff, thereby a loss of humeral head dynamic control, will result in the humeral head superiorly migrating (previously discussed in biomechanics), which may cause subacromial impingement.

Recently, scapular hypermobility has been cited as a possible cause of functional or secondary impingement.[193] Kibler[193] reported that individuals whose scapulae glided excessively laterally (protraction) during arm elevation had a correlation to subacromial impingement. This excessive protraction caused the glenoid fossa to "open up," which may contribute to excessive movement of the humeral head

Factors contributing to shoulder impingement

Structural

Acromioclavicular joint
  Joint abnormalities
  Degenerative spurs
  Sprains/separations
Acromion
  Unfused
  Abnormal shape
  Spurring
  Malunion of fracture
Abnormalities
  Nonunion of fracture
  Bursae
  Inflammation
  Chronic thickening
Rotator cuff
  Thickening
  Flap tears
  Irregularities
Humerus
  Congenital
  Malunion fracture

Functional

Humeral head
  Rotator cuff weakness
  Rotator cuff scar
Capsular
  Hypomobility
  Hypermobility
Scapulae
  Positional
  Muscular weakness
Neuromuscular control
Hypomobility

anteriorly and superiorly. Therefore, if the impingement is secondary to inadequate scapulae stability, the treatment must be focused on improving scapular stability and dynamic humeral head control.

Hence, the successful treatment of subacromial impingement is based on a careful examination that identifies the *causes* of the pathology. It would also appear that repetitive microtraumas are more of the causative factor for impingement than are macrotraumatic forces. Neer viewed impingement as a progressive degenerative process that often leads to failure of the rotator cuff.

Wilk[386] has developed a treatment cliche for subacromial impingement: "Treat anterior impingement posterior to anterior." This simply reminds the clinician to stretch the posterior structures, strengthen the posterior cuff muscles, and strengthen the scapular musculature, particularly the scapular retractors. The nonoperative treatment must also be directed toward diminishing the pain and inflammation present before an aggressive strengthening program can be initiated. The goal of the treatment plan is to balance the shoulder whereas there exists equal flexibility and strength of the posterior and anterior structures.

Nonoperative treatment for anterior or subacromial impingement has proven to be extremely effective in most patients. Neer et al.[254] state in the classic article that, "... many patients were suspected of having impingement, but responded well to conservative treatment." During the period of their report, Neer et al.[254] operated on an average of 10 shoulders a year with this diagnosis. However, if nonoperative treatment failed, then surgical intervention may be a viable option. Neer[251] reported that patients were advised not to have an acromioplasty until the stiffness of the shoulder had disappeared and the disability had persisted for at least 9 months. The surgical treatment for subacromial impingement is a decompression where the anterior and undersurface of the acromion is removed along with the coracoacromial ligament and possibly the distal end of the clavicle.

The surgical decompression may be accomplished through an open incision or arthroscopically. Once the acromion is exposed, an osteotome or a motorized burr is used to remove a layer of approximately 2 to 2.5 mm thickness from the 2.5 cm length of the anterior undersurface of the acromion, along with the entire coracoacromial ligament. If the acromioclavicular joint exhibits osteophytes, degeneration, etc., the distal 2.5 cm of the clavicle is also resected. The subacromial bursae may be removed entirely or partially, depending on the degree of the involvement. Numerous articles have documented the successful outcome of both the open decompression[254,354] and arthroscopic decompression,[119,131,235] with comparable results of 85% to 90% good to excellent.

The rehabilitation program following subacromial decompression varies slightly depending on whether the surgery was performed openly or arthroscopically. The rehabilitation of the arthroscopic decompression is detailed in the Box. Immediately after surgery the patient is initiated on active assisted range-of-motion exercises (usually the day after surgery). The patient also performs submaximal isometrics to minimize muscular atrophy, "cuff shutdown," and neuromuscular inhibition. Most patients reestablish full motion at approximately 10 to 14 days after the operation. During the second phase the program emphasis is on dynamic humeral head control, scapular strengthening, and maintaining flexibility. The last phase is directed toward reinitiation of functional activities, continuation of strengthening exercises (isotonics concentric/eccentric), and maintenance of shoulder flexibility. The patient may return to athletics usually at 3 to 4 months after surgery or when the following criteria have been met: (1) full nonpainful range of motion, (2) strength within 10% of

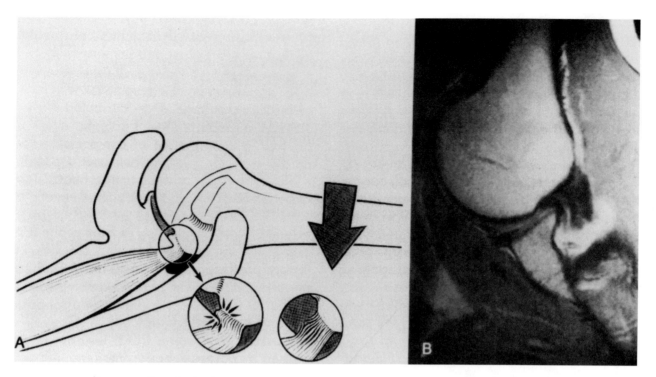

Fig. 15-20. Posterior impingement. **(A)** Illustration of posterior impingement and pain relief during relocation test. **(B)** CT scan illustrating the supraspinatus impingement against the posterosuperior aspect of glenoid rim. (From Walch G, Borleau P, Noel E, Donell T: Impingement of the deep surface of the supraspinatus tendon on the posterior glenoid rim: an arthroscopic study. *J Shoulder Elbow Surg* 1:239, 1992.)

the contralateral side, and (3) a satisfactory clinical examination. The rehabilitation program following an open subacromial decompression is similar to the arthroscopic program with a few exceptions. Immediately after surgery the patient may experience slightly more pain due to the larger surgical incision; thus the immediate motion phase may be slightly slower initially (although full motion usually occurs at 14 to 21 days). Additionally, some patients require the use of a sling for several more days to control shoulder soreness. The rehabilitation program following open decompression has been provided by Richard J. Hawkins, MD.

There are numerous other rotator cuff pathologies and types of impingement seen at the glenohumeral joint. Recently, posterior impingement has been described in the literature.[371] This type of impingement occurs when the arm is abducted and externally rotated (Fig. 15–20). During this movement, called the cocking phase in throwing, the supraspinatus and infraspinatus impinge on the posterosuperior edge of the glenoid, causing an undersurface abrasion of the rotator cuff and fraying of the posterior superior glenoid labrum. This lesion has been previously described by Andrews et al.[15] in the throwing athlete. We have noted this lesion frequently in the overhead athlete (i.e., thrower, swimmer, tennis player) as well as the fact that it may occur secondary to excessive anterior capsular laxity and/or

compromised dynamic stability. The nonoperative treatment for posterior impingement is to emphasize dynamic stabilization of the glenohumeral joint.

Another example of impingement is acute traumatic impingement, which occurs secondary to a fall or diving for a ball in sports. The arm is usually abducted, extended, and internally rotated so that the force of the fall jams the humerus into the acromion and causes acute inflammation of the rotator cuff, bursae, and surrounding tissues. This type of injury responds well to nonoperative treatment or active rest, gentle stretching and strengthening, antiinflammatory medications, and a gradual return to function. In the older patient a thorough examination is necessary to exclude the possibility of a rotator cuff tear or avulsion of the cuff due to the forceful abduction.

The rotator cuff is susceptible to injury in the overhead throwing athlete due to the tremendously large forces imparted on the shoulder joint during the acceleration and deceleration phases of the pitch. During the deceleration phase there is a significant distraction force at the glenohumeral joint, approximately one times that of body weight,[125] and the posterior cuff muscles must act to decelerate the arm through an eccentric muscular action. These repetitive microtraumatic forces and the eccentric muscular overload may cause failure of the rotator cuff seen as an undersurface cuff tear. This type of cuff injury has been

Arthroscopic subacromial decompression and/or partial rotator cuff debridement protocol

This rehabilitation program's goal is to return the patient/athlete to their activity/sport as quickly and safely as possible. The program is based on muscle physiology, biomechanics, anatomy, and healing response.

Phase I - motion phase

Goals: Reestablish nonpainful range of motion
    Retard Muscular Atrophy
    Decrease pain/inflammation
Range of Motion:
• pendulum exercise
• rope and pulley
• L-bar exercises
    - Flexion/Extension
    - Abduction/Adduction
    - ER/IR (Begin at 0° AB, progress to 45° AB, then 90° AB)
• self-stretches (capsular stretches)
Strengthening Exercises:
• isometrics
• may initiate tubing for ER/IR at 0° AB late phase
Decrease Pain/Inflammation:
• Ice, NSAIDS, Modalities

Phase II - intermediate phase

Goals: Regain & Improve Muscular Strength
    Normalize Arthrokinematics
    Improve Neuromuscular Control of Shoulder Complex
Criteria To Progress to Phase II
    1. Full ROM
    2. Minimal Pain & Tenderness
    3. "Good" MMT of IR, ER, Flex
• Initiate Isotonic Program with Dumbbells
    - shoulder musculature
    - scapulothoracic
• Normalize Athrokinematics of Shoulder Complex
    - joint mobilization
    - control L-bar ROM
• Initiate Neuromuscular Control Exercises
• Initiate Trunk Exercises
• Initiate UE Endurance Exercises
• Continue use of modalities, ice, as needed

Phase III - dynamic strengthening phase

Advanced Strengthening Phase
Goals: Improve Strength/Power/Endurance
    Improve Neuromuscular Control
    Prepare athlete to begin to throw, etc.
Criteria To Enter Phase III:
    1. Full nonpainful ROM
    2. No pain or tenderness
    3. Strength 70% compared with contralateral side
Emphasis of Phase III:
• High speed, high energy strengthening exercises
• Eccentric exercises
• Diagonal patterns
Exercises:
• Continue dumbbell strengthening (supraspinatus, deltoid)
• Initiate Tubing Exercises in the 90/90 degree position for
• ER/IR (slow/fast sets)
• Tubing exercises for scapulothoracic musculature
• Tubing exercises for biceps
• Initiate Plyometrics for RTC
• Initiate Diagonal Patterns (PNF)
• Initiate Isokinetics
• Continue endurance exercises: neuromuscular control exercises

Phase IV - return to activity phase

Goals: Progressively Increase Activities to prepare patient for full functional return
Criteria To Progress to Phase IV
    1. Full ROM
    2. No pain or tenderness
    3. Isokinetic Test that fulfills criteria to throw
    4. Satisfactory Clinical Exam
• Initiate Interval Program
• Continue all exercises as in Phase III
(Throw and Train on Same Day)
(LE and ROM on Opposite Days)
• Progress Interval Program
Follow-Up Visits:
    - Isokinetic Tests
    - Clinical Exam

---

referred to as a "tensile cuff failure."[16] This lesion is characterized by an undersurface fraying of the cuff or the supraspinatus and/or infraspinatus musculature.

Another common pathology seen in the general orthopedic population is calcifying tendinitis. Uhthoff and Sarkar[365] describe calcifying tendinitis of the rotator cuff as a common disorder of unknown etiology in which reactive calcification undergoes spontaneous resorption in the course of time with subsequent healing of the tendon. The calcium deposits may consist of calcium, phosphate, oxalate, carbonate, or calcium hydroxyapatite.[217] The most common site of calcific tendinitis in the shoulder is within the supraspinatus tendon in

the area of the critical zone but can develop in other muscle-tendon units. Although the etiology is not fully understood, it is believed the deposits may be the result of pressure at the avascular region or a decrease in oxygen supply to this area. These factors result in a transformation of tenocytes into chondrocytes, resulting in a dense homogeneous calcium deposit.[366] The disease process may silently progress, with symptoms developing once the deposit is large enough to cause impingement. It appears that the condition is self-limiting and self-healing (progresses from deposition to resorption). The overall incidence of calcifying tendinitis varies significantly from 3% to 20% of the general asymptomatic population.[57,58,379] The condition appears to affect females more than males and usually develops between the ages of 31 to 50 years of age.[104,365,379] There appears to be no relationship between calcifying tendinitis and trauma or rotator cuff failure. The condition may be divided into acute and chronic phases.[217] Malone et al.[217] suggest the following delineation: the acute phase occurs with resorption of the deposit; this phase is usually painful and lasts 3 to 7 days. The chronic phase is considered the time when the deposition is occurring and may last several months. Nonoperative treatment consists of ice, gentle motion, strengthening exercises, and pain medication. If discomfort persists, corticosteroid injections into the subacromial space may be beneficial. If symptoms persist, surgical resection of the calcium deposit may be indicated.

Conditions such as compressive cuff disease, tensile cuff failure, and/or posterior impingement may also develop secondary to glenohumeral joint instability.

Last, the rotator cuff tendon or tendons may exhibit frank failure. There are many terms used to describe cuff tendon failure. Almost always the cuff fails near its periphery, near the attachment of the cuff to the tuberosity.[221] Cuff failures are described as partial- or full-thickness tears. A full-thickness tear extends all the way through from the articular surface to the bursal surface of the rotator cuff. Conversely, a partial-thickness tear involves only the superficial surface, mid-substance, or deep surface. Acute tears occurring due to trauma account for approximately 3% to 8% of all rotator cuff tears.[221] Chronic tears are those that have existed for a long time and are often insidious in onset and degenerative in nature. In addition, tears are characterized according to the state of detachment from the humerus (retracted, atrophic, or absent). Tears are also classified according to size of tears—small, less than 1 cm, medium, 1 to 3 cm, large, 3 to 5 cm, and massive, greater than 5 cm.

Numerous factors contribute to cuff failure. Most full-thickness cuff tears appear to occur in tendons that have been weakened by some combination of age, repeated microtraumas, steroid injections, subacromial impingement, hypovascularity of the tendon, attrition, trauma, and previous partial tearing. The incidence of cuff tears begins to rise in the 50- to 60-year-old age group, and peaks in the 70-year and older age group.[26,151,255] DePalma and Kruper[104] noted cuff tears are uncommon before 40 years of age. Neer et al.[256] reported on 233 patients with cuff tears; all but eight were older than 40 years of age, and 70% occurred in sedentary individuals during light work. Once the cuff fails, even with a very small tear, the tendency is for the tear to enlarge or propagate when stresses are imparted onto the shoulder.

When a patient with cuff failure is being examined, he or she often reports persistent discomfort, especially with elevation, or abduction and external rotation. The patient usually experiences night pain, inability to lay on the shoulder, weakness, joint noise, and diminishing function. On physical examination crepitus, muscular weakness of the external rotators and abductors, shoulder muscular atrophy, and diminished active motion may be noted. Specific special tests, discussed earlier, may be beneficial. Imaging evaluation tests such as radiographs, arthrography, CT scans, and MRI may be used to confirm the diagnosis. The differentiation from rotator cuff tendinitis and rotator cuff tears may be accomplished through the previously mentioned imaging studies or through direct visual inspection (arthroscopy). In addition, care must be taken in the examination process to differentiate cuff tears from other causes of shoulder pain and weakness such as cervical spondylosis, suprascapular neuropathy, scapular pathologies, glenohumeral joint arthritis, acromioclavicular joint arthritis, and adhesive capsulitis.[220]

The treatment of documented cuff tears varies on the degree of disability exhibited by the patient. A nonoperative treatment approach should be attempted prior to any surgical repair. The goals of the rehabilitation program are to enhance the strength of the surrounding musculature, enhance the force couples of the glenohumeral joint to dynamically stabilize the joint, and eliminate stress on the injured cuff tissues. The challenge is to enhance the efficiency of the surrounding muscles to prevent the humeral head from migrating superiorly. Takagishi[350] reported that 44% of patients with a documented cuff tear responded well to nonoperative treatment. If the symptoms of pain and dysfunction persist, then surgical repair may become necessary.

SURGICAL REPAIR OF THE ROTATOR CUFF

There have been numerous indications identified for an operative rotator cuff tear. But most commonly the operative repair is performed because of the patient's persistent pain, discomfort, functional loss of arm, and a failed nonoperative treatment approach. The surgical approaches to the complete cuff tear vary substantially.[220] The surgical technique appears to vary the greatest with the technique to gain exposure to the rotator cuff. The traditional approach is one that utilizes a skin incision anteriorly, and the deltoid muscle is detached from the lateral clavicle,[84,120,151,289] whereas other approaches such as separating[282] or splitting[283,286] are being used. The rotator cuff tear can be identified and treated with these three surgical exposures. It should be noted, if the deltoid is retracted and then reattached to the acromion and clavicle, the postsurgical rehabilitation is usually slower to allow soft tissue healing.

The operative technique for dealing with full-thickness cuff tears include tendon-to-tendon repair and tendon advancement to bone,[220] although most physicians prefer tendon-to-bone repair, because this provides stronger repair fixation.

Once the acromioplasty and surgical exposure of the rotator cuff has been performed, the surgical repair may be continued. The subacromial bursa is identified and partially *resected* along with any other scar tissue for better definition of the rotator cuff defect. Uhthoff[364] has reported the undersurface of the bursa may contain regenerative cells; thus only enough bursa is excised to visualize the cuff tear. The torn cuff is identified, and torn edges are excised and cleaned. The cuff is then mobilized superiorly, anteriorly, and posteriorly to allow the torn tendon to be repaired to bone.[199] The area for repair into the bone is selected, near the greater tuberosity.[199,355] A high-speed burr is used to make a trough long enough to contain the torn tendon edge, approximately 3 to 4 mm deep. The tendon is then sutured to the bone using either absorbable or nonabsorbable sutures. Timmerman et al.[355] reported using suture anchors into the medial edge of the bony trough and *passing* and sewing the sutures within the rotator cuff tendon. The authors report this provides additional tissue attachment to bone.

Once completed, the shoulder is placed in a sling, or if excessive tension on the repair is noted intraoperatively, an abduction pillow or brace may be considered.

The actual rotator cuff repair operative technique varies based on the size of the tear, presence of other pathologies (biceps tendon pathology, acromial pathology, acromioclavicular joint degeneration), and tissue quality.

REHABILITATION FOLLOWING ROTATOR CUFF REPAIR

The rehabilitation program following rotator cuff repair is based on numerous factors. These factors include (1) size of the tear, (2) tissue quality, (3) type of repair process, (4) patient's age, (5) onset of injury, (6) desired activities, (7) rehabilitation potential, and (8) physician's philosophy and skill. We will briefly discuss each one of these factors to put forth an example for the reader. The size of the rotator cuff tear contributes to the rate of rehabilitation progression and aggressiveness. A repair of a small tear (<1 cm) may be more rapidly rehabilitated than that of a large (3 to 5 cm) or massive tear (>5 cm). Often massive or some large tear repairs are tenuous and require a period of time of guarded protection and possible immobilization.

The patient's tissue quality may provide the most important information regarding rate of progression. This variable takes into consideration the properties of the bone quality to which the muscle is going to be repaired and the remaining rotator cuff muscular tissue. In some cases the remnant of the rotator cuff is thin, flimsy, degenerated, and thus difficult for the suture to be "captured" or "secured" within the tissue. Occasionally, the bone is soft or fragile, and the suture anchors or sutures have a poor fixation point. In both these cases the tissue quality dictates a slower rate of progression in the rehabilitation to ensure time for soft tissue healing. In contrast, an individual whose tissues are strong, enabling excellent soft tissue and bony fixation, may pursue more aggressive rehabilitation compared with the inadequate tissue.

The type of repair, the surgical technique, plays a very significant role in the rehabilitation program. As previously discussed, the open repair and open acromioplasty require at least a partial take-down of the deltoid insertion from the acromion and lateral clavicle to complete the acromioplasty and to gain exposure to the rotator cuff. Thus the deltoid must be reattached following the rotator cuff repair, and many authors believe active motion should be restricted to prevent the deltoid from pulling off the bony reattachment sites. Conversely, the arthroscopic decompression with deltoid-splitting technique to gain exposure to the cuff tear enables an early advancement of the rehabilitation program in both motion (passive and active) and strengthening exercises.

The next factor, patient's age, may not be as important as the previously discussed factors. Typically, the older patient requires a more extensive rehabilitation program. This is related to degenerative osseous changes, rotator cuff degeneration, and an overall decrease in shoulder function.

The onset of the injury is important to consider. When an acute repair is performed, the residual rotator cuff tissue is viable, and a satisfactory tissue-to-bone repair is accomplished with little difficulty. When a large degenerative chronic tear is present, the repair process is often difficult, and thus the rehabilitation process is much slower than the acute tear. Bassett and Cofield[39] have reported that an early repair yielded a better functional outcome than a chronic repair.

The sixth and seventh factors are relative to the rehabilitation program and the activities to which the patient wishes to return. Most often, rotator cuff repairs are performed on individuals older than 45 years of age; consequently, these individuals may be involved in recreational activities such as golf, tennis, swimming, or gardening and may or may not be involved in strenuous work requirements. The patient who desires a higher functional (sport or work) level requires a different program than that of a sedentary worker with limited recreational interests. Bigliani et al.[46] reported on 23 tennis players who underwent rotator cuff repair. The authors reported 83% achieved painfree status and were able to return to play level, and 13% obtained satisfactory results and were able to play at less competitive levels. This documents patients with rotator cuff repair can participate in higher level functional activities. The rehabilitation potential addresses the patient's functional level and compliance to the rehabilitation program. We believe a possible contraindication to surgery is a patient who exhibits a behavior that is independent, unable to follow instructions, and an unwillingness to comply with the rehabilitation program. The rehabilitation program following rotator cuff repair is lengthy and somewhat strict, and adherence to the program is vital to the ultimate surgical success. Hawkins et al.[151] reported on 23 rotator cuff repairs. Only 2 of 14 patients on worker's compensation were able to return to work; whereas eight of nine patients not on workman's compensation were able to return to work.

Last, the surgeon's philosophy of the rehabilitation following rotator cuff repair contributes greatly to the postsurgical program. Some physicians believe a patient with rotator cuff repair should not attempt any active motions for 8 to 12 weeks, enabling adequate tissue healing. Other physicians believe the patient may perform early active motions that are carefully monitored and guarded. It is hoped that in time, the division in opinions will become narrower.

There have been numerous studies published discussing the results of rotator cuff repairs.[26,84,238,261,263,289,326,402] The results indicate 87% of all patients experience pain relief, and patient satisfaction is approximately 77%. Iannoti[164] reported on 40 large to massive repairs and reported the results are significantly affected by the size of tear, quality of tissue, difficulty of the repair, and presence of biceps tendon rupture. Recently, Rokito et al.[311b] have reported on 42 consecutive patients who have undergone rotator cuff repair surgery. The authors tested the patients' isokinetic strength every three months for one year. They noted the greatest amount of strength gain occurred in the first 6 months. In most cases, shoulder strength was 80% by 6 months and 90% by 12 months compared to the contralateral side.

We will briefly discuss several rehabilitation approaches following cuff repair. The first program is the more traditional approach following open acromioplasty and open cuff repair. Immediately following surgery, the repair is either protected with a sling or by an abduction bolster. The use of the abduction pillow or bolster is employed to protect the repair from maximum adduction, not because the arm is not able to reach the patient's side, but rather to avoid early tension on the repaired tendon. The sling or bolster length of use is variable and may be as short as 1 week or as long as 6 weeks, depending on tissue quality and size of the tear. The day after surgery passive motion is initiated for flexion, abduction, and external rotation. Early passive motion is critical to prevent adhesions, loss of motion, and motion compensations. Matsen and Arntz[222] have demonstrated the repair is the strongest immediately after surgery, and the weakest at approximately 3 weeks.

At 6 weeks gentle isometrics are permitted. At 12 weeks the patient is allowed to begin active use of the arm. No heavy lifting is permitted for 6 to 12 months after repair; actual length depends on the repair and rate of progression.

The rehabilitation program following rotator cuff repair utilizing the deltoid-splitting technique appears to allow an accelerated rehabilitation approach when compared with detachment of the deltoid. We have utilized this type of surgical repair and rehabilitation approach since 1989, with successful results. The rehabilitation approach is based on the factors discussed previously, and we employ three different rehabilitation programs based on these factors (see the Box). We refer to the rehabilitation program as type I, II, and III to delineate our progressiveness. The type I program is utilized for the small tears in younger patients with

excellent to good tissues. The type II program is employed for medium-sized tears in active individuals with good tissues. The type III rehabilitation program is designed for the large to massive size tear in patients with tenuous repair with fair to poor tissue quality. Thus the type I program is much more progressive than the type II or III program, with the program chosen as dictated by the patient's individual pathology at the time of surgery.

There are several areas unique to our rehabilitation program which we will briefly discuss. Reestablishing passive motion expeditiously and safely is of paramount importance. Immediately after surgery (next day) the patient's arm is passively moved through the range of motion (flexion, external, and internal rotation). We allow active assisted external rotation/internal rotation using an L-bar performed in the scapular plane. The patient will also perform pendulum exercises for motion but to also neuromodulate pain. At approximately 7 days after surgery we allow the patient to begin active assisted arm elevation in the scapular plane with an L-bar. Often the patient will experience discomfort or an inability to elevate or to control arm lowering from 20° to 50° of elevation; hence assistance can be performed by the therapist, or a support (pillow) is provided in this range. As motion improves, the arm is abducted to 75° to perform external rotation/internal rotation stretching and then last is lowered to arm at side for external rotation/internal rotation movements to control tension on the repair. Our goal is full passive motion in usually 6 to 8 weeks after surgery for our type II or III repairs and in 4 to 6 weeks for the type I. Active motion usually takes longer because of inhibition and weakness of the rotator cuff muscles. Passive motion should be obtained gradually but within an acceptable time frame to prevent stiffness, arthrofibrosis, or adhesive capsulitis.

We believe strengthening/active exercises should be performed immediately after the operation to prevent/minimize "cuff shutdown" (rotator cuff muscular inhibition). During the first several weeks the patient performs submaximal, painfree, multiangle isometrics for the external rotation/internal rotation, abductors, flexors, and elbow flexor muscle groups. At approximately 7 to 14 days after surgery we begin rhythm stabilization exercises in the supine position. These exercises are designed to promote dynamic stabilization of the glenohumeral joint through isometric cocontraction of the surrounding musculature. We begin these exercises in what Wilk refers to as the "balanced position" (which is defined as 100° to 110° of flexion and approximately 10° to 20° of horizontal abduction. In this position the therapist provides an isometric force to resist flexion/extension and horizontal abduction/adduction. Note the amount of force is low, usually 4 to 5 pounds, thus providing the stimulus to cause a submaximal isometric cuff contraction. We utilize this balance position because of the biomechanics of the shoulder joint. As previously discussed,

Type two - Rotator cuff repair (deltoid splitting) medium to large tear (greater than 1 cm and less than 5 cm)

Phase one - protective phase (week 0-6)

Goals: (1) Gradual increase in ROM
(2) Increase shoulder strength
(3) Decrease pain and inflammation

A. Week 0-3
1. Brace of Sling (Physician determines)
2. Pendulum exercises
3. Active Assisted ROM exercises (L-Bar Exercise)
a. Flexion to 125°
b. ER/IR (shoulder at 40° abduction) to 30°
4. Passive ROM to tolerance
5. Rope and Pulley - flexion
6. Elbow ROM and Hand gripping exercises
7. Submaximal Isometrics
a. Flexors
b. Abductors
c. ER/IR
d. Elbow Flexors
8. Ice and pain modalities

B. Week 3-6
1. Discontinue brace or sling
2. Continue all exercises listed above
3. AAROM exercises
a. Flexion to 145°
b. ER/IR (performed at 65° abduction) range to tolerance

Phase two - intermediate phase (week 7-14)

Goals: (1) Full, nonpainful ROM (Week 10)
(2) Gradual increase in strength
(3) Decrease pain

A. Week 7-10
1. AAROM L-Bar exercises
a. Flexion to 160°
b. ER/IR (performed at 90° shoulder abduction) to tolerance (Greater than 45°)
2. Strengthening exercises
a. Exercise tubing ER/IR arm at side
b. Initiate humeral head stabilizing exercise
c. Initiate *dumbbell strengthening exercises for:
- Deltoid
- Supraspinatus

- Elbow Flexion/extension
- Scapulae muscles

B. Week 10-14 (Full range of motion desired by Week 10-12)
1. Continue all exercises listed above
2. Initiate isokinetic strengthening (scapular plane)
3. Initiate sidelying ER/IR exercises (dumbbell)
4. Initiate neuromuscular control exercises for scapular
*Patient must be able to elevate arm without shoulder and scapular hiking before initiating isotonics; if unable, maintain on humeral head stabilizing exercises.

Phase three - advanced strengthening phase (week 15-26)

Goals: (1) Maintain full, nonpainful ROM
(2) Improve strength of shoulder
(3) Improve neuromuscular control
(4) Gradual return to functional activities

A. Week 15-20
1. Continue AAROM exercise with L-Bar - Flexion, ER, IR
2. Self Capsular stretches
3. Aggressive strengthening program
a. Shoulder Flexion
b. Shoulder Abduction (to 90°)
c. Supraspinatus
d. ER/IR
e. Elbow Flexors/Extensors
f. Scapulae Muscles
4. Conditioning program

B. Week 21-26
1. Continue all exercises listed above
2. Isokinetic test (modified neutral position) for ER/IR at 180° and 300°/sec
3. Initiate interval sport program

Phase four - return to activity phase (week 24-28)

Goals: (1) Gradual return to recreational sport activities

A. Week 24-28
1. Continue all strengthening exercises
2. Continue all flexibility exercises
3. Continue progression on interval programs

---

the deltoid acts as a compressor at 100° or greater of elevation; thus the superior shear force often generated by the deltoid is greatly diminished (Fig. 15-21). These rhythmic stabilization exercises are performed at 100° and 125° of elevation. In addition, these drills are performed for the external rotation/internal rotation in the plane of the scapula. As the patient reestablishes control of the glenohumeral joint, the drills can be performed at lower flexion angles (i.e., 30°, 60°, 90°). The progression is from supine

(with scapula support) to sidelying and finally seated. Usually by 3 to 4 weeks the patient can begin isotonic exercises using the weight of the arm, progressing to light weight by 4 to 6 weeks.

When the patient exhibits the inability to actively elevate the arm as illustrated in Fig. 15-22, we believe this is related to a lack of dynamic humeral head control. The individual may be able to elevate to 25° to 30°, but then the entire shoulder girdle begins to elevate. This is because the strong

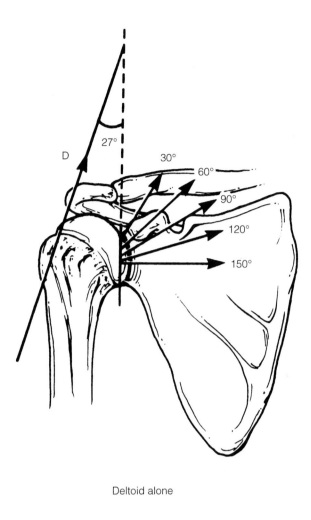

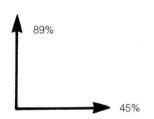

Deltoid alone

Fig. 15-21. Deltoid muscle angle of insertion and percentage of shear and compressive forces generated at neutral position. The direction of the resultant forces produced by the deltoid during abduction is illustrated. (From Kelley MJ: Biomechanics of the shoulder. In Kelley MJ, Clark WA, editors: *Orthopaedic therapy of the shoulder,* Philadelphia, 1995, JB Lippincott.)

deltoid overpowers the weaker cuff muscles, causing the humeral head to superiorly displace (Fig. 15-21). This is typically seen in patients with a cuff tear. Exercises that enhance dynamic stability attempt to alleviate this problem.

By 3 months the patient is progressed to a program of isotonic strengthening and flexibility exercises. We encourage patients to perform exercise bouts of low weight and high repetition to enhance endurance. Usually by 5 to 6

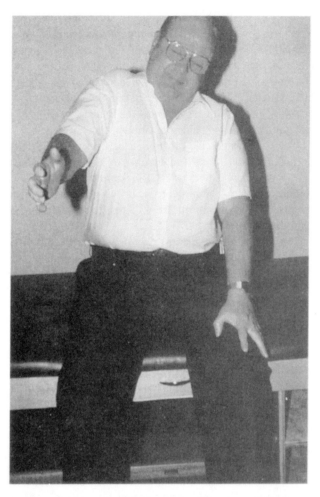

Fig. 15-22. This patient exhibits the inability to actively elevate his arm due to a loss of dynamic glenohumeral joint stability. Note the humeral head displacing superiorly during arm elevation.

months (depending on type of rehabilitation) the patient may play golf or other recreational sport activities.

It is important to realize that these are general rehabilitation guidelines; the specifics should be based on the individual characteristics and goals of the patient. We believe strongly on immediate motion and reestablishing voluntary dynamic stability of the glenohumeral joint—but it must be performed safely.

Quite possibly, one of the most challenging patients is the patient who presents with an irreparable rotator cuff tear related to size of tear or tissue quality, or he or she has retorn the original repair. Several investigations have noted significant improvement in comfort and function for these patients through acromial decompression and debridement of the frayed cuff tissue.[26,68,204,387] It is our experience that the posterior cuff is critical for these patients in controlling and stabilizing the glenohumeral joint. The principles of rehabilitation for these patients are the same as the postoperative rotator cuff repair patients utilizing dynamic control exercises.

GLENOID LABRUM LESIONS

In recent years, increasing attention has been paid to the glenoid labrum. As previously discussed, the glenoid labrum enhances the congruence of the glenohumeral joint by contributing to the depth of the glenoid by approximately 50% (Howell). This is evident in the detachment of the anterior labrum from the glenoid—the Bankart lesion, which results in anterior shoulder instability.[31]

There is considerable variation in the size and shape of the normal glenoid labrum. The labrum can range in width from 1 to 5 mm. Typically, the anterior labrum is triangular or rounded, whereas the posterior labrum is generally rounded in appearance. The inferior labrum tends to be much thicker than the superior aspect.[105,140]

Glenoid labrum lesions are extremely common and can be classified as either atraumatic or traumatic.[196] Injury to the glenoid capsulolabral complex is known to occur with dislocations and traumatic subluxations. A wide spectrum of glenoid labral injuries may occur, including a detachment of the labrum from the glenoid, a frank tear, or a combination of these lesions. Usually, a disruption of the capsulolabral complex results in recurrent anterior instability of the glenohumeral joint.

The shoulder joint is subjected to tremendous repetitive stresses during the throwing motion. Andrews et al.[13] have described a tear of the anterosuperior aspect of glenoid labrum near the origin of the long head of the biceps in the thrower. They theorized this lesion was secondary to the repetitive, forceful contraction of the biceps during the follow-through phase of the throw. Andrews et al.[12] reported on 73 throwers' shoulders arthroscopically with 83% of the cases exhibiting an anterosuperior labral lesion (60% isolated, 23% involved both the posterosuperior and antero-superior labrum).

Recently, Snyder et al.[339] have described an anterosupe-rior labral-biceps complex lesion through a four-type classification scheme. (Fig. 15-23) This superior labrum, anterior, and posterior (SLAP) lesion begins posteriorly and extends anteriorly, involves the "anchor" of the long head of the biceps brachii to the labrum, and is symptomatic relatively rarely (less than 5% of arthroscopically examined shoulders).[339] The mechanism injury producing this type of lesion has been described as one of a compressor force directly applied to the shoulder, usually as the result of a fall onto an outstretched arm. The second mechanism is due to a traction onto the arm frequently caused by the biomechan-ics of an overhead sport movement.

The recognition of labral lesions is often difficult to appreciate on clinical examination. Specific tests for the labrum have been discussed previously. Patients often complain of pain with specific activities, particularly overhead activities and movements. A "popping," "click-ing," or "catching" sensation may be described. CT arthrography or MRI is often required to make the diagnosis

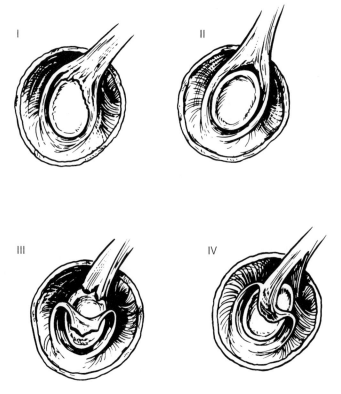

Fig. 15-23. Snyder's classification of SLAP lesions (Type I-IV). (From Guido EJ, Zuckerman JD: Glenoid labral lesions. In Andrews JR, Wilk KE, editors: *The athlete's shoulder,* New York, 1994, Churchill Livingstone.)

of a labral lesion. Several investigators have shown a sensitivity of 100% and a specificity of 97% in the diagnosis of anterior labral tears with CT arthrography.[195,399]

The treatment of glenoid labral lesions is based on numerous factors. In patients who complain of dysfunction related to pain, clicking, popping, or a locking sensation, arthroscopic resection is generally indicated. In these patients, resection of the labral tear usually results in significant symptomatic improvement. If the labral tear is associated with glenohumeral joint instability, excision of the torn labrum will probably result in resolution of the pain, but the dysfunction from the underlying instability will remain unchanged. However, in some cases the manifesta-tion of instability symptoms occur only after the labrum is excised.[8,12] Hence, the question should be asked, "Is the labral tear an isolated injury, or the result of instability?" In our experience, patients who exhibit an atraumatic labral tear may be suspect for subtle instability; thus the rehabilitation must be geared toward dynamic stabilization before and following the labral resection. Guidi and Zuckerman[140] note that an important principle to follow is that patients with labral tears with associated instability will not improve after simple excision of the labral tear. Therefore stabilization surgery should be considered in these instances.[339]

It should be strongly emphasized that following arthroscopic debridement or excision of labral tears the patient must be placed on a structured, supervised, and progressive rehabilitation program. The rehabilitation program must be designed differently for the debrided labral lesion compared with the reattached superior labral lesion. The patient with the reattached labrum requires a longer period of time of immediate postoperative guarded motion to allow adequate healing of the repaired tissue. Conversely, in the patient who undergoes debridement of the labrum, motion and strengthening may progress more rapidly, and rehabilitation is based solely on symptoms and signs. Each rehabilitation program must be tailored to meet the specific needs of the patient being treated.

NEUROVASCULAR COMPRESSION SYNDROMES

Neurovascular compression syndromes, also referred to as thoracic outlet syndromes, have been described as clinical disorders for several hundred years. In 1743 Hunald[162] was the first to describe cervical ribs as an anatomical anomaly causing thoracic outlet compression. In 1861 Coote[91] described a surgical procedure that advocated removal of the first rib. Several others have advocated first rib resection for thoracic outlet syndrome patients.[346,352,381] Adson and Coffey[3] in 1927 were the first to describe successful relief of thoracic outlet compression by sectioning the scalenus anticus muscle. These results were later confirmed by other investigators.[248,273] Lewis and Pickering[205] in 1934 were the first to discuss neurovascular compression at the costoclavicular level. Therefore numerous structures may contribute or cause neurovascular compression basically described as thoracic outlet.

There are several locations where compression of these neurovascular structures can occur with the diagnosis of neurovascular compression most often made after a detailed history, physical examination, and ancillary tests. Symptoms vary depending on the anatomical structures (nerve, artery, or vein) being compromised and on the site of compression. Compression of the lower trunk of the brachial plexus in the thoracic outlet frequently results in pain and paresthesia from the neck and shoulder down to the medial aspect of the hand, with associated hand weakness. Compression of the upper trunk of the brachial plexus results in more obscure symptoms, with proximal pain in the neck and shoulder region, similar to that of a cervical disk herniation.[27] Patients with vascular compression often present with complaints of upper limb heaviness, fatigue, and claudication. Arterial insufficiency usually produces symptoms of coolness, numbness, and exertional fatigue, whereas venous obstruction causes upper limb edema, heaviness, and cyanosis. If both blood vessels and nerves are being compressed, a mixed pattern of symptoms will normally be present.[27] Multiple tests have been described for evaluation of these structures,[27,184] and it should be carefully noted that these tests can result in both false-positive and false-negative findings. Several authors have reported that 50% of the normal population will exhibit a positive Adson test.[66,297,304,330] Therefore the test should be considered truly positive only when the maneuver reproduces the patient's symptoms. Specific tests such as nerve conduction studies and evoked potential stimulation have not proven reliable in the diagnosis of neurovascular compression syndrome.[66,297,304,312,330,344] Noninvasive studies such as Doppler sonography may be effective in measuring arterial blood flow, especially in the overhead athlete.[268]

The term thoracic outlet syndrome is an ill-defined, nonspecific diagnosis. There are many causes of neurovascular compression syndrome, both structural and functional. The role of the therapist is to determine the cause or causes of the compression, find the site of the lesion, and treat the specifically involved tissues.

The initial treatment for neurovascular compression syndrome should be a nonoperative physical therapy program. The patient may be treated with nonsteroidal antiinflammatory medications, massage, soft tissue mobilization, joint mobilization, stretching, and strengthening. The specific program is directed to address the problems associated with the tissues involved. Thus an elevated first rib may be treated with joint mobilization, soft tissue mobilization, stretching, etc. The patient's postural abnormalities can significantly contribute to neurovascular compression syndrome, and these findings must be treated.[65] Exercises to strengthen the scapular muscles (such as the trapezius, rhomboids, and serratus anterior) will assist in proper positioning of the scapulae. Stretching of the scalene muscles and pectoralis minor may also be helpful. If nonoperative treatment is unsuccessful, surgical decompression may become necessary to alleviate the patient's symptoms. Such surgical procedures are excision of a cervical rib, scalenotomy, or release of the fibromuscular bands causing the neurovascular compression.[27]

Axillary artery occlusion can produce numerous symptoms associated with neurovascular compression syndrome.[268,341,360] A clinical condition referred to as effort thrombosis is frequently associated with repetitive, vigorous activities or blunt trauma that produces a direct or indirect injury to the vein.[370] This condition is somewhat rare, accounting for less than 2% of the total venous thromboses.[1] Rest usually resolves the acute pain and swelling within 3 to 4 days. In most cases conservatively treated (60% to 85%) full resolution of symptoms occurs; however, some patients may experience residual symptoms due to occlusion of the vein. Medications such as anticoagulation therapy may be used to prevent the progression of the thrombus.[1,341] Surgical intervention has been advocated for this pathology with good results and no residual symptoms.[1,24]

Quadrilateral space syndrome involves compression of

the axillary nerve and the posterior humeral circumflex artery in the quadrilateral space.[71,72] For more detailed information regarding neurovascular compression syndromes of the shoulder, the reader is referred to the following written works.[28,146,312]

ADHESIVE CAPSULITIS

Adhesive capsulitis is a commonly encountered clinical condition seen by therapists. The condition is often referred to as "the frozen shoulder," which is an unfortunate term that is nonspecific, overused, and frequently misapplied. Adhesive capsulitis appears to be a more appropriate term for a specific clinical pathology; it describes a loss of active and passive range of motion due to capsular adhesions.

The pathophysiology of this condition remains poorly understood. The condition was first described by Duplay[113] in 1872 as "periarthritic scapulohumerale." Codman[83] in 1934 described the syndrome as tendinitis with secondary involvement of the bursae. Simmonds[335] reported the cause of the condition to be a vascular reaction around areas of degeneration within the supraspinatus tendon. The "frozen shoulder condition" has been referred to as many various clinical entities such as calcifying tendinitis, adhesive subacromial bursitis, bicipital tendinitis, supraspinatus tendinitis, and partial tears of the rotator cuff. Codman[83] summarized the condition as an entity that is . . . "difficult to define, difficult to treat, difficult to explain . . . from the point of view of pathology." Neviaser[258] in 1945 first introduced the term "adhesive capsulitis" due to the capsular thickening and contractions he observed on 10 frozen shoulder patients. Although the pathology has become better defined in recent years, considerable controversy remains concerning the etiology and what constitutes effective treatment.

It is generally accepted that the glenohumeral joint capsule becomes inflamed, thickened, and excessively scarred and that adhesions form to the humeral head.[260,264] In addition, cellular changes of chronic inflammation with fibrosis and perivascular infiltration in the subsynovial layer of the capsule consistent with an inflammatory process have also been noted in some patients.

The condition may develop in isolation or secondarily with another associated pathology. In secondary adhesive capsulitis the condition develops related to previous trauma such as overuse tendinitis, minor muscle soreness, immobilization, or guarded motion. In primary adhesive capsulitis, the onset is spontaneous without any particular trauma or injury. In other words, it truly has an unexplained origin.

Neviaser[262,264] has described four stages in the adhesive capsulitis disease process. In stage one the patient has mild signs and symptoms, and minimal restrictions in motion occur. This is often referred to as the preadhesive stage. The second stage is referred to as the adhesive stage. In this phase motion is restricted and painful, synovitis is present, and adhesions begin to form onto the humeral head. In stage three, the maturation stage, the adhesions are significant, and there is a significant loss of the axillary fold of the inferior glenohumeral joint capsule. In the last stage synovitis is no longer present, but the axillary fold is severely contracted, and range of motion is severely restricted. It has been noted that the affected shoulder demonstrates a significant loss of joint volume. In the normal shoulder the joint capsule can be injected with 20 to 30 ml of fluid, whereas the shoulder with adhesive capsulitis can accommodate only 5 to 10 ml.

The clinical diagnosis of adhesive capsulitis may be difficult because of associated pathologies that present with similar signs and symptoms.[292,305] Numerous authors have classified adhesive capsulitis into various conditions such as irritative capsulitis,[400] early capsulitis,[185] and posttraumatic stiff shoulders.[299] Neviaser[259] used a combination of arthrographic findings and clinical criteria to classify patients as either having adhesive capsulitis or a stiff and painful shoulder.

The condition is typically more common in women and frequently occurs during the fifth and sixth decades of life. Patients are usually middle-aged, with the mean age for males being 55 years and females 52 years.[213] In a study of more than 1000 patients, the incidence in the nondiabetic population was reported as 2.3%.[64] Seventeen percent may experience bilateral involvement.[213] There is a higher incidence of adhesive capsulitis in the diabetes mellitus patient, which appears to be approximately 10% to 20%.[64,203,278] Diabetic patients who are insulin-dependent have a higher incidence (36%) with a bilateral involvement up to 42%.[123,233] Other predisposing factors include minor trauma, cervical disk disease,[213] hyperthyroidism,[108,401] intrathoracic disorders,[23,179] and personality disorders.[93] Coventry[93] chose the term periarthritic personality, which may contribute to the patient developing adhesive capsulitis. He observed that most patients had "a peculiar emotional constitution in which the patient was unable to tolerate pain, expected others to get them well, and refused to take any personal initiative in their recovery."

On physical examination, patients demonstrate increased compensatory scapular motion with both active and passive motion grossly limited. Motion is limited in all directions, but most commonly a capsular pattern is present.[96] The capsular pattern at the glenohumeral joint involves external rotation being most limited, followed by lessening degrees by abduction, then internal rotation being least limited.[96] Active arm motion often reveals excessive scapular motion, shoulder girdle hiking, and occasional tenderness in the upper trapezius.

The clinical presentation of primary adhesive capsulitis has been described as progressing through a three-stage course. The first stage is referred to as the painful phase. There is usually a gradual onset of diffuse shoulder pain, which is worse at night, especially when lying on the shoulder. Because of the pain the patient does not use the arm, which renders the patient some satisfaction in the false belief that he or she is doing the right thing. The duration of this phase is variable and can last anywhere from 2 to 9 months.[93] The stiffening phase is a slowly progressing period of loss of shoulder movement. This phase may last 4 to 12 months.[300] The patient exhibits a significant loss of motion, especially overhead movements, reaching in the back pocket, dressing activities, and/or personal hygiene.[96] The final phase described is the thawing phase, in which the patient gradually regains shoulder motion. This phase is extremely variable. As motion slowly increases, there is a progressive lessening of shoulder discomfort. The time course required to return of shoulder motion is very unpredictable.

The treatment of the adhesive capsulitis patient is controversial. Some authors believe that this condition is a self-limiting disorder that lasts 12 to 18 months and that even the most severe cases recover with or without treatment in about 2 years.[138,141,213,378,400] In contrast, several authors have reported patients exhibiting a symptomatic adhesive capsulitis condition for 10 years.[50,78,93,331,335]

The major objectives of treatment are to relieve the discomfort and restore motion, thereby restoring function.[245] Because the pathophysiology is poorly understood, many different forms of treatment have been used empirically to manage this condition. The choice of treatment should be based on the clinical findings and the stage of the condition at the time the patient seeks treatment. The treatment should be cautiously modified based on the individual's response to the program and his or her rate of progression.

The treatment of a patient who presents with a painful shoulder (the painful stage) is directed toward prevention of adhesive capsulitis and patient education. In this situation the patient is instructed on range-of-motion exercises and gentle strengthening and is informed to use the arm for functional activities, even though there may be persisting discomfort. These treatment guidelines are especially important for individuals with predisposing factors for developing adhesive capsulitis. The patient is instructed to avoid immobilization. Binder et al.,[49] on questioning their adhesive capsulitis patients, found that 50% received no advice from the primary care physician on the need for early motion. And of those patients receiving advice, 75% were told to rest the shoulder, and only 25% were told to gently exercise.

The treatment of patients who present in stage two, the stiffening phase, consists of a passive stretching program. Passive stretching may include physiological stretching, joint mobilization techniques, and self-stretching by the patient. Passive stretching techniques are preferred over active techniques because they allow greater mechanical advantage than the patient's muscle alone.[217] Joint mobilization gliding techniques are often performed at the end range of the available motion to overcome stiffness by stretching the capsule.[216] The mobilization glides should be performed in the direction of capsular restrictions. The intensity of the stretching and/or mobilization glides should be modified based on the patient's pain response and inflammatory response. Prior to stretching, heating the tissues through a passive warm-up (moist hot pack) or active warm-up (active exercise) may be beneficial in increasing the extensibility of the collagen fibers and assist with patient relaxation. In addition, the patient is instructed to perform range-of-motion and stretching exercises at home as frequently as possible; patients who perform stretching for 5 to 10 minutes and do so 10 to 12 times per day appear to progress more rapidly than patients who exercise only a couple of times per day.

In patients who have reached a plateau regarding their motion progression or have had chronic adhesive capsulitis, we have noted that the use of low-load, long duration stretching techniques has been extremely beneficial in restoring motion. Several investigators have reported improved efficiency in improving motion by using a low load applied to the structure for a long duration (greater than 15 minutes).[207,374] Lentell et al.[203b] have noted greater effects of low-load, long duration (LLLD) stretching when performed with superficial heat applied. We believe the LLLD stretching techniques can be extremely beneficial in treating the adhesive capsulitis patient, because these techniques utilize a force that is more likely to induce permanent connective tissue changes. This technique (LLLD) may be performed as part of the home program; the home program is extremely important in restoring functional use of the arm. As the patient's motion improves, supervised physical therapy may be diminished to occasional visits and eventual discharge.

If all conservative measures fail, surgery may be necessary to restore full motion. In some cases a manipulation with the patient under anesthesia may be performed to restore motion but only in mature stage three patients. Often during this manipulation, the "popping' of adhesions may be felt.[264] If full motion is not obtained during the manipulation, then an arthrotomy or arthroscopic scar resection may be necessary. With this technique excessive scar tissue is resected from the anteroinferior capsule, subacromial space, etc. Immediately following the manipulation the patient is placed on a continuous passive motion device, and motion exercises with the therapist are instituted to prevent the condition from redeveloping. Other techniques such as distension of the capsule,[10,299] release of subscapularis trigger points,[359] and infiltration of the shoulder joint capsule[244] may be beneficial. Other techniques such as intraarticular injections,[210,293] oral corticosteroids,[95] radiotherapy,[93] and stellate ganglion block[283] have been shown to have no significant advantage in treating adhesive capsulitis.

THE SHOULDER JOINT IN SPORTS
Overhead throwing

Overhead throwing is a highly skillful, extremely stressful, and violent activity that requires flexibility, strength, power, endurance, coordination, and timing. The throwing action requires precisely coordinated movement and a synchronized muscular firing pattern, all of which must occur at an angular velocity faster than any other upper extremity sport movement.[126] The muscles most active during the arm cocking phase are the serratus anterior, subscapularis, infraspinatus, and teres minor.[109] During late cocking the internal rotators are eccentrically loaded and act to decelerate the end range of arm external rotation. In addition, these muscles are elastically stretched to provide a stretch stimulus, provoking a powerful shortening internal rotation acceleration muscular response. The rotator cuff muscles must also contract to stabilize the glenohumeral joint. In late cocking the anterior-inferior glenohumeral joint capsule acts to prevent the humeral head from subluxing anteriorly on the glenoid.

Once the arm reaches maximal external rotation, the elbow joint begins to extend, and the shoulder joint internally rotates, initiating the acceleration phase of throwing. During this phase the angular velocity at the shoulder joint exceeds 7000°/sec.[125] Regardless of what type of pitch is thrown or the style of the thrower (sidearm, overhead) at ball release, the shoulder is abducted between 90° to 100°. The difference between the "overhead" and the "sidearm" thrower is not the amount of shoulder abduction, but rather the degree of lateral tilt of the trunk.[110,126] During the acceleration phase the rotator cuff and deltoid muscles exhibit low to moderate levels of electromyographic activity (Table 15-2), whereas the internal rotators (subscapularis, latissimus dorsi, pectoralis major) exhibit higher levels of muscular activity (115%, 88%, and 54% MVIC, respectively).[109] These muscles act concentrically to accelerate the arm forward and downward during acceleration.[109] The serratus anterior also exhibits moderately high levels (60% MVIC) of muscular activity during this phase.[109]

After ball release, the arm continues to internally rotate and horizontally adduct at the shoulder joint while extending at the elbow. Because of this internal rotation, the hand appears to pronate. The distinctive forces at the glenohumeral joint are approximately equal to body weight.[110] The teres minor, posterior deltoid, middle deltoid, and infraspinatus exhibit the greatest amount of electromyographic activity.[109] During this phase the posterior shoulder musculature acts eccentrically to decelerate the arm, resists glenohumeral joint distraction, and dissipates the tremendous forces generated during the throwing motion (acting as a shock-absorber).

The energy generated during the acceleration and deceleration phases of throwing must be dissipated after ball release by follow-through, allowing the larger body parts to help dissipate the energy generated in the throwing arm. To reduce the distraction forces of deceleration, the throwing arm should exhibit a complete follow-through path that allows the energy to be dissipated over a longer period of time; thus the throwing hand should reach toward the opposite leg. A pitcher whose hand ends up directly toward the target is likely placing excessive stress on the posterior shoulder structures.

Hence, the thrower's shoulder joint capsule must be loose enough to allow excessive motion, especially external rotation, while maintaining dynamic joint stability. The joint stability is provided by the muscles about the shoulder and joint capsule. The shoulder musculature must be able to dynamically stabilize, act to accelerate the arm, and act to decelerate or dissipate the forces at the shoulder joint. Due to these tremendous demands occurring at extremely high angular velocities and the repetitive nature of throwing, the thrower becomes susceptible to a variety of shoulder joint injuries. The recognition of these injuries can be extremely difficult at times because of the adaptive hyperlaxity of the shoulder joint capsule. The most common injuries are overuse tendonitis, tensile tissue failure, shoulder capsular hyperlaxity, labral lesions, and posterior cuff impingement. The reader is referred to several recommended publications for a thorough description of these injuries and treatment options.[14,18,177]

Tennis strokes

Most arm movements during the tennis stroke require the significant muscular activity of specific shoulder muscles that occur at moderately high angular velocities. The tennis serve may be divided into four specific phases: the windup, cocking, acceleration, and follow-through phases much like that seen in throwing.[118,301] Several investigators have noted a significant difference in the electromyographic activity of skilled versus unskilled players when serving. The unskilled player exhibits significantly higher electromyographic activity during the serve.[232,368]

Similar to serving, the forehand and backhand ground strokes can be broken down into three phases: preparation, acceleration, and follow-through, with obviously significantly contrasting muscular actions seen in each.[118,301]

Biomechanical analysis of the forehand ground strokes indicates a peak internal rotation angular velocity ranging between 365°/sec and 700°/sec. To enhance ball velocity and shot accuracy, the proper biomechanics of the forehand stroke should be from a low to high position. This requires proper timing, coordination, flexibility, and strength. The unskilled player often exhibits an improper biomechanical movement in which the player attempts to put top spin on the ball by "rolling over" the ball.[116] This improper tennis stroke is achieved by excessive shoulder internal rotation and forearm pronation and may eventually lead to overuse injuries of the rotator cuff such as tendinitis, impingement, and possible tissue failures.

Peak external rotation angular velocities during the backhand stroke in the skilled tennis player range between 325°/sec to 1600°/sec.[139,301] The backhand stroke in a skilled player is one movement where a novice often experiences significant problems mastering the stroke and frequently exhibits improper mechanics.[116] The player

Table 15-2 EMG of muscle groups in the upper extremity during pitching*

	No. of pitchers	Windup	Early cocking	Late cocking	Acceleration	Deceleration	Follow-through
Scapular muscles							
Upper trapezius	11	18 ± 16	64 ± 53	37 ± 29	69 ± 31	53 ± 22	14 ± 12
Middle trapezius	11	7 ± 5	43 ± 22	51 ± 24	71 ± 32	35 ± 17	15 ± 14
Lower trapezius	13	13 ± 12	39 ± 30	38 ± 29	76 ± 55	78 ± 33	25 ± 15
Serratus anterior (sixth rib)	11	14 ± 13	44 ± 35	69 ± 32	60 ± 53	51 ± 30	32 ± 18
Serratus anterior (fourth rib)	10	20 ± 20	40 ± 22	106 ± 56	50 ± 46	34 ± 7	41 ± 24
Rhomboids	11	7 ± 8	35 ± 24	41 ± 26	71 ± 35	45 ± 28	14 ± 20
Levator scapula	11	6 ± 5	35 ± 14	72 ± 54	77 ± 28	33 ± 16	14 ± 13
Glenohumeral muscles							
Anterior deltoid	16	15 ± 12	40 ± 20	28 ± 30	27 ± 19	47 ± 34	21 ± 16
Middle deltoid	14	9 ± 8	44 ± 19	12 ± 17	36 ± 22	59 ± 19	16 ± 13
Posterior deltoid	18	6 ± 5	42 ± 26	28 ± 27	68 ± 66	60 ± 28	13 ± 11
Supraspinatus	16	13 ± 12	60 ± 31	49 ± 29	51 ± 46	39 ± 43	10 ± 9
Infraspinatus	16	11 ± 9	30 ± 18	74 ± 34	31 ± 28	37 ± 20	20 ± 16
Teres minor	12	5 ± 6	23 ± 15	71 ± 42	54 ± 50	84 ± 52	25 ± 21
Subscapularis (lower third)	11	7 ± 9	26 ± 22	62 ± 19	56 ± 31	41 ± 23	25 ± 18
Subscapularis (upper third)	11	7 ± 8	37 ± 26	99 ± 55	115 ± 82	60 ± 36	16 ± 15
Pectoralis major	14	6 ± 6	11 ± 13	56 ± 27	54 ± 24	29 ± 18	31 ± 21
Latissimus dorsi	13	12 ± 10	33 ± 33	50 ± 37	88 ± 53	59 ± 35	24 ± 18
Elbow and forearm muscles							
Triceps	13	4 ± 6	17 ± 17	37 ± 32	89 ± 40	54 ± 23	22 ± 18
Biceps	18	8 ± 9	22 ± 14	26 ± 20	20 ± 16	44 ± 32	16 ± 14
Brachialis	13	8 ± 5	17 ± 13	18 ± 26	20 ± 22	49 ± 29	13 ± 17
Brachioradialis	13	5 ± 5	35 ± 20	31 ± 24	16 ± 12	46 ± 24	22 ± 29
Pronator teres	14	14 ± 16	18 ± 15	39 ± 28	85 ± 39	51 ± 21	21 ± 21
Supinator	13	9 ± 7	38 ± 20	54 ± 38	55 ± 31	59 ± 31	22 ± 19
Wrist and finger muscles							
Extensor carpi radialis longus	13	11 ± 8	53 ± 24	72 ± 37	30 ± 20	43 ± 24	22 ± 14
Extensor carpi radialis brevis	15	17 ± 17	47 ± 26	75 ± 41	55 ± 35	43 ± 28	24 ± 19
Extensor digitorum communis	14	21 ± 17	37 ± 25	59 ± 27	35 ± 35	47 ± 25	24 ± 18
Flexor carpi radialis	12	13 ± 9	24 ± 35	47 ± 33	120 ± 66	79 ± 36	35 ± 16
Flexor digitorum superficialis	11	16 ± 6	20 ± 23	47 ± 52	80 ± 66	71 ± 32	21 ± 11
Flexor carpi ulnaris	10	8 ± 5	27 ± 18	41 ± 25	112 ± 60	77 ± 42	24 ± 18

*Means and standard deviations, expressed as a percentage of the maximal manual muscle test.
Reprinted with permission of DiGiovine NM, Jobe FW, Pink M et al. An electromyographic analysis of the upper extremity in pitching *J Shoulder Elbow Surg* 1992;1:15.

should utilize the legs, hips, and trunk to provide rotational torque rather than relying solely on the shoulders and arm motions. Improper mechanics during the backhand may lead to a variety of injuries such as overuse tendinitis, especially lateral epicondylitis of the elbow, or posterior rotator cuff tendinitis. Ellenbecker[117] and Kibler et al.[194] have described strength characteristics of tennis players.

Golf swing

Golf is one of the fastest growing sports in the world and is enjoyed by millions of people annually. Thus occasional shoulder injuries develop as a result of golf participation. The golfer is considered an overhead athlete because of the degree of motion required to accomplish the golf swing. Although the golf swing is a continuous motion, it can be divided into three phases: the backswing, downswing, and follow-through phases.[35]

The backswing muscle pattern demonstrates the supraspinatus, infraspinatus, and deltoid being moderately active in elevating the arm and stabilizing the glenohumeral joint.[176] The primary purpose of the backswing is to elastically load (muscular stretch) the golfer's musculature, placing the body in the correct position to initiate the downswing.

The downswing is initiated just prior to the end of the backswing. Preparation for the downswing begins with the action of the feet. Foot action creates a ground reaction force to stop the backswing rotation of the body and initiate downward club rotation. This reaction occurs as the rear foot begins to push away from the target with a lateral force.[35] At this time a force couple is created as the rear foot begins to push backward and the front foot pushes forward at the same time.

During the downswing phase the shoulders rotate toward this target at an angular velocity of approximately 725°/sec.[35] The latissimus dorsi, pectoralis major, and serratus anterior are the most active, with the subscapularis, deltoid, and other rotator cuff muscles also contributing to the swing.[61,176] At ball impact, the muscles of the shoulders and arms are forcefully contracting, allowing the arms to achieve over 1150°/sec of angular velocity.

The follow-through is an important phase of the golf swing. During this phase the body must decelerate gradually to prevent injury. During deceleration, the shoulders rotate in a counterclockwise direction (for a right-handed golfer); the lead arm externally rotates, and the rear arm internally rotates. Rotation of the lead arm is particularly important in dissipating the potentially harmful forces created during the swing. If the lead arm does not externally rotate, then elbow flexion and wrist extension must occur, which may lead to injury. The rear shoulder must horizontally adduct and internally rotate, a position that often produces discomfort in the mature golfer's shoulder due to impingement, especially when the shoulder is inflexible. The muscle activity of the shoulders and arms is gradually decelerated throughout the follow-through. Thus it is imperative for the golfer, especially the recreational golfer, to finish the golf swing with a fluent, well-coordinated, and complete follow-through to prevent injury.[178]

Many golf injuries, especially in the mature golfer, are due to poor physical condition. The golfer may exhibit poor flexibility, abdominal weakness, and weakness of the shoulder musculature. This combination often leads to a swing that utilizes shoulder rotation but minimal leg and trunk rotation. Commonly, this will lead to a variety of overuse injuries at the shoulders.

Swimming

The swimmer's shoulder is subjected to tremendous forces that are repetitively applied to the joint, which may lead to a variety of injuries. Most swimming strokes require overhead motions. There are four major swimming stroke techniques: the freestyle, the butterfly, the backstroke, and the breaststroke. We discuss the freestyle stroke because of its primary applications.

The freestyle stroke can be divided into two main phases—the pull-through and the recovery phase.[246] Each of these two phases can be further divided into three separate stages. The pull-through phase is divided into the hand entry, middle pull-through, and late pull-through stages, whereas the recovery phase consists of the elbow lift, middle recovery, and late recovery stages.

The pull-through phase is the propulsion phase of the swim. It may be thought of as the acceleration phase, similar to the throwing motion. The pull-through phase composes 65% to 70% of the entire swimming stroke.[303,329] During the pull-through the shoulder moves into adduction, internal rotation, and extension. It has been reported that electromyographic activity in experienced swimmers is significantly less compared to the novice swimmer, and selective activation of the latissimus dorsi and the teres minor than the novice swimmer.[166]

The recovery phase accounts for 30% to 35% of the total freestyle stroke. The purpose of this phase is to return the arm and body to the starting position for the next pull-through. Breathing typically occurs by turning the head to the side.

The swimmer often complains of a painful shoulder. This condition is often described as supraspinatus and/or biceps tendinitis.[192] Frequently, the swimmer's shoulder pain has been associated with mechanical impingement due to improper stroke mechanics, fatigue, muscular imbalances, and inflexibility. Numerous factors may contribute to the painful swimmer's shoulder. Proper stroke mechanics with an adequate body roll is vital in maintaining a healthy shoulder. The training schedule for most swimmers includes at least 7000 yards per day of training. This may lead to overuse syndromes, muscular fatigue, and glenohumeral joint instability. The swimmer's shoulder must exhibit muscular balance. As previously mentioned, the latissimus dorsi, teres minor, pectoralis major, and subscapularis all exhibit significantly high muscle activity during the pull-through phase. Therefore any strengthening or rehabilitation program should emphasize external rotation strengthening to balance the shoulder. Last, the swimmer's shoulder must be flexible enough to propel the swimmer through the water. However, although flexibility is important, the swimmer must not induce shoulder hyperlaxity or instability because of excessive or improper stretching. Muscular endurance is key for symptom-free swimming, thus ensuring dynamic stability of the glenohumeral joint.

Prevention

Prevention of shoulder injuries is the key to symptom-free function in the overhead athlete. The athlete should participate in a year-round conditioning program that utilizes the principle of periodization. Thus various exercises and intensity of exercises, would be phased into and out of the program at appropriate times of the year. The conditioning program must be sport-specific and based on the individual's unique characteristics, body type, and injury history. We have established numerous exercise programs for the overhead athlete, particularly the thrower. Plyometric exercise may also be initiated prior to and in preparation for the competitive season.[384,391,395,397] In addition, we have established an interval sport program that may be utilized following an injury or to prepare the athlete for the next season.

The overhead athlete represents a significant challenge to the medical team to accurately diagnose and appropriately treat this type of patient. In the overhead sport movements the shoulder joint is subjected to tremendous forces, and the muscles about the shoulder complex play a critical role in producing proper motion, stabilizing the joint, and dissipating joint force. All of these factors must be carefully considered in managing and rehabilitating the overhead athlete.

Acknowledgement

The author wishes to acknowledge Christopher Arrigo, MS, PT, ATC, Laura Timmerman, MD, and James R. Andrews, MD, for their assistance in writing this chapter, and Jerri Conner, Glenn Dortch, and The American Sports Medicine Institute staff for their assistance in manuscript preparation and illustrations.

REVIEW QUESTIONS

1. How can an impingement sign maneuver be used in the diagnosis of rotator cuff pathologies as well as for determining an impingement of the supraspinatus tendon?
2. What are the primary functions of the scapula?
3. What would be the similarities and differences in the rehabilitation program used for a Bankart versus Putti-Platt surgical procedure?
4. What is the difference between a structural and a functional shoulder impingement?
5. What is the nonoperative physical therapy treatment program for neurovascular compression syndrome?

REFERENCES

1. Adams JT, DeWeese JA: "Effort" thrombosis of the axillary and subclavian veins, *J Trauma* 11:923, 1971.
2. Adson AW: Cervical ribs: Symptoms, differential diagnosis of section of the insertion of the scalenus anticus muscle, *J Int Coll Surg* 16:546, 1951.
3. Adson AW, Coffey JR: Cervical rib: method of anterior approach for relief of symptoms by division of scalenus anticus, *Ann Surg* 85:839, 1927.
4. Alldredge, RH: Surgical treatment of acromioclavicular dislocation, *Clin Orthop* 63:262, 1969.
5. Allman FL Jr: Fractures and ligamentous injuries of the clavicle and its articulation, *J Bone Joint Surg* 49A:774, 1967.
6. Altchek DW, Schwartz E, Warren RF: *Radiologic measurement of superior migration of the humeral head in impingement syndrome,* Academy Orthopaedic Surgeons Meeting, New Orleans, 1990.
7. Altchek DW, Warren RF, Skyhar MJ: T-plasty modification of the Bankart procedure for multidirectional instability of the anterior and inferior types, *J Bone Joint Surg Am* 73A:105, 1991.

8. Altchek DW, Ortiz G, Warren RF, Wickiewicz T: Arthroscopiclabral debridement—a three year follow-up study, *Orthop Trans* 14:258, 1990.
9. American Academy of Orthopaedic Surgeons. *Joint motion: method of measuring and recording,* Chicago, 1965, American Academy of Orthopaedic Surgeons.
10. Andren L, Lundberg BJ: Treatment of rigid shoulders by joint distension during arthrography, *Acta Orthop Scand* 36:45, 1965.
11. Andrews JR: Personal communication, 1995.
12. Andrews JR, Carson WG: The arthroscopic treatment of glenoid labrum tears in the throwing athlete, *Orthop Trans* 8:44, 1984.
13. Andrews JR, Carson WG, McLeod WD: Glenoid labrum tears related to the long head of the biceps, *Am J Sports Med* 13:337, 1985.
14. Andrews JR, Carson WG, Zarins B: *Injuries to the throwing arm,* Philadelphia, 1985, WB Saunders.
15. Andrews JR, Kupferman SP, Dillman CJ: Labral tears in throwing and racquet sports, *Clin Sports Med* 10:901, 1991.
16. Andrews JR, Meister K: Classification and treatment of rotator cuff injuries in the overhead athlete, *J Orthop Sports Phys Ther* 18:413, 1993.
17. Andrews JR, Satterwhite YE: Anatomic capsular shift, *J Orthop Tech* 1:151, 1993.
18. Andrews JR, Wilk KE: Shoulder injuries in baseball. In Wilk KE, Andrews JR, editors: *The athlete's shoulder,* New York, 1994, Churchill Livingstone.
19. Arciero RA, Wheeler JH, Ryan JB, McBride JT: Arthroscopic Bankart repair versus nonoperative treatment for acute, initial anterior shoulder dislocation, *Am J Sports Med* 22.5:589, 1994.
20. Armstrong, JR: Excision of the acromion in treatment of the supraspinatus syndrome: report of ninety-five excisions, *J Bone Joint Surg Br* 31B:436, 1949.
21. Arntz CT, Matsen FA: *Partial scapulectomy for disabling scapulothoracic snapping,* Annual Academy Orthopaedic Surgeons Meeting, New Orleans, 1990.
22. Arrigo CA, Wilk KE: Shoulder exercise: a criteria based approach to rehabilitation. In Clark WA, Kelly MJ, editors: *Orthopaedic therapy of the shoulder,* Philadelphia, 1994, JB Lippincott.
23. Askey, JM: The syndrome of painful disability of the shoulder and hand complicating coronary occlusion, *Am Heart J* 22:1, 1961.
24. Aziz S, Straehley CJ, Whelan TJ: Effort related axillosubclavian vein thrombosis: a new theory of pathogenesis and a plea for direct surgical intervention, *Am J Surg* 152:57, 1986.
25. Bailey RW, O'Connor GA, Tilus PD, Baril JD: A dynamic repair for acute and chronic injuries of the acromioclavicular area (abstract), *J Bone Joint Surg Am* 54A:1802, 1972.
26. Bakalim G, Pasila M: Surgical treatment of rupture of the rotator cuff tendon, *Acta Orthop Scand* 46:751, 1975.
27. Baker CL, Liu SH, Blackburn TA: Neurovascular compression syndrome of the shoulder. In Andrews JR, Wilk KE, editors: *The athlete's shoulder,* New York, 1994, Churchill Livingstone.
28. Baker CL, Thornberry R: Neurovascular syndromes. In Zarins B, editor: *Injuries to the throwing arm,* Philadelphia, 1985, WB Saunders.
29. Baker CL, Uribe JW, Whitman C: Arthroscopic evaluation of acute initial anterior shoulder dislocations, *Am J Sports Med* 18.1:25, 1990.
30. Bankart ASB: The pathology and treatment of recurrent dislocation of the shoulder joint, *Br J Surg* 16:23, 1939.
31. Bankart ASB: Recurrent or habitual dislocation of the shoulder joint, *Br Med J* 2:1132, 1923.
32. Bannister GC, Wallace WA, Stableforth PG, Hutson MA: The management of acute acromioclavicular dislocation, *J Bone Joint Surg* 71B:848, 1989.
33. Barber, FA: Complete posterior acromioclavicular dislocation: a case report, *Orthopedics* 10.3:493, 1987.
34. Bargren JH, Erlanger S, Dick HM: Biomechanics and comparison of

452   REGIONAL CONSIDERATIONS

two operative methods of treatment of complete acromioclavicular separation, *Clin Orthop* 130:267, 1978.

35. Barrentine, SW: Biomechanics of the golf swing, In Wilk KE, Andrews JR, editors: *Golf,* Birmingham, 1995, Odysseus.

36. Barrett WP, Franklin JL, Jackins SE et al: Total shoulder arthroplasty, *J Bone Joint Surg Am* 69A:865, 1987.

37. Basmajian JV, Bazart FJ: Factors preventing downward dislocation of the adducted shoulder joint, *J Bone Joint Surg Am* 41A:1182, 1959.

38. Bassett RW, Browne AO, Morrey BF, An KN: Glenohumeral muscle force and moment mechanics in a position of shoulder instability, *J Biomech* 23:405, 1990.

39. Bassett RW, Cofield RH: Acute tears of the rotator cuff. The timing of surgical repair, *Clin Orthop* 175:18, 1983.

40. Bateman, JE: *The shoulder and neck,* ed 2, Philadelphia, 1978, WB Saunders.

41. Bearden JM, Hughston JC, Whatley GS: Acromioclavicular dislocation: method of treatment, *J Sports Med* 1.4:5, 1973.

42. Bearn, JG: Direct observation on the function of the capsule of the sternoclavicular joint in clavicular support, *J Anat* 101:159, 1967.

43. Bechtol, CO: Biomechanics of the shoulder, *Clin Orthop* 146:37, 1980.

44. Bergfeld JA, Andrish JT, Clancy WG: Evaluation of the acromio-clavicular joint following first- and second-degree sprains, *Am J Sports Med* 6.4:153, 1978.

45. Berson BL, Gilbert MS, Green S: Acromioclavicular dislocations: treatment by transfer of the conjoined tendon and distal end of the coracoid process to the clavicle, *Clin Orthop* 135:157, 1978.

46. Bigliani LU, Kimmel J, McCann PD, Wolf I: Repair of rotator cuff tears in tennis players, *Am J Sports Med* 20:112, 1992.

47. Bigliani LU, Norris TR, Fisher J et al: The relationship between the unfused acromial epiphysis and subacromial impingement lesions, *Orthop Trans* 7.1:138, 1983.

48. Bigliani LU, Pollock RG, Soslowsky LJ, Flatow EL, Pawluk RJ, Mow VC: Tensile properties of the inferior glenohumeral ligament, *J Orthop Res* 10:187, 1992.

49. Binder A, Hazleman BL, Parr G, Roberts S: A controlled study of oral prednisolone in frozen shoulder, *Br J Rheumatol* 25:288, 1986.

50. Binder AI, Bulgen DY, Hazleman DL, Roberts S: Frozen shoulder: A long term prospective study, *Ann Rheum Dis* 43:361, 1984.

51. Bjerneld H, Hovelius L, Thorling J: Acromioclavicular separations treated conservatively: a 5-year follow-up study, *Acta Orthop Scand* 54:743, 1983.

52. Blasier R, Burkus K: Management of posterior fracture-dislocations of the shoulder, *Clin Orthop* 232:197, 1988.

53. Blasier RB, Guldberg RE, Rothman ED: Anterior shoulder stability: contributions of rotator cuff forces and the capsular ligaments in a cadaveric model, *J Shoulder Elbow Surg* 1:140, 1992.

54. Boone DC, Azen SP: Normal range of motion of joints in male subjects, *J Bone Joint Surg Am* 61A:756, 1979.

55. Bost FC, Inman VT: The pathological changes in recurrent dislocation of the shoulder: a report of Bankart's operative procedure, *J Bone Joint Surg* 24:595, 1942.

56. Bosworth BM: Acromioclavicular separation: new method of repair, *Surg Gynecol Obstet* 73:866, 1941.

57. Bosworth, BM: Calcium deposits in the shoulder and subacromial bursitis: a survey of 12,122 shoulders. *JAMA* 116:2477, 1941.

58. Bosworth, BM: Examination of the shoulder for calcium deposits, *J Bone Joint Surg* 12:567, 1941.

59. Bowen MK, Deng XH, Warner JJP, Warren RF, Torzilli PA: The effect of joint compression on stability of the glenohumeral joint, *Trans Orthop Res Soc* 17:289, 1992.

60. Bowen MK, Warren RF: Ligamentous control of shoulder stability based on selective cutting and static translation experiments, *Clin Sports Med* 10:757, 1991.

61. Bradely JP, Tibone JE: Electromyographic analysis of muscle action about the shoulder, *Clin Sports Med* 10:789, 1991.

62. Brewer BJ: Aging of the rotator cuff, *Am J Sports Med* 7:102, 1979.

63. Brewer BJ, Wubben RG, Carrera GF: Excessive retroversion of the glenoid cavity, *J Bone Joint Surg* 68A:724, 1986.

64. Bridgeman JF: Periarthritis of the shoulder and diabetes mellitus, *Ann Rheum Dis* 31:69, 1972.

65. Britt LP: Nonoperative treatment of thoracic outlet syndrome symptoms, *Clin Orthop* 51:45, 1967.

66. Brown C: Compressive, invasive referred pain to the shoulder, *Clin Orthop* 173:55, 1983.

67. Browne AO, Hoffmeyer P, An KN, Morrey BF: The influence of atmospheric pressure on shoulder stability, *Orthop Trans* 14:259, 1990.

68. Burkhardt, SS: Arthroscopic treatment of massive rotator cuff tears, *Clin Orthop* 267:45, 1991.

69. Burkhead WZ, Rockwood CA: Treatment of instability of the shoulder with an exercise program, *J Bone Joint Surg Am* 74A:890, 1992.

70. Butters, KC: The scapula. In Matsen FA, Rockwood CA, editors: *The shoulder,* Philadelphia, 1990, WB Saunders.

71. Cahill BR: Quadrilateral space syndrome. In Spinner M, Omer GE, editors: *Management of peripheral nerve problems,* Philadelphia, 1980, WB Saunders.

72. Cahill BR, Palmer RE: Quadrilateral space syndrome, *J Hand Surg* 8:65, 1983.

73. Cain PR, Mutschler TA, Fu FH: Anterior stability of the glenohumeral joint. A dynamic model, *Am J Sports Med* 15:144, 1987.

74. Cameron H: Snapping scapulae: a report of three cases, *Eur J Rheumatol Inflamm* 7:66, 1984.

75. Cave AJE: The nature and morphology of the costoclavicular ligament, *J Anat* 95:170, 1961.

76. Chansky NA, Iannotti JP: The vascularity of the rotator cuff, *Clin Sports Med* 10:807, 1991.

77. Clark JC, Harryman DT: Tendons, ligaments, and capsule of the rotator cuff, *J Bone Joint Surg Am* 74A:713, 1992.

78. Clarke GR, Willis LA, Fish WW, Nichols PJR: Preliminary studies in measuring range of motion in normal and painful stiff shoulders, *Rheumatol Rehabil* 14:39, 1975.

79. Cleland J: On the actions of the muscles passing over more than one joint, *J Anat Physiol* 1:85, 1866.

80. Codman EA: Obscure lesions of the shoulder, rupture of the supraspinatus tendon, *Boston Med Surg J* 196:381, 1927.

81. Codman EA: Rupture of the supraspinatus, *Am J Surg* 42:603, 1938.

82. Codman EA: Rupture of the supraspinatus—1834-1934, *J Bone Joint Surg* 19:643, 1937.

83. Codman EA: *The shoulder.* Boston, 1934, Thomas Todd.

84. Cofield RH: Current concepts review rotator cuff disease of the shoulder, *J Bone Joint Surg Am* 67A:974, 1985.

85. Colachis SC, Strohm BR: Effect of suprascapular and axillary nerve blocks on muscle force in upper extremity, *Arch Phys Med Rehabil* 52:22, 1971.

86. Colachis SC, Strohm BR, Brechner VL: Effects of axillary nerve block on muscle force in the upper extremity, *Arch Phys Med Rehabil* 50:647, 1969.

87. Collins HR, Wilde AH: Shoulder instability in athletes, *Orthop Clin North Am* 4:759, 1973.

88. Cook FF, Tibone JE: *The Mumford procedure in athletes: an objective analysis of function (abstract),* Academy Orthopaedic Surgeons Annual Meeting, San Francisco, 1987.

89. Cooper DE, Arnoczky SP, O'Brien SJ et al: Anatomy, histology, and vascularity of the glenoid labrum: an anatomical study, *J Bone Joint Surg Am* 74A:46, 1992.

90. Cooper DE, O'Brien SJ, Arnoczky SP, Warren RF: The structure and function of the coracohumeral ligament: an anatomic and microscopic study, *J Shoulder Elbow Surg* 2:70, 1993.

91. Coote H. Pressure on the axillary vessels and nerve by an exostosis from a cervical rib; interference with the circulation of the arm, removal of the rib and exostosis; recovery, *Med Time* 2:108, 1861.

92. Cove EF, Burke JF, Boyd RJ: *Trauma management,* Chicago, 1974, Yearbook Medical Publishers.

93. Coventry MB: Problem of the painful shoulder, *JAMA* 151:177, 1953.

94. Cox JS: The fate of the acromioclavicular joint in athletic injuries, *Am J Sports Med* 9.1:50, 1981.

95. Cruess RL: Corticosteroid-induced osteonecrosis of the humeral head, *Orthop Clin North Am* 16.4:789, 1985.

96. Cyriax J: Diagnosis of soft tissue lesions. In *Textbook of orthopaedic medicine,* ed 8, Baltimore, 1970, Williams & Wilkins.

97. Cyriax J, Cyriax P: *Illustrated manual of orthopaedic medicine,* London, 1983, Butterworth.

98. Daniels L, Worthingham C: *Muscle testing: techniques of manual examination,* ed 5, Philadelphia, 1986, WB Saunders.

99. Davies GJ, Hoffman-Dickoff SD: Neuromuscular testing and rehabilitation of the shoulder complex, *J Orthop Sports Phys Ther* 18:449, 1993.

100. Dempster WT: Mechanisms of shoulder movement, *Arch Phys Med Rehabil* 46:49, 1965.

101. DePalma AF: The role of the disks of the sternoclavicular and acromioclavicular joints, *Clin Orthop* 13:7, 1959.

102. DePalma AF: *Surgery of the shoulder,* Philadelphia, 1973, JB Lippincott.

103. DePalma AF: *Surgery of the shoulder,* Philadelphia, 1983, JB Lippincott.

104. DePalma AF, Kruper JS: Long term study of shoulder joints afflicted with and treated for calcific tendinitis, *Clin Orthop* 20:61, 1961.

105. Detrisac DA, Johnson LL: *Arthroscopic shoulder anatomy: pathologic and surgical implications,* Thorofare, NJ, 1986, Slack.

106. Dewar FP, Barrington TW: The treatment of chronic acromioclavicular dislocation. *J Bone Joint Surg Br* 47B.1:32, 1965.

107. Dias JJ, Steingold RA, Richardson RA et al: The conservative treatment of acromioclavicular dislocation: a review after five years, *J Bone Joint Surg Br* 69B:719, 1987.

108. Dickson JA, Crosby EH: Periarthritis of the shoulder: an analysis of two hundred cases, *JAMA* 99:2252, 1932.

109. DiGiovine NM, Jobe FW, Park M et al: An electromyographic analysis of the upper extremity in pitching, *J Shoulder Elbow Surg* 1:15, 1992.

110. Dillman CJ: Proper mechanics of pitching, *Sports Med Update* 5:15, 1990.

111. Doody MS, Freedman L, Waterland JC: Shoulder movements during abduction in the scapular plane, *Arch Phys Med Rehabil* 51:595, 1970.

112. Dunn AW: Trapezius paralysis after minor surgical procedures in the posterior cervical triangle, *South Med J* 67:312, 1974.

113. Duplay ES: De La periarthrite scapulohumerale et des raideurs de l'epaule qui en son la consequence, *Arch Gen Med* 20:513, 1872.

114. Ehgartner K: Has the duration of cast fixation after shoulder dislocations an influence on the frequency of recurrent dislocation? *Arch Orthop Unfallchir* 89:187, 1977.

115. Ellenbecker TS: Muscular strength relationship between normal grade manual muscle testing and isokinetic measurement of the shoulder internal and external rotators, *J Orthop Sports Phys Ther* 19.1:72, 1994.

116. Ellenbecker TS: Shoulder injuries in tennis. In Wilk KE, Andrews JR, editors: *The athlete's shoulder,* New York, 1994, Churchill Livingstone.

117. Ellenbecker TS: A total arm strength isokinetic profile of highly skilled tennis players, *Isokinetics Exerc Si* 1:9, 1991.

118. Elliot B, Marsh T, Blanksby B: A three dimensional cinematographic analysis of the tennis serve, *Int J Sport Biomech* 2:260, 1986.

119. Ellman H: Arthroscopic subcromial decompression: analysis of one- to three-year results, *J Arthroscopic Rel Surg* 3.3:173, 1987.

120. Ellman H, Hanker G, Bayer M: Repair of the rotator cuff: end-result study of factors influencing reconstruction, *J Bone Joint Surg Am* 68A:1136, 1986.

121. Ferrari DA: Capsular ligaments of the shoulder: anatomical and functional study of the anterior superior capsule, *Am J Sports Med* 18:20, 1990.

122. Field LD, Warren RF, O'Brien SJ et al: Isolated closure of rotator interval defects for shoulder instability, *Am J Sports Med* 23:557, 1995.

123. Fisher L, Kurtz A, Shipley M: Association between cheiroarthropathy and frozen shoulder in patients with insulin dependent diabetes mellitus, *Br J Rheumatol* 25:141, 1986.

124. Flatow EL, Soslowsky LJ, Ticker JB et al: Excursion of the rotator cuff under the acromion, *Am J Sports Med* 22:779, 1994.

125. Fleisig GS, Andrews JR, Dillman CJ, Escamilla RF: Kinetics of baseball pitching with implications about injury mechanisms, *Am J Sports Med* 23:233, 1995.

126. Fleisig GS, Dillman CJ, Andrews JR: Biomechanics of the shoulder during throwing. In Wilk KE, Andrews JR, editors: *The athlete's shoulder,* New York, 1994, Churchill Livingstone.

127. Fleisig GS, Dillman CJ, Andrews JR: Proper mechanics for baseball pitching, *Clin Sports Med* 1:151, 1989.

128. Freedman L, Munro RH: Abduction of the arm in the scapular plane: scapular and glenohumeral movements, *J Bone Joint Surg Am* 48A:1503, 1966.

129. Galpin RD, Hawkins RJ, Granger RW: A comparative analysis of operative vs non-operative treatment of grade III AC separations, *Clin Orthop* 193:150, 1985.

130. Gardner R, Levy H, Lemak L: *Arthroscopic debridement and decompression in irreparable rotator cuff lesions: a long term follow-up,* presented at the Fellows Meeting, American Sports Medicine Institute, 1992.

131. Gartsman GM: *Arthroscopic treatment of Stage II subacromial impingement,* presented at the American Shoulder Elbow Society Meeting, Atlanta, 1980.

132. Germain NW, Blair SN: Variability of shoulder flexion with age, activity and sex, *Am Corr Ther J* 37:156, 1983.

133. Gibb TD, Sidles JA, Harryman DT et al: The effect of capsular venting on glenohumeral laxity, *Clin Orthop* 268:120, 1991.

134. Glick JM, Milburn LJ, Haggerty JF, Nishimoto D: Dislocated acromioclavicular joint: follow-up study of 35 unreduced acromioclavicular dislocations, *Am J Sports Med* 5(6):264, 1977.

135. Gohlke F, Essiskrus B, Schmitz F: The pattern of the collagen fiber bundles of the capsule of the glenohumeral joint, *J Shoulder Elbow Surg* 3:111, 1994.

136. Grant JCB: *Method of anatomy,* ed 7, Baltimore, 1960, William & Wilkins.

137. Gray H. *Anatomy of the human body,* ed 28, Philadelphia, 1966, Lea & Febiger.

138. Grey RG: The natural history of idiopathic frozen shoulder, *J Bone Joint Surg* 60:564, 1978.

139. Groppel JL: The biomechanics of tennis: an overview, *Int J Sport Biomech* 2:141, 1986.

140. Guidi EC, Zuckerman JD: Glenoid labral lesions. In Wilk KE, Andrews JR, editors: *The athlete's shoulder,* New York, 1994, Churchill Livingstone.

141. Haggart GE, Digman RJ, Sullivan TS: Management of the frozen shoulder, *JAMA* 161:1219, 1956.

142. Hardegger FH, Simpson LA, Weber BG: The operative treatment of scapular fractures, *J Bone Joint Surg Br* 66B:725, 1984.

143. Harryman DT, Mack LA, Wang KY et al: Repairs of the rotator cuff: correlation of functional results with integrity of the cuff, *J Bone Joint Surg Am* 73A:982, 1991.

144. Harryman DT, Sidles JA, Clark JM et al: Translation of the humeral head on the glenoid with passive glenohumeral motion, *J Bone Joint Surg Am* 72A:1334, 1990.

145. Harryman DT, Sidles JA, Harris SL, Matsen FA: Role of the rotator cuff interval capsule in passive motion and stability of the shoulder, *J Bone Joint Surg Am* 74A:53, 1952.

146. Hawkes CD: Neurosurgical considerations in thoracic outlet syndrome, *Clin Orthop* 207:24, 1986.

147. Hawkins RJ: The acromioclavicular joint. Paper prepared for AAOS Summer Institute, 1980.

148. Hawkins RJ, Angelo RL: Glenohumeral osteoarthritis: a late complication of the Putti-Platt repair, *J Bone Joint Surg Am* 72A:1193, 1990.

149. Hawkins RJ, Bokor DJ: Clinical evaluation of shoulder problems. In Matsen FA, Rockwood CA, editors: *The shoulder,* Philadelphia, 1990, WB Saunders.

150. Hawkins RJ, Hoebeika P: Physical examination of the shoulder, *Orthopedics* 6:1270, 1983.

151. Hawkins RJ, Misamore GW, Hobeika PE: Surgery of full thickness rotator cuff tears, *J Bone Joint Surg Am* 67A.9:1349, 1985.

152. Helfet AJ: Coracoid transplantation for recurring dislocation of the shoulder, *J Bone Joint Surg Br* 40B:198, 1958.

153. Henry JH, Genung JA: Natural history of glenohumeral dislocation—revisited, *Am J Sports Med* 10.3:135, 1982.

154. Hill NA, McLaughlin HL: Locked posterior dislocation stimulating a "frozen shoulder," *J Trauma* 3:225, 1963.

155. Hoppenfeld S: *Physical examination of the spine and extremities,* New York, 1976, Appleton-Century-Crofts.

156. Horowitz MT, Tocartins LM: An anatomic study of the role of the long thoracic nerve and the related scapular bursae in the pathogenesis of local paralysis in the serratus anterior muscle, *Anat Rec* 71:375, 1938.

157. Hovelius L, Akermark C, Albrektsson B, et al: Bristow-Latarjet procedure for recurrent anterior dislocation of the shoulder, *Acta Orthop Scand* 54:284, 1983.

158. Hovelius L, Eriksson K, Fredin H et al: Recurrences after initial dislocation of the shoulder: results of a prospective study of treatment, *J Bone Joint Surg Am* 65A:343, 1983.

159. Hovelius L, Thorling J, Fredin H: Recurrent anterior dislocation of the shoulder. Results after the Bankart and Putti-Platt operations, *J Bone Joint Surg Am* 61A:566, 1979.

160. Howell, SM, Galinet SJ: The glenoid labral socket: a constrained articular surface, *Clin Orthop* 243:122, 1989.

161. Howell SM, Galinat BJ, Renzi AJ, Marone PJ: Normal and abnormal mechanics of the glenohumeral joint in the horizontal plane, *J Bone Joint Surg Am* 70A:227, 1988.

162. Hunald (cited by Tyson RR, Kaplan GF): Modern concepts of diagnosis and treatment of the thoracic outlet syndrome, *Orthop Clin North Am* 6:507, 1975.

163. Hurley JA, Anderson TE, Dear W et al: Posterior shoulder instability: surgical vs conservative results with evaluation of glenoid version, *Am J Sports Med* 20:396, 1992.

164. Iannotti J, Bernot M, Kuhlman J, Kelley M: Prospective evaluation of rotator cuff repair. *J Shoulder Elbow Surg* (2) Abstract S9, 1993.

165. Iannotti JB, Swiontkowski M, Esterhafi J, Boulas HJ: Intraoperative assessment of rotator cuff vascularity using laser Doppler flowmetry. Abstract presented to American Academy of Orthopedic Surgeons Meeting, 1989.

166. Ikai M, Ishii M, Miyashita M: An electromyographic study of swimming, *Res J Phys Ed* 70:27, 1988.

167. Imatani RJ, Hanlon JJ, Cady GW: Acute complete acromioclavicular separation, *J Bone Joint Surg Am* 57A.3:328, 1975.

168. Inman VT, Saunder JR, Abbott LC: Observations on the function of the shoulder joint, *J Bone Joint Surg* 26:1, 1944.

169. Ito N: Electromyographic study of shoulder joint, *J Jpn Orthop Assoc* 54:53, 1980.

170. Jobe CM: Gross anatomy of the shoulder. In Matsen FA, Rockwood CA, editors: *The shoulder,* Philadelphia, 1990, WB Saunders.

171. Jobe FW, Giangaria CE, Kvitne RS et al: Anterior capsulolabral reconstruction of the shoulder in athletes in overhand sports, *Am J Sports Med* 19:428, 1991.

172. Jobe FW, Jobe CM: Painful athletic injuries of the shoulder, *Clin Orthop* 173:117, 1983.

173. Jobe FW, Kvitne RS, Giangarra CE: Shoulder pain in the overhead or throwing athlete: the relationship of anterior instability and rotator cuff impingement, *Orthop Rev* 18:963, 1989.

174. Jobe FW, Moynes DR: Delineation of diagnostic criteria and a rehabilitation program for rotator cuff injuries, *Am J Sports Med* 10:336, 1982.

175. Jobe FW, Moynes DR, Brewster CE: Rehabilitation of shoulder joint instabilities, *Orthop Clin North Am* 18.3:473, 1987.

176. Jobe FW, Perry J, Pink M: Electromyographic shoulder activity in men and women professional golfers, *Am J Sports Med* 17:782, 1989.

177. Jobe FW, Tibone GJE, Jobe CM et al: The shoulder in sports, In Matsen FA, Rockwood CA, editors: *The shoulder,* Philadelphia, 1990, WB Saunders.

178. Johnson H: The biomechanics of the golf swing, *Golfers' Newsletter.* Birmingham, 1993, American Sports Medicine Institute.

179. Johnston JTH: Frozen shoulder in patients with pulmonary tuberculosis, *J Bone Joint Surg* 41:877, 1959.

180. Johnston TB: The movements of the shoulder joint: a plea for the use of the "plane of the scapula" as the plane of reference for movements occurring at the humero-scapular joint, *Br J Surg* 25:252, 1937-38.

181. Kaltenborn FM: *Mobilization of the extremity joints: examination and basic treatment techniques.* Oslo, 1980, Olaf Bokhandel.

182. Kapandji I: *The physiology of joints,* Vol 1, Baltimore, 1970, Williams & Wilkins.

183. Kappakas GS, McMaster JH: Repair of acromioclavicular separation using a Dacron prosthesis graft, *Clin Orthop* 131:247, 1978.

184. Karas SE: Thoracic outlet syndrome, *Clin Sports Med* 9:297, 1990.

185. Kay N: The clinical diagnosis and management of frozen shoulders, *Practitioner* 225:164, 1981.

186. Kazar B, Relousky E: Prognosis of primary dislocation of the shoulder, *Acta Orthop Scand* 40:216, 1969.

187. Kelkar R, Flatow EL, Bigliani LU et al: A stereophotogrammetric method to determine the kinematics of the glenohumeral joint, *Adv Bioeng* 19:143, 1992.

188. Kelley MJ: Biomechanics of the shoulder. In Clark WA, Kelley MJ, editors: *Orthopaedic therapy of the shoulder,* Philadelphia, 1995, JB Lippincott.

189. Kendall FP, McCreary EK: *Muscle testing and function,* ed 3, Baltimore, 1982, Williams & Wilkins.

190. Kennedy JC, Cameron H: Complete dislocation of the acromioclavicular joint, *J Bone Joint Surg Br* 36B:202, 1954.

191. Kennedy JC, Cameron H: Complete dislocation of the acromioclavicular joint: 14 years later, *J Trauma* 8:311, 1968.

192. Kennedy JC, Craig AB, Schneider RC: Swimming. In Kennedy JC, Schneider RC, Plant ML, editors: *Sports injuries: mechanisms, prevention and treatment,* Baltimore, 1985, Williams & Wilkins.

193. Kibler BW: The role of the scapula in the overhead throwing motion, *Contemp Orthop* 22:525, 1991.

194. Kibler BW, McQueen C, Uhl T: Fitness evaluation fitness findings in competitive junior tennis players, *Clin Sports Med* 7:403, 1988.

195. Kieft GJ, Bloem JL, Rozing PM, Obermann WR: MR imaging of recurrent anterior dislocation of the shoulder: comparison with CT arthrography, *AJR* 150:1083, 1988.

196. Kohn D: The clinical relevance of glenoid labrum lesions, *Arthroscopy* 3:223, 1987.

197. Konin JG, McCue FC: Taping, strapping, and bracing of the shoulder complex, In Wilk KE, Andrews JR, editors: *The athlete's shoulder.* New York, 1994, Churchill Livingstone.

198. Kumar VP, Balasubramianium P: The role of atmospheric pressure in stabilizing the shoulder: an experimental study, *J Bone Joint Surg Br* 67B:719, 1985.

199. Kunkel SS, Hawkins RJ: Open repair of the rotator cuff. In Wilk KE, Andrews JR, editors: *The athlete's shoulder,* New York, 1994, Churchill Livingstone.

200. Lancaster S, Horowitz M, Alonso J: Complete acromioclavicular separations: a comparison of operative methods, *Clin Orthop* 216:80, 1987.

201. Larsen E, Bjerg-Nielsen A, Christensen P: Conservative or surgical treatment of acromioclavicular dislocation: a prospective, controlled, randomized study, *J Bone Joint Surg Am* 68A:552, 1986.

202. Leffart RD: Neurological problems. In Matsen FA, Rockwood CA, editors: *The shoulder,* Philadelphia, 1990, WB Saunders.

203. Lequesne M, Dang N, Bensasson M, Mery C: Increased association of diabetes mellitus with capsulitis of the shoulder and shoulder-hand syndrome, *Scand J Rheumatol* 6:53, 1977.

204. Levy HJ, Gardner RD, Lemak LJ: Arthroscopic subacromial decompression in the treatment of full thickness rotator cuff tears, *Arthroscopy* 7:8, 1991.

205. Lewis T, Pickering G: Observations upon maladies in which the blood supply to the digits ceases intermittently or permanently, *Clin Sci* 1:327, 1934.

206. Liberson F: Os acromiale—a contested anomaly, *J Bone Joint Surg* 19:683, 1937.

207. Lighe LE, Nuzik S, Personius W et al: Low-load prolonged stretch versus high load in treating knee contractures, *Phys Ther* 64:330-336, 1984.

208. Lindblom, K: On pathogenesis of ruptures of the tendon aponeurosis of the shoulder joint, *Acta Radiol* 20:563, 1939.

209. Lippett FG: A modification of the gravity method of reducing anterior shoulder dislocations, *Clin Orthop* 165:259, 1982.

210. Lloyd-Roberts GC, French PR: Periarthritis of the shoulder: a study of the disease and its treatment, *Br Med J* 1:1569, 1959.

211. Lombard SJ, Kerlan RK, Jobe FW et al: The modified Bristow procedure for recurrent dislocations of the shoulder, *J Bone Joint Surg Am* 58A:256, 1976.

212. Ludington NA: Rupture of the long head of the biceps flexor cubiti muscle, *Ann Surg* 77:358, 1923.

213. Lundberg, BJ: The frozen shoulder, *Acta Orthop Scand (Suppl)* 119:1, 1969.

214. MacConail MA, Basmajian JV: *Muscles and movements: a basis for human kinesiology,* Baltimore, 1969, Williams & Wilkins.

215. Magnuson PB: Bilateral habitual dislocation of the shoulders in twins, a familial tendency, *JAMA* 144:2103, 1945.

216. Maitland GD: Treatment of the glenohumeral joint by passive movement, *Physiotherapy* 69:3, 1983.

217. Malone TR, Richmond GW, Frick JL: Shoulder pathology. In Clark WA, Kelley MJ, editors: *Orthopaedic therapy of the shoulder,* Philadelphia, 1995, JB Lippincott.

218. Matsen F, Zuckerman J: Anterior glenohumeral instability, *Clin Sports Med* 2:319, 1983.

219. Matsen FA, Thomas SC, Rockwood CA: Anterior glenohumeral instability. In Rockwood CA, Matsen FA, editors: *The Shoulder,* Philadelphia, 1990, WB Saunders.

220. Matsen FA, Arntz CT: Rotator cuff tendon failure. In Rockwood CA, Matsen FA, editors: *The shoulder,* Philadelphia, 1990, WB Saunders.

221. Matsen FA, Arntz CT: Subacromial impingement. In Matsen FA, Rockwood CA, editors: *The shoulder,* Philadelphia, 1990, WB Saunders.

222. Matsen FA, Thomas SC, Rockwood CA: Anterior glenohumeral instability. In Matsen FA, Rockwood CA, editors: *The shoulder,* Philadelphia, 1990, WB Saunders.

223. McCluskey GM III, Biglianni LU: Scapulothoracic disorders. In Wilk KE, Andrews JR, editors: *The athlete's shoulder,* New York, 1994, Churchill Livingstone.

224. McKernan DJ, Mutschler TA, Rudert MJ et al: The characterization of rotator cuff muscle forces and their effect on glenohumeral joint stability: a biomechanical study, *Orthop Trans* 14:237, 1990.

225. McLaughlin, HL: Lesions of the musculotendinous cuff of the shoulder. I. The exposure and treatment of tears with retraction, *J Bone Joint Surg* 26:31, 1944.

226. McLaughlin, HL: Recurrent anterior dislocation of the shoulder. Morbid anatomy, *Am J Surg* 99:628, 1960.

227. McLaughlin HL, Cavallaro WU: Primary anterior dislocation of the shoulder, *Am J Surg* 80:615, 1950.

228. McLaughlin HL, MacLellan DI: Recurrent anterior dislocation of the shoulder. II. A comparative study, *J Trauma* 7:191, 1967.

229. Milch H: Partial scapulectomy for snapping in the scapula, *J Bone Joint Surg Am* 32A:561, 1950.

230. Milch H: Snapping scapula, *Clin Orthop* 20:139, 1961.

231. Milch H, Burman MS: Snapping scapula and humerus varus, *Arch Surg* 26:570, 1933.

232. Miyashita M, Tsunoda T, Sakurai S et al: Muscular activities in the tennis serve and overhand throwing, *Scand J Sports Sci* 2:52, 1980.

233. Moren-Hybbinette I, Moritz U, Schersten B: The clinical picture of the painful diabetic shoulder: natural history, social consequences and analysis of concomitant hand syndrome, *Acta Med Scand* 221:73, 1987.

234. Morrey BF, Chao EY: Recurrent anterior dislocation of the shoulder. In Black J, Dumbleton J, editors: *Clinical biomechanics,* London, 1981, Churchill Livingstone.

235. Morrison DS: *The use of magnetic resonance imaging in the diagnosis of rotator cuff tears,* Atlanta, 1988.

236. Moseley HF: The clavicle: its anatomy and function, *Clin Orthop* 58:17, 1958.

237. Moseley HF: *Ruptures to the rotator cuff,* Springfield, Ill, 1952, Charles C Thomas.

238. Moseley HF: *Shoulder lesions,* ed 3, Edinburgh and London: 1969, E & S Livingstone.

239. Moseley HF, Goldie I: The arterial pattern of the rotator cuff of the shoulder, *J Bone Joint Surg Br* 45B:780, 1963.

240. Moseley HF, Overgaard B: The anterior capsular mechanism in recurrent anterior dislocation of the shoulder, *J Bone Joint Surg Br* 44B:913, 1962.

241. Moseley JB, Jobe FW, Pink M et al: EMG analysis of the scapular muscles during a shoulder rehabilitation program, *Am J Sports Med* 20:222, 1992.

242. Mudge MK, Wood VE, Frykman GK: Rotator cuff tears associated with os acromiale, *J Bone Joint Surg Am* 66A:427, 1984.

243. Mumford EB: Acromioclavicular dislocation, *J Bone Joint Surg* 12:799, 1941.

244. Murnaghan GF, McIntosh D: Hydrocortisone in painful shoulder: a controlled trial, *Lancet* 269:798, 1955.

245. Murnaghan JP: Frozen shoulder. In Matsen FA, Rockwood CA, editors: *The shoulder,* Philadelphia, 1990, WB Saunders.

246. Murphy TC: Shoulder injuries in swimming, In Wilk KE, Andrews JR, editors: *The athlete's shoulder,* New York, 1994, Churchill Livingstone.

247. Murray MP, Gore DR, Gardner GM, Mollinger LA: Shoulder motion and muscle strength of normal men and women in two age groups, *Clin Orthop* 192:268, 1985.

248. Naffziger HC, Grant WT: Neuritis of the brachial plexus, mechanical in origin: the scalenus syndrome, *Surg Gynecol Obstet* 67:722, 1938.

249. Neer CS II: Anterior acromioplasty for the chronic impingement syndrome in the shoulder. A preliminary report, *J Bone Joint Surg Am* 54A:41, 1972.

250. Neer CS II: Fractures about the shoulder. In Green DP, Rockwood CA, editors: *Fractures,* Philadelphia, 1984, JB Lippincott.

251. Neer CS II: Impingement lesions, *Clin Orthop* 173:70, 1983.

252. Neer CS II: Involuntary inferior and multi-directional instability of the shoulder: etiology, recognition, and treatment, *Instruct Course Lect* 34:232, 1985.

253. Neer CS II: *Shoulder reconstruction,* Philadelphia, 1990, WB Saunders.

254. Neer CS II, Craig EV, Fukuda H: Cuff tear arthropathy, *J Bone Joint Surg Am* 65A:1232, 1983.

255. Neer CS II, Flatow EL, Lech O: *Tears of the rotator cuff: long term results of anterior acromioplasty and repair,* presented at American Shoulder Elbow Surgeons Meeting, Atlanta, 1988.

256. Neer CS II, Foster CR: Inferior capsular shift for involuntary inferior and multidirectional instability of the shoulder, *J Bone Joint Surg Am* 62A:897, 1980.

257. Neer CS II, Welsh RP: The shoulder in sports, *Orthop Clin North Am* 8:583, 1977.

258. Neviaser JS: Adhesive capsulitis of the shoulder, *J Bone Joint Surg* 27:211, 1945.

259. Neviaser JS: Arthrography of the shoulder joint: a study of the findings in adhesive capsulitis of the shoulder, *J Bone Joint Surg Am* 44A:1321, 1962.

260. Neviaser RJ: Lesions of the biceps and tendinitis of the shoulder, *Orthop Clin North Am* 11:343, 1980.

261. Neviaser RJ: Tears of the rotator cuff, *Orthop Clin North Am* 11:295, 1980.

262. Neviaser RJ, Neviaser TJ: The frozen shoulder diagnosis and management, *Clin Orthop* 223:59, 1987.

263. Neviaser RJ, Neviaser TJ: Reconstruction of chronic tears of the rotator cuff. In Welsh RP, Bateman JE, editors: *Surgery of the shoulder,* Philadelphia, 1984, BC Decker.

264. Neviaser TJ: Adhesive capsulitis, *Orthop Clin North Am* 18:439, 1987.

265. Nobuhara K, Ikeeda H: Rotator interval lesion, *Clin Orthop* 223:44, 1987.

266. Norris T: Fractures and dislocations of the glenohumeral complex. In Chapman M, editor: *Operative orthopedics,* Philadelphia, 1984, JB Lippincott.

267. Nuber GW, Bowman ID, Perry JP et al: EMG analysis of classical shoulder motion, *Trans Orthop Res Soc* 11:216, 1986.

268. Nuber GW, McCarthy WJ, Yao JST et al: Arterial abnormalities of the shoulder in athletes, *Am J Sports Med* 18:514, 1990.

269. O'Brien SJ: *Glenoid labrum lesions of the shoulder,* presented at the Advances in Shoulder and Knee Meeting, Hilton Head, 1994.

270. O'Brien SJ, Neves MC, Arnoczky SP et al: The anatomy and histology of the inferior glenohumeral ligament complex of the shoulder, *Am J Sports Med* 18:449, 1990.

271. O'Brien SJ, Warren RF, Schwartz E: Anterior shoulder instability, *Orthop Clin North Am* 18:395, 1987.

272. O'Connell PW, Nuber GW, Mileski RA, Lautenschlager E: The contribution of the glenohumeral ligaments to anterior stability of the shoulder joint, *Am J Sports Med* 18:579, 1990.

273. Ochsner A, Gage M, DeBakey M: Scalenus anticus (Naffziger) syndrome, *Am J Surg* 28:669, 1935.

274. Osmond-Clarke H: Habitual dislocation of the shoulder. The Putti-Platt operation, *J Bone Joint Surg Br* 30B:19, 1948.

275. Ovesen J, Nielsen S: Anterior and posterior shoulder instability, *Acta Orthop Scand* 57:324, 1986.

276. Pagnani MJ, Deng X-H, Warren RF et al: Effect of the long head of the biceps brachii on glenohumeral translation. Presented at The Hospital for Special Surgery, 1993.

277. Pagnani MJ, Warren RF: Stabilizers of the glenohumeral joint, *J Shoulder Elbow Surg* 3:173, 1994.

278. Pal B, Anderson J, Dick WC, Griffiths ID: Limitation of joint mobility and shoulder capsulitis in insulin and non-insulin dependent diabetes mellitus, *Br J Rheumatol* 25:147, 1986.

279. Park JP, Arnold JA, Coker TP, Harris WD et al: Treatment of acromioclavicular separations: a retrospective study, *Am J Sports Med* 8:251, 1980.

280. Paulos LE, Kody MH: Arthroscopically enhanced "mini" approach for rotator cuff repair, *Am J Sports Med* 22:19, 1994.

281. Pavlov H, Warren RF, Weiss CB et al: The roentgenographic evaluation of anterior shoulder instability, *Clin Orthop* 194:153, 1985.

282. Perthes G: Uber operationen bei habitueller schulterluxation, *Deutsch Ztschr Chir* 85:199, 1906.

283. Petersson CJ: The acromioclavicular joint in rheumatoid arthritis, *Clin Orthop* 223:86, 1987.

284. Petersson CJ: Degeneration of the acromioclavicular joint: a morphological study, *Acta Orthop Scand* 54:434, 1983.

285. Petersson CJ, Gentz CF: The significance of distally pointing acromioclavicular osteophytes in ruptures of the supraspinatus tendon, *Acta Orthop Scand* 54:490, 1983.

286. Podromos CC, Perry JA, Schiller JA et al: Histological studies of the glenoid labrum from fetal life to old age, *J Bone Joint Surg Am* 72A:1344, 1990.

287. Poppen NK, Walker PS: Forces at the glenohumeral joint in abduction, *Clin Orthop* 135:165, 1978.

288. Poppen NK, Walker PS: Normal and abnormal motion of the shoulder, *J Bone Joint Surg Am* 58A:195, 1976.

289. Post M, Silver R, Singh M: Rotator cuff tear: diagnosis and treatment, *Clin Orthop* 173:78, 1983.

290. Powers JA, Bach PJ: Acromioclavicular separations—closed or open treatment, *Clin Orthop* 104:213, 1974.

291. Price DD, McGrath PA, Rafii A, Buckingham B: The validation of visual analogue scales: a ratio scale measures for chronic and experimental pain, *Pain* 17:45, 1982.

292. Quigley TB: Indications for manipulation and corticosteroids in the treatment of stiff shoulders, *Surg Clin North Am* 43:1715, 1969.

293. Quin EH: Frozen shoulder: evaluation of treatment with hydrocortisone injections and exercises, *Ann Phys Med* 8:22, 1965.

294. Rao JP, Francis AM, Hurley J, Daczkewycz R: Treatment of recurrent anterior dislocation of the shoulder by duToit staple capsulorrhaphy. Results of long-term follow-up study, *Clin Orthop* 204:169, 1986.

295. Rathbun JB, Macnab I: The microvascular pattern of the rotator cuff, *J Bone Joint Surg Br* 52B:540, 1970.

296. Rawlings G: Acromioclavicular dislocations and fractures of the clavicle: a simple method of support, *Lancet* 2:789, 1939.

297. Rayan GM, Jensen C: Thoracic outlet syndrome: provocative examination maneuvers in a typical population, *J Shoulder Elbow Surg* 4:113, 1995.

298. Reagan WD, Webster-Bogaart S, Hawkins RJ, Fowler PJ: Comparative functional analysis of the Bristow, Magnusson-Stack, and Putti-Platt procedures for recurrent dislocation of the shoulder, *Am J Sports Med* 17:42, 1989.

299. Reeves B: Arthrographic changes in frozen and post traumatic stiff shoulders, *Proc R Soc Med* 59:827, 1966.

300. Reeves B: The natural history of the frozen shoulder syndrome, *Scand J Rheumatol* 4:193, 1975.

301. Rhu KN, McCormick J, Jobe FW et al: An electromyographic analysis of shoulder function in tennis players, *Am J Sports Med* 16:481, 1988.

302. Richards RR, McKee MD: Treatment of painful scapulothoracic crepitus by resection of the superomedial angle of the scapula, *Clin Orthop* 247:111, 1989.

303. Richardson AB: The biomechanics of swimming: the shoulder and knee, *Clin Sports Med* 5:103, 1986.

304. Riddell DH, Smith BM: Thoracic and vascular aspects of the thoracic outlet syndrome, 1986 update, *Clin Orthop* 207:54, 1986.

305. Rizk TE, Pinals RS: Frozen shoulder, *Arthritis Rheum* 11:440, 1982.

306. Rockwood CA: Disorders of the sternoclavicular joint, In Matsen FA, Rockwood CA, editors: *The shoulder.* Philadelphia, 1990, WB Saunders.

307. Rockwood CA, Matsen FA, editors: *The shoulder,* Philadelphia, 1990, WB Saunders.

308. Rockwood CA, Young DC: Disorders of the acromioclavicular joint. In Matsen FA, Rockwood CA, editors: *The shoulder,* Philadelphia, 1990, WB Saunders.

309. Rockwood CA Jr: Injuries to the acromioclavicular joint. In *Fractures in adults,* ed 2, vol 1, Philadelphia, 1984, JB Lippincott.

310. Rockwood CA Jr: Subluxation of the shoulder—the classification, diagnosis and treatment, *Orthop Trans* 4:306, 1979.

311. Rockwood CA Jr, Guy DK, Griffin JL: Treatment of chronic, complete acromioclavicular dislocation, *Orthop Trans* 12:735, 1988.

311b. Rokito AS, Zuckerman JD, Gallagher MA, Cuomo F: Strength after surgical repair of the rotator cuff. *J Shoulder Elbow Surg* 5(1):12, 1996.

312. Roos DB: The place for scalenectomy and first rib resection in thoracic outlet syndrome, *Surgery* 92:1077, 1982.

313. Rothman RH, Parke WW: The vascular anatomy of the rotator cuff, *Clin Orthop* 41:176, 1965.

314. Rowe C: Acute and recurrent anterior dislocations of the shoulder, *Orthop Clin North Am* 11:253, 1980.

315. Rowe C: Dislocations of the shoulder. In Rowe CR, editor: *The shoulder,* New York, 1988, Churchill Livingstone.

316. Rowe CR: Fractures of the scapula, *Surg Clin North Am* 43:1565, 1963.

317. Rowe CR: Prognosis in dislocations of the shoulder, *J Bone Joint Surg Am* 8A:957, 1956.

318. Rowe CR: *The shoulder,* New York, 1988, Churchill Livingstone.

319. Rowe CR, Patel D, Southmayd WW: The Bankart procedure—a long-term end-result study, *J Bone Joint Surg Am* 60A:1, 1978.

320. Rowe CR, Sakellarides HT: Factors related to recurrences of anterior dislocations of the shoulder, *Clin Orthop* 20:40, 1961.

321. Rowe CR, Zarins BR: Chronic unreduced dislocations of the shoulder, *J Bone Joint Surg Am* 64A:494, 1982.

322. Rowe CR, Zarins B: Recurrent transient subluxation of the shoulder, *J Bone Joint Surg Am* 63A:863, 1981.

323. Saha AK: Dynamic stability of the glenohumeral joint, *Acta Orthop Scand* 42:491, 1971.

324. Saha AK: Mechanism of shoulder movements and a plea for the recognition of "zero position" of the glenohumeral joint, *Clin Orthop* 173:3, 1983.

325. Saha AK: *Theory of shoulder mechanism: descriptive and applied,* Springfield, Ill, 1961, Charles C Thomas.

326. Samilson RL, Binder WF: Symptomatic full thickness tears of the rotator cuff: an analysis of 292 shoulders in 276 patients, *Orthop Clin North Am* 6:449, 1975.

327. Sarrafian SK: Gross and functional anatomy of the shoulder, *Clin Orthop* 173:11, 1983.

328. Schwartz E, Warren RF, O'Brien SJ et al: Posterior shoulder instability, *Orthop Clin North Am* 18:409, 1987.

329. Scovazzo ML, Browne A, Pink M et al: The painful shoulder during freestyle swimming: an electromyographic and cinematographic analysis of twelve muscles, *Am J Sports Med* 19:557, 1991.

330. Selke FW, Kelly TR: Thoracic outlet syndrome, *Am J Surg* 156:54, 1988.

331. Shaffer B, Tibone JE, Kerlan RK: Frozen shoulder: a long term follow-up. *J Bone Joint Surg* 74A5:738, 1992.

332. Shelvin MG, Lehman JF, Lucci JA: Electromyographic study of the function of some muscles crossing the glenohumeral joint, *Arch Phys Med Rehabil* 50:264, 1969.

333. Sigholm G, Styf J, Korner L, Herberts P: Pressure recording in the subacromial bursa, *J Orthop Res* 6:123, 1988.

334. Silliman JF, Hawkins RJ: Clinical examination of the shoulder complex. In Wilk KE, Andrews JR, editors: *The athlete's shoulder,* New York, 1994, Churchill Livingstone.

335. Simmonds FA: Shoulder pain with particular reference to the frozen shoulder, *J Bone Joint Surg Am* 31:834, 1949.

336. Simonet WT, Cofield RH: Prognosis in anterior glenohumeral joint dislocation, *Am J Sports Med* 12:19, 1984.

337. Sleeswijk Visser SV, Haarsma SM, Speeckaert MTC: Conservative treatment of acromioclavicular dislocation: Jones strap versus mitella (abstract), *Acta Orthop Scand* 55:483, 1984.

338. Smith-Petersen MN, Aufranc OE, Larson CB: Useful surgical procedures for rheumatoid arthritis involving joints of the upper extremity, *Arch Surg* 46:764, 1943.

339. Snyder SJ, Karzel RP, Del Pizzo W et al: SLAP lesions of the shoulder, *Arthroscopy* 6:274, 1990.

340. Soslowsky LJ, Flatow EL, Biglianni LU et al: Quantitation of in situ contact areas at the glenohumeral joint: a biomechanical study, *J Orthop Res* 10:524, 1992.

341. Sotta RP: Vascular problems in the proximal upper extremity, *Clin Sports Med* 9:379, 1990.

342. Speer KP, Hannafin JA, Altchek DW, Warren RF: An evaluation of the shoulder relocation test, *Am J Sports Med* 22:177, 1994.

343. Spurling RG, Scoville WB: Lateral rupture of the cervical intervertebral discs. A common cause of shoulder and arm pain, *Surg Gynecol Obstet* 78:350, 1944.

344. Stallworth JM, Horne JB: Diagnosis and management of thoracic syndrome, *Arch Surg* 119:1149, 1984.

345. Steindler A: Kinesiology of the human body under normal and pathologic conditions, 125, 1955.

346. Stopford JSB, Telford ED: Compression of the lower trunk of the brachial plexus by a first dorsal rib, *Br J Surg* 7:168, 1919.

347. Sunderland S: *Nerves and nerve injuries,* ed 2, Edinburgh, 1978, Churchill Livingstone.

348. Swiostkowski MF, Iannotti JB, Boulas HJ et al: Intraoperative assessment of rotator cuff vascularity of the shoulder. In Morrey BF, Post M, Hawkins RJ, editors: *Surgery of the shoulder,* St Louis, 1990, Mosby.

349. Taft TN, Wilson FC, Oglesby JW: Dislocation of the acromioclavicular joint: an end-result study, *J Bone Joint Surg Am* 69A:1045, 1987.

350. Takagishi N: Conservative treatment of the ruptures of the rotator cuff, *J Jpn Orthop Assoc* 52:781, 1978.

351. Tearse DS, Robinson A, Koch B et al: *Mechanoreceptors in the human shoulder capsule and labrum,* Academy Orthopedic Surgeons Meeting, New Orleans, 1994.

352. Telford ED, Mottershead S: Pressure at the cervicobrachial junction, *J Bone Joint Surg Am* 30:249, 1948.

353. Terry GC, Hammon D, France P, Norwood LA: The stabilizing function of the passive shoulder restraints, *Am J Sports Med* 19:26, 1991.

354. Thorling J, Bjerneld H, Halllin G, et al: Acromioplasty for impingement syndrome, *Orthop Scand* 56:147, 1985.

355. Timmerman LA, Andrews JR, Wilk KE: Mini-open repair of the rotator cuff, In Wilk KE, Andrews JR, editors: *The athlete's shoulder,* New York, 1994, Churchill Livingstone.

356. Torg JS, Balduini FC, Bonci C et al: A modified Bristow-Helfet-May procedure for recurrent dislocations and subluxaton of the shoulder: report of 212 cases, *J Bone Joint Surg Am* 69:904, 1987.

357. Tossy JD, Mead NC, Sigmond HM: Acromioclavicular separations: useful and practical classification for treatment, *Clin Orthop* 28:111, 1963.

358. Townley CO: The capsular mechanism in recurrent dislocation of the shoulder joint, *J Bone Joint Surg Am* 32A:370, 1950.

359. Travell JG, Simmons DG: *Myofascial pain and dysfunction: trigger point manual,* Baltimore, 1983, Williams & Wilkins.

360. Tullos HS, Erwin WD, Woods GW et al: Unusual lesions of the pitching arm, *Clin Orthop* 88:169, 1972.

361. Turek S: *Orthopaedics: principles and their applications,* Philadelphia, 1967, JB Lippincott.

362. Turkel SJ, Panio MW, Marshal JL: Stabilizing mechanisms preventing anterior dislocation of the glenohumeral joint, *J Bone Joint Surg Am* 63A:1208, 1981.

363. Tyurina TV: Age-related characteristics of the human acromioclavicular joint, *Arkh Anat Gistol Embriol* 89:75, 1985.

364. Uhthoff H, Sarkar K: Classification and definition of tendinopathies, *Clin Sports Med* 10:707, 1991.

365. Uhthoff HK, Sarkar K: Calcifying tendinitis. In Matsen FA, Rockwood CA, editors: *The shoulder,* Philadelphia, 1990, WB Saunders.

366. Uhthoff HK, Sarkar K, Maynard JA: Calcifying tendinitis, *Clin Orthop* 118:164, 1976.

367. Urist MR: Complete dislocation of the acromioclavicular joint (follow-up notes), *J Bone Joint Surg Am* 45A:1750, 1963.

368. VanGheluwe B, Hebbelinck M: Muscle actions and ground reaction forces in tennis, *Int J Sport Biomech* 1:88, 1986.

369. Vangsness CT, Ennis M: *Neural anatomy of the human shoulder ligaments and glenoid labrum,* Academy Orthopaedic Sugeons Meeting, Washington, DC, 1992.

370. Vogel CM, Jensen JE: "Effort" thrombosis of the subclavian vein in a competitive swimmer," *Am J Sports Med* 13:269, 1985.

371. Walch G, Boileau P, Noel E, Donell T: Impingement of the deep surface of the supraspinatus tendon on the glenoid rim: an arthroscopic study, *J Shoulder Elbow Surg* 1:239, 1992.

372. Warner JJP, Deng X-H, Warren RF et al: Static capsuloligamentous constraints to superior-inferior translation of the glenohumeral joint, *Am J Sports Med* 20:675, 1992.

373. Warner JJP, Micheli LJ, Arslaniai LE et al: Scapulothoracic motion in normal shoulders and shoulders with glenohumeral instability and impingement syndrome: a study using Moire topographic analysis, *Clin Orthop* 285:191, 1992.

374. Warren CG, Lehman JF, Koslonski NJ: Elongation of rat tendon: effect of load and temperature, *Arch Phys Med Rehabil* 52:465, 1971.

375. Warren R: Subluxation of the shoulder in athletes, *Clin Sports Med* 2:339, 1983.

376. Warren RF, Kornblatt IB, Marchand R: Static factors affecting posterior shoulder stability, *Orthop Trans* 8:89, 1984.

377. Warwick R, Williams PL, editors: *Gray's anatomy (British),* ed 35, Philadelphia, 1973, WB Saunders.

378. Watson-Jones R: Simple treatment of stiff shoulders, *J Bone Joint Surg* 45:207, 1963.

379. Welfling J, Kahn MF, Desroy M et al: Les calcifications de l'epaule. II. La maladie des calcifications tendineuses multiples, *Rev Rheum* 32:325, 1965.

380. Wheeler JH, Ryan JB, Arcerio RA: Arthroscopic versus nonoperative treatment of acute shoulder dislocations in young athletes, *Arthroscopy* 5:213, 1989.

381. Wheeler WI: Compression neuritis due to the normal first dorsal rib, *Practitioner* 104:409, 1920.

382. Wiley AM: Arthroscopic examination of the shoulder, In Kessel L, Bayley J, editors: *Shoulder surgery,* Berlin-Heidelberg, 1982, Springer-Verlag.

383. Wiley AM: Arthroscopy for shoulder instability and a technique for arthroscopic repair, *Arthroscopy* 1:250, 1988.

384. Wilk KE: Conditioning and training techniques. In Misamore GW, Hawkins RJ, editors: *Shoulder injuries in the athlete,* New York, 1996, Churchill Livingstone.

385. Wilk KE: The functional outcome results of rotator cuff patients: correlation between subjective and objective measurements, *J Orthop Sports Phys Ther,* Submitted for publication, 1995.

386. Wilk KE: *Treating shoulder impingement non-operatively,* Recent Advances in Rehabilitation American Sports Medicine Institute, Birmingham, 1995.

387. Wilk KE, Andrews JR: Arthroscopic subacromial decompression and aggressive rehabilitation in the treatment of full thickness unrepairable rotator cuff tears, *Phys Ther,* submitted for publication, 1995.

388. Wilk KE, Arrigo CA: Current concepts in the rehabilitation of the athletic shoulder, *J Orthop Sports Phys Ther* 18:365, 1993.

389. Wilk KE, Andrews JR, Arrigo CA: The abductor and adductor strength characteristics of professional baseball pitchers, *Am J Sports Med* 23:307, 1995.

390. Wilk KE, Andrews JR, Arrigo CA: The physical examination of the static stabilizers of the glenohumeral joint, *J Orthop Sports Phys Ther,* submitted for publication, 1995.

391. Wilk KE, Andrews JR, Arrigo CA et al, editors: *Preventive and rehabilitative exercises for the shoulder and elbow,* Birmingham, 1992, American Sports Medicine Institute.

392. Wilk KE, Arrigo CA: An integrated approach to upper extremity exercises, *Orthop Phys Ther Clin North Am* 9:337, 1992.

393. Wilk KE, Arrigo CA: Isokinetic testing and rehabilitation of microtraumatic shoulder injuries. In Davies GJ, editor: *A compendium of isokinetics in clinical usage,* ed 4, LaCrosse, Wis, 1992, S & S Publishers.

394. Wilk KE, Arrigo CA, Andrews JR: A comparison of individuals exhibiting a normal grade manual muscle test and isokinetic testing of the knee extensors/flexors, *Phys Ther* 76, 1992.

395. Wilk KE, Arrigo CA, Andrews JR: Functional training for the overhead athlete, *Sports physical therapy section home study course.* LaCrosse, Wis, 1995, SPTS.

396. Wilk KE, Arrigo CA, Andrews JR et al: The strength characteristics of internal and external muscles in professional baseball pitchers, *Am J Sports Med* 21:61, 1993.

397. Wilk KE, Voight M, Keirns MA et al: Plyometrics for the upper extremity: the theory and clinical application, *J Orthop Sports Phys Ther* 17:225, 1993.

398. Wilson AJ, Totty WG, Murphy WA et al: Shoulder joint: arthrographic CT and long-term follow-up with surgical correlation, *Radiology* 173:329, 1989.

399. Withers RJW: The painful shoulder: review of one hundred personal cases with remarks on the pathology, *J Bone Joint Surg* 31:414, 1949.

400. Wohlgethan JR: Frozen shoulder in hyperthyroidism, *Arthritis Rheum* 30:936, 1987.

401. Wolfgang GL: Surgical repair of tears of the rotator cuff of the shoulder, factors influencing the result, *J Bone Joint Surg Am* 56A:14, 1974.

402. Woo SLY: *Basic science of the ligaments and tendons around the glenohumeral joint,* Presented at the AOS Athlete's Shoulder Meeting, Vail, 1995.

403. Wvelker N, Brewer F, Sperveslage C: Passive glenohumeral joint stabilization: a biomechanical study, *J Shoulder Elbow Surg* 3:129, 1994.

404. Yergason, RM: Supination sign, *J Bone Joint Surg* 13:160, 1931.

405. Young D, Rockwood CA: Complications of a failed Bristow procedure and their management, *J Bone Joint Surg Am* 73A:969, 1991.

406. Zuckerman JD, Matsen FA: Complications about the glenohumeral joint related to the use of screws and staples, *J Bone Joint Surg Am* 66A:175, 1984.

SUGGESTED READINGS

1. Neer CS: *Shoulder reconstruction,* Philadelphia, 1990, WB Saunders.
2. Rowe CR: *The shoulder,* New York, 1988, Churchill Livingstone.
3. Rockwood CA, Matsen FA: *The shoulder,* Philadelphia, 1990, WB Saunders.
4. Hawkins RJ, Misamore GW: *Shoulder injuries in the athlete,* New York, 1996, Churchill Livingstone.
5. Andrews JR, Wilk KE: *The athlete's shoulder,* New York, 1995, Churchill Livingstone.
6. Kelley MJ, Clark WA: *Orthopedic therapy of the shoulder,* Philadelphia, 1995, JB Lippincott.

CHAPTER 16

The Hip

Paul Beattie

OUTLINE

Anatomy
  Osseous structures
  Arthrology
  Myology
  Neurology of the hip
  Vascular anatomy
Biomechanics
  Arthrokinematics
  The range of motion of the hip joint
  Kinetics
Summary: factors that provide stability and mobility to
  the hip
General concepts of hip joint dysfunction
Examination of the hip joint complex
  General principles
  The subjective examination
  The objective examination
  Standing position
  Sitting position
  Supine position
  The prone position
  The sidelying position
  Functional assessment
  Radiologic examination
Common hip disorders
  Osseous deformities involving the proximal femur
  Congenital and developmental conditions involving the
    hip joint
  Traumatic disorders that affect the hip and its associ-
    ated tissues
  Fractures of the hip and pelvis
Case 1
  Soft tissue disorders of the hip
Case 2
Degenerative and inflammatory conditions involving
  the hip
  Avascular necrosis of the femoral head
Case 3
  Arthritis of the hip
  Surgical management of end-stage arthrosis
Differential diagnosis
Summary

LEARNING OBJECTIVES

After studying this chapter, the reader should be able to:

1. Identify significant anatomical structures of the hip joint complex.
2. Describe the joint mechanics of the hip complex.
3. List the muscles responsible for performing the six motions of the hip joint.
4. State the normal range-of-motion values for the hip joint.
5. Describe and list all the components of a physical examination of the hip joint complex.
6. List and describe the four osseous deformities that affect the proximal femur.
7. State three congenital or developmental conditions that can affect the hip joint.
8. List and describe seven traumatic disorders that affect the hip joint as well as associated structures.
9. Describe the mechanism of degeneration and the conservative management of osteoarthritis.
10. State those factors that must be considered in the differential diagnosis of hip and buttock area pain.

KEY TERMS

hip joint	hip dysfunction
biomechanics	arthritis
examination	traumatic disorders
kinetics	

The ball-and-socket articulation of the hip and its associated soft tissues form the critical link between the lower extremity and the trunk. Critical for ambulation, the hip joint has been described by Radin as the "pivot upon which the body moves."[71]

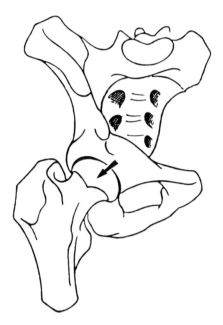

Fig. 16-1. The osseous components of the hip joint. (From Kapandji IA: *The physiology of joints,* vol 2, The lower limb, New York, 1970, Churchill Livingstone.)

The hip joint complex is a superbly organized array of tissues that must absorb and transmit enormous forces repeatedly throughout a lifetime. While meeting this task, the hip joint allows a large arc of motion necessary for such tasks as walking, sitting, squatting, and self-care. As such, the hip joint complex presents as a fascinating interplay of stability and mobility.

Clinically, dysfunction of the hip occurs at all ages in response to trauma as well as to a host of developmental, inflammatory, and degenerative conditions.[1,7,93,96] Pain perceived in the region of the hip not only can arise from many local sources but also can be referred from the lumbar spine and the lower abdomen.[14,16] Thus, the evaluation and treatment of people with problems involving the hip joint and its associated soft tissues require a strong understanding of the anatomy and mechanics of the hip, as well as the clinical manifestations of its pathologies. The purpose of this chapter is to provide the reader with an overview of the normal structure and function of the hip and the common abnormalities affecting the hip of the immature, mature, and aged skeleton. This information is then integrated into a scheme for evaluation and differential diagnosis for patients with hip problems.

ANATOMY
Osseous structures

The bony components that relate to the hip joint complex consist of the proximal femur and lateral aspect of the innominate bone or os coxae (Fig. 16-1).

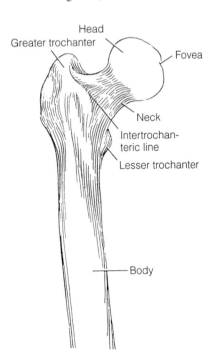

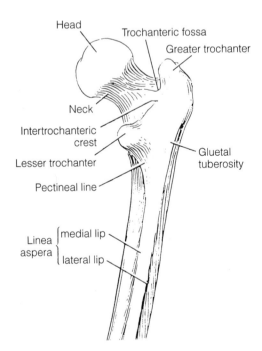

Fig. 16-2. The proximal femur. (Modified from Hollingshead WH, Rosse C, *Textbook of anatomy,* ed 4, Philadelphia, 1985, HarperCollins.)

The femur is the longest and strongest bone in the body.[98] Its great length and size contribute greatly to a person's height and potential stride length. It is almost completely covered with muscle, and thus great strength is required to resist the forces created by these structures.[84] The cylindric shaft of the femur is comprised primarily of dense, cortical bone and bows slightly in an anterior-lateral direction.[42,69,98] Its proximal portion, or metaphysis, is mainly cancellous bone and provides the bony arrangement that is critical to the

functioning of the hip.[31,63,65,87] The four major components of the proximal femur are the greater and lesser trochanter, the femoral neck, and the femoral head (Fig. 16-2).

Palpable at the lateral buttock, the greater trochanter is a large knob of reinforced trabecular bone. It provides the lateral attachment site of the muscles that abduct and externally rotate the hip.[50,65] The medial border of the greater trochanter marks the lateral margin of the hip joint capsule at the intertrochanteric line anteriorly and the

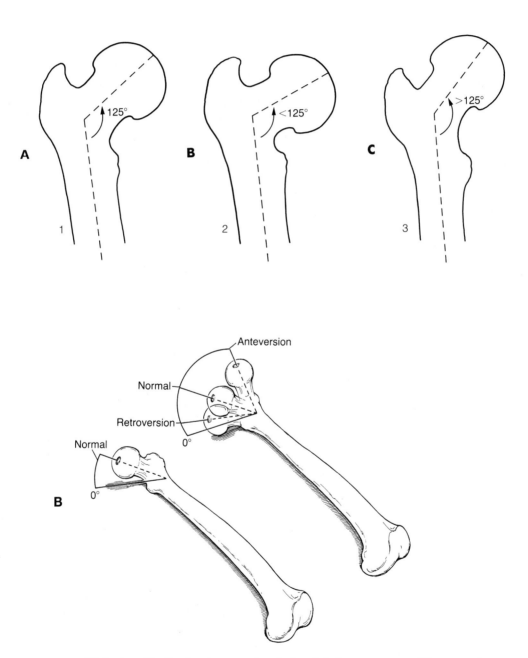

Fig. 16-3. (**A**) Angles of inclination, 1 = normal angle for adult, 2 = coxa vara, and 3 = coxa valga; (**B**) A representation of retroversion and anteversion of the femoral neck.

intertrochanteric crest posteriorly.[26,38] The lesser trochanter is a large, rounded, bony prominence that projects posterior-medially from the proximal shaft of the femur. It provides the distal attachment of the powerful hip flexor–external rotator muscle, the iliopsoas.[49,50,65]

Projecting superiorly, anteriorly, and medially from the proximal femur is the femoral neck. The femoral neck forms an "angle of inclination" with the femoral shaft on the frontal plane. In children, this angle may be up to 150 degrees; in adults, however, it is approximately 125 degrees.[1,31,38,49,63] Variations in this angle commonly occur: An increase in the angle of inclination is known as *coxa valga,* and a reduction in this angle is *coxa vara* (Fig. 16-3, *A*).[1,58,83] The femoral neck is typically aligned anterior to the femoral shaft on the transverse plane. This "angle of anteversion" is approximately 15 degrees in adults.[1,31,38] An increase in this angle is known as *excessive femoral anterversion;* a decrease is often called *femoral retroversion* (see Fig. 16-3, *B*).[7,74]

The shape of the femoral neck creates an overhang system that allows it to transmit enormous forces while positioning the femur far enough away from the pelvis to allow a large arc of motion of the hip.[49] Additionally, the transverse width of the femoral neck provides the moment arm acting on the hip abductor muscles.[31,63,71] The load-bearing capacity of the femoral neck is further enhanced by cancellous bone, the complex trabecular arrangement of which reinforces this structure to withstand compressive, tensile, and bending forces.[38,63] This principle is illustrated in Fig. 16-4. Originally described by Ward in 1838, the lamellae of trabecular bone are arranged parallel to the direction of the

compression and bending forces that are transmitted through the femoral neck.[38] By virtue of a complex latticework, these bony columns act to reinforce each other to withstand these forces. An area in the center of the femoral neck, Ward's triangle (see Fig. 16-4), often loses its trabecular bone in aged individuals and may be related to hip fractures.[38,49,66,87]

Medially, the femoral neck tapers and then thickens into the roughly spherical femoral head.[35,46,98] The femoral head is covered with articular cartilage that is thickest in its superior portion.[58,81] Its most medial aspect is devoid of articular cartilage and invaginates to form a fovea that is the lateral attachment site of the ligamentum teres.[42,49,98]

The medial component of the hip joint complex, the innominate or os coxae, is a broad, flat structure formed by the fusion of the ilium, ischium, and pubis (Fig. 16-5). The point of convergence of these three bones is a hemispheric socket, the acetabulum. The acetabulum is an incomplete cup whose articular surface is horseshoe-shaped.[57] It has a nonarticular fossa in its central portion and an opening, the acetabular notch, on its inferior portion. The outer margin, or rim, of the acetabulum is thickened, especially in its superior and posterior quadrants, to enhance its load-bearing capacity.[31,49,63] It is further reinforced by a fibrocartilaginous ring, the labrum acetabulare. The articular cartilage lining of the acetabulum is thickest in its superior and posterior margins, corresponding to the thickest areas of articular cartilage on the femoral head.[81] The remainder of the innominate bone provides a large surface area for the attachment of numerous muscles which span the hip. Important bony landmarks include the anterior superior iliac spine (ASIS), the anterior inferior iliac spine (AIIS), the posterior superior iliac spine (PSIS), the iliac crest, the pubic crest and symphysis, and the ischial tuberosity (see Fig. 16-5).

Arthrology

The convex femoral head articulates with the concave acetabulum to form a multiaxial, ball-and-socket type of synovial joint. According to Williams and Warwick, its joint center is approximately 1 to 2 cm, inferior to the middle third of the inguinal ligament.[98] Despite its great mobility, the hip joint is quite stable.

The femoral head faces superiorly, anteriorly, and medially within the acetabulum, with its geometric center traversed by the three axes of the joint.[49] The axis created by the acetabulum faces inferiorly 30 to 40 degrees because of the overhang of its superior rim, which Kapandji refers to as the "angle of Wiberg."[49]

The osseous components of the hip joint are surrounded by a large and complex joint capsule (Fig. 16-6). Formed by thick, fibrous tissue, the hip joint capsule surrounds not only the articular portion of the joint but much of the femoral neck as well.[26,38,69] Clinically, this is important because infections or fractures involving the femoral neck are intracapsular.[1,7,66] The superior and anterior portions of the capsule are the thickest corresponding to the areas of greatest force

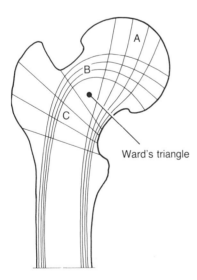

Fig. 16-4. Trabecular structure of proximal femur indicating (**A**) medical system; (**B**) arcuate system; (**C**) lateral system and the weak area of Ward's triangle. (Modified from Ramamurti C. In Tinker R, editor: *Orthopaedics in primary care,* Baltimore, 1979, Williams & Wilkins.)

concentration during load bearing.[26,31,64] Inferiorly, the hip joint capsule is thinner and similar to the shoulder in that it has a small redundancy that "unpleats" to allow abduction.[49] The anterior portion contains longitudinal bands, known as *reticula,* which contain important blood vessels to the femoral head.[64] The deep portion of the capsule contains circularly arranged fibers known as the *zona orbicularis,* which form a fibrous ring around the femoral neck.

The capsule of the hip is strongly reinforced by three ligaments: the iliofemoral, pubofemoral, and ischiofemoral.[42,69,97] These ligaments are thickest in the superior and anterior portion of the joint. An excellent description of their functions is reported by Fuss and Bacher (Table 16-1).[26]

In the midrange position of the hip, joint stability is primarily maintained by atmospheric pressure within the joint.[99] During hip extension, the capsule and medial portion of the iliofemoral ligament become twisted taut to strongly reinforce the hip.[71] The close-packed position of the hip is extension with some abduction and external rotation.[16,98] The synovial membrane that lines the joint capsule is very

large. Generally quite thick, it thins anteriorly where it is deep to the iliofemoral ligament. This change is of interest because the iliofemoral ligament at this location is pressed tautly against the femoral head during erect standing. The synovial membrane often communicates with the iliac or iliopectineal bursa, which is deep to the psoas major tendon. Lining the synovial membrane near the acetabulum is the acetabular fat pad. This structure increases the surface area of the synovial membrane and assists the distribution of synovial fluid.

The ligamentum teres consists of two bands that run from the fovea of the head of the femur to the center of the acetabulum. Although its function is unclear, it provides a pathway for the vessels supplying the head of the femur. Events that disrupt this ligament—for example, hip joint dislocations—may impair a portion of the blood supply to the head of the femur.[1,88]

Closely associated with the muscles of the hip is a complex arrangement of fascia. A specialized form of connective tissue, the fascia of the hip creates a low-friction

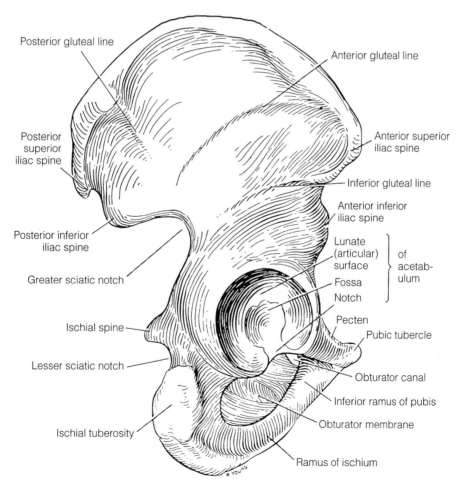

Fig. 16-5. The lateral view of the inominate (Os coxa) bone. (From Hollingshed WH, Rosse C, *Textbook of anatomy,* ed 4, Philadelphia, 1985, HarperCollins.)

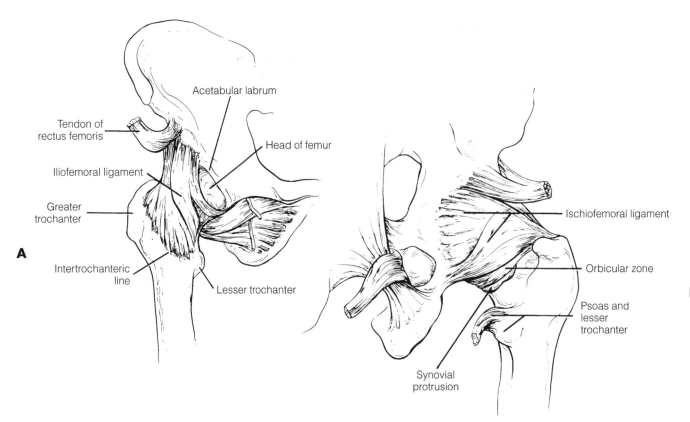

Fig. 16-6. The hip joint capsule and capsular ligaments, (A) anterior and (B) posterior views. (From Nicholas JA, Hershman EB, *Lower extremity & spine in sports medicine,* ed 2, St Louis, 1995, Mosby.)

Table 16-1. Hip joint motions restricted by ligaments

Motion	Ligament that restricts
Flexion	Inferior portion of ischiofemoral
Extension	Medial portion of iliofemoral
Abduction	Pubofemoral
Adduction	Superior ischiofemoral
Internal rotation	Superior portion of ischiofemoral
External rotation	Lateral portion of iliofemoral

From Fuss FK, Bacher A: New aspects of the morphology and function of the human hip joint fragments, *Am J Anat* 192:1, 1991; with permission.

plane to allow smooth gliding of adjacent tissues. The deep fascia of the buttock arises from the iliac crest, sacrotuberous ligament, and inguinal ligament and continues inferiorly as the fascia lata.[98] It joins with the tensor fasciae latae and gluteus maximus to form what Harty refers to as a "fibromuscular umbrella" around the hip joint.[38]

Myology

The hip joint complex is surrounded and reinforced by the thickest muscular system in the body. These muscles act to provide the tension required to control joint movement while concomitantly stabilizing the hip against externally applied forces.[44,60] Weakness and/or contracture of these muscles is a common sequela of hip joint dysfunction that must be addressed in planning a rehabilitation program.

Several of the muscles that span the hip act upon the knee or lumbar spine, illustrating the important interrelationship between the hip and its associated joints. An in-depth presentation of the attachments, actions, and innervation of the muscles of the hip is beyond the scope of this chapter; readers are referred to an anatomy text. Table 16-2 presents a summary of the muscles of the hip as they relate to the concentric activities on the cardinal planes.[50]

The gluteus maximus, the thickest muscle in the body, forms a soft tissue barrier to protect the posterior hip and the large neurovascular structures of the buttock region (Fig. 16-7). A powerful extensor, it works with the hamstring muscles to assist such activities as getting in and out of chairs, ascending and descending stairs, and lifting heavy objects.[22] Deep to the gluteus maximus, the posterior hip is spanned by several smaller muscles that act externally to rotate this joint (Fig. 16-8). The external rotation moment generated by these muscles stabilizes the hip by "driving" the head of the femur into the acetabulum during the stance phase of gait.[71]

Table 16-2. Muscle action and motion limiters referenced to the cardinal plane movements of the hip

Motion	ROM	Muscles active (agonists)	Motion limiters
Flexion	118-122	Iliopsoas Rectus femoris Sartorius Pectineus Adductor longus and brevis Tensor fasciae latae Gluteus minimus	Hip extensor muscles Posterior capsule Femoral neck on the acetabulum Medial ischiofemoral ligament
Extension	17-22	Gluteus maximus Gluteus medius Hamstrings Piriformis Adductor magnus (posterior)	Hip flexor muscles Anterior capsule Medial iliofemoral ligament
Abduction	39-44	Gluteus medius Tensor fasciae latae Gluteus minimus Piriformis Gluteus medius Iliopsoas Gemellus Obturatorius internus	Adductor muscles Inferior capsule Pubofemoral ligament Femoral neck on the superior rim of the acetabulum
Adduction	30	Adductor longus and brevis Adductor magnus Pectineus Gracilis Obturatorius externus	Abductor muscles Superior capsule Superior ischiofemoral ligament
Medial rotation	30-33	Tensor fasciae latae Gluteus medius (anterior) Adductor longus and brevis Gluteus minimus	Lateral rotation muscles Posterior capsule Superior ischiofemoral ligament
Lateral rotation	29-34	Piriformis Gemellus Obturatorius internus and externus Quadratus femoris Gluteus maximus Sartorius Biceps femoris, long head Iliopsoas Posterior gluteus medius	Medial rotation muscles Anterior capsule Lateral iliofemoral ligament

From Kapandji IA: *The physiology of joints,* vol 2, The lower limb, New York, 1970, Churchill Livingstone; Kendell FP, McCreary EK, Provance PG: *Muscles: test and function,* ed 4, Baltimore, 1993, Williams & Wilkins; and Roach KE, Miles T: Normal hip and knee active range of motion: the relationship to age, *Phys Ther* 71:656, 1991.

The iliopsoas muscle passes anterior to the hip joint and acts with the rectus femoris, sartorius, tensor fasciae latae, and anterior hip adductors to create a potential for flexion of the hip against strong resistance (Fig. 16-9). Although forceful hip flexion does not occur often during most daily activities, it is a component of many sports and some occupational activities. The medial aspect of the hip is spanned by the adductor muscles. Soderberg contends that, considering the large muscle mass of the adductors and the infrequent need for forceful hip adduction, these muscles primarily function as assisters of other movements, such as hip flexion and extension (Table 16-2).[87] The anterior lateral portion of the hip is occupied by the gluteus minimus and the

tensor fasciae latae, which act primarily as internal rotators.

Central to normal hip function, the gluteus medius, gluteus minimus, tensor fasciae latae, and piriformis muscles form the abductor mechanism of the hip. During weight bearing, this system counteracts the weight of the body to prevent excessive downward displacement of the pelvis on the frontal plane.[44,63,65,87] This system must be functioning adequately to allow normal load bearing through the hip.[44,60-62,67,68]

Neurology of the hip

Several nerves have important relationships with the hip. The buttock and lower extremity receive innervation from

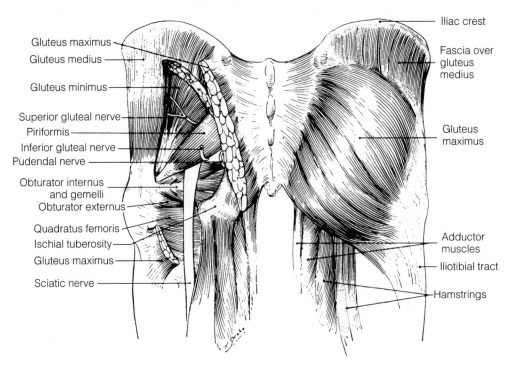

Fig. 16-7. Superficial muscles of the buttock and thigh: lateral. (From Nicholas JA, Hershman EB, *Lower extremity & spine in sports medicine,* ed 2, St Louis, 1995, Mosby.)

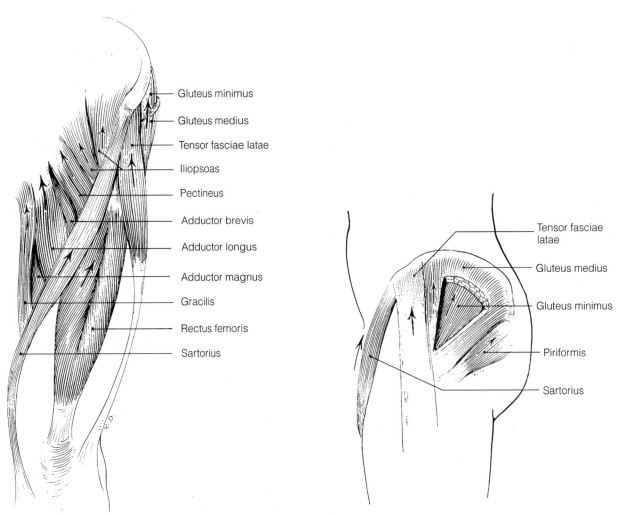

Fig. 16-8. Muscles of the anterior thigh. (From Nicholas JA, Hershman EB, *Lower extremity & spine in sports medicine,* ed 2, St Louis, 1995, Mosby.)

Fig. 16-9. Muscles of the lateral buttock. (From Nicholas JA, Hershman EB, *Lower extremity & spine in sports medicine,* ed 2, St Louis, 1995, Mosby.)

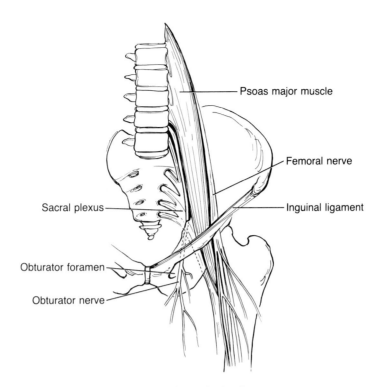

Fig. 16-10. Anterior hip, showing positions of related nerves and psoas major muscle.

branches of the lumbar plexus, lumbosacral trunk, and sacral plexus.[98] Because of the hip's central location, numerous nerves arising from these plexus must course near it as they travel to the buttock and lower extremity. Thus, injuries or infections of the hip can result in impairment of a variety of nerves.[1,96]

Entering the thigh through the femoral triangle and coursing anterior to the hip is the femoral nerve (Fig. 16-10). It innervates the muscles of the anterior compartment of the thigh and provides cutaneous innervation to most of the anterior thigh and medial leg. Coursing just posterior to the hip is the sciatic nerve, which innervates the muscles of the posterior compartment of the thigh and through its peroneal and tibial divisions, innervates the muscles of the leg and foot (Fig. 16-11). It provides cutaneous innervation to the leg and foot. Because of its location, the sciatic nerve can often be traumatized following a posterior dislocation of the hip. The obturator nerve is medial and somewhat distant from the hip as it courses into the medial compartment through the obturator foramen. The classic pain referral pattern from the hip to the medial knee is often attributed to this nerve, which supplies cutaneous innervation to the medial thigh. The lateral femoral cutaneous nerve enters the thigh deep to the inguinal ligament approximately 1 cm medial to the anterior superior iliac spine. It can become mechanically irritated by the pressure from the soft tissue of a protuberant abdomen or from an excessively tight lumbar orthosis. These events can result in pain and parasthesia over the lateral thigh, a

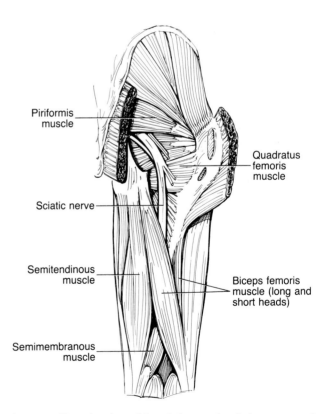

Fig. 16-11. Posterior view of the sciatic nerve in relation to external rotators and hamstring muscles. (Modified from Warwick R, Williams P, editors: *Gray's anatomy,* Br ed 35, Philadelphia, 1973, WB Saunders.)

condition known as *meralgia paraesthetica*. Occasionally this nerve can be entrapped in a lateral approach surgical incision to the hip. The superior and inferior gluteal nerves innervate the large muscles of the buttock.

The innervation of the hip joint follows Hilton's law, which states that a joint is innervated by the same nerves that innervate the muscles acting upon it. Thus, the hip joint is innervated by branches from the femoral, sciatic, obturator, and superior and inferior gluteal nerves, as diagrammed in Fig. 16-12. The sclerotomal reference for the hip joint is generally considered to be L3. The cutaneous innervation of the hip, buttock, and thigh can be referenced to peripheral nerves or dermatomes.

Vascular anatomy

The blood supply to the buttock is provided by the superior and inferior gluteal arteries; the hip joint and proximal thigh are perfused by branches from the femoral artery (Fig. 16-13).[38,42,86] These vessels communicate via the cruciate anastomosis in the inferior buttock and thus provide an excellent mechanism for collateral blood flow.[98]

Although the circulation to the buttock and thigh is abundant, the blood flow to the femoral head can, in certain circumstances, be tenuous.[38] Because the femoral neck and head are enclosed within the joint capsule, their blood supply is almost completely restricted to a pericapsular anastomosis and its retinacular branches (Fig. 16-14).[95] The pericapsular anastomosis is formed by branches from the medial femoral circumflex, obturator, and gluteal arteries. Small retinacular branches arise here and course proximally within the joint capsule near the femoral neck.[95] These branches provide the only source of blood flow to the femoral head in children and are the primary source of blood supply in adults.[1,7] Contributions of blood flow to the femoral head from the artery of ligamentum teres as well as perforating branches from the profunda femora artery are minimal.

BIOMECHANICS

The ball-and-socket articulation of the hip allows three degrees of freedom: movement of the femur and pelvis relative to one another on the sagittal, frontal, and transverse planes. The hip is well designed for repetitive load bearing; however, subtle abnormalities in the hip or lower extremity can lead to dysfunction of the hip and ultimately degenerative arthritis.[31,60,67,68]

In assessing movement at the hip joint during various activities, it is important to consider that hip joint movement can occur from the femur moving relative to the pelvis, from the pelvis moving relative to the femur, or from both moving relative to one another.[49,65] Additionally, the available range of motion of the hip is greatly influenced by the relative length of the biarthroidal muscles, such as the hamstrings or rectus femoris. Thus, the position of the lumbar spine and knee joint must be considered in evaluating the hip joint.

Arthrokinematics

The unique ball-and-socket shape of the hip allows joint movement in all directions.[87] At the joint surface, a gliding motion occurs as the femoral head and acetabulum move tangentially to one another around a central axis of motion. Alterations in the shape of the joint surfaces can impair this mechanism and cause abnormal compression and distraction to the articular cartilage.[58,68,92] Thus, discussing the biomechanics of the hip requires considering the joint geometry.

During load bearing in the upright position, the superior portion of the femoral head and the superior articular portion of the acetabulum sustain the largest concentration of the weight-bearing forces acting upon the joint.[31,81] These areas coincide with the thickest articular cartilage of the hip and are the most reinforced area of trabecular bone in the hip.[38,49,98] Hammond and Charnley have described the femoral head as "spheroid or slightly ovoid" rather than a smooth sphere.[35] This shape leads to a lack of precise fit, an

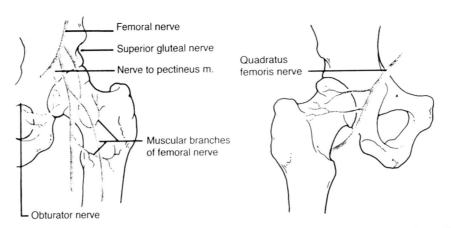

Fig. 16-12. Nerve branches supplying hip joint. (From Leveau B, The hip. In *Clinical orthopaedic physical therapy,* Philadelphia, 1994, WB Saunders.)

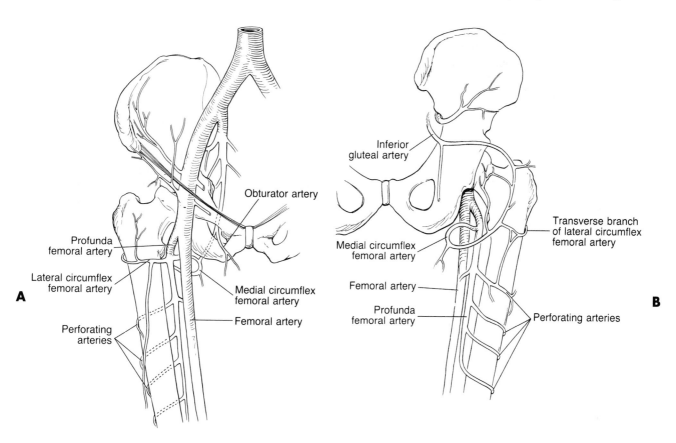

Fig. 16-13. Arterial pathways of the buttock and proximal femur, demonstrating (**A**) anterior and (**B**) posterior views. (Modified from Moore K: *Clinically oriented anatomy,* Baltimore, 1980, Williams & Wilkins.)

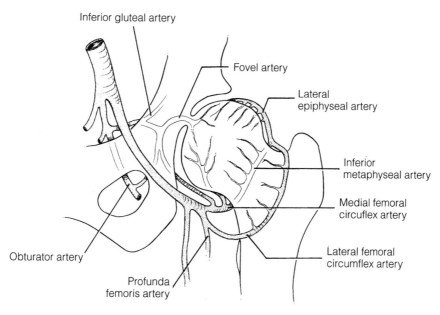

Fig. 16-14. Blood supply to the hip joint.

incongruity between the femoral head and the acetabulum when the hip is unloaded, for example, during the swing phase of gait.[31,71] When the normal hip becomes fully loaded in the midstance phase of gait, the joint surfaces become increasingly congruent because of deformation of the articular cartilage. This increases the surface area for weight bearing and thus minimizes excessive contact stress in any single portion of the femoral head.[31,71] This principle is illustrated in Fig. 16-15. The vacillation between incongruent/loose-packed and congruent/close-packed, which accompanies the cycle of unloading and loading of the hip during ambulation, provides very important mechanical force gradients to assist in the nutrition of the articular cartilage of the hip.[26,27]

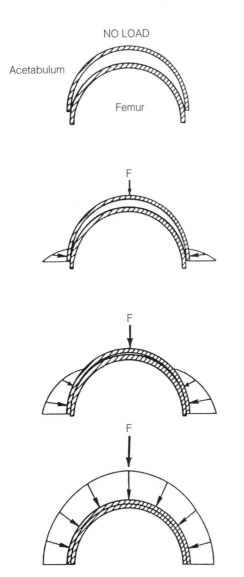

Fig. 16-15. The change in the congruency of the hip during load bearing. Note how the joint surfaces become more congruent with increasing load bearing. (From Greenwald AS: Biomechanics of the hip. In Steinberg ME, editor: *The hip and its disorders,* Philadelphia, 1991, WB Saunders.)

Arthrosis of the hip, characterized by alterations in joint geometry, alters this mechanism.[68]

The range of motion of the hip joint

The several normative values for hip range of motion (ROM) that have been described[50,53,65,77] have led to controversy regarding what should be considered a normal value. Additionally, there may be ROM differences related to age and body type. Considering the potential for age-related changes, Roach and Miles studied the hip joint ROM of 1892 healthy adults of various ages.[77] They reported that, despite a slight decrease in ROM associated with older individuals, any substantial loss should be regarded as abnormal and not attributed to aging. These values are listed in Table 16-3.

Limitations of hip joint ROM are quite common in individuals with hip pathology. They can often lead to functional limitations. In an attempt to determine the hip joint ROM requirements for various functional activities, Johnston and Smidt used electrogoniometry on 33 adult males who had no hip joint impairments (Table 16-4).[47] These values may prove useful for treatment plans that incorporate increasing the ROM of the hip to achieve functional goals.

Most hip joint disorders result in some form of gait impairment, thus analysis of gait is critical for evaluating a person with hip joint dysfunction. Additionally, restoration of normal gait is often the main goal of physical therapy treatment. The ROM of the hip required for normal gait reported by Murray is given in Table 16-5.[59]

Kinetics

The joint forces that act upon the hip are created both externally by gravity and inertia due to the acceleration of body parts and internally, primarily from the musculotendinous unit, with small contributions from the tension generated by ligaments and the joint capsule.[87,97] The result of internal and external forces is the joint reaction force (JRF).[75,79] The JRF has traditionally been studied with mathematical models.[6,67] Recently, data regarding the JRFs of the hip have been obtained from sensors contained in prosthetic hip implants in patients.[89] The following discussion illustrates clinical applications of the JRF.

When a person is standing with body balanced between the two legs, no muscle activity is required to stabilize the hip joints.[7,63] Because the person's body weight (BW) is distributed equally between the two lower extremities, the JRF for each hip is equal to half the superincumbent weight. Assuming that the person's lower extremities account for one third of the BW, then the remaining two thirds of the BW is borne by the hips; thus, each hip bears one third of the BW in this position.[63]

When a person moves to a single-leg standing position, the muscular activity in the abductor mechanism is required to prevent a downward displacement of the pelvis (Trende-

Table 16-3. Normal ROM of the hip excluding adduction

Motion	All ages (N = 1683)	Age Group (yr)		
		25-39 (N = 433)	40-59 (N = 727)	60-74 (N = 523)
Hip flexion				
X̄	121	122	120	118
SD	13	12	14	13
CI*	120-121	121-123	119-121	117-120
100%	160	150	160	150
75%	130	130	130	125
50%	120	120	120	120
25%	110	115	115	110
0%	0	55	0	0
Hip extension				
X̄	19	22	18	17
SD	8	8	7	8
CI	19-20	21-23	18-19	16-17
100%	45	45	40	40
75%	25	25	20	20
50%	20	20	20	15
25%	15	15	15	10
0%	0	0	0	0
Hip abduction				
X̄	42	44	42	39
SD	11	11	11	12
CI	42-43	43-45	41-43	38-40
100%	90	90	90	90
75%	50	50	50	45
50%	40	45	40	40
25%	35	35	35	30
0%	0	0	0	0
Hip internal rotation				
X̄	32	33	31	30
SD	8	7	8	7
CI	31-32	32-34	31-32	29-30
100%	60	60	55	50
75%	35	40	35	35
50%	30	30	30	30
25%	25	30	25	25
0%	0	10	0	5
Hip external rotation				
X̄	32	34	32	29
SD	9	8	8	9
CI	32-33	33-35	32-33	29-30
100%	65	65	60	55
75%	40	40	40	35
50%	30	35	30	30
25%	25	30	25	25
0%	0	10	0	5

From Roach KE, Miles T: Normal hip and knee active range of motion: the relationship to age, *Phys Ther* 71:656, 1991.
*CI = 95% confidence interval.

lenburg sign).[7,44,60-62] This movement causes the JRF to rise dramatically.[87] Fig. 16-16 is a free body diagram of the hip in single limb stance. This figure illustrates the relationship between the person's BW acting as the external force and the tension of the hip abductor muscles acting as the internal force. Notice that BW is acting through a longer moment arm than the hip abductors, which results in a great force demand on the abductors and then a JRF of approximately 2.5 times BW acting through the hip. Estimates of JRF acting upon the hip during the stance phase of walking have ranged from 2.5 to 4 times BW,[46] and running is said to cause up to 5 times BW.[82]

Because the JRF is primarily due to the force from muscular contractions, activities that increase the muscular activity around the hip increase the JRF.[63] Examples of factors that lead to increased JRF include obesity, carrying objects, and stair climbing.[60] Conversely, activities that reduce the muscular activity around the hip reduce the JRF. For example, a patient with a painful hip often deviates to the painful side during stance phase, which reduces the moment through which the BW acts and thus reduces abductor muscle contraction. The use of a cane shunts a portion of the BW through the upper extremity, thus reducing the BW acting upon the hip. This can lessen the joint forces by 60%.[6] Other factors that can reduce the JRF include reducing cadence to decrease the inertial forces or reducing the body weight of the individual.

SUMMARY: FACTORS THAT PROVIDE STABILITY AND MOBILITY TO THE HIP

To summarize hip anatomy and mechanics, in a clinical setting addressing the factors that provide mobility and stability to the hip is a fundamental concern of evaluation. The factors favoring stability follow:

1. The acetabulum forms a bony ring around the femoral head, which is reinforced by the capsule and labrum. Thus, the ball-and-socket structure of the hip creates a very stable joint.
2. The joint surfaces are nearly congruent during weight bearing (WB).
3. Bony trabeculae reinforce the femur and pelvis in the direction of WB.
4. A large muscle mass is acting through well-placed, bony lever arms.

The factors favoring mobility follow:

1. The hip joint has a large surface area, which allows for a large displacement between joint surfaces, resulting in a large ROM.
2. There are no barriers to motion from adjacent joints because the lower extremity is positioned away from the trunk by the femoral neck.
3. There is a slight capsular redundancy inferiorly to allow freedom of movement in abduction.

GENERAL CONCEPTS OF HIP JOINT DYSFUNCTION

Dysfunction of the hip joint and its associated tissues is common in all age groups. It is one of the major causes of

Table 16-4. Hip joint range of motion for various functional tasks (mean for 33 normal men)

Activity	Plane of motion	Recorded value (degrees)
Tying shoe with foot on floor	Sagittal	124
	Frontal	19
	Transverse	15
Tying shoe with foot across opposite thigh	Sagittal	110
	Frontal	23
	Transverse	33
Sitting down on chair and rising from sitting	Sagittal	104
	Frontal	20
	Transverse	17
Stooping to obtain object from floor	Sagittal	117
	Frontal	21
	Transverse	18
Squatting	Sagittal	122
	Frontal	28
	Transverse	26
Ascending stairs	Sagittal	67
	Frontal	16
	Transverse	18
Descending stairs	Sagittal	36

Data from Johnston RC, Smidt GL: Hip motion measurements for selected activities of daily living, *Clin Orthop* 72:205, 1970.

Table 16-5. Hip joint kinematics approximate values referenced to cardinal planes during gait

		Swing phase		
		Early	Middle	Late
	Sagittal	20 flexion	30 flexion	30 flexion
	Frontal	3 abduction	8 abduction	3 abduction
	Transverse	10 external rotation	2 external rotation	0 rotation

	Stance phase				
	Heel strike	Foot flat	Midstance	Heel off	Toe off
Sagittal	30 flexion	25 flexion	0 flexion	10-20 extension	0
Frontal	2 abduction	0 abduction	0-2 adduction	5 adduction	5 abduction
Transverse	0-2 internal rotation	2 internal rotation	2 external rotation	2 external rotation	10 external rotation

From Murray MP: Gait as a total pattern of movement, *Am J Phys Med* 46:290, 1967.

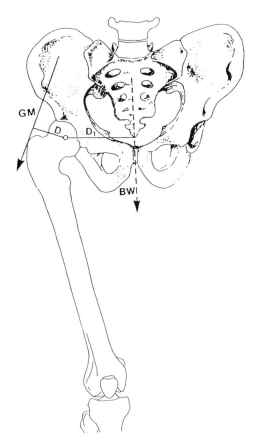

Fig. 16-16. Free body diagram of the hip in single limb stance where BW = body weight acting through moment arm D1, and GM = the force generated by the hip abductors (primarily gluteus medius) through moment arm D. (From Neumann DA, Cook TM. The effect of load and carry position on the electromyographic activity of gluteus medius during walking, *Phys Ther* 65:305, 1985.)

gait impairment in both pediatric and geriatric populations. In addition to pain, impairment of the hip joint and/or its associated soft tissues can predispose an individual to a considerable variety of functional limitations in gait and self-care.

Numerous anatomic factors can predispose the hip to dysfunction.[7,20] The hip relies on a precise bony alignment and is dramatically influenced by alterations in muscle tension and ligamentous support.* The hip joint transmits large forces repetitively throughout life, and therefore it is subjected to enormous wear and tear over time, which is typically related to a person's occupational demands and recreational pursuits. When combined with malalignment, this is probably a predisposing factor for arthrosis.[27] The blood supply to the femoral head is tenuous and can be compromised by trauma and disease, often leading to a very disabling condition known as *avascular necrosis* (AVN).[88] The bone tissue in the femoral neck is primarily cancellous. Loss of bone cells (osteopenia) in this area is common in

elderly people and can predispose to fractures.[1,66] The abductor muscle mechanism relies on a normally functioning hip joint, which, with dysfunction of the hip, is usually impaired. This alters the joint reaction forces acting upon the hip, which can then lead to further problems.[60]

Normal functioning of the hip joint system is based upon the complex interplay of all the tissues in the lower quarter. Because of its pivotal location, the tissues of the hip joint complex are susceptible to strain due to a variety of extrinsic causes. In addition, subtle malalignments of the lower extremity—for example, leg length asymmetries or torsional deformities—can adversely affect the hip.

Dysfunction of the hip joint typically presents as some combination of the following:

1. Pain perceived in the inguinal area, which can refer to the medial knee
2. Limited ROM of the hip
3. Gait disturbance

The following section consists of a detailed discussion of the strategies for the evaluation of people with disorders of the hip and its associated soft tissues.

EXAMINATION OF THE HIP JOINT COMPLEX
General principles

Planning for any clinical examination should include consideration of what information is necessary to make an accurate assessment of the patient's condition. Upon completion of the examination, the clinician should be prepared to decide whether to treat, treat and consult, refer, or discharge the patient. If the decision to treat is made, the clinician should have the information to develop a safe and effective treatment plan for the patient.[48] Numerous intake forms and checklists to assist the examination have been described. They are typically quite helpful; one example is shown in Fig. 16-17.

A useful way to categorize the information from the examination, which has been modified from Maitland, is described by the acronym SINS.[54] For the purposes of this chapter, it means:

S—Severity:	What is the degree of functional limitation and disability? How intense is the pain?
I—Irritability:	How easily are the patient's symptoms provoked? How long does it take for symptoms to ease after they have been provoked?
N—Nature:	What is the pathology? What tissues are abnormal, and how are they related to the patient's problem?
S—Stage:	Is the condition improving, worsening, or stable?

An enormous number of physical examination procedures have been described for the hip joint complex. To

* References 11, 24, 25, 46, 67, 68.

EVALUATION OF THE HIP

Date _____   # _____
Name _____ Age _____ Sex _____
Address _____ Occupation _____
Diagnosis or referral _____
Referring physician _____

A. SUBJECTIVE EXAMINATION OF THE HIP
1. Client's chief complaint _____
2. Location of symptoms _____

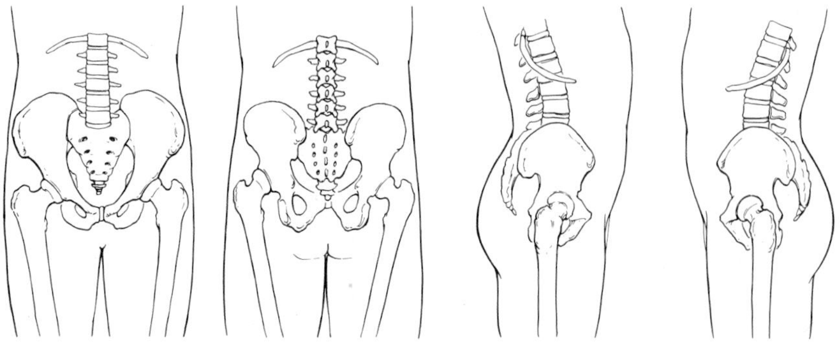

Front   Back   Side   Side

3. Onset of symptoms
    Date of injury/onset _____
    Nature and mechanism _____

4. Nature of symptoms _____
    _____
    Where did the symptoms start? _____
    Have they spread? _____ Where? _____
    Is there any tingling or numbness? _____
    Is the pain sharp, a dull ache, deep, etc.? _____

5. Previous history
    First episode in detail _____
    _____
    Successive episodes
      How frequently? _____
      Ease of onset _____
      How long to recover? _____
      Previous treatment and results _____

Fig. 16-17. An example of an examination form for the hip.

utilize each of these in every hip examination would be extremely time-consuming for the clinician and exhausting for the patient. Thus, clinicians have to select the most important procedures within the framework of the patient's symptoms, irritability, and precautions. The selection of a test should first be based upon the usefulness of the information that it yields, which, in turn, is based upon the reliability, validity, sensitivity, and specificity of the information (see Box).

The second primary concern of the utilization of a test relates to the potential harm to the patient. For example, although knowing the lifting capacity of a patient recovering from hip surgery might be useful, the performance of this test may harm the surgical site. Finally, one must consider issues of cost containment. For example, will the data from an expensive isokinetic test of the hip joint musculature be more useful in treatment planning than that obtained by less expensive means?

EVALUATION OF THE HIP—cont'd

6. Behavior of symptoms
   Constant or intermittent? _____
   What brings them on? _____
   What relieves them? _____
   What makes them worse? _____
   Is there associated stiffness? _____
   What is the effect of prolonged sitting? _____
   _____
   What is the effect of walking? _____
   _____

7. Previous treatment and results
   Treatment to date for present problem _____
   Effects? _____

8. Other medical history and family history
   Medications _____
   Radiographs _____
   Recent illnesses _____
   Family history _____
   General health _____

9. Hobbies and leisure-time activities _____
   Still able to do these activities? _____

B. OBJECTIVE EXAMINATION OF THE HIP
1. Initial observation
   Sitting posture _____
   Sitting to standing _____
   Gait _____
   Ease of movement _____

2. Standing
   Posture _____
   _____
   Detailed gait evaluation _____
   _____
   Balance
      Digital scale weight bearing   R_____ L_____
      Stork standing test: Standing on R leg_____ Standing on L leg_____
   Lumbar spine active movements
      Flexion _____
      Extension _____

Fig. 16-17, cont'd. For legend see opposite page.

There are three broad, overlapping scenarios in which clinicians may want to perform an examination of the hip:

1. The mobility-impaired patient with a well-defined diagnosis and a clearly outlined set of precautions. This category primarily refers to patients who have recently undergone joint replacement, osteotomy, or surgical stabilization of a fracture. In this case, the emphasis is on assessment of mobility and self-care rather than reproduction of symptoms. Because of the impaired stability of the hip joint complex, the majority of physical examination procedures are not used.

2. The patient whose primary complaint of pain is located elsewhere in the lower quarter. It is my belief that the hip should be examined in every patient who presents with a complaint of dysfunction in the lower extremity or thoracolumbar spine. In this instance, the hip joint complex needs to be examined to rule it out

Lateral flexion R _____

Lateral flexion L _____

Squat _____

3. Sitting

Lumbar spine active movements

    Rotation   R_____ L_____

Active, passive, and resisted internal and external rotation

    Internal rotation   R_____ L_____

    External rotation   R_____ L_____

Active and resisted hip flexion   R_____ L_____

Sartorius muscle test _____

Thomas test: R hip extended _____

             L hip extended _____

4. Supine

Palpations of anterior aspect _____

Leg-length measurements   R_____ L_____

SI joint compression and distraction _____

Fabere's test   R_____ L_____

Scouring   R_____ L_____

Distal and lateral traction   R_____ L_____

90-90 straight-leg raise   R_____ L_____

Knee clearing _____

Passive, active, and resisted hip movements

    Flexion   R_____ L_____

    Abduction   R_____ L_____

    Adduction   R_____ L_____

5. Side-lying position

Palpations of lateral and posterior aspects _____

_____

Active, passive, and resisted hip movements

    Extension   R_____ L_____

    Abduction   R_____ L_____

    Flexion   R_____ L_____

    Adduction: Ober test (knee extended)   R_____ L_____

             Knee flexed   R_____ L_____

             Hip and knee flexed (piriformis tightness test)   R_____ L_____

6. Prone

Palpations of posterior aspect _____

_____

Active, passive, and resisted hip movements

    Hip extension: Knee extended   R_____ L_____

              Knee flexed   R_____ L_____

    Internal rotation   R_____ L_____

    External rotation   R_____ L_____

Prone knee bend (femoral nerve stretch)   R_____ L_____

7. Miscellaneous

Other observations of tests _____

Subjective comments during objective examination _____

_____

_____

_____

8. Summary of findings

Fig. 16-17, cont'd. An example of an examination form for the hip.

Important concepts in the selection of a test

Reliability	The reproducibility of a test result
Validity	How well the measurement reflects what is to be measured
Sensitivity	The probability that a person who actually has the disorder will have a postitive response to the test
Sensitivity	The probability that a person who does not have the disorder will have a negative response to the test

as a source of both referred pain (e.g., the adolescent with medial knee pain arising from the hip) and as a contributor of mechanical forces that may result in pain elsewhere (e.g., hip abductor muscle weakness leading to a "Trendelenburg gait" that causes low back pain). In these instances, the examiner primarily employs "screening tests."

3. The patient whose primary complaint is pain in the hip or pelvic area. For these patients, the emphasis is on reproduction of the symptoms and identification of abnormalities of structure and movement. The choice of examination procedures is guided by the patient's degree of irritability and potential to tolerate load bearing within the hip. These patients typically require detailed examination of all structures within the hip joint complex.

4. The following section describes history and physical examination procedures that are useful to evaluate this third type of patient, the one with a complaint of pain in the hip or pelvic area.

The subjective examination

The most important component of any clinical examination is, in my opinion, the patient's own description of his or her problems and goals. Four major areas should be addressed during the oral history portion of the examination:

1. General patient information
2. Chief complaint symptoms
3. Past medical history and current medical and/or surgical problems
4. The patient's goals for treatment outcome

General patient information. The patient's age, occupation, and recreational pursuits and, when appropriate, information regarding home and work environment, such as stairs and other architectural barriers, should be obtained. Issues such as the need for prolonged standing, walking, or working in awkward postures should be identified. The goal is understanding the patient's daily physical challenges and their relationship to the hip problem. In addition, attempts

should be made to understand the patient's communication skills and unique cultural influences.

Chief complaint symptoms. Patients with hip disorders almost always complain of some combination of pain, stiffness, weakness, and gait disturbance.* In discussing pain with the patient, several issues should be clarified. The location of pain should be assessed by having the patient point to the area on his or her own body and fill in a body chart (Fig. 16-17). Frequently, pain arising in the hip joint is perceived in the inguinal area and is most commonly referred to the medial thigh. Local pain and tenderness are often due to bursitis, tendinitis, or apophysitis (e.g., inflammation at the point where a tendon inserts into bone). Pain that is referred is more likely to be caused by nerve entrapment, synovitis, or acute muscle injury. The intensity of the pain can be quantified with a visual analog scale (VAS) (Fig. 16-18), and the patient's interpretation of the pain can be identified with the modified McGill Pain Questionnaire (Fig. 16-19).[55] Perhaps the most important issue regarding pain is its behavior, that is, its response to activity. Clinicians should always ask, "What makes it better? What makes it worse?"[53,54] These questions help to identify not only the level of irritability of the disorder but also its nature or potential cause. For example, arthritic hip joints often are painful upon arising in the morning and then gradually loosen up, only to be painful again after prolonged standing or walking. A similar pattern is observed with tendinitis. A patient with a stress fracture of the femoral neck may report no symptoms during the day before running for a considerable length of time.[66] Pain in the midbuttock that is related to exertion may be due to vascular insufficiency.[86] Pain perceived in the middle of night often indicates hip joint effusion.[23] When a patient reports that activity or joint position fails to influence the pain, the clinician should consider more serious disorders such as infection or neoplasm.

Conditions such as joint stiffness, weakness, and gait disturbances are best clarified in reference to various activities. For example, does the patient report difficulty walking, standing, assuming or maintaining the sitting position, or moving from sitting to standing? Other frequent functional limitations reported by patients with hip joint problems include such activities as tying shoes or getting in or out of the bathtub.

Whenever a patient is complaining of muscle weakness, the potential of neurologic impairment should be considered. The examiner should plan to perform muscle testing, addressing both peripheral nerve and segmental innervation patterns as well as assessing cutaneous sensation and reflexes.

After a thorough understanding of the patient's current symptoms is achieved, the examiner should question the patient regarding the onset of symptoms. My opinion is that

---

* References 1, 7, 10, 14-16, 20, 37, 51, 85, 96.

The following line represents the intensity of your pain. The left end of the line indicates **no pain** while the right end represents the **worst pain** that you can imagine. Please put a slash through the part of the line which best represents your average pain over the last week.

No pain —————————————————————————————————————— Worst pain
                                                                                            imaginable

Fig. 16-18. The visual analog scale (VAS) used to measure pain intensity.

Please read each word below, and decide whether it describes what your pain has felt like over the last 3 days. If a word does not describe your pain, circle 0 (DOES NOT APPLY), and go to the next item. If a word does describe your pain, then rate how strongly you have felt that sensation (1=mild, 2=moderate, 3=severe).

	Does not apply	Mild	Moderate	Severe
1. Throbbing	0	1	2	3
2. Shooting	0	1	2	3
3. Stabbing	0	1	2	3
4. Sharp	0	1	2	3
5. Cramping	0	1	2	3
6. Gnawing	0	1	2	3
7. Hot-burning	0	1	2	3
8. Aching	0	1	2	3
9. Heavy	0	1	2	3
10. Tender	0	1	2	3
11. Splitting	0	1	2	3
12. Tiring-exhausting	0	1	2	3
13. Sickening	0	1	2	3
14. Fearful	0	1	2	3
15. Punishing-cruel	0	1	2	3

Fig. 16-19. The Modified McGill Pain Questionnaire. Choices 1-11 represent sensory descriptors while choices 12-15 are affective-cognitive descriptors. (From Melzack R: *Pain* 30:191, 1987.)

this topic should be discussed after the patient's current status has been determined rather than in the beginning of the history. If the examination is begun with the question "How did this all start?" then well-meaning but talkative patients may give very circuitous and perhaps confusing histories. The examiner who has first established the patient's current status can more easily guide that patient through the history. For identifying the onset of symptoms, the two primary concerns are when and how the symptoms began. In the case of a single traumatic episode, the examiner should carefully reconstruct the events to generate a mechanical hypothesis of the extent and nature of tissue injury. For example, information regarding radiographs, associated injuries, and care of associated injuries should be obtained. If the patient reports a gradual onset, the examiner should consider the presence of repeated stresses resulting from extrinsic causes such as irregular walking or running surfaces and inappropriate shoe type and from intrinsic causes such leg length differences or muscle "imbalances."[25] Additionally, patients who report a gradual, atraumatic onset of their symptoms potentially have serious disorders such as infection, neoplasm, or inflammatory disease.[30]

The stage of the disorder can be clarified by determining the behavior of the symptoms since their onset: Are the symptoms better, worse, or the same? Any previous

treatments that the patient has received for this problem, including the response to that treatment, should be identified.

Finally, the examiner should determine if the patient has had previous problems with the currently involved hip. If so, whether this current disorder is the same or different should be determined. If the problem is the same, a recurrent condition is implied.

Whenever a patient reports additional musculoskeletal problems such as dysfunction of other joints within the ipsilateral lower extremity, the examiner must consider the possibility of biomechanical problems within that limb. Patients' reports of atraumatic, multiple joint involvement should be evaluated for polyarthropathies such as lupus erythematosis and rheumatoid arthritis.[33,93]

Past and current medical status. As with all patients, individuals with hip joint dysfunction should be questioned regarding the presence of such disorders as diabetes mellitus, rheumatoid arthritis, cardiovascular disease, and lung disease. Additionally, the examiner should be aware of a patient's potential for osteoporosis.[7,96] In addition to elderly people and postmenopausal women, individuals with a history of long-term catabolic steroid usage, hyperparathyroidism, or prolonged bed rest are at great risk for osteoporosis. Individuals with a history of long-term catabolic steroid usage are also at risk to develop avascular necrosis of the femoral head, as are people with sickle cell anemia or those with a long history of excessive alcohol consumption.[30,88,96]

A list of the patient's medications should be obtained. Any medications for pain control are of particular interest because of their effect on masking the patient's symptoms. Individuals with a history of prolonged use of opiate-based analgesics may have chemical dependency. Prolonged use of nonsteriodal antiinflammatory medication may cause gastrointestinal or kidney problems.

The patient's goals for treatment outcome. A clear description of what the patient would like to achieve from the treatment is critical.[80] This understanding allows the clinician to target specific, functional goals toward which patient and therapist can work. These goals may range from putting on shoes and socks independently to running an ultramarathon. Without a clear agreement on goals between patient and clinician, the assessment of meaningful outcome becomes questionable.

Summary. Upon completion of the subjective examination, the examiner should form a preliminary hypothesis regarding the patient's condition. The following issues should be addressed in planning the next phase of the objective examination:

1. What physical examination procedures should be selected?
2. What are the precautions and contraindications?
3. How reliable is the patient as a historian?
4. What is the potential for this patient to have nonmusculoskeletal problems?
5. What is the patient's level of irritability?

The objective examination

In the broadest sense, the goals of the objective examination for patients with hip problems are to identify the patient's capacity for mobility and generate a hypothesis for the mechanisms of the patient's complaint of pain. Within this context, the clinician clarifies issues relating to the severity, irritability, nature, and stage of the patient's disorder. The specific tasks of this portion of the examination include:

1. Identifying structural abnormalities
2. Determining the joint ROM and muscle performance capacity of the lower quarter
3. Identifying movements and positions that reproduce the patient's symptoms
4. Identifying tissues that are "abnormal" to palpation

The physical examination maneuvers are described here for the following sequence of positions:

1. Standing
2. Sitting

Table 16-6. Common observed malalignments of the pelvis relative to the femur

Observation	Potential cause
Asymmetry of the iliac crest	Leg length difference
	Spasm of quadratus lumborum muscle
	Sacroiliac joint dysfunction
	Hip flexion contracture
	Dysplasia of the ilium
Internally rotated lower extremity	Femoral anteversion
	Internal femoral torsion
	Internal tibial torsion
	Primary or compensatory overpronation of the foot and ankle
	Contracture of the tensor fasciae latae muscle
Externally rotated lower extremity	Femoral retroversion
	External tibial torsion
	Uncompensated supinated foot
	Contracture of hip external rotator muscles
Thigh held in slight flexion	Hip joint pathology
	Contracture of hip flexors

3. Supine
4. Prone and, if indicated, sidelying

Because the examiner has to observe the pelvic area and lower extremity, the patient should wear loose-fitting gym shorts or a hospital gown during the examination.

Standing position. If the patient is full weight bearing in both lower extremities, the examination is begun in the standing position.

Inspection. The patient should be instructed to stand comfortably with feet a shoulder width apart while the examiner notes the ease of this stance. The alignment of the patient's lumbar spine and the symmetry of the lower extremities on the sagittal and frontal planes should then be assessed. An apparent lumbar scoliosis may actually be the result of lateral pelvic displacement due to pain or muscle weakness, or it may be caused by a leg length difference.[2,25] Asymmetry of the gluteal or lower extremity muscles should be noted. Observable atrophy of the gluteal muscles may indicate neuromuscular disease. Swelling over the lateral trochanter is often related to trochanteric bursitis. Swelling within the capsule of the hip joint is, however, very difficult to observe.

The relationship of the femur to the pelvis when the patient is standing is very important. The examiner should look for malalignment, which may indicate soft tissue contracture and/or bony asymmetry (Table 16-6). The examiner should then inspect the lower limb for deformities of the shank, foot, and ankle, as described in the chapters on those topics.

Many patients with hip joint dysfunction have coexisting medical problems; thus, the examiner should pay careful attention to the presence of pedal or pretibial edema as well as atrophic changes or discoloration of the skin.

When the inspection is complete, the patient should be asked to point to the painful area, which can be compared to the patient's verbal and diagrammed descriptions. The patient then is asked if the painful area is locally tender. If it is, the examiner should consider bursitis, tendinitis, apophysitis, or muscle strain. If the area is not tender and the pain is described as deep, hip joint pathology, bony problems, and referred pain are possibilities.

The patient remains standing while the iliac crests are palpated and the examiner observes their relative heights. If asymmetry is present, the leg lengths should be measured in the supine position.

Motion. The patient is then requested to perform ROM of trunk as follows: forward bending, backward bending, side bending, and the three-dimensional or quadrant positions. These movements are performed to rule out referred pain from the spine.

Special tests. The unilateral leg stand or Trendelenburg test is a useful procedure for detecting hip joint dysfunction. A positive Trendelenburg sign is identified when the patient is unable maintain the pelvis horizontal to the floor while standing first on one foot and then on the other foot (Fig. 16-20).[7,53] To perform the activity of unsupported single-limb standing requires innervation to the lower extremity muscles from the L4 and L5 nerve roots, adequate strength in the hip abductor muscles, and minimal or no pain in the hip joint region. A complaint of pain in the groin area during this procedure suggests hip joint pathology, whereas pain medial to the PSIS *may* indicate sacroiliac joint dysfunction.[5,13] After performing the unilateral leg stand, the patient is asked to unilaterally heel raise, thus establishing the strength of the triceps surae muscle group (S1, S2). Inability to perform this action may indicate impairment of the lumbosacral nerve roots and/or dysfunction of the foot and ankle system.

Patients who are reporting a minimum degree of pain and are not restricted in weight bearing should be asked to walk while the examiner performs a gait analysis. The use or misuse of assistive devices should be noted. Careful attention should be given to the symmetry of step length and the relative timing of each lower limb's stance phase. Any evidence of antalgia should be investigated.

Sitting position

Inspection. The examiner should note the ease with which the patient assumes and maintains the sitting position.

Motion and strength. The ROM of hip joint rotation can be assessed, but it is less significant than the ROM of hip joint rotation with the femur in relative extension. Manual muscle testing for hip flexion and rotation, knee extension, ankle dorsiflexion, inversion, and eversion can be performed in this position.[50,53] Muscle testing of the hip joint rotators on a patient with osteoporosis or recent surgery to the hip requires caution, however, because the high degree of torsion generated on the proximal femur may result in tissue injury. The examiner may want to assess the patient's capacity in the sitting position for certain self-care activities such as putting on shoes and socks.

Supine position

Inspection. The patient should be positioned with hips as close to the normal anatomic position as possible. Any surgical incisions, asymmetry of soft tissue, or lower extremity deformities should be identified. A leg length discrepancy is most effectively assessed by measuring the distance from the ASIS to the medial malleolus. This technique has been shown to be reliable and valid when careful palpation is performed.[2]

Motion and strength. Unless contraindicated, the ROM of the lower extremity should be assessed actively, followed by overpressure for the following motions:

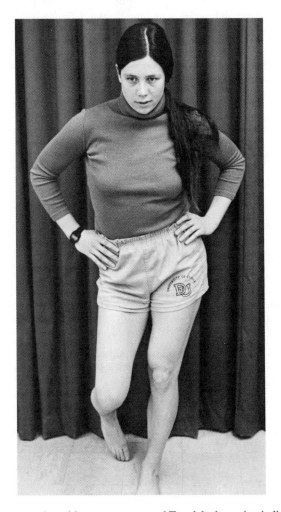

Fig. 16-20. A positive, uncompensated Trendelenburg sign indicating weakness of the left hip abductor mechanism.

1. Hip flexion, abduction, and adduction, rotation with hip in flexion, and rotation with the hip in anatomic neutral
2. Knee extension and flexion
3. Ankle dorsiflexion

The following motions should be resisted isometrically. Examiners should be aware of the selective tension techniques described by Cyriax[16] when they interpret the report of pain or weakness:

1. Hip flexion (L2, L3)
2. Knee extension (L3, L4)
3. Ankle dorsiflexion (L4, L5)
4. Subtalar eversion (L5, S1)
5. Great toe extension (L5)
6. Great toe flexion (S1)

If the examiner suspects neurologic impairment, the deep tendon reflexes and cutaneous innervation of the lower extremity should be assessed. This should also always be done on patients with a history of diabetes mellitus. Often overlooked during the hip examination is the presence of a positive Babinski sign and/or sustained clonus. Tests for these should always be performed for patients with a past history of injury to the brain or spinal cord and for any patients complaining of dizziness, loss of coordination, or

weakness of the extremities. These "long tract signs" may be the first indication of myelopathy, central nervous system ischemia, or neoplasm.

Palpation. Numerous structures may be palpated in the supine patient. Palpable tenderness associated with swelling is a very frequent finding with bursitis, tendinitis, and apophysitis.

A useful landmark to begin palpation of the hip is ASIS. Just inferior to it are the proximal attachments, the rectus femoris and sartorius muscles. Just medial to the ASIS, the iliopsoas muscle is palpable subcutaneously. Just superior and lateral to the ASIS is the iliac tubercle, the proximal attachment of the tensor fasciae latae muscle.

The crease between the ASIS and pubic tubercle is occupied by the inguinal ligament. It forms the superior border of the femoral triangle. This triangle, bounded laterally by the sartorius muscle and medially by the adductor longus, contains many structures (Fig. 16-21).[57] The inguinal lymph nodes are located superficially within the femoral triangle and may be tender to palpation. This finding may indicate the presence of an infection in the lower limb or abdomen and should always be investigated.[30] The pulse of the femoral artery is palpable within the femoral triangle. The large femoral vein is just medial to it. Any engorgement of this vein may indicate a very serious condition such as venous obstruction within the pelvis or

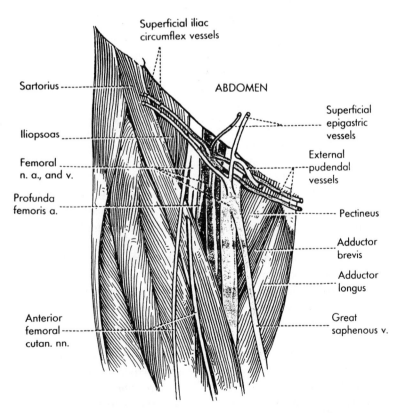

Fig. 16-21. The structure of the right femoral triangle. (From Hollingshead WH, Rosse C, *Textbook of anatomy,* ed 4, Philadelphia, 1985, HarperCollins.)

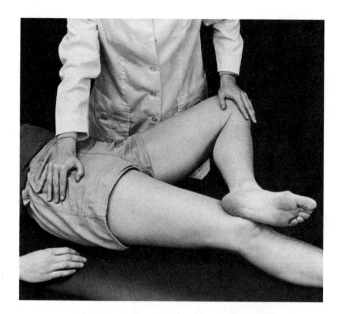

Fig. 16-22. The Patrick's, FABER, or figure-4 test.

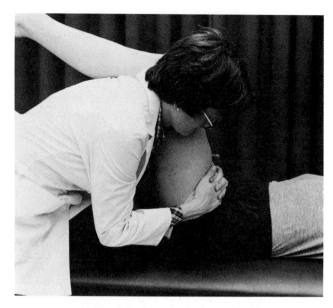

Fig. 16-23. "Perimeter scouring" of the hip.

lower abdomen. Deep to the bisection of the inguinal ligament is the hip joint. On thin individuals, the femoral head can be palpated when the hip is passively rotated and abducted. When evaluating this area in patients complaining of parasthesia over the anterior-lateral thigh, the examiner should tap a fingertip or reflex hammer medial to the ASIS to determine the presence of Tinel's sign over the lateral femoral cutaneous nerve. Finally, for individuals complaining of groin or medial thigh pain, the tendon of the adductor longus muscle should be palpated at its insertion on the pubic crest. For patients with suspected peripheral vascular impairment, the femoral, popliteal, posterior tibial, and dorsalis pedis pulses can be evaluated while the patient is in this position.

Special tests. Numerous special tests can be performed in the supine position to clarify the involved tissues. Gentle, manual spinal distraction may reduce low back pain and assist the examiner in differential diagnosis. The Patrick's test (FABER or figure-4 test) has long been advocated as a provocative test for hip joint pathology (Fig. 16-22).[53] This procedure is performed by passively flexing, abducting and externally rotating the supine patient's hip. Prior to over-pressure, the patient should point to any painful areas. If no pain is reported, the examiner then performs overpressure and again questions the patient regarding pain. Pain in or near the inguinal area suggests hip joint pathology such as arthrosis, avascular necrosis of the femoral head, or ligamentous sprains. Pain perceived in the sacroiliac area during this test may indicate SI joint dysfunction; however, the sensitivity and specificity of this finding are unclear. The nature of the passive motion of the hip can be further appreciated with inferior glide, lateral glide, and "perimeter" scouring (Fig. 16-23). The Thomas and modified Thomas tests are invaluable in determining the presence of

contracture of the iliopsoas and rectus femoris muscles (Fig. 16-24).[50] The straight leg raising test (SLR) should be performed to determine the extensibility of the hamstring muscles as the well the presence of tethering of the neuromeningeal pathway.

For patients who have dependent edema, calf pain, and/or a history of prolonged bed rest, the examiner should perform Homans' test (e.g., passive ankle dorsiflexion). If the patient complains of severe calf pain with this maneuver, deep vein thrombosis is a possibility.

Two maneuvers are described here to detect the presence of congenital hip dislocation in infants.[1,7,53] In Ortolani's test, the examiner passively flexes the supine infant's hips while applying gentle pressure to the greater trochanters and slight distraction to the hip. The femur is then slowly abducted. A positive sign occurs when the dislocated hip reduces and the examiner is aware of a hard click. This test is useful only for dislocated hips that are present within a few weeks of birth. Barlow's test is performed upon completion of the Ortolani's test by applying pressure against the inner thigh in an attempt to sublux the hip posteriorly. If the hip subluxes and then reduces when the examiner releases the pressure, the hip is classified as unstable. Both tests have the potential to damage the femoral head and should not be performed injudiciously.

Prone position. Many people, especially elderly individuals or patients who have recently undergone hip surgery, may be unable to assume or maintain the prone position. With care, the majority of the following procedures can be performed with the subject supine or sidelying.

Inspection. The examiner should observe the lumbar spine and buttock area for asymmetry of soft tissues.

Motion and strength. The passive ROM of knee flexion with the hip in anatomic neutral in the prone patient can be

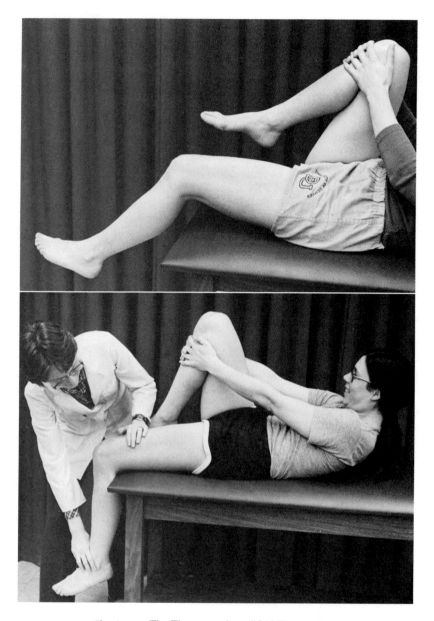

Fig. 16-24. The Thomas and modified Thomas test.

assessed. Limitations of the knee flexion that were not present with the hip flexed indicate contracture of the rectus femoris muscle. During this maneuver, a patient's hip may flex at the point where the contracted rectus femoris can no longer elongate (Ely's test). A provocation of sharp pain and/or parasthesia perceived in the anterior thigh during this maneuver may indicate excessive tension on the femoral nerve. (This test is also known as the femoral nerve stretch test.[16]) The strength of the hamstring and gluteus maximus muscles can be assessed in this position.

Palpation. Useful bony landmarks for palpation in the prone subject include the iliac crest, PSIS, sacrum, ischial tuberosity, and greater trochanter. Deep to the bisection of an imaginary line from the PSIS to the greater trochanter is the piriformis muscle. Tenderness in this area may indicate

strain of the piriformis or other lateral rotator muscles of the hip. Examiners should remember, however, that the gluteus maximus muscle that covers the posterior lateral buttock is extremely thick; thus, unobstructed palpation of the hip intrinsic muscles is not possible. Deep to the gluteus maximus, spanning from the inferior tip of the sacrum to the ischial tuberosity, is the sacrotuberous ligament. Tenderness here has been described as a sign of sacroiliac joint dysfunction, although the reliability and specificity of this sign are unclear. Tenderness inferior to the ischial tuberosity may be caused by ischial bursitis or tendinitis of the hamstring or adductor magnus muscle. Selective tension techniques may be useful to differentiate these disorders. Bursitis of the trochanteric bursa is usually accompanied by palpable tenderness and a mild, "boggy" type of swelling

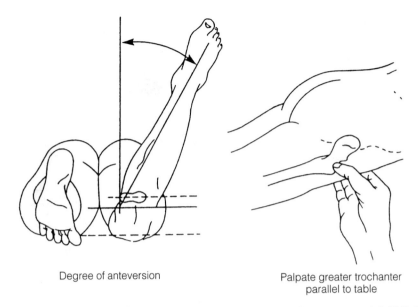

Degree of anteversion   Palpate greater trochanter
                                          parallel to table

Fig. 16-25. The Craig's test. (From Magee DJ: *Orthopedic physical assessment,* ed 2, Philadelphia, 1992, WB Saunders.)

over the lateral aspect of the greater trochanter. Finally, while the subject is in the prone position, palpation of the lumbar spine may be indicated.

Special tests. If a patient has an observable internal rotation of one or both lower limbs, excessive femoral anteversion may be present. There is also usually more ROM in internal than in external rotation of the hip in these patients.[53] The presence of excessive femoral anteversion can be corroborated by Craig's test (Fig. 16-25).[53] To perform this procedure, the prone patient's knee is flexed to 90 degrees. The examiner then rotates the hip while palpating the greater trochanter. When the greater trochanter is felt to be in a midposition, such as parallel to the floor, the examiner then views the angle of the tibia relative to the long axis of the body. In a normal adult hip, it should be roughly perpendicular to the floor. Excessive anteversion is present if the tibia is pointing outward, away from the midline of the patient's body.

Sidelying position

Motion and strength. The sidelying position allows an antigravity assessment of the hip abductor muscles.[50]

Palpation. For individuals who are unable to assume or maintain the prone position, palpation of the lateral and posterior buttock can be performed while the patient is sidelying. The uppermost lower extremity should be comfortably supported by pillows or bolsters to ensure relaxation of the soft tissues. Palpation is then performed as described for the prone position.

Special tests. Ober's test is quite useful for determining the presence of contracture of the tensor fasciae latae muscle and the iliotibial tract (Fig. 16-26).[50,53] To perform this test, the examiner stands behind the sidelying patient. While holding the knee in 90 degrees of flexion, the examiner

passively flexes the uppermost limb at the hip and then abducts it, extends it, and allows it to drop into abduction. The examiner carefully stabilizes the pelvis to prevent lateral trunk bending, which could result in downward displacement of the limb being tested. There is controversy over whether the knee should remain flexed or be allowed to extend. In my opinion, testing should done under both conditions. A positive Ober's sign is present if the limb remains in an abducted position. Passive rotation of the sacroiliac joints, as well as passive movements to the lumbar spine, can be performed.[14,54]

Functional assessment

Several published functional assessment protocols are specific for patients with hip joint problems. Two of the most commonly used are the Harris Hip Function Scale (Fig. 16-27)[37] and the Iowa Functional Hip Evaluation (Fig. 16-28).[51] These instruments are well known to clinicians and provide indexes that combine pain, physical impairment, functional limitations, and disability. The last several years have seen a growing acceptance of quality-of-life measures that target a patient's physical limitations and their psychosocial ramifications.[45] Examples that are not specific to hip disorders are the Sickness Impact Profile[3] and the Pain Disability Index.[12]

Radiologic examination

The standard radiographic series for the hip consists of the anteroposterior pelvis and true lateral (Figs. 16-29 and 16-30).[17] Other specific views may be ordered for clarification. The anteroposterior pelvis view visualizes proximal femur and acetabulum while allowing bilateral comparison. The examiner should appreciate the following:

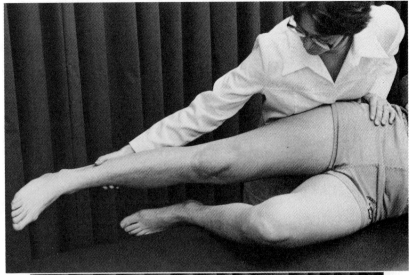

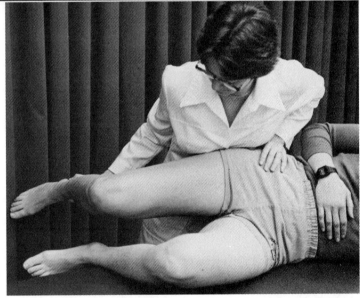

Fig. 16-26. The Ober's test.

1. The general appearance of the patient's bones; the presence or absence of osteopenia
2. The angle of inclination of the femoral neck
3. The presence of bone cysts, osteophytes, or both
4. Any disruptions of the bony cortex that may indicate a fracture
5. The joint space and shapes of the articular surfaces of the hips

The true lateral view is performed with the opposite hip flexed. It is primarily used to determine any displacement of the proximal femur on the sagittal plane.

COMMON HIP DISORDERS
Osseous deformities involving the proximal femur

Four common osseous deformities of the proximal femur are coxa vara, coxa valga, femoral anteversion, and femoral retroversion. They can occur as a primary problem or as a sequela to other problems, such as fractures or congenital hip dislocation.[58,68,74,83,92] Whether occurring unilaterally or bilaterally, each of these conditions can result in alterations in load bearing throughout the lower limb and spine and thus are of great importance.[11,92]

Coxa vara occurs when the angle between the femoral shaft and the femoral neck on the frontal plane (angle of inclination) is less than 125 degrees.[63] The source of this abnormality can be in the femoral neck, epiphysis, or both. This reduction in the angle of inclination not only results in ipsilateral limb shortening but also alters the biomechanics of the hip by shifting the concentration of weight bearing superiorly and laterally on the femoral head (Fig. 16-31).[58,68] The moment arm acting on the hip abductors is reduced, resulting in weakness of hip abduction (Fig. 16-32).[7,63] The developmental and acquired conditions that can result in

(Circle one in each group)

Pain (44 points maximum)

None/ignores	44
Slight, occasional, no compromise in activity	40
Mild, no effect on ordinary activity, pain after unusual activity, uses aspirin	30
Moderate, tolerable, makes concessions, occasional codeine	20
Marked, serious limitation	10
Totally disabled	0

Function (47 points maximum)

Gait (walking maximum distance) (33 points maximum)

1. Limp:
None	11
Slight	8
Moderate	5
Unable to walk	0
2. Support:
None	11
Cane, long walks	7
Cane, full time	5
Crutch	4
Two canes	2
Two crutches	0
Unable to walk	0
3. Distance walked:
Unlimited	11
Six blocks	8
Two to three blocks	5
Indoors only	2
Bed and chair	0

Functional Activities (14 points maximum)

1. Stairs:
Normally	4
Normally with banister	2
Any method	1
Not able	0
2. Socks and tie shoes:
With ease	4
With difficulty	2
Unable	0
3. Sitting:
Any chair, 1 hour	5
High chair, ½ hour	3
Unable to sit ½ hour any chair	0
4. Enter public transport
Able to use public transportation	1
Not able to use public transportation	0

Absence of Deformity (requires all four) (4 points maximum)

1. Fixed adduction <10°	4
2. Fixed internal rotation in extension <10°	0
3. Leg length discrepancy less than 1¼″	
4. Pelvic flexion contracture <30°	

Range of Motion (5 points maximum)

Instructions

Record 10° of fixed adduction as "−10° abduction, adduction to 10°"

Similarly, 10° of fixed external rotation as "−10° internal rotation, external rotation to 10°"

Similarly, 10° of fixed external rotation with 10° further external rotation as "−10° internal rotation, external rotation to 20"

Permanent flexion
(1) _____ °

Range	Index Factor	Index Value*
_____ °		
A. Flexion to		
(0–45°)	1.0	
(45–90°)	0.6	
(90–120°)	0.3	
(120–140°)	0.0	
_____ °		
B. Abduction to		
(0–15°)	0.8	
(15–30°)	0.3	
(30–60°)	0.0	
C. Adduction to _____ °		
(0–15°)	0.2	
(15–60°)	0.0	
D. External rotation in extension to _____ °		
(0–30°)	0.4	
(30–60°)	0.0	
E. Internal rotation in extension to _____ °		
(0–60°)	0.0	

*Index Value = Range × Index Factor

Total index value (A + B + C + D + E) _____

Total range of motion points (multiply total index value × 0.05) _____

Pain points: _____
Function points: _____
Absence of Deformity points: _____
Range of Motion points: _____
Total points _____
(100 points maximum)
Comments:

Fig. 16-27. The Harris hip function scale. (In Magee DJ: *Orthopedic physical assessment,* ed 2, Philadelphia, 1992, WB Saunders; modified from Harris WH: *J Bone Surg Am* 51:737, 1969.)

Chart 1	Chart 2

Chart 1

Date _____

Name _____ Age _____

100-Point Scale for Hip Evaluation

Total points _____

Function (35 points)

Does most of housework or job that
    requires moving about 5
Dresses unaided (includes tying shoes and
    putting on socks) 5
Walks enough to be independent 5
Sits with difficulty at table or toilet 4
Picks up objects from floor by squatting 3
Bathes without help 3
Negotiates stairs foot over foot 3
Carries objects comparable to suitcase 2
Gets into car or public conveyance unaided and rides
    comfortably 2
Drives a car 1

_____

Freedom From Pain (35 points) *(circle 1 only)*

No pain 35
Pain only with fatigue 30
Pain only with weight-bearing 20
Pain at rest but not with weight-bearing 15
Pain sitting or in bed 10
Continuous pain 0

_____

Gait (10 points) *(circle 1 only)*

No limp, no support 10
No limp, using cane 8
Abductor limp 8
Short leg limp 8
Needs two canes 6
Needs two crutches 4
Cannot walk 0

_____

Absence of Deformity (10 points)

No fixed flexion over 30° 3
No fixed adduction over 10° 3
No fixed rotation over 10° 2
Not over 1″ shortening (ASIS-MM)* 2

_____

Range of Motion (10 points)

Flexion-extension (normal 140°) .... _____ °
Abduction-adduction (normal 80°) .... _____ °
External-internal rotation (normal 80°) .... _____ °
            Total degrees .... _____ °
            Points (1 point/30°) .... _____ °

_____

Muscle Strength (no points)

Straight leg raising:
    Less than gravity _____ Gravity _____
    Gravity + resistance _____
Abduction:
    Less than gravity _____ Gravity _____
    Gravity + resistance _____
Extension:
    Less than gravity _____ Gravity _____
    Gravity + resistance _____
                    TOTAL (100 points maximum) _____

Chart 2

Name _____ Diagnosis _____
Age _____ Sex _____ Date of operation _____
Date of follow-up _____
Previous surgery: Date _____ Type _____
Subsequent surgery: Date _____ Type _____

Pain   40%

    None 40
    Pain with fatigue 35
    Pain with weight-bearing:
        Mild 30
        Moderate 20
        Severe 10
    Persistence with non-weight-bearing .... 10 (less than above)
    Continuous pain 0

Ability to Function   30%

    Work and household duties:
        Full day, usual occupation 10
        Modified work or duties 6
        Severe restriction of work or duties 2
    Walking tolerances:
        Long distances 10
        Short distances 6
        Two blocks or less 1
    Self-reliance:
        Dresses self unaided 3
        Help with shoes and socks 2
        Sit at table and toilet 3
    Stairs:
        Normal 2
        One at a time 1
        Gets into car or public conveyance without
            difficulty 2

Gait   15%

    No limp, no support 15
    No limp, with cane 12
    Limp, mild, without cane 12
    Limp, mild, with cane 9
    Limp, moderate, without cane or crutch 9
    Limp, moderate, with cane or crutch 6
    Limp, severe, without cane or crutch 3
    Limp, severe, with cane or crutch 2
    Two canes or crutches 1

Anatomic Assessment   15%

A. Motion:
    Flexion—up to 80° in range 0–100° × 0.1 8
    Abduction—up to 20° in range 0–30° × 0.1 ... 2
B. Shortening:
    None–½″ 3
    ½″–1″ 2
    1″–2″ 1
C. Trendelenburg—absent 2

_____

                                       100%

Fig. 16-28. The Iowa functional hip evaluation. (In Magee DJ: *Orthopedic physical assessment,* ed 2, Philadelphia, 1992, WB Saunders; modified from Larson CB, *Clin Orthop* 31:85, 1963.)

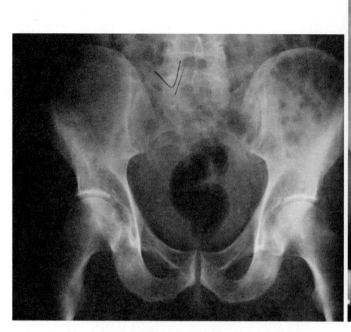

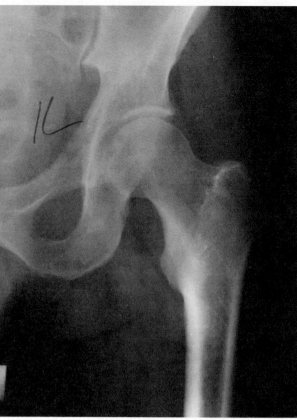

A

B

Fig. 16-29. (A) An anterior-posterior (A-P) radiograph of the pelvis. This standard film projection allows good visualization of both hip joints to allow bilateral comparison. Note the clearly visible joint spaces with some bilateral subchondral sclerosis of the superior rim of the acetabulum. **(B)** An A-P radiograph of the hip.

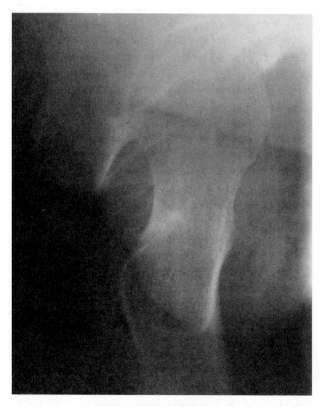

Fig. 16-30. A true lateral radiograph of the hip. Note the clear definition of the femoral head and neck.

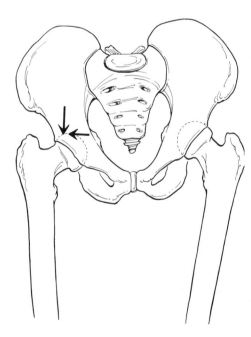

Fig. 16-31. Coxa vara of the right hip. Note that the weight-bearing area of the femoral head is more superior and lateral than the left hip.

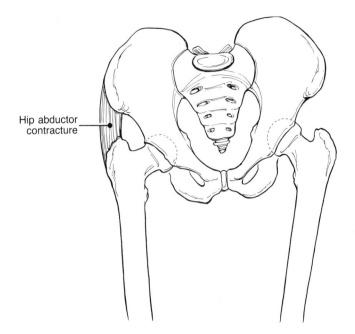

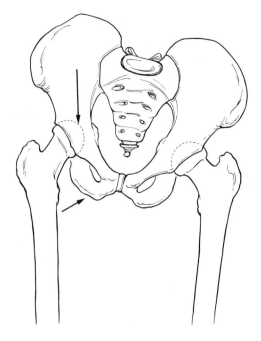

Fig. 16-32. Coxa vera of the right hip demonstrating an abductor contracture.

Fig. 16-33. Coxa valga of the right hip demonstrating ipsilateral lengthening and characteristic adducted position.

coxa vara include intertrochanteric fracture, slipped capital femoral epiphysis, Legg-Calvé-Perthes disease, congenital hip dislocation, rickets, and Paget's disease.[1,7,10,96]

The clinical findings of coxa vara typically include a leg length difference and a gait abnormality associated with a positive Trendelenburg sign. Hip abduction may be restricted by the superior portion of the femoral neck or greater trochanter as it prematurely impinges on the superior rim of the acetabulum. Hip abductor muscle contractures may also occur. Untreated, coxa vara potentially predisposes an individual to low back pain associated with standing or walking. Over long periods, persistent abnormal loading may lead to hip joint arthrosis.[58]

Physical therapy for this condition is limited. The use of a shoe lift to equalize leg lengths may be very helpful. Strengthening the hip abductors is difficult but should be attempted. Encouraging individuals to minimize prolonged standing and avoid high-impact sports is important.

In coxa valga, the angle between the femoral shaft and the femoral neck on the frontal plane is greater than approximately 125 degrees at skeletal maturity.[65] Coxa valga is normal in infants and gradually reduces to the normal angle as the skeleton develops. This condition may cause ipsilateral limb lengthening that then results in a characteristic adducted posture of the lower limb (Fig. 16-33). With weight bearing, the forces are shunted closer to the center of the head of the femur, which can potentiate the acetabulum to dysplasia or arthrosis.[58] The moment arm acting upon the hip abductors is reduced, resulting in weakness of abduction (Fig. 16-34). Coxa valga is often encountered with congenital hip dislocation and in people with spastic paralysis.[1,7,95]

The clinical findings of unilateral coxa valga typically include a leg length difference, with the involved side being longer. With either unilateral or bilateral involvement, there typically is a gait abnormality associated with a positive Trendelenburg sign. Untreated, coxa valga potentially predisposes an individual to low back pain associated with gait and, over long periods, to hip joint arthrosis.

Physical therapy for this condition is limited and very similar to that for coxa vara. A shoe lift to equalize leg lengths may be very helpful. Strengthening the hip abductors should be attempted. Encouraging individuals to minimize prolonged standing and avoid high-impact sports is important.

Excessive femoral anteversion is a condition in which the angle between the femoral neck and the femoral shaft on the transverse plane is greater than approximately 12 degrees in adults.[63] When this deformity is present, the ipsilateral lower limb appears to be excessively internally rotated when the femoral head is in the neutral position within the acetabulum (Fig. 16-35). This condition is typically bilateral and has been implicated in the etiology of numerous lower extremity disorders. Excessive stress may occur in the hip joint from altered rotational forces and from the effect of this deformity on the congruency of the hip joint during weight bearing.[11,92]

Clinically, patients may complain of pain in a variety of sites in the lower extremity of low back. Patients typically have a toe-in gait and may have concurrent malalignment of the lower limb; however, this may not always be present. Reikeras recently reported no correlation between the degree of femoral anteversion and external tibial torsion.[74] There is

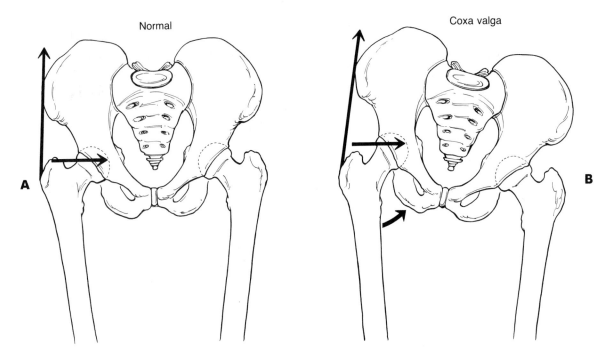

Fig. 16-34. The moment arm acting through the hip abductors in **(A)** a normal hip compared to **(B)**, a shortened moment arm with coxa valga.

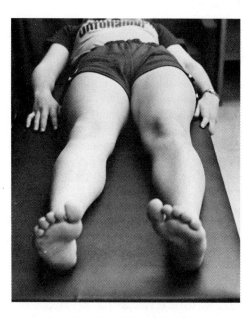

Fig. 16-35. A patient with bilateral femoral anteversion in a relaxed position. Note the lack of the normal out toeing.

usually a greater ROM of hip internal rotation than external rotation (Fig. 16-36).[53] Craig's test is typically positive.

Although physical therapy is unlikely to influence the degree of this deformity, foot orthotics can greatly improve the load-bearing dynamics of the lower extremity. General conditioning and flexibility exercises for the lower extremity may be useful in reducing the effect of lower extremity malalignment. Individuals with obvious femoral anteversion

who frequently engage in running or aerobics may be at increased risk to develop overuse syndromes in the lower extremity. These individuals should be encouraged to minimize these activities and to cross-train by cycling or perhaps swimming.

Femoral retroversion is essentially the opposite of femoral anteversion. With this disorder, there is a decrease in the angle between the femoral head and shaft on the transverse plane to the degree that an obvious outward rotation of the lower extremities is observable.[64] This condition can result in substantial malalignment and numerous compensations in the lower extremity.

In addition to the externally rotated appearance of the lower extremity, people with femoral retroversion tend to have a much greater ROM of hip external rotation than of internal rotation. Craig's test can also be used to evaluate a patient for this condition. A positive response is an inward pointing of the tibias in the prone subject.

Treatment for femoral anteversion is similar in concept to that for femoral anteversion. Foot orthotics, general conditioning, and flexibility exercises for the lower extremity may be useful in reducing the effect of lower extremity malalignment. Individuals with this condition should be encouraged to minimize repetitive lower extremity impact loading.

Congenital and developmental conditions involving the hip joint

Legg-Calvé-Perthes disease is an idiopathic form of osteonecrosis (i.e., avascular necrosis) of the femoral head in skeletally immature individuals.[1,7,10,21] Necrotic changes

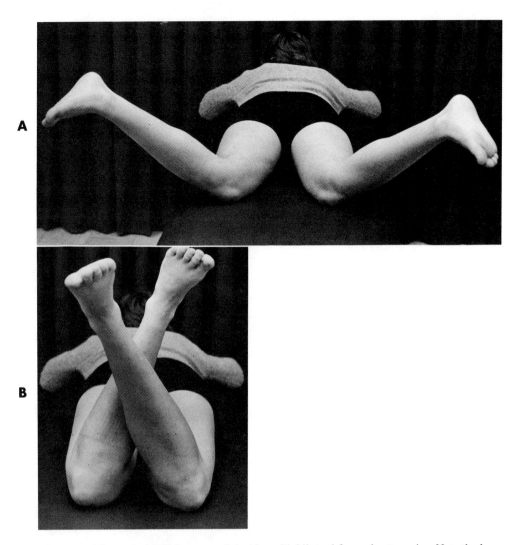

Fig. 16-36. The typical ROM pattern of the hips with bilateral femoral anteversion. Note the large angle of internal rotation (**A**) and the relatively small angle of external rotation (**B**).

within the epiphysis cause a collapse of the femoral head and alter its articular surface. This is followed by a slow re-formation of bone. The incidence of this disorder has been reported as 1 in 1200,[56] with 80% male and the typical age of onset 3 to 12 years. In approximately 85%, it is unilateral.[7,21]

The etiology of Legg-Calvé-Perthes disease is unknown. Although vascular injury with impairment of blood flow to the femoral head is presumed to be responsible for the osteonecrosis, this relationship has not been clearly documented.[7]

The classic diagnostic findings include an obvious limp and often a complaint of ipsilateral, medial thigh, and knee pain.[10] The affected hip is usually limited in internal rotation and abduction. The radiographic findings vary with the stage of the disorder. In the early stages, there may be no obvious findings, and patients may require a bone scan or diagnostic ultrasound.[24,90] In later stages, flattening of the femoral head

and reactive bone formation may be present (Fig. 16-37). The classic crescent sign of osteonecrosis—a thin radiolucent line inferior to the articular surface of the femoral head—may be observable.[10]

This disorder is often self-limiting, although severe cases may predispose to arthrosis in later years. The goal of treatment is to reduce the deforming forces of weight bearing and muscle tension by immobilizing the patient in abduction and slight internal rotation,[7] initially by traction and later by long leg casts or abduction types of braces, with patients allowed to ambulate with crutches. Patients wearing casts periodically have them removed to allow gentle ROM exercises. Pool therapy provides an optimal medium for these patients, but cycling or a Swiss ball has also been recommended.

A slipped capital femoral epiphysis occurs when shear forces lead to a displacement of the epiphysis of the femoral head and cause it to "slip" inferiorly and posteriorly relative

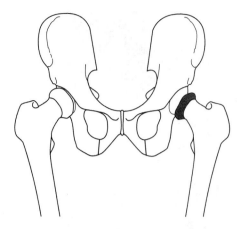

Fig. 16-37. A schematic A-P view of the hips demonstrating changes occuring with Legg-Calvé-Perthes disease. The darkened area in the left hip (on the right side of the drawing) represents necrosis and flattening of the femoral head.

to the neck of the femur (Fig. 16-38).[24] This condition is most common in children aged 10 to 16, more frequently boys than girls. Fifteen to 20% have bilateral involvement. Its onset may be sudden because of trauma, or it may be atraumatic and slow.[7,24]

The symptoms include a limp and a complaint of hip pain; however, in many instances, pain may be reported only in the medial knee, which illustrates the importance of evaluating the hip in the presence of knee pain. The hip joint may be limited in internal rotation and may move into external rotation and abduction when flexed. The radiographic findings are usually diagnostic, but lateral views are necessary because the primary displacement of the femoral head is often posterior.[1,7,96]

The treatment of a slipped capital femoral epiphysis is nearly always surgical stabilization. The postoperative physical therapy is quite similar to that of any other patients who have had surgical stabilization of fractures. Osteoarthrosis and osteoneciosos are occasional late complications of this disorder.[36] Issues such as weight control, and participation in sports activities must be considered.

Congenital dislocation of the hip can be due to a variety of conditions that result in dysplasia of the femur or acetabulum. Brashear and Raney[7] identify the following three conditions:

1. Congenital hip dysplasia, a dislocatable hip in a newborn
2. Acetabular dysplasia, abnormalities of the acetabulum that are radiographically evident at 3 to 4 months
3. Congenital subluxation, conditions in which the femur is subluxated relative to the acetabulum

Although few children are actually born with a dislocated hip, as many as 1% may be born with an unstable hip. Of them, 10% develop a dislocated hip; the overall incidence is between 1 and 2 per 1000 births.[7,20]

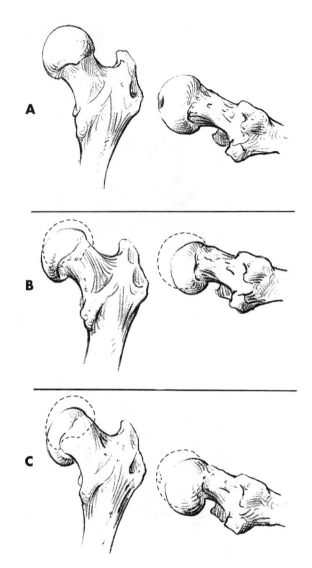

Fig. 16-38. Slipped capital femoral epiphysis (SCFE). **A,** mild; **B,** moderate; **C,** severe. (From Nicholas, Hershman, *Lower extremity & spine in sports medicine,* ed 2, St Louis, 1995, Mosby.)

The pathology associated with congenital hip dislocation progresses as the patient ages. At birth, the primary problem is excessive laxity of the hip joint capsule, as well as exaggerated femoral anteversion. If a baby's hips are maintained in the position of extension and adduction, further stretching of the capsule as well as dysplasia of the acetabulum can occur. This condition may occur in certain neuromuscular diseases and may also be observed in cultures where infants are kept in restrictive holders. If the condition is untreated when the patient begins weight bearing, upward subluxation of the femoral head can occur, resulting in the formation of a pseudoarthrosis.

When diagnosing congenital hip dysplasia, the following age-related procedures are useful[1,7]:

1. Neonatal (birth to 1 month): Barlow's test, Ortolani's test
2. Infancy (1 month to 2 years): limited hip abduction with

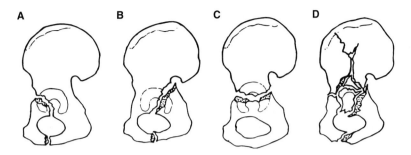

Fig. 16-39. Types of acetabular fractures. **A,** simple; **B,** posterior; **C,** transverse; and **D,** composite. (From Apley AG, Solomon L: *Apley's system of orthopaedics and fracture,* ed 6, Boston, 1982, Butterworths.)

the hips flexed to 45 degrees; shortening on the affected side with hips and knees flexed (Galeazzi's sign); Trendelenburg sign

3. Age 2 to 6 years: obvious limp, Trendelenburg sign, limb shortening if unilateral.
4. Older than 6 years: limp, limited hip abduction

To summarize, in very young patients the hip has limited abduction and can be passively dislocated or subluxed; in older patients, limb shortening, a positive Trendelenburg sign, and limited abduction are the obvious signs.

With early recognition, patients typically respond very well to splinting or surgical correction. Once the hip morphology has been established, however, these interventions are much less effective. Therapy is often indicated for gait training, ROM exercises, and developmental activities.

Traumatic disorders that affect the hip and its associated tissues

Traumatic disorders of the hip and its associated tissues are common in all age groups. Hip dislocations as well as fractures of the pelvis and femur are frequently caused by high-velocity trauma such as motor vehicle accidents.[1,100] In athletes and laborers, intense muscle contractions can lead to muscle strains and avulsion of tendinous insertions, and repetitive loading can result in stress fractures. In the elderly population, hip fractures are common because of the combination of bone weakened by osteoporosis and an increased predisposition for falls.

Fractures of the hip and pelvis

Acetabular fractures occur from high-velocity trauma such as motor vehicle accidents. They are most commonly encountered in young adults. The common fracture patterns are illustrated in Fig. 16-39. These fractures may be associated with a hip dislocation, sciatic nerve injury, and/or trauma to the pelvic and abdominal viscera. Because of the disruption of the articular surface and their inherent instability, these fractures often require open reduction with internal fixation (ORIF).[19]

Postoperatively, these patients are started on early ROM

exercise; however, non–weight-bearing periods of up to 3 months are often necessary, especially if the fracture involves the superior portion of the acetabulum. It is often difficult for patients to appreciate this need because the pain subsides within several weeks and ambulation is painless. If excessive weight bearing is sustained through the acetabulum before a stable union is achieved, disruption of the joint surface can occur, thus predisposing the patient to early arthrosis. Restoration of the abductor mechanism is critical to allow normal gait and load distribution through the hip. Dickinson and colleagues reported that nearly 2 years following injury patients demonstrated a 50% deficit of hip abduction torque.[19]

Femoral shaft fractures are also high-energy fractures and are most common in young adults. These fractures are nearly always treated by internal fixation with an intramedullary rod.[1] Because of the stability of the fixation, patients are typically allowed early weight-bearing and ROM exercises of the entire lower extremity. In evaluating these patients postoperatively, it is important to be aware of the potential for associated knee and hip injuries that may not have been previously identified. With advances in surgical technique, shortening of the affected limb is now less frequently encountered; however, the examiner should carefully measure leg length. The copious hemorrhage that occurs with these fractures can increase the possibility of compartment syndromes in the thigh that can lead to substantial loss of muscle tissue and impair the patient's capacity for postoperative strengthening.

Pelvic ring fractures are classified as stable or unstable. Stable pelvic ring fractures are usually nondisplaced fractures of the superior or inferior pubic ramus or of both. Patients with these fractures are usually treated with bed rest, followed by ambulation with crutches. Unstable pelvic ring fractures result from very high-energy trauma and are frequently associated with serious injuries to brain, spine, and pelvic viscera. Patients who sustain these fractures are often impaired by the associated injuries and represent a great challenge for mobility training. Unless the acetabulum has been disrupted, these fractures are typically not treated with internal fixation. If diastasis pubis (a separation of the pubic symphysis) is present, stabilization is achieved with an external fixator while the patient remains wheelchair-dependent.

Hip joint dislocations are due to high-energy trauma and are most common in young adults.[1,7,96,100] The most frequent direction of dislocation is with the femoral head displacing posteriorly (80%). The hip, however, may also dislocate anteriorly and centrally.[18] The posterior dislocations are often associated with injury to the common peroneal division of the sciatic nerve, and all dislocations create a high risk of osteonecrosis due to vascular trauma. Hip dislocations are commonly encountered in the multiply traumatized patient and may not be diagnosed acutely in comatose individuals. Therapists who evaluate patients with acute trauma who are communication-impaired should pay careful attention to the position and ROM of the hip.

The typical deformity of a posterior hip joint dislocation is an adducted internally rotated position of the lower limb. The patient is unable to bear weight, and there is typically a severe loss of ROM. Both anteroposterior and lateral view radiographs of the hip are necessary to determine the displacement of the femoral head. Following successful reduction of the hip, the patient should begin early ROM exercises within a restricted range and ambulate without bearing weight for several weeks.

Hip fractures, one of the most common orthopedic disorders, account for half of all people with fractures who require admission to the hospital. Approximately 250,000 occur each year in the United States.[66,70] The incidence of hip fractures is expected to increase noticeably as the population ages. Although surgical reductions and fixations of hip fractures are usually successful, Craik has reported a high proportion of these patients have permanent functional limitation and disability.[15]

Hip fractures in the elderly are related to demineralization of bone and the potential for falls. The numerous risk factors for sustaining a fracture to the hip include the following:

1. Elderly
2. Female
3. White
4. Sedentary
5. History of prior fracture
6. Use of psychotropic drugs
7. Alcoholism
8. Dementia

Fractures of the hip may be broadly classified as intracapsular and extracapsular. Parker and Pryor have proposed an expanded classification based upon the location of the fracture (Table 16-7).[66] The two most common fractures in elderly people are subcapital and intertrochanteric.

Subcapital femoral neck fractures are within the capsule of the hip (Fig. 16-40). They frequently occur in elderly people whose femoral neck has been weakened by osteoporosis. Relatively minor trauma, such as twisting while weight bearing, can result in fracture. It is estimated that 1 of every 1000 women over the age of 70 years will sustain this fracture.[66] Prior to the acceptance of ORIF, patients with femoral neck fractures were often treated with prolonged bed rest. Complications such as pneumonia resulted in a very high mortality rate. Currently, these fractures are stabilized operatively to allow early weight bearing.

If this fracture is impacted, cannulated screws are used for fixation.[1,66] Fractures near the head with an associated deformity are more problematic.[1,7,66] Because these fractures are intracapsular and in an area of high shear forces, there is a high potential for osteonecrosis or nonunion. Thus, prosthetic replacement of the femoral head may be performed. Because many elderly patients have difficulty maintaining a non–weight-bearing status during transfers and gait, the goal of the surgery is to provide the patient with

Table 16-7. Classification of hip fractures	
Intracapsular fractures	**Extracapsular fractures**
Femoral neck fracture	Lateral femoral neck fracture
Medial femoral neck fracture	Basal
Subcapital	Trochanteric
Transcervical	Intertrochanteric
Midcervical	Pertrochanteric
Basicervical	Subtrochanteric
Basal	

From Parker MJ, Pryor GA: *Hip fracture management,* Boston, 1993, Blackwell.

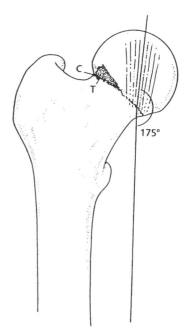

Fig. 16-40. Intracapsular femoral neck fracture with angulation of fracture indicated.

a hip that tolerates some degree of weight bearing postoperatively. As a result, prosthetic implants are cemented rather than porous-coated.[9,66]

Postoperative care of these patients is critical and typically includes treatment in the hospital and later in the patient's residence.[70] These patients are often challenged by health and communication problems common in the elderly population. Despite the many guidelines for weight bearing and exercise progression, the therapist should discuss each patient with the surgeon because variations in the extent of the fracture, the stability of remaining bone, and the nature of the fixation all influence the patient's postoperative course.

Intertrochanteric fractures can have a variety of patterns (Fig. 16-41).[66] These fractures are occasionally treated with closed reduction but usually are treated with open reduction and internal fixation with a sliding compression screw. This type of internal fixation is designed to allow early weight bearing.

The high degree of residual disability for patients sustaining intracapsular or extracapsular hip fractures should be of great concern to physical therapists. Although anatomic reduction is usually present, many patients fail to regain their preinjury range of motion, strength, and functional capacity,[15] an indication of the need to reevaluate rehabilitation strategies and criteria for discharge.

Stress fractures occur because of fatigue failure in bone that has been subjected to repetitive loading.[24] They can occur in a variety of sites in and around the hip, including the femoral neck, femoral shaft, greater trochanter, and pubic ramus.[24] The groups of people most often affected by stress fractures are those who are progressively increasing the duration of repetitive impact loading in the lower extremities, for example, long-distance runners and military recruits.

One frequent site of stress fractures of the hip is in the medial femoral neck (Fig. 16-42). This fracture may occur in athletes who do a considerable amount of downhill running. Presumably, the high-impact loading with the hip in a relatively extended position can lead to bone injury. Risk factors for the development of stress fractures include amenorrhea and the nutritional deficiencies of some people who are on a vegetarian diet.

The diagnosis of a stress fracture of the femoral neck can be problematic. Local tenderness over bone is generally a sign that makes an examiner consider the presence of a stress fracture. The femoral neck, however, is typically not

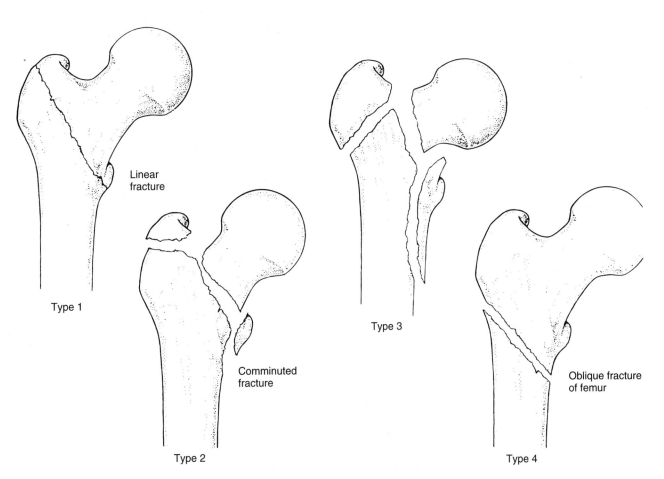

Fig. 16-41. Four common types of trochanteric fractures. (From Parker MJ, Pryor GA: *Hip fracture management,* Boston, 1993, Blackwell.)

CASE 1

C.M. was a 19-year-old college student and recreational long-distance runner. She presented with a complaint of a deep, sharp pain in her right inguinal area that had been present for 2 weeks. This pain was typically not present early in the day; however, it was noticeable each day after she had run approximately 4 miles. C.M. was seen by a student health medical practitioner who diagnosed her problem as a strained hip muscle and referred her to physical therapy (PT). No radiographs were obtained.

During her PT examination, C.M. indicated that she had recently substantially increased her running mileage and had begun training runs on a 7-mile downhill mountain trail. She was unable to recall any trauma or previous history of pain in her lower extremity. She stated that her pain was now coming on much sooner in her run than when she had seen her the student health physician. Her goal was to return to running for fitness and recreation.

On physical examination, she had no obvious lower extremity asymmetries. The ROM of her lower extremities was normal and pain-free, with the exception of slight pain during passive overpressure of right hip extension. Her muscle strength was tested isometrically with manual resistance and was thought to be normal. She did not complain of pain during this test. C.M. reported slight tenderness to palpation of the right inguinal area 5 cm medial to the ASIS.

Based on the patient's reports of the nature of her pain and the examination findings, the therapist felt that C.M. was a candidate for a stress fracture of the right femoral neck. She was referred to an orthopedist who concurred. A bone scan revealed an increased uptake of the right femoral neck.

C.M. was referred back to PT with a diagnosis of a stable stress fracture of the femoral neck. She was advised to avoid running for 8 weeks. During this time she performed cycling and lower extremity resistive exercises using accommodative resistance exercise equipment with light weights. At 8 weeks following her diagnosis, she was begun on walk-run progression on a treadmill. At 12 weeks, she was allowed to run outside on level surfaces.

At 1 year after the onset of her pain, she is currently running 25 miles per week on a level surface and alternating her running with cycling and step aerobics. She has reported no inguinal pain with these activities.

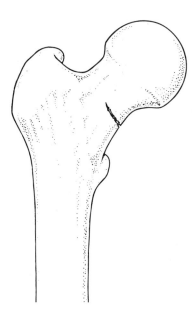

Fig. 16-42. Stress fracture of the femoral neck. (From Parker MJ, Pryor GA: *Hip fracture management,* Boston, 1993, Blackwell.)

palpable, and thus groin pain that worsens with activity in individuals with risk factors may be the most obvious early indication. A bone scan is often required for early diagnosis.

The treatment consists of greatly reducing or eliminating the offending activity for several weeks. For individuals who are unwilling to do this, such activities as running short distances in a pain-free manner on a level treadmill may be psychologically useful. Cardiovascular fitness can be maintained by riding a stationary bicycle. Swimming or water-walking has been advocated. However, the torsion on the femoral neck during the frog or flutter kick may be harmful.

Soft tissue disorders of the hip

Muscle strains frequently occur in the pelvis and thigh. The two primary causes of muscle injury are acute trauma and overuse trauma.

There are two common mechanisms of acute trauma: The first results from single traumatic events, which are usually high-velocity eccentric contractions in which the muscle is rapidly forced into an elongated position,[27] the so-called pulled muscle. It is common in all age groups and frequently seen in middle-aged athletes. A classic example is the softball player who strains a hamstring muscle while forcibly increasing stride length to beat out a ground ball. Because of their potential to be forced through large length changes, the biarthrodial muscles of the hip—hamstrings, rectus femoris, tensor fasciae latae, and iliopsoas—are often injured in this way.[24,76] Additionally, the adductor longus is also frequently injured by forced adduction.

A second common mechanism of injury to muscles around the hip is contusion resulting from blunt trauma. These injuries are commonly encountered in sports, such as the football player who is "speared" with a helmet in the thigh or buttock or the baseball pitcher who is hit by a line drive (Fig. 16-43).[24,28] Injuries caused by acute trauma can range from minor to very severe, resulting in a substantial loss of muscle contractility.

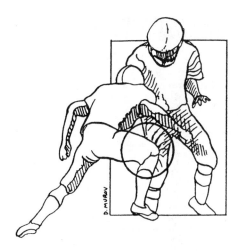

Fig. 16-43. Blunt trauma to muscle. (From Nicholas JA, Hershman EB: *Lower extremity & spine in sports medicine,* ed 2, St Louis, 1995, Mosby.)

Often, considerable hemorrhage occurs at the time of the injury. Thus, patients should be instructed to avoid aspirin for at least 24 hours because of its anticoagulant effect. With the more severe injuries, large hematomas can result, potentiating pain and in some cases predisposing an individual to heterotopic bone formation, such as myositis ossificans. Thus, therapists planning treatments should be very careful to avoid activities such as early stretching that may enhance or cause recurrence of bleeding in the injured area.

The clinical picture of acute muscle strains in the pelvis or thigh area usually includes a history of an acute onset of pain during some activity. The patient often experiences a tearing or popping sensation in the area of the injury. There is typically a diffuse area of pain with palpable tenderness at the site of the injury. Often, a palpable mass representing a hematoma is present. Patients often have great difficulty contracting the involved muscle due to pain. This condition must be differentiated from a tendon rupture or avulsion.[16]

The treatment of acute muscle strains is centered around patient comfort and avoidance of reinjury.[28] Frequent administration of ice is very helpful. Compression bandages help to control swelling and may reduce pain; however, they are somewhat difficult to apply to the buttock and proximal thigh.

Transverse friction massage can be an excellent treatment for regaining contractility and length of injured muscle, but it should not be attempted until several days after the injury. There are no clear guidelines for the transition from ice to heat. Anecdotally, when the pain progresses from a "sharp" sensation to "dull ache and stiffness," moist heat, warm whirlpool, and ultrasound may be helpful. Isometric contractions can be started when the patients are comfortable with a progression to isotonic, concentric, and finally eccentric contractions. Passive stretching of the muscle must be carefully applied and, in more serious injuries, may not

be indicated for several weeks.[29] Patients should be instructed to use care when exercises increase pain at the site of the injury. This problem is common in athletes who attempt to return to competition too quickly. Electrical stimulation may be quite useful for pain control and to assist strengthening exercises.

The second major cause of muscle injury in the pelvis and thigh, overuse trauma, occurs when muscle tissue and its connective tissue elements become strained from repetitive use. Although the degree of tissue damage from overuse is typically less extensive than that sustained in moderate or severe acute trauma, the insidious nature and notoriously slow healing of these disorders make them problematic for both the patient and the clinician.

The mechanism of overuse trauma around the pelvis and thigh is typically multifactoral. Usually, lower extremity malalignment and muscle performance deficits are combined with issues such as inappropriate footgear, irregular terrain, and, most important, repetitive activity. Although most overuse trauma of the hip muscles is seen in runners, other repetitive activities such as kicking sports, martial arts, and dance can predispose a person to injury in this area. Among the muscles most commonly subjected to overuse injury in the hip area are the rectus femoris, tensor fasciae latae, and hip external rotators.

The diagnosis of overuse muscle injuries can be difficult. If the injured muscle has a high degree of irritability, active contractions and passive stretching should reproduce the symptoms.[16,53] Careful palpation often reveals areas of tenderness and occasionally causes referred pain.[94] For example, with a strain of the rectus femoris, the patient may complain of pain with straight leg raising and with the modified Thomas test while reporting tenderness just inferior to the AIIS.

Many patients, however, have no symptoms at the time of the examination and may require a prolonged reproduction of the offending activity, for example, running on the treadmill, to develop symptoms. The treatment is focused on reducing any injurious forces acting upon the tissues by correction of malalignment through foot orthotics and modification of the repetitive activity when possible. Unfortunately, reducing the repetition of activity is often quite difficult because this activity is almost always associated with an important recreational or occupational pursuit. Improved muscle performance through stretching and strengthening exercises is important. After the symptoms have subsided, the patient must be instructed to maintain a normal degree of muscle and joint flexibility by engaging in a routine stretching program. Patients must be instructed that to improve flexibility several bouts throughout the day of 2-minute stretch holds are important.

Bursitis around the hip area can be extremely painful and potentially disabling. Located throughout the body near areas of gliding tissue, bursa sacs act as shock absorbers. In response to acute or overuse trauma, these sacs can develop

CASE 2

A.M. was a 41-year-old computer programmer and marathon runner. He was referred to PT with a diagnosis of low back pain and sciatica. During his initial evaluation, he complained of pain in his left midbuttock that referred posteriorly to his left thigh and left calf. He indicated that these symptoms were worsened when he attempted to run. He denied muscular weakness or loss of sensation in the lower extremities. He was unable to recall any trauma to his spine or lower extremities and stated that his pain developed gradually over the last 4 months. His goal was to return to running 50 miles per week.

On examination, A.M. stood with an erect posture; the ROM of his lumbar spine was normal and did not reproduce pain. He did, however, complain of a mild reproduction of his symptoms during single-leg standing on the left. The ROM of both lower extremities was normal, with the following exceptions: left hip flexion was 110 degrees, left hip adduction

was 15 degrees, and left hip internal rotation was 5 degrees. Left straight-leg raising reproduced his pain at 50 degrees. Inspection of his lower extremities showed an obvious left forefoot varus. He was moderately tender to palpation of the left buttock.

The PT classified this condition as piriformis syndrome. The patient was instructed to avoid running past the onset of pain. He was instructed in a vigorous stretching program of the hip extensors, hip abductors, and hip external rotators. He received an orthotic device to compensate for his left forefoot varus.

Six weeks after the initial PT visit, the patient was pain-free and reported running 50 miles in the last week without symptoms. Six months following the initial PT visit, the patient was continuing a maintenance stretching program, asymptomatic, and continuing to run 50 miles per week.

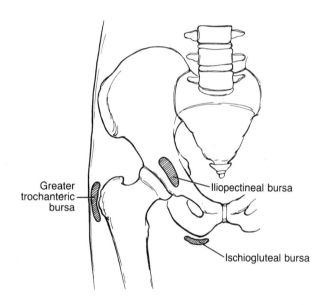

Fig. 16-44. Bursa of the hip and external pelvis. (Modified from Raney R, Brashear H, Shands A, editors: *Shands' handbook of orthopaedic surgery,* St Louis, 1971, Mosby.)

a considerable amount of swelling, which results in acute pain. The three most common types of bursitis around the hip area are greater trochanteric, ischial, and iliopectineal bursitis.

The greater trochanteric bursa separates the tendon of the gluteus maximus from the superior portion of the greater trochanter; the trochanteric bursa lies between the tendon of the gluteus medius and the anterior-superior portion of the greater trochanter (Fig. 16-44).[98] Most frequently involved, the greater trochanteric bursa is often irritated by friction from a shortened iliotibial band, via its attachment to the gluteus medius, as it slides back and forth over the lateral thigh during gait.[24,34] Another cause of irritation of this bursa

may be from excessive pelvic displacement on the horizontal plane. This could result from leg length discrepancies, a Trendelenburg gait caused by weakness of the gluteus medius muscle, and/or running on an irregular or banked surface. An individual with a broad pelvis and associated femoral anteversion may be at risk for this disorder, as may an individual who performs repetitive hip adduction activities.

During the clinical examination, the patient typically indicates a localized area of tenderness near the superior-posterior tip of the greater trochanter. This area is often quite tender, and the patient may be unable to lay on the affected side for prolonged periods. A positive Ober's sign is often present, as is weakness of the hip abductors when tested in an antigravity position. A careful evaluation for the presence of lower extremity malalignment should be conducted.

The treatment of this disorder consists of stretching any tight tissues, for example, the tensor fascia and iliotibial tract, as well as strengthening the hip abductors. Correction of malalignment and training errors like a poor running surface is usually quite helpful. Phonophoresis using hydrocortisone may be useful, and steroid injection is an excellent treatment for more severe cases.

The ischial or ischial-gluteal bursa lies between the gluteus maximus muscle, where it acts to reduce friction between these two structures (Fig. 16-45).[98] This bursa can become irritated, a condition once known as weaver's bottom, in people who sit for prolonged periods of time on firm surfaces. It also can be traumatized when a person lands directly on the ischial tuberosity after a fall.

Clinically, patients complain of pain on the inferior surface of the ischial tuberosity that is noticeably increased with sitting and occasionally with climbing stairs or walking. Generally, palpable tenderness is reported near the ischial tuberosity, but it may be difficult to appreciate in individuals with well-developed gluteal muscles. According to Williams and Warwick,[98] this bursa is frequently absent; thus, examiners must consider tendinitis of the hamstrings or adductor magnus muscle as a possible source of these symptoms.

The treatment consists of the use of an inflatable ring or padded seat cushion to reduce the compressive loading on the irritated tissues. Patients should be instructed to stand frequently throughout the day. Ice, heat, and electrical stimulation may be useful for pain control. Individuals with shortened hamstring, gluteus maximus, or adductor magnus muscles should be instructed in proper stretching.

The iliopectineal bursa, also referred to as the *iliac* or *psoas bursa* lies on the anterior portion of the hip joint capsule deep to the iliopsoas muscle (Fig. 16-45). It may become irritated with contracture of the iliopsoas or because of capsular changes associated with hip joint arthrosis. Because this bursa often communicates with the hip joint capsule, it can become involved in hip joint infections.[95]

Patients with this disorder often complain of inguinal pain that is worsened with active hip flexion. Palpable tenderness may be present over the anterior portion of the hip joint capsule and must be differentiated from other disorders. Frequently there is a positive Thomas test.

Thermal or electrical agents may be used for pain relief. Stretching of a contracted muscle, especially the iliopsoas, is important.

Piriformis syndrome is a condition in which the piriformis muscle contributes to entrapment or irritation of the adjacent nerves.[8] Numerous pain-sensitive structures course in the small interval created by the inferior margin of the piriformis and the superior gemellus muscles (Fig. 16-45).[42,57,98] In up to 30% of people, the common peroneal division of the sciatic nerve pierces the piriformis muscle.[52] Presumably, blunt trauma to buttock or repetitive internal rotation of the hip can cause a strain of the piriformis, resulting in irritation of the structures.

The clinical picture of piriformis syndrome includes a complaint of buttock pain, which often refers posteriorly to the ipsilateral thigh and occasionally to the calf.[8] The patient may describe a history of acute trauma or repetitive strain to the buttock muscles. Prolonged sitting with a thick wallet in one's back pocket may also precipitate these symptoms, the so-called wallet sciatica. During the physical examination, the patient often has substantial limitation of hip internal rotation. The symptoms may be provoked with passive internal rotation, flexion, and adduction of the affected hip. Passive straight-leg raising also often reproduces the symptoms. Tenderness to palpation of the midbuttock area may be present. The patient may be observed to overpronate during walking or running. The differential diagnosis includes radiculopathy of the lumbosacral nerve roots, strain of the gluteus maximus, trochanteric bursitis, hematoma in the buttock area, and thrombosis of the gluteal arteries.

The treatment for piriformis includes ultrasound for pain relief and frequent stretching of the hip external rotator

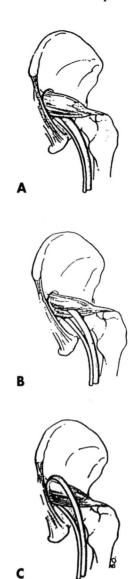

Fig. 16-45. Relationship of the sciatic nerve to the piriformis muscle. Usually it passes inferior to the muscle (**A**). In 12.2% of 640 limbs studied, the sciatic nerve divided before it entered the gluteal region and the common fibular (peroneal) division passed through the piriformis muscle (**B**). In 0.5% of cases the common fibular division passed superior to the muscle (**C**), where it is vulnerable to injury during gluteal intramuscular injections. (From Moore K: *Clinically oriented anatomy,* Baltimore, 1980, Williams & Wilkins.)

muscles (Figs. 16-46 and 16-47). Patients may benefit from orthoses to control overpronation. Runners should be instructed to avoid banked surfaces. Weakness of hip abduction, extension, or external rotation should be addressed by strengthening exercises.

DEGENERATIVE AND INFLAMMATORY CONDITIONS INVOLVING THE HIP

Chronic dysfunction of the hip joint typically results in osteoarthrosis, whereas ischemia to the femoral head often causes avascular necrosis (AVN). Either condition can be

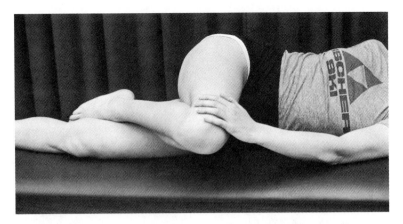

Fig. 16-46. Stretch for the right piriformis muscle in sidelying position.

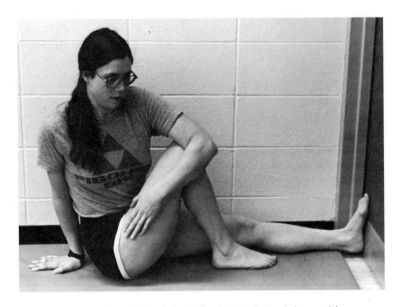

Fig. 16-47. Stretch for right pirifomis muscle in sitting position.

disabling and difficult to treat. As such, an understanding of these disorders can assist the practitioner in early recognition and proper intervention for patients who are at risk.

Avascular necrosis of the femoral head

Death of the subchondral bone of the femoral head due to vascular impairment is known as *avascular necrosis* (AVN), *aseptic necrosis,* or *osteonecrosis.*[1,7] This severely disabling condition can affect individuals of all ages.[88]

The blood supply to the femoral head is tenuous and can be impaired by trauma, by thrombosis, or idiopathically. Death of the subchrondral bone can result from prolonged ischemia. Conditions in which AVN is a potential sequela include femoral neck fractures and hip joint dislocations. Avascular necrosis is also a frequent occurrence in individuals with sickle cell anemia, systemic lupus erythematosus, alcoholism, or a history of prolonged use of catabolic steroids such as prednisone.[1,7,33,40,88]

As the subchrondral bone of the femoral head gradually necroses, the articular cartilage loses its normal base and deforms in response to the change in the shape of the subchondral bone. A loss of congruency of the hip joint results, as well as an impaired ability to tolerate joint reaction forces.[88]

The clinical picture typically includes persistent inguinal pain and limping. In many cases, the patient is unable to report a recent injury or precipitating event but, when questioned in detail, may report one or more of the risk factors mentioned previously.

During the clinical examination, the patient may report a reproduction of pain when the examiner exerts overpressure at various extremes of the hip joint's motion, for example, Patrick's test or perimeter scouring.[53] The diagnosis is confirmed with radiographic evaluation. In many cases, the classic finding of the crescent sign is apparent on antero-posterior films (Fig. 16-48). Magnetic resonance imaging is

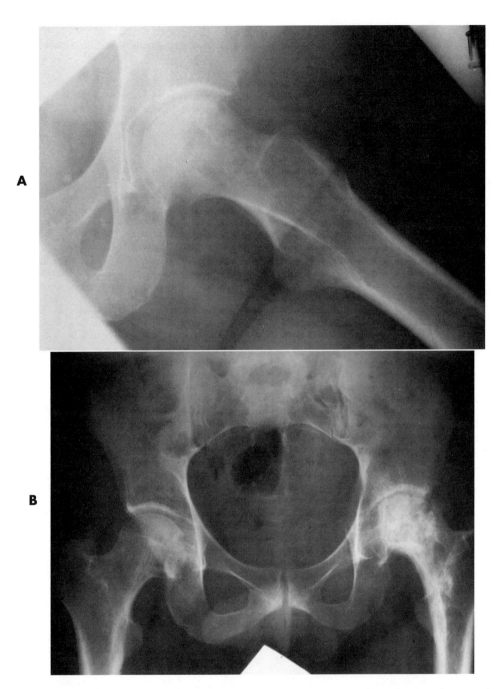

Fig. 16-48. (A), "Frog leg view" radiograph of the hip in a patient with early avascular necrosis (AVN) of the femoral head. The small, dark line in the head of the femur corresponds to the area of osteonecrosis. **(B),** An A-P pelvis view of a patient with severe AVN of the left hip. Note the extensive disruption of the joint surface of the femoral head.

also quite useful for diagnosing AVN.[41] In adults, this condition typically requires surgical intervention by core decompression, bone grafting, or arthroplasty.

Arthritis of the hip

Numerous conditions can result in the process of destruction of the hip joint surface, a process known as *arthrosis*. It is usually referred to clinically as *arthritis*, even though there is often no inflammatory or infectious component. The Box on p. 502 identifies diseases that can result in arthrosis of the hip.[96]

In clinical practice, the two most frequently encountered disorders that result in arthrosis of the hip are osteoarthritis and rheumatoid arthritis.

Osteoarthritis (OA) is a degenerative disorder of joints characterized by a series of events leading to loss of articular

---

CASE 3

J.R. was a 39-year-old unemployed laborer who was referred to PT with a chief complaint of low back pain and chronic pain syndrome. J.R. stated that he had injured his back while lifting a heavy box on the job 3 years ago and that he had been out of work since that time. He had unsuccessfully undergone two previous courses of rehabilitation. J.R. stated that his left groin area had recently become very sore and that he frequently limped from pain. He stated that he was told that this was referred pain. He was unable to recall any trauma. J.R. had a long history of alcoholism and admitted to drinking a pint to a quart of whiskey per day for the last several years.

On examination J.R. had a positive Trendelenburg sign on the left. The ROM of his hip was 105 degrees of flexion, 0 degrees of extension, 20 degrees of abduction, 5 degrees of adduction, 0 degrees of internal rotation, and 25 degrees of external rotation. He complained of a reproduction of his hip pain during the Patrick's test and perimeter movements on the left.

Despite J.R.'s history of chronic pain syndrome, the examining therapist felt that there was substantial evidence of left hip pathology that had not been diagnosed. An orthopedic consultation was obtained. Radiographs and magnetic resonance imaging of the left hip revealed avascular necrosis. Because of the advanced degree of tissue damage, J.R. underwent arthroplasty of the femoral head. In addition, J.R. successfully completed an alcoholism rehabilitation program and has recently become employed as a radio talk show host.

A classification of diseases resulting in arthrosis of the hip

Infectional arthritis

Acute (*Streptococcus, Staphylococcus,* gonococcus)
Chronic (tubercle bacillus)

Probably infectional

Rheumatic fever
Rheumatoid arthritis (atrophic arthritis, proliferative arthritis, chronic infectious arthritis)
Ankylosing spondylitis (Marie-Strümpell disease)
Psoriatic arthritis

Toxic arthritis

Arthritis associated with various infections

Degenerative arthritis (osteoarthritis, hypertrophic arthritis, osteoarthrosis)

Generalized
Localized
    Secondary to previous trauma
    Secondary to structural abnormality
    Secondary to rheumatoid arthritis
    Cause unknown

Arthritis associated with metabolic diseases

Gout
Other metabolic diseases

Neuropathic joints

Tabes dorsalis
Syringomyelia

Neoplasms of joints (cyst, xanthoma, hemangioma, giant cell tumor, synovioma)

Traumatic arthritis

Direct trauma
Indirect trauma (secondary to postural strain)

Systemic disease manifestation

Serum sickness
Hemophilia
Intermittent hydrarthrosis
Pulmonary osteoarthropathy

Local joint disturbances

Aseptic necrosis
    Known etiology (fracture, dislocation, air embolism)
    Unknown etiology (juvenile osteochondritis or Legg-Calvé-Perthes disease, Köhler's disease, Freiberg's disease, Osgood-Schlatter disease)
Osteochondritis dissecans (aseptic necrosis?)
Osteochondromatosis
Pigmented villonodular synovitis

From Turek SL: *Orthopaedics: principles and their application,* ed 4, Philadelphia, 1984, JB Lippincott.

---

cartilage and reactive bone formation, resulting in pain, deformity, and disability. Osteoarthritis can be classified as primary or secondary.[1] Primary OA has no obvious cause, but secondary OA occurs in response to a known cause such as a history of an intraarticular fracture. Although OA is often referred to as *degenerative joint disease* (DJD), this reference may not be appropriate because DJD encompasses a spectrum of disorders, not just OA. The large, weight-bearing joints are the most frequently involved, with OA being the most frequent painful problem of the hip.[8]

The etiology of primary arthritis of the hip remains unclear. Although often attributed to the aging process, it may relate more to the summation of microtrauma rather than to an age-specific process. Repeated loading within *normal* limits of the hip has not been shown to wear out the joint. Emerging evidence identifies genetic markers that may predispose certain individuals to OA. Numerous factors can cause secondary OA; for example, destruction of articular cartilage can be potentiated by macrotrauma, hemarthrosis, intraarticular infections, and synoviolytic diseases such as rheumatoid arthritis. Whenever patients present with a history of any of these conditions, clinicians should consider the potential for hip joint arthrosis.

The mechanical events that cause physical injury to cartilage or subchondral bone can be divided into microtrauma and macrotrauma. Microtrauma can occur with excessive impact loading on subchondral bone and is potentiated by inadequate neuromuscular control or abnormal joint angle of loading, such as occurs with a leg length difference.[25,32] Excessive shearing on articular cartilage due to joint instability, as well as prolonged compressive loading—for example, standing for long periods—can also result in cartilage injury. Macrotrauma or a single trauma that disrupts the articular cartilage or subchrondral bone can be due to intraarticular fractures, osteochondral injuries, or dislocation. Prolonged immobilization or non–weight-bearing periods can lead to arthrosis due to the disruption in the normal nutritional mechanisms of articular cartilage.[91]

Several other factors can predispose a joint to arthrosis. From a biochemical perspective, an alteration of proteoglycan aggregates within the matrix of the articular cartilage results in a loss of bound water that impairs its mechanical properties.[43] An alteration of synovial fluid; the presence of lytic enzymes, blood, or infectious material in a joint; intraarticular injections of cortisone; and lytic agents associated with a variety of systemic inflammatory diseases all have adverse effects on articular cartilage. The common disorders of the hip that can predispose a patient to secondary OA are listed in the Box.[1]

Another proposed mechanism of arthrosis is increased stiffness of the subchondral bone that impairs the ability of the articular cartilage to deform, thus leading to breakdown of articular cartilage and further abnormal loading on subchrondral bone. It can be caused by mechanical or chemical injury to articular cartilage or subchondral bone as described previously. The sequence of pathologic changes in articular cartilage is:

1. Disruption of tangential layer (fibrillation)
2. Formation of large defects (fissuring)
3. Exposed subchondral bone (eburnation)

As the articular cartilage deteriorates, small pieces of cartilage become free within the joint and are absorbed by the synovial membrane. This process results in synovial hyperplasia and capsular fibrosis. The alterations of the joint surfaces and accompanying deformity further alter the mechanics of the hip and lead to additional degenerative changes (Fig. 16-49).

The source of pain in osteoarthritis remains controversial. Articular cartilage is aneural.[98] As the disease progresses,

Various causes of secondary arthritis
Malalignment
Coxa vara
Coxa valga
Acetabular dysplasia
Leg length difference
Femoral anteversion
Cartilage abnormalities
Infection
Rheumatoid disease
Intraarticular fracture
Cortisone injections
Joint dislocation
Bony abnormalities
Avascular necrosis
Subchondral fracture
Paget's disease
Subchondral sclerosis

From Apley AG, Solomon L: *Apley's system of orthopaedics and fractures,* ed 6, Boston, 1982, Butterworth.

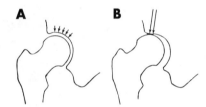

Fig. 16-49. Abnormal loading due to hip arthrosis. Note how the altered joint surface has reduced the area of contact resulting in cencentrated stress. (From Apley AG, Solomon L: *Apley's system of orthopaedics and fracture,* ed 6, Boston, 1982, Butterworths.)

capsular fibrosis and shortening occur; the typical pattern results in limited extension, abduction, and internal rotation of the hip. Then the capsule can be painfully stretched during the middle and late stance phases of gait, which require the hip to assume these positions. This may result in muscle guarding by the hip intrinsic muscles, further restricting motion and causing pain.

The clinical presentation of hip OA varies, depending on the stage of its progression. Initially, patients may be aware of only an occasional dull ache in the groin area after vigorous activity. At this time, patients may have a positive Patrick's test or report increased pain during passive joint compression or "perimeter movements." As the condition worsens, the pain may refer to the medial thigh and be provoked during daily activities such as getting in and out of bed or after prolonged weight-bearing activity. Patients at this stage often develop a progressive loss of extension, abduction, and internal rotation of the hip as described previously. Cyriax has described this pattern as capsular.[16] It often leads to the characteristic deformity of hip flexion, adduction, and external rotation. When the degree of pain and deformity reaches a critical threshold, the patient often requires assistive devices for ambulation. Because the hip joint is difficult to palpate, one can rarely appreciate swelling or crepitus. Upon radiographic examination, the femoral head often assumes a flattened appearance. The other classic radiographic findings of hip osteoarthritis include loss of joint space, sclerosis of subchrondral bone of the femoral head, osteophytes around the joint margins, especially the superior rim of the acetabulum, and bone cysts in the subchondral bone (Fig. 16-50).

The treatment options for arthrosis are numerous and based on the stage of the disorder. Prevention is certainly an optimal goal. Although supporting data are minimal, maintenance of ROM and muscle strength and avoidance of prolonged standing are presumably useful. Carefully prescribed foot orthoses are potentially very valuable to assist

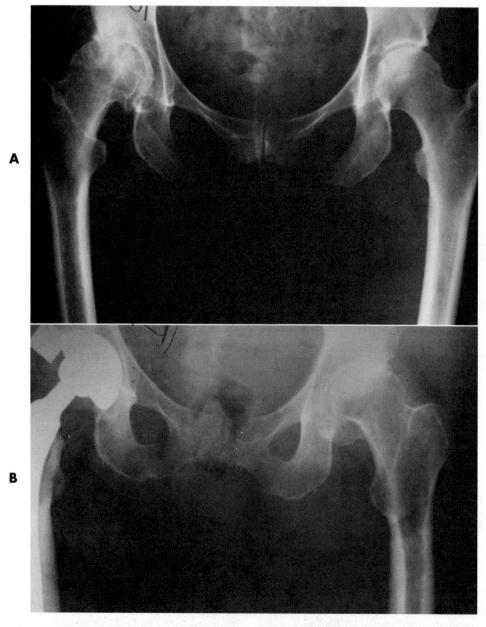

Fig. 16-50. Arthrosis of the hip. **(A)** In this A-P pelvis view, the patient's left hip demonstrates early radiographic signs of arthrosis, that is, subchondral sclerosis in the superior rim of the acetabulum. The patient's right hip demonstrates advanced signs of arthrosis including loss of joint space, subchondral sclerosis, bone cysts in the femoral head and obvious deformity of the hip joint. **(B)** In this A-P pelvis view of a different patient, radiographic signs of severe arthrosis are present in the the left hip. Note the obliteration of the joint space coupled with severe deformity of the femoral head. This patient has undergone a prosthetic replacement of the right hip.

symmetric loading. Once the disease has developed, several treatment options are available. Although physical therapy has not been shown to reverse the effects of arthrosis, carefully followed exercise programs may slow the progression or at least buy the patient some time.

Individuals with minimal or moderate arthrosis should be counseled to reduce high-risk activities such as running or carrying heavy loads. Joint mobilization procedures such as inferior and lateral glides are useful for gaining motion and pain control. When an individual begins to limp frequently due to pain, reduced load bearing through the use of an assistive device such as a cane is very important. Overweight individuals must work diligently on weight loss. For individuals whose pain becomes disabling, the spectrum of available surgical procedures is discussed in a subsequent section of this chapter.

Rheumatoid arthritis (RA) is a disabling, autoimmune, systemic connective tissue disease that is present to different degrees in more than 3.6 million Americans.[7,93] This disease is characterized by chronic swelling of the synovial membranes, leading to diffuse swelling, pain, and progressive deformity of multiple joints.

The hips joints are very frequently involved in patients with RA. In the early stages of the disorder, synovitis results in swelling and thickening of the synovial membrane. There is a gradual alteration of the nature of the synovial fluid, with proteolytic enzymes becoming active in destroying the articular cartilage. In later stages, the destruction of the articular surface, combined with capsular fibrosis and chronic muscle spasm, leads to joint deformities. Usually there is bilateral involvement in the hips. Reducing load bearing by crutch ambulation is helpful but can be problematic because of upper extremity involvement. Conservative treatment such as strengthening and mobility exercises, combined with pharmacologic intervention, can be useful. Patients who become disabled often require synovectomy or total hip arthroplasty.

Surgical management of end-stage arthrosis

In the advanced stages of arthrosis, chronic pain and joint deformity can be extremely disabling. In the last 30 years, enormous advances have been made in the surgical options available to these patients. Although the outcomes from arthroplasty continue to improve, this procedure is for end-stage arthosis and is not a panacea for everyone with chronic joint pain. Once a prosthesis has been implanted, the duration of its function is based upon numerous factors such as metal fatigue and loosening. Thus, arthroplasty is avoided until it is the last resort. As a result, numerous surgical alternatives have been described to extend the "life" of the hip joint. Wedge osteotomy of the proximal femur may be performed to correct skeletal malalignment due, for example, to coxa valga.[1] Synovectomy is often performed in individuals with rheumatoid arthritis.[93] Arthroscopic debridement and chondroplasty may also be undertaken in

attempts to prolong the life of the joint.[39] Finally, fusion (arthrodesis) of the hip is still considered to be a useful procedure in select cases.

When other surgical procedures are no longer an option, or in elderly patients who presumably will not outlive the prosthesis, total joint arthroplasty of the hip is performed. Numerous implants are available. One of the most frequently utilized systems consists of metallic femoral and acetabular components with a polyethylene cup interposed between the two. This is referred to as a total hip arthroplasty.[9]

The two principal forms of fixation of the prostheses are cemented and porous coated. A cemented fixation uses strong adhesives that fixate quickly and generally allows early weight bearing. A porous-coated prosthesis relies on ingrowth of bone to provide fixation. Thus it becomes well fixated over time, but it requires non–weight-bearing activity during the early stages postoperatively.

As with any major surgical procedure, many complications can occur. They are summarized in the Box.

Following total hip arthroplasty, the most serious complications include infection and loosening or dislocation of the prosthesis.[4,72] Although infrequent, infections at the site of the arthroplasty can be catastrophic.[72] A polysaccharide coating forms around the prosthesis and acts as a barrier to antibiotics. Thus, enormous precautions are taken to prevent infections. For example, following total joint arthroplasty, patients are instructed to take antibiotics before any subsequent invasive procedures, including dental work. Wound care postoperatively is critical, and any signs of infection should be taken seriously.

Complications of total hip arthroplasty

Early complications

Local vascular problems
Deep vein thrombosis
Ectopic ossification
Trochanteric bursitis
Dislocation of the hip
Leg length inequality
Wound infection

Late complications

Aseptic loosening
Sepsis
Dislocation
Heterotopic ossification
Femoral fracture
Leg length inequality
Metal toxicity
Chronic pain

From Bierbaum BE et al: Late complications of total hip replacement and Ranawat CS, Figgie MP: Early complications of total hip replacement, in Steinberg ME, editor: *The hip and its disorders*, Philadelphia, 1991, WB Saunders; and Cameron HU: *The technique of total hip arthroplasty*, St Louis, 1992, Mosby.

Table 16-8. Differential diagnosis for pain in the hip or buttock area

Pain distribution	Potential cause

Groin area	Hip joint pathology
	   AVN
	   Arthrosis
	   Fracture
	   Subluxation
	   Dislocation
	   Synovitis
	   Infection
	Loosened prosthesis
	Inflamed lymph nodes
	Muscle strain
	   Adductor
	   Iliopsoas
	   Lower abdominal
	Iliopectineal bursitis
	Inguinal hernia
	Referred pain from Viscera
	   or L3 spinal nerve

Pubic area	Sprain of pubic symphysis Osteitis pubis Abdominal muscle strain Bladder infection

Lateral buttock area	Trochanteric bursitis
	Tendinitis of abductors or
	   external rotators
	Strain of abductors or external
	   rotators
	Apophysitis of greater trochanter
	Referred pain from mid or
	   lower lumbar spine
	Thrombosis of gluteal arteries

Anterior and lateral thigh	Strain of quadriceps
	Meralgia paresthetica
	Entrapment of femoral nerve
	Thrombosis of femoral
	   artery or great saphenous
	   vein
	Stress fracture of femur
	Referred pain from hip or
	   midlumbar spine

Medial thigh	Strain of adductor muscles
	Entrapment of obturator
	   nerve
	Referred pain from hip
	   or knee

ASIS	Apophysitis or sartorius or rectus femoris

Iliac crest	Strain of gluteal, oblique
	   abdominals, tensor fasciae
	   latae, quadratus lumborum
	Entrapment of iliohypogastric
	   nerve
	Referred pain from upper
	   lumbar spine

Loosening of a prosthesis can occur from bone resorption, inadequate fixation, or excessive loading of the hip.[4] The signs of loosening usually include pain or perhaps reported instability at the hip. Revision arthroplasty, a technically very difficult procedure, is often necessary to correct this problem; thus, physical therapists must be acutely aware of the potential for prosthetic loosening. This condition can often be prevented by accurate communication with the surgeon to determine motion and activity limitations. For example, many patients may have a great reduction in symptoms postoperatively and decide to play basketball. The impact loading from this sport can rapidly impair the functioning of the prostheses. Thus, therapists must counsel patients not to go beyond their limitations.

Dislocation of the prosthetic hip is an occasional but serious complication. A common mechanism is exceeding the safe range of motion for the hip. Careful patient education and great care in performing ROM of the hip are very important to prevent it. External supports such as abduction pillows and knee immobilizers can appreciably reduce the occurrence of dislocation.[73]

Rehabilitation of patients following arthroplasty of the hip is a major portion of orthopedic physical therapy. Much has been written regarding movement and activity precautions. Note that the maximum available motion of hip is determined at the time of implantation of the prostheses. The shape of the prostheses, the angle of implantation, and the type of surgical approach dictate the potential for postoperative motion. The nature of the fixation and bone stock dictate the potential stability of the joint. Thus, physical therapists must communicate with the referring surgeon regarding each patient and should never make unilateral judgments regarding ROM or load-bearing goals.

DIFFERENTIAL DIAGNOSIS

Numerous causes of symptoms and problems in the hip area are possible. Table 16-8 lists common sources of hip pain.

SUMMARY

Central to normal gait and most activities of daily living, the hip joint plays a critical role in human existence. Considering its predisposition for developmental anomalies, coupled with the lifetime of load bearing to which the hip is subjected, that the pain and disability arising from hip joint dysfunction are a common clinical entity is not surprising. This chapter summarizes the salient features of the structure, function, and dysfunction of the hip.

REVIEW QUESTIONS

1. What are the early- and late-stage complications of total hip arthroplasty that could affect the postoperative rehabilitation program?

2. How does the treatment and prognosis differ between Legg-Calvé-Perthes disease and avascular necrosis of the hip joint?
3. What are the five factors that should be considered when examining radiographs of the hip joint?
4. What could be the potential causes of an internally rotated lower extremity?
5. What factors provide stability and mobility to the hip joint complex?

REFERENCES

1. Apley AG, Solomon L: *Apley's system of orthopaedics and fractures,* ed 6, Boston, 1982, Butterworths.
2. Beattie P et al: Validity of derived measurements of leg-length differences obtained by the use of a tape measure, *Phys Ther* 70:150, 1990.
3. Bergner M et al: The sickness impact profile: development and final revision of a health status measure, *Med Care* 19:787, 1981.
4. Bierbaum BE et al: Late complications of total hip replacement. In Steinberg ME, editor: *The hip and its disorders,* Philadelphia, 1991, WB Saunders.
5. Blower PW, Griffin AJ: Clinical sacroiliac tests in ankylosing spondylitis and other causes of low back pain, *Ann Rheum Diseases* 43:192, 1984.
6. Brand RA, Crowninshield RD: The effect of a cane on hip contact force, *Clin Orthop* 147:181, 1980.
7. Brashear HR, Raney RB: *Handbook of orthopaedic surgery,* ed 10, St Louis, 1986, Mosby.
8. Calliet R: *Low back pain syndrome,* ed 5, Philadelphia, 1995, FA Davis.
9. Cameron HU: *The technique of total hip arthroplasty,* St Louis, 1992, Mosby.
10. Catterall M: Perthes disease. In Steinberg ME, editor: *The hip and its disorders,* Philadelphia, 1991, WB Saunders.
11. Chao EY et al: Biomechanics of malalignment, *Orthop Clin North Am* 25:379, 1994.
12. Chibnall JT, Tait R: The pain disability index: factor structure and normative data, *Arch Phys Med Rehabil* 75:1082, 1994.
13. Cibulka MT, Delitto A, Koldehoff RM: Changes in inominate tilt after manipulation of the sacroiliac joint in patients with low back pain, *Phys Ther* 68:1359, 1988.
14. Corrigan B, Maitland GD: *Practical orthopaedic medicine,* Boston, 1983, Butterworths.
15. Craik RL: Disability following hip fracture, *Phys Ther* 74:387, 1994.
16. Cyriax J: *Textbook of orthopedic medicine,* vol 1, ed 7, Bailliere Tindall, London, 1981.
17. Dalinka MK, Neustadter LM: Radiology of the hip. In Steinberg ME, editor: *The hip and its disorders,* Philadelphia, 1991, WB Saunders.
18. Dawson I, van Rijn AB: Traumatic anterior dislocation of the hip, *Arch Orthop Trauma Surg* 108:55, 1989.
19. Dickinson WH, Duwelius PJ, Colville MR: Muscle strength following surgery for acetabular fractures, *J Orthop Trauma* 7:39, 1993.
20. Ellis MI, Stowe J: The hip, *Clin Rheumat Dis* 8:655, 1982.
21. Fisher F: An epidemiological study of Legg-Perthes disease, *J Bone Joint Surg Am* 54:769, 1972.
22. Fleckenstein SJ, Kirby RL, MacLeod DA: Effect of limited knee flexion range on peak hip moments of force while transferring from sitting to standing, *J Biomech* 21:915, 1988.
23. Foldes K et al: Nocturnal pain correlates with effusions in diseased hips, *J Rheumatol* 19:1756, 1992.
24. Fox JM: Injuries to the pelvis and hip in athletes: anatomy and function. In Nicholas JA, Hershman EB, editors: *The lower extremity and spine in sports medicine,* St Louis, 1986, Mosby.
25. Friberg O: Clinical symptoms and biomechanics of the lumbar spine and hip joint in leg length inequality, *Spine* 8:643, 1983.
26. Fuss FK, Bacher A: New aspects of the morphology and function of the human hip joint ligaments, *Am J Anat* 192:1, 1991.
27. Gamble JG: *The musculoskeletal system: physiological basics,* New York, 1988, Raven.
28. Garrett WE: Muscle injuries and inflammation, *Ann Sports Med* 3:71, 1987.
29. Garrett WE et al: The effect of muscle architecture on the biomechanical properties of skeletal muscle under passive tension, *Am J Sports Med* 16:7, 1988.
30. Goodman CG, Synder TE: Systemic origins of musculoskeletal pain: associated signs and symptoms. In *Differential diagnosis in physical therapy,* Philadelphia, 1990, WB Saunders.
31. Greenwald AS: Biomechanics of the hip. In Steinberg ME, editor: *The hip and its disorders,* Philadelphia, 1991, WB Saunders.
32. Grofton J, Trueman G: Unilateral idiopathic osteoarthritis of the hip, *Can Med Assoc J* 97:1129, 1967.
33. Halland AM et al: Avascular necrosis of the hip in systemic lupus erythematosus: the role of magnetic resonance imaging, *Br J Rheumatol* 32:972, 1993.
34. Haller CC et al: Traumatic trochanteric bursitis, *Kans Med* 90:17, 1989.
35. Hammond BT, Charnley J: The sphericity of the femoral head, *Med Biol Eng* 5:445, 1967.
36. Hansson G et al: Radiographic assessment of coxarthrosis following slipped capital femoral epiphysis, *Acta Radiol* 34:117, 1993.
37. Harris WH: Traumatic arthritis of the hip after dislocation and acetabular fracture: treatment by mold arthroplasty, *J Bone Joint Surg Am* 51:737, 1969.
38. Harty M. Hip anatomy. In Steinberg ME, editor: *The hip and its disorders,* Philadelphia, 1991, WB Saunders.
39. Hawkins RB: Arthroscopy of the hip, *Clin Orthop* 249:44, 1989.
40. Hernigou P et al: Deformities of the hip in adults who have sickle-cell disease and had avascular necrosis in childhood, *J Bone Joint Surg* 73:91, 1991.
41. Hiehle JF, Kneeland JB, Dalinka MK: Magnetic resonance imaging of the hip with emphasis on avascular necrosis, *Rheum Dis Clin North Am* 17:669, 1991.
42. Hollingshead WH, Rosse C: *Textbook of anatomy,* ed 4, Philadelphia, 1985, Harper & Row.
43. Inman VT: Functional aspects of the abductor muscles of the hip, *J Bone Joint Surg Am* 29:607, 1947.
44. Inerot S et al: Proteoglycan alterations during developing experimental osteoarthritis in a novel hip joint model, *J Orthop Res* 9:658, 1991.
45. Jette AM: Using health-related quality of life measures in physical therapy outcomes research, *Phys Ther* 73:528, 1993.
46. Johnston RC: Mechanical considerations of the hip joint, *Arch Surg* 107:411, 1973.
47. Johnston RC, Smidt GL: Hip motion measurements for selected activities of daily living, *Clin Orthop* 72:205, 1970.
48. Jones M: Clinical reasoning in manual therapy, *Phys Ther* 72:875, 1992.
49. Kapandji IA: *The physiology of joints, vol 2, The lower limb,* New York, 1970, Churchill Livingstone.
50. Kendell FP, McCreary EK, Provance PG: *Muscles: testing and function,* ed 4, Baltimore, 1993, Williams & Wilkins.
51. Larsen CB: Rating scale for hip disabilities, *Clin Orthop* 31:85, 1963.
52. Lee CS, Tsai TL: The relation of the sciatic nerve to the piriformis muscle, *J Formos Med Assoc* 73:75, 1974.
53. Magee DJ: *Orthopedic physical assessment,* ed 2, Philadelphia, 1992, WB Saunders.
54. Maitland GD: *Vertebral manipulation,* ed 4, Boston, 1984, Butterworths.
55. Melzack R: The short-form McGill Pain Questionnaire, *Pain* 30:191, 1987.

56. Molley M, MacMahon B: Birthweight and Legg-Calvé-Perthes disease, *J Bone Joint Surg Am* 49:498, 1967.

57. Moore KL: *Clinically orientated anatomy,* ed 3, Baltimore, 1985, Williams & Wilkins.

58. Moore RJ et al: The relationship between head-neck-shaft angle, calcar width, articular cartilage and bone volume in arthrosis of the hip, *Br J Rheumatol* 35:432, 1994.

59. Murray MP: Gait as a total pattern of movement, *Am J Phys Med* 46:290, 1967.

60. Neumann DA, Hase AD: The electromyographic analysis of the hip abductors during load carriage: implications for hip joint protection, *J Orthop Sports Phys Ther* 19:296, 1994.

61. Neumann DA, Soderberg GL, Cook TM: Electromyographic analysis of hip abductor musculature in healthy right-handed persons, *Phys Ther* 69:431, 1989.

62. Neumann DA et al: An electromyographic analysis of hip abductor muscle activity when subjects are carrying loads in one or both hands, *Phys Ther* 72:207, 1992.

63. Nordin M, Frankel VH: *Basic biomechanics of the musculoskeletal system,* ed 2, Philadelphia, 1989, Lea & Febiger.

64. Noriyasu S et al: On the morphology and frequency of Weitbrecht's retinacula in the hip joint, *Okajimas Folia Anat Jpn* 70:87, 1993.

65. Norkin CN, Levangie PK: *Joint structure and function: a comprehensive analysis,* ed 2, Philadelphia, 1992, FA Davis.

66. Parker MJ, Pryor GA: *Hip fracture management,* Boston, 1993, Blackwell.

67. Paul JP: Forces transmitted by joints in the human body, *Proc Inst Mech Engrs* 181:8, 1967.

68. Pauwels F: *Biomechanics of the normal and diseased hip,* Berlin, 1976, Springer-Verlag.

69. Pratt NE: *Clinical musculoskeletal anatomy,* Philadelphia, 1991, JB Lippincott.

70. Pryor GA, Williams DR: Rehabilitation after hip fractures: home and hospital management, *J Bone Joint Surg Br* 71:471, 1989.

71. Radin EL: Biomechanics of the human hip, *Clin Orthop* 152:28, 1980.

72. Ranawat CS, Figgie MP: Early complications of total hip replacement. In Steinberg ME, editor: *The hip and its disorders,* Philadelphia, 1991, WB Saunders.

73. Rao JP, Bronstein R: Dislocation following arthroplasties of the hip: incidence, prevention and treatment, *Orthop Rev* 20:261, 1991.

74. Reikeras O: Is there a relationship between femoral anteversion and leg torsion? *Skeletal Radiol* 20:409, 1991.

75. Reilly DT: Dyanamic loading of joints, *Rheum Dis Clin North Am* 14:497, 1988.

76. Renstrom P, Peterson L: Groin injuries in athletes, *Br J Sports Med* 14:30, 1980.

77. Roach KE, Miles T: Normal hip and knee active range of motion: the relationship to age, *Phys Ther* 71:656, 1991.

78. Rogers AW: *Textbook of anatomy,* New York, 1992, Churchill-Livingstone.

79. Rogers M, Cavanagh P: Glossary of biomechanical terms, concepts and units, *Phys Ther* 64:1866, 1984.

80. Rothstein JM, Echternach JL: Hypothesis-oriented algorithm for clinicians: a method for evaluation and treatment planning, *Phys Ther* 66:1388, 1986.

81. Rushfield PD, Mann RW, Harris WH: Influence of cartilage geometry on the pressure distribution in the human hip joint, *Science* 204:413, 1979.

82. Rydell N: Biomechanics of hip joint, *Clin Orthop* 92:6, 1973.

83. Saji MJ, Upakhyay SS, Leong JCY: Increased femoral neck-shaft angles in adolescent idiopathic scoliosis, *Spine* 20:303, 1995.

84. Seireg A, Arvikar RJ: A mathematical model for evaluation of forces in the lower extremities of the musculoskeletal system, *J Biomech* 6:313, 1973.

85. Smidt GL: Hip motion and related factors in walking, *Phys Ther* 51:9, 1971.

86. Smith G et al: Hip pain caused by buttock claudication: relief of symptoms by transluminal angioplasty, *Clin Orthop* 284:176, 1992.

87. Soderberg G: *Kinesiology: application to pathological motion,* Baltimore, 1986, Williams & Wilkins.

88. Steinberg ME, Steinberg DR: Avascular necrosis of the femoral head. In Steinberg ME, editor: *The hip and its disorders,* Philadelphia, 1991, WB Saunders.

89. Strickland E et al: In vivo contact pressures during rehabilitation, part 1: acute phase, *Phys Ther* 1992, 72:691.

90. Terjesen T: Ultrasonography in the primary evaluation of Perthe's disease, *J Pediatr Orthop* 13:437, 1993.

91. Teshima R, Otsuka T, Yamamoto K: Effects of nonweight bearing on the hip, *Clin Orthop* 279:149, 1992.

92. Tetsworth K, Paley D: Malalignment and degenerative arthropathy, *Orthop Clin North Am* 25:367, 1994.

93. Thabe H: *The rheumatoid hip,* New York, 1990, Springer-Verlag.

94. Travel J: The myofascial genesis of pain, *Postgrad Med* 11:425, 1952.

95. Trueta J, Harrison MHM: The normal vascular anatomy of the femoral head in adult man, *J Bone Joint Surg Br* 35:442, 1953.

96. Turek SL: *Orthopaedics: principles and their application,* ed 4, Philadelphia, 1984, JB Lippincott.

97. Vrahas MS et al: Contribution of passive tissues to the intersegmental moments at the hip, *J Biomech* 23:357, 1990.

98. Williams PL, Warwick R: *Gray's anatomy,* ed 36, Philadelphia, 1980, WB Saunders.

99. Wingstrand H, Wingstrand A, Krantz P: Intracapsular and atmospheric pressure in the dynamics and stability of the hip, *Acta Orthop Scand* 61:231, 1990.

100. Yang RS, Tsuang YH, Liu TK: Traumatic dislocation of the hip, *Clin Orthop* 265:218, 1991.

CHAPTER 17

The Spine

Carl DeRosa and James A. Porterfield

OUTLINE

Clinical anatomy
   General concepts
   Bony elements
   Ligaments
   Articulations of the spine
   Musculature of the spine
Evaluation of the spine
   Clinical evaluation
      History
      Physical examination: functional assessment
Treatment of activity-related spine disorders
   Modulating pain
   Generation of controlled forces in order to promote
     reactivation
   Enhancing neuromuscular efficiency
   Biomechanical counseling
   Objectives of treatment: commonly used treatment
     techniques
Treatment plans for selected medical conditions: matching
  the functional assessment to objectives of treatment
   Instability of low back/neck
   Instability of posterior support structures to tolerate
     ground and trunk forces such as occurs with degen-
     erative process, stenotic spine, spondylolisthesis
   Sprain and strain
Summary

LEARNING OBJECTIVES

After studying this chapter, the reader should be able to:

1. Identify the significant bony elements of the cervical, thoracic, and lumbar vertebra, as well as the sacrum.
2. List and describe the components of the major spinal articulations.
3. Discuss the function of the low back, upper back, neck, and abdominal musculature.
4. Describe and perform a comprehensive physical examination of the lumbosacral and cervicothoracic spinal regions.
5. List ten major diagnostic categories derived from the Quebec Task Force Report.
6. List the physical therapy working assessment classifications for activity related to low back and neck pain.
7. Describe active, passive manual, and mechanical techniques for the generation of controlled forces to promote patient reactivation.
8. List five principles that must be considered when prescribing resistance exercises for the spine.
9. State five functions of the abdominal wall mechanism.
10. Describe the treatment plan for low back and neck instability, stenotic spine conditions, spondylolisthesis, spinal sprains, and spinal strains.

KEY TERMS

spine	examination
vertebra	spinal disorders
sacrum	treatment
intervertebral disc	

Spinal pain is a nearly ubiquitous musculoskeletal problem in physical therapy practice. Disorders of the spine outrank all other musculoskeletal problems in both total numbers and total costs dedicated toward evaluation and treatment. Spinal pain and, in particular, low back pain are the most frequent causes of activity limitation in people younger than 45, the second most common reason for physician visits, and the fifth most frequent reason for hospitalization.[1]

Activity-related spinal pain is a term that refers to spinal disorders involving the connective tissues and muscular or neural elements as a result of injury, the aging process, or adaptive changes to the tissues. Such a classification focuses attention to the biomechanics of injury and the healing process as opposed to those spinal disorders occurring as a result of lesions to the abdominal or pelvic viscera and as opposed to back pain resulting from medical conditions such as infection, systemic disease, or neoplasm. The primary emphasis of this chapter is activity-related spine pain.

This chapter is divided into three primary sections: clinical anatomy, the evaluation process, and treatment considerations. Clinical anatomy is especially important because comprehensive understanding of the functional anatomy guides the evaluation and treatment process. The focus in treatment is restoration of function, and an active approach to exercise is the treatment philosophy that most often results in cost-effective outcomes. Throughout each of the sections, relevant medical considerations related to the spine are mentioned as clinical examples. However, a complete discussion of medical disorders of the spine is beyond the scope of this chapter. For a detailed analysis of medical and surgical considerations, the reader is referred to texts detailing these subjects.[14,35]

CLINICAL ANATOMY
General concepts

The spine is a segmented column forming the axial skeleton. Through a series of specialized articulations, it meets the conflicting demands of stiffness and flexibility. These intervertebral articulations are primarily the apophyseal joints and the intervertebral disks. Serving as the central core of the human body, the spine houses and protects the spinal cord and related neural tissues, affords a stable foundation from which the appendages can act, and provides attachment sites for cervical, thoracic, abdominal, and pelvic visceral structures.

The entire column consists of 33 vertebrae (Fig. 17-1). The movable segments of the spine consist of 7 cervical vertebrae, of which the first two, the atlas and the axis, have evolved into highly specialized structures; 12 thoracic vertebrae; and 5 lumbar vertebrae. The last lumbar vertebra articulates with the first sacral vertebra and forms the lumbosacral junction. Typically, the 5 sacral vertebrae are fused as one sacrum. In certain conditions, the last lumbar vertebra fuses with the sacrum, a condition referred to as *sacralization of the fifth lumbar vertebra;* or the first sacral vertebra fails to fuse with the rest of the sacrum, which is referred to as *lumbarization of the first sacral vertebrae.* Caudal to the sacrum, four or five irregularly shaped bones form the coccyx.

Bony elements

The typical vertebrae. Although the phrase *typical vertebra* is often used in textbooks of anatomy, differences between individual vertebrae abound, not only between different regions of the spine but also within the same region. In addition, asymmetry between two sides of a vertebra are the rule rather than the exception. Despite such constraints, describing several of the multiple bony processes of a vertebra is a worthwhile way to explain the attachment sites for the ligamentous and muscle-tendon elements.

A vertebra consists of two distinct parts: the vertebral body and the posteriorly positioned vertebral arch (Fig. 17-2). The vertebral body is a cylindrical mass with a cancellous core of bony trabeculae and a cortical shell of compact bone (Fig. 17-3). Three unique attachments to the vertebral body are the cartilaginous end plates, the annulus fibrosus, and, in the thoracic spine, the ribs.

In contrast to the vertebral body, the vertebral arch is a complex bony structure (Fig. 17-4). It is attached to the posterior aspect of the vertebral body by the two pedicles. Between each two vertebrae, the spinal nerve exits via the intervertebral foramen, a space formed above and below the adjacent pedicles of opposing vertebrae. The path that the nerve root takes as it makes its exit through the intervertebral foramen is especially important. Compromise of the nerve root canal or the foraminal opening is referred to as *lateral recess stenosis.* Factors that contribute to lateral recess stenosis include thickening of the pedicle, disk space narrowing, and degenerative changes of the apophyseal joints.

Extending posteriorly from the pedicles are the laminae, and the laminae of the two sides are joined centrally by the spinous process. A bony ring is formed by the posterior aspect of the vertebral body, pedicles, laminae, and spinous process, forming the spinal canal or vertebral foramen, through which the spinal cord and lumbosacral nerve roots, the cauda equina, traverse. *Spinal stenosis* refers to conditions in which the diameter of the spinal canal is decreased and thus compromises tissues housed in the canal, such as the dura mater, spinal cord, and nerve roots. Decompression laminectomies are surgical procedures designed to relieve this compromise of the spinal canal.

At the junction of the pedicle and lamina are two specialized structures, the transverse processes and the articular processes. The articular processes are covered with hyaline cartilage, which forms the facet surface of the apophyseal joint. There are two articular processes on each side, the superior and inferior articular processes. All of the superior articular processes in the spine face posteriorly to

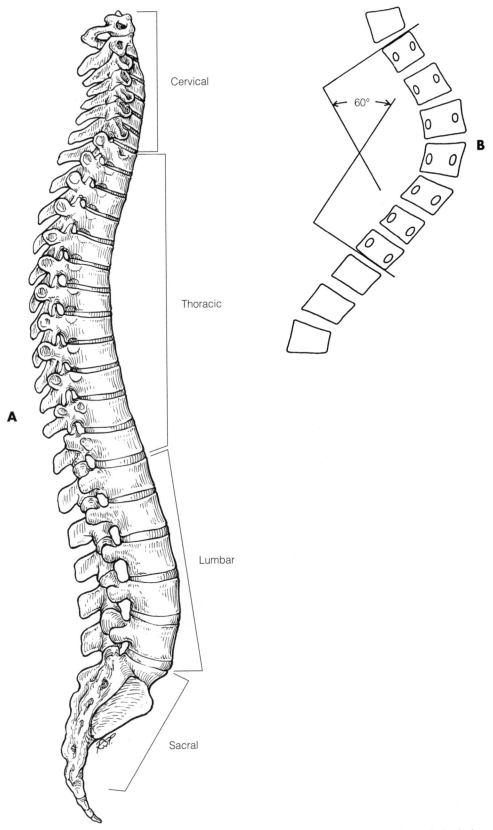

Fig. 17-1. A, The regions of the spinal column. The cervical and lumbar regions feature a lordosis; the thoracic and sacral regions feature a kyphosis. **B,** Scoliosis is a lateral curvature of the spine, most often occurring in the thoracic region. Vertebral rotation accompanies the lateral curvature. The Cobb method is used to assess the angle of scoliotic curvature.

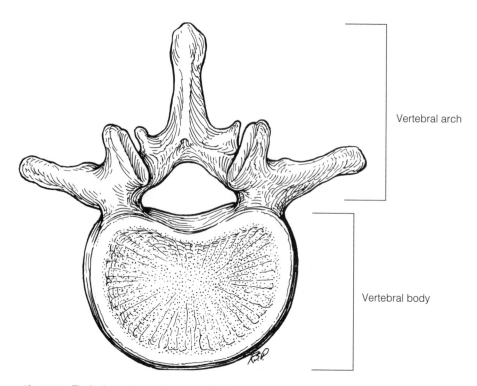

Fig. 17-2. Typical vertebra with its two divisions: the vertebral body and the vertebral arch.

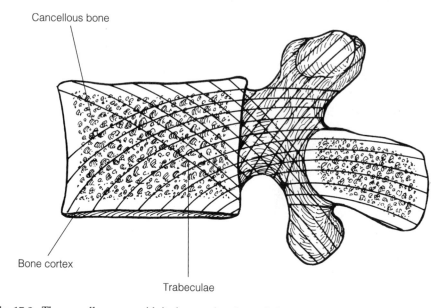

Fig. 17-3. The cancellous core with its bony trabeculae and the cortical shell of the vertebral body.

some degree, whereas the inferior articular processes have some degree of anterior inclination. Developmentally, the transverse processes are associated with a costal element and, in the mature spine, either articulate with a rib or embody the rib component of the vertebra. The transverse

and articular processes serve as important sites for muscle attachments.

Regional considerations. Each region of the spine features a typical curve in the sagittal plane (see Fig. 17-1). The cervical and lumbar regions are marked by a lordosis

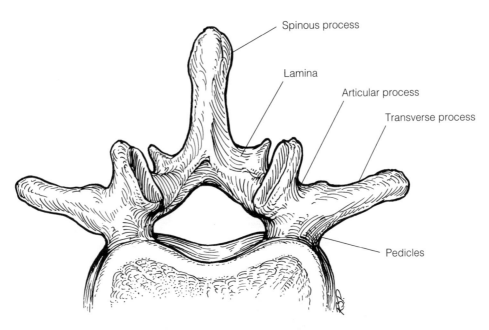

Fig. 17-4. The vertebral arch. Elements of the arch include the pedicles, lamina, spinous process, transverse process, and the articular process with its facet surface.

(convexity facing anteriorly) and the thoracic spine and sacrum by a kyphosis (convexity facing posteriorly). *Scoliosis* refers to the clinical diagnosis of lateral curvature, which is accompanied by rotational, shear, and compressive stresses of the vertebrae involved in the lateral curvature.

Proceeding from a cranial to a caudal direction, the vertebrae of specific regions take on unique characteristics. For the purposes of this chapter, those differences that are primarily related to functional adaptations are the primary focus. For example, moving from the cervical region to the lumbar region, the increase in mass of the vertebrae is the functional adaptation made as a result of increased weight-bearing demands in the upright, antigravity posture. Also relevant is the gradual transition between regions of the spine. The seventh cervical vertebra is a transitional vertebra between the cervical and thoracic regions, the first thoracic vertebra can be considered a transitional vertebra between the thoracic and cervical regions, and the twelfth thoracic vertebra is a transitional vertebra between the thoracic and lumbar regions.

The cervical vertebrae. Two highly specialized vertebrae, the atlas (first cervical vertebra) and the axis (second cervical vertebra), have evolved in the cervical spine. The atlas occupies the space between the occiput and the axis and is thus involved in two primary articulations, the atlantooccipital articulation and the atlantoaxial articulation. These are the only two movable spinal articulations that do not have an intervertebral disk interposed between the vertebrae. In contrast, the third through seventh cervical vertebrae are relatively uniform.

The vertebral bodies of C3 to C7 are comparatively small,

with a greater transverse than anteroposterior diameter. They present a modified beveled appearance, with the raised lateral ridges of the superior plateau of the vertebral body forming uncinate processes (Fig. 17-5). Uniform joints, uncovertebral joints, or joints of Luschka are formed when the lateral region of the inferior plateau of the vertebral body articulate with the unciform process of the subjacent vertebral body. The unciform processes are not considered synovial joints by most sources because they lack the hyaline cartilage, subchondral bone, synovium, and joint capsule.[16]

A unique aspect of the cervical vertebrae is the presence of the transverse foramen through which the vertebral artery, a plexus of veins, and nerves course. The vertebral artery is the first branch from the subclavian trunk and travels to the transverse process of C6 (Fig. 17-6). Accompanying the artery are the vertebral plexus of veins and the sympathetic nerve fibers arising from the stellate (inferior cervical) ganglion. They pass upward through each transverse foramen, make a sharp lateral bend between the transverse process of the axis and atlas owing to the extremely wide profile of the transverse process of the atlas, and then curve around the posterolateral aspect of the atlas to lie on its superior surface, from which point it runs through the foramen magnum into the cranial cavity. On the lower border of the pons, the ipsilateral vertebral artery meets with the contralateral vertebral artery to form the basilar artery. Evaluation of the cervical spine often includes vertebral artery testing, especially if vigorous stretching or manipulation is being considered. In this test, the cervical spine is positioned into end range extension and rotation. This position is maintained to determine if nystagmus, vertigo, or

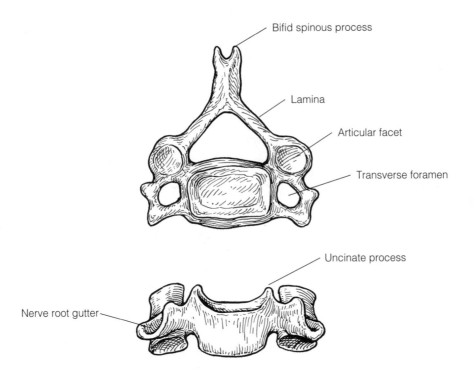

Fig. 17-5. Components of a typical cervical vertebra. The raised ridges of the cervical vertebral body are referred to as uncinate processes, which contribute to the formation of the uniform joints.

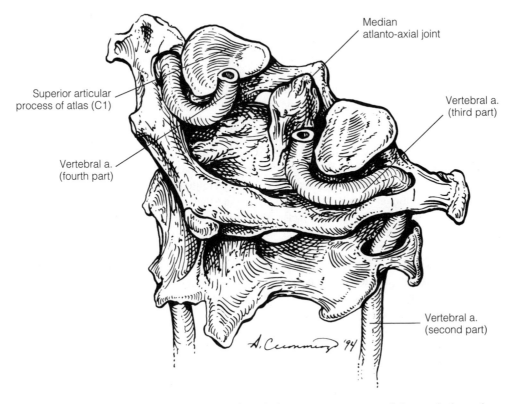

Fig. 17-6. Course of the vertebral artery through the transverse process of the cervical vertebra.

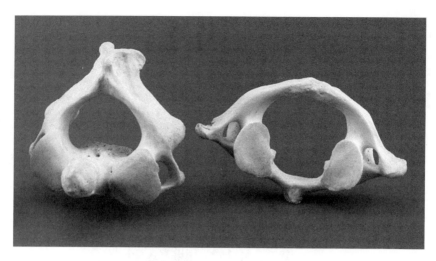

Fig. 17-7. The first two cervical vertebrae, the atlas and the axis.

cognitive changes are elicited, in which case further referral may be indicated and treatment techniques into this end range should be avoided.

The apophyseal joints of the cervical spine are oriented approximately 45 degrees to the horizontal plane. The superior articular process faces posteriorly and upward, whereas the inferior articular process faces anteriorly and downward. The transverse processes arise laterally and project anteriorly and inferiorly. A distinct groove is present along their superior surface, over which the cervical nerves pass in their path from the spinal cord to the periphery.

The spinal canal in the cervical region houses the spinal cord, proximal portion of the nerve root complex, vasculature, and meningeal coverings. Compromise of the spinal cord is referred to as *myelopathy*. The most common clinical complaint in cervical myelopathy is gait disturbance. The syndrome occurs insidiously and is often accompanied by upper motor neuron signs below the level of the compromise, lower motor neuron signs at the level of the compromise, loss of hand dexterity, and a deep burning in the spine. The myelopathic condition can be caused by any pathology decreasing the diameter of the spinal canal, such as intervertebral disk protrusion into the canal, osteophytes associated with the vertebral bodies or unciform processes, thickening of the lamina and ligamentum flavum, or abnormal translation of one vertebra on another due to instability between the segments (segmental instability).

The atlas and axis. The first two cervical vertebrae, the atlas and axis, are highly specialized.[33] Through a sophisticated articular system, they allow primarily a "nodding" (flexion-extension motion) at the atlantooccipital articulation and rotation between the atlantoaxial articulation. The rotation between the atlas and axis is especially significant, as it accounts for nearly half of the total rotation in the cervical spine.

The atlas is primarily a bony ring consisting of an anterior and posterior arch (Fig. 17-7). It is devoid of a vertebral body, which appears to have been absorbed into the superior aspect of the vertebral body of the subjacent vertebrae (C2), now appearing as the dens (odontoid process). The superior articular facets of the atlas are deeply concave and accept the convex condyles of the occiput in the formation of the atlantooccipital joints. Direct blows to the head, as in falling or direct trauma, may produce compressive loads through the occipital condyles to the lateral facets of the atlas, which result in a type of "explosive" fracture—known as *Jefferson's fracture*—of the ring of the atlas. The transverse processes of the atlas are wider than those of any other cervical vertebra, which affords the muscles attached to these processes an excellent mechanical advantage for rotation.

The distinctive characteristic of the axis is the upwardly projecting dens. The dens articulates with the anterior arch of the atlas, and it is around the pivot of the dens that the atlas moves in rotation. The anterior surface of the dens has a facet that articulates with the arch of the atlas. The posterior surface of the dens also features a facet for articulation with the ligament maintaining the stability of this complex, the cruciate ligament complex, of which the transverse ligament is a key component (Fig. 17-8). The inferior articular processes of the atlas and the superior articular process of the axis are both convex. These synovial articulations, in conjunction with the relationship of the ring of the atlas to the dens, are designed to allow significant rotary motion between the two segments.

On the inferior surface of the axis are the right and left articular pillars, which articulate with the third cervical vertebra. From the dens arise the alar ligaments, which connect the second cervical vertebra to the occiput. This ligamentous connection assures that motion of the occiput

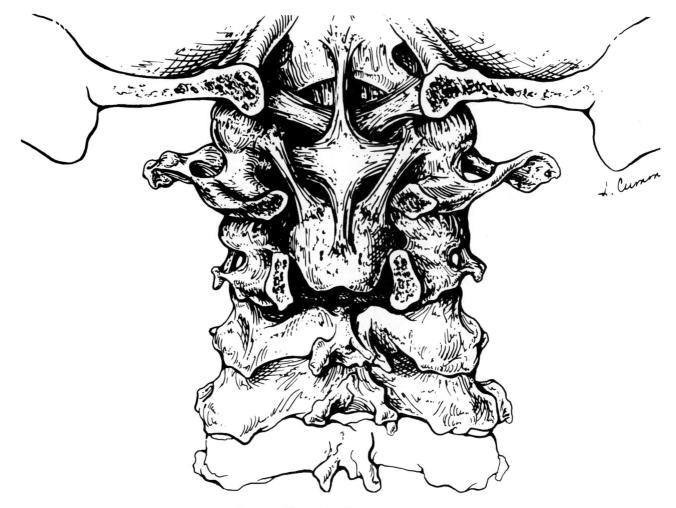

Fig. 17-8. The cruciate ligament complex.

results in immediate movement of the second cervical vertebra as well. As a result, it is instructive to think of the occiput-atlas-axis complex as one functional unit.

The thoracic vertebrae. One of the unique features of the thoracic vertebrae is the articulating surface for the ribs. In the midthoracic spine, one rib articulates with two adjacent vertebrae and the intervening intervertebral disk. Thus, on the inferior aspect of the thoracic vertebral body, a demifacet is present, and on the superior aspect of the subjacent vertebral body is located another demifacet. One rib articulates with these two demifacets at the costovertebral joint (Fig. 17-9). On the anterior side of the thoracic transverse processes, a facet is present that also serves as another articulation with the rib, the costotransverse joint.

The superior articular processes arise from the junction of the lamina and pedicles. They face posteriorly and slightly laterally and thus describe a slight convex arc. The inferior articular process faces anteriorly and slightly laterally, complementing the geometry of the superior articular process. This joint plane allows for slight rotation and lateral bending of the thoracic spine, but the motion is markedly limited owing to the resistance to movement provided by the rib cage. The spinous processes of the thoracic spine are very long and typically slope downward at an angle between 40 and 60 degrees to the horizontal.

The spinal canal in the thoracic spine is smaller than that of the lumbar and cervical spine. With such a small diameter, there is very little free space between the spinal cord and the spinal canal, which renders the cord susceptible to myelopathy.

Idiopathic scoliosis, the most common spinal deformity, is most common in the thoracic spine. Three types are found: Infantile appears before age 3, juvenile between 3 and puberty, and adolescent after puberty. Growth plays a major

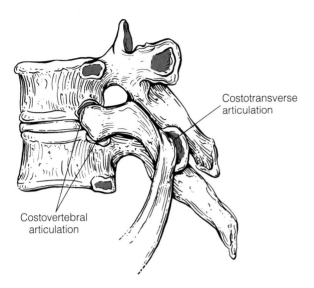

Costotransverse
articulation

Costovertebral
articulation

Fig. 17-9. Articulation of one rib with two adjacent demifacets of the thoracic spine at the costovertebral joint and the articulation of the rib with the transverse process, the costotransverse joint.

role in curve progression. Scoliotic curves tend to progress rapidly during the adolescent growth spurt, which occurs at approximately age 12 in girls and 1 or 2 years later in boys.

Curve progression can occur even after skeletal maturity.[40] The etiology of idiopathic scoliosis is most likely multifactorial rather than due to one single cause. Genetic, neuromuscular, biochemical, and central nervous system theories have been suggested as etiologic factors.

School screening has helped in the early identification of scoliosis. Students are checked using the Adams position, a forward-bent position allowing the clinician to detect the presence of a rib hump on one side in the thoracic region. The rib hump occurs because of vertebral rotation which displaces the attached ribs. A complete examination includes assessment for pelvic asymmetry, scapula height, waist asymmetry or unilateral fullness, and spine mobility. Radiographic examination allows the curve to be measured with the Cobb method (see Fig. 17-1). With this method, the cranial and caudal vertebrae are identified, and a line parallel to their end plates drawn. A perpendicular to each line is then drawn, and the angle of intersection determines the scoliotic angle.

Nonsurgical management of scoliosis consists of observation in order to assess how rapidly the curve is progressing, posture principles, trunk strengthening, flexibility, and orthotic treatment (Milwaukee brace, TSLO thoracic-lumbar-sacral orthosis, Boston brace). Operative management, which includes spinal instrumentation such as Harrington rods, is considered when curves exceed approximately 45 degrees and show evidence of curve progression; it becomes essential to consider treatment not

only for cosmesis but also because of the potential for compromise of cardiopulmonary function.

Lumbar vertebrae. The five lumbar vertebrae are characterized by the stoutness of their bony elements. The vertebral body is massive, with the width greater than the anterior-posterior diameter. The last two lumbar vertebrae are slightly wedge-shaped, with greater anterior than posterior height.

The articular processes of the lumbar spine are primarily oriented in the sagittal plane but have a distinct concave-convex arrangement (Fig. 17-10). The inferior articular process is convex and faces anteriorly and laterally. It is medial to the subjacent concave superior articular process, which faces posteriorly and medial. Such an arrangement markedly limits rotation of the lumbar spine. The superior articular processes of the lumbar spine also feature distinct mamillary processes, which serve as bony attachments for the powerful multifidus muscles of the lumbar spine.

The sacrum. The sacrum consists of five fused vertebrae forming a singular bony mass. As a result of the fusion of the sacral vertebrae, a distinct intervertebral foramen is not present. Instead, separate anterior and posterior foramina exist for the anterior and posterior divisions of the sacral nerves, respectively. The anterior divisions of the sacral nerves, exiting through the large anterior sacral foramen, are especially important because they give rise to the major components of the sciatic nerve.

An intervertebral disk is interposed between the sacrum and the fifth lumbar vertebra at the lumbosacral junction. Because of the lumbar lordosis and the kyphotic shape of the sacrum, the lumbosacral angle is formed at this junction (Fig. 17-11). The lordosis is largely due to the wedge shape of this intervertebral disk, with the anterior height of the disk often twice the height of the posterior aspect of the disk.

The superior articular processes of the first sacral vertebra, which articulate with the inferior articular processes of the fifth lumbar vertebrae, are directed posteriorly and are thus oriented in the frontal plane. They are oriented to resist an anterior displacement of the fifth lumbar vertebra on the sacrum. An increase in the lumbar lordosis or an increased anterior tilt of the pelvis results in an increased lumbosacral angle, whereas a decrease in the lumbosacral angle is a consequence of decreased lumbar lordosis or posterior tilt of the pelvis.

Because the center of gravity of the human body lies anterior to the lumbosacral joint, there is a gravitational force promoting a tendency toward anterior displacement (anterior shear) of L5 on the sacrum. It is largely resisted by the sacral articular processes. *Spondylolisthesis* refers to an anterior displacement of one vertebra upon the subjacent vertebra and is often seen at the lumbosacral articulation (Fig. 17-12). There are several causes of spondylolistheses, the most common of which are a defect in the bony region between the superior and inferior articular processes of the vertebrae

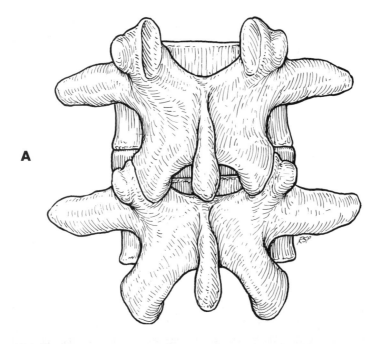

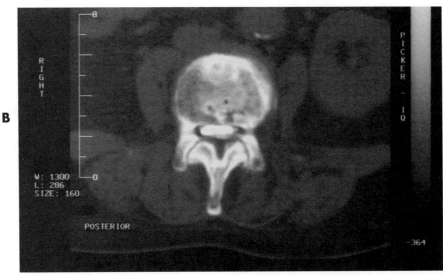

Fig. 17-10. Articulation of the lumbar spine. **A,** Posterior view showing how the inferior articular process sits medial to the superior articular process. **B,** Transverse plane view (computed tomography scan view) showing medial placement of inferior articular process and the concave/convex arrangement.

(pars interarticularis), a fracture, and an elongated pedicle. The lytic defect in the pars interarticularis is referred to as *spondylolysis.*

The laterally projecting surfaces of the sacrum (sacral alae) exhibit a roughened articular surface that meets with the ilium at the sacroiliac joint.[39] Primarily the first three fused sacral vertebrae contribute to the sacroiliac joint. Contrary to movements in other regions of the spine, motion at the sacroiliac joint is unique, owing to this specialized anatomy. Movement of the sacrum on the ilium is referred

to as *nutation* (flexion) or *counternutation* (extension). Movement of the ilium on the sacrum, however, is referred to as *torsion.* These motions are described around an imaginary horizontal axis through the sacroiliac joint. Anterior torsion occurs when the anterior superior iliac spine moves forward and down; posterior torsion occurs when the anterior superior iliac spine moves upward and back.[32]

Although the description of these motions has some clinical utility, the important biomechanical application is the attenuation of ground reaction and gravitational forces by

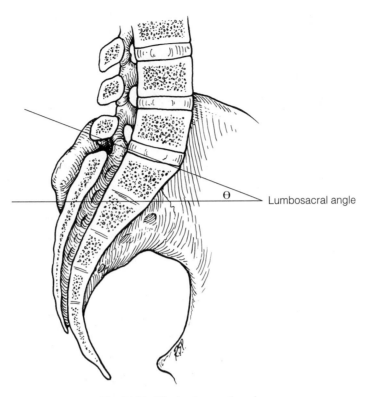

Fig. 17-11. The lumbosacral angle.

the sacroiliac articulations. The gravitational force traversing downward through the spine results in a flexion moment of the sacrum on the ilium (sacroilial moment), whereas the ground reaction force (that force traversing upward through the lower extremity as a result of the impact at initial contact during the gait cycle) results in a posterior torsional moment of the ilium on the sacrum (iliosacral moment).[17] The thick cartilaginous surface of the sacrum and the dense interosseous ligament work in combination with the sacrotuberous and sacrospinous ligaments to provide an extremely effective mechanism of force attenuation.

During pregnancy, ligamentous laxity increases as a result of hormonal changes. As the infant passes through the pelvic portion of the birth canal, great stress is placed over the sacroiliac joints, and ligamentous injury can occur during difficult deliveries. The ligamentous laxity in combination with injury can render the joint hypermobile and unable to adequately attenuate ground and trunk forces during upright activities. A sacroiliac orthosis is often used in an attempt to stabilize the joint. When the patient is in extreme discomfort, the treatment plan should include crutches to avoid weight bearing and instructions regarding avoidance of such activities as squatting, taking stairs two at a time, prolonged sitting or standing on the painful side, ballistic jumping, and sexual positions that increase shear or torsion of the sacroiliac joint.

Motion of the complete pelvis—both ilia and the intervening sacrum—is referred to as upward (posterior) or downward (anterior) *tilt*. Upward tilt of the pelvis decreases the lumbosacral angle, and downward tilt increases the angle.

On the posterior surface of the sacrum, a bony ridge appears at the region of the fused sacral apophyseal joints. This ridge terminates caudally at the sacral cornua, a region that is typically utilized to provide needle access to the spinal canal of the sacrum.

The coccyx. The coccyx is usually composed of three or four small bones bearing slight resemblance to the vertebral body but displaying no evidence of a vertebral arch. The first coccygeal vertebra is the largest and articulates with the sacrum at the sacrococcygeal junction. The coccyx serves as a bony origin for muscles of the pelvic diaphragm. Falls can result in fracture of the coccyx, which may necessitate coccyx excision for pain relief.

Ligaments

The spine is served by numerous ligaments, several of the most important of which are discussed here. Two ligaments serve to link the vertebral bodies: the anterior and posterior longitudinal ligaments. The anterior longitudinal ligament extends along the anterior surface of the spine from the region of the foramen magnum to the sacrum. It is narrow

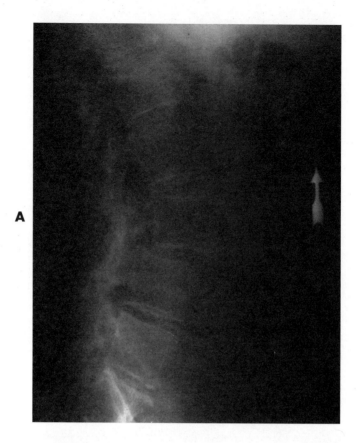

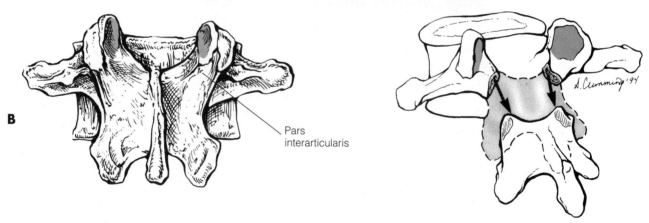

Pars
interarticularis

Fig. 17-12. A, Radiograph of spondylolisthesis. **B,** Fracture of the pars interarticularis resulting in spondylolisthesis.

in the cervical region, increases in width in the lower spinal column, and is especially wide in the lumbar region. It is strongly attached to the vertebral bodies, blending with the periosteum, and less strongly attached to the intervertebral disks.

The posterior longitudinal ligament also extends from the skull to the sacrum and is widest in the cervical region. The hourglass shape of this ligament is especially notable as it fans out over the posterior aspect of the intervertebral disk and narrows over the vertebral bodies. It is not firmly attached to the vertebral bodies but instead spans the concavity of the posterior aspect of the vertebral body. Such an arrangement permits the ingress of blood vessels to the vertebrae by allowing them to course under the posterior longitudinal ligament and into the bone. A rich venous plexus surrounds the posterior longitudinal ligament, and the ligament is also connected to the dural tissue by loose connective tissue.

Several key ligaments are related to the vertebral arch of the vertebrae. The ligamentum flavum bridges the space between adjacent laminae. These ligaments extend as far laterally as the articular pillars, at which point they

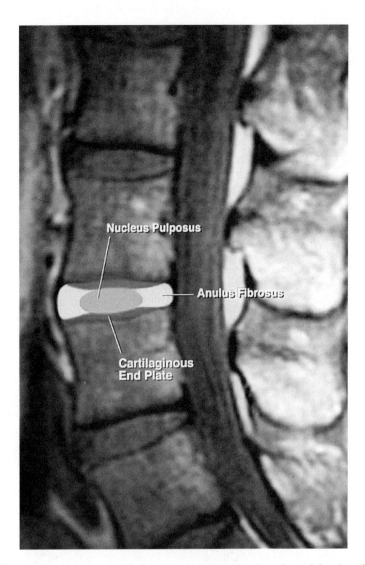

Fig. 17-13. The major components of the intervertebral disk. Note how the peripheral portions of the intervertebral disk (annulus fibrosus) have strong attachments to the vertebral body, whereas the nucleus pulposus is covered on its superior and inferior surface by the cartilaginous end plate.

contribute to the apophyseal joint capsule and medially to the midline. The ligamentum flavum is attached to the anterior surface of the upper lamina and the superior surface of the lamina below. A unique feature of this ligament is its high proportion of elastic fibers. This feature is of clinical importance as the elasticity of the ligament helps minimize the chance that the ligament will buckle into the spinal canal by infolding during extension movements of the spine.[41]

The supraspinous ligament is a continuous band that courses over the spines of the vertebrae from the seventh cervical to the upper sacral spinous processes. In the cervical region, the supraspinous ligaments are represented by the very thick and prominent ligamentum nuchae. The interspinous ligaments are fibrous tissue interposed between adjacent spinous processes; the intertransverse ligaments course between vertebral transverse processes.

Articulations of the spine

The major articulations of the spine include the vertebral body–intervertebral disk interface, the facets of opposing articular process surfaces forming apophyseal joints, the atlantoaxial articulation, the costotransverse and costovertebral articulations in the thoracic spine, the lateral surface of the sacrum and the ilium, and the pubic symphysis. Diarthrodial (true synovial) joints are primarily limited to the apophyseal, costovertebral, costotransverse, and atlantoaxial joints, and the sacroiliac joints are a combination of synovial and fibrous joints.

The intervertebral disk. The intervertebral disk helps form a fibrocartilaginous union between two opposing vertebral bodies (Fig. 17-13). Although the size of the intervertebral disks varies within the complete spinal column (i.e., the lumbar disks are significantly thicker and have a greater cross-section than the cervical intervertebral disks), the essential molecular components of the intervertebral disks are very similar throughout the spine. The intervertebral disks comprise approximately one fourth the length of the spinal column. In the cervical spine, the disks provide one fifth of the cervical spine length, one fifth of the thoracic spine length, and one third of the lumbar spine length.

An intervertebral disk is present between each pair of vertebrae, including the fifth lumbar and first sacral, but is absent between the articulations between the occiput and atlas and between the atlas and axis. From both anatomic and functional standpoints, three components of the intervertebral disk need to be recognized: the nucleus pulposus, the annulus fibrosus, and the cartilaginous end plate.

The nucleus pulposus. The nucleus pulposus occupies a central or eccentric position within the intervertebral disk and is characterized by its large water content and smaller proportions of collagen fibers and ground substance. The mucopolysaccharide content of the ground substance has a strong affinity for water, and a biochemical bonding occurs between the water molecule and the various mucopolysaccharides. Because of this affinity for water, the nucleus pulposus is often referred to as a *hydrophilic* structure. During the aging process, both the quantity and type of mucopolysaccharide changes, and as a result the nucleus pulposus decreases in its water content.[3]

The ability of the nucleus pulposus to bind chemically to the water molecule results in the development of an internal disk pressure. One can think of the nucleus pulposus as exerting a force against the vertebrae articulating with it (pushing the vertebrae apart), as well as a force against the inner walls of the annulus fibrosus that surrounds the nucleus pulposus. Thus, a major function of the nucleus pulposus is to redistribute compressive forces tangentially to the annulus fibrosus.[6]

Pathology related to this nuclear pressure includes herniation of the nuclear material through the cartilaginous end plate and into the vertebral body (Schmorl's nodes) and herniation of nuclear material against a weakened annulus fibrosus (diskal protrusion or herniation) (Fig. 17-14). The most common spinal levels for diskal protrusion or herniation are the L4 to L5 and L5 to S1 segments in the low back and the C6 to C7 segment in the neck. The water content of the young nucleus demonstrates consistent ability to rebound from compressive forces applied to it. This further demonstrates the strength of the chemical bond between water and the molecules of the ground substance.

The loose collagen fibers of the nucleus pulposus are randomly arranged, but a significant portion of fibers are oriented to attach to the thin cartilaginous end plate that covers the central region of the plateaus of the vertebral body. The most central region of the nucleus pulposus has a greater concentration of mucopolysaccharides and less fibrous matter, whereas the peripheral aspect of the nucleus is more fibrous. As noted in the next section, the annulus fibrosus is largely a fibrous structure. There is a gradual transition of increasing fibrous tissue from the most central region of the intervertebral disk toward the most peripheral aspect. Therefore there is no clear demarcation between outer nucleus pulposus and the inner annulus fibrosus.

Annulus fibrosus. The distinguishing feature of the annulus fibrosus is the presence of concentric fibrous rings with alternating fiber direction in successive lamellae (Fig. 17-15). These rings are firmly attached to the vertebral body and serve as one of the primary motion restraints between two vertebrae. The posterior lamellae are thinner than the anterior, primarily because the nucleus pulposus is positioned slightly posterior and the complete intervertebral disk is essentially kidney-shaped. The structure of the annulus fibrosus affords resistance to all motions that create forces to the spinal unit. Movements that generate compression,

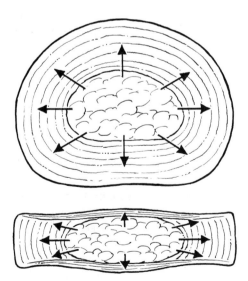

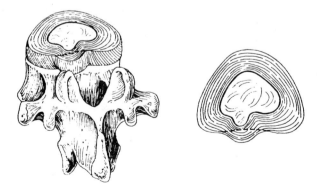

Fig. 17-14. Protrusion of nuclear material against the weakened annular wall.

Fig. 17-15. Concentric rings of the annulus and the increase in ring tension as a result of nuclear pressure.

torsion, or shear to the spinal segment result in an increase in tension to the collagenous fibers of the annulus.

Because the annulus fibrosus is essentially a collagenous structure, any force that increases tension of the annular rings offers resistance to movement of the spinal segment and enhances stability. This is one of the reasons why intradiskal pressure, generated by the nucleus pulposus against the annular rings, is so important. Such a pressure mechanism maintains tension of the annular rings, which enhances the stability between adjacent vertebrae.[6]

The intervertebral foramen. The spinal nerves exit from the intervertebral foramen and serve as the transition between the central and peripheral nervous system. In the cervical region, the spinal nerves exit above their corresponding vertebrae; that is, the C1 nerve root exits between the occiput and the first cervical vertebrae, the C2 spinal nerve exits between the C1 and C2 vertebrae, and so on. There are eight pairs of cervical spinal nerves, with the C8 spinal nerve exiting between the C7 and T1 vertebrae. In the remainder of the spine, the spinal nerve exits below its corresponding vertebra. Because the spinal cord ends at approximately the first lumbar vertebra, the lumbar and sacral nerve roots must course a great distance in order to exit from their associated intervertebral foramina. This cluster of elongated lumbosacral nerve roots that occupies the lower region of the spinal canal is the cauda equina (Fig. 17-16).

The intervertebral foramen serves as a portal for vessels and nerve branches that exit as well as enter the spinal canal to supply the bone and soft tissues. The boundaries of the intervertebral foramina are essential to understand in order to comprehend pathomechanics (see Fig. 17-16). The superior and inferior boundaries are primarily the pedicles of the vertebra, the posterior boundary the apophyseal joints, and the anterior boundary is the intervertebral disk. Thus, pathologies related to the apophyseal joints such as degenerative joint disease or diskal degeneration can profoundly affect the spinal nerve or nerve root complex in the region of the intervertebral foramen.

The nerve root complex is formed as the dorsal and ventral roots pass through the subarachnoid space and converge to form the spinal nerve (Fig. 17-17). At the region of this juncture, the small sinuvertebral nerve courses back through the intervertebral foramen to innervate structures within the spinal canal such as the dural tissue, posterior longitudinal ligament, and outer aspect of the intervertebral disk.

A significant portion of the nutrients supplying the nerve roots are derived from the cerebrospinal fluid via diffusion.[31] Nerve root health is potentially compromised with inflammatory states within the spinal canal, such as that caused by disk degeneration. The nutrient supply is adversely affected because it interferes with this diffusion mechanism. When the nerve root is thus irritated, its sensitivity to mechanical stresses such as compression or tension is increased.[22] The

intervertebral disk, in particular, nucleus pulposus material that has escaped from the confines of the annulus fibrosus, is considered to be a key inflammatory agent affecting the mechanosensitivity of the nerve roots.[24] Pain due to irritation of the nerve root is referred to as *radicular pain*. Involvement of the nerve roots in spinal conditions often results in reflex, sensory, or motor changes in the extremity innervated by that nerve root.

The vertical diameter of the intervertebral foramen is much greater than the transverse diameter. Thus, the potential for compromise of the neural structures at the region of the intervertebral foramen is greater when the positional relationship between vertebrae is altered, such as that which would occur with excessive anterior translation of one vertebra on the subjacent vertebra. Shear force resulting in translation has a greater influence on the nerve root complex and spinal nerve than axial loading.

Apophyseal joints. The apophyseal joints are true synovial joints with joint capsules and articular processes lined with hyaline cartilage forming the facet surface. These joints are innervated by branches of the posterior primary ramus (Fig. 17-18). The capsules are lax posteriorly and allow limited movement in specific planes of motion. The anterior aspect of the joint capsule is typically represented by the ligamentum flavum. Degenerative joint disease of the apophyseal joints is often accompanied by hypertrophic-ligamentum flavum because the ligamentum flavum is an integral part of the joint (Fig. 17-19).

The primary function of the apophyseal joints is to guide the movement in the various cardinal planes. The cervical spine facet surfaces are oriented to allow for flexion and extension, lateral bending, and rotation. Because of their orientation, flexion and extension motions of the cervical spine are coupled to anterior and posterior translation, respectively. Lateral flexion of the cervical spine is coupled to rotation; that is, when the cervical spine is laterally flexed to the right, there is an obligatory rotation of the same vertebral segments to the right as well (Fig. 17-20).

In the thoracic spine, the facet surfaces are oriented to allow lateral bending and rotation, but this movement is very small owing to the presence of the rib cage. In the lumbar spine, the primary movement is flexion and extension. There is a very small degree of lumbar rotation and lateral flexion at each segment in the lumbar spine, and the lumbar spine motions are not as strongly coupled as the cervical spine motions. In the lumbar spine, the lumbosacral junction and the L4 to L5 region account for approximately 25 and 20 degrees of sagittal plane motion, respectively. Fig. 17-21 depicts the segmental motion of the spinal column.

Both the intervertebral disk and the apophyseal joints bear the compressive loads of the spine. Typically, the intervertebral disk bears the greater proportion of this compressive load. However, as the disk space narrows, there is a "settling" or increased compression between the facet

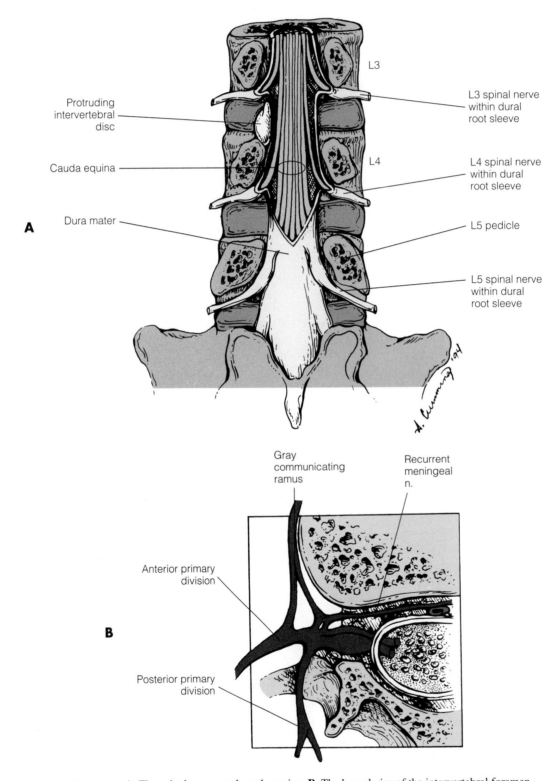

Fig. 17-16. **A,** The spinal nerves and cauda equina. **B,** The boundaries of the intervertebral foramen.

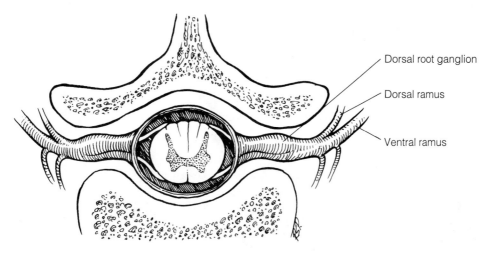

Fig. 17-17. The formation of the spinal nerve. The dorsal and ventral roots converge at the region of the intervertebral foramen to give rise to the spinal nerve. The nerve roots are bathed by the cerebrospinal fluid that occupies the subarachnoid space. A significant portion of the nutrients to the nerve root are derived from the cerebrospinal fluid.

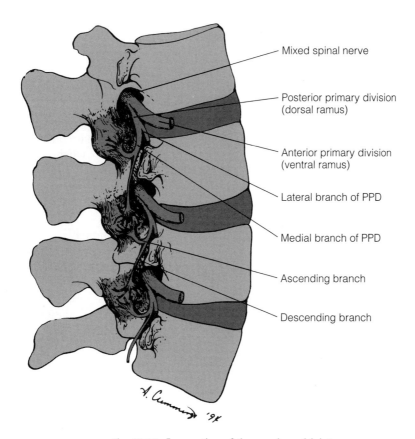

Fig. 17-18. Innervation of the apophyseal joints.

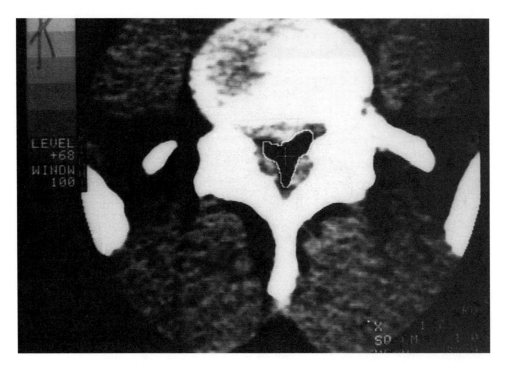

Fig. 17-19. Computerized tomography of lumbar spine showing degeneration of apophyseal joints and hypertrophic ligamentum flavum.

surfaces.[15,42] Due to this change in spine mechanics, increased stress is placed over the apophyseal joints, and the cartilaginous surface begins to erode, eventually exposing the subchondral bone.[18] Spondylosis is the age-related, degenerative changes of the apophyseal joints and the intervertebral disk; essentially, it is degenerative joint disease of the spine.

Musculature of the spine

At first appearance, the musculature of the spine appears highly complex, with uncertain functional implications. However, recent advances in the study of the anatomy of the spine have greatly clarified the role of several key muscles. This section focuses on aspects of the muscular system considered essential in the evaluation and treatment of spinal disorders.

The low back musculature

Thoracolumbar fascia. This fascial complex is considered important in the dynamic stability of the low back. Besides attaching to the transverse and spinous processes of the spine, it serves as an attachment site for several key muscles of the trunk: the latissimus dorsi, internal oblique, and transversus abdominis (Fig. 17-22).[5] In addition, the thoracolumbar fascia forms a fascial envelope and encases the erector spinae and multifidi muscles of the low back. Hypertrophy of these muscles encased in the thoracolumbar fascia potentially "fills" this fascial envelope. Thus, tension can be placed through the thoracolumbar by either the "pull" of the muscles (latissimus dorsi, internal oblique, and transversus abdominis) or a "push" of the muscles (contraction of the erector spinae and multifidi, which results in broadening of the muscles as they contract).[12,32]

Erector spinae muscles of the low back. The erector spinae muscles of the low back can be divided into a

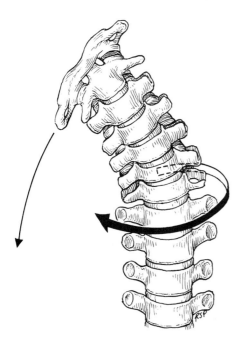

Fig. 17-20. Coupled motions of the cervical spine. Lateral flexion is coupled to rotation in the same direction.

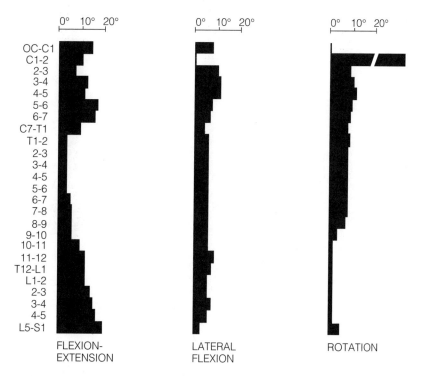

0° 10° 20°   0° 10° 20°   0° 10° 20°

OC-C1
C1-2
2-3
3-4
4-5
5-6
6-7
C7-T1
T1-2
2-3
3-4
4-5
5-6
6-7
7-8
8-9
9-10
10-11
11-12
T12-L1
L1-2
2-3
3-4
4-5
L5-S1

FLEXION-   LATERAL   ROTATION
EXTENSION   FLEXION

Fig. 17-21. Segmental motion of the spinal column in the three cardinal planes. (From White AA, Panjabi MM: *Clinical biomechanics of the spine,* ed 2, Philadelphia, 1990, JB Lippincott.)

superficial component, which can be further divided into a lateral iliocostalis portion and a medial longissimus portion, and a deep component, which can also be further divided into the same two components, iliocostalis and longissimus.[6]

The superficial erector spinae takes its origin from a broad, extensive tendon—the erector spinae aponeurosis—on the lumbar and sacral spinous processes and posterior iliac crest; it courses superiorly to attach to the ribs. Although it does not attach directly to the lumbar spine, it acts to extend it secondarily via its attachment to the posterior aspect of the thorax.

The deep erector spinae takes origin primarily from the iliac crest in a region adjacent and lateral to the posterior superior iliac spine of the pelvis. From this origin, it courses superiorly and anteriorly to attach to the lumbar transverse processes. Because the axis of motion for sagittal plane motion of the lumbar spine is located in the region of the intervertebral disk, this transverse process attachment results in a poor lever arm for extension of the lumbar spine. However, the anterior inclination of the muscle allows it to exert a posterior shear force to the lumbar vertebrae via the transverse process attachment (Fig. 17-23). This dynamic function is especially important when the anterior shear force over the lumbar spine due to the lumbar lordosis and gravitational pull is considered. Although there are several ligamentous restraints to anterior shear of the lumbar spine, the deep erector spinae muscle offers a dynamic restraining force.[32]

The multifidus muscles. Although the multifidi muscles span the complete spine, they are much more prominent and extensive in the lumbar spine. Taking their origin from the dorsal surface of the sacrum and the transverse and mamillary processes of the lumbar vertebrae, they course superiorly and medially to attach to the spinous processes. By attaching to the spinous processes, they benefit by being afforded a long lever arm for lumbar hyperextension (Fig. 17-24). The cross-sectional area of the multifidus muscle in the lumbar spine is greater than most of the low back muscles, and it is frequently the muscle seen to undergo the most severe degenerative changes with chronic low back pain.[34] Therefore, attention should be given to incorporating resistance extension exercises of the lumbar spine, which help to recondition these muscles in active rehabilitation programs for the low back pain patient.

The multifidi muscles are primarily concerned with extension of the spine. Although textbooks of anatomy refer to a function of rotation due to the "transversospinous" orientation, very little rotation is available between the lumbar vertebral segments. The multifidi muscles are covered by the erector spinae aponeurosis and the superficial layer of the thoracolumbar fascia.

Quadratus lumborum muscles. The quadratus lumborum muscles are thin, flat muscles spanning the space between the iliac crest and the last (twelfth) rib and lumbar transverse processes. The muscles are immediately deep to the deep erector spinae muscles and oriented to function in a similar manner. There is a noticeable absence of quadratus lumborum muscle fibers over the last two lumbar segments.

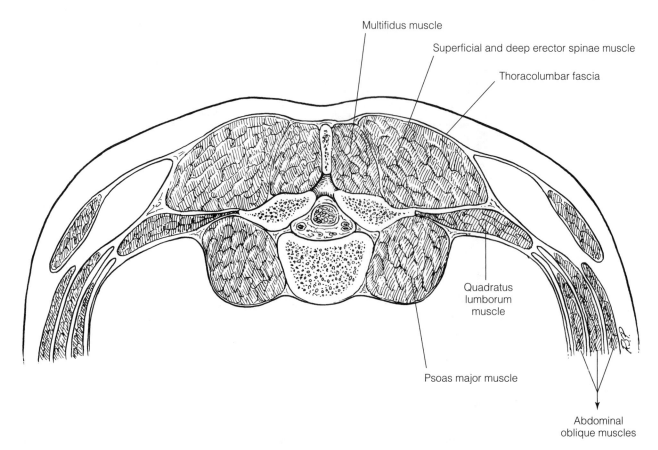

Fig. 17-22. Cross-section of the lumbar spine showing the muscular attachments to the thoracolumbar fascia.

It has been suggested that the lowest fibers of the quadratus lumborum muscle undergo metaplasia to form the broad, dense iliolumbar ligament.[20]

The iliolumbar ligament runs from the iliac crest to the fifth and often the fourth lumbar transverse process. It is so extensive that it also reinforces the anterior aspect of the sacroiliac joint. It is an extremely strong ligament and one of the primary stabilizers of the lumbosacral junction because it "squares" the fifth lumbar vertebra on the sacrum. The iliolumbar ligament and the quadratus lumborum muscle work to passively and dynamically stabilize the lumbar spine in the frontal plane.

Psoas major muscles. The psoas major muscles attach to the anterior aspect of the lumbar transverse processes, the vertebral bodies, and the intervertebral disks. From this extensive attachment, the muscle courses inferiorly, where it joins the iliacus and travels over the pubic ramus to then attach to the lesser trochanter of the femur. How movements of the lower extremity affect the lumbar spine is important to recognize. For example, internal rotation of the femur or hyperextension of the femur increases the tension within the psoas major, which, in turn, increases the anterior shear force over the lumbar spine due to the anteriorly placed psoas major attachment.

This is perhaps best illustrated in the gait of a woman during the last months of a pregnancy. Because growth of the infant in the uterus has resulted in the center of gravity of the body assuming a new position markedly anterior to the lumbar spine, there is a significantly increased anterior shear force to the lower lumbar spine. In order to avoid an even greater anterior shear of the lumbar spine, the pregnant female often maintains a toe-out, externally rotated hip gait pattern. By placing the hips in external rotation, the psoas major has less passive tension to it and thus does not exert an anterior shear force to the lumbar spine.

An overlooked aspect of psoas major function is the compressive force it exerts between two vertebral segments when it contracts. Compression by muscle contraction increases the stability of the lumbar segments for two primary reasons:

1. It further engages the lumbar joints, which helps to provide more of a locking mechanism between the two vertebrae.
2. It increases intradiskal pressure, an extremely important means to increase stability because it causes the nucleus pulposus to exert force against the inner aspect of the annulus fibrosus in a direction tangential to the

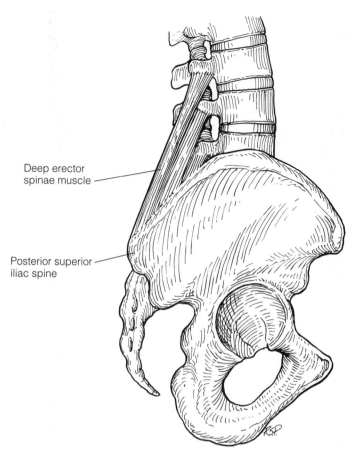

Deep erector
spinae muscle

Posterior superior
iliac spine

Fig. 17-23. Sagittal view of deep erector spinae that illustrates the potential for dynamic posterior shear force.

compressive force, that is, laterally against the annular walls. This internal pressure increases the tension of the connective tissue in the annular walls, which results in an increased stiffness of the annular rings. With such increased stiffness, the annulus is better able to stabilize the vertebral segments.

The importance of the psoas major in its role as a major stabilizer of the lumbar spine is evident from the fact that the muscle is electromyographically active in nearly all postures and movements of the lumbar spine.[28]

The abdominal muscles. The length, strength, endurance, and coordination of the abdominal muscles are extremely important in overall function of the low back. There are four important abdominal muscles to consider. The rectus abdominis is primarily a flexor of the lumbar spine, and it also causes an upward-tilting motion of the pelvis. The external oblique runs in an anterior-inferior direction and assists with flexion of the spine as well as rotation. The internal oblique fibers are nearly perpendicular to the external oblique and are primarily seen in the posterior and lateral aspects of the abdominal wall. The transversus abdominis is the deepest muscle and runs like a horizontal

girdle from its attachments to the thoracolumbar fascia. There is a dense fascial arrangement anteriorly—the rectus sheath—into which the oblique muscles blend and the rectus muscles are encased.

Several functions have been ascribed to these important muscles.[2,30,36] From a functional viewpoint, the abdominal muscles serve to support the abdominal and pelvic viscera by lifting and pushing the abdominal contents up and against the lumbar spine. As a result, the anterior shear force of the lumbar spine that is due to the lumbar lordosis is partially held in check.

The abdominal muscles also provide the muscular framework for the anterior and lateral walls of a trunk "cylinder," with the posterior wall of the cylinder being formed by the spinal extensors, the superior roof by the diaphragm, and the inferior floor by the pelvic diaphragm. When preparing for a heavy lift, or exerting a Valsalva maneuver, the cylinder allows the abdominal cavity to be momentarily "pressurized" and thus keeps the spine relatively rigid (Fig. 17-25).

The abdominal muscles also play a key role in controlling the forward head and neck posture so often seen in patients with upper quarter problems. With a weakened abdominal

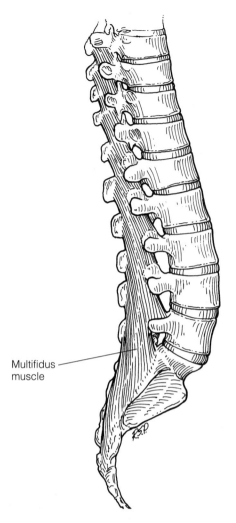

Multifidus
muscle

Fig. 17-24. Sagittal view of the multifidus muscle that illustrates the lever arm for extension/hyperextension of the lumbar spine. The multifidus muscle of the low back has nearly the same mechanical function as the semispinalis capitis muscle of the cervical spine; they are the primary extensors of the lumbar and cervical spine, respectively.

wall, the diaphragm is no longer pushed up by the supported abdominal contents. The chest wall descends inferiorly, the scapulae protract around the collapsed chest, and the humerus assumes an internally rotated posture. Training of the abdominal muscles helps place the thorax, abdomen, and pelvis in proper relationship and thus minimizes abnormal stresses placed upon otherwise normal tissues.[33]

The upper back and neck musculature

Trapezius muscle. This broad flat muscle has attachments extending from the occiput down to the last thoracic spinous process and, laterally, to the spine of the scapula, acromion, and lateral aspect of the clavicle. Over the cervicothoracic junction, it is usually very tendinous instead of muscular.[33] It has multiple actions over the scapulothoracic articulation as well as the occiput.

Of special clinical note for evaluating upper back and neck pain is the relationship that the trapezius muscle has with the deep neck flexors, the longus colli and longus capitis. For the upper trapezius to elevate the shoulder girdle, it must pull from a fixed point of origin, namely, the occiput. Stabilization of the occiput occurs via contraction by the longus capitis muscles. If there is injury to these deep neck flexors, as typically occurs during whiplash injuries to the neck, contraction of the anterior neck flexors is difficult and painful. Consequently, the occiput and cervical spine cannot be adequately stabilized to allow the trapezius to smoothly and effectively work over the scapulothoracic articulation.

Splenius capitis. The splenius capitis is also a broad, flat muscle coursing from the spinous process of the upper back and neck to the transverse processes of the cervical vertebrae and the mastoid process of the occiput. Acting unopposed, its orientation allows it to position the head and neck in the combined position of extension and ipsilateral rotation.

The mastoid process attachment is especially clinically significant. It is a large bony prominence into which three powerful neck muscles insert: the splenius capitis, longissimus capitis, and sternocleidomastoid. The orientation of these muscles allows them to serve as stabilizers or movers of the occiput and neck in all three cardinal planes. With injury to the neck, the mastoid process is often extremely tender to palpation, in part because all three of these muscles increase their state of activation in order to provide the muscle guarding that occurs after injury or painful conditions of the cervical spine.

Semispinalis capitis and cervicis. The semispinalis muscle groups are extremely important muscles of the cervical spine. They are fusiform in shape and present as the large, rounded muscle masses just lateral to the cervical spinous processes. Although many of the other cervical muscles are flat, these muscles are much more prominent owing to their impressive cross-sectional areas.

Like the multifidi muscles of the lumbar spine, these muscles have an optimal lever arm for neck extension (see Fig. 17-24). By attaching to the occiput and the cervical spinous processes, the attachments are at a distance from the center of rotation for cervical spine motions and therefore can exert a powerful extension moment. These muscles are the primary ones responsible for dynamic maintenance of the cervical lordosis. The semispinalis capitis and cervicis muscles are perhaps the most important extensor muscles of the occiput and cervical spine because their muscle fibers are oriented to generate a line of force that results in nearly pure extension of the cervical spine and the occiput.[29]

Suboccipital muscles. The suboccipital muscles are concerned with the motor control of the occiput, atlas, and axis. They are important because they allow for motion of the occiput, atlas, and axis, independent of motion of the rest of the cervical spine. This adaptation of the cervical spine is important because it allows the upper cervical spine to move independently of the rest of the cervical spine and optimally

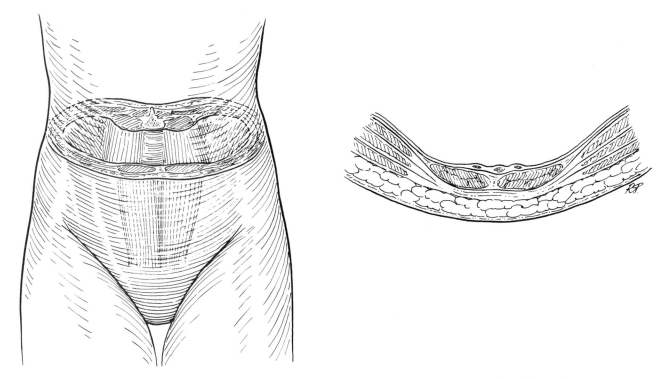

Fig. 17-25. The abdominal wall serves an important dynamic role as the muscular walls of the trunk cylinder. In addition to maintaining pelvic position and helping to control the distribution of compressive force in the bone-disk interface in the lumbar spine, it also works in maintaining the postural relationships between the thorax and abdomen, helping to counter the rounded-shoulder, forward-head posture.

positions the sense organs of vision, hearing, and equilibrium.

There are four suboccipital muscles: the superior oblique, inferior oblique, rectus capitis posterior major, and rectus capitis posterior minor (Fig. 17-26). All except the rectus capitis posterior major, which travels from the second cervical spinous process to the occiput, span one segment.

The inferior oblique muscle is especially important because it is responsible for rotation of the atlas on the axis. It courses from the spinous process of the axis to the transverse process of the atlas. Contraction of the inferior oblique causes the atlas to pivot around the dens of the axis. The superior oblique muscle travels from the transverse process of the atlas to the occiput and helps extend the occiput. The rectus capitis posterior minor travels from the spinous process of the atlas to the occiput and also assists with occipital extension. All four of these muscles form the suboccipital triangle in which the vertebral artery is located.

The suboccipital muscles are important in that they are often involved in cervical spine syndromes occurring as a result of forward head postures. In the forward head posture, the head is positioned well ahead of the shoulder girdle. In order to keep the eyes looking forward, the patient must keep the occiput tilted back into extension. This position is maintained by contraction of the suboccipital muscles. The suboccipital region is often tender to palpation and a source of head and neck discomfort in patients with prolonged forward head positioning, such as occurs with reading and computer work.

Levator scapulae. The levator scapulae muscles take their origin from the superomedial corner of the scapula and course superiorly, medially, and anteriorly to attach to the transverse processes of the upper cervical vertebrae. The anterior inclination toward their point of insertion is very similar to the anterior inclination of the deep erector spinae of the lumbar spine. Thus, contraction of the levator scapulae not only results in elevation of the scapula over the scapulothoracic articulation or lateral bending of the cervical spine but also a posterior shear force to the cervical spine.

Very often, patients with cervical pain are tender to palpation over the superomedial border of the scapula. This focal point of tenderness may be the result of prolonged and continuous muscle contraction of the levator scapulae as they work to minimize the anterior shear force in order to counter the anterior shear of the cervical lordosis.[33]

Sternocleidomastoid muscles. The sternocleidomastoid muscles are long strap muscles placed on the anterior and lateral aspects of the cervical spine. They are extremely important clinically, as they are often injured with resultant hemorrhages during acceleration injuries in which the head and neck are forced into rapid and excessive hyperextension.[21]

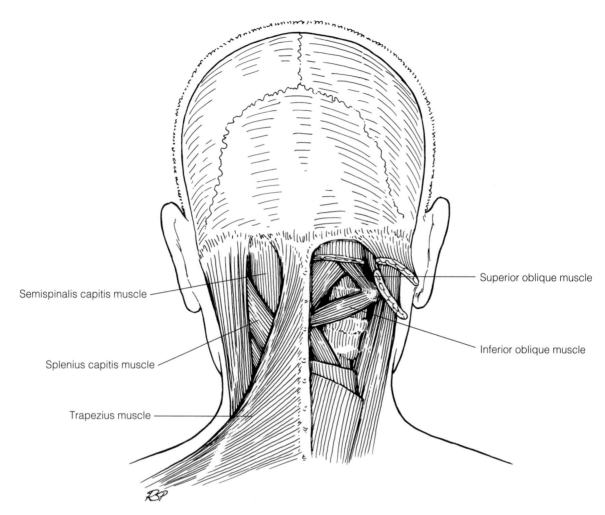

Semispinalis capitis muscle

Splenius capitis muscle

Trapezius muscle

Superior oblique muscle

Inferior oblique muscle

Fig. 17-26. The suboccipital muscles.

Congenital torticollis is a condition usually discovered during the first 3 months of life. It is caused by contracture of the sternocleidomastoid muscle, which leaves the head and neck tilted toward the involved side with the head rotated contralaterally. This muscular torticollis is thought to be due to local compression of the soft tissues of the neck during delivery, especially with breech or difficult deliveries.[19]

The scalene muscles. There are three scalene muscles: the anterior, middle, and posterior. All of the scalene muscles attach to the anterior and lateral aspects of the cervical transverse processes and then course inferiorly, with the anterior and middle scalenes attaching to the first rib and the posterior scalene attaching to the second rib. The scalene muscles are important to consider in forward head and neck postures. Such prolonged postures put these muscles in a shortened position and invite adaptive changes to the muscle tissue.

The anterior and middle scalene muscles are separated by the neurovascular bundle of the brachial plexus and

subclavian artery (Fig. 17-27). The scalene anterior is thought to occasionally encroach upon this neurovascular bundle and give rise to vascular and neurologic symptoms in the upper extremity, one of several causes of thoracic outlet syndrome. In some cases, the anterior scalene must be surgically resected to minimize this encroachment. Prolonged forward head posturing shortens the scalene musculature and decreases the space between the first rib and clavicle, which is also often associated with signs and symptoms of thoracic outlet syndrome.

EVALUATION OF THE SPINE

A thorough evaluation is the essential first step to establish the treatment process in the management of the patient with spine pain. The evaluation provides both the clinician and the patient with information that not only can be used to establish short- and long-term treatment goals but also can be used in the establishing the self-management strategies necessary for successful outcomes. The patient must become part of the treatment process and take an active

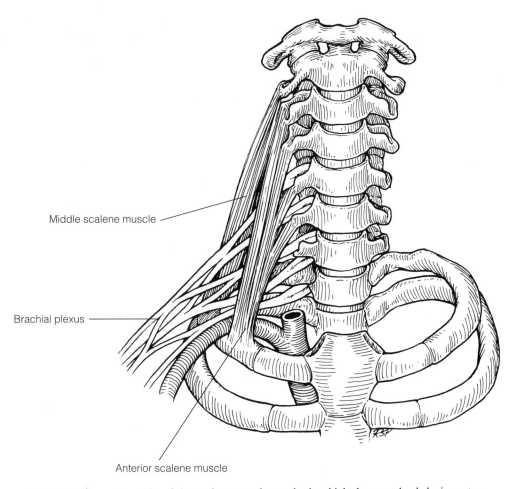

Middle scalene muscle

Brachial plexus

Anterior scalene muscle

Fig. 17-27. The relationship of the scalene muscles to the brachial plexus and subclavian artery.

role in self-management, which can take place only if the results of the examination are clearly and effectively communicated.

In most activity-related low back disorders, the precise anatomic structure cannot be identified. In some cases, irritation of the nerve root complex is identifiable because the patient presents with leg pain greater than back pain, arm pain greater than neck pain, reflex changes of musculature related to the extremity, sensory deficits, or motor weakness and atrophy. In such cases, the nerve root complex as the source of pain is highly probable. Unfortunately, most activity-related spinal pain does not present with such signs and symptoms. This lack of clarity invites speculation, often based on examiner bias, as to the anatomic lesion causing the pain. Many patients receive several different "diagnoses" based on such examiner bias, which leads the patient to develop fear that the injury is more severe than originally thought.[9]

Unfortunately, the uncertainty of diagnosis leads to a multiplicity of treatment efforts that have questionable

---

Diagnostic categories from the Quebec Task Force Report

1. Localized spinal pain
2. Pain radiating to extremity proximally
3. Pain radiating to extremity distally
4. Pain radiating to extremity + neurological signs
5. Radicular compression presumed
6. Radicular compression confirmed
7. Spinal stenosis confirmed
8. Post surgery <6 months
9. Post surgery >6 months
10. Chronic pain syndrome
11. Other

From Nachemson A et al: *Spine* 12 (suppl): 59, 1987.

value. To assist with such a dilemma, the Quebec Task Force suggested meaningful diagnostic categories that have the potential to be reliable between examiners (see Box).[28] This diagnostic scheme can be adapted to facilitate a working

Table 17-1. Physical therapy working assessment classifications for activity-related spine pain

Working assessment: low back pain	Working assessment: neck pain
Low back pain without radiation	Neck pain without radiation
Low back pain with proximal referral	Neck pain with proximal referral
Low back pain with distal referral	Neck pain with distal referral
Leg pain greater than back pain	Arm pain greater than neck pain
Leg pain greater than back pain with neurologic signs	Arm pain greater than neck pain with neurologic signs
Postsurgery less than 6 months	Postsurgery less than 6 months
Postsurgery greater than 6 months	Postsurgery greater than 6 months
Chronic pain syndrome	Chronic pain syndrome

Modified from Quebec Task Force recommendations; Nachemson A et al: *Spine* 12(suppl):59, 1987.

assessment for patients with activity-related spinal pain seen in the physical therapy clinic, as suggested in Table 17-1.

Last, many prospective and retrospective studies have confirmed that psychosocial factors inside and outside the patient significantly influence the evaluation process and treatment results.[8] Workplace factors are also important to consider during the evaluation process. Factors such as workers' perception of the workplace, their jobs, their relationship with their supervisors, and their interactions with their workers play a major role in their perception of the problem and response to injury. In some instances, the influence of psychosocial factors outweighs the pathomechanics of injury.[4]

Clinical evaluation

The essentials of the evaluation of the spine include a problem-oriented history, an understanding of the patient's perception of the problem and how it alters work or activities of daily living (ADL) status, a physical examination that analyzes the response of the patient to specific stresses of the spinal structures, a neurologic screen, and special questions or tests that may alert the examiner that further referral or diagnostic testing is indicated.

History. A carefully taken history should include the patient's primary complaint, a discussion of this complaint, and a past history of any general orthopedic or medical conditions and past spine problems. When reviewing the present complaint with the patient, a discussion of how the present complaint started, its effect on activity, and how its pattern is affected with activity is important.

The most common complaint in spine problems is pain, and it is important to localize the pain, determine its onset and pattern since the onset, and ascertain what makes the pain worse. It is extremely important to ascertain whether the pain pattern being described resembles radicular or referred pain. Radicular pain, or nerve root irritation, is characterized by pain in the leg being more intolerable than pain in the back or by pain in the arm being much more disconcerting than pain in the neck. This extremity pain is often described as deep, piercing, and intolerable, with burning intensity that is highly unpleasant

and over a clearly demarcated dermatomal distribution (Fig. 17-28).

Referred pain is the perception of discomfort felt distally due to irritation of injured spinal tissues. Any tissue of the spine—muscle, joints, ligaments, intervertebral disk—can refer pain distally when injured. As the injured spinal tissue becomes less irritated, the referral pattern tends to be more centralized with less distal referral. For example, a complaint of right-sided low back pain that occasionally spreads into the right buttock and even less often into the midthigh is most likely referred pain from tissues in the lower lumbar or pelvic region. A general rule of thumb is that, with referred pain, the spine discomfort is the primary complaint, whereas in the radicular pain pattern, the primary complaint is the extremity.

The clinician should also attempt to gain an understanding of the pain by the descriptors the patient uses. Patients should use their own words to describe the type and intensity of pain. A pain rating scale and body chart provide objective data for comparison at a later date (Fig. 17-29). The goal of this history is to make the patient aware of the pain pattern.

The chronologic development of spinal pain provides valuable information in helping to determine activity-related spinal pain from other types of pain. Such information alerts the examiner as to whether the complaint is due to an acute injury or to an exacerbation of a previous injury. A graph depicting intensity versus time can be used to record the history.[32,33] This graph can serve as a valuable tool to analyze changes in the frequency, intensity, or duration of pain at a later date.

Pain worse with movement or brought on following lifting, twisting, or prolonged postures should be distinguished from spine pain with a more insidious onset, especially pain that is not made worse with activity. Such pain descriptions should alert the examiner to further investigate or seek another referral to rule out medical causes of spinal pain, such as tumor or infection. Sample questions for the history are provided in the Box. Note carefully that patients are asked to rate their activity, pain, and stress on a scale and that they are also asked for *their* goals for treatment.

Physical examination: functional assessment. The

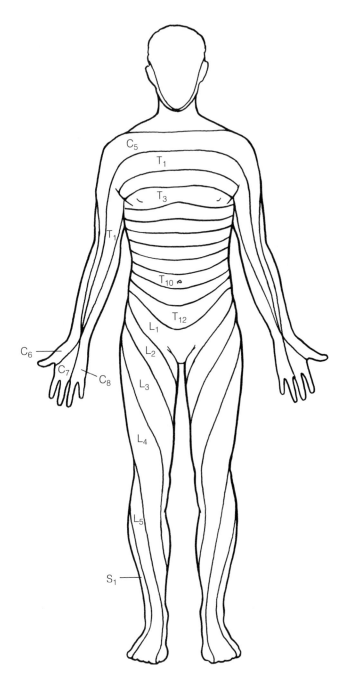

Fig. 17-28. Dermatomes of the upper extremity and lower extremity. Radicular pain tends to follow more clearly defined dermatomal patterns, while referred pain into the extremity is more diffuse.

goal of functional assessment of the spine is to determine those stresses that reproduce familiar pain. Through a series of active patient movements and with the application of passive movements and overpressures by the examiner, an attempt is made to reproduce familiar pain. The examiner asks the patient whether the maneuver "reproduces the familiar pain," not "does this cause pain?" Stresses such as shear, compression, and tension are introduced into the spine in a controlled and sequential manner in order to determine the patient's response to such stresses.

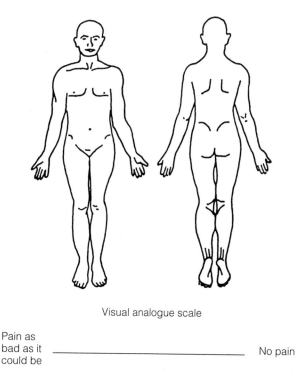

Visual analogue scale

| Pain as bad as it could be | _____ | No pain |

Fig. 17-29. Body chart and pain rating scale for spinal pain.

In general, the antigravity positions (standing for the low back patient; sitting or standing for the upper back and neck patient) are the positions in which to start the functional assessment. From these antigravity positions, pain should first be elicited and the stresses that reproduce the painful response analyzed. The patient is subsequently placed in a gravity-eliminated position (supine, prone, sidelying) to substantiate the results that were found in the antigravity postures. With a comprehensive understanding of the three-dimensional anatomy of the spine, the examiner can visualize how similar stresses (compression, tension, or shear) reach the spine regardless of the position. By starting with the antigravity posture, the examiner is able to begin analyzing the posture that is typically the most difficult to tolerate for activity-related spine problem.

The examiner should continually inform the patient of the test procedures being used. The application of stresses should be careful and precise. The point in the range of motion, the position of the spine, and the position of the extremities should all be noted when familiar pain is reproduced. The information gained from this part of the examination is critical because it forms the foundation for self-management strategies given to the patient concerning positions of rest, activity modification, movements, and positions that might exacerbate the problem. The greater the understanding patients have in this regard, the better chance they have of becoming part of the treatment process. Utilizing information from the examination in this way and applying it to treatment are the basis for biomechanical counseling, one of the four primary treatment objectives.

The Box outlines the low back evaluation. It is organized to avoid excessive turning and position changes of the patient. This allows the examiner to proceed expeditiously with the examination, yet carry out a movement assessment as well as a neurologic screen. The examination sequence chosen by the examiner should be consistent from patient to patient. A systematic examination assures comprehensiveness of the exam, and, more important, a consistent and standardized approach allows an examiner to make comparisons between patients. The box should be studied carefully to note the application of forces to the lumbar spine and sacroiliac joint and the assessment of the hip, which

---

Questions for patient history

Questions: Low back pain/neck pain

How old are you?/What is your occupation?

> Women: Are you working outside the home? Do you have any children? If yes, how old? Have you had any surgeries? Cesarean sections?
>
> Men: Have you had any surgeries?

How long have you had back/neck pain?

What position were you in when you were initially hurt?

Show me where you have pain. Do you ever have pain or numbness or tingling into your thighs or legs/arm or hand?

Describe previous episodes of back pain/neck pain and how long these episodes have lasted.

What positions or activities increase your pain? What activities are limited by this problem?

How would you rate your level of activity?

How would you rate your level of pain?

How would you rate your level of stress? Is there a relationship between your level of stress and level of pain?

Is your pain worse in the morning upon awakening or is it worse toward the end of the day? Are you stiffer or sorer in the morning as compared to the end of the day?

Are you currently taking any medications for your pain?

What do you think is the cause of your back pain/neck pain?

What would be your goals as a result of treatment?

Special questions related to low back pain

Have you had any recent weight loss?

Are you experiencing any bowel or bladder disturbances? Numbness in this area?

Does your pain prevent you from sleeping? Is it worse at night?

Special questions related to neck pain

Have you any associated dizzy spells?

Do you regularly experience headaches along with your neck pain?

Do you experience pain or numbness in or about your face?

Does your pain prevent you from sleeping? Is it worse at night?

Do you have tingling in your hands or feet, or any gait disturbance?

---

plays a key role in the attenuation of ground forces through the pelvis and lumbar spine. Note especially how the examiner must carefully separate hip ROM from sacroiliac stresses and lumbar stresses.

Several aspects of the low back examination should be mentioned. In the standing assessment, an asymmetry of posture as viewed in the frontal plane should be carefully ascertained by looking at the patient's waist angle and the pelvic bony prominences. A frontal plane asymmetry leads to increased compressive loading of the lumbar apophyseal joints, increased shear stress at the sacroiliac joint, and increased compressive loading of the femoral head on the long leg side of the asymmetry (Fig. 17-30).[13,32] Often, correction with a heel lift, which subtly changes the distribution of the weight line through the lumbopelvic region, helps unload injured tissue.

The application of compressive load in the extension quadrants during the standing exam is also an important test. Most patients, when asked to bend backward, simply extend at the hip joints, and the ability of the lumbar spine to accept loads in extension is not assessed. As can be seen in Fig. 17-31, the examiner retracts the patient's shoulders and then applies a downward compressive force to the lumbar spine through the shoulders. The examiner can then assess tolerance to loading by gradually moving the patient throughout the extension quadrants. The response to extension and shear is also assessed through posterior-anterior stresses to the lumbar spine from the prone position. These stresses, as well as any other passive intervertebral stresses, can also be used as treatment techniques. By varying the excursion and points in the range of motion at which the stress is applied, a grading scheme for classifying such passive intervertebral stresses can then be used to document the technique applied.[23]

Assessing the range of motion of the hip is extremely important. If the hip is tight in the Fabers position and is limited in hyperextension, an assumption can be made that the patient has minimal hip hyperextension available for pushoff during the gait cycle. Instead, the lower extremity is placed behind the body at this point of the gait cycle by extending and rotating the pelvis and lumbar spine, which increases the compressive load to the apophyseal joint support structures. Patients with pain due to inability to tolerate compressive loads to the lumbar apophyseal joints frequently need to bend forward and rest with their hands on their thighs, especially after walking short distances. Their posture is also seen as "tucking the buttocks under the spine" (posterior tilting the pelvis). Both of these maneuvers are attempts by the patient to maintain a flexed lumbar spine, thereby unloading the compressive force to the painful posterior joint structures (Fig. 17-32).

The Box outlines the cervicothoracic evaluation. The evaluation begins with an assessment of shoulder girdle function because the forward head posture is often accompanied by excessive protraction of the scapulae, an internally

Examination of the lumbosacral spine

A. Standing evaluation
  1. Posture analysis: note at least two postural "planes":
    a. Sagittal plane: envision the weightline (postural line) traversing the lumbosacral tissues. Consider that in the standing, upright posture, weight is borne 85% by the bone-disk-bone interface, and 15% by the apophyseal joints. Note how the degree of lumbar flexion or extension or pelvic tilt potentially alters this.
    b. Frontal plane: envision the weightline, and note the closed-pack position on one side (compression) and tensile stress on the opposite side with frontal plane assymetry. Note the compression and shear at the sacroiliac joint. Note the relative abduction or adduction at the hip joints. Is there a list?
    c. Palpation points for visualizing pelvic base:
      i. Waist angle
      ii. ASIS
      iii. Iliac crest
      iv. PSIS
      v. Greater trochanter
    d. With these postural points assessed, complete the skeletal exam with analysis of foot and ankle, knee, and upper quarter with the ultimate goal of determining if these might play a factor in the mechanical disorder of the low back.
B. Gross movement testing: standing position
  1. Forward bending
  2. Backward bending
  3. Forward and backward quadrant testing: various combinations of three planes of movement.
  4. Application of overpressure: stabilize the pelvis and sacral base to apply tensile forces in forward-bending combinations. Using the extension quadrant, direct the line of force to load tissues posteriorly in backward-bending combinations.
  5. Standing neuro screen: walk on toes (S1-S2), walk on heels (L4).
  6. Seated neuro screen: gastroc-soleus reflex (S1-S2)
    a. Quadriceps reflex (L3-L4)
    b. Posterior tibialis reflex (L5)
    c. Extensor hallucis longus manual muscle test (L5)
    d. Anterior tibialis manual muscle test (L4)
    e. Peroneals manual muscle test (S1-S2)
    f. Sensory assessment (dermatomes of lower extremity)
C. Supine lying exam
  1. Hip ROM: note when the movement ceases to be iliofemoral and becomes iliosacral accommodation and then lumbar flexion.
  2. Figure 4 (Faber test): note when this tests hip ROM, then becomes a gapping stress to the sacroiliac joint, and then initiates rotation of pelvis on lumbar spine.
  3. Straight leg raise (SLR): add femoral adduction and internal rotation to further increase stretch to sciatic nerve and associated nerve roots.
  4. Stresses to the sacroiliac joint:
    a. With long axis of femur aligned with plane of sacroiliac joint, a shear stress is imparted to sacroiliac joint via femur.
    b. "Gapping" of posterior aspect of sacroiliac joint by placing femur in slight adduction, pushing down through long axis of femur, and, while maintaining this slight compression, slightly adduct femur.
  5. Although not a routine part of every low back exam, the pubic tubercles can be palpated for tenderness, which often accompanies true sacroiliac problems.
D. Prone lying exam
  1. Passive knee flexion: note if tightness of the rectus femoris causes anterior tilt of pelvis during knee flexion.
  2. Passive femoral extension: first stabilize ilium to assess true hip hyperextension. With slack taken up in hyperextension, continue to pull the femur toward hyperextension to begin to allow the test to impart an anterior torsional stress of ilium on sacrum, and then an extension stress of the pelvis to the lumbar spine.
  3. Sacroiliac stresses: posterior to anterior directed force centrally over sacrum and over the sacral sulcus. If the sacroiliac joint is suspect, the sacrum can be stabilized and ilium pulled "upward" (sheared posteriorly) on sacrum by the examiner.
  4. Posterior-anterior (P-A) stress over lumbar spine: this is a powerful compression stress to the lumbar support joints as well as a shear stress to the bone-disk interface and apophyseal joints. Patient can also prop up in extension (support on elbows) and P-A pressures can again be applied.
  5. Posterior-anterior stresses over paraspinal area: this is a rotary force that increases the compression on the same side to the unilateral to the apophyseal joint structures.
  6. Complete neuro screen: quadriceps muscle test, hamstring muscle test, gluteus maximus set.
E. Palpation from prone
  1. Tissues above the iliac crest up to the last rib
  2. Tissues below the iliac crest
  3. Supraspinous ligament
F. Sidelying exam: lumbar stresses can be done to assess response to flexion and extension, side bending, or rotation.

rotated humerus, and a decreased ability to elevate the arm over the head. Careful active and passive testing of the range of motion and ability of the tissues of the cervical spine and upper thoracic region to tolerate compression, tension, and shear are key components of the exam. These same stresses can be applied in the supine position as well, and the neck is then palpated from a supine and/or prone to determine areas of muscle guarding and tenderness, potential apophyseal joint irritation by palpating the articular pillars, and muscle attachment sites at key bony prominences. This

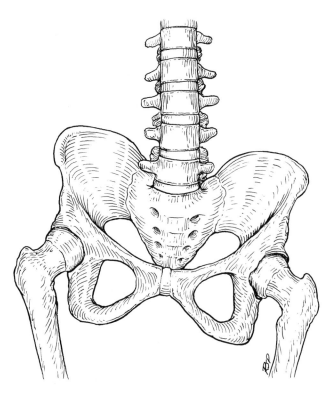

Fig. 17-30. Frontal plane asymmetry. This posture results in increased compressive loading to the apophyseal joint, increased shear of the sacroiliac joint, and increased compression of the hip on the long leg side.

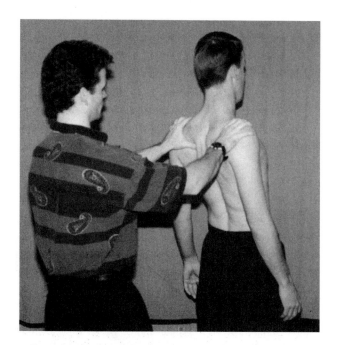

Fig. 17-31. Application of extension-loading stress to the spine from the standing position. The examiner must retract the shoulders to direct the force into the lumbar spine.

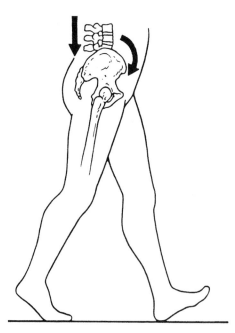

Fig. 17-32. A tight hip joint results in increasing the compression of the apophyseal joint structures during pushoff phase of gait. Because the hip cannot move into hyperextension, the pelvis and lumbar spine are extended and rotated, excessively loading the lumbar joints.

evaluation sequence also allows the upper cervical spine (occiput, atlas, and axis) to be differentiated from the lower cervical spine.

Several key points should be briefly mentioned regarding the evaluation of the neck. Again, the examiner must direct a compressive stress to the cervical spine in the extension quadrants to determine how easily and where this stress reproduces familiar pain. In addition, the overpressure to the cervical spine must be carefully applied, with the shoulders and thoracic spine stabilized, so that a true rotary force with overpressure is localized to the cervical spine. Care must be taken to apply the overpressure through the occiput rather than the mandible, which stresses the temporomandibular joint (Fig. 17-33).

Neural tension testing assesses the ability of the cervical nerve root complex to tolerate tensile stresses via maneuvers that stress peripheral nerves of the brachial plexus.[7,11] Fig. 17-34 shows positioning of the upper extremity utilizing a median nerve bias.

Palpation of the cervical spine is an extremely important part of the examination. The mastoid process, occipital line, and superior medial corner of the scapula are important points to palpate because of their muscle attachments. Muscle irritability and contractile state are also important to ascertain with palpation. Cervical spine injuries are often accompanied by prolonged and excessive muscle guarding, which leads to symptoms of muscle irritation with or without

Examination of the cervicothoracic spine

A. Inspection
   1. Head and neck posture. Key that forward head posture is present is "vertical" Sternocleidomastoid muscle.
   2. Angle of head on neck, and angle neck makes with cervicothoracic junction.
   3. Spasm, hypertrophy, or any contour change.
   4. Cervical list, position of upper quarter.
   5. Activity of facial muscles or muscles of mastication.
   6. Overall pelvic base.
B. Active ROM of shoulder girdle, overpressure applied at end ROM by examiner.
C. Seated examination: active movements give an idea of range but also willingness to move. Why is there a limit to movement? Pain, muscle spasm, stiffness, etc. Capsular pattern for the neck: Flexion is usually full range and painful while extension is limited; rotation and side bending are equally limited.
   1. Upper cervical spine
      a. Flexion and extension of occiput on atlas (nodding).
      b. Rotation of A-A: maintain cervical side bending to one direction (this locks lower cervical spine), and have the patient rotate opposite way ("Turn and look up to my finger").
   2. Lower cervical spine and cervicothoracic junction.
      a. Flexion.
      b. Extension.
      c. Rotation.
      d. Lateral bending.
      e. Quadrants: move in and out of the plane to examine rotary and lateral flexion movements in varying positions of flexion and extension.
      f. Application of overpressure to active movements by examiner. When applying overpressure, recognize if stretching or compression force is being imparted. Spurling test is extension-sidebending-rotation quadrant with compressive pressure through top of occiput to assess neuroforaminal encroachment.
   3. Thoracic spine.
      a. Flexion: "slump sit."
      b. Extension: raise arms overhead.

   c. Deep inspiration/expiration to assess potential irritation at costovertebral junctions.
   4. Neurologic screen
      a. Reflexes
         i. Biceps—C5.
         ii. Brachioradialis—C6.
         iii. Triceps—C7.
      b. Myotomes
         i. Deltoid, biceps—C5.
         ii. Biceps, wrist extensors—C6.
         iii. Triceps, wrist extensor—C7.
         iv. Extensor pollicis longus, finger flexors—C8.
         v. Interossei, abductor digit minimi—T1.
      c. Dermatomes
         i. Lateral brachium—C5.
         ii. Lateral antebrachium, thumb, first finger—C6.
         iii. Middle finger—C7.
         iv. Little finger, medial antebrachium—C8.
         v. Medial arm—T1.
      d. Neural tension testing.
         i. Thoracic outlet tests.
         ii. Median nerve bias neural tension test.
         iii. Ulnar nerve bias neural tension test.
         iv. Neck flexion or slump sit to assess dura.
D. Supine lying examination.
   1. Palpation of paracervical soft tissues, bony elements of occiput, spinous processes, and articular pillars.
   2. Active ROM.
   3. Passive ROM in all cardinal planes as well as combinations of movements in all quadrants.
   4. Test resting length of anterior chest muscles and glenohumeral joint. Specific stretches of cervical musculature, such as scalenes, levator scapulae, sternocleidomastoid, and upper trapezius, can also be done in this position.
   5. Vertebral artery test, if indicated.
E. Prone lying examination.
   1. Reassess palpation if necessary.
   2. Gentle posterior-anterior stresses can be applied to assess response to anterior shear of vertebrae.

underlying connective tissue (bone, ligament, joints structure) involvement. The Box lists the typical referred pain patterns involved with lesions of the cervical spine musculature.[37] Increased states of muscle contraction and irritability are common when individuals are under emotional stress, a factor the examiner must recognize. Palpation should also allow for careful assessment of the involvement of the apophyseal joint structures, which are best palpated just lateral to the spinous process and are represented by ridges and valleys of bone. The "valleys" represent the articular pillars of the cervical vertebrae, and the "ridges" are the apophyseal joint lines (Fig. 17-35).

TREATMENT OF ACTIVITY-RELATED SPINE DISORDERS

More than 80% of all people in industrialized countries suffer pain in the spine at some time in their lives. Spine pain is so common that it might even be considered a normal aspect of being human.[38] Most cases of spinal pain have a favorable prognosis and a natural tendency toward spontaneous resolution. However, two issues are of concern: First, even though there is a tendency toward spontaneous resolution, there is also a high frequency of recurrent attacks of similar pain. Second, although the incidence of spine pain has not changed significantly over the past years, disability

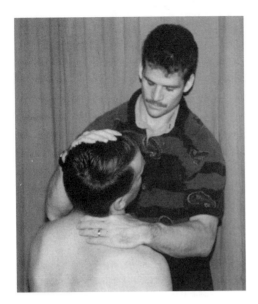

Fig. 17-33. Application of overpressure stress to the cervical spine. Note that the force is placed through the occiput, and the examiner is stabilizing the shoulders and thoracic spine.

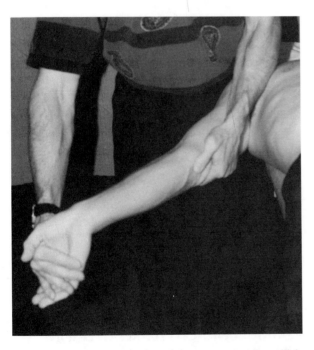

Fig. 17-34. Neural tension testing of the upper extremity, utilizing the median nerve.

from spine pain has dramatically increased, and it has become clear that a new challenge of the clinician is to distinguish spinal pain from disability and to treat accordingly.

As a consequence of these factors and in recognition of the need to better control costs for spinal care, an active approach toward rehabilitation that emphasizes education for self-management and restoration of function has replaced

Location of referred pain from cervical muscle involvement

Trapezius—temporal headache pattern
Sternocleidomastoid—temporomandibular joint area, autonomic responses
Levator scapula—posterior shoulder, paracervical spine
Semispinalis—greater occipital nerve entrapment, posterior and top of occiput
Suboccipitals—headache
Scalenes—C5-C6 dermatomal region

From Travell JG, Simons DG: *Myofascial pain and dysfunction*, Baltimore, 1983, Williams & Wilkins.

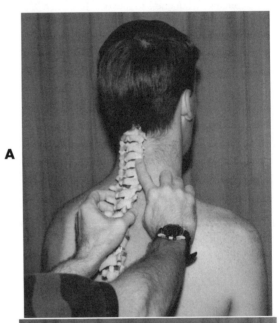

A

B

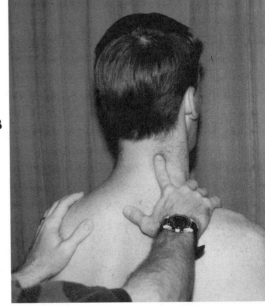

Fig. 17-35. Palpation of the articular pillars and ridges between these pillars provides an indication of the irritability of the apophyseal joints.

most other treatment strategies, especially those emphasizing passive manual and mechanical modalities. This section follows such a philosophy by organizing treatment along the four primary objectives of treatment for spinal disorders: modulation of pain, generation of controlled forces to promote reactivation of the patient, enhancing neuromuscular efficiency, and biomechanical counseling.[9]

Modulating pain

Numerous interventions are available to modulate pain including thermomodalities, electromodalities, and medications. It is essential to understand symptomatic relief and natural progression of the problem. It is ethical to treat pain in the appropriate patient, especially with the intent of progressing the patient to the active phase of the rehabilitation process. Pain is an excellent indicator of overuse or further injury. However, directing treatment with pain relief as the *primary* intent is appropriate for only a small, selected group of patients. In most situations, pain can be used as a guide to activity and exercise level.

Generation of controlled forces in order to promote reactivation

Early return to activity has the most significant impact in the long-term management of low back problems. This objective refers to the ability of the physical therapist to place controlled, nondestructive stresses through the low back or neck regions to facilitate and encourage movement by the patient and expedite the return to physical activity. Techniques that can be included under this objective are noted in the Box. The goal of any of these techniques should be to generate a state of well-being that promotes the patient's active movement.

In the past, explanations of each of the various techniques focused on their purported effects and dissimilarities with other techniques. These reports were largely anecdotal and biased. Most of these techniques can be explained on the basis of current scientific knowledge by the following mechanisms and thus their similarities:

1. *Influence fluid dynamics.* Fluid stasis and an altered chemical environment of the tissues propagate the nociceptive response and impede the healing process. It is difficult to find any manual, mechanical, or active technique that does not facilitate tissue fluid movement.

2. *Generate afferent input into the central nervous system.* Each manual, mechanical, or active technique sends a barrage of afferent input into the central nervous system. Although the details of reflex connections are relatively unknown, two common results of this input are modulation of pain and alteration in the state of muscle contraction. Whenever a change is realized in a patient's movement pattern or postural positioning of the spine or pelvis following any technique, it should be intuitively obvious that bones

---

Common techniques for generation of controlled forces in order to promote patient reactivation
Passive manual
Joint mobilization and manipulation
Soft tissue mobilization, massage traction
Mechanical
Traction
External supports
Spinal pillows, rolls, wedges
Heel lifts
Active
Muscle energy
Strain-counterstrain
Extension flexion protocols
Contract/relax proprioceptive neuromuscular facilitation

---

are not "put back in place" or connective tissue structurally altered. Rather, the difference is most likely due to a new and different resting tension of the muscle that results in a change in the active or passive motion pattern.

3. *Modify connective tissue.* Connective tissue can be altered only if the force is applied in a continuous and prolonged manner that alters the structural characteristics of the tissue. Of the three effects, this is probably the most difficult to accomplish in the clinical setting, owing to the strength of connective tissue.

Enhancing neuromuscular efficiency

Training of the neuromuscular system is essential because muscles act as shock absorbers for the skeleton and act as the motors that generate forces into and through the spine. Training also entails teaching patterns of movement to minimize stresses to the injured region. The passive approaches of the previously discussed objectives must be undertaken with the goal of moving the patient quickly and rapidly toward the objective of enhancing neuromuscular performance. Many different techniques are available to meet this objective, such as stabilization exercises, Feldenkrais techniques, progressive resistance exercises, work hardening, and functional restoration programs. Despite the variety of techniques, however, resistance exercises are the mainstay of treatment for deconditioned patients. Only when overload training principles are applied is it possible to induce the anatomic and biochemical changes necessary for increasing strength, hypertrophy, and endurance.

When this active approach is initiated promptly, return to activity is optimized and the potential for disability is lessened. This objective is extremely important in the management of spinal patients because increasing their function results in altering their perception of disability. More important, this objective promotes self-management of the low back pain problem.

Biomechanical counseling

Education of the patient is a critical component of any treatment program. The patient must realize the importance of setting activity limits in work or activities of daily living. With significant tissue injury of the spine or the onset of age-related changes in the tissues, accepting the fact that a percentage of back function is lost and perhaps cannot be restored may be more reasonable, and the goal then becomes teaching the person how to maximize activity within new limits. Tissue that is significantly injured or degenerated cannot attenuate stresses with the same efficiency as normal, uninjured tissue, which is often difficult for the patients to accept because of their expectations for a permanent "cure." Not only is this expectation unreasonable but also it leaves the onus of responsibility for care on the clinician rather than on the patient.

Objectives of treatment: commonly used treatment techniques

Historical perspective. A brief historical perspective is necessary in order for the reader to appreciate how past treatment philosophies have influenced current treatment strategies. In the 1930s and 1940s, a great deal of attention was focused on two anatomic and pathologic entities: (1) the degenerative joint disease process and its influence on the spatial relationships of the intervertebral foramen and (2) the dynamics and pathology of the intervertebral disk. Paul Williams combined an understanding of the mechanics of the vertebrae, especially at the region of the intervertebral foramen, with the concept of the trunk as a closed cylinder pressurized by the abdominal muscles to propose the Williams flexion exercise program:

1. Posterior pelvic tilting exercises
   a. Supine
   b. All fours—the typical "cat arch"
   c. Standing
2. Abdominal strengthening exercises
   a. Isometric trunk curls
   b. Isometric trunk curls with rotation
   c. Unilateral and bilateral leg lifts
3. Low back stretching exercises
   a. Single knee to chest
   b. Double knees to chest

Note the intent of these exercises: Increase the height of the intervertebral foramina and strengthen the abdominal wall. Why was there such a focus on the nerve root? At that time, the concept of referred pain was not completely understood, and it was logically deduced that all pain into the hip and thigh or leg was most likely due to nerve root

irritation. Movements were thus prescribed with the intended effect of increasing intervertebral foramen opening.

In 1934, Mixter and Barr published their classic paper on disk protrusion (Rupture of the intervertebral disc with involvement of the spinal canal, N Engl J Med 211:210)—the first paper that recognized that material removed from the spinal canal during surgery was, in fact, intervertebral disk material and not cartilaginous neoplasm. This paper began the era of the disk, which initially increased the use of Williams flexion protocols primarily because most disk protrusions were posterolateral and potentially impinged upon the nerve root at the region of the intervertebral foramen. Therefore, the intent of the exercises was still valid: Open the intervertebral foramen and strengthen the abdominal wall to help "unload" the intervertebral disks.

During this same period, James Cyriax published a series of classic papers as well as a textbook that began to describe more clearly the difference between referred pain and radicular pain. It was recognized that any low back structure, if injured, could refer pain into the lower extremity, and pain in the lower extremity was not necessarily from nerve root irritation. Instead, he suggested that most low back pain was caused by the intervertebral disk impinging upon the posterior longitudinal ligament, dura mater, or the nerve root. He recognized the pulplike structure of the nucleus pulposus and advocated (1) complete extension-hyperextension exercises to compress the posterior aspect of the disk and "push" the nuclear contents anteriorly as a method of treatment or (2) the use of heavy traction to accomplish this same result. Disk lesions that were thought due to annular (cartilaginous) lesions were treated by manipulation to reduce the cartilaginous displacement.

In New Zealand, Robin McKenzie began to review the writings of Cyriax and Kapandji and his own clinical results to develop the McKenzie system of evaluation and treatment (further described later in this chapter). McKenzie initially presented a case for intervertebral disk mechanics and advocated extension exercises to centralize the pain. He initially felt that the centralization of pain phenomena was due to the anterior migration of the nucleus during the exercise, which redirected the "pressure" from the structure that happened to be impinged upon.[24,25]

The initial zeal for the intervertebral disk subsided slightly over time, although it still remained in the forefront. Physical therapists began to expand their treatment approaches because of an increased understanding of joint mechanics, in particular, intervertebral joint motion. Primarily through the influence of two physical therapists, Geoff Maitland and Stanley Paris, techniques of joint mobilization and manipulation were developed as logical clinical applications of intervertebral joint mechanics.

This historical synopsis is intended to show the continued progress made toward developing successful management strategies. These schools of thought remain significant influences. The remainder of this section provides several examples of treatment techniques for the spine that can be used in treatment. It is not possible to detail the myriad of treatment techniques available to the clinician; more important is understanding the four objectives, which assume greater importance than individual techniques. Treatment techniques vary because of the needs of the patient, equipment availability, and personality of the patient and clinician. The key to successful management, however, is always restoration of function and education for self-management.

The McKenzie method of treatment. The McKenzie method of treatment is an excellent way to meet the goals set out in the second objective: introduction of controlled forces in order to promote reactivation of the patient.[26] One of the most important contributions made by McKenzie was the concept of centralization, the phenomenon in which the lower extremity pain associated with low back pain or the upper quarter pain associated with neck pain begins to diminish with specific repeated maneuvers, and the pain becomes more centralized to the low back or neck, respectively. Centralization allows the clinician to monitor the effects of treatment. As the patient improves, pain should centralize. If it peripheralizes, then there is a good chance that the treatment techniques or activities of the patient are aggravating the spine problem. The concept is also important for patients to understand, as they can monitor their work and activities of daily living by becoming cognizant of peripheralization and then initiating motions or positions of rest that centralize pain.

Three syndromes are identified through the evaluation process: dysfunction, postural, and derangement. *Dysfunction* refers to the adaptive changes of tissues that, when subjected to tensile stresses, give rise to pain. These patients often have a history of repeated episodes of pain. The tissue repair that occurs following injury results in adaptively shortened scar tissue that does not tolerate tensile stress as would uninjured tissue. Treatment of this group, identified in part by pain being reproduced at the end ranges of spinal movement and an easing of pain when the patient moves away from end range, is to attempt to increase the extensibility of the tissue with controlled stretching maneuvers into the painful range.

In the *postural* syndrome, the patient typically does not have pain in the neutral standing position, does not present with postural deformities, and has nearly the full range of spinal motion. Pain occurs with prolonged positioning, such as prolonged postures at work. Such prolonged postures begin to stress the connective tissue elements of the spine and result in pain. Treatment is designed around postural instruction and exercise to provide the strength and endurance to maintain pain-free postures and minimize end-range loading during the course of the day. Identification of this syndrome becomes easier if the patient helps to graphically illustrate the pain during the course of the day. The patient

who awakens with little pain or stiffness and who then has a gradual increase in pain as the day progresses may be an excellent candidate for postural instruction and exercise to train the musculoskeletal system.[32]

The *derangement* syndrome is characterized by sudden onset, and the patient is markedly incapacitated due to the pain. The term *derangement* is used because of the suggestion that the pain is due to displacement within the intervertebral disk.[25] McKenzie further classifies the derangement syndrome into seven subcategories. The patient has not only painful obstruction of movement but also postural changes such as a lateral shift. Treatment of this syndrome first focuses on attempting to correct the lateral shift with side-gliding maneuvers of the spine, followed by exercises that centralize the pain. For example, a patient whose pain increases centrally and peripheralizes with repeated forward bending is a candidate for extension exercises, beginning with prone positioning of patient and progressing through lying prone on elbows, and press-ups (Fig. 17-36). This progression is designed to have patients learn to self-manage their pain. If necessary, the clinician can also add extension mobilization maneuvers to the spine with a series of posterior to anterior pressures over the spine.

Stretching, soft tissue mobilization, joint mobilization. Stretching, soft tissue mobilization, and joint mobilization are treatment techniques that are also included under the second treatment objective. Owing to the different demands of the neck and low back, stretching and mobility exercises assume a high priority for neck problems. Neck mobility is essential to optimally position the sense organs of vision and hearing. In addition, motion of the neck results in a significant barrage of afferent input to the central nervous system because some of the highest concentrations of muscle spindles per gram of muscle are found in the paraspinal muscles of the cervical region.[10] In contrast, stability is essential for the successful management of low back problems; thus, the primary emphasis is on strengthening, with secondary emphasis on mobility.

Specific stretches for the neck take advantage of the ability to pre-position the head and neck in order to apply the stretch (Fig. 17-37). Instead of applying the stretching force over the small joints between the cervical vertebrae, the force is applied to the much larger scapula. It is often useful to apply contract-stretch techniques to the musculature to further increase the mobility. Isometric contraction can be of the muscle itself, followed by stretch, or contraction of the antagonistic muscle followed by stretch of the involved muscle tissue.[32]

Mobilization maneuvers of the neck affect both the muscle-fascia system and joint structures. Gentle passive mobility maneuvers applied by the clinician in a controlled manner decrease fluid stasis and diminish muscle guarding. Mobilization maneuvers of the cervical spine are effective because controlled forces are easily applied through the occiput, and various regions of the spine can be stabilized to

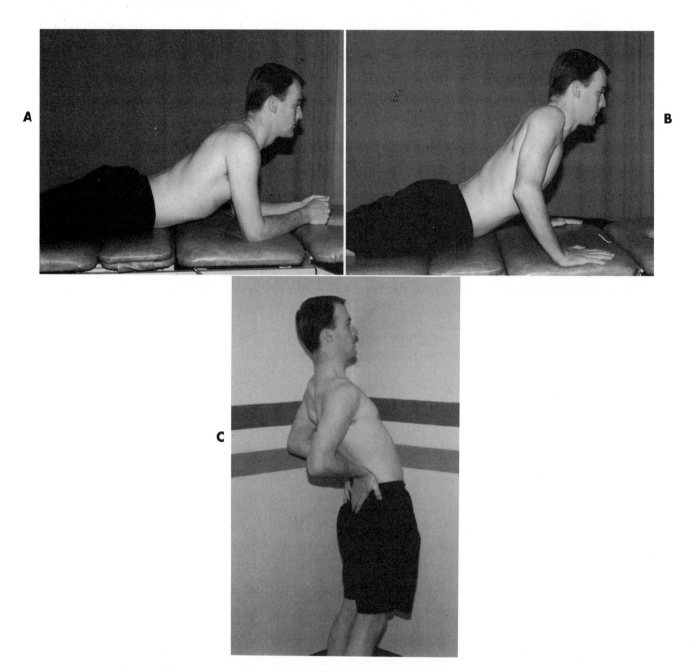

Fig. 17-36. A, Positioning the patient in prone on elbows; **B,** press-up position; **C,** standing extension.

focus the forces to specific cervical levels (Fig. 17-38). The cervical spine can be easily mobilized using general anterior, posterior, or lateral gliding motion, in addition to rotation, lateral bending, or flexion-extension motions. Rotary motions are often the most comfortable mobilization maneuvers tolerated by the patient, and increases in rotation mobility often result in an increase in other motions. The clinician should carefully monitor pain during and after treatment. Techniques need to be modified not only if there is an increase in the intensity or duration of pain but also if the pain peripheralizes.

Although stretching of the low back is important in order to maintain some degree of flexibility, strengthening often assumes greater importance because of the need to enhance the stability of the trunk with most low back disorders. With patients in acute distress, however, it is often necessary to gently mobilize the soft tissues and joints prior to initiating any active exercises. Gentle passive, active assistive, and active side bending from the sidelying position can be used very effectively in decreasing pain and increasing mobility (Fig. 17-39).

Mobility of the hip plays a key role in directing forces

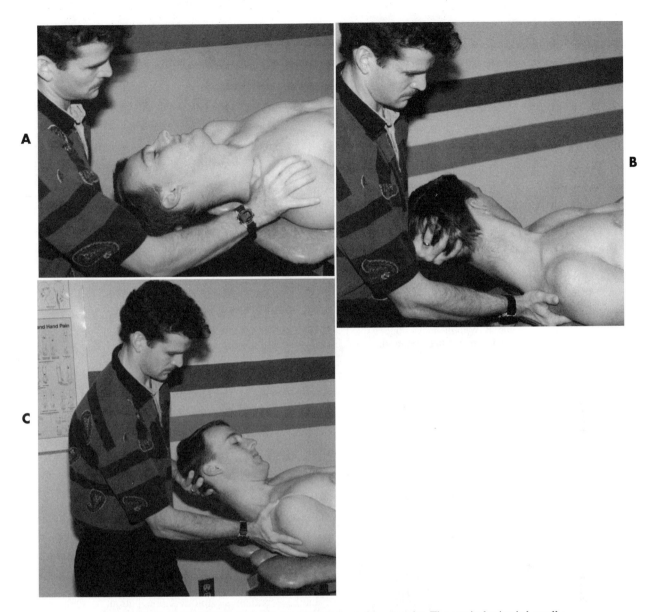

Fig. 17-37. A, Stretch of the right anterior and middle scalene muscles. The cervical spine is laterally flexed to the left, rotated to the right and pulled toward a more "retracted" head and neck posture. **B,** Stretch of the right levator scapulae. The neck is laterally flexed to the left, rotated to the left, and pulled toward a more forward head and neck position. The arm can also be abducted, which upwardly rotates the scapula and consequently moves the superior medial border of the scapula away from the cervical transverse processes. The stretching force is applied by pushing the scapula in an inferior direction. **C,** Stretch of the right upper trapezius. The occiput is flexed, the cervical spine laterally flexed to the left and rotated to the right, and the head and neck moved anteriorly. The stretching force is applied by pushing the scapula in an inferior direction.

through the pelvis and lumbar spine during upright postures. Therefore, stretching of the hip, especially the anterior hip musculature and the hip joint capsular tissues, assumes great importance. Fig. 17-40 shows two ways of stretching the hip joint without increasing the extension and compressive stress to the lumbar spine.

Traction. Both mechanical and manual traction techniques are used for spinal disorders; they also fit under the second objective of treatment. *Traction* is defined as a separation of joint surfaces. Traction for spinal disorders is typically used to "decompress" the bone-disk-bone interface. Due to the relative sizes of the cervical and lumbar vertebrae, traction forces are easier to apply to the cervical spine than to the lumbar spine. Cervical traction is best applied if compression of the temporomandibular joint is avoided. It is better tolerated if the mechanical or manual

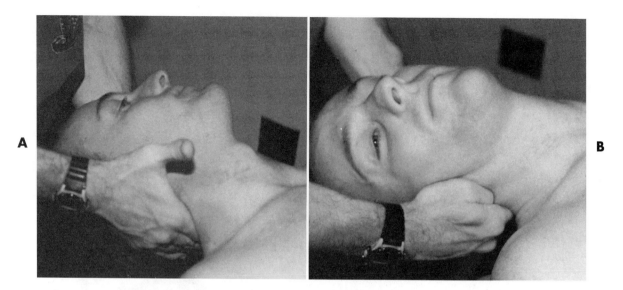

Fig. 17-38. Mobilization maneuvers of the cervical spine. **A,** Applying the force over the articular pillar in an anterior-superior direction in the plane of the facets places a slight rotary force to the cervical spine. **B,** With the index finger fixated at a specific cervical level, the cervical spine can be laterally flexed over this fixed point, thereby localizing the mobilizing force.

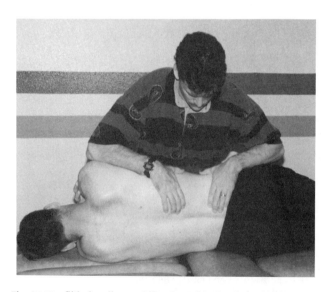

Fig. 17-39. Side-bending mobilization of the lumbar spine. A gentle distraction force applied through the rib cage and the pelvis by the clinician's elbows occurs simultaneously with an upward pull of the hands on the lumbar paraspinal muscles. This results in gentle side bending of the lumbar spine.

traction force is placed solely through the occiput. By gradually increasing the degree of cervical spine flexion, the traction force is transmitted to lower regions of the cervical spine.

Because of the plane of the apophyseal joints in the cervical spine, traction forces result in an unweighting between the bone-disk-bone interface as well as the cervical facet surfaces. This is not the case in the lumbar spine. Due

to the plane of the lumbar facets, a traction force simply causes gliding between the joint surfaces. Decompression between the lumbar facets occurs with rotation maneuvers. Rotation of the lumbar spine *increases* compression between the facet surfaces on one side and *decreases* compression between facets on the opposite side. Patients with unilateral low back pain, who have an increase in pain with extension and rotary stresses, can often use sidelying positions in slight rotation to decompress and temporarily unload the facet surfaces (Fig. 17-41).

Exercise training: stabilization exercises. The use of spinal stabilization exercises requires that the evaluation process determine those ranges of motion and positions that increase patient symptoms. The patient is then passively positioned in pain-free ranges and the trunk muscles given a series of challenges to isometrically hold those positions. As the patient develops the neuromuscular coordination to actively position the spine through pain-free ranges, the same isometric challenges to the trunk musculature are given via movement of the extremities, changes of position, or external challenges by the clinician. The intent is to develop the strength, coordination, and endurance of the trunk muscles to allow painless spinal positioning during activities of daily living and work. Thus, there is no "standard" posture position that is taught, but rather the most pain-free, asymptomatic position one as determined in the evaluation.

Stabilization exercises for the low back are often begun by simply teaching the patient the anterior and posterior pelvic tilt in order to provide proprioceptive feedback to the patient regarding lumbopelvic position. Similarly, exercises for the neck are begun by teaching the patient movement into and away from the forward head posture. Isometric holds are

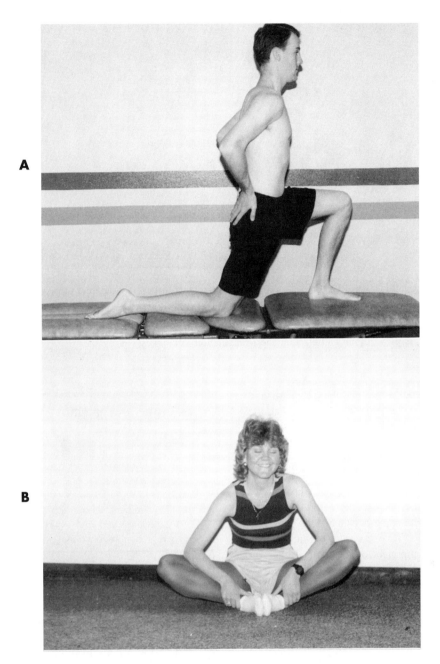

Fig. 17-40. **A,** Stretching of the right hip from the kneeling position. **B,** Stretching of the hip capsule from the seated position. Both positions stretch the hip without placing increased extension and compressive stresses to the lumbar apophyseal joints.

then used to increase proprioceptive awareness of spine positioning.

Resistance exercise training. One of the limitations of stabilization exercises is their inability to place the requisite challenge to the neuromuscular system to stimulate hypertrophy and muscle power. A stimulus of overload to the muscles is necessary in order to make substantive changes. Often the education gained by the patient with stabilization exercises can be used as an important starting point because

the patient understands the difference between vulnerable and invulnerable positions of the spine, and resistance exercises can then be tailored to the patient's spine problem.

The Box lists important points to consider in a resistance exercise program for patients with spine pain. Strengthening exercises are an essential component in the management of spinal disorders because they stimulate muscle growth and minimize the chance of reinjury. The pushing and pulling effect of the muscles on the fascial system, the ability of the

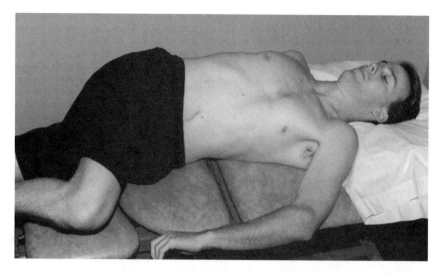

Fig. 17-41. In the left sidelying position, the thorax is rotated to the right, and the pelvis is rotated to the left. This decreases the compressive stress between the right lumbar apophyseal joints but increases the compressive force between the left lumbar apophyseal joints. Such a decompression maneuver for right-sided back pain, made worse with compression stresses to the right side of the low back, is used in joint mobilization and manipulation techniques.

muscles to act as the true shock absorbers of the skeleton and control the weight-bearing pattern through the spine, and the deconditioned state that is typical of patients imply that the most successful strategy in dealing with long-term management of activity-related spine pain is increased awareness of health and fitness and a healthy, trained muscular system.

The abdominal muscles. The abdominal muscles are essential muscles to exercise in both the patient with low back pain and the patient with upper back and neck pain. The Box lists the key reasons why training the abdominal muscles is an essential component of spine rehabilitation.

Maintenance of spine and pelvis position while performing resistance exercises with the upper or lower extremities is one way to begin stimulating abdominal muscle contraction. Another effective exercise is to have the patient pull the stomach in, away from the belt line, repeatedly and hold this position. Resistance exercises utilizing body weight can be done with curl-ups, curl-ups with a modified twisting motion, and single or bilateral leg lifts done with the pelvis continuously being maintained in an upwardly tilted position. Resistance through use of a pulley system can also be an effective means to provide resistance to the abdominal muscles (Fig. 17-42). The Box lists several exercises that focus a training effect to the abdominal muscles.

Training the extensor mechanism. The extensor mechanism includes the spinal extensors (superficial erector spinae and multifidi muscles), gluteus maximus, and hamstrings acting as extensors over the hip joints, the quadriceps, and the ankle plantar flexors. When considering the upper quarter, the scapula retractors and shoulder extensors are also included in the extensor mechanism. Many of the most effective ways to train these muscles mirror the requirements

---

Principles of resistance exercises: spine

1. Work in movement patterns and positions that have the least chance of causing reinjury or exacerbating pain.
2. Utilize submaximal workloads in leading to progressive resistance exercises.
3. Exercise until momentary fatigue, defined as repetition until movement substitution patterns become evident.
4. Vary the loads and angles of resistance.
5. Progress to more functional positions.

From Porterfield JA, DeRosa C: *Principles of mechanical neck pain: perspectives in functional anatomy,* Philadelphia, 1995, WB Saunders.

---

of these muscles for work and activities of daily living, such as squatting, lifting, and pulling exercises, including one-arm and two-arm pulls from different angles.

Resistance exercises for the spinal extensors were neglected in rehabilitation programs for spinal problems in the past because of a concern that hyperextension motion of the spine, especially against resistance, compromised the nerve root complex at the region of the intervertebral foramina. However, resistance exercises for the spinal extensors can be safely applied in a variety of ways, and exercises can be easily modified to meet the needs of the patient. Resistance exercises for the spine extensors are essential because of the essential role these muscles play in spine mechanics. They are also noted to display atrophic and degenerative histologic changes in chronic low back conditions.[34] There are several excellent ways to provide resistance to the extensor mechanism of the trunk and extremities, some of which are listed in the Box.

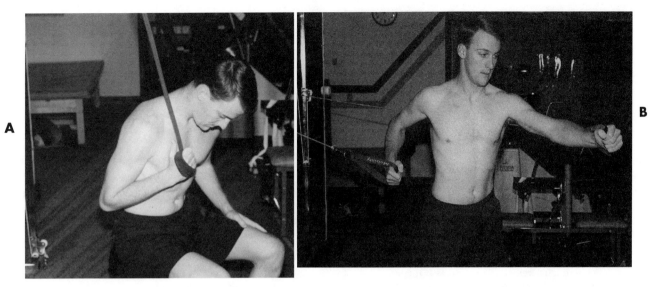

Fig. 17-42. Use of pulley system to train the abdominal muscles. **A,** Seated position to perform abdominal crunch with pulley resistance; **B,** standing rotary torso exercises between two pulleys.

Functions of abdominal wall mechanism

1. Provides anterior and anterolateral structural support to closed cylinder of abdominal cavity
2. Provides laterally directed forces via attachment to lateral raphe, potentially increasing tension of thoracolumbar fascia
3. Controls sagittal plane position of pelvis, thereby checking anterior shear at lumbosacral junctions and L4-L5 segments
4. Serves as dynamic check to control rate and amplitude of torsional stresses imparted to spine
5. Controls relationship of abdominal wall and abdominal wall contents to thorax, minimizing forward shoulder and head positioning

TREATMENT PLANS FOR SELECTED MEDICAL CONDITIONS: MATCHING THE FUNCTIONAL ASSESSMENT TO OBJECTIVES OF TREATMENT

This section is designed to provide suggestions for treatment for three common spine problems. Treatment emphasizes an active approach toward rehabilitation and is meant to serve as a working template rather than an all-inclusive list of treatment options. Findings that might be encountered from the functional assessment are used to formulate treatment strategies.

Instability of low back/neck

1. Considered when:
   a. Pain occurs *during* forward bending quadrants, but full forward-bending position with overpressure is
tolerated reasonably well. End range positions result in increased connective tissue tension, which potentially offers segmental stability.
   b. Pain with extension/compression quadrant is reproduced as result of shear force imparted.
   c. Pain with posteroanterior (P-A) stresses from prone position.
   d. Less pain with P-A shear stress from prone when person is prone on elbows or neck is "supported" in extension, which is also an end range position.
   e. Tenderness over PSIS/superior medial border of scapula. Pain over the region of the PSIS may be due to reflex muscle guarding by deep erector spinae muscle to minimize resultant shear force at lumbar spine due to instability. Pain over the superomedial border of scapula may be due to reflex muscle guarding of levator scapulae muscle to minimize anterior shear over cervical spine.
   f. Greater stiffness and soreness in morning upon awakening.
2. Intent of treatment
   a. Stability utilizing trunk and abdominal muscles.
   b. Education regarding torsion and shear occurring during ADLs and work.
   c. Correlating the pain pattern to ADLs and work and/or the result of the assessment regarding forces that reproduce familiar pain.
   d. Developing power and strength in the hip and thigh muscles, which are the primary motors for raising and lowering body (squatting, stooping, lifting, etc.).
3. Treatment progression
   a. Start: Goal is exercises to begin conditioning and teaching patient vulnerable and invulnerable positions

---

Exercises for abdominal muscles

A. Training focus to *lower abdominal region*
  1. Upward pelvic tilt
  2. Maintenance of upward pelvic tilt while leg lowering (low back remains fixed against surface at all times)
     a. One leg lowering
     b. Two legs lowering with hips and knees remaining bent
     c. Two legs lowering with knees nearly fully extended
  3. Reverse "crunch"—pelvis rolled posteriorly and slightly elevated off table at end of range via abdominal contraction
  4. Supine over gymnastic ball, one foot fixated on floor
B. Training focus to *oblique muscles*
  1. Cross-crunch (supine)—upper thorax is rotated while maintaining flexed position of hips and knees
  2. Reverse cross-crunch (supine)—pelvis is rotated while thorax is fixated and lumbar spine is firmly held against surface
     a. Hips and knees flexed to 90 degrees and maintained during rotary motion
     b. Knees extended and hips flexed toward 90 degrees and maintained in that position
  3. Simultaneous cross-crunch and reverse crunch (supine)
  4. Alternating bicycle motions with lower extremities (supine)
  5. Rotary resistance through use of pulley system (sitting)
  6. Medicine ball rotations with partner (standing)
C. Training focus to *upper abdominal region*
  1. Curl-up enhanced by increasing lever arm via position of hands at side, across chest, or lightly touching head
  2. Sagittal plane crunch with hips and knees flexed
  3. Resistance exercise using pulleys (sitting)
  4. Medicine ball catches and throws with partner
  5. Supine curl-ups on gymnastic ball

---

of low back and the concept of anterior shear of the spine.

  i. Exercise/conditioning general principles (education that maximizes the training effect).
    (a) Gradually deemphasize the focus on the number of repetitions and instead incorporate concept of repetition to substitution.
    (b) Overload without reinjury.
    (c) Morning stiffness should be a key indicator of overtraining or reinjury.
  ii. Specific exercises.
    (a) General conditioning such as stationary cycling.
    (b) Abdominal set—pulling "stomach" away from belt line.
    (c) Pulling exercises from supine, if very acute.
    (d) Pulling exercises from sitting (away from quadrant reproducing pain).
    (e) Partial low back extension from prone (emphasize chin tuck, scapular retraction during motions).
    (f) Partial wall squats (emphasize scapular retraction during motion and tracking of patella over second toe).
    (g) Standing hip pivots attempting to completely avoid torsion of back during pivots.
    (h) Deemphasis on modalities: avoid joint mobilization or manipulation.
  b. Progression.
    i. General conditioning.
    ii. Abdominal sets—pulling "stomach" away from belt line; progress to more aggressive abdominal muscle challenges.
    iii. Pulling exercises from seated (toward but not into pain quadrant).
    iv. Low back partial extensions—increases range (avoiding end range of extension) but still with emphasis on chin tuck and scapular retraction during motions.
    v. Squat exercises (lowering body center of gravity).
    vi. Standing hip pivots avoiding torsion in back; progress to pulley or resistance exercise tubing for resistance.
    vii. Partial compound lift—gluteal/hamstring emphasis with "stomach" pulled in.
    viii. Prone, with low back supported in partially flexed positions with pillows/gymnastic ball—alternate arm raises.
    ix. Standing alternate arm raises—maximal emphasis on minimizing trunk torsion and lumbar postures of anterior shear.
    x. Leg pressing exercise.
    xi. Modalities as appropriate for pain relief following exercise.
  c. Biomechanical counseling emphases for this problem.
    i. Avoid torsion in back.
    ii. Avoid ballistic "return to back extension" type of motions due to shear, for example, returning from forward bent position.
    iii. Minimize times of heavy loads above head level.
    iv. Minimize times of asymmetrical lifts.

Inability of posterior support structures to tolerate ground and trunk forces such as occurs with degenerative process, stenotic spine, spondylolisthesis

1. Considered when:
   a. Frontal plane asymmetry with pain on the long leg side.

Exercises for training the extensor mechanism

A. Squat exercise—teaching the patient to raise and lower body weight
  1. Be sure the patient can accept vertical loading of the spine.
  2. Key aspects of instruction:
     a. Keep the eyes forward and head up.
     b. Pinch scapula together—strong active retraction and upper spine extension.
     c. Feet turned out (usually about 30 degrees of hip external rotation).
     d. Push through heels during the move rather than toes ("sitting back" during the descent phase rather than shifting). Descent of the squat dependent on ankle dorsiflexion ROM.
     e. During the descent, the patella should "track" over second toe.
     f. If a bar is placed across the upper back, the weight line of the bar should fall through the midfoot.
  3. Begin with multiple repetitions without weight to encourage proper mechanics.
B. Functional lift training
  1. Considerations
     a. Can be broken out into compound lifting or focused toward gluteals/hamstrings or spinal extensors.
     b. Be certain that caution is utilized when treating patients with forward bending injury.
     c. Closely monitor position and movement of hip joints, pelvis, and spine during the motion.
  2. Compound lift instructions
     a. Keep feet parallel and approximately a shoulder-width apart, flex the knees to about 20 degrees. Flexing knees to about 20 degrees increases tension of the fascia lata–iliotibial tract passively, which is the structure that the gluteus maximus pulls on and quadriceps push against.
     b. Push through the complete foot and not just through toes when moving toward the upright position.
     c. Back is straight at start of the ascent.
     d. During the ascent, the knees and back move synchronously.
     e. Roll the shoulders back during the ascent, which helps bring the lumbar spine toward a neutral lordotic position by the end of the lift.
  3. Hamstring and gluteal focus: If the focus is on the hamstrings and gluteals, then the instruction is such that the individual "fixes" spine via abdominal and spine extensor cocontraction, and it is the pelvis that moves around the hips in both the controlled descent and the controlled ascent. The focus should be on the ischial tuberosities going "upward" as one bends forward and downward as one returns to the upright position.
  4. Spinal extensor focus: The pelvis is fixed via the hamstrings and the gluteals, i.e., the ischial tuberosities do not move during the descent or the ascent. Over the fixed pelvis, the lumbar spine gradually flexes in a controlled manner, and then the individual returns to the upright position by extending the lumbar spine to restore the neutral lordosis. Note that range of movement in the lumbar spine is small and controlled. If you see the back "round out" excessively, the lumbar joints' maximal end-range motion is reached and placed in a vulnerable position.
C. Kneeling extensions: Same exercises (hamstring and gluteal focus and the spinal extensor focus) can also be performed from the kneeling position. A slightly elevated surface for knees is less stressful to the feet and ankles. The same attention to the motion pattern or fixation of the ischial tuberosities is then the focus of the exercise motion. Hands at the side is a short lever, but hands outstretched forward, result in an increased lever arm. With the arms outstretched forward, the upper extremity should be externally rotated. This increases lower trapezius activity.
D. Prone extension exercise: This exercise can be done to focus training effects to the hamstrings and gluteals and/or the spinal extensors. This focus can be achieved by fixing the pelvis (having table or gymnastic ball compressed to the anterior superior iliac spine). With fixed pelvis, the dynamic motion focused to spinal extension via the spinal extensors; with pelvis free to rotate, the extension maneuver results in posterior pelvic rotation by the hamstrings and gluteals as well as extension by the spinal extensors.
  1. Tuck chin toward chest.
  2. Do not put the hands behind the neck but rather leave the arms in front of the body.
  3. When the ascent is begun, the arms move toward the body (extend and adduct the shoulder via a strong latissimus contraction).
  4. As the upper trunk extends, chin remains tucked and elbows are pulled in close to the body.
E. Lunge: Be certain that the patient has the spinal extensor strength to counter a forward bend of the trunk during the motion. It is also essential that the individual not "arch the back" and simply rest on the posterior arches of the lumbar joints, as this places those joints in the close-packed position and renders them vulnerable to injury. The exercise focuses the forces to the quadriceps and the deep gluteal muscles.
  1. Keep head up and the back straight. The tendency is to lean too far forward during the exercise. This substitution "unloads" the quads and lessens the effectiveness of gaining a training effect to the quads.
  2. Step forward so that the patella tracks over the second toe with the goal of moving toward the position of the upper thigh being nearly parallel with the floor.
  3. The opposite leg has only a slight to moderate bend associated with it at the end of the lunge.
F. Step-ups
G. Latissimus pull-downs
H. Seated rows
I. One arm pulls/rows

b. Pain with extension quadrant overpressure (compression and shear), especially if this test reproduces familiar pain on same side as long leg side.

c. "Flat buttocks" due to tucking of pelvis; "loss" of abdominal wall; flat cervical spine.

d. Pain with P-A stress over imaginary line over joints (compression-rotation stress).

e. Pain with prone on elbows position; made worse with P-A overpressure from prone on elbows position. This position close-packs the joints, and then a compression overpressure is applied.

f. Adaptive changes in hips (cannot be changed with contract-relax techniques), such as asymmetrical (marked difference between right and left hips) with Fabers test.

2. Intent of treatment: Rational treatment for abnormalities within the segment includes exercise programs that offer stabilization of the range of motion by muscle activity and improved nutrition of the joint by mechanical activity.

3. Treatment progression (back).

a. Start.

   i. "Balance" frontal plane with heel lift if indicated.

   ii. Stretch hip in figure-4 position from sitting; avoid stretching hamstrings. The hamstring force flexes the lumbosacral junction and thus decreases the compressive load to posterior lumbar joints.

   iii. Pull "stomach" away from belt line; focus on abdomen below the umbilicus.

   iv. General conditioning—seated cycling.

   v. Begin leg pressing activities.

   vi. Begin low back extension repetitions in range available; monitor where pain occurs in the ROM in order to determine safe range.

   vii. Physiologic mobilization—sagittal plane primarily and supplemented with techniques for frontal plane motion, begun passive but rapidly progressed to active.

   viii. Walking, but with an emphasis on "pulling in" abdominal wall, squeezing buttocks, and working to maintain such postural control.

b. Progression.

   i. Continue with general conditioning.

   ii. Self-stretching of hips and low back; self-mobilization of back.

   iii. Continue with and increase leg pressing activities.

   iv. Increase range of low back extension exercises from increasingly flexed position.

   v. Supine lying upper trunk lifts (scapula clear), progressing to medicine ball overhead, hips and knees flexed. When medicine ball is used, the rib cage must move toward pelvis (true lumbar flexion motion).

   vi. Alternate shoulder flex/extend from sitting with stomach away from belt line; strong emphasis on abdominal control during alternate shoulder flexions.

   vii. Begin lowering of COG exercises: squat, compound lift, lift with gluteal and hamstring focus.

c. Biomechanical counseling emphases.

   i. The importance of pain-free range of motion.

   ii. Rest postures instructed in positions to decompress apophyseal joints.

   iii. Minimize overhead pushing activities as much as possible.

4. Treatment progression (neck)

a. Progression.

   i. Assess adaptive changes in soft tissues and in muscles: scalenes, sternocleidomastoid, occipital extensors.

   ii. Segment connective tissues: Is flexion and rotation away from the side of pain both limited and painful? Is extension and rotation toward the side of pain limited and painful?

   iii. Joint and soft tissue mobilization.

   iv. Instruct patient in cervical stretches and cervical ROM with emphasis on rotations.

b. Biomechanical counseling.

   i. Educate in regard to cervical postural positions, especially those that minimize cervical apophyseal joint compression, such as emotional stress and muscle contraction, which loads cervical spine and forward head postures.

Sprain and strain

1. Considered when:

a. History "intensive"; not insidious or gradual-onset history.

b. Pain worse in any of forward bending quadrants made worse with tensile overpressure.

c. Tenderness to palpation lateral to spinous processes, above or below pelvis/spine of scapula.

d. Difficulty in tolerating sitting (low back pain); prolonged antigravity postures (neck).

e. May feature disproportionate radiation into extremities with forward bending assessment.

2. Intent of treatment: Functional healing recognizing limits of soft tissue repair capabilities, especially in regards to the aging process.

3. Treatment progression (back).

a. Start.

   i. Instruct in postural positioning for rest if acute (first 7 days following injury); patient must understand the concept of active and passive rest.

ii. Active mobilization—prone hyperextension, press-ups, especially if pain is reproduced or peripheralizes with forward bending tests.

iii. Active flexion and extension of lumbar spine from "all fours" position.

iv. Leave "tight" anterior hip structures alone initially, as this helps minimize the flexion force at the lumbosacral junction.

v. Isometric low back extension progressing to unresisted low back hyperextension.

vi. Overhead pressing activities against light resistance from sitting or standing (medicine ball).

vii. Active proprioceptive neuromuscular facilitation (nonresisted) diagonals for lower extremities.

b. Progression (when pain decreased in morning upon awakening).

i. Soft tissue/joint mobilization.

ii. Overhead pressing activities against moderate resistance from standing.

iii. Seated rowing exercises.

iv. One-arm rowing exercises from semiquadruped position.

v. Controlled range compound lifting, gluteal and hamstring emphasis maximizing lumbar isometric activity.

vi. Leg press activities.

vii. Lumbar hyperextension exercises.

c. Biomechanical counseling emphases.

i. Tissue healing—time constraints and natural course of healing events.

ii. Keep loads close to center of gravity.

iii. Avoid pulling, jerking motions.

4. Treatment progression (neck)

a. Start.

i. Active mobilization into limited range of motion pattern from supine.

ii. Assess barrier of movement. Isometric contractions into the barrier followed by passive stretch further into barrier.

iii. Soft tissue/joint mobilization in physiologic motion pattern.

b. Progression.

i. Assess barrier of movement. Isometric contraction in direction opposite of motion barrier, then stretch further into the barrier. Use specific muscle contractions emphasizing direction of movement rather than intensity of contraction.

ii. Active postural exercises.

c. Biomechanical counseling emphases with this problem.

i. Understand time constraints of healing when comparing hyperextension injuries (take longer time) to hyperflexion injuries.

ii. Early use of collar with frequent non–weight-bearing cervical ROM exercises, especially in rotation.

iii. Sleep postures that allow positions to have a completely supported cervical spine (pillow fills in complete space between occiput and shoulder).

SUMMARY

This chapter introduces the anatomy and biomechanics of the spine and provides a framework for evaluation and treatment. It emphasizes understanding the impacts of age, the degenerative process, injury history, and adaptive changes in order to establish reasonable and realistic outcome goals. Evaluation and treatment of many activity-related spinal disorders are hampered by the fact that the precise anatomic lesion is often impossible to diagnose, and the repair process of injured tissue does not typically result in tissue that can tolerate the same intensity, frequency, and duration of applied forces. Consequently, reinjury is common, and exacerbations of familiar spine pain are frequent features of a patient's history. Therefore, this chapter stresses an active treatment process emphasizing patient education for self-management and exercise programs to promote active, healthy lifestyle.

REVIEW QUESTIONS

1. What examination components should be included in school screenings conducted for the early identification of scoliosis?

2. What is the difference between a Schomorl's node and a diskal protrusion or herniation?

3. What was the theoretical basis for Williams' flexion exercises versus the McKenzie method of treatment?

4. What would be an appropriate progression of exercises for training the spinal extensor mechanism?

5. How would the biomechanical counseling program differ for a patient with low back instability in comparison to a patient with a low back strain?

REFERENCES

1. Andersson G: The epidemiology of spinal disorders. In Frymoyer J, editor: *The adult spine,* New York, 1991, Raven Press.

2. Bankoff ADP, Furlani J: Electromyographic study of the rectus abdominis and external oblique muscles during exercises, *Electromyogr Clin Neurophysiol* 24:501, 1984.

3. Beard HK, Stevens RL: Biochemical changes in the intervertebral disc. In Jayson MIV, editor: *The lumbar spine and backache,* ed 2, London, 1980, Pitman.

4. Bigos SJ et al: A retrospective study: III, employee related factors, *Spine* 11:252, 1986.

5. Bogduk N, Macintosh JE: The applied anatomy of the thoracolumbar fascia, *Spine* 9:164, 1984.

6. Bogduk N, Twomey LT: *Clinical anatomy of the lumbar spine,* New York, 1987, Churchill Livingstone.

7. Butler D: *Mobilisation of the nervous system,* Melbourne, 1991, Churchill Livingstone.

8. Crawford WC, Yang JC, Janal MN: Altered pain and visual sensitivity in humans: the effects of acute and chronic stress, *Ann N Y Acad Sci* 467:116, 1986.

9. DeRosa C, Porterfield JA: A physical therapy model for the treatment of low back pain, *Phys Ther* 72:261, 1992.

10. Dvorak J, Dvorak V: *Manual medicine: diagnostics,* New York, 1990, Thieme.

11. Elvey R: Brachial plexus tension tests and the pathoanatomical origin of arm pain. In *Proceedings, aspects of manipulative therapy,* Melbourne, 1979, Lincoln Institute of Health Sciences.

12. Farfan HF: *Mechanical disorders of the lowback,* Philadelphia, 1973, Lea & Febiger.

13. Friberg O: Clinical symptoms and biomechanics of lumbar spine and hip joint in leg length inequality, *Spine* 8:643, 1983.

14. Frymoyer J: *The adult spine,* New York, 1991, Raven Press.

15. Gotfried Y, Bradford DS, Oemgema TR: Facet joint changes after chemonucleolysis induced disc space narrowing, *Spine* 11:944, 1986.

16. Hoyashi K, Yabuki T: Origin of uncus and of Luschka's joint in the cervical spine, *J Bone Joint Surg Am* 67:7, 1987.

17. Kapandji IA: *The physiology of the joints,* vol 3, Edinburgh, 1974, Churchill Livingstone.

18. Lewin T: Osteoarthritis in lumbar synovial joints: a morphologic study, *Acta Orthop Scand Suppl* 73:1, 1964.

19. Ling CM, Low YS: Sternomastoid tumor and muscular torticollis, *Clin Orthop* 86:144, 1972.

20. Luk KDK, Ho HC, Leong JCY: The iliolumbar ligament: a study of its anatomy, development, and clinical significance. *J Bone Joint Surg Am* 68:197, 1986.

21. MacNab I: Acceleration injuries of the cervical spine, *J Bone Joint Surg Am* 46:1797, 1964.

22. MacNab I: The mechanism of spondylogenic pain. In Hirsch C, Zotterman Y, editors: *Cervical pain,* Oxford, 1972, Permagon.

23. Maitland GD: *Vertebral manipulation,* ed 5, London, 1986, Butterworths.

24. McCarron RF et al: The inflammatory effect of the nucleus pulposus: a possible element in the pathogenesis of lowback pain, *Spine* 12:760, 1987.

25. McKenzie RA: Prophylaxis in recurrent low back pain, *N Z Med J* 627:22, 1979.

26. McKenzie RA: *The lumbar spine: mechanical diagnosis and therapy,* Waikanae, New Zealand, 1981, Spinal Publications.

27. Nachemson A: The possible role of the psoas major for stabilization of the lumbar spine, *Acta Orthop Scand* 39:47, 1968.

28. Nachemson A et al: Scientific approach to the assessment and management of activity related spinal disorders: a monograph for clinicians. Report of the Quebec Task Force on Spinal Disorders, *Spine* 12 (suppl) S1, 1987.

29. Nolan JP, Sherk HH: Biomechanical evaluation of the extensor musculature of the cervical spine, *Spine* 13:9, 1988.

30. Ortengren R, Andersson GBJ: Electromyographic studies of the trunk muscles with special reference to the functional anatomy of the lumbar spine, *Spine* 2:44, 1977.

31. Parke WW, Watanabe R: The intrinsic vasculature of the lumbosacral nerve roots, *Spine* 10:508, 1985.

32. Porterfield JA, DeRosa C: *Mechanical low back pain: perspectives in functional anatomy,* Philadelphia, 1991, WB Saunders.

33. Porterfield JA, DeRosa C: *Mechanical neck pain: perspectives in functional anatomy,* Philadelphia, 1995, WB Saunders.

34. Rantanen J, Hurme M, Falck B: The lumbar multifidus muscle five years after surgery for a lumbar intervertebral disc herniation, *Spine* 18:568, 1993.

35. Rothman RH, Simeone FA: *The spine,* ed 3, Philadelphia, 1992, WB Saunders.

36. Tesh KM, Dunn JS, Evans JH: The abdominal muscles and vertebral stability, *Spine* 12:501, 1987.

37. Travell JG, Simons DG: *Myofascial pain and dysfunction,* Baltimore, 1983, Williams & Wilkins.

38. Waddell G: A new clinical model for the treatment of low back pain, *Spine* 12:632, 1987.

39. Walker JM: Age related differences in the human sacroiliac joint: a histologic study; implications for therapy, *J Orthop Sports Phys Ther* 7:325, 1986.

40. Weinstein SL, Zavala DC, Ponseti IV: Ideopathic scoliosis: long term followup and prognosis in untreated patients, *J Bone Joint Surg Am* 63:702, 1981.

41. White AA, Panjabi MM: *Clinical biomechanics of the spine,* Philadelphia, 1978, JB Lippincott.

42. Yang KH, King AI: Mechanism of facet load transmission as a hypothesis for low back pain, *Spine* 9:557, 1984.

CHAPTER 18

The Temporomandibular Joint

Anne Leath Harrison

OUTLINE

Functional anatomy
    Osseous structures
    The disc and attachments
    The capsule and ligaments
    Osteokinematics
    Musculature
    Innervation
    Biomechanics and arthrokinematics
    Function
Temporomandibular Disorders
    Pathomechanics
    Hypermobility
    Capsular fibrosis
    Masticatory muscle disorders
    The role of dental occlusion
    Growth and development considerations
    Cervical spine considerations
    Differential diagnosis
Evaluation of TMJ and Associated Structures
    Patient history and subjective report
    Physical exam
    Psychologic considerations
    TMJ imaging
Physical therapy approach to TMJ disorders
    Treatment of joint derangement
    Treatment for masticatory muscle disorders
    Exercises for the patient with TMD
    Treatment of the cervical spine
    Surgical approaches for TMD
Case 1
Case 2
Conclusion

LEARNING OBJECTIVES

After studying this chapter, the reader should be able to:

1. Describe the articular components of the temporomandibular joint.
2. Describe the musculature that serves to move and stabilize the temporomandibular joint.
3. Describe the biomechanics of temporomandibular joint movements.
4. Define and discuss the pathomechanics associated with disk lesions of the temporomandibular joint.
5. Define and discuss the pathomechanics associated with soft tissue and capsular disorders affecting the temporomandibular joint.
6. Define and discuss the pathomechanics associated with masticatory muscle disorders affecting the temporomandibular joint.
7. List and describe all the components of a physical examination and evaluation of the temporomandibular joint.
8. Discuss factors to consider in assessing the findings of the physical examination of the temporomandibular joint.
9. Describe the treatment program used for the management of acute inflammatory disorders affecting the temporomandibular joint or associated structures.
10. Discuss the rationale for various exercise approaches to treating patients with temporomandibular joint dysfunction.

KEY TERMS

temporomandibular	pain
biomechanics	evaluation
joint derangement	masticatory muscle disorders
craniomandibular	

The temporomandibular joint (TMJ) was one of the last synovial joints in the body to escape scrutiny by the physical therapy (PT) profession. For many years, people with temporomandibular disorders (TMD) were treated by the few dentists who had developed expertise in the area, or they were misdiagnosed and perhaps left untreated. It is fortunate for the many patients who suffer from disorders of the TMJ and its associated structures that many professionals, including physical therapists, have begun to add new and necessary dimensions to the assessment and treatment of this area.

The TMJ is a link in the chain of synovial joints connecting the body. It interrelates anatomically and kinesiologically with adjacent joints in this chain, particularly those of the cervical spine. It is responsible for performing functions basic to life, such as chewing and swallowing, and participates in important functions such as speech and emotional expression. Dysfunction in this area has been associated with visual, auditory, and balance disturbances. Pain in this area can be unrelenting and often requires a multidisciplinary team approach. The physical therapist plays an integral role in providing treatment for the patient with TMD.

In spite of the need for more research validating PT approaches, much progress has been made in providing effective treatment for patients with TMD through transfer of our knowledge base and experience in treating other areas of the body. Therefore, we must continue judiciously and with a commitment to increasing our knowledge base about therapeutic interventions in this area.

FUNCTIONAL ANATOMY

The temporomandibular joint is the synovial articulation between the cranium and the mandible (Fig. 18-1). The joint represents an impressive interplay among bone, disc, ligament, and muscle and is driven by a well-organized neurologic system to perform functions basic to life, such as mastication, swallowing, speaking, and emotional expression. It influences and is influenced by the cervical spine. A thorough understanding of the normal functional anatomy and biomechanics of the joint is necessary for comprehension of pathology and therapeutic interventions.

Osseous structures

The TMJ articulation occurs between the convex condylar head of the mandible as it relates through an interposed disc to the mandibular fossa and articular eminence of the temporal bone. The concave fossa blends anteriorly with the articular eminence, which is varied in its convexity and steepness, and posteriorly with the postglenoid spine.[43] Anterior and medial to the temporal bone is the maxillary bone, which houses the upper 16 adult teeth (see Fig. 18-1).

The convex head of the mandibular condyle is ellipsoidal from its superior aspect, with the medial-lateral aspect wider and less convex than the anterior-posterior aspect.[26] It can be easily palpated just anterior to the ear while the mouth is opening and closing. Inferior to the head is the condylar neck, which blends with the ramus to initiate the body of the mandible. The coronoid process projects from the ramus anterior to the condyle; it serves as an attachment for the temporalis muscle. The body of the mandible houses the lower 16 adult teeth (see Fig. 18-1).

The mandibular fossa, the articular eminence, and the head of the condyle are distinguished as articular surfaces during dissection by the presence of avascular and aneural fibrocartilage, rather than hyaline cartilage, on their surfaces.[26] The TMJ is a load-bearing joint with thousands of repetitive movements daily. The presence of fibrocartilage on its joint surfaces allows for flexibility in the repair and remodeling process that occurs throughout the life span in response to changes in the quality and quantity of functioning.

The arthrology of the joint is not complete without consideration of the dentition. The maxilla and the mandible house the upper and lower teeth, respectively. The end point of mandibular elevation comes with mouth closure and occurs when the teeth are occluded. The posterior teeth have cone-shaped projections known as *cusps* and depressions known as *fossae*. During normal occlusion, the cusps fit into the fossae. The anterior teeth are known as *central incisors*. During normal occlusion, the maxillary teeth slightly overlap the mandibular teeth in a vertical and horizontal direction (see Fig. 18-1).

The teeth are attached to the alveolar bones through periodontal ligaments (Fig. 18-2). The afferent innervation of the ligaments influences the firing of the muscles of mastication by relaying proprioceptive information to the central nervous system (CNS) about tooth positioning and occlusion. Although it seems logical to conclude that the attributes of the occlusal position have implications for the health and stability of the TMJ, recent research suggests that occlusion is not as predictably influential in pain and dysfunction of the TMJ as was once thought.[33] This relationship is further considered in the discussion of pathology.

The disc and attachments

The articular disc of the TMJ is composed of dense fibrous connective tissue in anterior, intermediate, and posterior zones. It is essentially avascular and aneural at its articulating intermediate zone and, like the vertebral disc, receives its primary nutrition through movement. Although flat at birth, the adult disc is described in *Gray's Anatomy* as a peaked cap, with its upper surface concavoconvex to articulate with the fossa and the articular eminence and its inferior surface concave to articulate with the condylar head.[43] It is thinnest in its intermediate zone and thickest in its posterior zone, with a slight thickening of its medial and anterior aspects. This variation in thickness plays an important role in maintaining disc positioning on the condyle during normal function.[33]

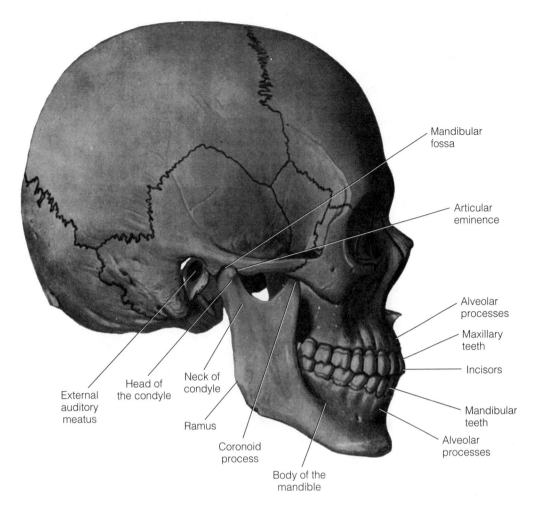

Fig. 18-1. Adult skull, lateral aspect. Note the slight overlap of the mandibular teeth by the maxillary teeth. (From DuBrul EL: *Sicher's oral anatomy,* ed 7, St Louis, 1980, Mosby.)

The disc has attachments around its perimeter. It is firmly attached to the medial and lateral poles of the condyle by collateral ligaments. These ligaments, also known as *discal ligaments,* assure that the disc moves with the condyle while allowing some mobility of the disc on the condyle in an anterior-posterior direction. The disc is attached posteriorly to a thick layer of highly vascularized and well innervated retrodiscal tissue, which fills with blood and fluid during depression of the mandible. The retrodiscal tissue, also called the *posterior attachment,* is bilaminar, with the superior lamina attaching to the posterior aspect of the fossa and the glenoid spine, and the inferior lamina attaching to the mandibular condyle. The superior component has elastin fibers and is thought to play a role in maintaining disc position on the condyle during exaggerated end-range movements of mouth opening (Fig. 18-3).[33]

Anteriorly, the disc is attached to the joint capsule and to the tendon of the superior lateral pterygoid muscle. The circumferential nature of the discal attachments results in the TMJ being a compound joint with distinct superior and inferior joint cavities, with the superior cavity having a larger volume than the inferior (see Fig. 18-3).[26]

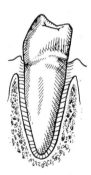

Fig. 18-2. Periodontal ligaments of the tooth stimulate afferent nerves, which deliver information about tooth positioning during function. (From Okeson J: *Management of temporomandibular disorders and occlusion,* St Louis, 1993, Mosby.)

The capsule and ligaments

Up to this point, the discussion has focused on intracapsular structures. The TMJ capsule and extracapsular ligaments are stabilizers of the joint. The fibrous capsule encompasses the joint with the superior attachment around the articular area of the temporal bone and the inferior attachment to the neck of the condyle. It prevents displacement of the condyle medially, laterally, and inferiorly[26] and has connections to the retrodiscal tissue and to the anterior disc attachments. A synovial lining covers the inner wall of the capsule, producing synovial fluid to lubricate and bring nutrition to the joint surfaces.[43] This lubrication is most effective in the presence of normal mobility.

Wyke describes the presence of mechanoreceptors in the capsule that deliver information about position and movement of the joint, resulting in facilitory and inhibitory effects on the motor neurons that power the masticatory muscles.[25,44] As with all synovial joints, the response of the

mechanoreceptors is important during dysfunctions of the capsule, such as capsular inflammation or fibrosis.

The lateral aspect of the capsule thickens to become the temporomandibular ligament (Fig. 18-4). It travels from the zygomatic process to the posterior neck of the condyle and has two bands: the outer oblique portion and the inner horizontal portion. The oblique portion prevents inferior displacement of the condyle at rest and tightens after 20 to 25 mm of mandibular opening to influence anterior displacement of the condyle at that range (Fig. 18-5). The horizontal portion protects the retrodiscal tissue from posterior displacement of the condyle.[33] The intimate relationship

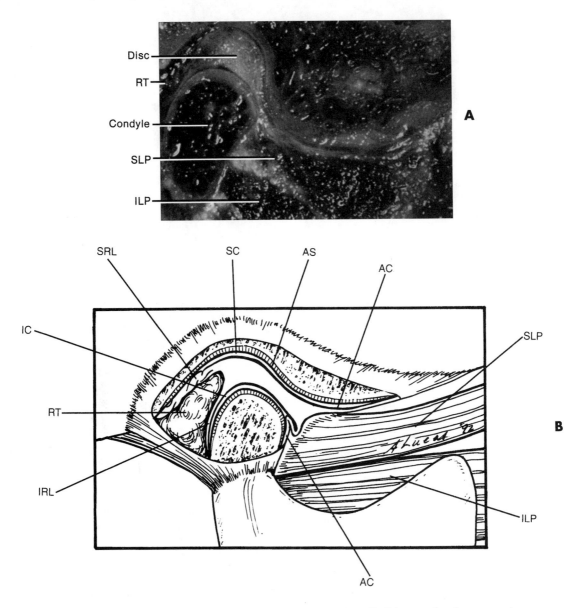

Fig. 18-3. Temporomandibular joint, lateral view. **A,** Dissection. **B,** Diagram showing anatomic components. *RT,* Retrodiskal tissues; *SRL,* superior retrodiskal lamina; *IRL,* inferior retrodiskal lamina; *AC,* anterior capsule; *SLP* and *ILP,* superior and inferior lateral pterygoid muscles; *AS,* articular surface; *SC* and *IC,* superior and inferior joint cavity; the diskal ligament has not been drawn. (**A,** Courtesy of Dr. Julio Turrell of University of Montevideo, Uruguay; B, from Okeson J: *Management of temporomandibular disorders and occlusion,* St Louis, 1993, Mosby.)

between this ligament and the capsule should be considered when dysfunction of the capsule is present.

The sphenomandibular and the stylomandibular ligaments are considered accessories to joint function. They are extracapsular, medial to the joint, and thought to play a role in end-range mouth opening.[33,43]

Osteokinematics

The three osteokinematic motions of the TMJ are mandibular depression and elevation, right and left lateral excursion, and protrusion and retrusion. Opening and closing

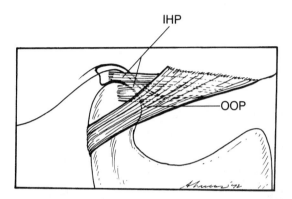

Fig. 18-4. Temporomandibular ligament, lateral view. *OOP*, outer oblique portion limits normal rotational opening; *IHP*, inner horizontal portion limits posterior movement of the condyle and disk. (Modified from DuBrul EL: *Sicher's oral anatomy,* ed 7, St Louis, 1980, Mosby.)

the mouth in the sagittal plane are functions of mandibular depression and elevation (Fig. 18-6, *A*). Lateral movement of the mandible to the right or the left in the horizontal plane is termed *lateral excursion* or is variously referred to as *lateral deviation, laterotrusion,* or *mediotrusion* (Fig. 18-6, *B*). Anterior and posterior movements of the mandible in the horizontal plane are called *protrusion* and *retrusion* (Fig. 18-6, *C*).

Musculature

Muscles of mastication. The four primary muscles of mastication are the temporalis, the masseter, the medial pterygoid, and the lateral pterygoid (Fig. 18-7). They are responsible for powerful functional activities, such as chewing and tearing, and for the fine, detailed movements needed in speaking and swallowing. Afferent information from receptors in the TMJ capsule and ligaments stimulate reflexive firing of the muscles to guard against dysfunction at the end range of mandibular movements.[18] The muscles of mastication are also responsible for activities of the mandible that are outside normal function, such as clenching, grinding, and gum chewing. These parafunctional activities are often performed on a habitual or involuntary basis.

The muscles of mastication function as dynamic stabilizers of the joint by maintaining a degree of intraarticular pressure with their resting muscle tone. This positive pressure assures constant contact between the articular surfaces and the interposed disc, which is necessary for joint stability during joint mobility.[33] If muscle tone or activity of

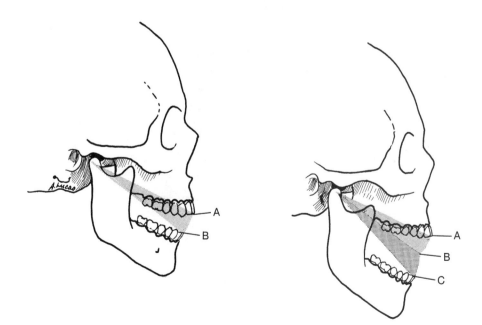

Fig. 18-5. Effect of the outer oblique portion of the temporomandibular ligament. As the mouth opens, the teeth can be separated 20-25 mm (**A** to **B**) without the condyles moving from the fossa. At **B,** the TM ligament is lengthened, and, as the mouth opens wider, the ligament moves the condyles anteriorly and downward onto the articular eminence, to position **C.** (From Okeson J: *Management of temporomandibular disorders and occlusion,* St Louis, 1993, Mosby.)

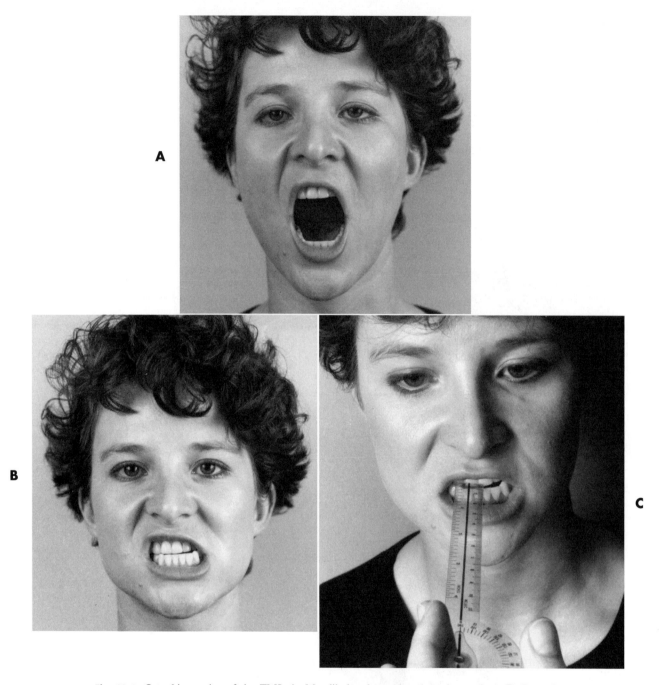

Fig. 18-6. Osteokinematics of the TMJ. **A,** Mandibular depression (mouth opening). **B,** Lateral excursion; **C,** protrusion.

the mandibular elevators is abnormally increased during rest, then increased intraarticular pressure occurs at rest.

The temporalis muscle is fan-shaped, with palpable superior tendinous attachments to the temporal bone and inferior attachments to the coronoid process and the anterior ramus of the mandible. The orientation of its fibers is easily palpated, with the anterior fibers vertical, the intermediate fibers oblique, and the posterior fibers horizontal.[26,33,43] Orientation influences function; thus, the anterior fibers are involved in mandibular elevation, the intermediate fibers in mandibular elevation and retrusion, and the posterior fibers in retrusion. The temporalis also functions during ipsilateral lateral excursion.[2] The broad origin and narrow insertion of the muscle as a whole contribute to its role of positioning the condyle on the fossa during functional activities such as tearing and chewing and parafunctional activities such as clenching. Overuse of the muscle during these activities can result in palpable tenderness in its muscle belly in the

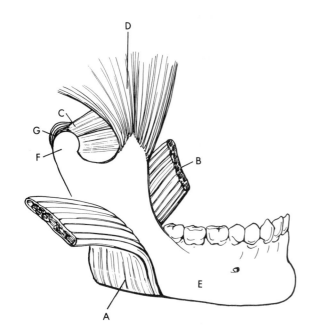

Fig. 18-7. The muscles of mastication. **A,** Masseter muscle. **B,** Medial pterygoid muscle. **C,** Lateral pterygoid muscle. **D,** Temporalis muscle. **E,** Lateral surface of mandible. **F,** Mandibular condyle. **G,** Articular disk.

temporal fossa and intraorally at its tendinous insertion along the anterior aspect of the ramus.

The powerful masseter muscle is rectangular, with deep and superficial fibers running from the zygomatic arch obliquely posteriorly to the angle of the mandible. It provides the main force in chewing[43] and unilaterally functions in ipsilateral lateral excursion of the mandible.[2] It is easily palpable when clenching and hypertrophies in people who habitually perform this parafunctional activity.[26]

The medial pterygoid is medial to the mandible and travels posteriorly and inferiorly from the pterygoid fossa to attach to the medial aspect of the angle of the mandible. It functions in mandibular elevation and protrusion and unilaterally in contralateral excursion.[2] Its participation in parafunctional activities that move the teeth from side to side, such as grinding, results in hypertrophy.[26] It is difficult to isolate for clinical palpation and is evaluated through its function.

The lateral pterygoid muscle is functionally divided into superior and inferior components, with the superior portion originating from the sphenoid and the inferior portion originating from the lateral pterygoid plate. The inferior lateral pterygoid inserts primarily on the neck of the condyle. The superior lateral pterygoid attaches to the neck of the condyle and also has attachments to the anterior capsule and the disc.[26,33] The inferior portion glides the condyle anteriorly during mouth opening and mandibular protrusion, and it unilaterally participates in contralateral excursion. The superior lateral pterygoid is electrically silent during mouth opening and fires in conjunction with the mandibular

elevators,[2] playing a role in positioning the disc on the condyle at the end range of closure and during resistance to closure, as in chewing or clenching. Its role in parafunctional activities such as clenching and grinding can result in microtrauma to the muscle or tendon through overuse. It is not distinctly palpable and must be evaluated through its functioning.

Other relevant musculature. The digastric muscle is responsible for opening the mouth wide or against resistance and works in tandem with other suprahyoid and infrahyoid muscles to position the hyoid during activities such as swallowing and speaking.[2]

Other cervical spine muscles play a critical role in the health of the craniomandibular complex. The stabilizers of the cervical spine are essential players during mandibular movements (Fig. 18-8). One need only palpate the posterior cervical musculature during the mandibular activity of yawning or shouting to confirm its participation. The postural positioning of the head by the cervical spine joints and muscles influences mandibular posture.[25,44] Trigger points in the sternocleidomastoid, trapezius, and suboccipital muscles are known to refer pain to the face,[40] sometimes causing diagnostic confusion for the inexperienced practitioner. The greater occipital nerve pierces the suboccipital tendinous tissue as it carries afferent information from the posterior cranium, and compromise of this nerve by the suboccipital tissue can result in pain in the posterior cranium, a symptom sometimes associated with TMD.[25] Cervical spine influences on craniomandibular pain and TMD are discussed in subsequent sections of this chapter.

The equilibrium of forces around the mouth is maintained intraorally by the muscles that power the tongue and extraorally by the orbicularis oris muscle and the buccinator. Weakness or dysfunction in these muscles can result in developmental changes and dysfunction of the masticatory system. Rocabado states that the normal rest position of the middle portion of the tongue is on the roof of the mouth; when the tongue rests abnormally on the floor of the mouth, the intraoral forces pushing outward on the mandible may result in increased firing and overuse of extraoral muscles. His pediatric work has resulted in further proposals connecting the detrimental developmental effects of parafunctional activities such as thumb sucking and fingernail biting to TMD.[35]

Innervation

Afferent innervation of joint structures, including the capsule and the retrodiscal tissue, and efferent innervation of the muscles of mastication are primarily supplied by the trigeminal nerve. This nerve also supplies afferent information for the lateral aspect of the face. Sensory input, in the form of proprioception or pain from afferent receptors in the joint structures or periodontal ligaments of the teeth, can influence masticatory motor function and resting tone through facilitation or inhibition.[44]

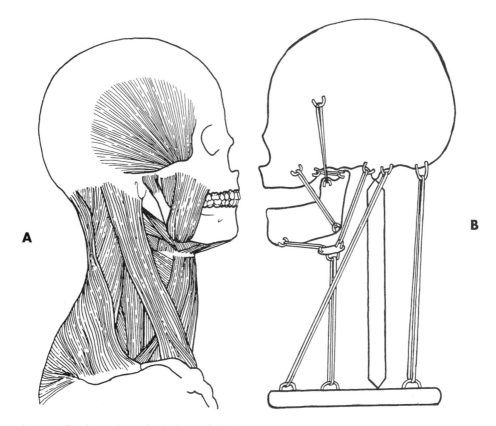

Fig. 18-8. Precise and complex balance of the head and neck muscles must exist to maintain proper head position and function. **A,** The musculature. **B,** Schematic of tension provided by the musculature. Imbalances in one part of this system can influence imbalances in other parts of the system. (From Okeson J: *Management of temporomandibular disorders and occlusion,* St Louis, 1993, Mosby.)

The nucleus of the trigeminal nerve begins in the medulla and extends in the upper dorsal horn of the spinal cord to the level of C5. There is an influential relationship between the trigeminal nucleus and the cell bodies of the cervical nerves secondary to their convergence in the dorsal horn. This convergence has been demonstrated to result in pain referral patterns among the structures innervated by the trigeminal nerve and the cervical nerves.[23,33] In other words, sensory information from cervical spine structures may have secondary influences on the structures innervated by the trigeminal nerve on the same side by influencing them at the spinal cord level.

The upper cervical nerve roots supply afferent information to the posterior-lateral aspect of the cranium, including the area just inferior to the ear, another area commonly symptomatic in patients with TMD (Fig. 18-9).

The facial nerve (cranial nerve VII) supplies efferent innervation to the muscles of facial expression.

Biomechanics and arthrokinematics

Position of rest. The stable rest position of the mandible represents an equilibrium between the resting muscle tone of the mandibular elevators and the forces of gravity. Joint stability demands continual contact between the fossa, the disc and the condyle, and the slight positive pressure provided by the muscle tone of the mandibular elevators assures this. When the head is held erect in a relaxed state, opposing teeth do not contact. The gap between occlusal surfaces in this resting posture, called the *freeway space,* varies from 2 to 4 mm.[25,33,35] People with abnormally increased activation of the mandibular elevators may have no freeway space at rest.

Centric occlusion. When the teeth contact maximally, the intercuspal position of centric occlusion has been reached. Complete mouth closure is dependent on the positioning of the teeth, which has led many to assume that faulty occlusion plays a role in TMJ dysfunction.[25,33,35] Stability in the position of centric occlusion is characterized by each posterior tooth interdigitating with two opposing teeth, a symmetrical increase in activity in the mandibular elevators, a symmetrical increase in intraarticular pressure, articulation of the condyle with the posterior aspect of the intermediate zone of the disc, and articulation of the condyle-disc complex with the anterior-superior aspect of the mandibular fossa. Deviations in the joint such as a bony anomaly, disc derangement, or muscle imbalance may alter the stable occlusal position.[33] Deviations in the occlusion itself, such as loss of posterior teeth or an increased overbite,

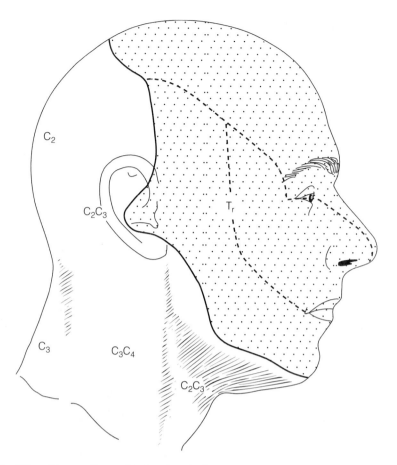

Fig. 18-9. Afferent innervation to skin by trigeminal nerve *(Tr)* and cervical nerves *(C₂C₃C₄)*. (From DuBrul EL: *Sicher's oral anatomy,* ed 7, St Louis, 1980, Mosby.)

may alter the stable position of the joint during occlusion. Physical therapists frequently must work as a team with a dentist to define and treat occlusal factors that are influential in TMD.

Mouth opening and closing. The inferior joint cavity of the TMJ is a hinge joint where the primary motion occurs during the first half of mouth opening and involves rotation of the condyle on the disc, with an accessory anterior glide. The anterior glide of the condyle-disc complex on the articular eminence occurs in the superior joint cavity and completes the process of opening the mouth.

Initial opening occurs as a hinge-type movement in the inferior joint cavity when the mandibular elevators relax enough to allow gravity to depress the mandible. The condyle rotates on the disc, and glides to the middle of its intermediate zone. The inferior lateral pterygoid muscle contracts early in this process to initiate slight anterior translation of the condyle.[2] The hinging motion predominates over the gliding motion for approximately 20 to 25 mm of opening. The rotation and anterior translation of the condyle makes the superior lateral pterygoid slack as the condyle approaches the anterior aspect of the intermediate zone of the disc during midopening. As the condyle translates anteriorly, the anterior disc thickness and the firm

attachment of the collateral ligaments result in anterior movement of the disc (Fig. 18-10, parts *1* to *3*).

At approximately 25 mm of opening, the oblique portion of the temporomandibular ligament tightens, resulting in anterior translation of the condyle-disc complex on the articular eminence of the temporal bone. This function is unique to humans and prevents encroachment by the mandible on anterior structures of the neck.[33] The inferior lateral pterygoids continue to contract, resulting in continued anterior translation. Bilateral contraction of the digastrics achieves full mandibular depression. At full mouth opening, the condyle resides in a slightly anterior position on the disc, the disc-condyle complex resides on the articular eminence, the superior lateral pterygoid is slack, and the retrodiscal tissue is lengthened (Fig. 18-10, parts *4* and *5*).

Closing is initiated by the mandibular elevators. Gliding of the condyle and disc occur in the posterior direction. Initially, the disc lags behind, but disc morphology and tightening of the collateral ligaments quickly result in posterior movement of the disc as the condyle moves posteriorly. When the mandible reaches the rest position, the normal muscle tone of the superior lateral pterygoid exerts a slight anterior pull on the disc, and the condyle is once

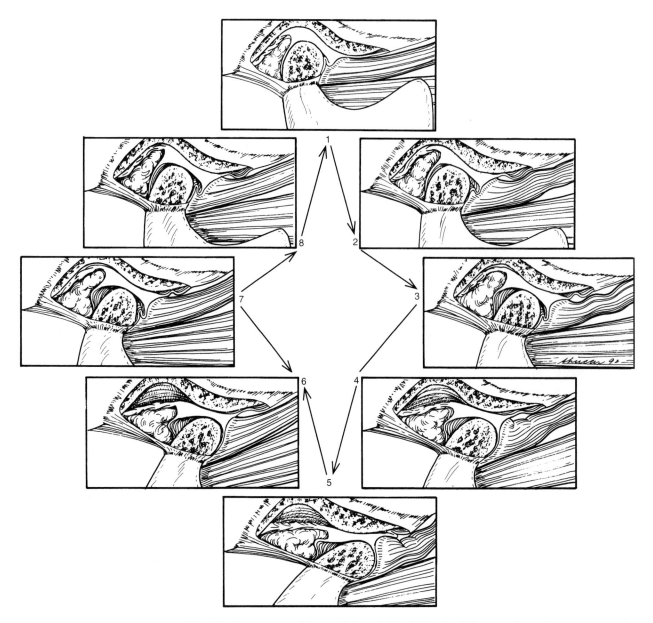

Fig. 18-10. Normal functional movement of the condyle and disc during the full range of opening *(1-5)* and closing *(5-8)*. (From Okeson J: *Management of temporomandibular disorders and occlusion,* St Louis, 1993, Mosby.)

again relating to the posterior aspect of the intermediate zone of the disc (Fig. 18-10, parts *5* to *8*).[33]

A *power stroke* of the mandible is defined as biting against resistance, as in biting down on a bolus of food. This action causes a fulcrum effect on the mandible, which results in increased intraarticular pressure in the TMJ on the side opposite the food and decreased intraarticular pressure in the ipsilateral joint. In order to maintain the constant contact necessary between the condyle, the disc, and the fossa, the superior lateral pterygoid contracts to achieve optimal positioning of the disc in an attempt to compensate for the pressure changes.[33] The superior lateral pterygoid is par-

ticularly active in contracting on the side where the bolus of food is present, thus bringing the posterior thickness of the intermediate zone of the disc to occupy the joint space created by the decrease in joint pressure. This is an excellent example of how the superior lateral pterygoid functions during the power stroke to maintain the optimal disc position on the condyle. When the power stroke is habitually performed in a parafunction such as clenching, the excessive anterior forces on the disc by the superior lateral pterygoid may put the disc in a position to be damaged by the increased intraarticular forces, although further research is needed to verify this theory.

Lateral excursion. The movements that occur at the right and left TMJs during lateral excursion are asymmetric. As the mandible moves laterally, the ipsilateral condyle rotates around a vertical axis, while the contralateral condyle-disc complex glides anteriorly, medially, and downward on the articular eminence. This movement is powered primarily by the contralateral medial and lateral pterygoids and the ipsilateral temporalis and masseter.[2]

Protrusion. Protrusion of the mandible is accomplished by simultaneous contraction of the inferior lateral pterygoids. The arthrokinematic result is a symmetric anterior glide of the condyle-disc complex on the articular eminence. Mandibular retrusion results from the contraction of the digastric and posterior fibers of the temporalis muscles.[2] It is significantly limited by the posterior aspect of the fossa, the highly innervated retrodiscal tissue, and the posterior thickness of the disc.

Function

Arthrokinematic and osteokinematic movements of the TMJs combine to produce chewing, swallowing, and speaking and are involved in other important functions such as emotional expression and respiration. Tearing and chewing involve not only mandibular elevation against resistance but also combinations of protrusion-retrusion and lateral deviation. Intraarticular pressure can be significantly increased on the side opposite the food and can result in pain if intraarticular inflammation is present.

Chewing food is the initial stage of digestion. The average number of chewing movements in one person per day is approximately 1800.[33] Eating harder foods such as steak or carrots requires stronger contractions from the muscles of mastication, resulting in increased intraarticular pressure as those muscles pull across the TMJ. In pathologies involving joint inflammation or musculotendinous dysfunction, eating such hard foods can result in pain. Temporary dietary restrictions to soft food are often utilized in management of these dysfunctions.

TEMPOROMANDIBULAR DISORDERS

Dysfunctions that involve the temporomandibular joint or the muscles of mastication are called *temporomandibular disorders,* or TMD. A clear understanding of the potential pathomechanics of the major systems implicated in TMD is essential to accurate diagnosis and implementation of a rational treatment approach. The three major systems discussed here are the joints, the muscles, and the dentition, with a summary of potential cervical spine conditions and systemic pathologies that can contribute to temporomandibular pain.

Pathomechanics

Joint derangements. Derangement of the relationship between the condyle and the disc is often seen in the patient with TMD. The passive stability in the relationship between the disc and the condyle is maintained in part by the firm attachment of the disc to the condyle by the collateral ligaments and also by disk and condyle morphology. This passive stability changes if the collateral ligaments become lengthened or if the shape of the disc or the condyle changes.

The collateral ligaments can lengthen through macrotrauma that results in condylar displacement. Examples of macrotrauma include a blow to the mandible, medical intubation, and forced mandibular depression during procedures such as molar extraction. Even yawning may cause macrotrauma in a person with a short, steep articular eminence. When the disc is no longer tightly attached to the condyle by the collateral ligaments, the disc tends to displace anteriorly and medially. Such an anterior displacement may result in thinning of the posterior aspect of the disc, especially in the presence of increased intraarticular pressure, such as clenching or chewing. The thinning of the posterior aspect of the disc contributes to the facilitation of the lengthening of the collaterals, and vice versa.

Microtrauma may also change the relationship between the condyle and the disc. A form of microtrauma in some patients with TMD is habitual parafunctional activities. Parafunction of the masticatory system involves nonfunctional and often subconscious or habitual activities, such as clenching and grinding of the teeth, bruxing (rhythmic grinding), nail biting, and chewing on the cheek. These activities involve nonfunctional use of the power stroke. Habitual parafunctional use of the power stroke results in increased occurrence of elevated intraarticular pressure and thus increased compressive forces to the disc. The result may be a change in disc morphology, particularly if the disc is positioned anteriorly on the condyle.[10]

Disc displacement/dislocation with reduction. A change in disc morphology and an increase in the length of the collateral ligaments can result in anterior displacement of the disc in relation to the condyle. The causal factors contribute to a cycle in which each perpetuates the other. The effect of these factors may be heightened by the anterior forces on the disc created if there is overactivity of the superior lateral pterygoid. A disc that is resting anteriorly to its original position but still relating to the condylar head at rest is considered displaced (Fig. 18-11, *A*). When a disc is displaced anteriorly, functional or parafunctional intraarticular forces may result in thinning of the posterior aspect of the disc.[10] Clinically, one of the first signs of displacement is the presence of a click upon opening or closing as the disc accesses the intermediate aspect of the disc during opening and glides off the intermediate aspect during closing. This condition is called *disc displacement with reduction,* and studies indicate its presence in significant numbers of the asymptomatic population.[22,24,36]

When the disc is anterior to the condyle and is no longer positioned on the condylar head, it is said to be dislocated (Fig. 18-11, *B*). Opening or closing clicks are also signs of disc dislocation. During opening, a click occurs as the

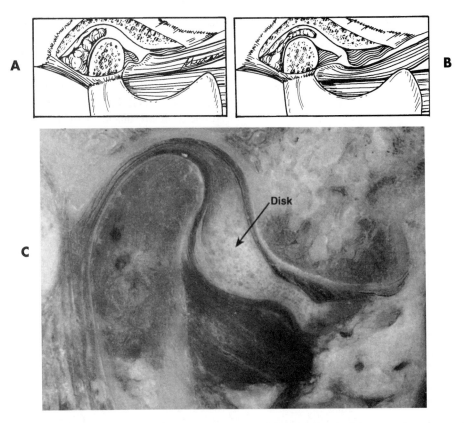

Fig. 18-11. A, Displaced disc. **B,** dislocated disc. In the dislocated disc the joint space has narrowed and the disc is trapped anteriorly. **C,** Specimen in which disc is dislocated anterior to the condyle. (**A** and **B** from Okeson J: *Management of temporomandibular disorders and occlusion,* St Louis, 1993, Mosby; **C,** courtesy of Dr. Per-lennart Westesson, University of Rochester, Rochester, NY.)

condyle accesses the posterior aspect of the disc. A reciprocal or closing click may also occur as the condyle glides off the disc during closing (Fig. 18-12). This combination of opening and closing clicks is referred to as a *reciprocal click* and is a diagnostic sign for an anterior disc displacement or dislocation. Such clicks are characterized by their intensity, their location during the movement of the mandible, and their association to the patient's pain. An opening click tends to be increased in intensity compared to the closing click. The location of the click in the range of movement can give information about the degree of anterior displacement or dislocation, with a late opening click and an early closing click indicating increased anterior positioning of the disc. The association that the clicks have with the patient's pain is important in determining the cause of the patient's pain.

The clinician utilizes palpation to detect clicks. (Specific procedures are discussed in the evaluation section.) The practitioner must understand two important facts when diagnosing disorders by clicks: The disc itself is essentially aneural, and compression resulting in altered morphology does not produce pain signals from the disc. In addition, numerous studies demonstrate the presence of reciprocal clicking or other TMJ sounds in up to 30% of the

asymptomatic population, implying that other processes must occur to cause pain when these pathomechanics are present.[22,24,33,36]

What is the outcome of the anteriorly displaced or dislocated disc? Studies indicate that in a portion of this population the joint sounds disappear with no intervention because of the compensatory remodeling capabilities present in the TMJ.[41] Another portion of this population may continue to have clicking for some time with no pain or dysfunction, and people in this population who progress to pain or dysfunction may find their way to the physical therapist's office.

Disc dislocation without reduction. Progression of anterior disc dislocation may proceed to the point where the condyle can no longer glide onto the disc during opening and the disc impedes anterior translation of the condyle during function (Fig. 18-13). This condition is known as *disc dislocation without reduction* or *closed lock.* Anterior translation of the condyle is necessary for full range of motion in the movements of mandibular depression, protrusion, and contralateral lateral excursion, and the range of these movements is decreased in the joint with this problem. Joint sounds disappear initially because the condyle is no

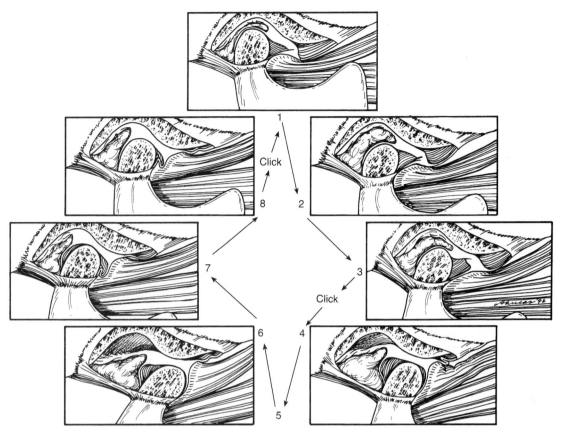

Fig. 18-12. Disc dislocation with reduction. During opening, the condyle passes over the posterior border of the disc onto the intermediate zone of the disc, thus reducing the dislocated disc. A click occurs with disc reduction and with disc dislocation. (From Okeson J: *Management of temporomandibular disorders and occlusion,* St Louis, 1993, Mosby.)

longer "clicking" onto the disc. The condylar head is articulating with the retrodiscal tissue throughout the range. This tissue was not designed to withstand continual compressive forces and responds to this trauma with the normal processes of inflammation, proliferation, and remodeling. In some individuals, the tissue remodels sufficiently to withstand such forces. In others, the retrodiscal tissue remains in a chronic state of inflammation that can progress to deterioration and perforation of the retrodiscal tissue.

Inflammatory processes

Retrodiscitis. As mentioned previously, anterior displacement or dislocation of the disc can contribute to other processes in the joint. When the disc is anteriorly displaced, the condyle begins its movement in mouth opening by rotating on the posterior aspect of the disc. Thinning of the disc posteriorly can result in further anterior displacement of the disc. When the condyle begins to articulate on the retrodiscal tissue, the disc is dislocated. Unlike the disc, the retrodiscal tissue is highly innervated and vascularized, and the trauma of compression during articulation by the condyle can result in an inflammatory process known as *retrodiscitis* (Fig. 18-14, *A*).

Capsulitis and synovitis. Displacement or dislocation of the disc or condyle through microtrauma or macrotrauma can also result in trauma to the capsule and/or synovium, resulting in capsulitis or synovitis. Chemicals released during the inflammatory process activate nociceptors, resulting in pain signals to the CNS. Joint effusion may also stimulate nociceptors mechanically through distention of the capsule. It is difficult to delineate clinically between retrodiscitis, capsulitis, and synovitis.[25,33] Each of these diagnoses can result in pain just anterior to the ear, known as *preauricular pain.* Chronic capsular inflammation can result in capsular fibrosis and scarring, decreasing capsular mobility and further altering the biomechanics of the joint.[25]

Arthritis. If retrodiscal tissue erodes, then erosion of the fibrocartilaginous surfaces of the condyle, fossa, and articular eminence may follow. An active inflammatory process during deterioration of joint surfaces is known as *arthritis;* in the absence of inflammation, this process is known as *arthrosis.* Joint sounds, known as *crepitus,* can result as the condyle articulates with the irregular eroding surfaces of the retrodiscal tissue and fibrocartilage of the fossa and eminence. As in most arthritic processes that progress, continued

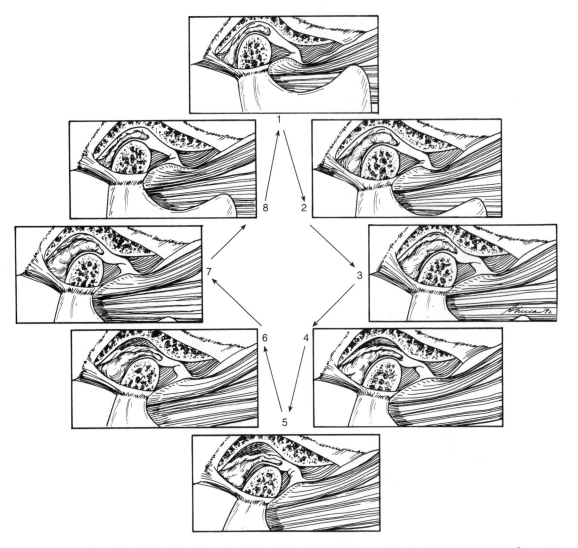

Fig. 18-13. Disc dislocation without reduction (closed lock). The condyle never assumes a normal relationship with the disc. The disc impedes anterior translation of the condyle. (From Okeson J: *Management of temporomandibular disorders and occlusion,* St Louis, 1993, Mosby.)

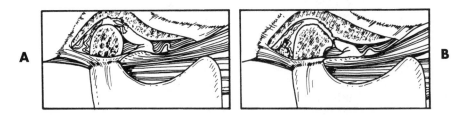

Fig. 18-14. Two potential dysfunctions resulting from internal derangement of the TMJ. **A,** Retrodiscitis and tissue breakdown. **B,** Osteoarthritis. (From Okeson J: *Management of temporomandibular disorders and occlusion,* St Louis, 1993, Mosby.)

erosion of the cartilage can result in exposure of the subchondral bone, development of bone spurs, and flattening of the condylar head (Fig. 18-14, *B*). Inflammation can result in preauricular pain. Further degeneration in the presence of chronic inflammation can lead to fibrous adhesions or bony ankylosis between the joint surfaces.

Research into TMJ arthritis and arthrosis continues. It is seen in women at a much higher rate than in men,[3] and researchers are beginning to study the gender-related aspects of this phenomenon. It has been suggested that primary osteoarthritis may be the cause of disc displacement rather than the result of it.[9]

The discerning practitioner must recognize that the patient may present anywhere in the outline of events described previously for joint derangement, inflammation, and degeneration and that the initiation of dysfunction does not imply a continued progression through these events. Although restriction of movement is often the end result of an arthritic process, such a restriction may not be painful or dysfunctional.[10] The patient's physiologic ability to remodel and adapt to changing relationships in the joint is the primary determinant of pain and dysfunction for the individual. Individual variation in this adaptability over time demands a conservative approach to treatment.

Hypermobility

If the condyle translates anteriorly to the articular eminence during mouth opening, TMJ hypermobility is considered to occur. This phenomenon is not always accompanied by pain or dysfunction, but it may be a perpetuating factor in some cases of capsulitis and retrodiscitis because of the increased stress to these tissues during an excessive anterior glide of the condyle. During an activity such as yawning, the patient with a hypermobile TMJ occasionally displaces the condyle anterior to the articular tubercle of the eminence and is unable to close his or her mouth. This condition is known as *open-lock* or *dislocation* and represents a form of macrotrauma that can be an initiating event for joint dysfunction.

Capsular fibrosis

Capsular fibrosis is not known to be a common problem in patients diagnosed with TMD. When it does occur, it is usually related to (1) capsular trauma, as in the surgical procedure of arthrotomy; (2) prolonged immobilization, as in osteotomy procedures that require wiring the mouth closed; or (3) infection in the joint. (Active and passive range of motion procedures for this problem are discussed in the treatment section.) In cases of multiple trauma from surgical procedures, infection, or chronic inflammation, fibrous ankylosis in the superior or inferior joint space can occur. In severe cases involving deterioration of intracapsular structures, a bony ankylosis is possible.

Masticatory muscle disorders

Temporomandibular disorders may be a function of a disorder of the masticatory muscles, which may or may not be accompanied by a joint derangement. The three diagnostic categories of masticatory muscle dysfunction most commonly seen clinically are protective cocontraction (muscle guarding), local muscle soreness, and myofascial pain with trigger points.

Protective cocontraction. Protective cocontraction, also known as *muscle guarding,* is a state of increased activation of the masticatory muscles by the central nervous system. This increased activation can occur in response to (1) afferent input from joint receptors during joint dysfunc-

tion,[44] (2) prolonged deep pain, as in chronic inflammatory processes,[23] (3) sympathetic nervous system response to emotional stress,[6] (4) habitual parafunction such as clenching, or (5) local masticatory muscle or tendon injury.

Most of the primary muscles of mastication are mandibular elevators, and increased activation results in increased intraarticular pressure of the TMJ. Normal fluctuation in intraarticular pressure during functional movement is the method by which synovial lubrication of the joint occurs. A prolonged abnormal increase in intraarticular pressure is inhibitory to the lubrication function of the synovial fluid and results in decreased nutrition to the intracapsular structures. Increased pressure on the disc in combination with decreased nutritional processes may be excessive for the tissue tolerance of the disc, resulting in structural damage such as perforation.

Local muscle soreness. Protective cocontraction is often a temporary functional response to trauma to the mandibular area. Protective cocontraction can result in a prolonged isometric contraction of the muscle, which contributes to decreased blood flow to the muscle and tendon. The tissue tolerance of the muscle or tendon may be exceeded, resulting in an inflammatory response and local muscle or tendon pain. This pain can stimulate further muscle guarding, exacerbating the cycle.

Local muscle or tendon soreness may also result from the microtrauma of repetitive stresses, as occurs in parafunction, or from macrotrauma to the muscle or tendon, as in dislocation of the joint because of a blow to the face.

Myofascial pain. Another common form of muscle dysfunction seen in patients with TMD is myofascial pain. Janet Travell defined *myofascial pain* in the early 1950s as regional involvement of the muscle, characterized by the presence of taut, hypersensitive bands known as *trigger points.* Trigger points have the ability to refer pain to areas away from the muscle location, confusing the inexperienced practitioner as to the source of the problem. Active trigger points in the upper trapezius and the sternocleidomastoid muscles refer pain to the temporal area and the eye. Active trigger points in the masseter and temporalis muscles refer pain to the eye or the teeth. The origin of trigger points is not well understood; they are thought to be related to a history of microtrauma or macrotrauma to the muscle.[40] Another theory suggests that they are related to central sensitization of peripheral nerves.[34] Successful approaches to their treatment are discussed in following sections.

In all of these muscle disorders, muscle pain or guarding may result in decreased range in movements that lengthen the mandibular elevators, such as mouth opening. Pain may inhibit movements that require firing of the muscles against resistance, as in chewing hard foods. The range of movement of lateral excursion and protrusion is not usually limited in the presence of a masticatory muscle disorder if a capsular or intracapsular dysfunction is not present.

The role of dental occlusion

When the mandible is elevated, the mouth is closed and contact is made at both TMJs and at the teeth. As discussed earlier, normal occlusion of the teeth involves convex surfaces complementing concave surfaces. In the position of TMJ stability during occlusion, the condylar heads are relating to the intermediate zone of the disc, and are in a superior-anterior position in the mandibular fossa. As seen in anterior disc dislocation, TMJ instability may result in instability in the occlusion. Instability in the occlusion can also result from such malocclusions as a deep overbite, a loss of overbite, or an anterior open bite, and this can contribute to TMJ instability (Fig. 18-15). The relationship between occlusal and TMJ instability is not linear, however, and each form of instability may exist without contributing to temporomandibular pain or dysfunction.[33] When there is a question about the role of occlusion in a patient with TMD, referral to a dentist experienced in treating TMD is essential.

Growth and development considerations

The most common forms of growth and development disorders of the TMJ are of the bones or muscles. Hypoplasia is a condition of decreased growth of bone, whereas hyperplasia implies too much growth. These conditions are manifested in the mandible by a significantly recessive chin (bilateral hypoplasia) or a significantly protruded chin (bilateral hyperplasia).[33] Unilateral occurrences can result in striking asymmetries and compensatory positioning. Given the body's natural tendencies toward healthy compensations, these conditions may be more aesthetically problematic than functionally disturbing. Treatment, if necessary, is usually with orthognathic surgery.

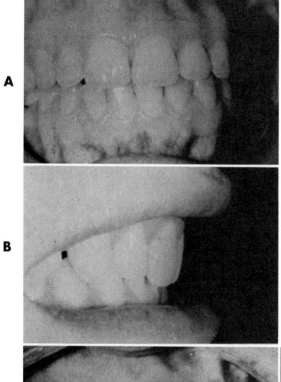

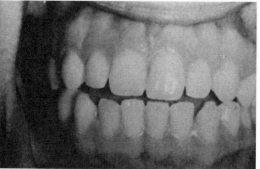

Fig. 18-15. Various types of occlusions. **A,** Normal. **B,** Deep overbite. **C,** Loss of overbite. **D,** Anterior open bite. (From Okeson J: *Management of temporomandibular disorders and occlusion,* St Louis, 1993, Mosby.)

Hypotrophy of muscle is usually related to a disorder such as multiple sclerosis causing muscle atrophy. Hypertrophy of muscle is often secondary to a chronic parafunction such as bruxism and may be treated with techniques to facilitate muscle relaxation.

Cervical spine considerations

The cervical spine may be a primary source of pain referral to the craniomandibular region or a contributing source to TMJ or masticatory muscle disorder. In one study, approximately one third of 215 TMD patients reported known history of trauma or injury to the cervical spine.[3] Pain contributions to the craniomandibular area come from cervical structures such as muscle, tendon, ligament, facet joints, and peripheral nerves, whose dysfunction may result from microtrauma such as work positions or from macrotrauma such as whiplash.

Contributions to temporomandibular pain from muscles of the cervical spine through trigger points and central sensitization have been discussed elsewhere in this chapter. One animal study illuminates the concept of central sensitization by demonstrating reflex activation of jaw muscles in response to irritation of deep cervical paraspinals.[19] Another study demonstrates that stimulation of the dorsal roots of C1 through C4 results in excitation of the muscles innervated by the trigeminal nerve.[21] Kraus discusses the mechanism of irritation of the greater occipital nerve (C2, C3) by suboccipital musculotendinous tissue, resulting in pain referral to the posterior cranium, a symptom often associated with TMD.[25]

Studies demonstrate facet joint pain referral patterns from C1 through C5 to the craniomandibular area, demonstrating the capacity of pain referral from the facet joint to mimic the location of pain found in TMD.[12]

Several authors discuss and demonstrate the importance of the posture and function of the cervical spine to the posture and function of the TMJ. The reader is referred to these authors for more thorough treatises on the subject.[14,20,25,27,35] In evaluating a patient with suspected TMD, the cervical spine must be screened for its contributions to the problem. See the Box for a discussion of headache disorders.

Differential diagnosis

Temporomandibular disorder is only one diagnosis under the classification system for headaches. The competent clinician must be able to determine when a referral to a headache specialist, or a neurologist, is warranted (see the Box).

Temporomandibular disorders can originate in systemic problems. Rheumatologic diseases such as rheumatoid arthritis or Reiter's syndrome cause inflammation of the synovium and deterioration of joint structures and are known to affect the TMJ. Diagnosis of these diseases is through serologic testing by a rheumatologist, and their management includes working as a team with the rheumatologist.

Fibromyalgia is a chronic muscle disorder involving multiple sites of pain throughout the body. Its origin is not well understood, and it is currently characterized by the presence of defined tender spots in multiple muscles throughout the body, accompanied by other specific symptomatology such as sleep disturbances. As with many dysfunctions, it is thought to be aggravated by emotional stress.[15] The diagnosis can be confused by the additional

---

Headache disorders

The International Headache Society's classification system for headache disorders, cranial neuralgias, and facial pain includes TMJ disorders and masticatory muscle disorders as components of this system.[16] Among many other components to the classification, three of the more common headache diagnoses encountered by the clinician are the migraine headache, the tension-type headache, and the cervicogenic headache. The presenting symptoms can be similar for all three: a feeling of a tight band around the head, a pulsing or throbbing pain, a feeling of pressure outward or inward on the eyes, nausea, tinnitus, visual and auditory disturbances, and dizziness. Migraine headaches result from vasodilation of intracranial or extracranial arteries and are treated with vasoconstrictor medications. Although plausible theories have been proposed, research on the etiology of the vasodilation is still inconclusive. Migraine headaches are usually associated with triggers such as light, sounds, certain foods, alcohol, and emotional stressors, but these triggers are individual to each patient. For a patient presenting with both migraine headaches and TMD, the TMD may be a trigger for the migraine. Eliminating the TMD can result in improved management of the migraine headaches.

Tension-type headaches and cervicogenic headaches overlap in many respects.[13] A tension-type headache implies symptoms whose etiology is secondary to increased muscular tension in the craniocervical areas. Headaches of cervicogenic etiology are referred from the muscles, the joints, the peripheral nerves or their roots, or the arteries of the cervical spine. The demonstration of influences between the cervical structures and the facial structures through central convergence in the cervical component of the trigeminal nucleus in the spinal cord leaves little doubt about the possibility of a relationship between cervicogenic or tension-type headaches and TMD.[14,38] They may also coexist with migraine headaches, rendering them potential triggers for migraines. Physical therapy may have much to offer this patient in terms of treating the muscle or joint problems and their origins.

presence of a masticatory muscle disorder or TMJ derangement. The patient with this diagnosis is best treated with a multidisciplinary team approach, with a rheumatologist as part of the team.

Benign or malignant tumors may present in or in close proximity to the structures associated with the temporomandibular joint. They may mimic TMD symptomatology as a secondary consequence to their location. Symptoms such as unrelenting pain of unexplained origin or neurologic deficits always require additional medical referral and diagnostic imaging.

Pathologies affecting intracranial structures such as neoplasms, aneurysms, abcesses, or hemorrhage must always be considered in the presence of CNS signs and symptoms such as nausea, balance disorders, visual changes, and cranial nerve disorders.

Compression of the facial nerve (cranial nerve VII) in Bell's palsy results in paralysis of the muscles of facial expression innervated by this nerve.

Trigeminal neuralgia, also known as *tic douloureux,* is a rare condition causing intermittent sharp, shooting pain in a unilateral distribution of the trigeminal nerve (cranial nerve V), that is triggered by stimuli such as light touch, cold, and wind. Its onset appears to be spontaneous, and its origin is related to posterior fossa pathology. It is treated pharmacologically and with nerve blocks.

EVALUATION OF THE TMJ AND ASSOCIATED STRUCTURES

Evaluating the patient with craniomandibular pain requires remembering that 50% to 60% of the general population presents with symptoms present in the TMD population, such as joint sounds, intermittent masticatory muscle pain, and deviations in mandibular mobility.[33] Many of these people do not have pain or dysfunction of enough significance to prompt them to seek treatment. Such statistics accentuate the necessity for thoroughness in evaluation and amplify the need for caution in basing diagnosis on limited evaluations.

Patient history and subjective report

A thorough history defines the course of the evaluation. Specific concerns integral to evaluating the patient presenting with TMD symptoms include gaining information about dental history, cervical spine history, psychologic stressors, previous treatment, and previous physical therapy. The history is often the key factor in determining if referral for further medical, dental, or psychological evaluation is needed.

A complete assessment of the patient's pain, which is essential in the final diagnosis, includes understanding the location, onset, frequency, intensity, nature, and daily patterns. Although a discussion about the physiology of pain is beyond the scope of this chapter, an understanding of the complexity of pain mediation and of the difficulty in

individual evaluation is necessary for the clinician who attempts to treat patients with TMD.[4,11,29,33,38]

The patient with pain involving joint pathology usually presents with preauricular pain, with or without reference to the temporalis or masseter area, which changes (increases or decreases) with jaw function (Fig. 18-16). If pain referral exists, the patient may describe unilateral or bilateral generalized headache pain. Other associated symptoms may involve ear symptoms such as tinnitus, vertigo, ear pain, or ear stuffiness. As mentioned in the section on pathomechanics, joint pathology is often accompanied by dysfunction of the muscles of mastication.

The patient with pain originating from the muscles of mastication may also report pain in the temporalis or masseter area, frequently described as a generalized or local headache, depending on the muscles involved. Trigger points in the muscles of mastication can refer pain to the teeth, to the posterior aspect of the eye, and to other locations in the posterior and superior aspects of the skull.[40] Pain originating in the lateral pterygoid muscle or tendon is preauricular in location. Pain originating from temporalis tendinitis presents around the tendinous insertion on the coronoid process and anterior ramus of the mandible.

If a patient's pain occurs primarily upon waking in the morning, the therapist should be concerned that an activity such as bruxing may be occurring intermittently throughout the night. Morning pain due to nocturnal bruxing is often felt in the area of the temporalis muscle. If the pain occurs only after normal jaw function throughout the day, then tissues involved in function, such as the joint or the muscles of mastication, should be considered. If the pain is most evident during or after activities requiring cervical function, but is not associated with mandibular function, the discerning

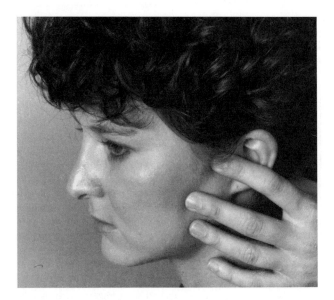

Fig. 18-16. Index finger is on location of preauricular pain resulting from joint pathology. Pain resulting from the lateral pterygoid muscle may also be preauricular in location.

therapist defines the role of the cervical spine with a thorough cervical evaluation. If the patient is having pain in other areas of the body, the therapist may consider systemic possibilities, such as fibromyalgia or rheumatic disease, which require evaluation by a physician such as a rheumatologist.

In addition to craniomandibular and cervical pain, other symptoms sometimes reported by patients with TMD include joint sounds, visual disturbances, balance problems, ear stuffiness, a feeling of an altered occlusion, and difficulty opening or closing the mouth.[25,33,35]

The therapist should note activities of daily living involving use of the mouth, such as singing or playing a wind instrument, or activities that involve ergonomically compromised positions of the neck, such as telephone work. Particular note should be taken of habitual parafunctional activities, such as nail biting, cheek biting, gum chewing, and clenching, which may cause muscle dysfunction through overuse or joint pain by increasing intraarticular pressure. Patients are often unaware of habitual parafunction such as clenching or grinding, particularly if it occurs primarily at night. Careful questioning may not reveal such activities, and other signs or symptoms such as morning headaches in the temporal region must be considered. Examples of pain and history presentations for TMD is most commonly seen clinically are presented in the Box on p. 571.

Physical exam

Inspection of facial symmetry and posture. Inspection of facial symmetry gives the therapist information about alterations in the bony and/or soft tissue structures. An anterior view of facial symmetry can best be assessed by comparing the transverse planes of the eyes, the ears, and the mouth. These three planes are parallel in normal structure.[35] Significant deviations from this relationship should be noted.

A thorough postural assessment gives the clinician information about influences from the spine and shoulder girdle. Scoliosis or upper thoracic kyphosis may have significant effects on the cervical spine and thus secondarily contribute to facial pain. Significant forward head postures may play a role in cervical spine joint and soft tissue dysfunction, and head posture can influence mandibular posture.[25,27,35,44]

Inspection of cervical and TMJ guarding patterns during the interview gives the clinician information about compensatory or dysfunctional posturing. The rest position of the mandible should allow for a slight space between the upper and lower teeth. Shallow, rapid breathing patterns may also be observed; they can contribute to or be a result of increased dysfunction in the area secondary to increased sympathetic nervous system activation.[6]

Mobility assessment: range of motion. During mobility assessments, the therapist is evaluating quantity and quality of mobility, as well as pain production and, if possible, end feel.

Mandibular depression. Mandibular depression or mouth opening is measured with a millimeter ruler from mandibular incisor edge to maxillary incisor edge (Fig. 18-17, *A*). Given the variability in facial development, the prevalence of altered mandibular biomechanics in the asymptomatic population, and variations with age, absolute norms cannot be established. Openings of 40 to 55 mm are considered within normal limits, and a measure as low as 35 mm is often considered functional in the absence of pain and dysfunction.[25,33,35] A screen for functional restriction is performed by evaluating the patient's ability to place two flexed proximal interphalangeal joints horizontally between the incisors (Fig. 18-17, *B*).

Restrictions in mouth opening may be caused by capsular tightness, protective cocontraction of the masticatory muscles, anteriorly displaced disc(s), or pain. End-range mouth opening stresses by lengthening the elevator muscles and their tendons, the capsule and the TM ligament, and the retrodiscal tissue. Restrictions in mouth opening due to pain may occur from such pathologies as retrodiscitis, capsulitis, temporalis tendinitis, TMJ arthritis, and masticatory muscle disorder.

Asymmetry of function between right and left TMJs in mouth opening may result in a deflection or a deviation in opening. A deflection is movement of the mandible laterally at the end range of opening; it may indicate the unilateral presence of one of the mechanical or painful restrictions mentioned previously (Fig. 18-18, *A*). A deviation occurs if the mandible deviates laterally during opening and then returns to the midline at the end range of opening (Fig. 18-18, *B*). Deviations suggest such conditions as disc dislocation with reduction unilaterally or bilaterally, an asymmetry in muscle firing due to a masticatory muscle dysfunction, or an asymmetry in bony structure.

When evaluating mouth opening, the therapist compares the measure of comfortable mouth opening with the measure of opening into the painful range in order to discriminate between a mechanical restriction, such as a shortened capsule, and a painful restriction, such as soreness in the mandibular elevators. If the restriction is due to pain in the mandibular elevators, the patient can usually open further into the painful range. A mechanical restriction allows little to no movement once the block has been reached.

The antagonistic movement to mandibular depression is mandibular elevation, or mouth closing. Mouth closing against resistance, as in chewing hard foods or clenching, stresses the mandibular elevators and increases intraarticular pressure. Such movements can reproduce pain in the presence of joint or muscle dysfunction. The location of the pain may help to discriminate between joint and muscle if both are not in dysfunction. Inability to close the mouth (open-lock) may occur if the condyle dislocates anteriorly to the articular tubercle or if the rare event of a posteriorly dislocated disc occurs.

Lateral excursion. Lateral excursion of the mandible is

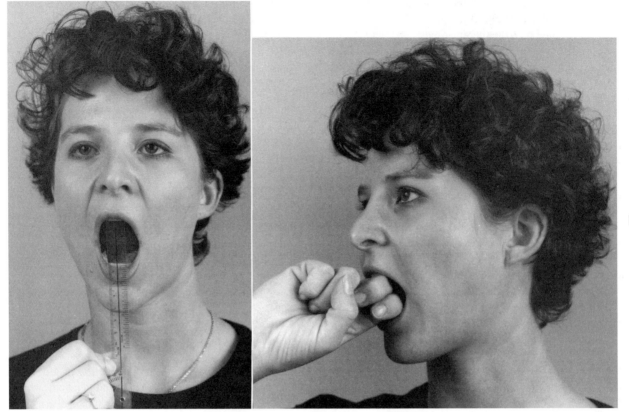

Fig. 18-17. **A,** Measurement of mandibular depression (mouth opening) using a mm ruler. **B,** Screen for functional mouth opening.

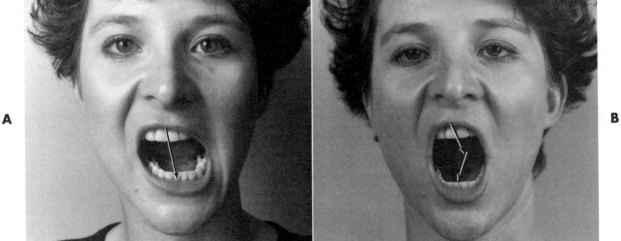

Fig. 18-18. **A,** Deflection of mandible during mouth opening indicating a unilateral restriction in range of motion on the side of the deflection. **B,** Deviation of mandible during mouth opening indicating asymmetry in function from right to left TMJ. Note the mandible returns to the midline with a deviation.

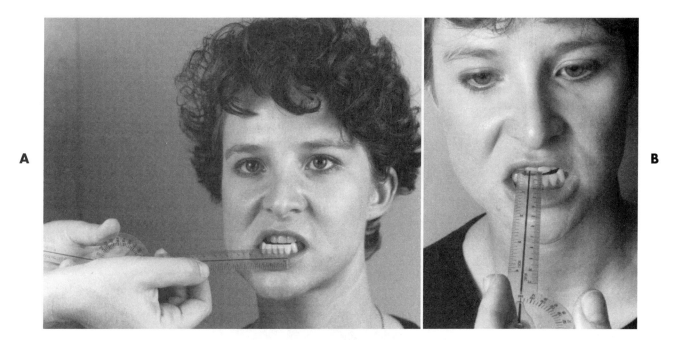

Fig. 18-19. A, Measurement of lateral excursion. **B,** Measurement of protrusion.

measured by placing a millimeter ruler on the maxillary teeth at the midline of the mandibular incisors. The patient is asked to move the mandible laterally and the distance moved by the mandibular incisor midline is measured (Fig. 18-19, *A*). Less than 8 mm of lateral excursion is considered restricted.[33] Lateral excursion can be restricted by inability of the contralateral condyle to translate anteriorly. Mechanical restrictions to anterior translation include disc derangement and capsular tightening. Painful restriction of anterior translation of the condyle can be caused by retrodiscitis and capsulitis. The inferior lateral pterygoid participates in active anterior condylar translation, and problems with this muscle or tendon may restrict contralateral lateral excursion.

Protrusion. Most people have the ability to protrude the mandibular incisors 5 to 10 mm past the maxillary incisors.[25] The minimal range recommended for functional protrusion is the ability to bring the tip of the mandibular incisors to the tip of the maxillary incisors. The horizontal distance is measured with a millimeter ruler (Fig. 18-19, *B*). Restrictions are due to an inability of the condyle(s) to translate anteriorly, which may be due to mechanical blocks (dislocated disc, shortened capsule) or pain (retrodiscitis, capsulitis, dysfunction of the lateral pterygoid). A deflection in one direction at the end of the range indicates the probability of a unilateral restriction on the side of the deflection. Protrusion is not limited by guarding of the mandibular elevators and is used to differentiate involvement of these muscles. For example, a restriction in opening that is not accompanied by a restriction or deviation in protrusion is suggestive of a dysfunction in the masseter, the temporalis, or the medial pterygoid.

A unilateral capsular pattern of the TMJ, indicating a dysfunction of the entire capsule, is characterized by decreased mouth opening with deflection to the restricted side, decreased protrusion with deflection to the restricted side, and decreased lateral excursion to the side opposite the restriction.

Joint sounds. The presence of joint sounds during mandibular function is related to intracapsular alterations in function. Joint sounds may be detected through palpation of the lateral aspect of the condyles, just anterior to the tragus of the ears, during opening or closing (Fig. 18-20, *A*). An alternative method involves gentle placement of the therapist's little fingers in the ear canal during opening and closing (Fig. 18-20, *B*). Use of a stethoscope over the preauricular area during opening and closing increases the auditory component for the therapist (Fig. 18-20, *C*).

A click is a single sound that may occur during opening, closing, or both (reciprocal click) as the condyle glides over the posterior aspect of the displaced or dislocated disc (see Fig. 18-12). The location of the opening click gives information about the magnitude of anterior displacement, with a minimal displacement resulting in an early click as the condyle regains access to the intermediate aspect of the disc early in translation. Generally, if reciprocal clicks are present, the opening click is more pronounced than the closing click. Clicking may also occur with protrusion or lateral excursion, as both involve anterior translation of the condyle. The therapist should note if pain is associated with clicking. Nevertheless, a significant percentage of the asymptomatic population reports clicks, and diagnosis based only on joint sounds is not prudent.

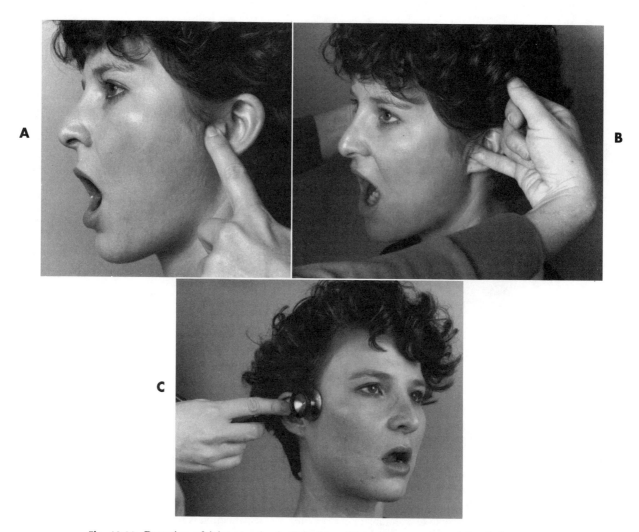

Fig. 18-20. Detection of joint sounds. **A,** Palpation of lateral aspect of condyles during mouth opening. **B,** Gentle placement of therapist's little fingers in ear canals during mouth opening. **C,** Use of a stethoscope to increase the auditory component.

Crepitus sounds like movement across gravel and is usually the result of changes resulting from deterioration of the disc, retrodiscal tissues, or joint surfaces. Crepitus may occur when the condyle articulates for prolonged periods of time on deteriorated retrodiscal tissue. This condition may progress to the point of articulation of the joint surface of the condyle with the fossa or articular eminence, resulting in erosion of the fibrocartilage and arthritis (see Fig. 18-14, *B*).

Palpation. A thorough knowledge of the anatomy is essential in palpating structures of the craniomandibular area. Because of their vulnerability to overuse during parafunction or to increased tone in response to joint dysfunction, the muscles of mastication and their tendons should be palpated for tenderness, active trigger points, and a change in tissue texture or temperature.

The temporalis muscle is large and fanlike and is palpated along its posterior horizontal fibers, its middle oblique fibers, and its anterior vertical fibers (Fig. 18-21, *A*). The anterior fibers may be tender in response to overuse in bruxing or

clenching. Patients who brux during sleep often report temporal headaches upon waking. The proximity of the anterior fibers to the orbit of the eye may result in pain referral around the eye. The insertion of the temporalis tendon on the coronoid process and anterior ramus is palpated intraorally by the therapist placing the finger on the ramus of the mandible and traveling to its superior aspect (Fig. 18-21, *B*). The tendon is stressed during the microtrauma of parafunction and can develop inflammation proceeding to tendinitis when its tissue tolerance is exceeded.

The masseter muscle has a superficial portion that can be palpated with bilateral manual palpation beginning inferior to the zygomatic arch and traveling inferiorly and posteriorly to the angle of the mandible (Fig. 18-21, *C*). The patient's masseter is easily viewed when the patient clenches. The deep portion of the masseter is palpated intraorally deep to the anterior aspect of the superior portion. Both muscle bellies may exhibit tenderness or trigger points in response to microtrauma such as bruxing or to macrotrauma.

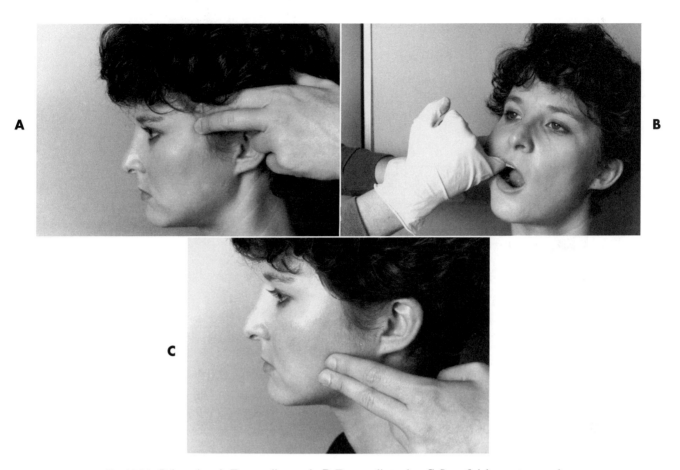

Fig. 18-21. Palpatation. **A,** Temporalis muscle. **B,** Temporalis tendon. **C,** Superficial masseter muscle.

Reliably palpating the medial pterygoid muscle is difficult, and the lateral pterygoid is not palpable. Special tests to discern their involvement are discussed in a following section.

Palpation of the posterior cervical muscles, such as upper trapezius, levator scapulae, semispinalis, and splenius capitis, and of the anterior and lateral muscles, such as the sternocleidomastoid, scalenes, and the suprahyoids, is an essential element of the exam. Trigger point referral and reproduction of facial pain are possible during palpation of the cervical spine tissues. Palpation of tendinous insertions along the occiput and mastoid processes frequently results in reproduction of local tenderness or pain in the symptomatic patient. Palpation of the articular pillar of the cervical spine gives information about pain, tenderness, and swelling in the facet joints.

Extraoral palpation of the TMJ is performed bilaterally in the open- and closed-mouth positions with the therapist's fingertips on the lateral and posterior aspects of the head of the condyle (Fig. 18-22). If there is difficulty discerning the area, the therapist should palpate the moving condyle while the patient is performing small movements of opening and closing the mouth. Pain to palpation in the lateral aspect of the TMJ may indicate inflammation in the capsule or

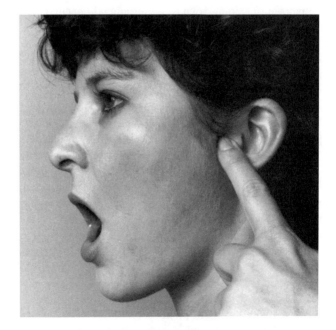

Fig. 18-22. Palpation of TMJ. Pain in the lateral aspect may indicate capsular or synovial inflammation; pain in the posterior aspect may indicate inflammation in the retrodiscal tissues or posterior capsule.

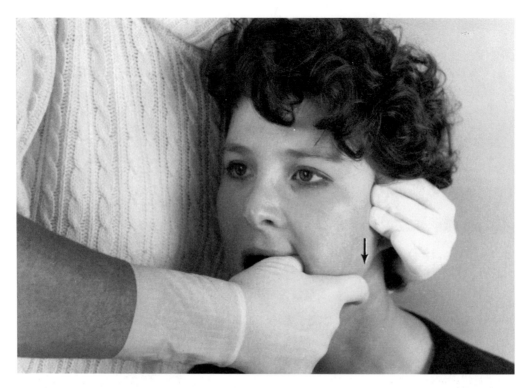

Fig. 18-23. Special test: applying distractive force to the TMJ. The therapist's mobilizing thumb is placed over the mandibular molars, the patient's head is stabilized, and the therapist's stabilizing hand is palpating movement at the joint. The force is gentle and directed caudally. This technique is also employed in joint mobilization.

synovium in this area. Pain to palpation in the posterior aspect may indicate inflammation in the posterior capsule or retrodiscal tissues. This point in the evaluation is appropriate to palpate for joint sounds during mouth opening and closing.

Special tests: Application of distractive and compressive forces. Special tests to apply distractive or compressive forces to the joints will give information about the joint's response to unloading (distraction) and loading (compression). Distractive forces are applied with the therapist standing at the sitting patient's contralateral side, with thumb placed over the mandibular molars and pressing caudally (Fig. 18-23). Distraction here does not imply an actual separation of joint surfaces, but rather a decrease in the intraarticular pressure of the joint. This decrease in pressure may relieve pain associated with intracapsular inflammatory processes of the joint. It may stress the joint capsule and reproduce pain in the presence of capsulitis. Application of distractive forces may be used to evaluate accessory motion and capsular mobility.

Loading the joint can be achieved actively or passively. Pain secondary to synovitis, retrodiscitis, and arthritis is increased with loading. The masseter muscle is a powerful mandibular elevator, and dynamic loading of the joints occurs bilaterally during clenching. Selective dynamic

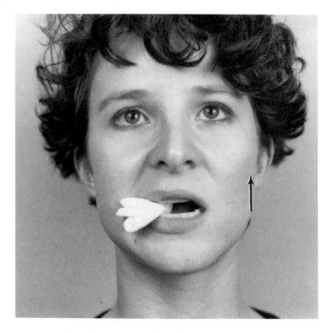

Fig. 18-24. Special test: dynamic loading (increased intraarticular pressure) occurs to the TMJ opposite the cotton roll secondary to the torque of the mandible that occurs. Intraarticular pressure decreases on the ipsilateral side.

loading occurs when the patient bites down on a cotton roll. The mandibular torque produced results in increased intraarticular pressure (loading) of the contralateral TMJ and decreased intraarticular pressure (unloading) of the ipsilateral TMJ (Fig. 18-24). Pain on the side contralateral to the

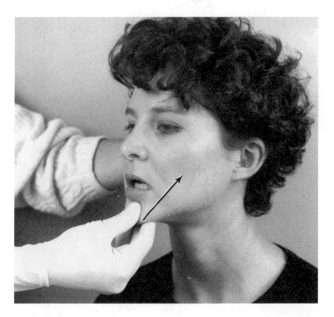

Fig. 18-25. Special test: passive loading of the posterior aspect of the TMJ to screen for inflammation in retrodiscal tissues or in posterior joint structures.

cotton roll may indicate an inflammatory process in the joint, particularly if pain is not produced on the ipsilateral side. The superior lateral pterygoid muscle is activated during this maneuver, particularly on the ipsilateral side, and may cause ipsilateral preauricular pain if these musculotendinous fibers are in dysfunction.

Pain in the mandibular elevators or their tendons may also occur on either side with this maneuver if they are in dysfunction. Passive joint loading is necessary to further differentiate between joint and musculotendinous sources of pain. The therapist loads the posterior aspect of the joint, which causes compression of the retrodiscal tissue, by grasping the patient's chin and applying pressure posteriorly and superiorly (Fig. 18-25). The therapist loads the superior aspect of the TMJ by pressing down on the anterior aspect of the mandible and up on the border of the mandible (Fig. 18-26).

Manual muscle testing. Muscle testing of the mandibular elevators (masseter, medial pterygoid, and temporalis) may be done by resisting mouth closure (Fig. 18-27, *A*). Detectable weakness in these muscles is not common in the patient with TMD, and pain with resistance may be due to the increase in intraarticular pressure if intraarticular problems are present, resulting in limited usefulness in this testing. Resistance to lateral excursion stresses the contralateral medial and lateral pterygoid, and resistance to mouth opening stresses the suprahyoid muscles, giving limited

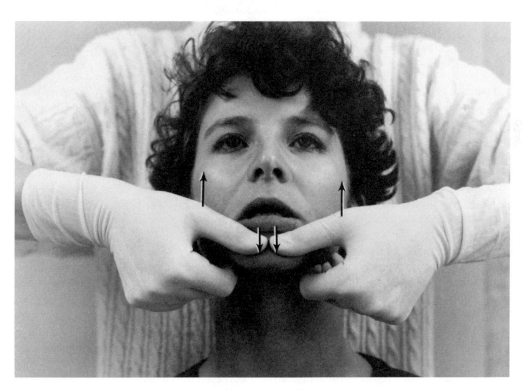

Fig. 18-26. Special test: passive loading of the superior aspect of the TMJ to screen for inflammation in superior joint structures, including the capsule and synovium.

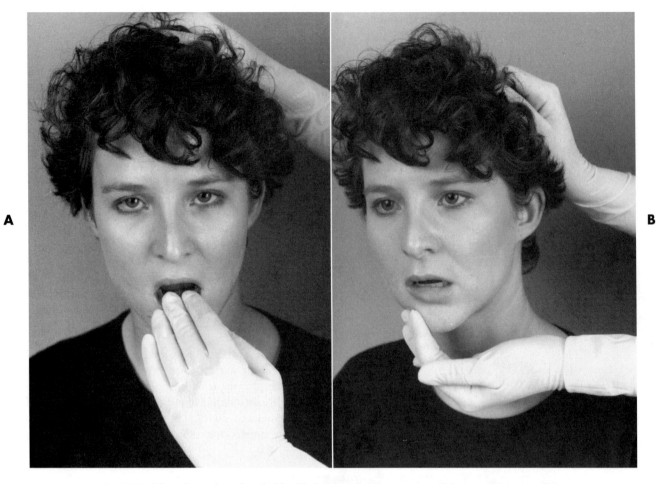

Fig. 18-27. Manual muscle testing. **A,** Mandibular elevation (masseter, medial pterygoid, temporalis).
B, Lateral excursion (contralateral medial and lateral pterygoid).

information about pain reproduction from these tissues (Fig.
18-27, *B* and *C*).

Accurately palpating or stretching the lateral pterygoid is
difficult. Therapist resistance to mandibular protrusion is an
identifying exam for dysfunction of the lateral pterygoid
(Fig. 18-27, *D*). The procedure described for biting down on
the cotton roll accentuates the contraction of the ipsilateral
superior lateral pterygoid, giving additional information
about its ability to reproduce pain (see Fig. 18-24).

Neurologic screen. A neurologic screen of the cranial
nerves is important in determining the presence of neurologic involvement. With practice, a screen is quick and gives
essential information about the need for further medical
input. The reader should have access to various texts to
review the evaluation of the cranial nerve system. The
trigeminal nerve (cranial nerve V) is the primary sensory
nerve to the face, nose, and mouth; it provides efferent
innervation to the muscles of mastication. Sensory input can
be evaluated by comparing patient responses to bilateral
stroking of the face with cotton or gauze. Evaluation of the
motor function of muscles innervated by the trigeminal
nerve is completed with resisted muscle testing as described

previously. The myotactic tendon reflex test for the masseter
muscle is performed by tapping the mandible, either directly
or through a tongue depressor (Fig. 18-28). This reflex test
gives information about the functional innervation of the
masseter by the trigeminal nerve, and may give information
about the activation of this muscle in terms of its established
tonicity.

The facial nerve (cranial nerve VII) innervates the
muscles of facial expression and is evaluated with a screen
of these muscles.

The therapist also must note the dermatomal distribution
for cervical nerve roots C2 through C4 (see Fig. 18-9).
Dysfunction involving the nerve roots of the upper cervical
spine may contribute to sensory alterations in the posterior
or lateral cranium.

Cervical spine evaluation. The therapist who is evaluating the patient with suspected TMD should always
evaluate the cervical spine to ascertain its contributions to
the problem. The evaluation should pay special attention to
daily postures and functions, range of motion, soft tissue
mobility, facet joint mobility, soft tissue response to
palpation, neurologic signs, and vertebral artery signs. The

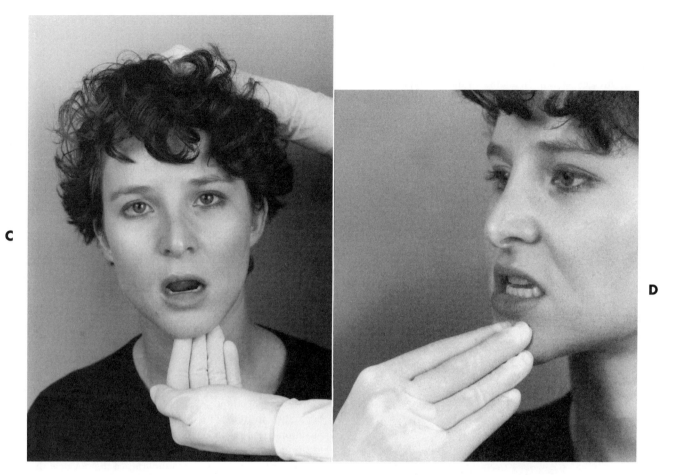

Fig. 18-27, cont'd.   C, Mandibular depression (suprahyoid muscles). **D,** Protrusion (lateral pterygoid). Note that resistance to protrusion is the most useful screen for detecting pain coming from the lateral pterygoid muscle.

therapist evaluates specifically for reproduction of craniomandibular pain. Cervical pain of significant intensity or duration, however, may contribute to sensitization at a central nervous system level and contribute to pain and muscle hyperactivity in structures of the craniomandibular area.[11,14,25,33]

Screening of the oral cavity. The physical therapist cannot perform a full dental evaluation and should refer to a dentist for specific information about occlusion, tooth wear, dental health, and occlusal contacts during mandibular movements. However, the physical therapist can perform a cursory screen of the oral cavity for the patient who has not seen a dentist. The screen entails taking a general dental-history about problems and procedures, noting the patient's association between dental history and pain and the patient's report of alterations in normal occlusion, observing the occlusion, particularly obvious abnormalities such as an anterior open bite, a significant overbite, or an asymmetry of occlusion (see Fig. 18-15), and evaluating pain with jaw function. The assessment made as a result of the entire evaluation determines the appropriateness of referral to the dentist.

Psychologic considerations

Pain and suffering are interpreted by the higher centers of the brain, which determine a person's response to dysfunction. Carlson and colleagues note several features of facial pain that highlight the importance of psychological factors, including the psychologic meaning for the patient of facial and oral pain, the role of physiologic sympathetic overreaction to psychologic trauma, and the potential psychologic trauma experienced during the development of the physical dysfunction. The variation in patient beliefs about the interaction between the mind and the body, as well as the varied beliefs of health care practitioners, requires that this area be addressed with caution and skill.[6]

TMJ imaging

Various approaches to imaging the TMJ complement or clarify clinical evaluation findings. The panoramic radiograph is widely used by dentists to give an adequate screening view of the condition of the condyles (Fig. 18-29). The lateral transcranial view and the anterior-posterior (A-P) views are sometimes utilized, but the imposition of bony surfaces makes these views more difficult to interpret for condylar defects. Tomograms are a type of radiograph that gives a clearer view of the condyles both laterally and in the A-P view. Their expense and higher dosage of radiation make them less practical for the typical patient. Radiographic images such as flattening of the condylar head and lipping at its margins are utilized to determine the degree of deterioration of subchondral bone in a diagnosis of TMJ arthritis. Arthritis implies an active inflammatory process

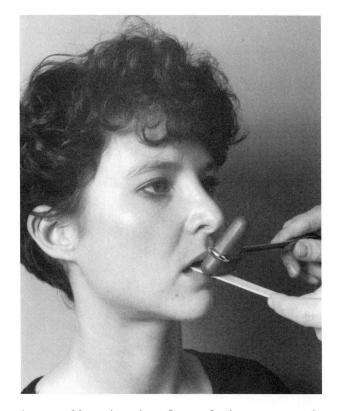

Fig. 18-28. Myotactic tendon reflex test for the masseter muscle.

and cannot be discriminated from arthrosis in radiographic imaging. Arthrosis is frequently asymptomatic.[10] Other suspected conditions such as calcification of the ligaments attaching to the styloid process, elongation of the coronoid process, or bony developmental anomalies may also be confirmed through radiology.

Radiographs view bony contours and are not useful in further defining suspected soft tissue problems, such as an anterior disc dislocation. Arthrograms involve fluoroscopic imaging of a TMJ that has been injected with a radiopaque medium. The injection, which is usually into the lower joint space, can delineate disc position or perforations. These findings are tempered, however, because the introduction of dye can alter joint relationships minimally. The precision needed and the resultant discomfort for the patient require a highly skilled practitioner in performing the procedure.

Computerized tomography and magnetic resonance imaging (MRI) are increasing in popularity as tools for imaging soft tissue disorders of the TMJ. According to one study, the MRI was found to be more reliable in detecting soft tissue pathology such as disc deterioration and tendinitis than an arthrogram, whereas the arthrogram was found to be more reliable than the MRI for determining disc position.[37]

Nevertheless, these tools should not be used alone in diagnosing pathology. Moreover, the TMJ may have a deviation in form with no symptoms, which emphasizes the caution required in pursuit of the diagnosis with imaging techniques.

Refer to the Boxes for summaries of the physical therapy evaluation and case studies of three TMD diagnoses commonly seen in the clinic.

PHYSICAL THERAPY APPROACH TO TMD

The objectives of the physical therapist in treating the patient with TMD may include the following: (1) patient

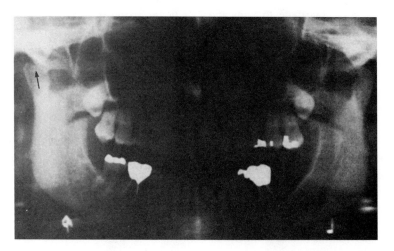

Fig. 18-29. The panoramic radiograph is widely used by dentists to screen for condylar defects such as flattening of the condylar head, osteophyte formation, or lipping. Note flattening of right condyle *(arrow)* secondary to osteoarthritic changes. (From Okeson J: *Management of temporomandibular disorders and occlusion,* St Louis, 1993, Mosby.)

education, (2) management of inflammation, (3) modulation and/or management of pain, (4) restoration of normal function, (5) evaluation and treatment of adjacent areas as appropriate, and (6) referral to other medical resources as needed.

This chapter has discussed the evaluation of the patient's joints and muscles. Screening of psychologic stressors, accomplished through the subjective history, gives information about the need for further psychologic evaluation and support. Screening the oral cavity, oral history, and occlusion gives the therapist information regarding the need for a dental referral. A multidisciplinary team, including a dentist and a psychologist, is frequently necessary for the proper care of the patient with TMD. Differential diagnosis screening leads to referral to medical specialists such as a neurologist or a rheumatologist, as appropriate.

Improper sequencing of treatment or overtreatment are common criticisms heard of treatment approaches for the patient with TMD. An emphasis on prioritizing and proper

sequencing of treatment helps to confirm the diagnosis and increases the possibility of success, even with a team involving only two medical professionals. The approach must be driven by a skillful assessment or reassessment and tailored to the needs of the individual patient and the patient's response to treatment.

Treatment of joint derangement

As mentioned previously, many people have TMJ sounds and evidence of joint abnormalities but do not seek treatment unless pain is present. Most medical teams consider the presence of pain to be a decisive criterion in determining the magnitude of intervention with the TMD patient. Given the masticatory system's efficient ability to remodel, erring on the side of conservative care is wise in approaching treatment for this patient.

If the patient with a joint derangement has symptoms, they are usually related to inflammation of the retrodiscal tissue, the capsule, the synovium, or the subchondral bone or

---

Evaluation summary

Chief complaint and history

Pain
- Location
- Nature, character, intensity
- Onset, frequency, duration, change over time
- Increased by ?
- Decreased by ?

Dysfunction
- Interference with daily or nightly activities
- Sleep interference
- Eating interference

Associated symptoms
- Headache, numbness, tingling, neck pain, earache, auditory disturbances, visual disturbances, mouth or tooth pain, dizziness, nausea

Activities of daily and nightly living
Habitual activities/parafunction
Life stressors
Past medical history, medication, past trauma
Dental history
Treatment history
Patient's goals

Physical exam

Inspection
- Cranial structure: facial development, symmetry
- Posture: axial, shoulder, mandibular
- Skin color, scars
- Splints

Function: mobility (restriction, pain, deflection, deviation, asymmetry)
- Mouth opening and closing
- Lateral excursion
- Protrusion, retrusion

Joint sounds (opening click, closing click, crepitus)
- Does protruding while opening change joint sounds?

Palpation (tenderness, tissue texture, trigger point referral of pain)
- Temporalis muscle and tendon
- Masseter muscle and tendon
- TMJ, lateral and posterior: mouth open, mouth closed
- Cervical spine musculature and facets
- Occiput and mastoid process

Special tests
- Passive application of distractive forces by therapist
- Passive compression of posterior joint space by therapist
- Passive compression of superior joint space by therapist
- Dynamic simultaneous compression and distraction (biting on a cotton roll)

Muscle testing (strength, pain, function)
- Resistance to mouth opening and closing
- Resistance to lateral excursion
- Resistance to protrusion (lateral pterygoid)
- Function of muscles of facial expression
- Function of tongue and lips

Neurologic screen
- Sensory (face, scalp, posterior cranium, C-spine, upper extremities)
- Reflexes (include masseter reflex)
- Motor
- Cranial nerves

Cervical spine evaluation

Oral cavity screen
- Overall oral health
- Malocclusions

Psychological considerations
Diagnostic imaging

Samples of evaluation findings for patients with TMD

Diagnosis: retrodiscitis, right TMJ; anterior disc dislocation with reduction, right TMJ

History and chief complaint

    Right preauricular pain with recent increase in intensity

    Pain prevalent after periods of jaw functioning, particularly mastication

    Pain decreases with rest of TMJ, antiinflammatories, ice, or heat

    Pain interferes with eating

    History of popping and clicking, insidious onset

    Upon further questioning may remember trauma such as dislocation during a yawn or problem during dental work

Physical exam

    Mobility: normal ROM, may see deviation on opening, right preauricular pain with retrusion

    Joint sounds: reciprocal click on right; click disappears with opening while protruded

    Special tests: increased right preauricular pain with passive compression of posterior joint space; increased right preauricular pain when biting on cotton roll placed on left

    Palpation: tender in posterior joint area with mouth open and closed

    Muscle test: negative

(Note: If accompanied by masticatory muscle disorder, evaluation findings may differ.)

Diagnosis: synovitis, right TMJ; anterior disc dislocation without reduction, right TMJ

Chief complaint and history

    Right preauricular pain

    Pain increases with jaw usage

    Pain decreases with rest, antiinflammatories, heat, or ice

    Pain and loss of mobility interfere with eating

    History of popping, now gone or changed to crepitus-like sounds

    Prior history of macrotrauma may be remembered

    May have history of habitual parafunction

    May note change in occlusion

Physical exam

    Mobility: ROM: decreased opening with deflection to right,

decreased left lateral excursion, decreased protrusion with deflection to right

Joint sounds: may have none or crepitus on right

Special tests: passive application of distractive force elicits pain on right, passive compression of superior or posterior joint space elicits right preauricular pain, biting on cotton roll on left elicits right preauricular pain

Palpation: tender in lateral joint space

Muscle testing: negative

(Note: If accompanied by masticatory muscle disorder, evaluation findings may differ.)

Diagnosis: masticatory muscle disorder

Chief complaint and history

    Unilateral or bilateral masseter or temporalis pain, pain anterior to TMJ if lateral pterygoid involved

    Increases with jaw usage

    Decreases with rest, unless subconscious parafunction occurs at rest

    Interferes with eating and, if parafunction, sleep

    May have morning temporal headaches if nocturnal bruxism

    Patient or patient's significant other may note parafunctional activity

    Patient may note increased life stressors

    May note cervical spine problems.

Physical exam

    Mobility: ROM: decreased pain-free opening, can increase opening into painful range, normal lateral excursion and protrusion

    Joint sounds: may or may not be present

    Special tests: Biting on cotton roll may reproduce pain in involved muscle secondary to use of the muscle; passive application of distractive and compressive forces are negative

    Palpation: tender in affected muscles

    Muscle testing: may have pain with resistance to mouth closing; pain with resistance to protrusion if lateral pterygoid is in dysfunction

    Cervical spine screen may have positive findings

(Note: If accompanied by joint derangement, evaluation findings may differ.)

---

to a secondary masticatory muscle disorder. The PT goals are to decrease pain, manage inflammation, and restore comfortable function.

Patient education. The first approach to treatment involves educating the patient about the nature of the problem and how to decrease intraarticular pressures by decreasing the intensity of the activity of the muscles of mastication. Inflammation around the joint is frequently exacerbated by muscular activities that significantly increase intraarticular pressure, such as eating hard foods, biting fingernails, chewing ice, clenching, and bruxing. Advising the patient to eat soft foods and refrain from parafunctional

activities in order to decrease the intraarticular pressure is the initial approach to treatment. It should be accompanied with education about the rest position of the mouth (teeth slightly apart) and the importance of breathing fully during respiration. Education often gives patients enough reassurance to help them manage their pain and decreases barriers to healing by decreasing intraarticular pressures.

Parafunctional activities performed during waking hours may be resolved with increased cognitive awareness by the patient or with biofeedback techniques to decrease masseter and temporalis activity. Nocturnal parafunctional activity is more difficult to decrease, with biofeedback for relaxation

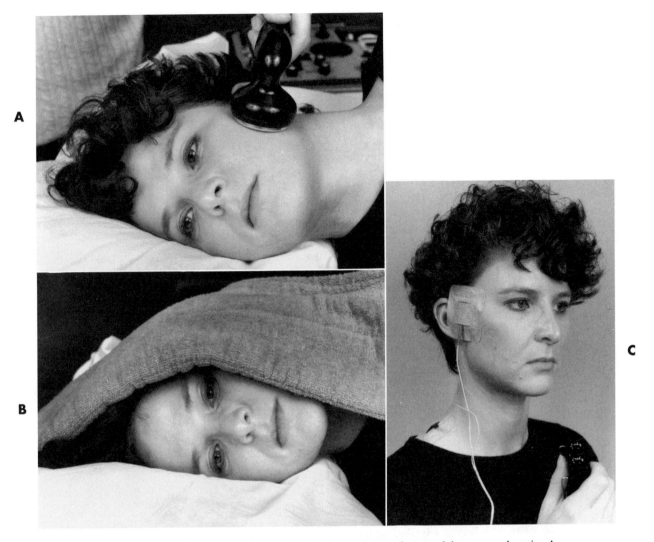

Fig. 18-30. Modalities used to manage joint inflammation or decrease joint or muscle pain. **A,** Ultrasound to the joint or muscles. **B,** Heat to muscles of mastication. **C,** Transcutaneous electrical stimulation for preauricular pain.

prior to sleep having only minimal success.[31] Referral to a psychologist or other professional trained in treating sleep disorders may be necessary.

Occasionally an inflammatory response is related to a hypermobile TMJ. Education then includes information about restricting excessive mouth opening during activities such as yawning. The patient can decrease the extent of opening by placing a hand under the mandible during opening.

Modalities. In some patients, modalities may be added as an adjunct to education or precursor to manual techniques or exercise. Research regarding the effectiveness of modalities in decreasing pain and restricting inflammation is increasing.[17,30] Research specific to the masticatory system is needed, mandating judicious utilization of modalities.[31]

Modalities such as ice, nonthermal ultrasound, phonophoresis, and iontophoresis have been used to deal with inflammation of the TMJ. Electrical stimulation, ultrasound,

ice, and heat are often used to decrease pain produced by inflammatory processes within the joint (Fig. 18-30).

If the inflammation is the result of an anteriorly displaced disc, and these conservative measures are not successful, the dentist may fabricate a splint, a resin appliance that covers the maxillary or mandibular teeth and repositions the mandible anteriorly during closing, bringing the condyle to rest on the displaced disc (Fig. 18-31). Such repositioning allows tissue healing by decreasing stress on the retrodiscal tissue but is not considered conservative because of the potential for permanent changes in the occlusion. The long-term success of anterior repositioning splints has been questioned in the literature,[39] although they may give enough short-term relief to interrupt the cycle of pain and inflammation.

Treatment for disc dislocation without reduction. The patient with this diagnosis has usually progressed from a disc displacement with reduction to a dislocation. If inflammation

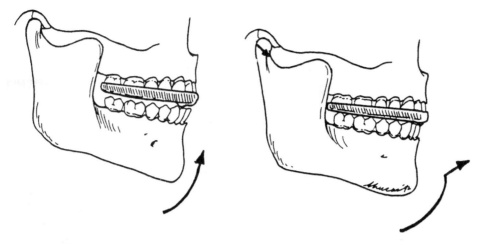

Fig. 18-31. The anterior repositioning appliance causes the mandible to assume a more forward position during closure, creating a more favorable condyle-disc relationship and decreasing pressures on retrodiscal tissues if the disc is dislocated anteriorly. (From Okeson J: *Management of temporomandibular disorders and occlusion,* St Louis, 1993, Mosby.)

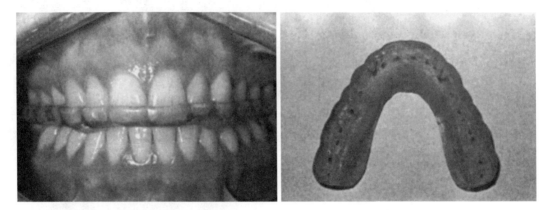

Fig. 18-32. The muscle relaxation appliance does not reposition the mandible. It decreases hyperactivity of the masticatory muscles by interrupting habitual parafunction and is often used only during sleeping hours. (From Okeson J: *Management of temporomandibular disorders and occlusion,* St Louis, 1993, Mosby.)

is a problem, then the goals are to manage inflammation and pain and to restore as much normal functioning as possible within pain-tolerant limits. Hyperactivity in the masticatory muscles may result in response to the joint dysfunction, and muscle hyperactivity must be treated with education and relaxation techniques.

The dental approach to decreasing offending stressors on the retrodiscal tissues may include use of antiinflammatory medication and an anterior repositioning splint. If masticatory muscle hyperactivity is causing increased pain and intraarticular pressure, the dentist may fabricate a resting mouth splint for use at night to interrupt habitual bruxing patterns. A resting splint (sometimes called a *muscle relaxation splint*) does not reposition the mandible (Fig. 18-32).

In response to decreased TMJ mobility in the patient with disc dislocation without reduction, the capsule and ligamentous structures may begin to exhibit tissue changes, such as increased viscosity of ground substance, increased binding between collagen fibers, decreased extensibility, and shortening. Grades III and IV mobilizations are used to lengthen connective tissue and can be performed to the TMJ capsule if inflammation is not significant. Mobilizations using distractive force are performed with the patient sitting, the therapist's thumb on the molars, and the therapist pressing caudally (Fig. 18-23). Lateral mobilizations to the capsule are performed in a similar position, with the force of the thumb directed slightly caudally and laterally. To ascertain patient response, initial mobilizations to the capsule should be grades I and II.

If shortening of connective tissue or muscle is limiting mobility, the patient may perform self-stretching techniques after mobilizations (Fig. 18-33). Another stretching technique for connective tissue uses tongue depressors to provide a sustained stretch to the capsule (Fig. 18-34). Instead of reversing the problem, some of these treatments are designed

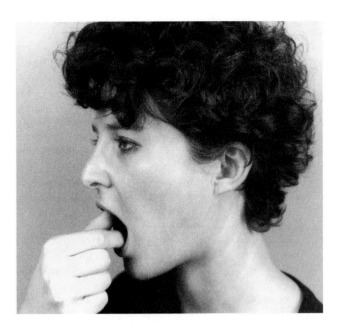

Fig. 18-33. A self-stretching technique to lengthen connective tissue or muscle.

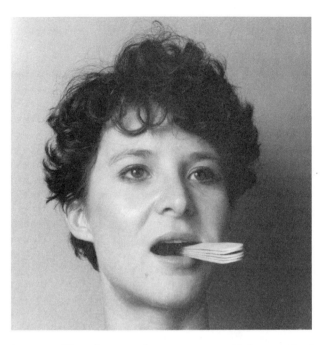

Fig. 18-34. Use of tongue depressors to provided a sustained distractive stretch to the capsule.

to restore as much function as possible by eliminating inflammation and increasing range of mouth opening without disc reduction; they are particularly useful to the patient who is able to adapt well to the dislocated disc by functional remodeling of the retrodiscal tissue. In the presence of chronic pain and inflammation, however, deterioration of the retrodiscal tissue may occur, and more aggressive approaches to treatment, such as surgery, may be recommended.

Treatment for masticatory muscle disorders

Protective cocontraction of the primary muscles of mastication may occur in response to joint derangements. Hyperactivity or hypertonicity of the muscles of mastication results in increased intraarticular pressure that may exacerbate local muscle soreness, tendinitis, trigger points, and joint inflammation. The PT goals for the patient diagnosed with a masticatory muscle disorder include decreasing parafunction, decreasing pain, inactivating trigger points, and restoring comfortable function through restoring functional muscle length and coordination.[7]

Education. Education is the initial and ongoing approach for treatment of masticatory muscle disorders. Education begins with an explanation of the problem to reassure the patient about the source of the pain. Education continues with information about decreasing conscious parafunctional activity. If nocturnal bruxing is a primary determinant of pain for this patient, consultation with a professional trained in dealing with sleep disorders may be appropriate.

Dentists often fabricate a resting night splint to interrupt the activity of nocturnal bruxing (Fig. 18-32). The goal of

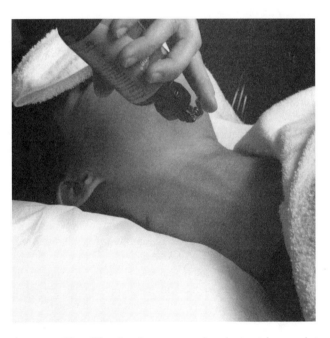

Fig. 18-35. Use of fluorimethane spray to inactivate a trigger point from the sternocleidomastoid, which is referring pain to the temporal area.

this splint is to facilitate muscle relaxation. It is hypothesized that relaxation occurs as a result of altering sensory and proprioceptive feedback to the brain, thus interrupting habitual firing patterns in the brain. These splints seem to be most effective if used intermittently rather than continuously.[33]

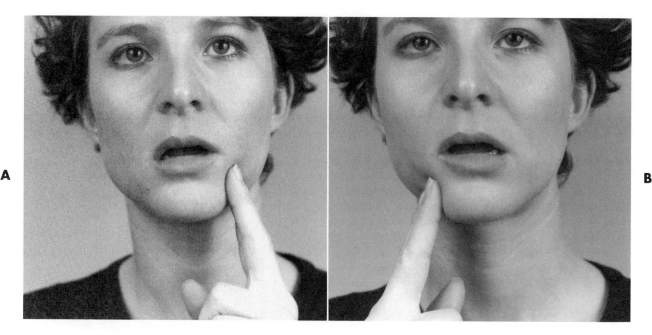

Fig. 18-36. An exercise using short, alternating, submaximal isometric contractions for each range of mandibular movement is thought to increase normal function in these muscles. **A,** Left lateral excursion. **B,** Right lateral excursion.

Medications are sometimes successfully utilized to facilitate better sleep patterns in patients who have excessive nocturnal parafunction. Mild antidepressants have improved sleep quality for some patients.

Modalities. Moist heat, ultrasound, or electrical stimulation to the muscles in dysfunction may decrease pain and facilitate muscular relaxation in the short term. Patients often note the lack of carryover with these modalities, which emphasizes the need for combining them with education, soft tissue mobilization, or exercise, as indicated.

Overuse of the temporalis muscle frequently occurs with parafunction and sometimes results in temporalis tendinitis. The pain and inflammation of tendinitis may respond positively to modalities such as iontophoresis, phonophoresis, ice, or ultrasound.

The use of fluorimethane spray while the muscle is stretched has been successful in decreasing trigger point activity in the masticatory and cervical spine muscles.[40] Care must be taken to shield the patient's face while using this chemical (Fig. 18-35). Ultrasound phonophoresis and electrical stimulation to trigger points have potential success with decreasing trigger point activity. Dentists frequently employ anesthetic injections to trigger points to decrease their activity. Such injections may also be diagnostic in differentiating the source of the patient's pain.

Manual therapy to the facial muscles. Soft tissue mobilization to the masseter or temporalis has been advocated to relax the muscle and treat trigger points.[5] Some therapists recommend the use of hold-relax techniques with the mandibular elevator muscles to facilitate agonist relaxation through autogenic inhibition or with the mandibular depressors to facilitate reciprocal inhibition of the masticatory muscles. Care must be taken not to increase muscle activity with this technique.

Exercises for the patient with TMD

The primary purpose of utilizing facial exercises in the patient with TMD is neuromuscular reeducation, with the goals of normalizing muscle tone, enhancing coordination and TMJ awareness, and the restoration of comfortable function through retraining normal movement patterns. Strength training is employed when significant weakness results from such diagnoses as Bell's palsy or facial nerve neuropathy resulting from surgery or a tumor.

Submaximal isometric exercises to the mandible—alternately resisting opening, closing, lateral excursion, and protrusion—are useful in increasing blood flow to the muscles and increasing patient awareness of the muscles (Fig. 18-36). An exercise of opening the mouth repetitively while maintaining the tongue on the roof of the mouth provides exercise to the muscles and nutrition to joint structures while controlling the magnitude of opening (Fig. 18-37). It may prevent the deteriorating effects of immobility and can promote relaxation and neuromuscular reeducation in the muscles of mastication.

Active range-of-motion exercises for lateral excursion and protrusion can be initiated when anterior condylar translation no longer puts undue stress on healing tissues and increased capsular and myofascial mobility is the goal.

An aerobic exercise program has been found to decrease

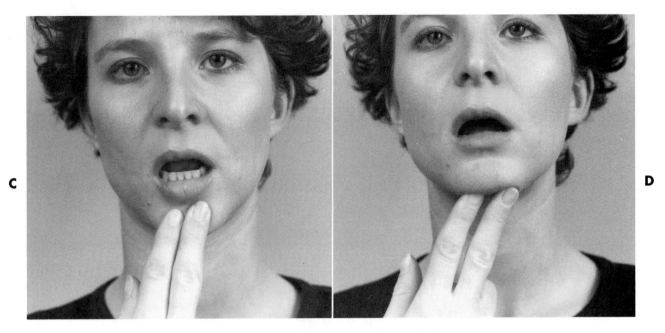

Fig. 18-36, cont'd.   C, Mandibular elevation. **D,** Mandibular depression.

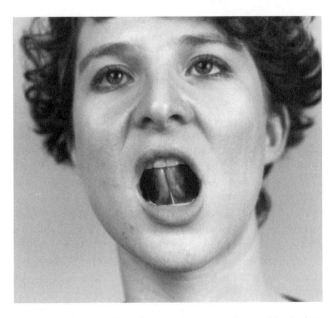

Fig. 18-37. An exercise of opening the mouth repetitively into midrange is thought to increase nutrition to joint structures and normalize functions in the muscles of mastication. Note that the tongue remains on the roof of the mouth during opening, which decreases the possibility of opening into a painful range.

pain perception ratings and increase overall feelings of well-being in patient and nonpatient subjects. It has been used with limited success in treating patients diagnosed with fibromyalgia.[28]

A full upper quarter screen can dictate the initiation of exercises for postural correction, for lengthening cervical spine muscles or tendons, and for strengthening.

Treatment of the cervical spine

The importance of treatment for cervical spine dysfunction in the patient with TMD cannot be overemphasized. Dysfunction in the cervical spine may be the source of craniomandibular pain or an exacerbating factor. Frequently the only member of the team with sufficient knowledge and experience to treat the spine is the physical therapist.

Surgical approaches for TMD

Surgical approaches to treating TMD have evolved significantly during the last decade. The two primary types of surgery performed to treat TMD are arthroscopy and arthrotomy. Orthognathic surgery is less frequent, and all surgeries are considered only after appropriate conservative approaches to treat pain and dysfunction have failed. Postoperative physical therapy may be necessary to treat the effects of presurgical and postsurgical immobilization, inflammation, pain, and weakness.

Arthroscopy. Arthroscopy has evolved dramatically in the last decade in treating TMD because of its success and because it is less invasive than other surgical approaches. This procedure involves two 2-mm incisions in the posterior and lateral joint areas. The oral surgeon utilizes a small-diameter needle-scope to view the superior joint space for adhesions, inflammatory debris, irregularities in the soft tissue, and disc positioning. In addition to its evaluative capacity, arthroscopy is utilized to perform surgical procedures, including lavage of the superior joint space to eliminate inflammatory by-products, lysis of adhesions in the superior joint space and anterior capsular attachments, and disc repositioning. It has a high success rate in the short term for decreasing pain and increasing function in the

CASE 1 ▼ Chief Complaint and History

A 38-year-old woman presented with a complaint of right preauricular pain and right temporal headaches that were worse in the morning and at the end of the day. Pain level fluctuated between 7 and 9 on a 10-point scale. She is the chief financial officer for a large company who performs long periods of desk and phone activity. Pain began 4 weeks ago after a particularly lengthy dental procedure requiring full-mouth opening for a prolonged period. Patient's spouse reported that patient has a long history of bruxing at night. Patient decreased pain with aspirin in the morning and heat at night, but it was present upon waking each morning.

Physical Exam (Positive Findings)

Mobility: ROM is within normal limits, with deviation on opening mouth

Joint sounds: reciprocal click on right reproduced right preauricular pain

Special tests: passive joint compression of posterior joint space was painful; biting on cotton roll on left was painful in right preauricular area

Clenching: painful in right preauricular and right temporal areas

Palpation: painful right temporalis muscle, right posterior TMJ space

Cervical screen: negative for reproduction of facial pain, although patient reported intermittent cervical problems related to work positions

Assessment

Retrodiscitis; anterior disc dislocation with reduction; masticatory muscle disorder right temporalis.

Treatment

Dentist ordered regimen of antiinflammatories and referred to PT, who provided education about decreasing parafunction, keeping teeth apart at rest, eating softer foods for 1 to 2 weeks, and using heat or ice on the temporalis at home.

Patient's preauricular pain decreased to 3 in 1 week; temporalis pain still at a level of 6; nocturnal bruxing continues.

Ultrasound and soft tissue mobilization to temporalis muscle began at 3 times a week, with education about postural improvement and cervical spine care during activities of daily living. Her dentist fabricated a resting night splint for her. In 2 weeks her preauricular pain was at a level of 1, and her temporal pain fluctuated between 2 and 4, depending on the amount of emotional stress in her day. Patient was referred to a psychologist for stress reduction education. She continued in PT twice a week with an emphasis on aerobic exercise and a gradual decrease in ultrasound and soft tissue mobilization. She reported only negligible pain in 2 weeks and was discontinued from PT with a home exercise program.

---

appropriate patient. This success does not seem to be related to improved positioning of the disc on the condyle but rather to improved joint mobility.[8,32] Further research regarding long-term effects continues.

Arthrotomy and orthognathic surgery. Arthrotomy, or open joint surgery, involves a face-lift type of incision just anterior to the ear and surgical entry into the joint through the lateral aspect of the capsule. It has been used to treat disc dislocations and soft tissue perforations when conservative means have failed. Procedures that have been performed during arthrotomy include disc plication (relocation with suturing), discectomy with replacement using allogenic materials (Teflon, Proplast), discectomy using autogenic material (ear cartilage, fascia), discectomy with no replacement, suturing of perforated discs, and shaving of debris from the condylar head. Surgical success depends in part on stringent criteria in patient selection and exhaustion of more conservative approaches. The evolution of arthroscopy seems to be decreasing the need for this more invasive approach.

Orthognathic surgery is occasionally indicated for the patient with TMD when bony abnormalities result in malalignment of teeth and joints in a patient whose masticatory system is unable to adapt. It is usually considered the most invasive of the surgical approaches and often involves osteotomy and repositioning of the mandible or maxilla.

Postsurgical physical therapy. Physical therapy is utilized postoperatively to decrease the continuation of inflammation and pain and to promote normal TMJ function. Positive relationships are documented in the literature for postsurgical patients receiving PT and their rate of return to normal function.[1] Other PT goals may involve normalizing posture and decreasing dysfunction of the cervical spine, as needed.

Communication with the oral surgeon about the surgical procedure is imperative in order to understand the tissues involved in the surgery and the original diagnosis. A preoperative evaluation is extremely beneficial in understanding the status of the tissues prior to surgery and in educating the patient about postoperative procedures. A thorough understanding of the normal stages of inflammation, proliferation, and remodeling guides the therapist through the appropriate protocols and helps delineate deviations from the normal healing process.

In the first 1 to 2 weeks, during the acute inflammatory phase, the therapist may use cryotherapy and electrical stimulation to decrease pain and muscle guarding and to

CASE 2 ▼ Chief Complaint and History

A 44-year-old man presented with pain in the area of the right temporalis, around the cranium superior to the ear, and in the right mastoid and suboccipital area. It has fluctuated between 4 and 8 for the last 2 years. In the last month, it has stayed at a level of 8. He has worked as a car mechanic for 15 years, spends long working days in positions stressful to the cervical spine, and reported a long history of neck pain and stiffness. His pain increased at the end of the working day and was decreased upon waking in the morning. He can decrease his pain temporarily with heat and massage.

Physical Exam (Positive Findings)

TMJ mobility: within normal limits

Joint sounds: reciprocal clicking noted on right and left

Special tests: TMJ compression and unloading tests negative

Palpation: tenderness right temporalis, masseter, suboccipital, mastoid, right sternocleidomastoid (SCM), right and left upper trapezius, all cervical facet joints on right, lower left cervical facet joints. Trigger point referral of pain from trapezius and SCM to suboccipital, mastoid, and temporal areas.

Cervical spine evaluation: decreased ROM in all directions, with reproduction of symptoms upon left side bending, right rotation, flexion, and extension. Accessory motion testing reveals decreased extension of the upper and lower right cervical facets and decreased extension of the left lower facets. Pain reproduction with extension of upper cervical facets on right.

Assessment

Cervical spine dysfunction; decreased facet mobility, particularly in right upper cervical; trigger point pain referral in right upper trap, right SCM, and right suboccipital muscles.

Treatment

PT initiated moist heat, electrical stimulation, and ultrasound to the right and left cervical areas, with emphasis on trigger point areas, followed by low-grade mobilizations to upper and lower right cervical spine facets and mild soft-tissue mobilization to posterior cervical spine muscles. Exercises for postural improvement and cervical range of motion were initiated in the first week. After three visits the first week, the patient reported pain decreased to a level of 6, although he continued to have significant pain by the end of the work day.

The PT modalities continued in week 2, with joint mobilizations increased to grade IV, and soft tissue mobilization continued, 3 times weekly. The PT also performed passive stretching using fluorimethane spray to both upper trapezius and SCM. Exercises increased to include passive stretching techniques for the lateral cervical muscles and strengthening for the cervical and thoracic extensors. The patient reported pain at a level of 4 by end of week 2.

The PT used moist heat prior to manual therapy in week 3, but stopped administering ultrasound and electrical stimulation. Manual therapy continued. Exercises continued to increase to include more upper body strengthening, an aerobic component, and job simulation activities. After ergonomic evaluation of the patient's workplace, PT recommended modifications to decrease the degree of stress on patient's spine. Patient reported pain at a level of 3 by end of week.

In week 4, manual therapy continued prior to exercise and job simulation activities, 3 times weekly. The patient was educated about use of equipment in a neighborhood gym. He reported his pain fluctuating between 1 and 2. In weeks 5 and 6 he is seen once for follow-up, exercise review, and reevaluation. He was then discharged.

---

restrict inflammation. Pulsed ultrasound may be helpful in restricting the progression of inflammation. A progression to submaximal isometrics and controlled mouth opening with the tongue maintained against the roof of the mouth may be initiated during or at the end of this period.

With decreased inflammation and progression into the proliferation and remodeling stage, active, passive, and resistive exercises may be gradually increased. In the patient who is progressing well through the inflammatory phase but having difficulty regaining motion, low-grade joint mobilizations may be initiated, with progression to grades III and IV as the tissue tolerates it.[42] The therapist treats masticatory muscle guarding and cervical spine dysfunction concomitantly.

Education about progression of diet is done in tandem with the surgeon's recommendations. Education about rest position of the mandible, proper breathing techniques, use of

ice at home to decrease pain, and decreased parafunctional activities continues. Home exercises for increasing range, function, and neuromuscular control can be progressed as tissue healing allows.

CONCLUSION

The physical therapist is an essential member of the team in treating the patient with TMD. This chapter gives an overview of anatomy and pathology to help the physical therapist make critical decisions about treatment approaches. It delineates evaluation techniques and discusses treatment options for a variety of problems, while emphasizing the importance of coordination and prioritization of treatments. Further research and delineation of appropriate treatment approaches for the patient with TMD are essential as we piece together the complex puzzle often presented by our patients.

REVIEW QUESTIONS

1. What are the similarities and differences in the treatment approaches for patients with temporomandibular joint derangements versus those with masticatory muscle disorders?

2. What evaluation findings differentiate between a diagnosis of a masticatory muscle disorder and a diagnosis of temporomandibular joint derangement?

3. What procedures can the clinician use to differentiate between cervical spine and temporomandibular joint sources of craniomandibular pain?

4. What is the role of the physical therapist in treating the postsurgical temporomandibular joint patient?

5. What is the rationale for the use of various physical therapy interventions, including modalities, joint mobilization, and exercise, in the treatment of the patient with temporomandibular joint dysfunction?

ACKNOWLEDGMENTS

The author wishes to thank and acknowledge Sharon Ruble, medical photographer, and Stacie Milam, patient model. Special thanks goes to Jeffrey Okeson, DMD, Director of the Orofacial Pain Center at the University of Kentucky College of Dentistry, for his mentoring and his commitment to continued development of the knowledge base necessary for proper care of patients with TMD.

REFERENCES

1. Austin BD, Shupe SM: The role of physical therapy in recovery after temporomandibular joint surgery, *J Oral Maxillofac Surg* 51:495, 1993.

2. Basmajian JV, DeLuca CJ: *Muscles alive: their functions revealed by electromyography,* Baltimore, 1985, Williams & Wilkins.

3. Bates RE, Gremillion HA, Stewart CM: Degenerative joint disease: part 1, diagnosis and management considerations, *The Journal of Craniomandibular Practice* 11:284, 1993.

4. Calliet R: *Head and face pain syndromes,* Philadelphia, 1992, FA Davis.

5. Cantu RI, Grodin AJ: *Myofascial manipulation theory and clinical application,* Rockville, Md, 1992, Aspen.

6. Carlson CR, Bertrand PM, Okeson JP: The role of behavioral medicine in the treatment of chronic temporomandibular disorders: neuromuscular reeducation in the dental setting. In Kall NR, Schtark M, Sokhadzi T, editors: *Encyclopedia of applied psychophysiology and behavioral medicine,* Salem, Pa, Future Health Press (in press).

7. Clark GT: Examining temporomandibular disorder patients for craniocervical dysfunction, *The Journal of Cr-anioman Prac* 21:56, 1984.

8. Clark GT, Moody DG, Sanders B: Arthroscopic treatment of temporomandibular joint locking resulting from disc derangement: two year results, *J Oral Maxillofac Surg* 49:157, 1991.

9. De Bont LGM, Stegenga B: Pathology temporomandibular joint internal derangement and osteoarthrosis, *Int J Oral Maxillofac Surg* 22:71, 1993.

10. DeLeeuw R: Temporomandibular joint osteoarthrosis clinical and radiographic characteristics 30 years after non-surgical treatment: a preliminary report, *J Craniomandib Pract* 11:15, 1983.

11. Dubnar R: Introductory remarks: basic mechanisms of pain associated with deep tissues, *Can J Physiol Pharmacol* 69:607, 1991.

12. Dwyer A, Aprill C, Bogduk N: Cervical zygoapophyseal joint pain patterns 1: a study in normal volunteers, *Spine* 15:453, 1990.

13. Edeling J: *Manual therapy for chronic headache,* Oxford, 1994, Butterworth-Heinemann.

14. Edmeads J: The cervical spine and headache, *Neurology* 38:1874, 1988.

15. Goldenberg DL: Fibromyalgia, chronic fatigue syndrome, and myofascial pain syndrome, *Curr Opin Rheumatol* 5:199, 1993.

16. Headache Classification Committee of the International Headache Society: Classification and diagnostic criteria for headache disorders, cranial neuralgias and facial pain, *Cephalalgia* 8(suppl 7):11, 1988.

17. Hecox B, Mehreteab TA, Weisberg J: *Physical agents: a comprehensive text for physical therapists,* East Norwalk, Conn, 1994, Appleton & Lange.

18. Hesse JR, Hansson TL: Factors influencing joint mobility in general and in particular respect of the craniomandibular articulation: a literature review, *J Craniomandib Disord Facial Oral Pain* 2:19, 1988.

19. Hu JW et al: Excitatory effects on neck and jaw muscle activity of inflammatory irritant applied to cervical paraspinal tissues, *Pain* 55:243, 1993.

20. Kendall HO, Kendall FP, Wadsworth GE: *Muscles testing and function,* Baltimore, 1971, Williams & Wilkins.

21. Kerr FWL, Olafson RA: Trigeminal and cervical volleys, *Arch Neurol* 5:171, 1961.

22. Kircos LT et al: Magnetic resonance imaging of the TMJ disc in asymptomatic volunteers, *J Oral Maxillofac Surg* 45:852, 1987.

23. Kojima Y: Convergence patterns of afferent information from the temporomandibular joint and masseter muscle in the trigeminal subnucleus caudalis, *Brain Research Bulletin* 24:609, 1990.

24. Kozeniauskas JJ, Ralph WJ: Bilateral arthrographic evaluation of unilateral temporomandibular joint pain and dysfunction, *J Prosthet Dent* 6098, 1988.

25. Kraus SL, ed: *Temporomandibular disorders,* New York, 1994, Churchill Livingstone.

26. Langton DP, Eggleton TM: *Functional anatomy of the temporomandibular joint complex,* Tucson, 1992, IFORC.

27. Mannheimer JS: Acute and chronic postural abnormalities as related to craniofacial pain and temporomandibular disorders, *Dent Clin North Am* 35:185, 1991.

28. McCain G et al: A controlled study of the effects of a supervised cardiovascular fitness training program on the manifestations of primary fibromyalgia, *Arthritis Rheum* 31:1135, 1988.

29. Mense S: Review article: nociception from skeletal muscle in relation to clinical muscle pain, *Pain* 54:241, 1993.

30. Michlovitz SL: *Thermal agents in rehabilitation,* Philadelphia, 1990, FA Davis.

31. Mohl ND et al: Devices for the diagnosis and treatment of temporomandibular disorders: part III, thermography, ultrasound, electrical stimulation, and electromyographic biofeedback, *J Prosthet Dent* 63:472, 1990.

32. Montgomery MT et al: Arthroscopic TMJ surgery: effects on signs, symptoms, and disc position, *J Oral Maxillofac Surg* 47:1263, 1989.

33. Okeson JP: *Management of temporomandibular disorders and occlusion,* St Louis, 1993, Mosby.

34. Quintner JL, Cohen ML: Referred pain of peripheral nerve origin, *Clin J Pain* 10:243, 1994.

35. Rocabado M, Iglarsh ZA: *Musculoskeletal approach to maxillofacial pain,* Philadelphia, 1991, JB Lippincott.

36. Salonen L, Hellden L: Prevalence of signs and symptoms of dysfunction in the masticatory system: an epidemiologic study in an adult, Swedish population, *J Craniomandib Disord Facial Oral Pain* 4:241, 1990.

37. Schellhas KP et al: The diagnosis of temporomandibular joint disease: two compartment arthrography and MR, *Am J Neuroradiol* 9:579, 1988.

38. Sessle BJ: The neurobiology of facial and dental pain: present knowledge, future directions, *J Dent Res* 66:962, 1987.
39. Solberg WK: Temporomandibular disorders: management of internal derangement, *Br Dent J* 160:379, 1986.
40. Travell JG, Simons DG: *Myofascial pain and dysfunction: the trigger point manual,* Baltimore, 1983, Williams & Wilkins.
41. Wabeke KB et al: Temporomandibular joint clicking: a literature review, *J Craniomandib Disord Facial Oral Pain* 3:163, 1989.
42. Waide FL et al: Clinical management of a patient following temporomandibular joint arthroscopy, *Phys Ther* 72:355, 1992.
43. Williams PL et al: *Gray's anatomy,* ed 37, New York, 1989, Churchill Livingstone.
44. Wyke BO: Neuromuscular mechanisms influencing mandibular posture: a neurologist's review of current concepts, *J Dent* 2:111, 1973.

SUGGESTED READING

1. Langton DP, Eggleton TM: *Functional anatomy of the temporomandibular joint complex,* Tucson, 1992, IFORC.
2. Okeson JP: *Management of temporomandibular disorders and occlusion,* St Louis, 1993, Mosby.
3. Kraus SL, ed: *Temporomandibular disorders,* New York, 1994, Churchill Livingstone.
4. Travell JG, Simons DG: *Myofascial pain and dysfunction: the trigger point manual,* Baltimore, 1983, Williams & Wilkins.
5. Rocabado M, Iglarsh ZA: *Musculoskeletal approach to maxillofacial pain,* Philadelphia, 1991, JB Lippincott.
6. Hecox B, Mehreteab TA, Weisberg J: *Physical agents: a comprehensive text for physical therapists,* East Norwalk, Conn, 1994, Appleton & Lange.

PART FOUR

Special Areas

CHAPTER 19

Industrial Physical Therapy

Susan J. Isernhagen

OUTLINE

Rationale
    Kinesiology
    Relationship to injury or illness
    FunctionPhysical therapist's role in industrial rehabilitation
    Acute musculoskeletal/cumulative trauma injury treatment
    Functional capacities evaluation: work task testing
    Work rehabilitation
    Future issues
The therapist in work injury prevention
    Education
    Injury prevention ergonomics
    Prework screening
    Summary
Future perspectives

KEY TERMS

industrial
rehabilitation
work place
acute injury

cumulative trauma
functional capacity
evaluation

LEARNING OBJECTIVES

After studying this chapter, the reader should be able to:

1. Describe the nine work tasks assessed in a functional capacity evaluation.
2. Discuss the primary body systems and segments required to perform the nine work tasks.
3. Define and perform a functional capacity evaluation.
4. Define the terms *work hardening* and *work conditioning.*
5. List and describe the four steps required to determine return to work outcome.
6. Correlate the findings of a functional capacity evaluation and the functional job analysis.
7. Describe the different types of functional capacity evaluations, including those based on patient reports of pain and those based on functional criteria.
8. Discuss the legal issues—including ADA, OSHA guidelines, and workers' compensation laws—that can affect the evaluation of work function.
9. Discuss the role of the physical therapist in industrial rehabilitation.
10. Discuss the contribution of the physical therapist to work injury prevention.

RATIONALE

Physical therapy has always been a pivotal profession in the management of the injured worker.* Not only is the physical therapist able to treat injured workers, measure functional abilities, and rehabilitate chronically injured workers but also the therapist can understand the physical demands of work from a physiologic perspective. The

* References 4-6, 15, 16, 20, 21, 24, 34, 37.

physical therapist's education lends itself to this functional evaluation, restoration, and injury prevention model because of the sciences in which the profession is grounded.

Kinesiology

Physical therapy involves science and the art of analyzing human movement patterns (kinesiology). A background in anatomy, physiology, and neurology allows the therapist to understand the components of motion and their relationship to specific movement patterns. The physical therapist is

uniquely qualified to use movement science to evaluate
levels of work ability for productivity and safety. The
physical therapist can also break down overall patterns into
the individual components that comprise movement. The
therapist understands angles and arcs that are stressful on the
musculoskeletal system, patterns of movement that produce
greatest forces, angles of joints that produce greatest
strength, and principles of neuromuscular control.

Relationship to injury or illness

The physical therapist's background also includes knowledge of the pathology of the musculoskeletal or neuromuscular system that impairs movement function. Principles of
illness or disease, including cumulative trauma, allow the
therapist to understand their effect on movement and
function. For example, back injuries are common in workers,
and carpal tunnel syndrome is increasing in prevalence. The
physical therapist with anatomic and physiologic knowledge
of pathology understands their causes from either sudden
injury or repetitive strain. In addition, primary disease
processes are present in workers who have osteoarthritis,
diabetes, and multiple sclerosis. They require the physical
therapist's ability to evaluate the relationship of the stress of
the job to the ability of the worker. Therefore, the physical
therapist puts into a work perspective the condition of the
body relating to injury, illness, or disease.

Function

Basic kinesiologic movement patterns are related to overall body function. In occupational rehabilitation, physical
therapists deal specifically with work function. Functional
evaluation of a worker correlates the physical resources of
the body in performing specific tasks with the physical demands of work. It makes understandable to the therapist the
balance between the worker who produces the work and the
work that creates responses in the worker's body.

The physical therapist is uniquely positioned in science,
clinical skills, and movement evaluation to understand the
relationship of the worker and the demands of the job.

PHYSICAL THERAPIST'S ROLE IN INDUSTRIAL REHABILITATION

The continuum of physical therapy interventions is
broad.[12] Four primary components form the link between
intervention and establishment of safe work.

- *Acute care:* As long as physical therapists have been
  involved in acute musculoskeletal treatment, they have
  treated the outcomes of work injury. Patients with back
  strains, shoulder sprains, and cumulative traumas have
  always been treated clinically by therapists. For many
  years there was no differentiation between the work-
  injured patient and other patients. However, this
  delineation is now required, as the goal for an injured
  worker, to return to work, requires specific goal setting.

- *Functional capacity evaluation:* In the early 1980s,
  physical therapists became involved with functional
  capacity evaluation, a subset of functional evaluation
  specifically oriented to identify ability to perform in
  work categories as defined by the Department of
  Labor or in specific jobs through a functional job
  description. The work tasks utilized in a functional
  capacity evaluation include lifting, carrying, bending,
  stooping, squatting, reaching, walking, and hand activities (Table 19-1).
- *Work conditioning/work hardening:* Because some
  workers cannot return to work after acute care or
  functional capacity evaluation, a longer, more intense
  rehabilitation process was developed. Physical therapists were involved in the development of the work
  conditioning and work hardening models described by
  the American Physical Therapy Association.
- *Injury prevention:* In the early 1980s, "back schools"
  became prevalent in industry. Professionals often
  involved in presenting back schools were physical
  therapists. Because of therapists' teaching abilities and
  their detailed knowledge of how the spine functions and
  how injuries to the back occur, back schools became a
  large part of injury prevention education. However, as
  time elapsed, other methods of work safety became
  more recognized. Injury prevention education is now
  only one component of the injury prevention spectrum.
  Physical therapists integrate education with a more

Table 19-1. Relationship of functional and physical components

Work requirements	Primary body systems/segments
Lift (from floor)	Knees, hips, spine, hands, cardiopulmonary system, coordination, balance
Lift (overhead)	Shoulder, elbow, wrist, hand, scapula, cardiopulmonary system, coordination, balance
Carry	Hand-wrists, shoulder, spine, lower extremities, cardiopulmonary system, coordination, balance
Reach	Shoulder, elbow, wrist, spine, coordination
Trunk bend	Spine (lumbar and cervical), hips, balance
Squat, kneel	Ankles, knees, hips, spine, balance
Climb	Knees, hips, ankles, hands, shoulders, cardiopulmonary system, balance
Walk	Ankles, knees, hips, balance, cardiopulmonary system
Hand use	Finger-thumb, wrist, elbow, shoulder, neck, coordination, sensation

complete spectrum of prework screening, ergonomic analysis, job modification, and reasonable accommodations, as well as cumulative trauma prevention education.

Acute musculoskeletal/cumulative trauma injury treatment

Physical therapy principles. Proactive methods of early, active intervention are critical with injured workers. In acute work injury intervention, the physical therapist uses traditional skills to decrease pain and inflammation, increase motion, increase strength and endurance, increase overall function, and educate the injured worker in exercise and injury prevention. The aspects of physical therapy treatment that are important in effective work injury management are the following:

Algorithmic/critical pathway care. Rather than using random, nonspecific, or untargeted methods, the physical therapist must realize that work injury management requires treatment for a specific outcome. The outcome desired is early return to work in a safe, productive mode. Therefore, study of the literature regarding back injuries, carpal tunnel syndrome, and the like can help the clinician design focused algorithms of care.[3,7,32,33]

- Limited use of passive modalities
- Postural and body mechanics education
- Fostering of self-responsibility on the part of the patient (worker)
- Activation and strengthening
- Functional matching with job requirements

In this way, initial physical therapy treatment is prompt, active, and focused on education, self-empowerment, functional outcomes, and return to work as the goal.

Return to work outcome. Setting specific goals of treatment starts physical therapy care on a directed course. It is important to acknowledge that the patient is a "worker" and that the therapist is seeing the patient as a result of a physical injury that is limiting "work function." Those limitations may be caused by stiffness, discomfort, swelling, or muscle spasm, which physical therapists treat in order to assist the worker back to full, safe function.

Contrast this with the medical provider who, instead, treats the injured worker with a "patient in pain" approach. The medical provider can send the injured worker down the road of chronicity by focusing on the pain issue. For example, "Where does it hurt? How much does it hurt? Rate your pain on a scale of one to ten" may seem to be an important part of the examination, but pain as the primary focus gives the worker the wrong impression. They are led to believe that their pain is the primary concern of the practitioner, rather than their function.

To avoid the pain focus, patient education should indicate that discomfort is merely one of the effects of a musculoskeletal problem that needs to be addressed. A medical practitioner's focus on inability to move (due to stiffness, spasm, weakness, or discomfort) in the context of a movement dysfunction is far preferable in patient management than focus on the sensation of pain. The messages that physical therapists give to patients regarding function (rather than pain) are critically important to return to work outcome (Table 19-2).

The four-step process

Step One. Retain the worker role: Acknowledge that the patient is a worker and the medical provider's goal is to provide a return to work. At the initial stage, workers still see themselves as nurses, truck drivers, and construction workers. Keep that context.

Step Two. Identify functional goals: The physical therapist, on the first visit, should establish what work tasks the worker performs, what physical requirements are necessary to return the person to work, and whether any modifications can be made in the work to allow early return to work. This outlook establishes a framework of sequential functional testing that allows measurement toward return-to-work goals.

Step Three. Determine if modified or partial duty is an interim step: If fully modified work is available (the traditional "light duty" concept), the person may be able to return to work to a transitional job in which few to none of the original job tasks are required. The availability of this alternative should be established at the outset so that even while receiving physical therapy treatment the worker may return to alternative work doing productive activities.

Table 19-2. How to encourage a patient	
To lead toward chronic pain	**To become functionally oriented**
• Ask about pain first • Make pain the focus of treatment questions	• Ask about functional limitation • Utilize descriptions of discomfort as only one indicator of treatment (along with tightness, stiffness, numbness, and the like)
• Use elimination of pain as the treatment outcome • Be the "reliever of pain" for the patient • Say, "When it hurts, stop!"	• Utilize return to safe productivity as treatment outcome • Teach the worker how to control and relieve discomfort • Perform objective functional evaluation to determine/demonstrate safe work activity

Step Four. Target and measure full return to work status: For an injured worker, a return to light duty is usually not an end in itself. Return to full original duty is always the primary target and should not be forgotten even if a temporary light duty return is accomplished. Therefore, the physical therapist must understand the hierarchy of return-to-work options and not discharge the patient until the final goals are fully met. Intensive ongoing therapy may not be necessary; the requirement is, rather, following the workers' recovery and slowly increasing their functional capabilities through testing and matching with job tasks, until the highest level of return-to-work goal is obtained.

Functional capacities evaluation: work task testing

Functional capacity evaluation is well established in medical parameters and in the medical literature. Functional capacity evaluation (FCE) components can be used in several ways: as single specific tests, grouped for directed testing needs, or as a comprehensive whole-body test to establish work ability.[15,16,20,21,24]

For example, if a truck driver with a shoulder injury is being treated, and job analysis indicates truck loading is essential, then safe, effective lifting is an important goal. Lifting evaluations designed to match the job requirements and demonstrate that the injured part can function safely are important prior to work return. This objective functional matching not only promotes a return to work but also is critical in prevention of reinjuries. It utilizes targeted specific functional task testing.

If the truck driver has been off work for 12 weeks, however, there are secondary questions about deconditioning and safety in all aspects of work. There is a question regarding his ability to even return to his former job. In this case, a comprehensive FCE is required.

Method. Objective, clear, physical-based, expert-assessed function of the worker. Functional capacity evaluation requires the following:

- Objective evaluation of work function. The evaluator must know how the physical demands stress a worker's body during the physical aspects of work. This necessitates criteria for evaluating body movement, physiologic signs, and safety parameters.
- Competent neuromusculoskeletal evaluation prior to FCE, identifying impairments and ability to undertake FCE safely.[11]
- Linking of the physical deficiencies of the worker with the physical demands of the job. This issue becomes important because defining whether an injury is amenable to treatment leads to the most appropriate case resolution. Endurance, limitations, neuromusculoskeletal ability, degenerative changes, and disease must be fully identified in order to discuss accommodations and make job matching more accurate.

- Expert evaluation. The skilled physical (or occupational) therapist is the expert. The background is in science, movement analysis, kinesiology, and pathology. The evaluator must take charge of the test, report observations clearly, and take responsibility for the safety of the injured worker. Clear, objective documentation makes legal case resolution possible.[35,39]
- Worker confidence. Rapport with the injured worker must be established. It is important that the worker fully participate in the testing. It is the evaluator's responsibility to set the professional tone and gain the confidence and cooperation of the injured worker.
- Professional basis. Injured workers told to be responsible for stopping their own tests "before they get injured" become defensive, afraid, and reluctant to put forth full effort. Trust in the competence of the evaluator is more likely to result in full cooperation than is placement of responsibility on the patient.
- Safe function. The evaluator must work with the client to understand full safe function. Workers will need to monitor their own safety upon return to work. It is also important for the employer that the FCE evaluate limitations and document them in clear terms backed by objective medical evidence so that the worker is not forced into doing unsafe activities once back on the job.
- Ability to define maximum effort. Although isometric "consistent scores" may indicate that the person is performing similarly on repetitive tests, they are not necessarily an indication of full effort. Similarly, inconsistent scores do not necessarily indicate that the person is faking, malingering, or magnifying. Rather, the evaluator's skill and measurement of other objective data must be applied to numerous indicators such as consistency/inconsistency scores through observable signs to give a fuller interpretation of effort. Indicating compliance with test protocols is serious, and therapists should exert every effort to be comprehensive in this judgment, look for physical problems that could have caused deviations, and then put compliance (consistency) in the proper context.
- Clear, concise reporting. Objective medically and legally credible reports are paramount. All parties in a workers' compensation case must be able to clearly read a report. The physician will look for medical backup for the functional items; the attorney will look for criteria and expert witness testimony; the employer will look for clear language that clearly matches the worker to the job with or without modifications; insurance companies and managed care organizations will look at return to work outcomes.

Job matching. This FCE information, once gathered, is only half of the issue. The second component is the functional requirements of the job, which must be obtained by evaluation of the physical job demands. These critical physical issues involve weighted activities such as:

Lifting (from where to where, repetition, type of weight lifted)
Endurance activities
Manual materials handling tasks
Ambulation activities
Repetitious hand movement
Positional tolerances
    Spine forward bending
    Neck forward bending
    Rotation spine
    Joint compressions
    Overhead work activities
    Sitting
    Standing
Coordination activities
    Hand coordination
    Balance and coordination (standing and walking)

Frequency. Once the critical demands are identified, the repetitiousness and other environmental factors surrounding these activities must be identified. The frequency with which the activity is performed during the workday can be matched exactly with the functional capacity abilities of the client (Table 19-3).

Indications for functional capacity evaluation. Because many workers referred to FCE are chronically off work, there has been a tendency to relegate the FCE to the chronic population. However, the purpose of FCE is to find a worker's safe functional abilities and match them to job demands, which may be done any time in the return-to-work process when the following issues occur.

The client must be:

- Medically stable (for safety reasons)
- Plateaued in progress (so that FCE results do not change significantly with increased healing or treatment)

Issues that precipitate FCE are:

- Can the worker return to work (level)?
  At what level (former, modified, or new job)?
  With what modifications?
- Can the worker return to work (timeliness)?
  Now?
  After further treatment?
  Not at all?
- Is there a match between the job and the worker?
  Appropriate when this is a reinjury of the same person at the same job
  In the case of a condition or disease that is progressing (not related to work injury such as multiple sclerosis, rheumatoid arthritis)
- Is the physical condition diagnosed responsible for the functional limitation? (Available *only* with a function-based test complete with history, neuromusculoskeletal assessment, and physical movement pattern analysis.)

See the Box for a summary of the different types of FCE.

The legal issues. Sending an injured worker back to work has ethical, legal, medical, and financial implications. Three laws (and common sense) are forcing a match between the worker and the work. The evaluator of work function

Table 19-3. Matching worker and work demands		
Critical job demands	**Physical work strengths**	**Job match**
1. Use of long handled tools: occasionally	R hand grip = 40# occasionally L hand grip = 90# occasionally	Yes
2. Painting and cleaning surfaces with whole body reach: occasionally	Forward bend standing = continuously	Yes
3. General inspection of school areas	Walking = continuously	Yes
4. Floor to waist lift of boxes and pails: 1#-35# occasionally	Floor to waist lift = 40# occasionally	Yes
5. Front carry of boxes, tools, etc. 1-40# occasionally	Front carry = 60# occasionally	Yes
6. One handed carry of pails (R or L) 1-40# = rarely	R = 20# L = 55#	Yes
7. Stand-frequently	Standing to tolerance: continuously	Yes
8. Walk-frequently	Walking tolerance: continuously	Yes
9. Squat-occasionally	Repetitive squat: continuously	Yes
10. Forward bend-occasionally standing	Forward bend in standing: continuously	Yes
11. Waist to over shoulder lift-1-40# occasionally	Waist to overhead lift: 5# occasionally	No
12. Overhead painting and cleaning = occasionally	Elevated work: occasionally	Yes
13. Use of hand tools-frequently	R & L upper extremity coordination: continuously	Yes

Copyright: Isernhagen & Associates, Inc, 1992.

Types of FCE

Patient report/pain based

Asks client to stop test when they wish

- Is subjective—may not stand up in court as objective evidence of ability. Expert witness testimony mandates the therapist acts as an expert evaluator with objective data, not as a person documenting what the client says.
- When client does not put forth full effort, there is no way to determine *objectively* any functional capacities.
- Gives clients the impression *they* are in charge—not the evaluator—which may actually facilitate lack of effort.

Evaluator does ensure safety or body mechanics

- Client may get injured during the test. If information gained is incorrect, injury may occur when the client returns to work.
- Client assumes that unsafe body mechanics are okay because the evaluator does not correct them.
- If a therapist documents "unsafe" or "poor" body mechanics and yet lets the client continue, there is written evidence of negligence.

Does not identify the physical problem

- No initial history or physical is given by the therapist.
- Therapist is unable to know of undiagnosed or unidentified physical problems before testing—injury (negligence) may be a consequence.
- Unable to correlate physical limitations with injury.
- Lacks reliability.
- Takes the therapist out of the "expert" role. Could be criticized in a courtroom situation.

Functional/criteria based

Therapist is an educated evaluator who is in charge of the test

- With *criteria-based testing,* the evaluator observes and identifies performance levels.
- If client does not put forth full effort, there is confrontation in a positive manner, which most often facilitates a better effort. If not, the objective signs of lack of effort are documented.
- Evaluator is "professional" and communicates with client in a manner that fosters trust and cooperation.

Evaluator monitors safety in testing

- Evaluators know that safety during testing is linked with safety on return to work.
- Evaluators want to *assure* safety in testing for the client's sake as well as because of the malpractice issue.
- Results given are accurate and based on specific criteria of safe maximum function.
- The client is empowered to perform both during the test and at work when safety is assured.

Follows professional protocols of physical assessment to functional evaluation results

- Initial history is taken by the therapist in addition to medical records review.
- Initial physical assessment is performed to establish physical status that will be related to functional limitations.
- Allows any contraindication to testing to be identified.
- Recommendations are backed by credible objective physical evidence.

---

must take into consideration the responsibility and liability that these legal standards dictate.

The Americans with Disabilities Act (ADA) indicates that all people must be given equal opportunity to work based on their abilities.[8] If disability exists, reasonable accommodations must be made to ensure the fit of the work and worksite to the worker. It stresses that each individual must be matched to the individual job, which leads evaluators away from norms and generic formulas and toward individual evaluation and matching with individual job demands.

OSHA Cumulative Trauma Guidelines propose that a worker with cumulative trauma should be placed at work tasks that match their abilities and conditions and do not cause or aggravate cumulative trauma.[36] Doing so again necessitates individual functional evaluation matched with individual job demands.

Workers' compensation laws promote the return-to-work process through matching the worker to job demands. There is a strong movement in workers' compensation hearings to facilitate matching objective functional capacity and the job. Discontinuing workers' compensation benefits is often based upon providing job offers that are within the worker's capability. This fact also forces FCE with job matching.

The three laws mandate matching the worker and the work. Each law was created for different purposes, and, therefore, the course of action professionals take will differ. However, the direction and action that satisfy one law often satisfy all. Table 19-4 delineates the laws for comparison. These are important responsibilities for all involved. Both ADA and OSHA litigate or fine if worker and work do not match. Therefore, the functional evaluator is in a highly responsible position. The functional evaluator must use objective methods for worker evaluation, match the evaluation results to work requirements, and be able to defend this match!

The science of functional evaluation. The following issues are often misunderstood or misused. Science directed toward the wrong goal can lead to noncompliance with the relevant laws.

Reliability. Reliability indicates that the results of functional evaluations are reproducible. The likelihood of scientific reproducibility is higher if functional tests are:

- Standardized
- Based on defined objective findings

Table 19-4. Evaluation responsibility/liability

	Employer	Employee	Medical-functional evaluator
ADA	Avoid discrimination in hiring	Be qualified for duty	Do only job-related, nondiscriminatory screening
	Make reasonable accommodations after evaluation	By physically able to perform essential functions	Develop functional job descriptions and accommodations
	Remove architectural barriers	Ask for accommodation	Suggest work and worksite modification
WC	Avoid expensive claims	Comply with state workers' comp law	Match evaluation with work requirements
	Manage claims effectively	Comply with workers' comp rehabilitation plan	Do functional, job-related screening
	Provide modified or full-duty positions after injury	Return to work as facilitated and approved	Be objective in recommending modified work
OSHA	Have commitment to avoid back injuries or cumulative trauma	Report nonergonomic conditions	Assist with ergonomic risk analysis
	Provide cumulative trauma and ergonomic education	Work smart	Provide worker education on ergonomic principles
	Do monitoring of injury resulting from poor worker-work match	Perform work as designated through education	Evaluate early symptoms and provide work modifications
	Utilize therapists for early intervention	Report symptoms/injury early	Make ergonomic changes that facilitate safe work-worker fit
	Provide modified duty after evaluation	Adjust work site to self	Provide effective early intervention

- Performed on 2 or more days
- Facilitate a cooperative rather than an adversarial approach

Reliability in itself, however, does not make a test useful unless it looks at a useful outcome. For example, if 10 therapists all verify that a patient says, "I can't lift more than 10 pounds," reliability would be demonstrated. However, whether the patient is correct regarding actual lifting ability is the FCE issue. Reliability based on subjective data still remains subjective.

It is better to design real-world tests and then ensure reproducibility. When one utilizes reliability studies on tests that measure actual function, then objectivity and reliability are directed at information desired by more than just the scientist. It will be appreciated by worker, employer, doctor, and insurer as well.

External validity. In functional worker-work matching terms, external validity indicates that the functional and work capacity conclusions (either in prework screening or in full FCE and WCE testing after injury) will hold true on the work site. In other words, if John is found to be able to lift 60 lb, carry 50 lb, and work overhead in an FCE, then these capacities will hold true when he is subjected to the stresses of the work that will demand those performance levels from him.

Content validity. A test that directly matches the real-life activity has content validity. Therefore, the closer the test is to the actual work, the greater the content validity. Without content validity, statistical analysis must be done to show that a test is valid; with content validity (test matches tasks), statistical analysis is not required.

Normative data. Norms in facilitating workers' return to work are almost completely useless. It matters not whether John has 25% or 75% of normal strength, lift, or range of motion. What is important is whether John can do the specific requirements of his own job.

Norms rank us, and norms can demean us. In the three laws discussed earlier, the impetus is on facilitating safe full work for the worker. There is no implication that a worker should meet an artificial norm. This is the basis of the ADA: All tests required for a worker getting or keeping a job must be "job related."

Scientifically, norms are interesting, and they can assist in workplace design. To match *one* worker with *one* job, however, all the evaluator needs to know is whether there is a match (and whether a modification would be needed for that match to occur).

Outcome studies. The validity measure that is most important to people other than researchers is "Did the FCE accomplish what was intended?" In most cases the FCE is intended as a return-to-work mechanism. If therapists do not measure the outcome (whether the person returned to work), there is no accountability in the system. Physical therapists must be responsive to the necessity for the payer, referral source, and patient to obtain what is needed.

Following is an outcome study that identifies and measures APTA-recommended outcomes and other case resolution variables.

FCE outcome study. Retrospective audits of consecutive clients who were referred for FCE were reviewed for outcome. These reviews consisted of medical record chart audits combined with telephone surveys 6 months after FCE,[38] a time chosen to represent enough time to ensure that a sustained return to work was viable.

- 114 clients were identified as having received no PT intervention other than FCE.
- Time off work from date of injury to FCE was calculated to be an average of 8.8 months (thus classifying these clients as in a "chronic state").

Note: Once a client has been off work beyond 6 months and is considered "chronic," statistics indicate a very low likelihood of returning to work, and then only with extensive and expensive rehabilitation. Analysis of the return-to-work process indicates that there must be agreement by all three primary parties:

- The doctor, who must sign the release
- The employer, who must accept the employee back at work
- Most important, the worker, who must make the decision that he or she feels capable of returning to work and that the FCE information is correct

Returned to work after one FCE. Of these clients, 64% returned to work based on the results and recommendations of the FCE, with no other intervention, and were still at work 6 months later (36% went on to case settlement of a workers' comp or legal nature). Of the clients who returned to work after FCE,

1. 29%—Same company, previous job
2. 49%—Same company, previous job but modified
3. 11%—Same company, new job
4. 11%—New company, new job

A total of 78% returned to their previous jobs with the same employer (either at the same or a modified format), which is considered the best result by insurance companies. In total, 89% returned to work at the same place of employment. The combination of the FCE's clarity in defining modifications and the employer's willingness to modify the job based on objective information creates a positive outcome.

Of those clients who returned to work, work load was indicated to be:

1. 71%—Full-time
2. 26%—Part-time (4 to 8 hours per day)
3. 3%—Part-time (1 to 3½ hours per day)

More than two thirds of clients who returned to work were full-time status. This placement result is excellent, considering duration of time off work.

Of those clients who returned to work, the job satisfaction level was:

1. 70%—Satisfied with work level
2. 15%—Wish to work harder
3. 15%—Wish to work not as hard

More than two thirds of these clients were satisfied with their work level at 6 months after FCE, and several wished to work harder. When returned to work at appropriate functional levels, clients can satisfactorily perform their tasks, which contributes to employee morale and work performance.

Clients indicated their discomfort level to be:

1. 15%—Had no limiting discomfort
2. 62%—Clients indicating "having pain but worked through it"
3. 23%—Pain stopped the clients from working hard

Pain and *function* are not the same, and FCEs that focus on pain rather than function can limit return-to-work capability. An approach that focuses on safe function, however, allows for differentiation between pain and function and focuses on the *ability* of the person to functionally perform the job tasks required. After working at a level in which discomfort may have been present but could be tolerated, all of these workers indicated they would continue to work, as they could manage their discomfort level adequately.

Work rehabilitation

If a functional capacity evaluation shows that the worker is physically unable to return to work safely and adequately, and if modified return to duty is not a choice, then the modifications that must take place would be in the worker.

Ethically and under workers' compensation law, the worker has the right to be rehabilitated to work status. Given that the worker has suffered a work injury that leaves her or him unable to do the physical requirements of the job, most workers' compensation systems provide reimbursement for a specific amount of money or period of time to increase the functional capability of the worker to return to the original or next-best level of work.

Maximum medical improvement (MMI) is also an issue in settling workers' compensation cases in the aspect of permanent partial disability settlements. Theoretically, MMI should not be designated until full functional capacity has been reached. Otherwise, true maximum medical improvement has not been reached. This factor is often an issue of workers' compensation litigation. Therapists must recognize that workers ought to be rehabilitated before maximum medical improvement is established. Then, MMI has a functional as well as a medical outcome that can be utilized for absolute return-to-work determination.

The Box contains excerpts from the American Physical Therapy Association statement on types of work rehabilita-

Guidelines for programs for injured workers[22]

Preface

For those who are not able to return to work because of unresolved physical problems following acute care, treatment focus changes to restoration of function. Defined as WORK CONDITIONING these programs address the physical issues of flexibility, strength, endurance, coordination, and work-related function for the goal of return to work.

For the limited number of clients with behavioral and vocational dysfunction, WORK HARDENING may be indicated. WORK HARDENING programs are interdisciplinary and address the physical, functional, behavioral and vocational needs of the injured worker, with the goal of returning to work. Physical therapists provide the physical and functional components within both of these programs.

Guidelines for programs for injured workers (program comparison)

Work conditioning program

Addresses physical and functional needs which may be provided by one discipline (single discipline model).

Requires Work Conditioning assessment.

Utilizes physical conditioning and functional activities related to work.

Provided in multi-hour sessions up to:
- 4 hours/day
- 5 days/week
- 8 weeks

Work hardening program

Addresses physical, functional, behavioral, vocational needs within an interdisciplinary model.

Requires Work Hardening assessment.

Utilizes real or simulated work activities.

Provided in multi-hour sessions:
- up to 8 hours/day
- 5 days/week
- up to 8 weeks

Work conditioning guidelines

Client eligibility

To be eligible for Work Conditioning, a client must:
(a) Have a job goal.
(b) Have stated or demonstrated willingness to participate.
(c) Have identified systemic neuro-musculoskeletal physical and functional deficits that interfere with work.
(d) Be at the point of resolution of the initial or principal injury that participation in the Work Conditioning program would not be prohibited.

Provider responsibility
- The Work Conditioning provider shall develop and utilize an outcome assessment system designed to evaluate at a minimum, patient care results, program effectiveness, and efficiency.

Work hardening guidelines

Client eligibility

To be eligible for Work Hardening, a client must:
(a) Have a targeted job or job plan for return to work at the time of discharge.
(b) Have stated or demonstrated willingness to participate.
(c) Have identified physical (systemic neuro-muscular-skeletal), functional, behavioral and vocational deficits that interfere with work.
(d) Be at the point of resolution of the initial or principal injury that participation in the Work Hardening program would not be prohibited.

Provider responsibility

This is similar to that of work conditioning intent, but in work hardening there is a "team" of providers. In addition to a PT, there are other members, OT, psychology professional, and vocational professional.

The team members must evaluate the client to determine needs and goals regarding physical, psychosocial, and voca-

- The Work Conditioning providers should be appropriately familiar with job expectations, work environments, and skills required of the client through means such as site visitation, videotapes, and functional job descriptions.

Program content
- Techniques to improve strength, endurance, movement, flexibility, motor control, and cardiopulmonary capacity related to the performance of work tasks.
- Practice, modification, and instruction in work-related activities.
- Education related to safe job performance and injury prevention.
- Promotion of client responsibility and self management.

tional attributes. Team members involved must participate in evaluation, treatment, and discharge planning.

Program content. This has the same content as work conditioning but adds:

Practice, modification, and instruction in simulated or real work activities.

Provision of behavioral and vocational services as determined by the respective Work Hardening provider.

Promotion of client responsibility and self management.

Provision in multi-hour sessions with a minimum of 4 hours and up to 8 hours, 5 days a week, for a duration up to 8 weeks.

Assist the client to obtain as appropriate:
(a) Alcohol and other drug dependency counseling
(b) Engineering and ergonomic services
(c) Medical services
(d) Nutrition and weight control services
(e) Orthotic and prosthetic services
(f) Smoking cessation counseling

tion. The entire document can be obtained from the American Physical Therapy Association (1-800-999-APTA). These excerpts explain the hierarchy of the two main types of work rehabilitation, work conditioning, and work hardening.[1]

In both types of work rehabilitation, outcome studies are recommended. The APTA guidelines incorporate outcome data that include:

- Type of injury
- Time after injury before program starts
- Definition of rehab program as work conditioning or work hardening
- Duration and cost of program
- Return-to-work outcome

This study is designed to be used on a nationwide basis to collect data regarding effectiveness.

As the industrial rehabilitation field has developed, there has been a transition in program usage. Because early referral and effective functional evaluation were not highly utilized initially, the focus was on management of chronic cases. As more effective treatment and evaluation are utilized, there has been a shift from work hardening toward work conditioning. However, there will always be those cases that need more intensive help, and thus there will always be a need for work rehabilitation.

Future issues

The future for the physical therapist in the work injury management field revolves around excellent management of the injured worker. Physical therapists who expect to succeed for their patient, the employer, and themselves must realize that because the system is fraught with inadequacies and pitfalls, they must ensure that the worker does not fall through the cracks. Therefore, communication with the physician, employer, and rehabilitation consultant is extremely important to make sure that functional information is thoroughly understood by all team members and that the outcome for the worker is the return to work.

As physical therapists' referrals and reimbursement depend upon outcomes, the physical therapist must understand that the outcome desired in the workers' compensation system is return to work of the injured worker. Measuring this outcome and assuring that the return-to-work outcome happens are the new challenge for therapists.

THE THERAPIST IN WORK INJURY PREVENTION

The physical therapist may play a primary role in the prevention of work injuries. Education, experience, and study beyond entry level are required to develop expertise in many of the injury prevention modules (such as in ergonomics). Physical therapists participating in work injury prevention may undertake additional education in ergonomics, occupational health, safety and health, engineering,

industrial hygiene, and industrial psychology to enhance their ability to work with industry.

Because of physiology, anatomy, and kinesiology skills, a physical therapist can analyze external work stresses on the body that create the occasion for injury. The two primary causes of workers' compensation claims are back injuries and upper extremity cumulative trauma. The physical therapist is well schooled in spinal conditions and risk factors for back injury, as well as upper extremity cumulative trauma such as carpal tunnel syndrome, rotator cuff injury, tendinitis/tendinosis and epicondylitis.

The physical therapist takes knowledge of the factors that create these injuries, analyzes how these factors may be present in a work setting, and provides education to supervisors and workers regarding elimination of these risks. The three primary components of work injury prevention in the advanced professional realm of the physical therapist are (Fig. 19-1):

1. Injury prevention education
2. Ergonomic adaptation of work and work site
3. Functional prework screening

Education

Expertise in making educational principles meaningful to workers and supervisors is the "art" of effective education. Because the therapist often does not understand the job thoroughly, it is extremely important that the workers communicate with the therapist and that the program is interactive.[2,5,13,17,18]

The two primary areas for the therapist's participation in injury prevention education are back injury prevention[13,18] and cumulative trauma prevention.[2] The therapist may learn the principles of prevention through continuing education, commercially available programs, and study of safety programs.

Educational principles indicate that learners retain information best when they have participated in the "discovery" process; for instance, if a therapist is educating workers on how to prevent back injury, lecturing the workers on the do's

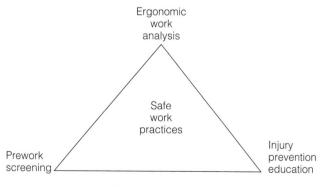

Fig. 19-1. The effective prevention model.

and don'ts of back position and methods of handling loads is not particularly effective. In fact, workers may view a therapist-educator, brought in without their specific invitation, as an outsider who could not understand their job as well as they do. There may be no way an outsider could tell them how to do their job better than they already do it, and this attitude is what the therapist must overcome. The interactive approach conversely allows both therapist and workers to discuss cumulative trauma and productivity issues. The therapist can present the science and safety part, and the workers take these concepts and discuss how to apply them to their actual work.

It is far better practice for principles to be discussed and an opportunity given to the workers to "solve" their own issues. For example, there is often a "discounting" of previous back school information on proper body mechanics. If asked at the beginning of a back school class, "Do you know the principles of proper lifting?" the group usually states, "Yes." Participants are almost always able to state the "rules":

- Use your legs, not your back.
- Keep the load close.
- Use controlled motions.
- Keep your back straight; do not bend or twist.

Nevertheless, when workers are asked whether they are able to apply these rules, the most common answer is "No." The problem is not that no one taught them proper lifting methods; it is that they ignore those rules because "we can't do it that way on our job."

With such a common finding in industry, the therapist must adopt an alternative method of teaching: Describe the principles needed for back safety, and then look at the job requirements with the workers. The workers then are the experts in evaluating how to apply these basic rules to the requirements of doing the job. In this way, the methods and needs of the worker and the workplace can be brought together through a problem-solving approach. The workers may decide that "the conveyor belt must be raised" or that "I should use a cart rather than carry the load that far" or "I should move the materials off the floor to a higher shelf." Then it is much easier to get those issues resolved.

Similarly, this type of education process can be used for upper extremity cumulative trauma. The risk factors tend to be somewhat different and, therefore, the solutions go in a different direction. Often, with cumulative trauma, what is causative is excessive hand gripping and pinching, highly repetitive work without breaks, poor design of work so that there are extraneous movements and distances, lack of task rotation, and lack of job rotation.

The interactive problem-solving approach here often leads to group discussion on the need for interventions such as hourly 2-minute rests or stretch breaks or changing tasks every half hour rather than every 3 hours (which is in their

control), designing an acceptable job rotation schedule, and more ergonomic seating and placement of work tasks.

In both back and upper extremity injury prevention, the important issues the physical therapist-educator must consider are:

- Having the workers take ownership in the solutions
- Making the solutions realistic so that management can assist in their accomplishment
- Encouraging management and workers to participate in the same educational session so that their input and comments are made as a "team"
- Creating a hierarchy of solutions regarding expense. For example, repositioning items on the loading dock may be an immediate solution, whereas the long-term solution is the purchase of two additional forklifts.

Injury prevention ergonomics

Ergonomics is the science of matching the work and work site to the worker. Underlying its concepts is the philosophy that the worker is a human being with certain inherent capabilities and susceptibilities. In the past, expecting the worker to adapt to the design of a machine or the rigors of a task has led to poor productivity and safety concerns. By changing the work site and the work to fit the worker instead, the focus is on changing the inanimate, changeable objects to meet the needs of the human worker.[14,26] Properly applied ergonomic principles should reduce injury and should also increase productivity.

Therefore, the physical therapist using ergonomic philosophy in the work force should look at productivity issues as well as safety issues in making recommendations. Although a primary reason for a physical therapist to go to the work site regarding ergonomics is often to reduce work injury, nevertheless, the uninformed physical therapist may inadvertently make recommendations that negatively affect productivity. Therefore, additional study may be needed on the physical therapist's part to understand industrial needs, the work site psychology, and specific ergonomic principles that are inferred but generally not taught specifically in physical therapy education.

The basic concepts, however, of ergonomic recommendations in the workplace fall into 10 categories of forces and stresses that must be understood.

Force. Force must be measured accurately and compared with the physical abilities of the workers. When force is an issue in cumulative or sudden trauma, one answer is to reduce the amount of force the worker needs to produce. It can be done through mechanical-assist devices (tools, mechanical lifts, pulleys, and so on) or by making ergonomic changes so that the worker is positioned in the most efficient and strongest way to do the work. (For example, a tool handle that is too large reduces the worker's gripping force. Making the grip match the optimum grip span of the worker's hand automatically increases the force that can be produced by the worker.) Mechanical lifts in manual material handling can also be utilized in workplaces to reduce the load on the spine and thus reduce back injury.

Repetition. Again, the ergonomist therapist reduces repetitions when they are a trauma factor by redesigning the work task or by changing the distances or forces moved so that repetitions are less stressful on the body. This category also includes designing physiologic rest breaks, which take the form of stretch and exercise pauses in the work pace.

Excessive hold time. This time can be measured and monitored by videotape in the workplace. Muscles that must contract and hold over time restrict the oxygen supply to the muscle and the elimination of waste products.[28,30] The remediations for hold time are to reduce the amount of force that must be held (which reduces the maximum voluntary capacity of the muscle being utilized) or to ergonomically change the activity to provide more rest time in comparison to hold time.

Angle/twist. Whether the spine is undergoing twisting and bending, which are ergonomically stressful on the spine,[23,31] or wrist flexion and deviation, which increase the pressure in the carpal tunnel,[27] the therapist evaluates the safest and most physiologically correct position of working joints and muscles.

Design of the work and the work site creates the need to twist or bend the body. Lack of education may also play a role, as the worker who does not understand the noxious effects of these bent postures will not be able to effect a change. A therapist defines whether the work site or the worker is creating the bend and twist by analyzing whether all workers on the job are forced to angulate and twist or whether some can perform their activities in neutral postures and only others use bent or twisted positions. The analysis of the reason behind the angle or the twist leads the therapist to the correct intervention.

Impact. Whether the cause is jumping down from a height (impact on spine, hip, and knee) or using the hand as a hammer (as in pounding boards into place with a fist) impact is damaging on the physiologic components of joints. It creates damage to the joint, nerves, muscles, or blood vessels. Possible remediation is education, substituting mechanical assistance, and, when impact cannot be ergonomically designed out, utilizing impact absorbers.

Vibration. Noxious vibration to the spine can be a result of vehicle driving, and vibration to the upper extremities may be associated with use of vibrating hand tools; both indicate the need for ergonomic change.[19,29]

The therapist may address reduction of vibration, both through better equipment (tools with less vibration, a vehicle seat with vibration absorption) and through education in the use and positioning for the work site structures.

Acceleration. At times it is not the actual movement pattern but the acceleration and velocity of that movement pattern that are most damaging to joint and muscle

structures.[22] Structures can undergo high stresses as tissues respond to sudden muscle contraction or speed change. Therefore, analysis of the motion patterns utilized by workers can lead to changes in work motion to allow better control at all angles and avoid heavy acceleration as much as possible. Acceleration examples would be that in flipping heavy objects (such as a seamstress) or starting momentum on an object (such as pushing a heavy swinging door open quickly). Both modifications to the work and to the worker's education are usually needed.

Work time duration. Two types of duration appear to be problematic. One is the piece work concept in which pay is dependent upon production. Repetition may go beyond what can safely be tolerated by the body. For this, the therapist must analyze the piece work production and compare it with injury rates. In this case, the therapist must work closely with team members and supervisors at the work site to change the incentive from a destructive one to a constructive one. This issue is complicated and not one that can be managed by a health care provider alone. It is an administrative issue.

The therapist may also note that workers state that since 10- or 12-hour days or mandatory overtime was started, that injury rates have gone up. If the therapist is working with an on-site medical professional or the workers' compensation administrator, this relationship (long hours to increased injury) should be verified and studied. The therapist provides the "physiologic" analysis of the issue.

Often, workers desiring either more income or more days off are resistant to ending overtime or long days. To be objective, the therapist must look at the effect of fatigue and injury rate created by the long duration so that there can be objective information given to workers and administration regarding duration of work.

Cold. Cold temperatures can constrict the blood vessels and decrease flexibility of structures, often creating an occasion for injury. The therapist must understand the physiologic effects of the cold and how they may be added factors in cumulative trauma. This is not to say that working outdoors or in cold weather is necessarily prohibited. Rather, the therapist can measure flexibility changes, sensation changes, and productivity changes in an objective way to look at the effects of cold on the overall stress factors.

Individual risk factor identification. The therapist should understand the pathologic risk factors that may be prevalent in workers that will create a susceptibility for work injury. These factors might include arthritis (of all types), other systemic diseases such as diabetes or multiple sclerosis, or the effect of age and gender on work abilities.[27] In addition, risk factors of stature and anthropometric measures may be identified by the therapist as being factors in mismatching the worker with the worksite. When quantified, they will be of help in the ergonomic identification. Each type of injury has personal risk and stress factors associated with it. It is the responsibility of the prevention-

Table 19-5. Functional prework screening

Job title: stock room attendant	
Critical demands	**Functional screen**
1. Lift lower 25-60 lb 6 in. to 5 ft Package dimensions: 2 in. × 12 in. to 2 ft × 3 ft Repetitions: 20 objects in 10 min.	1. Lift (6 in. to 5 ft) 5 repetitions with safe body mechanics 25 lb ☐ Met ☐ Not met 40 lb ☐ Met ☐ Not met 50 lb ☐ Met ☐ Not met 60 lb ☐ Met ☐ Not met _____ time (target 10 minutes or less) Note: Safe body mechanics (stable spine, use arms and legs) enforced by employer
2. Climb 30-ft ladder 25-40 times per shift (no carrying)	2. Climb 30-ft ladder 5 repetitions ☐ Met ☐ Not met
3. Push dolly with inventory throughout storeroom (average travel 30 ft, 4 corners, moderate speed) 68-lb force required to begin movement and at corners	3. Push weight sled set at 68 lb resistance 30 ft, 4 corners ☐ Met ☐ Not met

oriented therapist to know, understand, and utilize current research on the conditions.

Overall, the therapist working with ergonomic changes understands the relationship of the work and work site to the worker. In this way ergonomics becomes part of the prevention triad.

Prework screening

If the worker does not have the strength or functional capability to perform the work safely, this may lead to work injury. It is legal and ethical to screen workers after the offer of hire in order to find if they have capabilities matching the job. This is called functional prework screening. The Americans with Disabilities Act is specific, however, that the screening must be job related. Also, if one individual is screened, all incoming applicants for that same job must be subject to the same screening. The ADA also gives specific guidelines for job relatedness and the circumstances under which medical screenings are legal. The therapist performing prework screens must be well versed in the ADA.

The therapist often evaluates the functional components of the job and designs the functional prework screen to measure the physical aspects of job demands. This work leads to related development of nondiscriminatory functional testing to match the capacities of the worker with the physical demands of the job (Table 19-5).

Screening results are also used as a baseline so that, if injury happens after work is commenced, the worker can again be rehabilitated and evaluated for return to the job. Baseline information also demonstrates capacities and impairments as an employee is beginning a job so that any changes can be compared to original data after an injury.

The ADA mandates that prework screening for a "qualified disabled individual" necessitates a reasonable accommodation, which is an ergonomic modification that the skilled therapist can implement in the workplace. This is a proactive utilization of screening combined with ergonomics.

Summary

Screening completes the triad of injury prevention.[9,10,25] The physical therapist can be pivotal in all three aspects and should prepare to analyze and utilize all three as necessary. One important issue surrounding the safe worker issue transcends all three interventions: The work must be safe. The work must provide a setting where safety standards are identified and monitored. Then, the therapist's intervention will have the foundation of safer, more productive work.

FUTURE PERSPECTIVES

The physical therapist is uniquely qualified to make an important impact on the management of work injury and the prevention of injures and accidents at the work site. Therefore, work injury management and prevention are areas of opportunity for service.

Because work injury is a specific entity that involves function, a therapist is the pivotal professional who can link the physical status of a worker to the workplace. A strong functional background and the specialty skills to match worker and work make a significant impact on bringing together all the participants in work injury management. Although employers, workers, doctors, psychologists, and ergonomists are also pivotal, without the therapist, this circle of matching functional capabilities of the worker with functional demands of the job is not complete.

Physical therapists are important members of the team. As a result, work injury management is a satisfying and appropriate use of the skills of the physical therapist.

REVIEW QUESTIONS

1. What are the three primary components of work injury prevention? Describe each component.
2. What is the underlying philosophy of injury prevention ergonomics?
3. Can the physical therapist contribute to the development of chronic pain behaviors in clients? How can these behaviors be redirected?
4. When assessing the findings of the functional capacities evaluation, should the client, doctor, or therapist determine the level of medically safe functional performance?
5. What issues related to reliability and validity must be considered in performing a functional capacity evaluation?

REFERENCES

1. American Physical Therapy Association: *Guidelines for programs for injured workers,* Alexandria, Va, 1992, The Association.
2. Anderson M: Ergonomics: analyzing work from a physiological perspective. In Isernhagen S, editor: *The comprehensive guide to work injury management,* Gaithersburg, Md, 1995, Aspen.
3. Benz LN: Carpal tunnel syndrome measurement and surveillance management. In Isernhagen S, editor: *The comprehensive guide to work injury management,* Gaithersburg, Md, 1995, Aspen.
4. Bryan J, Geroy G, Isernhagen S: Nonclinical competencies for physical therapists consulting with business and industry, *J Orthop Sports Phys Ther* 18:673, 1993.
5. Bullock M: Health education in the workplace. In Isernhagen S, editor: *Work injury: management and prevention,* Gaithersburg, Md, 1988, Aspen.
6. Darphin L: Work-hardening and work-conditioning perspectives. In Isernhagen S, editor: *The comprehensive guide to work injury management,* Gaithersburg, Md, 1995, Aspen.
7. DeRosa C, Porterfield J: A physical therapy model for the treatment of low back pain, *Phys Ther* 72:4, 1992.
8. Equal Employment Opportunity Commission: *Americans with Disabilities Act technical assistance manual,* Washington DC, 1992, The Commission.
9. Fearon H: Prework screening. In Isernhagen S, editor: *Orthopaedic physical therapy clinics of North America,* Philadelphia, 1992, WB Saunders.
10. Gray R, Campbell S: Case studies: prework screening. In Isernhagen S, editor: *The comprehensive guide to work injury management,* Gaithersburg, Md, 1995, Aspen.
11. Hart D, Matheson L, Isernhagen S: Guidelines for functional capacity evaluation of people with medical conditions, *J Orthop Sports Phys Ther* 18:682, 1993.
12. Isernhagen D: The continuum of care. In Isernhagen S, editor: *Orthopaedic physical therapy clinics of North America,* Philadelphia, 1992, WB Saunders.
13. Isernhagen S: Back schools. In Isernhagen S, editor: *Work injury: management and prevention,* Gaithersburg, Md, 1988, Aspen.
14. Isernhagen S: Ergonomics and cumulative trauma. In Isernhagen S, editor: *Work injury: management and prevention,* Rockville, Md, 1988, Aspen.
15. Isernhagen S: Functional capacity evaluation. In Isernhagen S, editor: *Work injury: management and prevention,* Gaithersburg, Md, 1988, Aspen.
16. Isernhagen S: Functional capacity evaluation and work hardening perspectives. In Mayer T, Mooney V, Gatchel R, editors: *Contemporary care for painful spinal disorders,* Philadelphia, 1991, Lea & Febiger.
17. Isernhagen S: General program paramaters, *Spine* 5:463, 1991.
18. Isernhagen S: *Principles of prevention for cumulative trauma: spine,* Philadelphia, 1991, Hanley & Belfus.
19. Isernhagen S: Ergonomic basics. In Isernhagen S, editor: *Orthopaedic physical therapy clinics of North America,* Philadelphia, 1992, WB Saunders.
20. Isernhagen S: Advancement in functional capacity evaluation. In D'Orazio B, editor: *Back pain rehabilitation,* Fredericksburg, Va, 1993, Orthopedic and Sports Physical Therapy Associates.
21. Johnson L: The kinesiophysical approach matches worker and employer needs. In Isernhagen S, editor: *The comprehensive guide to work injury management,* Gaithersburg, Md, 1995, Aspen.
22. Marras WS, Mirka GA: Trunk responses to asymmetric acceleration, *J Orthop Res* 8:824, 1990.
23. Marras WS et al: The role of dynamic three-dimensional trunk motion in occupationally related low back disorders: the effects of workplace factors, trunk position, and trunk motion characteristics on risk of injury, *Spine* 18:617.
24. Miller M: Functional assessments, *Work* 1:6, 1991.
25. Miller M: Functional prework screening. In *The comprehensive guide to work injury management,* Gaithersburg, Md, 1995, Aspen.
26. Mistal MA: Establishing an industrial prevention program. In Isernhagen S, editor: *The comprehensive guide to work injury management,* Gaithersburg, Md, 1995, Aspen.
27. Pfalzer LA, McPhee B: Carpal tunnel syndrome research. In Isernhagen S, editor: *The comprehensive guide to work injury management,* Gaithersburg, Md, 1995, Aspen.
28. Pheasant, S: *Ergonomics, work and health,* Gaithersburg, Md, 1991, Aspen.
29. Pope M, Andersson G, Chaffin D: The workplace. In Pope M et al, editors: *Occupational low back pain,* St Louis, 1991, Mosby.
30. Rodgers S: Job evaluation in worker fitness determination. In Himmelstein J, Pransky B, editors: *Worker fitness and risk evaluation,* Philadelphia, 1988, Hanley & Belfus.
31. Saunders D: *Evaluations, treatment and prevention of musculoskeletal disorders,* Minneapolis, 1985, Educational Opportunities.
32. Saunders R: Physical therapy early intervention. In Isernhagen S, editor: *The comprehensive guide to work injury management,* Gaithersburg, Md, 1995, Aspen.
33. Saunders R, Anderson M: Early treatment intervention. In Isernhagen S, editor: *Orthopaedic physical therapy clinics of North America,* Philadelphia, 1992, WB Saunders.
34. Smith RL: Integrated work therapy in small practice. In Isernhagen S, editor: *The comprehensive guide to work injury management,* Gaithersburg, Md, 1995, Aspen.
35. Sommerness WD: Testifying in court: you and your records. In Isernhagen S, editor: *The comprehensive guide to work injury management,* Gaithersburg, Md, 1995, Aspen.
36. U.S. Department of Labor, Occupational Safety and Health Administration: *Ergonomics program management guidelines for meatpacking plants,* Washington, DC, 1991, U.S. Government Printing Office.
37. Vance SR, Brown AM: On-site medical care and physical therapy impact. In *The comprehensive guide to work injury management,* Gaithersburg, Md, 1995, Aspen.
38. Wiklund M: Quality outcomes in work rehabilitation. In Isernhagen S, editor: *The comprehensive guide to work injury management,* Gaithersburg, Md, 1995, Aspen.
39. Wise D: The functional capacity evaluation summary report. In Isernhagen S, editor: *Orthopaedic physical therapy clinics of North America,* Philadelphia, 1992, WB Saunders.

INDEX

Note: Page numbers in italics indicate figures; Page numbers followed by *t* indicate tables.

A

Abdominal muscles, 529
  exercises for, 550
  training of, 530, 548
Abdominal wall, functions of, 549
Abduction stress test, 153, *154*
Abductor digiti minimi (ADM), 328
Abductor pollicis brevis (APB), 335
Acceleration, 76
  in injury prevention ergonomics, 608
  law of, 77
Accessory bones, 4
Accessory movements
  of elbow, 388, 391-393
  of knee, 314-315, 319
  of shoulder, 414
Acetabulum, 462, 472
Achilles tendon, 137
  rupture of, *137*
  tendinitis of, 151-152
Acromioclavicular joint, 405-406, *406, 408*
  injuries of, 423 424
  palpation of, 419
Acromioplasty, 439
Across–fiber pattern coding, 56-57
Activation, eccentric, 218
Active movements, 177-178
  of elbow, 385
Active range of motion (AROM) analysis, 178
Active–resistive exercise, 211
Activities of daily living (ADL), 534
Activity performance profile, establishing, 212, *212*
Activity–related spinal pain, 510
Acute care, role of physical therapist in, 559
Adams position, 517
Adductor pollicis, 335
Adductor stretch, 145, *147*
Adenosine triphosphate (ATP), 212
Adhesive capsulitis, 404, 446-447
Adson maneuver, 418
Age
  as factor in bone strength, 33-35, 34*t*
  and shoulder disorders, 411
Alar ligaments, 515
Allograft, 132
AMBRI (atraumatic, multi–directional instability, bilateral shoulders, rehabilitation, inferior capsular shift), 426

American Academy of Orthopaedic Surgeons (AAOS), 413
American Dietetic Association, requirements on prework screening, 609, 609*t*
American Physical Therapy Association statement on work rehabilitation, 604-606
Americans with Disabilities Act (ADA)
  and job matching, 602
  and prework screening, 609, 609*t*
Amphiarthroses, 82
Analastic, 74
Anatomical snuffbox, 348
Anatomic motion barrier, 387
Angiology
  of hip, 469, *469*
  of wrist and hand, 336-338
Angle/twist in injury prevention ergonomics, 608
Anisotropic, 11, *12*
Ankle. *See also* foot
  assessment and management, 282-283
  common disorders of
    chronic overuse conditions, 289-292
    joint sprains, 287, 289
    orthopedic trauma, 287
  examination, 271-273
    active, passive, and resistive tests, 274-275, *276*
    final gait analysis, 281-282
    history and subjective exam, 273-274
    mobility testing, 275
    neurological tests, 276
    objective, 274, *275*
    palpation, 275-276
    screening, 274
    special tests, 276-281
  joint sprains, 287, 289
  orthoses, 283-284, *284*
    fabrication methods, 284-286, *285, 286*
Ankylosing spondylitis, 99, 185
Annulus fibrosus, 510, *522, 522-523*
Anterior drawer test
  for foot, 276-277, *277*
  for knee, 316
  for tibia, 195
Anterior stability assessment, *415,* 415-417, *416, 417*
Apatites, 18
Apophyseal joints, 510, 515, 521, 523, *525, 526, 526, 527*
Apophyses, 16
Apparent density, 18

Appendicular joints, 49
Arch supports, 283
Arcuate ligament, 153
Arteries. *See* Angiology
Arthritis
  degenerative, 125-126
  of hip, 501-506
  rheumatoid, 170, 505
  and temporomandibular joint, 567-569, 578, 582
  traumatic, 111
Arthrogenic lesion, 178-179
Arthrography of ligament injuries, 141-142, *142*
Arthrokinematics, 195, *196*
  of hip joint, 468, 470, *470*
  of knee, 306-308
  of temporomandibular joint, 562-565, *564*
Arthrology
  of elbow complex, *381*, 381-385, *382, 384*
  of hip, 462-464, *463*
  of wrist and hand, 329-331, *331*
Arthroscopy
  in diagnosing ligament injuries, 142-144, *143, 144*
  in treating temporomandibular disorders, 589-590
Arthrosis, 501-506, 567, 582
  surgical management of end–stage, 505-506
Arthrotomy for treating temporomandibular disorders,
  590
Articular cartilage
  composition of, 102-103
  functions of, 104-106
  metabolic activity of, 104
  nutritional supply, 103
  reaction to injury
    capacity for repair, 106-107
    complete fracture of, 108-109
    degenerative arthritis, 125-126
    osteoarthritis, 109
    partial–thickness and full–thickness defects, 107-108,
      108
    pathology and pathogenesis, 109-110, *111*
    symptoms and treatment, 111
    traumatic arthritis, 111
  stress applied to, 105
Articular conditions, 324
Articular eminence, 556
Articular endplates, 82
Articular processes, 510-511
Articular tissues, 48
Articulation
  atlantoaxial, 513, 521
  atlantooccipital, 513, 521
Ash density, 18
Ash weight, 18
Association for the Scientific Investigation of Fractures (ASIF),
  124
Atlantoaxial articulation, 513, 521
Atlantoaxial joint, 521
Atlantooccipital articulation, 513
Atlas, *515*, 515-516, *516*
Atypical haversian systems, 15

Autograft, 132
Avascular necrosis (AVN), 328, 473, 499-500
  of femoral head, 500-501, *501*
Axial loading, 20
Axillary artery occlusion, 445
Axis, *515*, 515-516, *516*

B

Babinski's sign, 183
Ball–and–socket articulation of hip, 460
Ballottement, 318
Bankart lesion, 425, 428
Bankart procedure, 427-428
  rehabilitation following, 430-431
Barlow's test, 482
Barton's fracture, 364
Basic/fundamental measurements, 231
Bells' palsy, 588
Bending loads, 20
Bending moment of inertia, 8-9
Benediction attitude, 335, *336*
Biaxial joints, 328, 331
Biceps brachii muscle, 403, 411
  assessment, 418
  palpation of, 419
Biceps tendinitis, 450
Biochemical activity of calcium, 23
Bioelectrical stimulation, 127, *129, 130*
Biomechanics
  creep, 74
  fatigue, 74
  force, 66-68, *66, 67, 68, 69*
  frictional force, 69
  of hip, 468, *470*, 470-472, *471t, 472t*
  of knee, 306-308
  load, 70
  of orthopedic and sports therapy, 66-79
  power, 70
  pressure, 70
  reasons for, 65-66
  resilience and toughness, 73-74
  of shoulder, 407-409
  strain, 70-72
  strength, 70
  strength of materials, 72-73, *73*
  stress, 70-72
  of temporomandibular joint, 562-565, *564*
  terminology in, 66-74
Blood, classification of, as connective tissue, 9
Blood supply to joint capsule, 99-100
B & L pinch gauge, 344, *347*
Bone–compression plating, 124-126, *125, 126, 127*
Bones, 3. *See also* Fractures; *specific bones*
  cancellous, 18, 26
  capacity for load bearing, 116-117
  categories of, 3-4
    accessory, 4
    flat, 4
    irregular, 4

Bones, 3.—cont'd
  categories of—cont'd
    long, 3-4
    pneumatic, 4
    sesamoid, 4
    short, 4
  classification of, as connective tissue, 9
  compact, 26
  composition of, 9, *10,* 11-12, *12*
  cortical, 18
  growth and loading patterns of lower extremity bones, 36*t,* 36-37
    femur, 37-38, *37, 38t, 39*
    fibula, 38-39, *41*
    foot, 41-42, *42*
    tibia, 38-39, *41*
  growth of, 12, *13*
    membranous, 17-18
    sequential, 13-17, *13, 14, 15, 16,* 17*t*
  haversian, 24
  mechanical properties of
    adaptation of, to exercise stress, 35-36
    age–associated differences in, 33-35, 34*t*
    areas of, and weakness, 23-28, *24,* 26*t, 27t, 28, 28t*
    differences in men's and women's, 33, 33*t,* 35
    healing, 31, 33
    stresses and strains related to shape, 18-23, *19, 20, 21, 22*
    stresses at epiphyseal plates, 28-29
    yielding and failure, *29,* 29-31, *30,* 32*t*
  osteoarthrosis and osteoporosis, 42-43
  porosity of, 18
  purpose of modeling, 21
  resorption, 21-22
  stiffness of, 24
  strength of materials, 4*t,* 4-9, *5,* 5*t, 6, 7, 8, 9*
  subchondral, 48-49
  subperiosteal, 33
  trabecular, 18
Bonesetters, 192
Boosted lubrication, 106
Boston brace, 517
Boundary lubrication, 106
Boutonniere deformity, 334, *335,* 359
Brachial plexus compression test, 182
Bristow procedure, 428
Brittle material, 6
Brudzinski's test, 182
Brunnstrum, Signe, 228
Bruxing, 576
BTE Work Simulator, 342
Bunnell–Littler test, 344, 346
Buoyant force, 67
Burned hand, 367-368, 370
Bursa, 305-306
  greater trochanteric, 498, *498*
  infrapatellar, 302, 305
Bursitis, 306
  around hip area, 497-498
  scapulothoracic, 423

C

Cable tensiometers, 228
Calcaneofibular ligament, 287
Calcaneus, 41
Calcifying tendinitis, 438-439
Calcium, 11
  biochemical activity of, 23
Callus formation, 317
Callus stage, 31
Canaliculi, 18
Cancellous bone, 15, 18, 26, 33
Cantilever bending, 72, *72*
Capitate, 328
Capitellum, 380
Capsular end feel, 387
Capsular fibrosis, 569
Capsular hypermobility, 435
Capsular hypomobility, 412, 413
Capsular patterns, 201, 386
Capsular problems, passive joint mobilization for, 319, 319*t*
Capsular shift, 429
  rehabilitation following, 431-432
Capsular treatment techniques, 319
Capsulitis, 567, 578
  adhesive, 404, 446-447
Carbonate fluoride, 11
Cardiovascular conditioning, limiting factors in, 212-213, *213*
Carpal arch, 329
Carpal bones, 4
Carpal joints, 329
Carpal navicular bone, nonunion fractures in, 132
Carpal tunnel syndrome, 169, 170, 181, 182, 329, 332, 361, *361,* 598
Carpometacarpal joint, 330
Carpus, 328, *328*
Carrying angle, 382
Cartilage
  articular, 102
    capacity for repair, 106-107
    complete fracture of, 108-109
    composition of, 102-103
    degenerative arthritis in, 125-126
    functions of, 104-105
    lubrication of, 106
    metabolic activity of, 104
    nutritional supply to, 103
    osteoarthritis, 109
    partial–thickness and full–thickness defects, 107-108, *108*
    pathology and pathogenesis, 109-110, *111*
    symptoms and treatment, 111
    traumatic arthritis in, 111
    zones of, 103-104, *104, 105*
  classification of, as connective tissue, 9
Cartilaginous plates, 15-16
Cast braces, 123, *124*
Cement lines, 15, 18
Central incisors, 556
Centric occlusion, 562-563
Cervical myelopathy, 183
Cervical nerve, 562

Cervical nerve root pressure, 336
Cervical spine
  evaluation of, 580-581
  influences on crandiomandibular pain, 561
  motion in, 197
  palpation of, 538-539, *540*
  screening, 413
  as source of temporomandibular joint pain, 571
  treatment of, 589
  vertebrae in, 510, 513, *514, 515*
Cervical traction, 545-546
Cervicogenic headache, 571
Cervicothoracic junction, 530
Chaddock's sign, 183
Chemotaxis, 84-85, 86
Children, fractures in, 120, *120, 121*
Chondroblasts, 13
Chondrocytes, 102, 104
Chondromalacia, 117
Chondromalacia patellae, 323
Circle stability concept, 409-410
Circuit weight training, 221-222
Citrate, 11
Clavicle, 12
Clearing examination, 172-173
Clicking, 565-566, *567,* 575, 576
Closed kinetic chain computerized isokinetic testing, versus
    open kinetic chain computerized isokinetic testing, 230
Closed kinetic chain exercise, 216
Closed kinetic chain isokinetic testing, 232
Closed kinetic chain–squat isokinetic testing, 233
Closed lock, 566-567, *568*
Closed reduction of fracture, *122, 123,* 123-124, *124*
Cobb method, *511,* 517
Coccyx, 519
Coefficient of friction, 69
Cold in injury prevention ergonomics, 608
Colitis, 99
Collagen, 9, 11, *11, 12,* 105
Collagenous fibrils, 11
Collateral ligament, 304
  spring test for tearing of, 216
  tests for, 315
  treatment of injuries, 152-154, *154, 155*
Colles' fracture, 364
Comminuted fracture, 119
Compact bone, 26
Comparable sign, 180
Compensatory hypermobility, 203
Composite material, 11
Composition
  of bone, 9, *10,* 11-12, *12*
  of forces, 68
Compound articulation, 330
Compound fractures, 116, 119
Compression plating, 125
Compression stress, 71
Compression test, 277
Compressive fractures, 37
Compressive stress, 9, 37

Computed tomography (CT) scan in assessing temporomandibu-
    lar joint, 582
Computerized closed kinetic chain isokinetic dynamometer
    strength assessment, 230
Computerized eccentric isokinetic dynamometer strength assess-
    ment, 229
Computerized isokinetic dynamometer strength assessment, 229
Concave fossa, 556
Concentric contraction, 216, 218
Concentric muscle loading, 227
Condyles, 296, 298, 563
Congenital muscular torticollis, 532
Connective tissue
  blood as form of, 9
  components of, 9-10
  ligaments as form of, 136
  mechanical properties of, 9
  tendons as form of, 136
Conservation of momentum, law of, 78
Contractile elements, 200
Contractile lesions, 395
  treatment of, 395, 397-398
Contractile tissues, dysfunction of, 395, 397-398
Contraction
  concentric, 216, 218
  eccentric, 216
Contusions, 136, *150,* 150-151
Convex–concave rule, 195-196, *197*
Coracoacromial ligament, 405
Coracoclavicular ligaments, 406
Coracohumeral ligament (CHL), 405
Coronary ligaments, 302
Coronoid fossa, 380
Coronoid process, 556
Corpus Hippocrates, 192
Cortical bone, 18, 25, 27*t*, 30, 31
  fracture of, 31
Costoclavicular ligament, 406
Costotransverse articulation, 521
Costotransverse joint, 516, 521
Costovertebral articulation, 521
Costovertebral joint, 521
Counternutation, 518
Coxa valga, 489
Coxa vara, 485
Craig's test, 484, *484,* 490
Cranial nerves
  examination, 183-184
  neurologic screen of, 580
Craniosacral rhythm (CSR), 206
Craniosacral technique, 206
Cranium, 556, *557*
Crawford Small Parts Dexterity, 342
Creep, 74, 105
Crepitus, 567, 576
Cruciate ligaments, 304-305
  anterior and posterior testing of, 315
  injuries to anterior, 155
    diagnosis of, 155-156, *155, 156*
    treatment of, 156-158, *157, 158*

Cruciate ligaments—cont'd
   injuries to posterior, 158
      diagnosis of, *158,* 158-159
      treatment of, 159, *159, 160*
Crush injury to hand, 362-363
Cryotherapy, 86
   for sprained ligaments, 149
   in treating inflammation, 111, 359
Cubital complex, treatment of, 389
   accompanying dysfunction of capsule and accessory
      ligaments, 393-394
   dysfunction of capsule and accessory ligaments, 390-391
   dysfunction of contractile tissues, 395, 397-398
   dysfunction of noncontractile tissues, 389-390
   hypomobility, 394-395, *395, 396*
   of hypomobility associated with connective tissue dysfunc-
      tion, 391-393, *392, 393*
   noncontractile lesions, 395
Cusps, 556
Cyriax, James, 193, 203-204, 542
Cytokines, 84

D

Daily adjusted progressive resistance exercise (DAPRE), 223
Deceleration, 76
Decompression laminectomies, 510
Deep tendon reflex (DTR), 182-183
Defects
   full–thickness, 107
   partial–thickness, 107
Deformation, units of measure for, 4*t*
Degenerative arthritis, 125-126
Degenerative joint disease (DJD), 67, 110, 173, 502-503, 523
Delayed–onset muscle soreness (DOMS), 220-221
Deltoid muscle, contraction of, 410-411
Dennen, Marjorie, 228
Dental occlusion, 570, *570*
de Quervain's syndrome, Finklestein test for, 344, *348,* 361-362
Diapedesis, 84
Diarthrodial joint, 521
Diathermy in treating inflammation, 111
Diathroses, 82. *See also* Synovial joints
Diffuse tenderness, 141
Digastric muscle, 561
Digital balance evaluator, 232
Diploës, 18
Direct trauma, 83
Discal ligaments, 557
Disc dislocation without reduction, 566-567, *568,* 585-587, *586*
Disc displacement with reduction, 565-566, *566*
Discharge rate, 49
Diskal protrusion or herniation, 522
Distal interphalangeal (DIP) joint, 331
Distal radioulnar joint, 329, *330*
Distal ulnar syndrome, 361
Distal ulnar tunnel, 329
Distal upper extremity testing, 251
Dorsal glide, 373
Double–contrast arthrogram, 141

Double crush phenomenon, 181
Drawer test
   for knee assessment, 318
   and shoulder stability assessment, 415, *416*
Ductile material, 6
Dupuytren's contracture, 332
Dupuytren's disease, 362, *362*
Dural stretch signs, 182
Duration, 216
Dynamics, 66
Dynamometry, handheld, 228
Dysfunction, 543

E

Eburnation, 109-110
Eccentric activation, 218
Eccentric contraction, 216
Eccentric muscle loading, 227
Ecchymosis, 117
Edema
   as complication of fracture healing, 132
   rest in reducing, 86
Elastic deformation range, 5
Elastic limit, 73
Elastic range, 73
Elastin fibers, 9
Elastohydrodynamic lubrication, 106
Elbow, *381,* 381-382
   arthrology, *381,* 381-385, *382, 384*
   examination of, 385
      functional, 385-389, 388*t*
   extension/flexion, 251
   golfer, 398
   lateral tennis, 398
   osteology, 380-381
   supporting structures of, 382-383
   treatment of cubital complex
      accompanying dysfunction of capsule and accessory liga-
         ments, 393-394
      dysfunction of capsule and accessory ligaments, 390-391
      dysfunction of contractile tissues, 395, 397-398
      dysfunction of noncontractile tissues, 389-390
      hypomobility, 394-395, *395, 396*
      of hypomobility associated with connective tissue dysfunc-
         tion, 391-393, *392, 393*
      noncontractile lesions, 395
Elderly
   bone–related problems in
      osteoarthrosis, 42-43
      osteoporosis in, 42-43
   fractures in, 120-121
      hip, 494
Electrical stimulation, 588
Electrophysiologic testing, 185
Emergency splinting, 118-119, *119*
End feels, 179, 201, 318, 387
   abnormal, 201-202
   bone-to–bone, 179
   capsular, 179

End feels—cont'd
  empty, 179
  normal, 201
  springy block, 179
  tissue approximation, 179
Endothelium, microvascular, 90-91
Endurance, 309-310
Endurance limit, 74
Energy, 78-79
  kinetic, 78
  mechanical, 78
  potential, 78
  role of muscle in absorption of, 117
  storage of, 5
Enthesitis, 101
  clinical application of, 101
Epicondyles, 296, 380
Epicondylitis, 398
Epiphyseal plates
  and bone growth, 15, 16
  calcaneal, 41
  of the femur, 37
  Salter–Harris system for classification of injuries, 120
  stresses at, 28-29
  of the tibia, 39
Erector spinae muscles, 526-527, *529*
Ergonomics injury prevention, 607-609
Excessive femoral anteversion, 462
Excessive hold time in injury prevention ergonomics, 608
Excessive lateral compressive syndrome, 306
Exercises
  active–resistive, 211
  closed kinetic chain, 216
  designing program for, 221-224, *222t, 223t*
  isokinetic, 216, 218
  isometric, 215, 227
  isotonic, 215-216, 218, 227
  limiting factors in, 211-213
    cardiovascular, 212-213, *213*
    neuromuscular, 213, *214*
    physiologic, 213-215, *215t*
    skills, 212, *213*
  negative resistance, 216
  open kinetic chain, 216
  for patient with temporomandibular disorders, 588-589
  progressive resistance, 215
  resistance, 221, 227, 547-548
  stabilization, 546-547, *548*
Exercise stress, adaptation of bone to, 35-36
Extension, 382
Extensor mechanism
  exercises for training, 551
  training, 548
Extensor pollicis longus (EPL), 328
Extensor tendon central slip avulsion, 365
Extensor tendon lacerations, 367, *367, 368, 369*
External oblique, 529
Eye dominance, 202

F

Fabellofibular ligaments, 153, 304
Facial muscles, manual therapy to, 588
Facial nerve, 562, 580
  neuropathy, 588
Fasciae, classification of, as connective tissue, 9
Fat, classification of, as connective tissue, 9
Fatigue, 74
Fatique fractures, 31, 74
Fatiguing muscle weakness phenomenon, 182
Fat pads, 101
  injury to, 102
Feedback, utilization of visual in strength assessment, 238
Femoral anteversion, 489-490, *491*
Femoral condyle, 296
Femoral nerve stretch, 182
Femoral quadriceps muscle, 306
Femoral retroversion, 462, 490
Femoral triangle, 467
Femur, 4, *37,* 37-38, *39,* 296, 461
  fracture of, 37, 126, 493
  gender changes in, 35
  material strengths of portions of, 38*t*
  nonunion fractures in, 132
  osseous deformities involving proximal, 485, *488, 489,* 489-490, *490*
Fibers
  collagen, 9
  elastin, 9
Fiber spectrum, 55
Fibrinogen, 98
Fibrinopeptides, 84
Fibroblasts, 11
Fibrocartilage, 556
Fibrocytes, 11
Fibromyalgia, 571-572, 589
Fibrous capsule, 82, 382
Fibula, 38-39, *41*
  material strengths of portions of, 40*t*
Finkelstein's test for DeQuervain's syndrome, 344, *348,* 361
First metatarsophalangeal joint (FMTPJ) extension range of motion, 278, *278*
5–5 examination scheme, 173
Flat bones, 4
Flexibility, 310
Flexion–rotation drawer test, 316
Flexor carpi radialis (FCR), 328
Flexor carpi ulnaris (FCU), 328
Flexor digiti minimi (FDM), 335
Flexor digitorum profundus (FDP), 332-333
  avulsion, 365
Flexor digitorum sublimis (FDS), 332-333
Flexor pollicis brevis (FPB), 4, 335
Flexor pollicis longus (FPL), 335
Flexor tendon lacerations, 365-367, *366*
Fluid lubrication, 106
Fluorimethane spray, 588

Foot, 41-42, *42*, 261-262. *See also* Ankle
  anatomy of, 262
    ligamentous components, 262-263
    osseous components, 262
  assessment and management, 282-283
  common disorders of
    chronic overuse conditions, 289-292
    joint sprains, 287, 289
    orthopedic trauma, 287
  dysfunctions of, 316
  examination, 271-273
    active, passive, and resistive tests, 274-275, *276*
    final gait analysis, 281-282
    history and subjective exam, 273-274
    mobility testing, 275
    neurological tests, 276
    objective, 274, *275*
    palpation, 275-276
    screening, 274
    special tests, 276-281
  functions of, 269-271
  joint mechanics, 263
    closed chain movement of articulations, 268-269, *269, 270*
    intertarsal region, 266, *266*
    rays, 266-267, *267, 268*
    terminology, 263-264
    windlass mechanism of plantar fascia, 267-268, *268*
  orthoses, 283-284, *284*
    fabrication methods, 284-286, *285, 286*
  typical pattern of rearfoot motion during walking, 271, *272*
Force, 66-68, *67, 68, 69,* 77
  buoyant, 67
  characteristics of, 66-67, *66*
  composition of, 68
  frictional, 69
  gravitational, 67
  in injury prevention ergonomics, 607-608
  moments of, 74-76, *75, 766*
    torque, 74-76, *75, 766*
  resolution of, 67, *67*
  resultant, 68
  units of measure for, 4*t*
Force couples, 409
Force sensitivity, 56, 56*t*
Forearm, joints of, 383-385
Forgione–Barber pain production device, 171, *173*
Fossae, 556
Fractures. *See also* Bones
  Barton's, 364
  in children, 120, *120, 121*
  Colles', 364
  comminuted, 119
  complete, of articular cartilage, 108-109
  complications of healing, 130
    edema, 132
    joint stiffness, 132
    neurologic, 132
    nonunion, 130, 132
  compound, 116, 119

Fractures—cont'd
  compressive, 37
  cortical bone, 31
  definition of, 115
  definitive management of, 122-123
    bioelectrical stimulation, 127, *129, 130*
    closed reduction, *122,* 123-124
    open reduction, 124-127, *125, 126, 127, 128*
    rehabilitation, 127-130, *131*
    rigid external fixation, 127, *128*
    traction, 124
  in elderly, 120-121
  emergency care of, 118
    splinting, 118-119, *119*
  fatigue, 31, 74
  of femur, 37
  healing of, 117-118
  of hip and pelvis, *493,* 493-496, 494*t, 495, 496*
  Jefferson's, 515
  of knee, 120
  march, 31, 116
  Monteggia, 383
  pathomechanics of, *116,* 116-117
  of radius, 364, *365*
  of scaphoid, 348, 364-365
  shear, 37
  and soft tissue damage, 116
  spiral, 72
  stress, 116, *121,* 121-122, 289
  tibial, 39
  types of, 119-122
Free nerve endings, 52*t,* 53, *54*
Freestyle stroke, 450
Freeway space, 562
Frequency, increased, 216
Friction, coefficient of, 69
Frictional force, 69
Froment's sign, 346
Fryette, 197
Fryette's laws, 198
Fulcrum test and shoulder stability assessment, 415-416, *416*
Full–thickness defects, 107
Functional capacities evaluation, role of industrial physical
    therapist in, 598, 598*t,* 600-601, 601*t*
Functional evaluation of musculoskeletal disorders, 175,
    177-178
Functional hop test (FHT), 233
Functional jump test, 233, 233*t*
Functional progression, 324
Functional testing
  algorithm for, 231, *231*
  of knee, 243-247

G

Gait analysis, 76
  of foot, 274, 281-282
  of knee, 317
Galen, 192

Gastrocnemius muscle, 306
Gender as factor in bone strength, 33, 33t, 35
Gerdy's (lateral tibial) tubercle, 153
Glenohumeral joint, *402,* 402-405, *403, 404,* 408
    instability of, 424-427
    ligaments of, 409-410
    palpation of, 419
    testing, 248
    testing positions, 250-252
Glenoid fossa, 403
Glenoid labrum, 403
    lesions, *444,* 444-445
Gliding, 180, 195
Gluteus maximus, 464
Glycosaminoglycans (GAGs), 9
Golfer's elbow, 398
Golf swing, 449-450
Golgi ligament endings, 52t, *54,* 57-58
Golgi–Mazzoni corpuscles, 52t, 53, *54*
Golgi–Mazzoni receptors, 56, 57
Grafting, bone, 132
Granulation tissue, 390
Gravitational forces, 67
Greater trochanteric bursa, 498, *498*
Growth of bone, 12, *13*
    membranous, 17-18
    sequential, *13,* 13-17, *14, 15, 16,* 17t
Guyon's canal syndrome, 361
Gyration, radius of, 8

H

Hallux limitus, 292
Hallux rigidus, 292
Halstead's test, 418
Hamate, 328
Hamstrings, 306
Hamstring stretch, 145-146, *148*
Hand. *See* Wrist and hand
Hand grip dynamometer, 226
Handheld dynamometry, 228
Harrington rods, 517
Haversian bone, 24, 30
Haversian canal, 15, *16*
Haversian systems, 15
    atypical, 15
Headache, 571
Heel spur, 289
Hemarthrosis, 139, 155
Hemorrhagic effusions, synovial fluid in, 98-99
Hemosiderin, 92-93
Hilton's law, 468
Hinge joints, 331
Hip, 263-264, 460
    anatomy
        arthrology, 462-464, *463*
        myology, 464-465
        neurology of, 465, 467-468, *468*
        osseous structures, *460,* 460-462, *461, 462*
        vascular anatomy, 468, *469*

Hip—cont'd
    arthrokinematics of, 468, 470, *470*
    biomechanics, 468, *470,* 470-472, 471t, 472t
        arthrokinematics, 468, 470, *470*
    common disorders
        congenital and developmental conditions involving
            joint, 490-493, *492*
        fractures of pelvis and, *493,* 493-496, 494t, *495,*
            496
        osseous deformities involving proximal femur, 485,
            488, 489-490, *489, 490*
        soft tissue, 496-499, *497, 498, 499*
        traumatic, that affect hip and associated tissues,
            493
    degenerative and inflammatory conditions involving,
        499-506, *500, 501, 502, 503, 504*
    differential diagnosis, 506, 506t
    examination of
        functional assessment, 484, *486, 487*
        general principles, 473-475, *474-476*
        objective, 479t, 479-484, *480, 481, 482, 483, 484*
        radiologic, 484-485, *488*
        subjective, 477-479, *478*
    factors that provide stability and mobility, 472
    general concepts of, 472-473
    range of motion, 278
Hippocrates, 192
Histamine, 84
History
    in ankle evaluation, 273-274
    in clinical spine evaluation, 534, *535*
HLA–B27, testing for, 185
Hoffmann's sign, 183
Homans' sign, 277
Hooke's law, 5, 23
Hughston system, 138
Humeroradial joints, *381,* 381-382
Humeroulnar joint, *381,* 381-382
Humerus, 4
    fracture of, 126
Humphrey ligament, 305
Hyaline cartilage, 16-17, 82
Hyaluronate, 95, 96-97, 106
Hyaluronic acid, 96-97
Hydrophilic structure, 522
Hydroxyapatite, 11, 18
Hydroxyapatite crystals, 19
Hydroxyl ions, 11
Hyperextension, 313, 382
Hypermobility, 203, 282, 569
    capsular, 435
    compensatory, 203
    of elbow, 393-395, *395, 396*
    scapular, 435-436
Hyperreactivity, 182
Hypomobility, 203, 282
    capsular, 412, 413
    of joint, 319
Hypoplasia, 570-571
Hyporeactivity, 182

I

Idiopathic scoliosis, 516-517
Iliofemoral ligament, 463
Iliolumbar ligament, 528
Iliopectineal bursa, 463, 499, *499, 500*
Iliopsoas muscles, 306, 465
Ilizarov method of external fixation, 127
Impact in injury prevention ergonomics, 608
Impingement sign, 418, *418*
Impingement syndrome of shoulder, 170
Impulse, 77-78
Indirect trauma, 83
Individual risk factor identification, 608-609
Industrial physical therapy, 598*t*, 598-599. *See also* Physical
    therapy
    function, 598
        in acute muscoloskeletal/cumulative trauma injury treat-
            ment, 598*t*, 599*t* 598-600
        capacities evaluation, 600-601, 601*t*
        future issues, 606
        work rehabilitation, 604, *605,* 606
    future perspectives, 609
    kinesiology, 597-598
    relationship to injury or illness, 598
    role of therapist in, 598*t*, 598-599
    work injury prevention, *606,* 606-609
        prework screening, 609
Inertia, 67
    bending moment of, 8-9
    law of, 77
    mass moment of, 8
    polar moment of, 9, 25
Inferior glenohumeral ligament complex (IGHLC), 404, *404,*
    410
Inferior oblique, 531
Inferior stability assessment, 414-415, *414, 415*
Inflammation, 221
    causes of, 83
    definition of trauma, 83
    effects of trauma, 84-85
    of elbow complex, 390-391
    outcomes of, 86
    phagocytosis, 85-86
    repair, 86
    types of trauma to joints, 83-84
Infrapatellar bursa, 302, 305
Infraspinatus muscle, 411
Injuries
    prevention, 598-599
    prevention ergonomics, 607-609
    reaction of articular cartilage to, 106-111, *108, 111*
    reaction of intraarticular structures to, 101-102
    reaction of joint capsule to, 100
    reaction of synovial fluid to, 97-100
    reaction of synovial membrane to, 91-95, *94t, 95, 96*
Innervation density, 354
Innervation of temporomandibular joint, 561-562, *563*
Inspection of hip joint, 479-480, 482-483
Instability of glenohumeral joint, 424-427
Interclavicular ligament, 406

Intercondylar region, 297-298
Interdigital neuroma, 291
Interleukin–1, 84
Intermedullary rodding, 126-127, *128*
Internal oblique, 529
Internal rotation, 313
International Knee Documentation Committee (IKDC), 233
International Knee Documentation Form, 310, *311-312*
Interphalangeal (IP) joints, 328, 331, *331*
Interspinous ligaments, 521
Intertarsal region of foot, 266, *266*
Intertrochanteric fractures, 495, *495*
Intervertebral articulations, 510
Intervertebral disk, 517, *521,* 521-522
Intervertebral foramen, 523, *524, 525*
Intima, 87
Intraarticular damage and osteophytes in osteoarthritis, 102
Intraarticular disk ligament, 406
Intraarticular fibrocartilage and fat pads
    fat pads, 101
    functions, 101
    menisci, 101
Intraarticular ligament injuries, 154-160, *155, 156, 157, 158,*
    159, 160
    anatomy of, 154-155
    anterior cruciate, 155
        diagnosis of, 155-156, *155, 156*
        treatment of, 156-158, *157, 158*
    posterior cruciate
        diagnosis of, *158,* 158-159
        treatment of, 159, *159, 160*
Intraarticular structures
    damage and osteophytes in osteoarthritis, 102
    injury of fat pads, 102
    reaction to injury, 101-102
        meniscus, 101-102
Intrinsic minus hand, 335
Inversion stress test, 277, *277*
Irregular bones, 4
Irritability, 193
Isokinetic exercise, 216, 227
    disadvantages of, 230
    testing, 236
        closed kinetic chain, 232
        of knee, 236-240, *237, 238, 239, 240*
        relationship of, to functional performance, 252
    in upper extremity, strength assessment, 247*t,* 247-248
Isolation of muscle, 217, *217, 218*
Isometric exercise, 215, 218, 227
    advantages of, 227
    disadvantages of, 227
Isotonic exercise, 215-216, 218, 227, *228*
    advantages of, 228, 229
    disadvantages of, 229
Isotonic muscle assessment, 228-229

J

Jamar dynamometer, 344, *344*
Jebsen–Taylor Hand Function, 342

Jefferson's fracture, 515
Jendrassik's maneuver, 183
Jerk test in shoulder assessment, 417
Job matching, role of industrial physical therapist in, 600-601
Joint afference, 59
Joint bodies, 102
Joint capsule
  composition, 99
  enthesitis, 101
  functions, 100
  nerve and blood supply, 99-100
  and reaction to injury, 100
    sprains, 100
  redundancy, 100
Joint cavity, 82
Joint congruency, positions of, 196, *197*
Joint effusion, 318
Joint fiber afference, efferent modulation of, 58
Joint laxity, degree of, 141
Joint lubrication, 89-91
Joint reaction force (JRF), 470-472
Joint receptors, 50, 52*t*, 53, 55
Joint replacement arthroplasty, 360
Joint restriction, 204
Joint(s). *See also* Synovial joints
  acromioclavicular, 405-406, *406,* 408
    injuries of, 423-424
    palpation of, 419
  acute inflammation in, 84
  apophyseal, 510, 515, 521, 523, *525,* 526, *526, 527*
  appendicular, 49
  atlantoaxial, 521
  biaxial, 328, 331
  carpal, 329
  carpometacarpal, 330
  classification of, 82
  complex, 194
  compound, 194
  costotransverse, 516, 521
  costovertebral, 521
  diarthrodial, 521
  distal interphalangeal, 331
  distal radioulnar, 329, *330*
  of forearm, 383-385
  functional implications, 58
    postural and equilibrium mechanisms, 59
    proprioceptive and kinesthetic awareness, 59-60
    spinal reflex action, 58-59
  general functional anatomy, 48-50, *50, 52t*
  glenohumeral, *402,* 402-405, *403, 404,* 408
    instability of, 424-427
    ligaments of, 409-410
    palpation of, 419
    testing, 248
    testing positions, 250-252
  hinge, 331
  humeroradial, *381,* 381-382
  humeroulnar, *381,* 381-382
  and inflammation, 83
  instability resulting from ligamentous injury, 138

Joint(s)—cont'd
  interphalangeal, 328, 331, *331*
  manual methods for assessing dysfunction
    abnormal end feels, 201-202
    contractile and noncontractile elements, 200
    normal end feels, 201
    selective tissue assessment, 200
    systematic evaluation techniques, 200-201
  mechanics, of foot, 263-271
  metacarpophalangeal, 328, 330-331
  midcarpal, 329-330
  mobilization of, 82, 543-545
  motion of
    barriers to movement, 198-200, *199*
    convex–concave rule, 195-196, *197*
    laws of vertebral, 196-198, *198*
    positions of joint congruency, 196, *197*
  occipitoatlanto, 198
  patellofemoral, 68, 71, 296, 302, 307
  pisiform–triquetral, 330
  proximal interphalangeal, 363-364
  sacroiliac, 518, 521
    dysfunction of, 167
  scapulothoracic, 406-407, *407,* 420, 422-423
  simple, 194
  stability of, 60, 82
    shoulder, 409-411
  sternoclavicular, 406, 407-408
    palpation of, 419
  stiffness as complication of fracture healing, 132
  structural specialization of, 48
  temporomandibular, 556
    disorders
      capsular fibrosis, 569
      cervical spine consideration, 571
      differential diagnosis, 571-572
      growth and development considerations, 570-571
      hypermobility, 569
      masticatory muscle disorders, 569-570, *570*
      pathomechanics, 565-569, *566, 567, 568*
    evaluation of
      patient history and subjective report, *572,* 572-573
      physical exam, 573, *574, 575,* 575-591, *576, 577*
    functional anatomy, 556, *557*
      biomechanics and arthrokinematics, 562
      capsule and ligaments, 557-559, *559*
      disc and attachments, 556-557, *558*
      function, 565
      innervation, 561-562, *563*
      musculature, 559-561, *561*
      osseous structures, 556, *557*
      osteokinematics, 559, *560*
    imaging, 581-582
    physical therapy approach to, 582-583
      exercises for patient with, 588-589
      surgical approaches for, 589-591
      treatment of cervical spine, 589
      treatment of derangement, 583-587, *585, 586*
  tibiofemoral, 296, *296,* 302, 306-307
    examination of, 313-314

Joint(s)—cont'd
   tibiofemoral—cont'd
      intraarticular disorders of, 310
   trapeziometacarpal, 330
   types of trauma to, 83-84
   vertebral, 49

K

Kaltenborn, 193, 204
Keinbock's disease, 363
Kendall, Florence, 228
Kendall, Henry, 228
Kenny, Elizabeth, 228
Kernig's test, 182
Kibler's test, 180
Kinematics, 194
   measurement of motion, 76-77
   motion, 76
   motion and injury, 77
Kinesiology, 597-598
Kinesthetic awareness, 59-60
Kinetic chain, 307-308
Kinetic energy, 78
Kinetics
   energy, 78-79
   of hip joint, 470-473, *473*
   impulse and momentum, 77-78
   Newton's first law, 77
   Newton's second law, 77
   Newton's third law, 77
   work, 78
Knee, 296
   anatomy
      bursae, 305-306
      capsule, *302,* 302-305, *303, 304*
      menisci, *300-301,* 301-302
      musculature, 306
      osteology, 296-298, *297, 298, 299,* 300-301
   assessing and treating range–of–motion deficiencies, 318-319, 319*t,* 320*t*
   biomechanics/arthrokinematics
      kinetic chain, 307-308
      patellofemoral joint, 307
      tibiofemoral joint, 306-307
   fracture of, 120
   functional testing of, 243-247
   injuries
      arthrographic evaluation of, 142
      environmental factors, 310
      functional predisposition, 309
      ligamentous, 139, *140*
      macrotrauma, 308
      mechanisms of, 308
      muscular factors, 309-310
      prevention, 308-309
      previous injury, 309
      proprioception, 310
      shoes, 310
      structural predisposition, 309

Knee—cont'd
   interpretation of test data, 240-243, 241*t,* 242*t,* 243*t*
   isokinetic testing of, 236-240, *237, 238, 239, 240*
   joint stability, 236
   lateral ligamentous stabilizers of, 153
   macrotraumatic injuries, 296
   physical examination of
      anterior and posterior cruciate ligament testing, 315
      evaluation form, 310, *311-312*
      foot, 316-317
      functional assessment, 316
      gait evaluation, 317
      objective, 313-315
      posture, 317
      reexamination, 317
      referral, 317
      rotational, 315-316
      specialized, by physical therapists, 317-318
      specific tests, 315
      spring test, 316
      subjective, 310, 313
   superficial medial side of, 152-153
   surgical management, 323-324
   testing, 240, *241*
   treatment, 319-320
   unacceptable results, 320-323
Korr, 207
KT1000 testing, 231
Kyphosis, 513
   thoracic, 573

L

Labrum, role of, as stabilizing structure, 403
Labrum–biceps tendon, 403
Lachman's test, *155,* 155-156, 315, 318
Lacuna, 18
Lamellae, 18
Laminae, 510
Laminectomies, decompression, 510
Lateral capsule sign, 153, *155*
Lateral deviation, 559
Lateral epicondylitis, 398
Lateral excursion of mandible, 573, 575, *575*
Lateral knee pain, 307
Lateral pterygoid, 559, *561*
Lateral recess stenosis, 510
Lateral tennis elbow, 398
Laterotrusion, 559
Legg–Calvé–Perthes disease, 489, 490
Lesion, Bankart, 425, 428
Lesions
   glenoid labrum, *444,* 444-445
   meniscus, 323-324
Leukocytes, 84
Levator scapulae, 531
Levator scapulae tendinitis, 423
Lever arm of load, 74
Ligament injuries and instabilities
   classifying, 138

Ligament injuries and instabilities—cont'd
  diagnosis
    arthroscopy, 142-144, *143, 144*
    history, 138
    loss of function, 139
    magnetic resonance imaging, 142
    mechanism of, 138
    physical examination, 139, *140,* 141
    radiographic evaluation, *141,* 141-142
    symptoms, sounds, and swelling, 138-139, *140*
  treatment of, 144-145
    collateral, 152-154, *154, 155*
    contusions, *150,* 150-151
    intraarticular, 154-160, *155, 156, 157, 158, 159, 160*
    muscle–tendon unit injuries, 145
    tendinitis, 151*t,* 151-152, *152*
Ligament of Humphrey, 302
Ligament of Wrisberg, 302
Ligamentous components, of foot, 262-263
Ligamentous repairs, 323-324
Ligaments, 82, 136
  arcuate, 153
  classification and grading of injury to, 137-138
  discal, 557
  fabellofibular, 153
  in joint capsule, 99
  periodontal, 556, *557*
  rehabilitation program for strains, 149-150, 150*t*
  for spine, 519-521
Ligamentum flavum, 520-521
Ligamentum teres, 463
Limb–length difference and knee injuries, 308
Linea, 232
Listner's tubercle, 328
Load, biomechanical, 70
Load carriage, 104-106
Locking, 313
Long bones, 3-4
Longissimus capitis, 530
Longitudinal arch, 329
Lordosis, 512-513, 517
Lovett, Robert, 197, 227
Lower extremity
  bone growth and loading patterns of, 36*t,* 36-37
    femur, *37,* 37-38, 38*t, 39*
    fibula, 38-39, *41*
    foot, 41-42, *42*
    tibia, 38-39, *41*
  muscle strength assessment for, 234-236
    functional testing, 243-247
    interpretation of test data, 240-243, 241*t,* 242*t,* 243*t*
    isokinetic testing of knee, 236-240, *237, 238, 239, 240*
    knee testing, 240, *241*
  strength assessment for, 234-236
    functional testing, 243-246
    interpretation of test data, 240-243, 241*t,* 242*t, 243*
    isokinetic testing of knee, 236-240, *237, 238, 239, 240*
    knee testing, 240, *241*
Lower extremity functional test, 233-234, *234,* 234*t, 235, 235t*
Lowman, Charles, 227-228

Lubrication, 106
  boosted, 106
  boundary, 106
  cartilage, 106
  elastohydrodynamic, 106
  fluid, 106
  self–pressurized hydrostatic, 106
  squeeze–film, 106
  weeping, 106
Ludington test, 418
Lumbarization of first sacral vertebrae, 510
Lumbar spine, motion in, 197
Lumbar vertebrae, 510, 517, *518*
Lumbrical muscles, 334
Lumbrical plus deformity, 334
Lunate, 328
  dislocation, 363
Lysosomes, 85

M

Macrophages, 85
Macrotrauma
  of knee, 296, 308
  and temporomandibular joint, 565
Magnetic resonance imaging (MRI)
  in assessing avascular necrosis, 500-501
  in assessing ligament injuries, 141, 142
  in assessing temporomandibular joint, 581-582
Magnuson–Stack procedure, 429
Maigne, Robert, 193, 205
Maitland, Geoff, 193, 204, 205, 542
Malleolar torsion, 278, *279*
Mallet finger, 333
Mandible, 556, *557*
  lateral excursion of, 573, 575, *575*
  power stroke of, 564
  stable rest position of, 562
Mandibular condyle, 556
Mandibular depression, 575, 576
Mandibular elevators, 563-564
Mandibular fossa, 556
Mandibular retrusion, 565
Manipulation, 192
Manipulation/mobilization, 203-205, *204,* 204*t*
Manipulative techniques, 204
Manual muscle testing (MMT), 226, 227-228, 236, 247
  of knee, 236
  of mandibular elevator, 579-580, *580*
  in upper extremity strength assessment, 247
Manual therapy to facial muscles, 588
Marathon running, 213
March fractures, 31, 116
Margination, 84
Massage, 192
Masseter muscle, 559, 561, *561,* 576
Mass moment of inertia, 8
Mastication, muscles of, 559-560
Masticatory muscle disorders, 569-570, *570*
  treatment for, 587-588

Mastoid process, 530
Material creep, 74
Material fatigue, 74
Materials
    brittle, 6
    composite, 11
    ductile, 6
    strength of, 72-73, *73*
Maxillary bone, 556
Maximal compressive stress, 4
Maximal tensile stress, 4
Maximum medical improvement (MMI), 604
McGill Pain Questionnaire, 477, *478*
McGill Short Form Questionnaire, 171, *172*
McKenzie, Robin, 542
McKenzie method of treatment, 543
McMurray test, 316
Measurement of motion, 76-77
Mechanical creep, 74
Mechanical energy, 78
Mechanical strain, 70
Mechanical stress, 70
Medial and lateral collateral ligament testing, 315
Medial epicondylitis, 398
Medial facet, 300
Medial pterygoid, 559, *561*
Mediotrusion, 559
Medullary cavity, 4
Membranous bone growth, 17-18
Meniscal tearing, 316
Meniscectomy
    partial, 143
    total, 143
Menisci, 101, *300-301, 301-302*
    functions, 101
Meniscopatellar ligaments, 303
Meniscus, 82-83
    injury to, 101-102
    lesions in, 323-324
Mennel, 193
Meralgia paraesthetica, 468
Mesenchymal cells, 13, 17
Mesenchyme, 12
Mesoderm, paraxial, 12
Metabolic activity of articular cartilage, 104
Metacarpal arch, 329
Metacarpals, fracture of, 365
Metacarpophalangeal joints, 328, 330-331
Metacarpus, 328, *328*
Metatarsalgia, *291,* 291-292, *292*
Metatarsus primus elevatus, 292
Microdamage, 29-30
    accumulation, 31
Microtrauma
    of knee injuries, 296, 308
    and muscle soreness, 220-221
    and temporomandibular joint, 565
Microvascular endothelium, 90-91
Midcarpal joint, 329-330
Middle glenohumeral ligament (MGHL), 404, *404,* 410

Migraine headache, 571
Milking, 314, 318
Milwaukee brace, 517
Minimal effective strain (MES), 23
Minnesota Manual Dexterity, 342
Mitchell, 206
Mobility testing of foot, 275
Mobility training, 211
Mobilization, 192
    maneuvers, 543-544
Modulus of elasticity, 5
Modulus of resilience, 74
Modulus of toughness, 74
Moments, 7
    of force, 74-76
Momentum, 77-78
Monocytes, 85
Monteggia's fractures, 383
Morphology, 87
Morton's neuroma, 291
Morton's toe, 291
Motion, 76
    assessment of, in hip joint, 480-481
    assessment of shoulder, 413-414
    of hip joint, 482-483
    and injury, 77
    measurement of, 76-77
Motion barrier
    appraisal of, for elbow, 387-388
    relationship of pain to, 388
Motor examination, 183
Mucin, 96
Mucopolysaccharides, 9
Multifidus muscles, 527, 530, *530*
Muscle energy, 206
    technique, 206
Muscle fatigue, 30, *30,* 220
Muscle fibers
    classification of, 213
    condition of, 215
Muscle guarding, 569
Muscle loading
    concentric, 227
    eccentric, 227
Muscle performance, modifying factors in, 213, *213*
Muscle relaxation splint, 586, *586*
Muscle(s). *See also specific*
    biomechanics of, 66
    isolation of, 217, *217, 218*
    isotonic assessment, 228-229
    mode of action, 226-227
    role of, in energy absorption, 117
Muscle stretch reflex (MSR), 182
Muscle–tendon techniques for noncapsular problems,
        319-320
Muscle–tendon unit, 136
    injuries
        running–functional progression program, 146, 147*t,* 148
        stretching program, 145-146, *146, 147*
        treatment of, 145-146, *146, 147,* 147*t,* 148-149, 149*t*

Muscle–tendon unit—cont'd
  injuries—cont'd
    weight program, 148-149, 149t
      ligament sprains, 149-150, 150t
Muscular endurance, 218
Muscular strength
  importance of, 309
  physiological factors limiting, 213, 214
Musculature of spine, 526-532
Musculoskeletal disorders
  diagnosis, 185-186
  documentation, 166-167
  evaluation schemes for, 166
  interpretation of test procedures, 188
  objective examination, 173
    additional medical, 184-185
    function, 175, 177-180
    neurologic tests, 181-184
    observation, 173, 175
    palpation, 180-181
  standard examination procedure, 167
    case history, 167-171, 169, 170
    clearing, 172-173
    measurement of pain, 171, 171, 172, 173, 174-175, 176-177
    planning, 171
  trial treatment, 186-187
Musculoskeletal evaluation, goals of, 165-166, 166
Myelopathy, 515
Myofascial pain, 569
Myofascial release, 205-206
Myology of hip, 464-465, 465t, 466

N

Neck injuries, emergency treatment of, 118-119
Negative resistance exercise, 216
Nerve conduction velocity (NCV) studies, 185
Nerve supply, to joint capsule, 99-100
Nerve trunk, examination of, 182-183
Neural system, basic relevance, 47-48
Neural tension testing, 538, 540
Neurobiology for orthopedic and sports physical therapy, 47-60
Neurogenic inflammation, 181
Neurological disease, 291
Neurologic complication of fracture healing, 132
Neurologic screen of cranial nerves, 580
Neurologic tests, 181-184
  of the foot, 276
Neurology
  of hip, 465, 467-468, 468
  of wrist and hand, 335-336, 336
Neuromuscular control, 409
Neuromuscular performance parameter, 242
Neuron population response, 56-57
Neurovascular compression syndromes, 445-447
Neutral zero method, 346
Neutropenia, 86
Neutrophils, 85
  reaction to injury, 92, 92

Newton
  first law of motion, 67, 77
  second law of motion, 77
  third law of motion, 77
Nocturnal parafunctional activity, 584-585
Noncapsular pattern, 386
Noncapsular problems, muscle–tendon techniques for, 319-320
Noncontractile elements, 200
Nonunion fractures, 130, 132
Normal shear strain, 4
Nucleus pulposus, 522
Nutation, 518

O

Ober's sign, 484
Ober's test, 484, 485
Oblique retinacular ligaments, 334
Observation in evaluation of musculoskeletal disorders, 173, 175
Occipitoatlanto joint, 198
Occlusion, centric, 562-563
Occupational Safety and Health Administration (OSHA) and job matching, 602
Olecranon fossa, 380, 387
Olecranon process, 387
One–repetition maximum (RM), 226
Open kinetic chain (OKC)
  versus closed kinetic chain computerized isokinetic testing, 230
  computerized isokinetic testing versus closed kinetic chain computerized isokinetic testing, 230
  exercise, 216
  isokinetic test, 226
  testing, 232-233
Open–lock, 569
Open reduction and internal fixation (ORIF), 124
Open reduction of fracture, 124-127, 125, 126, 127, 128
Opponens digiti minimi (ODM), 335
Opponens pollicis (OP), 335
Opsonins, 85
Oral cavity, screening of, 581
Orthognathic surgery for treating temporomandibular disorders, 590
Orthopedic and sports physical therapy. See also Physical therapy
  biomechanics of therapy, 66-79
  efferent modulation of joint fiber afference, 58
  functional implications in, 58-60
  general functional anatomy in, 48-50, 50, 52t8
  joint receptors in, 50, 52t, 53, 55
  neural system in, 47-48
  neurobiology for, 47-60
  role of frictional force in, 69
  stimulus–response relationships in, 55-58
Orthopedic manual therapy, 192
  arthrokinematics, 195, 196
  classification of synovial joints, 194, 194
  concepts and rules of joint motion
    barriers to movement, 198-200, 199
    convex–concave rule, 195-196, 197

Orthopedic manual therapy—cont'd
  concepts and rules of joint motion—cont'd
    laws of vertebral motion, 196-198, *198*
    positions of congruency, 196, *197*
  contraindications, 207-208, 208*t*
  history of, 192-194
  methods of assessing joint dysfunction
    abnormal end feels, 201-202
    contractile and noncontractile elements, 200
    normal end feels, 201
    selective tissue assessment, 200
    systematic evaluation techniques, 200-201
  nontraditional techniques, 205
    craniosacral, 206
    muscle energy, 206
    myofascial release, 205-206
    strain counterstain, 207, *207*
  osteokinematics, 194-195, *195*
  palpation techniques, 202-203
  traditional treatment techniques, 203
    manipulation/mobilization, 203-205, *204, 204t*
Orthopedic trauma in foot and ankle, 287
Orthosis
  foot, 283-284, *284*
  sacroiliac, 519
Ortolani's test, 482
Os acromiale, 422
Os coxae, 462
Osseious components
  of foot, 262
  of temporomandibular joint, 556, *557*
Osseous deformities involving proximal femur, 485, *488,*
    489-490, *489, 490*
Ossification, 298
  primary centers of, 13-14, 16, 17*t*
  secondary centers of, 16, 17*t*
Osteoarthritis (OA), 109, 501-502, 598
  of acromioclavicular joint, 424
  intraarticular damage and osteophytes in, 102
Osteoarthrosis, 42-43
Osteoblasts, 11-12
Osteochondritis, 167
Osteochondromatosis, secondary synovial, 110
Osteoclasts, 11
Osteocytes, 15
Osteoid, 17
Osteokinematics, 194-195, *195,* 407, 559, *560*
Osteology
  for elbow, 380-381
  for knee, 296-298, *297, 298, 299,* 300-301
  for wrist and hand, 328-329, *329*
Osteons, 19, 26, 33
  primary, 18
Osteopathy, 192-193
Osteophytes, 109
  in osteoarthritis, 102
Osteophytic growth, 109
Osteoporosis, 37, 42-43, 120-121, 220, 478
Osteoprogenitor cells, 12
Oswestry Disability Index for Low Back Pain, 171, *174-175*

Overhead exertion test, 418-419
Overhead throwing, 447-448
Overuse injuries
  diagnosis of muscle, 497
  knee, 296
  special tests for, 277-281, *278, 279, 280, 281*
Overwork, 220
Oxford technique, 221

P

Pacinian corpuscles, 52*t,* 53, *54*
Paget's disease, 489
Pain
  guidelines for assessment, 186-187
  in knee disorders, 313
  measurement of, 171, *171, 172, 173, 174-175, 176-177*
  myofascial, 569
  patellofemoral, 49
  preauricular, 567, 568
  radicular, 523
  referred, 168, 534
  spinal, 510
Painful arcs, 178, 200-201
Palmar aponeurosis, 332
Palmaris brevis, 335
Palmar metacarpal arteries, 337
Palmer, Daniel David, 193
Palpation
  in assessing biceps brachii, 418
  in assessing cervical spine, 538-539, *540*
  in assessing clicks, 566
  in assessing foot injuries, 275-276
  in assessing hip joint, *481,* 481-482, 483-484
  in assessing knee injuries, 314
  in assessing musculoskeletal disorders, 180-181
  in assessing shoulder injuries, 419-420, 420*t*
  in assessing temporomandibular joint, *576,* 576-578
  in assessing wrist and hand injuries, 348, *354*
  techniques in, 202-203
Palsy, Bells, 588
Paraxial mesoderm, 12
Pare, Ambrose, 192
Paris, Stanley B., 193, 205, 542
Partial–thickness defects, 107
Passive joint mobilization for capsular problems, 319, 319*t*
Passive movements, 178
  of elbow, 385-386
Passive range of motion, 178, 192, 199-200
Patella, 25, 296, 298, 300-301, 307
  palpation of, 314
Patellar facet, 300
Patellar ligament, 298, 300
Patellar pain, 307
Patellar stabilization, 307
Patellar tendinitis, 307
Patellar tendinosis, 307
Patellar tendon, 300
Patellofemoral articulation, 298-299
Patellofemoral joint, 68, 71, 296, 302, 307

Patellofemoral ligaments, 303
Patellofemoral pain, 49
Patellofemoral pain syndrome, 48
Patellofemoral problems, 323-324
Pathomechanics of fracture, *116,* 116-117
Patient education
    role of physical therapist in, 606-607
    and temporomandibular joint pain, 584-585
    in treating masticatory muscle disorders, 587-588
Patrick's test, 482, 500-501, 503
Peak torque, assessing, 241
Pedicle, 510
Pelvic ring fractures, 493-494
Periarticular receptors, 53
Perichondrium, 13, 14
Perimeter scouring, 500-501
Periodontal ligaments, 556, *557*
Periosteum, 14, 16-17
Peripheral nerve entrapment, 353
Peripheral nerve injuries to wrist and hand, 370
Pes anserinus bursa, 303, 305
Pes anserinus expansion palpation, 314
Phagocytosis, 85-86
Phalanges, 328, *328*
    fracture of, 365
Phalen's test, 182, 353, *354*
Phonophoresis, 498
Phosphorus, 11
Physical examination
    of elbow complex, 385
        functional, 385-389, 388*t*
    of hip
        functional, 484, *486, 487*
        general principles, 473-475, *474-476*
        objective, 479*t,* 479-484, *480, 481, 482, 483, 484*
        radiologic, 484-485, *488*
        subjective, 477-479, *478*
    of knee
        anterior and posterior cruciate ligament testing, 315
        evaluation form, 310, *311-312*
        foot, 316-317
        functional assessment, 316
        gait evaluation, 317
        objective, 313-315
        posture, 317
        reexamination, 317
        referral, 317
        rotational, 315-316
        specialized, by physical therapists, 317-318
        specific tests, 315
        spring test, 316
        subjective, 310, 313
    of ligament injuries and instabilities, 139, *140, 141*
    of shoulder, 412
    of spine, 535-539, *538, 540*
    of temporomandibular joint, 573, *574, 575, 575-591, 576, 577, 578, 579, 580, 581*
    of wrist and hand, *342,* 342-344, *343, 344, 345, 346,* 346-349, *347,* 347*t, 348,* 348*t, 349, 349, 350-351, 352, 353, 354, 354, 355, 356,* 356*t,* 356-357, *357*

Physical therapist
    approach to temporomandibular disorders, 582-583
    neurobiology for, 47-60
    role in industrial rehabilitation, 598*t,* 598-599
        in acute musculoskeletal/cumulative trauma injury treatment, 599*t,* 599-600
        functional capacities evaluation, 600-601, 601*t*
        future issues, 606
        work, 604, *605,* 606
    specialized examination by, 317-318
Physical therapy. *See also* Industrial physical therapy; Orthopedic and sports physical therapy.
    for temporomandibular joint disorders, 590-591
Physiologic movement, 319
    of elbow complex, 393
Piezoelectric effect, 21
Pigmented villonodular synovitis, 94-95, *95, 96*
Pinocytosis, 87
Pisiform–triquetral joint, 330
Pivot–shift test, 316
Plantar fasciitis, 289, 291
Plastic deformation range, 5
Plastic range, 73
Plyometric exercise, 451
Pneumatic bones, 4
Point tenderness, 139
Polar moment of inertia, 9, 25
Polymorphonuclear leukocytes (PMN), 85
Popliteal muscles, 306
Popliteal tendon, 304
Posterior attachment, 557
Posterior fulcrum test in shoulder assessment, 417, *417*
Posterior oblique ligament, 152-153, 303
Posterior stability assessment, 417, *417*
Posttraumatic synovitis, 91-94, 94*t*
    synovial fluid in, 98
Postural syndrome, 543
Potential energy, 78
Power, 218, 309
    biomechanical, 70
Power stroke of mandible, 564
Preauricular pain, 567, 568
Prefabricated splints, 123
Pregnancy, ligamentous injury in, 519
Prepatellar bursa, 305
Pressure, biomechanical, 70
Prevention, 450-451
Prework screening, role of physical therapist in, 609, 609*t*
Primary afferent fibers, stimulus–response relationships, 55-58
    fiber spectrum, 55
    force sensitivity, 56, 56*t*
    neuron population response and across–fiber pattern coding, 56-57
    quantitative stimulus–response functions, 57-58
    receptive fields, 55-56
    temporal response patterns, 57
Primary osteons, 15, 18
Principal stresses, 4
Problem–oriented medical record method, 166

Progressive resistance exercise (PRE), 215, 227
  isotonic testing, 226
Pronation, 383
  factors limiting, 384
Pronator teres syndrome, 182
Proportional limit, 73
Proprioception, 322
Proprioceptive awareness, 59-60
Proprioceptive receptors, 47
Prostaglandin release, 31
Protective gear in injury prevention, 117
Proteoglycans, 105
Protrusion, 559, 575, *575*
  of mandible, 565
Provocative elevation test, 418-419
Proximal interphalangeal joints, 363-364
Proximal radius, 380
Proximal ulna, 380-381
Psoas major muscles, 528-529
Psychological factors in temporomandibular joint pain,
    581
Pterygoid muscle, 557, *558,* 561
Purdue Pegboard, 342
Push–pull test in shoulder assessment, 417
Putti–Platt procedure, 429

Q

Quadratus lumborum muscles, 527-528
Quadriceps muscle contusions, 150
Quadriceps stretch, 145, *146*
Quadriceps tendon, 298, 300
Quadrilateral space syndrome, 445-446
Quantitative stimulus–response functions, 57-58
Quebec Task Force Report, 533-534

R

Radial collateral ligament, 383
Radial fossa, 380
Radial nerve, 335-336
Radicular pain, 523
Radiocarpal joint, 329
Radiographs
  in assessing fractures, 118, 120
  in assessing hip injuries, *484,* 484-485
  in assessing ligament injuries, 141
  in assessing temporomandibular joint, 582
Radius, 328
  fracture of, 126
  of gyration, 8
Range–of–motion, 217-218
  active, 178
  assessing and treating deficiencies, 318-319, 319*t,* 320*t*
  of elbow, 386-387
  exercises for temporomandibular disorders, 588
  of hip, 470, 471*t,* 472*t,* 536
  passive, 178, 192, 199-200
  for shoulder, 413
  for temporomandibular joint, 573

Rate of movement, increased, 216, *217*
Rays of foot, 266-267, *267, 268*
  mobility of, 278, *279*
Reaction, law of, 77
Receptive fields, 55-56
Recessus sacciformis, 329
Reciprocal click, 566, 575, 576
Rectus abdominis, 529
Rectus capitis posterior major, 531
Rectus capitis posterior minor, 531
Referred pain, 168
  in spine, 534
Reflex sympathetic dystrophy, 342
Regeneration, 86
  of synovium, 95
Regional acceleratory phenomenon, 31
Rehabilitation
  following rotator cuff repair, 440-443
  following shoulder stabilization, 429-430
  goal of, 211
  of knee injuries, 320-323
  for ligament sprains, 149-150, 150*t*
  training, 216
Reiter's syndrome, 99, 571
Reorganization process, 31, 33
Repair, 86
Repetition, 221
  in injury prevention ergonomics, 608
Repetition maximum, 221
Repetitions/sets, increased, 216
Replacement, 86
Resilience, 73-74
Resistance exercise, 227
  terminology of, 227
  training, 547-548
Resisted movements, 179
  responses to testing, 201-202
Resisted tests for elbow, 388*t,* 388-389
Resistive and overload training, 215, 221
  methods of, 216-218, *217, 218, 219*
  precautions and contraindications, 220-221
  principles of strength, power, and muscular endurance, *219,*
      220, 220*t*
  types of exercise in, 215-216
Resolution of force, 67, *67*
Rest
  interval, 216-217
  in reducing edema, 86
Resting standing foot posture (RSFP), 279-280, *280, 281*
Resultant force, 68
Reticula, 463
Retrodiscitis, 567, *568,* 578
Retrusion, 559
  mandibular, 565
Rheumatoid arthritis, 170, 291, 357-362, *358, 359, 361, 362,*
    505, 571
Ribs, 510
Rickets, 489
Rigid external fixation, 127, *128*
Roll–gliding, 408

Rolling, 195
Rotary open kinetic chain (OKC) isokinetic test, 226
Rotator cuff, 413, 439
    pathologies, 432, 434-439
    rehabilitation following repair of, 440-443
    surgical repair of, 439-440
    susceptibility to injury, 437-438
    cuff tendinitis, 411
Rotatory instabilities, 316
    classification of, 138
Ruffini receptor endings, 52t, 54, 56, 57
Running, resolution of force in, 67-68
Running–functional progression program for muscle–tendon unit
        injuries, 146, 147t, 148

S

Sacralization of fifth lumbar vertebra, 510
Sacral vertebrae, 510
Sacroiliac joint, 518, 521
    dysfunction of, 167
Sacroiliac orthosis, 519
Sacrum, 510, 517-519
Sagittal bands, 333
Salter–Harris system for classification of epiphyseal plate inju-
        ries, 120
Scalene muscles, 532
Scaphoid, fracture of, 328, 348, 364-365
Scapula, 4
    evaluating, 422
    mobility of, 420, 422
    primary functions of, 420
    snapping, 422
Scapular hypermobility, 435-436
Scapulohumeral rhythm, 407, 420
Scapulothoracic articulation, 530
Scapulothoracic bursitis, 423
Scapulothoracic joint, 406-407, 407, 420, 422-423
Scapulothoracic testing, 251
Schaffer and Whitman plates, 283-284, 284
Scheuermann's disease, 167
Schmorl's nodes, 522
Sclerotome, 13
Scoliosis, 513, 573
    idiopathic, 516-517
    nonsurgical management of, 517
    school screening for, 517
Secondary (lamellar) osteons, 15
Secondary synovial osteochondromatosis, 110
Self–pressurized hydrostatic lubrication, 106
Semispinalis capitis and cervicis, 530, 530
Semmes–Weinstein monofilaments, 356
Sensation examination, 183
Sensorineural theory, 57
Serotonin, 84
Serratus anterior paralysis, 423
Sesamoid bones, 4
Set, 221
Severity, 193
Shear fractures, 37

Shear modulus of elasticity, 6
Shear stress, 4, 20, 71
Short bones, 4
Shoulder
    acromioclavicular joint injuries, 423-424
    adhesive capsulitis, 446-447
    anatomy, 402
        acromioclavicular joint, 405-406, 406
        glenohumeral joint, 402, 402-405, 403, 404
        scapulothoracic joint, 406-407, 407
        sternoclavicular joint, 406
    anterior stability assessment, 415, 415-417, 416, 417
    biceps brachii assessment, 418
    biomechanics of, 407-409
    evaluation, 411-412
        physical examination, 412
    glenoid labrum lesions, 444, 444-445
    impingement syndrome of, 170
    inferior stability assessment, 414, 414-415, 415
    inspection, 412-413
        cervical spine screening, 413
    instability, 424-427
        Bankart procedure, 427-428
        Bristow procedure, 428
        capsular shift, 429
        historical overview, 427
        Magnuson–Stack procedure, 429
        Putti–Platt procedure, 429
        surgical approach to, 427
    joint in sports
        golf swing, 449-450
        overhead throwing, 447-448
        prevention of, 450-451
        swimming, 450
        tennis strokes, 448-449
    joint stabilization
        basic muscle function, 410-411
        dynamic/stabilizers, 409
        static stabilizers, 409-410
    motion assessment, 413-414
    neurological assessment, 419
    neurovascular compression syndromes, 445-447
    observation, 412
    palpation, 419
        functional performance testing, 420, 420
        muscular performance testing, 419-420, 420t
    posterior stability assessment, 417, 417
        impingement sign, 418, 418
    rehabilitation following rotator cuff repair, 440-443
    rehabilitation following stabilization, 429-430
        following Bankart procedure, 430-431
        following capsular shift procedures, 431-432
    resisted movements, 419
    rotator cuff pathologies, 432, 434-439
    scapulothoracic joint, 420, 422-423
    surgical repair of rotator cuff, 439-440
    vascular examination, 418-419
Shoulder abduction/adduction, 250
Shoulder flexion/extension and horizontal abduction/adduction,
        250-251

Shoulder internal/external rotation strength testing, *248,*
    248-249, *249*
Siderosomes, 92-93
Single–contrast arthrogram, 141
Single leg standing (SLS), measurement of tibiofibular varum
    during, 281
Skull, 4, 12
Slipped capital femoral epiphysis, 491-492
Snapping scapula, 422
Soft tissue
    disorders of hip, 496-499, *497, 498, 499*
    injury to, in fractures, 115-116
    mobilization, 543-545
    significance of damage, 116
Solitary nodular synovitis, 95
Somatic dysfunction, 205
Somatic exteroceptive receptors, 47-48
Somites, 12, 13
Speed, 76
    increased, of movement, 216, *217*
Speed's test, 418
Sphenomandibular ligament, 559
Spin, 194
Spinal canal, 515, 516
Spinal motion, rules of, 197
Spinal nerve exits, 510
Spinal pain, 510
Spinal reflex action, 58-59
Spinal stenosis, 510
Spine, 510
    articulations of, *521,* 521-523
    cervical screening, 413
    clinical anatomy
        bony elements, 510, *512,* 512-513, *513, 514, 515,* 515-519,
            516, 517, 518, 519, 520
        general concepts, 510, *511*
        ligaments, 519-521
    evaluation of, 532-534, 534*t*
        biomechanical counseling, 542
        clinical, 534-539
        enhancing neuromuscular efficiency, 541-542
        generation of controlled forces in order to promote reacti-
            vation, 541
        modulating pain, 541
        objectives of treatment, 542-548
    musculature of, 526-532
    treatment of activity–related disorders, 539-541
    treatment plans for selected medical condition
        instability of low back/neck, 549-552
        sprain and strain, 552-553
Spiral fractures, 72
Splenius capitis, 530
Splinting, emergency, 118-119, *119*
Splints, prefabricated, 123
Spondylolisthesis, 517, *520*
Spondylolysis, 518, 526
Sports, shoulder joint in
    golf swing, 449-450
    prevention of, 450-451
    swimming, 450

Sports, shoulder joint in—cont'd
    tennis strokes, 448-449
Sprains, 83, 100, 136, 137-138
    ankle joint, 287, 289
    clinical application of, 101
    first–degree, 83
    second–degree, 83
    third–degree, 83
Spring test
    for knee assessment, 318
    for tearing of collateral ligaments, 216
Squeeze–film lubrication, 106
Squeeze technique in emergency splitting, 118
Stability assessment
    anterior, *415,* 415-417, *416, 417*
    inferior, *414,* 414-415, *415*
    posterior, 417, *417*
Stabilization exercises, 546-547
Standing in subtalar joint neutral (SSJN), 280-281
Statics, 66
Stenosis
    lateral recess, 510
    spinal, 510
Sternoclavicular joint, 406, 407-408
    palpation of, 419
Sternocleidomastoid muscle, 530, 531-532, 561
Sternum, 4, 12
Stiffness, 5, 73
Still, Andrew Taylor, 192, 206
Stimulus intensity, 356
Stimulus–response relationships, 55
    across–fiber pattern coding, 56-57
    fiber spectrum, 55
    force sensitivity, 56, 56*t*
    neuron population response, 56-57
    quantitative functions, 57-58
    receptive fields, 55-56
    temporal response pattern, 57
Stork test, 310
Straight leg raise test, 182
Strains, 4, 100, *136,* 136-137, *137*
    counterstain technique, 207, *207*
    first–degree, 136
    mechanical, 70
    second–degree, 136
    third–degree, 136-137
    units of measure for, 4*t*
Stratum fibrosum, 99, 100
Stratum synoviale, 99
Strength, 218
    biomechanical, 70
    of bone, 4*t,* 4-9, *5, 5t, 6, 7, 8, 9*
    of hip joint, 482-483
    of materials, 72-73, *73*
Strength assessment, 226
    basic/fundamental measurements, 231
    closed kinetic chain isokinetic testing, 232
    closed kinetic chain–squat isokinetic testing, 233
    computerized closed kinetic chain isokinetic dynamometer,
        230

Strength assessment—cont'd
  computerized eccentric isokinetic dynamometer, 229
  computerized isokinetic dynamometer, 229
  digital balance evaluator, 232
  functional hop test (FHT), 233
  functional jump test, 233, 233*t*
  functional testing algorithm, 231, *231*, 231*t*
  in hip joint, 480-481
  isometric exercise, 227
  isotonic exercise, 227, *228*
  isotonic muscle, 228-229
  KT1000 testing, 231
  for lower extremity, 234-236
    functional testing, 243-246, 243-247
    interpretation of test data, 240-243, 241*t*, 242*t*, *243*, 243*t*
    isokinetic testing of knee, 236-240, *237, 237, 238, 239, 240*
    knee testing, 240, *241*
  lower extremity functional test, 233-234, *234*, 234*t*, *235*, 235*t*
  methods of, 227
    cable tensiometers, 228
    handheld dynamometry, 228
    manual muscle testing, 227-228
  mode of muscle action in, 226-227
  open kinetic chain testing, 232-233
  purpose of, 226
  subjective examination, 231
  terminology of resistance exercise, 227
  for upper extremity
    glenohumeral joint testing positions, 248, 250-252
    interpretation of shoulder IR/ER testing, 249-250, 250*t*
    rationale for utilization of isokinetics in, 247, 247*t*
    reliability of isokinetics, 247-248
    shoulder internal/external rotation testing, *248*, 248-249, *249*
Stress
  bone, 4
  compressive, 9, 37, 71
  at epiphyseal plates, 28-29
  maximal compressive, 4
  mechanical, 70
  principal, 4
  shear, 71
  tensile, 9, 37
  tension, 70-71
  units of measure for, 4*t*
Stress fractures, 116, *121*, 121-122
  of foot and ankle, 289
Stress radiographs of ligament injuries, 141
Stress risers, 29
Stress–strain curve, 73, *73*
Stretch
  hamstring, 145-146, *148*
  quadriceps, 145, *146*
Stretching, 543-545
Structural specialization of joints, 48
Stylomandibular ligament, 559
Subcapital femoral neck fractures, *494*, 494-495
Subchondral bone, 48-49
Subchrondral tissue, proliferation of bone in, 109
Subjective, Objective, Assessment, and Plan (SOAP), 166-167

Subjective examination, 231
Suboccipital muscles, 530-531, *532, 561*
Subperiosteal bone, 14-15, 33
Subscapularis, 411
Subsynovial tissue, 82, 88-89, *91*
Superior articular processes, 516
Superior glenohumeral ligament (SGHL), 404, *404*, 405, 410
Superior oblique, 531
Supernumerary bones, 4
Supination, 383
  factors limiting, 384
Suprapatellar bursa, 305
Supraspinatus muscle, 411
Supraspinous ligament, 521
Surface energy, 29
Surgical management
  of end–stage arthrosis, 505
  of knee injuries, 323-324
  of rotator cuff injury, 439-440
    rehabilitation following, 440-443
  of shoulder instability, 427
    Bankart procedure, 427-428
    Bristow procedure, 428
    capsular shift, 429
    historical overview, 427
    Magnuson–Stack procedure, 429
    Putti–Platt procedure, 429
  of temporomandibular disorders, 589-591
Sutherland, William G., 206
Swan neck thumb deformity, 334, 358-359, *359*
Swimming, 450
Swing, 194-195, *195*
Synarthroses, 82
Synergistic response, 217
Synovectomy, 505
Synovia, 95
Synovial articulation, 556, *557*
Synovial cells, 88
Synovial fluid, 92, 95
  cloudy, 99
  composition and characteristics of, 95-96
  containing fat globules, 99
  functions of, 97
  in hemorrhagic effusions, 98-99
  in posttraumatic synovitis, 98
  and reaction to injury, 97-100
  viscosity of, 96-97
Synovial joints, 48
  classification of, 194, *194*
  inflammatory response
    causes of inflammation, 83
    definition of trauma, 83
    effects of trauma, 84-85
    phagocytosis, 85-86
    repair, 86
    types of trauma, 83-84
  structure and functions, 82-83, *83*
Synovial lining, 87-88, *88*
Synovial membrane, 82, 86-87, *87, 382*
  functions, 89

Synovial membrane—cont'd
  intima, 87
  joint lubrication, 89-91
  lining, 87-88, *88*
  morphology, 87
  reaction to injury, 91
    pigmented villonodular synovitis, 94-95, *95, 96*
    posttraumatic synovitis, 91-94, *94t*
  regeneration of synovium, 95
  solitary nodular synovitis, 95
  subsynovial tissue, 88-89, *91*
  type A and B cells, 88, *89, 90, 91*
Synovial regeneration, 95
Synovial transport, 90-91
Synovianalysis, 96, *97t*
Synoviocytes, 82, 87
Synovitis, 567, 578
  pigmented villonodular, 94-95, *95, 96*
  posttraumatic, 91-94, *94t*
    synovial fluid in, 98
  solitary nodular, 95
Synovium, 86, 89
  regeneration of, 95
Systemic lupus erythematosus (SLE), 168

T

Talocrural joint range of motion, 278-279, *280*
Tarsal bones, 4
Tears, 100
Temporal bones, 4
Temporalis muscle, 559, 560-561, *561*, 576
  overuse of, 588
Temporal response pattern, 57
Temporomandibular joint (TMJ), 556
  disorders, 556, 561
    capsular fibrosis, 569
    cervical spine consideration, 571
    differential diagnosis, 571-572
    growth and development considerations, 570-571
    hypermobility, 569
    masticatory muscle disorders, 569-570, *570*
    pathomechanics, 565-569, *566, 567, 568*
  evaluation of
    patient history and subjective report, *572*, 572-573
    physical exam, 573, *574, 575*, 575-591, *576, 577*
  functional anatomy, 556, *557*
    biomechanics and arthrokinematics, 562
    capsule and ligaments, 557-559, *559*
    disc and attachments, 556-557, *558*
    function, 565
    innervation, 561-562, *563*
    musculature, 559-561, *561*
    osseous structures, 556, *557*
    osteokinematics, 559, *560*
  imaging, 581-582
  physical therapy approach to, 582-583
    exercises for patient with, 588-589
    surgical approaches for, 589-591
    treatment of cervical spine, 589

Temporomandibular joint—cont'd
  physical therapy approach to—cont'd
    treatment of derangement, 583-587, *585, 586*
Temporomandibular ligament, 558, *559*
Tendinitis, 136
  Achilles, 151-152
  biceps, 450
  calcifying, 438-439
  conditions, 324
  rotator cuff, 411
  treatment of, *151t*, 151-152, *152*
Tendinosis, 136
Tendon(s), 136
  Achilles, 137
    rupture of, *137*
    tendinitis of, 151-152
  classification of, as connective tissue, 9
  injuries to, in wrist and hand, 365-370
  labrum–biceps, 403
  patellar, 300
  popliteal, 304
  quadriceps, 298, 300
  rotator cuff, 439
Tennis strokes, 448-449
Tensile loads, 4, 19
Tensile stress, 9, 37
  maximal, 4
Tension sign, 418
Tension stress, 70-71
Tension–type headache, 571
Teres minor muscle, 411
Terminal extensor tendon avulsion, 365
Thomas splint, 118
Thompson test, 137, *137*, 277
Thoracic kyphosis, 573
Thoracic outlet syndrome, 445
Thoracic spine
  motion in, 197
  vertebrae in, 516-517
Thoracolumbar fascia, 526, *528, 529*
3–D motion analysis, 77
Thumb dysfunction, 359
Tibia, 38-39, *41*, 296-298
  anterior drawer test for, 195
  external rotation of, 315-316
  fracture of, 126
  material strengths of portions of, *40t*
Tibial collateral ligament, 303
Tibial fractures, 39
Tibial plateau, 296-297, *298*
Tibia valga, 296
Tibia vara, 296
Tibiofemoral joints, 296, *296*, 302, 306-307
  examination of, 313-314
  intraarticular disorders of, 310
Tic douloureux, 572
Tidemark, 107
Tinel's sign, 182, 277, *278*, 349
Tissues, articular, 48
Toed–out gait, 309

Torque, 74-76, *75, 76*
Torque curve shape, 242
Torque measurements, interpreting, 241
Torsion, 518
Torsional loads, 20, 72, *72*
Torticollis, 532
    congenital muscular, 532
Total energy absorbed, 5
Toughness, 73-74
Trabeculae, 18, 25, 38
Trabecular bone, 14, 18, 25
Traction, 124, 545-546
Traction epiphyses, 16
Traction splints, 118
Training, rehabilitation, 216
Training error, 121
Transcutaneous electrical nerve stimulation (TENS), 390
Translation glide, 195
Transmigration, 84
Transverse processes, 510, 512
Transverse retinacular ligaments, 334
Transversus abdominis, 529
Trapeziometacarpal joint, 330
Trapezius muscle, 530, 561
Trapezius paralysis, 423
Trapezoid, 328
Trauma
    definition of, 83
    direct, 83
    effects of, 84-85
    indirect, 83
    inflammatory response to, 85-86
    types of, to joints, 83-84
Traumatic arthritis, 111
Traumatic effusions, reabsorption of, 99
Triangular fibrocartilage complex (TFCC), 329
Trigeminal nerve, 562
Trigeminal neuralgia, 572
Trigger finger/thumb, 333, 362, *362*
Trigger points, 569
Triplane motion of foot, 263-264
Triquetrum, 328
Trochanter, greater, 461-462
Trochlea, 380
Tropocollagen, 11, *11*
TSLO thoracic–lumbar–sacral orthosis, 517
TUBS (Traumatic, Unidirectional, Bankart Lesion, requiring surgery), 426
Tubular bone, 25
Tumor necrosis fiber, 84
2–D motion analysis, 76
Two–point discrimination (2PD) tests, 354, 356, *356*
Type A cells, 88
Type B cells, 88
Type C cells, 88

U

Ulna, 328
Ulnar artery, 337
Ulnar collateral ligament, 382-383
Ulnar nerve, 335
Ulnar styloid process, 328
Ulnomeniscotriquetral joint, 330
Ultimate failure point, 5
Ultimate strain, 6
Ultimate stress, 6
Ultrasound in treating inflammation, 111
Ultrasound phonophoresis, 588
Unilateral muscle ratios in interpreting torque measurements, 241
Unilateral strength ratios, 249-250
Upper extremity, strength assessment for
    glenohumeral joint testing positions, 248, 250-252
    interpretation of shoulder IR/ER testing, 249-250, 250*t*
    rationale for utilization of isokinetics in, 247, 247*t*
    reliability of isokinetics, 247-248
    shoulder internal/external rotation testing, *248,* 248-249, *249*

V

Valsalva maneuver, 220, 529
Varus disorder, 313
Vascular anatomy of hip, 468, *469*
Vastus medialis atrophy, 306
Vastus medialis obliquus, 306
Veins. *See* Angiology
Velocity, 76
Vertebrae, 510
    cervical, 510, 513, *514,* 515
    lumbar, 510, 517, *518*
    sacral, 510
    thoracic, 516-517
Vertebral arch, 510, 513, 520
Vertebral body, 510
Vertebral joints, 49
Vertebral motion, laws of, 196-198, *198*
Vibration in injury prevention ergonomics, 608
Viscosity of synovial fluid, 96-97
Visual Analog Scale, 171, *171*
Volkmann's canals, 18, 24
Volkmann's ischemic contracture, 130
Volkmann's systems, 15

W

Walking
    resolution of force in, 67-68, *68, 69*
    typical pattern of rearfoot motion during, 271, *272*
Wartenberg's sign, 361
Weeping lubrication, 106
Weight problem for muscle–tendon unit injuries, 148-149, 149*t*
Weight/resistance, increased, 216
Weight training, 227
White blood cells, 84
    and phagocytosis, 85-86
    reaction to injury, 92, *92*
Williams, Paul, 542

Wolff's law, 21-22
  and bone remodeling, 130
  and osteoporosis, 43
Work, 78
Work conditioning/work hardening, role of physical therapist in, 559
Workers' compensation laws and job matching, 602
Work hardening, 370-371, *371*
Work injury prevention, role of physical therapist in, *606,* 606-609
Work task testing, role of industrial physical therapist in, 600-601, 601*t*
Work time duration in injury prevention ergonomics, 608
Wrisberg ligament, 305
Wrist and forearm testing, 251
Wrist and hand
  burned, 367-368, 370
  case study, 374, *375, 376, 377,* 377*t*
  clinical anatomy and mechanics of
    angiology, 336-338
    arthrology, 329-331, *330*
    neurology, 335-336, *336*
    osteology, 328-329
    and soft–tissue relationships, 331-334, *332, 334, 335*

Wrist and hand—cont'd
  examination procedures specific to, 338, *338*
    history, 338-339, *339, 340, 341,* 341-342
    physical, *342,* 342-344, *343, 344, 345, 346,* 346-349, *347,* 347*t, 348,* 348*t, 349, 349, 350-351, 352, 353,* 354, *354, 355, 356,* 356*t,* 356-357, *357*
  joint mobilization techniques for, 371, *371, 372, 373, 373*
  pathologic conditions and treatment guidelines
    acute injuries, 362-368, *363, 364, 365, 366, 367, 368, 369,* 370
    rheumatoid, 357-362, *358, 359, 361, 362*
    work hardening, 370-371, *371*

Y

Yergason test, 418
Yield point, 5
Young's modulus, 5, 34

Z

Zero instability, 138
Zona orbicularis, 463
Zones of articular cartilage, 103-104, *104, 105*